D1162652

Imaging *of the* Wrist *and* Hand

Imaging *of the* Wrist *and* Hand

Edited by

Louis A. Gilula, M.D.
Professor of Radiology
Department of Radiology
Mallinckrodt Institute of Radiology
St. Louis, Missouri

Yuming Yin, M.D.
Department of Radiology
Beijing Ji Shui Tan Hospital
Beijing, People's Republic of China

Currently
Research Fellow
Musculoskeletal Section
Mallinckrodt Institute of Radiology
St. Louis, Missouri

W.B. SAUNDERS COMPANY
A Division of Harcourt Brace & Company
Philadelphia London Toronto Montreal Sydney Tokyo

W.B. SAUNDERS COMPANY

A Division of Harcourt Brace & Company

The Curtis Center
Independence Square West
Philadelphia, Pennsylvania 19106

Library of Congress Cataloging-in-Publication Data

Gilula, Louis.
Imaging of the Wrist and Hand / Louis A. Gilula, Yuming Yin.—
1st ed.
p. cm.
Includes bibliographical references and index.
ISBN 0-7216-5125-9
1. Hand—Radiography. 2. Wrist—Radiography. I. Yin, Yuming.
II. Title.
[DNLM: 1. Hand—radiography. 2. Wrist—radiography. WE 830
G489r 1996]
RC951.G55 1996
617.5′7507572—dc20
DNLM/DLC 95-5453

IMAGING OF THE WRIST AND HAND ISBN 0–7216–5125–9

Printed in the United States of America

Last digit is the print number: 9 8 7 6 5 4 3 2 1

To our wives, Debbie and Yali, and children, Tanya, Ian, and Yue, who tolerated the tremendous time commitment necessary to bring this book to completion.

CONTRIBUTORS

DUFFIELD ASHMEAD IV, M.D.

Assistant Clinical Professor, Departments of Orthopaedic Surgery and Plastic Surgery, University of Connecticut. Instructor in Surgery, Plastic and Reconstructive Surgery, Yale University, New Haven, Connecticut. Associate in Surgery, University of Massachusetts, Worcester, Massachusetts. Staff, Connecticut Combined Hand Surgery Fellowship, Hartford, Connecticut.

Examination of the Hand and Wrist

MARK EVERETT BARATZ, M.D.

Assistant Professor, Department of Orthopaedic Surgery, Medical College of Pennsylvania and Hahnemann University, Allegheny Campus, Pittsburgh, Pennsylvania. Senior Attending Physician, Allegheny General Hospital, Pittsburgh, Pennsylvania.

Wrist and Hand Measurements and Classification Schemes

RICHARD A. BERGER, M.D., Ph.D.

Associate Professor of Orthopaedic Surgery, Associate Professor of Anatomy, Mayo Graduate School of Medicine, Rochester, Minnesota. Consultant in Orthopedic Surgery, Division of Hand Surgery, Department of Orthopedic Surgery, Mayo Clinic/Mayo Foundation, Rochester, Minnesota.

Physical Examination and Provocative Maneuvers of the Wrist, Ligamentography: A Method of Imaging Intracapsular Wrist Ligaments

ALAIN BLUM, M.D.

Assistant of Radiology, Department of Radiology, Centre Hospitalier Universitaire Nancy-Brabois, Nancy, France.

CT–Arthrography of the Wrist

FRANCK BRESLER, M.D.

Assistant of Orthopaedic Surgery, Centre Hospitalier Universitaire Nancy, Nancy, France. Assistant of Orthopaedic Surgery, Clinique de Traumatologie, Nancy, France.

CT–Arthrography of the Wrist

ALAN CHRISTENSEN, M.D.

Chairman, Orthopedic Surgery, Wilford Hall Medical Center, Lackland Air Force Base, Texas.

Miscellaneous Surgical Entities of the Hand and Wrist

DAVID J. CURTIS, M.D.

Staff Radiologist, Veterans Administration Medical Center, Durham, North Carolina. Assistant Clinical Professor, Duke University, Durham, North Carolina.

Radiography of Soft Tissues in Trauma to the Hand and Wrist

MICHAEL D. DAKE, M.D.

Assistant Professor, Stanford University Medical Center, Stanford, California. Chief, Cardiovascular and Interventional Radiology, Department of Radiology, Stanford University Medical Center.

Angiographic and Interventional Procedures in the Hand

JAMES H. DOBYNS, M.D.

Professor of Orthopedic Surgery, Emeritus, Mayo Clinic, Mayo Medical School, Rochester, Minnesota. Professor of Orthopedic Surgery, Clinical, University of Texas Health Science Center, San Antonio, Texas. Consultant, The Hand Center, The University Medical System, The Baptist Memorial Medical System, San Antonio, Texas.

Physical Examination and Provocative Maneuvers of the Wrist

GEORGES Y. EL-KHOURY, M.D.

Professor of Radiology, Professor of Orthopaedic Surgery, The University of Iowa College of Medicine, Iowa City, Iowa. Director of Diagnostic Clinical Services, Department of Radiology, University of Iowa Hospitals and Clinics, Iowa City, Iowa.

Conventional Tomography of the Wrist and Hand

JÜRGEN FREYSCHMIDT, M.D.

Professor of Radiology, Director, Department of Radiology and Nuclear Medicine, Central Hospital, St.-Jürgen Straße, Bremen, Germany.

Normal Variants

LOUIS A. GILULA, M.D.
Professor of Radiology, Director, Musculoskeletal Section, Mallinckrodt Institute of Radiology, Washington University School of Medicine, St. Louis, Missouri.
History of Imaging of the Hand and Wrist, Anatomy Affecting the Metacarpal and Phalangeal Bones of the Hand, Positions and Techniques, Indications for Wrist Instability Series and Its Cost-Effectiveness, Roentgenographic Interpretation of Ligamentous Instabilities: Static and Dynamic Instabilities, Roentgenographic Approach to Complex Bone Abnormalities, Computed Tomography: Applications and Tailored Approach, Miscellaneous Conditions of the Wrist, Algorithmic Approach to Wrist Pain

JACQUELINE C. HODGE, M.D.
Instructor, Musculoskeletal Section, Mallinckrodt Institute of Radiology, Washington University School of Medicine, St. Louis, Missouri.
Roentgenographic Interpretation of Ligamentous Instabilities: Static and Dynamic Instabilities, Roentgenographic Approach to Complex Bone Abnormalities, Miscellaneous Conditions of the Wrist

MARGARETHA HÖGLUND, M.D.
Assistant Professor, Department of Radiology, Södersjukhuset, Stockholm, Sweden.
Ultrasound

LAWRENCE E. HOLDER, M.D., F.A.C.R.
Professor of Radiology, University of Maryland School of Medicine, Baltimore, Maryland. Director, Division of Nuclear Medicine, University of Maryland Medical Systems, Baltimore, Maryland.
Bone Scintigraphy

JOHN M. G. KAUER, M.D. Ph.D.
Professor of Anatomy and Embryology, Department of Anatomy and Embryology, Faculty of Medical Sciences, University of Nymegen, Nymegen, the Netherlands. Chairman, Department of Anatomy and Embryology, University of Nymegen.
The Wrist Joint: Anatomic and Functional Considerations

GRAHAM J. W. KING, M.D., M.Sc., F.R.C.S.C.
Assistant Professor, Division of Orthopaedic Surgery, University of Western Ontario, London, Ontario, Canada. Active Staff, Hand and Upper Limb Centre, London, Ontario, Canada. Co-Director, Musculoskeletal Research Laboratory, St. Joseph's Health Centre, London, Ontario, Canada.
Physical Examination of the Wrist

BRUCE A. KRAEMER, M.D.
Assistant Professor of Plastic and Reconstructive Surgery, Division of Plastic Surgery, Washington University School of Medicine, St. Louis, Missouri.
Anatomy Affecting the Metacarpal and Phalangeal Bones of the Hand

CLAUS FALCK LARSEN, M.D., Ph.D.
Consultant Hand Surgeon, Department of Orthopedic Surgery, National University Hospital, Rigshospitalet, Hand Surgery Section, Copenhagen, Denmark.
Wrist and Hand Measurements and Classification Schemes

KEVIN W. McENERY, M.D.
Assistant Professor of Radiology, Department of Radiology, Mallinckrodt Institute of Radiology, Washington University School of Medicine, St. Louis, Missouri.
Computed Tomography: Applications and Tailored Approach

ROBERT Y. McMURTRY, M.D., F.A.C.S., F.R.C.S.C.
Dean, Faculty of Medicine, Health Sciences Centre, University of Western Ontario, London, Ontario, Canada. Consultant Orthopaedic Surgery, St. Joseph's Health Centre, London, Ontario, Canada.
Physical Examination of the Wrist

F. A. MANN, M.D.
Associate Professor of Radiology, University of Washington School of Medicine, Seattle, Washington. Director, Emergency and Trauma Radiology, Harborview Medical Center, Seattle, Washington.
Positions and Techniques, Indications for Wrist Instability Series and Its Cost-Effectiveness, Roentgenographic Interpretation of Ligamentous Instabilities: Static and Dynamic Instabilities, Roentgenographic Approach to Complex Bone Abnormalities, Algorithmic Approach to Wrist Pain.

MICHEL MERLE, M.D.
Professor of Plastic and Reconstructive Surgery, Nancy Medical School, Vandoeuvre, France. Chief of the Department of Plastic and Reconstructive Surgery, Centre Hospitalier Universitaire Nancy, Hôpital Jeanne d'Arc, Dommartin les Toul, France.
CT–Arthrography of the Wrist

VIKTOR M. METZ, M.D.
Associate Professor of Radiology, Department of Radiology, University of Vienna Medical School, Vienna, Austria.
Arthrography of the Wrist and Hand

RICHARD J. MILLER, M.D.
Associate Professor, Department of Orthopaedics, University of Rochester, Rochester, New York.
MRI of the Wrist and Hand

WILLEM R. OBERMANN, M.D., Ph.D.
Radiologist, Department of Radiology, University Hospital Leiden, Leiden, The Netherlands.
Ligamentography: A Method of Imaging Intracapsular Wrist Ligaments

DANIEL J. PERELES, M.D.
Assistant Clinical Professor of Orthopaedic Surgery, George Washington University, Washington, D.C. Director of Sports Medicine, Montgomery Orthopaedics and Spine Center, Rockville, Maryland.
Arthroscopic Findings of Ligaments Around the Wrist

DENIS REGENT, M.D.
Professor of Radiology, Radiology Department, Centre Hospitale Universitaire Brabois, Vandoeuvre-les-Nancy, France.
CT–Arthrography of the Wrist

FRANÇOIS SCHERNBERG, M.D.
Professor of Reconstructive Surgery, Chief, University of Medicine, Service d'Orthopédie et de Traumatologie I, Hôpital Maison Blanche, Centre Hospitalier Universitaire de Reims, Reims Cedex, France.
Radiography for Wrist Instabilities

DOUGLAS K. SMITH, M.D.
Assistant Clinical Professor, University of Texas Health Science Center, San Antonio, Texas. Chief, Musculoskeletal Radiology, Wilford Hall Medical Center, Lackland Air Force Base, Texas.
Miscellaneous Surgical Entities of the Hand and Wrist

PAUL TORDAI, M.D.
Assistant Professor, Department of Hand Surgery, Södersjukhuset, Stockholm, Sweden.
Ultrasound

SAARA M. S. TOTTERMAN, M.D., Ph.D.
Associate Professor of Radiology; Director, MR Center, Department of Radiology, University of Rochester Medical School, Rochester, New York.
MRI of the Wrist and Hand

NHAN P. TRUONG, M.D.
Department of Radiology, St. Francis Hospital, Tulsa, Oklahoma.
Indications for Wrist Instability Series and Its Cost-Effectiveness

SYLVIA VENZKE, M.D.
Resident in Radiology, Central Hospital, St.-Jürgen Straße, Bremen, Germany.
Normal Variants

PHILIPPE VOCHE, M.D.
Assistant Professor, University of Nancy 1, Medical School, Nancy, France. Medical Doctor; Hand and Plastic Surgeon, Unit of Plastic and Hand Surgery, Hôpital Jeanne d'Arc, Dommartin les Toul, France.
CT–Arthrography of the Wrist

H. KIRK WATSON, M.D.
Clinical Professor, Department of Orthopaedic Surgery, University of Connecticut, Farmington, Connecticut. Assistant Clinical Professor of Surgery (Plastic), Yale University, New Haven, Connecticut. Associate Professor of Orthopaedics and Physical Rehabilitation, University of Massachusetts, Worcester, Massachusetts. Chief of Hand Surgery, Newington Children's Hospital, Newington, Connecticut, Senior Staff, Hartford Hospital, Hartford, Connecticut. Director, Connecticut Combined Hand Surgery Fellowship, Hartford, Connecticut.
Examination of the Hand and Wrist

TERRY L. WHIPPLE, M.D., F.A.C.S.
Clinical Professor of Orthopaedic Surgery, Bowman Gray School of Medicine, Wake Forest University, Winston-Salem, North Carolina. Clinical Associate Professor of Orthopaedic Surgery, University of Virginia School of Medicine, Charlottesville, Virginia. Clinical Associate Professor of Orthopaedic Surgery, Medical College of Virginia. Richmond, Virginia. Director, Orthopaedic Research of Virginia, Richmond, Virginia.
Arthroscopic Findings of Ligaments Around the Wrist

CAMELIA G. WHITTEN, M.D.
Musculoskeletal Radiologist, St. Cloud Radiology, P.A., St. Cloud, Minnesota.
Conventional Tomography of the Wrist and Hand

WAYNE F. J. YAKES, M.D.
Clinical Professor, University of Colorado Health Sciences Center, Denver, Colorado. Director, Interventional Radiology and Interventional Neuroradiology, Radiology Imaging Associates, P.C., Englewood, Colorado.
Angiographic and Interventional Procedures in the Hand

YUMING YIN, M.D.
Radiologist, Beijing Ji Shui Hospital, Beijing Institute of Tramatology and Orthopaedics, Beijing, People's Republic of China. Currently: Research Fellow, Mallinckrodt Institute of Radiology, Washington University School of Medicine, St. Louis, Missouri.
History of Imaging of the Hand and Wrist, Positions and Techniques, Roentgenographic Interpretation of Ligamentous Instabilities: Static and Dynamic Instabilities, Roentgenographic Approach to Complex Bone Abnormalities, Algorithmic Approach to Wrist Pain, Computed Tomography: Applications and Tailored Approach, Miscellaneous Conditions of the Wrist

PREFACE

There are two major reasons for my creation of this multi-authored text. First, techniques for imaging the human body have changed dramatically in the hundred years since Roentgen's discovery of x-rays. Indeed, there are so many imaging modalities now available that tailoring an economical and suitable imaging approach to diagnosis and treatment has truly become a challenge. Second, some wrist and hand disorders are both so complicated and so common that specialized knowledge is a widespread requirement in dealing with these problems. Hence, hand and wrist surgeons have developed their own subspecialized field within general surgery. This book not only presents the currently available, state-of-the-art imaging techniques, but also provides basic diagnostic tools for any person dealing with patients who have diagnostic problems in the wrist and hand.

Imaging of the Wrist and Hand is the result of my personal work over many years in the field of wrist and hand disorders. My serious interest in the wrist was prompted by the publication of my first two major articles on the subject (Gilula LA, Weeks PM. Post-traumatic ligamentous instabilities of the wrist. *Radiology* 1978;129:641–651, and Gilula LA. Carpal injuries: Analytic approach and case exercises. *AJR* 1979;133:503–517). During many teaching sessions with medical students, this interest continued to evolve as I realized that these students could interpret wrist radiographs even better than my radiology residents, surgical residents, and other personnel. Empirically I had developed an approach to the analysis of complex carpal trauma that worked well. Since then, there has been increasing interest in the wrist and hand, leading to the emergence of a new subgroup of surgeons, biomedical experts, and a few imagers within the already-specialized group of hand surgeons. This new group, the International Wrist Investigators' Workshop (IWIW), meets regularly (annually or more frequently) to discuss diagnostic, treatment-related, and biomechanical problems in the wrist.

Diagnosing and treating wrist and hand abnormalities can range from being somewhat easy to relatively difficult. Indeed, many problems can be found that may not sufficiently explain patient symptomatology. As mentioned above, various techniques are available for imaging, and equally numerous are approaches to the use of these techniques. As knowledge and experience increase and change, such approaches to diagnosis and treatment will also continue to evolve.

The major goal of this book is to summarize the current state of knowledge of wrist and hand imaging. Other important information for evaluation is also included. I have attempted to provide material on all aspects of imaging of the wrist and hand, contributors being selected on the basis of their recognized expertise. Detailed information is presented about clinical evaluation of the wrist and hand, including material from three different expert sources. Because people have various approaches to physical examination, the more that is learned about effective examination, the better such an exam can be performed. Therefore, some repetition within the text by the different chapter authors is a helpful method of learning physical examination and certain tests. Such repetition actually stresses the value of specific parts of the examination process of the painful wrist and hand.

This book also provides basic information that those interested in understanding, diagnosing, and treating the problematic wrist and hand via various imaging techniques will find useful. Sections are included on basic anatomy and biomechanics. A special chapter on radiographic techniques for the wrist and hand is designed to present all the different radiographic positions published to date. However, it is impossible to capture every technique, and we expect there may be some inadvertent omissions. An algorithmic approach to the painful wrist represents the state of our current knowledge. Of course, this will continue to change as, again, the general information increases in this complex area: the wrist and hand.

Three sections from my first book, *The Traumatized Hand and Wrist: Radiographic and Anatomic Correlation* (Philadelphia: WB Saunders, 1992), are repeated here with slight modifications, as those chapters are important to this book. (These chapters appear in the current text as "Anatomy Affecting the Metacarpal and Phalangeal Bones of the Hand," by Bruce A. Kraemer and Louis A. Gilula (the latter part of Chapter 4); "Radiography of Soft Tissues in Trauma to the Hand and Wrist," by David J. Curtis (Chapter 6); and "Bone Scintigraphy," by Lawrence E. Holder (Chapter 12).) Although some other concepts and additional case material are borrowed elsewhere from my first book, most of the remainder of *Imaging of the Wrist and Hand* does not appear there.

Finally, this work would have been completely impossible without the help of my colleague, Dr. Yuming Yin. His coming to work with me at the Mallinckrodt Institute of Radiology in St. Louis from the Beijing Ji Shui Tan Hospital (Beijing Institute of Traumatology and Orthopaedics) at the recommendation of his former mentor, Yunzhao Wang, Professor of Radiology, has provided me with the necessary support to bring this work to closure. I also thank all of the contributing authors and my secretaries, Linda Macker and Mary Keller, for their untiring support, without which this book would not have been possible.

LAG

CONTENTS

CHAPTER 1

HISTORY OF IMAGING OF THE HAND AND WRIST

Yuming Yin and Louis A. Gilula

On November 8, 1895, the first radiograph of a human was created. That radiograph was of a hand and represented the beginning of radiology; however, the first formal announcement of this discovery of x-rays did not take place until December 28, 1895. This caused a great interest in the field of medicine.[1–3] Just a few days later, in January 1896, Jastrowitz first described the clinical application of a roentgen plate. It was the hand of a patient who had been injured 1 year earlier. The radiograph showed the "point of a glass splinter" in the epiphyseal area of the distal phalanx of the left long finger.[4] In the early days of the x-ray's development, a great effort was made to explore the capability of x-rays to show human anatomic structures. A few days after Jastrowitz's work, Haschek and Lindenthal performed the first angiogram on a cadaver. They injected "Teichmann's mass," a radiopaque material, into the arteries of the wrist. This was the first reported successful imaging demonstration of the digital and interosseous arteries and their anastomoses.[5]

The first recorded application of roentgen rays for preoperative evaluation was by Mosetig-Moorhof in the last week of January 1896. His patient had a gunshot wound that had entered the left palmar area. Radiography showed clearly a small, dark bullet projecting in part over the middle of the radial side of the fifth metacarpal. It barely projected over the interosseous space. This demonstrated the exact bullet location and helped the surgeon plan his subsequent operation.[6]

Wertheim-Salomonson described a hand roentgenogram of a 2-year-old child in February 1896 and discovered that cartilage allows x-rays to pass freely through it, even easier than through fingernails or skin. He concluded that "the degree of ossification may be determined in living individuals. This could also be of help in the study of rickets."[7] He also described for the first time the roentgenographic appearance of hypertrophic pulmonary osteoarthropathy (clubbed fingers) encountered in chronic respiratory infections and other long-standing hypoxemic states. Hoppe-Seyler first recognized hand arterial calcifications in April 1896 on a hand radiograph.[8] On July 6, 1896, Bryce published a paper in which he described in detail the radiographic appearance of the wrist and hand articulations for the first time.[9] He also described the changes of these bones in different positions of the hand, such as pronation in neutral position, pronation with adduction and abduction, and supination in neutral position.

As can be seen, within several months after discovery of the x-ray, many applications of x-rays for use in the hand comparable with those used today had been identified; however, those demonstrations were in a preliminary stage of development. The hand was one of the main body parts studied in the early developmental stages of radiology. This occurred because the x-ray machine had a relatively low output in those days, the skeletal system provided a good natural contrast with soft tissue in roentgenography, and the hand was a part of the body thin enough to be easily radiographed.[10]

Most early applications of roentgenograms were concentrated around bone trauma, and this was mainly in the wrist and hand. In 1896 there were about 1000 papers dealing with roentgenograms; most of these concerned the hand. During those years the exposure times were lengthy, lasting from several minutes to even 30 minutes.[1,11]

In 1928, Alessandro Vallebona described a method to enlarge radiographic images that he called "microradiografia."[12] This technique still makes visible certain kinds of lesions that may not be as easily shown on ordinary films. In 1935, Wright studied wrist movement using stereoscopic x-ray films. This was a relatively detailed study of wrist movement. He came to the conclusion that radial deviation occurs entirely at the transverse carpal joint and ulnar deviation is almost wholly a sliding movement of the radiocarpal joint. He also showed that flexion and extension are composed of both radiocarpal and transverse carpal joint movements, with the latter the more extensive. He also recognized that the scaphoid bone shows a wide range of movement in relation to the other bones of the proximal carpal row.[13]

Until this time, all the imaging studies evaluated the static condition of the wrist and hand. Because the wrist is a complex joint, the standard radiographic views in various projections may show some potentially unstable conditions but the abnormal dynamic interactions of the carpal bones will not be shown on static examinations. In 1966, using cineradiography Arkless studied dynamic interactions of the carpal bones in normal and abnormal states. This method of examination helped demonstrate how distribution of stress within the carpus is altered in abnormal states, predict the possibility and location of future arthritis, and determine the type of treatment that could be used.[14]

In 1961, Kessler and Silberman reported their results with both experimental and clinical applications of radiocarpal joint arthrography.[15] Using this technique, communication between the radiocarpal and the distal radioulnar joints was recognized to identify triangular fibrocartilage (TFC) defects, but the precise location, orientation, and dimensions of the defect were not readily determined. They indicated that details are obscured by overlapping bones, intraarticular contrast media, and contrast medium extravasated into adjacent tendon sheaths and soft tissue. In 1969, Weston applied this technique to the metacarpophalangeal, metatarsophalangeal, and interphalangeal joints and described normal arthrography of those joints.[16]

In 1969, Brewerton was the first to use tenography to study the tendon sheaths in rheumatoid hands. Using this technique he demonstrated the presence of tenosynovitis in rheumatoid disease radiologically.[17]

The first successfully performed thin-section nuclear magnetic resonance (NMR) images on a human were performed on a wrist by Hinshaw et al in 1977.[18] By the next year they had successfully performed a systematic study of thin-section forearm and hand anatomy using NMR on a cadaver.[19] This was the beginning of magnetic resonance imaging (MRI) applications in humans. At that time only proton-density imaging was obtained. That technique barely demonstrated the variable contrast of different tissues.

In 1977, Gilula presented an enlarged radiographic carpal instability series based on previously mentioned or reported instability views at the annual Radiologic Society of North America (RSNA) meeting. This series of views was designed to stress a systematic approach to identification of static types of wrist instabilities.[20]

Although many descriptions about complex carpal trauma cases had been reported in previous studies, no systematic approach to analysis of the traumatized wrist on radiographs had been published or described prior to Gilula's 1979 article.[21] In that article he presented an approach to analyzing the disorganized carpus and described three normal arcs (subsequently called Gilula's arcs by various authors in other reports) that can be drawn. He also stressed the concepts of parallelism and joint symmetry between normally articulating wrist bones (see Chapter 11).

Computed tomography (CT) was first used to image the head. In 1981, Zucker-Pinchoff, Hermann, and Srinivasan used CT to study and publish the cross-sectional anatomy of the carpal tunnel.[22] They found that variation of CT numbers as manifested by different densities allowed identification of the median nerve in the carpal tunnel as a nonhomogeneous structure with lower attenuation values than the adjacent flexor tendons. Thereafter, several articles described the role of CT in the diagnosis of wrist disease. Such articles described normal soft tissues of the wrist,[23] diagnosis of subluxation and dislocation of the distal radioulnar joint,[24] normal and pathologic conditions of the hand,[25,26] and detection of a wooden foreign body in the hand.[27] As more CT machines became available, CT became increasingly popular for use in the hand and wrist.

In 1984, Tirman et al described an alternative method of arthrography that was believed to better demonstrate the scapholunate and lunotriquetral ligaments. They first reported injection of the midcarpal joint to produce midcarpal wrist arthrography.[28] In their opinion this method improved the diagnosis of communication between the radiocarpal and midcarpal compartments. In addition this technique demonstrated the distal surfaces of the scapholunate and lunotriquetral ligaments.

At first the standard wrist arthrographic technique consisted of an initial radiocarpal injection with radiopaque contrast material and subsequent plain-film radiography before and after exercise, using a series of routine projections. In the early 1980s, some modifications of this technique were reported. These included fluoroscopic monitoring,[29] magnification and stress radiography,[30] and conventional tomography.[31] In 1983, Berger, Blair, and El-Khouri combined the arthrogram with tomography, calling it arthrotomography.[31] Using this technique, they divided TFC defects into three patterns. Type I defects involve the radial side of the TFC with a long, narrow, posteroanterior fissure that has thick regular borders. Type II defects are usually centrally located, wide defects with irregular margins. Type III defects are communications between the prestyloid recess and the distal radioulnar joint.

In 1984 Resnick et al reported that digital radiography applied during wrist arthrography using subtraction may demonstrate subtle abnormalities hard to see by nondigital techniques.[32] In 1987 Levinsohn et al developed and popularized the three-compartment wrist arthrography injection technique.[33] They injected the radiocarpal, distal radioulnar, and midcarpal joints separately and strongly encouraged injection of all three compartments. This was based on their finding that some communicating defects were seen only by injecting one compartment and not the other. They suggested that these one-way defects were due to a ball-valve or flap-type one-way defect; therefore three-compartment arthrography identifies many abnormalities not seen with injection of only one compartment.

Today many kinds of imaging techniques are available for evaluation of various wrist conditions. Although CT and MRI are superior in certain aspects to conventional radiography, the basic method of examination remains plain film radiography. Because the history of imaging of the wrist begins with plain radiography, we suggest that any kind of imaging examination of the hand and wrist should also begin with plain film screen radiography.

REFERENCES

1. Bruwer AJ. *Classic descriptions in diagnostic roentgenology,* Vol. 1. 1st ed. Springfield, IL: Charles C Thomas, 1964;47–67.
2. Murphy WA. Radiologic history exhibit: Introduction to the history of musculoskeletal radiology. *RadioGraphics* 1990; 10:915–943.
3. Cipollaro AC. The earliest roentgen demonstration of a pathological lesion in America. *Radiology* 1945;45:555–558.
4. Jastrowitz M. Die Röntgen'schen Experimente mit Kathodenstrahlen und ihre diagnostische Verwerthung. *Dtsch Med Wochenschr* 1896;22:65–67.
5. Haschek VE, Lindenthal OT. Ein Beitrag zur praktischen Verwerthung der Photographic nach Röntgen. *Wien Klin Wochenschr* 1896;9:63–64.
6. Mosetig-Moorhof AR. Officielles protokoll der k. k. Gesellschaft der Arzte in Wein. *Wien Klin Wochenschr* 1896;9:83.
7. Wertheim-Salomonson JKA. Röntgen's X-stralen. *Ned Tijdschr Geneeskd* 1896;32:241–249.
8. Hoppe-Seyler G. Über die Verwendung der Röntgen's-Strahlen zur diagnose der Arteriosklerose. *München Med Wochenschr* 1896;43:316–317.
9. Bryce TH. On certain points in the anatomy and mechanisms of the wrist-joint reviewed in the light of a series of roentgen ray photographs of the living hand. *J Anat Physiol* 1896; 31:59–79.
10. Grigg ERN. The first clinical roentgen plate and related "firsts" from the year 1896. In: Grigg ERN, ed. *The trail of the invisible light.* Springfield, IL: Charles C. Thomas, 1965: 3–46.
11. Rigler LG. Development of roentgen diagnosis. *Radiology* 1945;45:467–502.
12. Vallebona A. Radiography with great enlargement (microradiography) and a technical method for the radiographic dissociation of the shadow. *Radiology* 1931;17:340–341.
13. Wright RD. A detailed study of movement of the wrist joint. *J Anat* 1935;70:137–143.
14. Arkless R. Cineradiography in normal and abnormal wrists. *AJR* 1966;96:837–844.
15. Kessler I, Silberman Z. An experimental study of the radiocarpal joint by arthrography. *Surg Gynecol Obstet* 1961;111: 33–40.
16. Weston WJ. The normal arthrograms of the metacarpal-phalangeal, metatarso-phalangeal and inter-phalangeal joints. *Aust Radiol* 1969;13:211–218.
17. Brewerton DA. Radiographic studies of tendons in the rheumatoid hand. *Br J Radiol* 1969;42:487–492.
18. Hinshaw WS, Bottomley PA, Holland GN. Radiographic thin-section image of the human wrist by nuclear magnetic resonance. *Nature* 1977;270:722–723.
19. Hinshaw WS, Andrew ER, Bottomley PA, Holland GN, Moore WS, Worthington BS. An in vivo study of the forearm and hand by thin section NMR imaging. *Br J Radiol* 1979;52: 36–43.
20. Gilula LA, Weeks PM. Post-traumatic ligamentous instabilities of the wrist. *Radiology* 1978;129:641–651.
21. Gilula LA. Carpal injuries: Analytic approach and case exercises. *AJR* 1979;133:503–517.
22. Zucker-Pinchoff B, Hermann G, Srinivasan R. Computed tomography of the carpal tunnel: A radioanatomical study. *J Comput Assist Tomogr* 1981;5:525–528.
23. Cone RO, Szabo R, Resnick D, Gelberman R, Taleisnik J, Gilula LA. Computed tomography of the normal soft tissues of the wrist. *Invest Radiol* 1983;18:546–551.
24. Mino DE, Palmer AK, Levinsohn EM. The role of radiography and computerized tomography in the diagnosis of subluxation and dislocation of the distal radioulnar joint. *J Hand Surg* 1983;8:23–31.
25. Hauser H, Rheiner P, Gajisin S. Computed tomography of the hand. Part 1: Normal anatomy. *Medicamundi* 1983;28:90–94.
26. Hauser H, Rheiner P. Computed tomography of the hand. Part 2: Pathological conditions. *Medicamundi* 1983;28:129–134.
27. Rhoades CE, Soye I, Levine E, Reckling FW. Detection of a wooden foreign body in the hand using computed tomography: Case report. *J Hand Surg* 1982;7:306–307.
28. Tirman RM, Weber ER, Snyder LL, Koonce TW. Midcarpal wrist arthrography for detection of tears of the scapholunate and lunotriquetral ligaments. *AJR* 1985;144:107–108.
29. Gilula LA, Totty WG, Weeks PM. Wrist arthrography: The value of fluoroscopic spot viewing. *Radiology* 1983;146:555–556.
30. Schwartz AM, Ruby LK. Wrist arthrography revisited. *Orthopedics* 1982;5:883–888.
31. Berger RA, Blair WF, El-Khouri G. Arthrotomography of the wrist: The triangular fibrocartilage complex. *Clin Orthop* 1983;172:257–264.
32. Resnick D, Andre M, Kerr R, Pineda C, Guerra J, Atkinson D. Digital arthrography of the wrist: A radiographic-pathologic investigation. *AJR* 1984;142:1187–1190.
33. Levinsohn EM, Palmer AK, Coren AB, Zinberg E. Wrist arthrography: The value of the three compartment injection technique. *Skeletal Radiol* 1987;16:539–544.

CHAPTER 2

PHYSICAL EXAMINATION OF THE WRIST AND HAND

I. PHYSICAL EXAMINATION OF THE WRIST — *Graham J. W. King and Robert Y. McMurtry*

II. EXAMINATION OF THE HAND AND WRIST — *Duffield Ashmead IV and H. Kirk Watson*

I. PHYSICAL EXAMINATION OF THE WRIST

Graham J. W. King and Robert Y. McMurtry

GENERAL CONSIDERATIONS

The evaluation of a patient who has complaints related to the wrist primarily relies on a careful history and physical examination. This should include a methodical search for both intrinsic and extrinsic pathology to guide further investigation and treatment.

The initial history should include the age of the patient, handedness, sex, vocation, and avocations. The date of onset of the patient's dysfunction and any association with a specific injury should be sought. The mechanism of injury should be clearly understood because this is often helpful in evaluating the extent of potential damage to the patient's wrist. Past history of injuries to the extremity should also be determined. The ergonomics and precise job description of patients who have work disorders are helpful in making this diagnosis and in planning treatment.

Pain is the most common presenting complaint in patients with wrist disorders. Less commonly, patients may complain of wrist stiffness or instability. It is essential to clarify the nature, location, onset, and characteristics of the patient's pain. Pain severity is difficult to quantify, but the extent of the patient's dysfunction can often be inferred by knowing the type and quantity of analgesics used. The presence of night pain is often a sign of more disabling pain. Aggravating and relieving factors should be specifically identified where possible. The radiation of pain either into the digits or proximally toward the shoulder is helpful in distinguishing any radicular distribution of pain. The location of the patient's pain is an important diagnostic feature in directing the physical examination and subsequent imaging studies. The patient should be carefully questioned to localize the area of maximal pain in the wrist. It is often useful to have the patient indicate the point of maximal discomfort, so that this area can be avoided until the latter portion of the physical examination. Functional limitations can also be evaluated on the basis of work history. Patients who are continuing to work usually have less dysfunction than those who must stop. Motivational factors can sometimes be inferred from the work history. Interference with sports and daily activities should also be sought.

During the interview the patient should be specifically questioned with regard to numbness, tingling, and weakness, if these have not already been volunteered. The position of the patient's hand, wrist, elbow, shoulder, or neck should be considered, as they relate to complaints of pain or sensory deficits.

Limitation of wrist flexion and extension, while often present with significant wrist pathology, is not a common presenting complaint. Restricted forearm rotation is much less well tolerated and a more common source of patient disability. Patients with a loss of supination often complain of an inability to accept coins, while patients who lack pronation may complain of problems with writing. Abnormalities of the proximal or distal radioulnar joint (DRUJ) are the most common cause of reduced forearm rotation.

Complaints of weakness in the wrist are occasionally due to extrinsic neurologic causes that can be determined by a careful neurologic examination. More commonly, patients have functional weakness caused by pain. This type of weakness is characterized by the patient "giving way" with an irregular jerky pattern at variable levels of strength. Finally, patients may complain of weakness due to wrist instability. Patients prevent symptomatic joint subluxation by avoiding excessive wrist loading, which may be manifested as weakness. Some patients with carpal or

DRUJ instability may complain of a feeling of giving way or a painful clunk, click, or snap.

Complaints of swelling should be carefully evaluated to determine the site, extent, and frequency as well as any aggravating or relieving factors. Dorsal wrist swelling aggravated by repetitive activity that improves with rest can usually be attributed to overuse tendonitis. A history of a slowly enlarging mass is more consistent with the presence of a tumor or tumorlike condition such as a wrist ganglion.

Complaints of fever, chills, night sweats, and weight loss often indicate systemic disorders such as diabetes or collagen vascular disease. The presence of multiple joint complaints in both the upper and lower extremities suggests the possibility of a systemic arthropathy. Bilateral symmetric symptoms may indicate overuse syndromes or a systemic polyarthritis. Family history of nodular osteoarthritis or rheumatoid arthritis may be helpful in selected cases.

After careful documentation of the patient's history, a methodical physical examination should be performed directed to some extent by the patient's presenting complaint and localization of discomfort. Of all the aspects of wrist examination, localization of the point of maximal tenderness correlates best with a treatable surgical pathology. An inconsistent point of maximal tenderness and diffuse areas of tenderness are more often associated with systemic disorders or repetitive overuse syndromes that respond poorly to surgical treatment.

INSPECTION OF THE WRIST

As the patient enters the room the examiner should note any abnormal motion patterns or use of the upper extremities. Similar observations during history-taking and physical examination are important in detecting pathology and evaluating the extent of a patient's disability. Because wrist symptoms are commonly referred from extrinsic sites, the neck, shoulder, arm, elbow, forearm, and hand should also be inspected and subsequently routinely examined. As the patient is asked to undress normal motion patterns of the hand and wrist should be observed.

The Dorsal Aspect

The skin of the wrist and hand should be inspected for evidence of previous traumatic or surgical scars. The presence or absence of hair should be noted as it may relate to the vascular supply of the hand. The color of the fingers, extent of sweating, and appearance of the nails should be evaluated. Certain workers may have dirty fingernails due to the nature of their jobs. Deformities of the nails may indicate previous trauma or systemic diseases such as psoriatic arthritis. Wasting of the interossei muscles should be looked for as they lie between the metacarpal shafts and in the first web space. Attention should be paid to each of the six extensor compartments, specifically looking for evidence of a focal tubular swelling as seen in tenosynovitis. Central dorsal swellings that are well circumscribed are most commonly wrist ganglions. The general contour and alignment of the wrist should also be evaluated. Posttraumatic deformities such as radial shortening and loss of radial inclination are often evident in patients with a malunion of a distal radial fracture. Patients with rheumatoid arthritis often have a radially deviated posture of the wrist as well as a dorsal prominence of the ulnar head.

The Radial Aspect

Prominence of the radial styloid and the overlying first extensor compartment should be examined. Patients with DeQuervain's tenosynovitis often have swelling localized to this area. Patients with scaphoid nonunions, trapeziometacarpal osteoarthritis, and scaphotrapezial osteoarthritis often have a fullness in the snuff box. Dorsal prominence of the ulna is often best seen from the radial aspect of the wrist in patients with subluxation or dislocation of the DRUJ. Dorsal translation of the carpus may be seen with malunited distal radial fractures and static midcarpal instability.

The Ventral Aspect

Traumatic or operative scars, callouses, and atrophy of the skin should be noted. Patients who use their hands often will have well-developed callouses, while those not using the hands much will have minimal callous formation. In advanced cases of disuse, atrophy of the pulp of unused digits may be noted. The normal pattern of palmar creases should be identified. Atrophy of the thenar or hypothenar eminence should be noted. The normal position of the pisiform and scaphoid tubercle can often be identified by inspection. Radial deviation and extension of the wrist brings the scaphoid tubercle into more prominence. Focal swelling of the flexor carpi radialis, the common flexors, or flexor carpi ulnaris are often difficult to identify by observation alone, due to their deep locations.

The Ulnar Aspect

Examination of the ulnar aspect should include an evaluation of the pisiform and position of the ulna relative to the radius. Patients with dorsal subluxation of the DRUJ have a dorsal prominence of the ulna relative to the radius. An increase in carpal supination, often seen in early rheumatoid arthritis, is also manifested as an increase in the prominence of the distal ulna. In addition, ventral subluxation of the extensor carpi ulnaris tendon can be seen in patients with a deficient sixth extensor compartment retinaculum.

PALPATION

Palpation of the wrist is performed on a regional basis in a systematic manner to ensure all areas are addressed. Specific attention should be paid to the area identified by the patient as the primary source of their pain or dysfunction. Palpation is executed with a precise knowledge of the normal wrist anatomy. It includes skin, subcutaneous tissues, tendons, tendon sheaths, and the underlying osseous and ligamentous structures. The sequence of examination should be tailored to the patient's area of maximal complaint. The point of maximal tenderness should be palpated last and other areas of abnormality excluded prior to examining the area in which the patient localizes his or her pain.

The Dorsal Aspect

Tendons and Other Soft-Tissue Structures

The dorsal aspect of the wrist has 6 extensor compartments containing a total of 12 extensor tendons. Extension of the fingers and wrist brings these structures into prominence (Fig. 2–1). Beginning radially over the first extensor compartment, one can palpate the abductor pollicis longus and extensor pollicis brevis as they pass over the radial styloid. Crepitus, swelling, and focal tenderness along the tendon sheath of the first extensor compartment is seen in patients with DeQuervain's tenosynovitis. The second extensor compartment containing the extensor carpi radialis longus and brevis can be felt more dorsoulnarly and deeper, especially with resisted wrist extension. Focal areas of swelling or tenderness may indicate a tendonopathy of these tendons. The pulsation of the dorsal branch of the radial artery may be felt as it winds around the scaphoid from ventral to dorsal between the first and second extensor compartments. The third extensor compartment, containing the tendon of extensor pollicis longus, can be palpated just ulnar to Lister's tubercle, a dorsal prominence of the distal radius. Hyperextension of the thumb accentuates the pathway of this tendon as it wraps around Lister's tubercle en route to the thumb. The tendons of the fourth extensor compartment are comprised of the extensor indices proprius and extensor digitorum comminus. These tendons are often involved with extensor tendon tenosynovitis. As the fingers are flexed and extended the dorsal tenosynovium may bunch up against the extensor retinaculum to give the so-called tuck sign with digital extension. More ulnarly the fifth extensor compartment can be palpated by flexing and extending the small finger to reveal the extensor digiti minimi. Resisted small finger extension brings this tendon into further prominence. The sixth extensor compartment is the most ulnar structure in the wrist and contains the extensor carpi ulnaris, a common site of tendonitis. Dorsal inspection while supinating the wrist brings this structure into prominence (Fig. 2–2). Asymmetry from side to side may indicate ventral subluxation of the tendon with a retinacular tear—the so-called empty sulcus sign.[1]

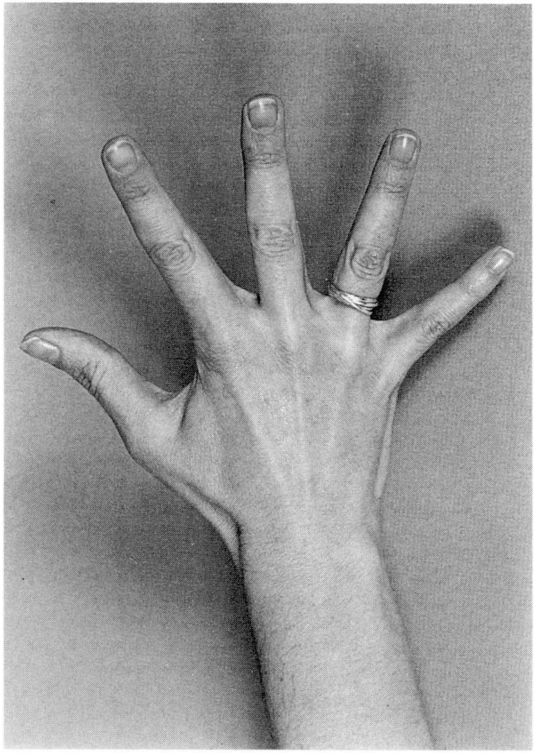

FIGURE 2–1. The dorsal aspect of the wrist. Extension of the wrist and fingers brings the extensor tendons into prominence.

Distal Radius and Ulna

The margins of the distal radius and ulna can be palpated using the landmarks of the extensor tendons. The "snuff box" can be defined by hyperextending the thumb and radially deviating the wrist. The abductor pollicis longus and extensor pollicis brevis lie ventrally while the extensor pollicis longus defines the dorsal border. Within the snuff box the radial styloid can be palpated as well as the dorsal radial aspect of the radius. Point tenderness may indicate a fracture or nonunion of the scaphoid as well as a radioscaphoid arthritis. The remainder of the dorsal margin of the distal radius can be palpated in the soft spot just ulnar to the second and third extensor compartments. The articulation of the distal radius with the proximal pole of the scaphoid and the radial margin of the lunate can be felt in this location. Proceeding more ulnarly, beneath the fourth extensor compartment, the remainder of the radiolunate articulation as well as the articulation of the radius with the radial margin of the triquetrum can be palpated. Deep to the extensor digiti minimi, in the fifth extensor compartment, one can palpate the dorsal aspect of the DRUJ and just distal to this

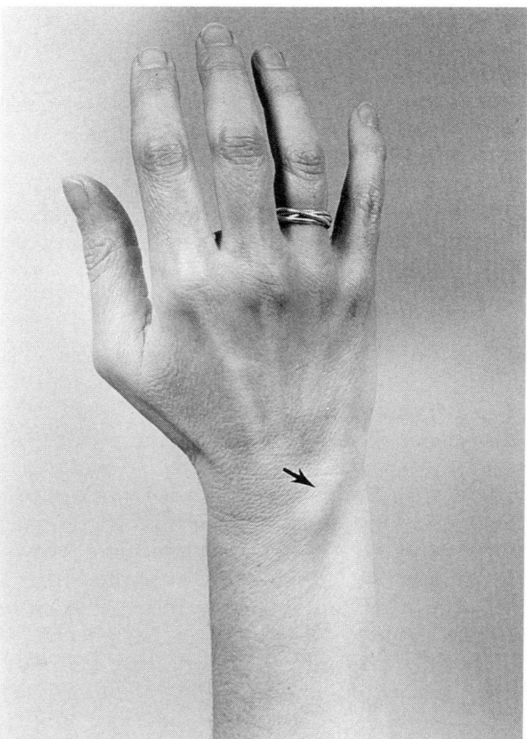

FIGURE 2–2. The extensor carpi ulnaris. Supination of the wrist brings the tendon of the extensor carpi ulnaris into prominence along the ulnar border of the wrist (arrow). Ventral subluxation of this tendon may produce the so-called empty sulcus sign.

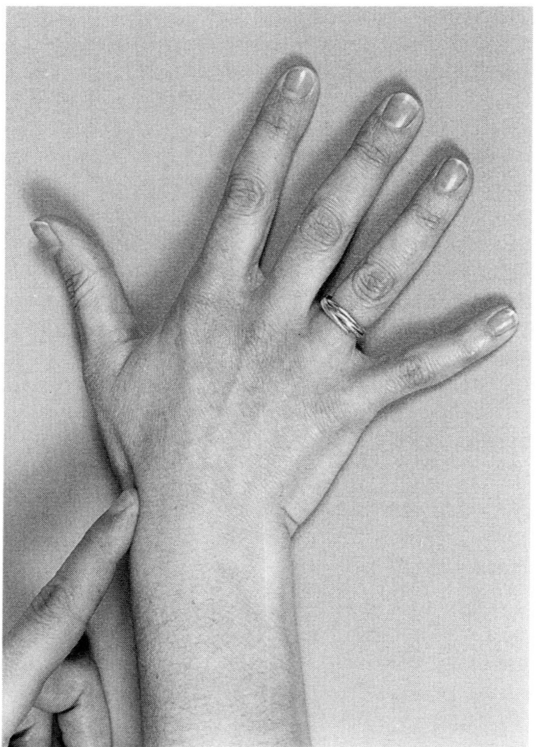

FIGURE 2–3. The scaphoid. The finger is palpating the scaphoid in the snuff box just distal to the radial styloid.

articulation, the triangular fibrocartilage. Pronosupination of the wrist helps to define this articulation. Point tenderness in this region may indicate a tear of the triangular fibrocartilage.[2] More ulnarly the ulnar styloid can be identified, especially with the wrist in pronation. Tenderness over this site may indicate an ulnar avulsion of the triangular fibrocartilage or a nonunion of the ulnar styloid.

Proximal Carpal Row

The scaphoid can be felt in the snuff box extending from the scaphotrapezial joint to the proximal pole (Fig. 2–3). Firm pressure over the scaphoid is often uncomfortable and therefore side-to-side differences should be noted. More ulnarly the scapholunate articulation and the dorsal portion of the scapholunate ligament can be identified by flexing the wrist and palpating between the third and fourth extensor compartments in the soft spot on the back of the wrist. Point tenderness at this site may indicate a scapholunate ligament tear. A little more radially this discomfort could be consistent with nonunion of the scaphoid or avascular necrosis of the proximal pole of the scaphoid. Palpating more ulnarly, just distal to Lister's tubercle the lunate can be palpated (Fig. 2–4). Tenderness at this site may indicate avascular necrosis of the lunate as seen in Kienböch's disease. The lunotriquetral articulation can be felt just distal to the DRUJ and deep to the extensor digiti minimi. Radial deviation of the wrist combined with slight

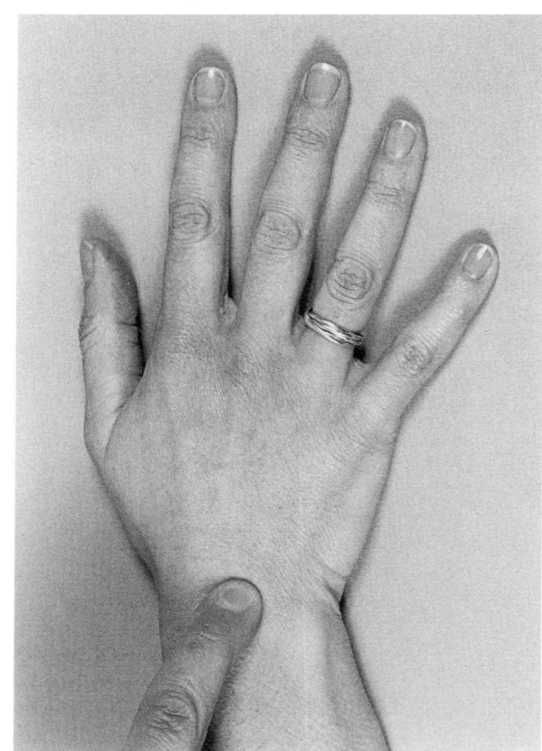

FIGURE 2–4. The lunate. The lunate can be felt just ulnar and distal to Lister's tubercle. Flexion of the wrist brings it out from underneath the dorsal lip of the distal radius.

flexion brings these structures into further prominence. The ulnar margin of the triquetrum is easily palpated beneath the extensor carpi ulnaris (Fig. 2–5).

Midcarpal Joints

The scaphotrapezial and scaphotrapezoidal joint can be palpated at the distal margin of the snuff box. This articulation can also be felt at the base of the index metacarpal as a deep indentation, sometimes called the pretrapezoid fossa, between the extensor pollicis longus and the extensor carpi radialis longus (Fig. 2–6). Motion of the thumb ray should be performed to distinguish this articulation from the basal joint of the thumb. Ulnar deviation of the wrist brings these joints into more prominence. Moving ulnarly the lunocapitate articulation can be felt in the soft spot between the third and fourth extensor compartments. The ridge between the lunate and the capitate can be accentuated by flexing and extending the wrist. The articulation of the triquetrum with the hamate can be felt as a prominent notch along the ulnar border of the wrist distal and ventral to the ulnar styloid (Fig. 2–7).

Distal Carpal Row

The trapezium is easily identified radially by circumducting the thumb and noting the differential motion between the thumb metacarpal and the adjacent trapezium. Moving just ulnar to this the trapezoid can be felt in line with the index metacarpal. Further

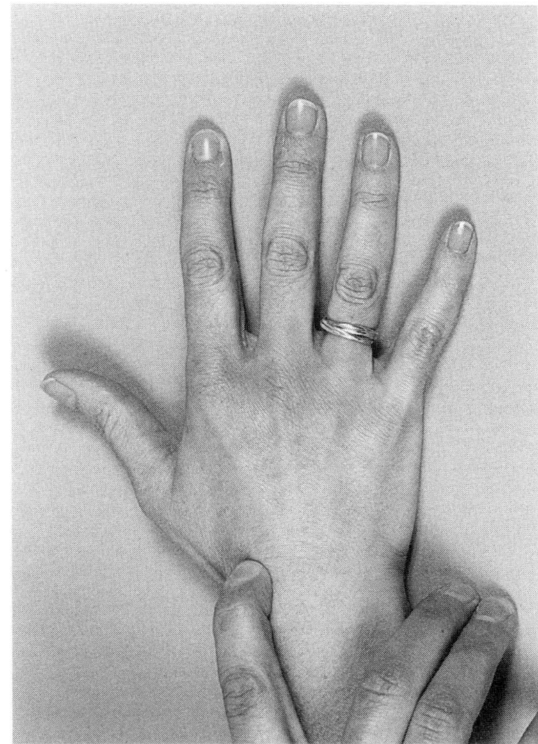

FIGURE 2–6. The scaphotrapeziotrapezoidal joint. This articulation can be felt at the base of the second metacarpal as a deep indentation sometimes referred to as the pretrapezoid fossa.

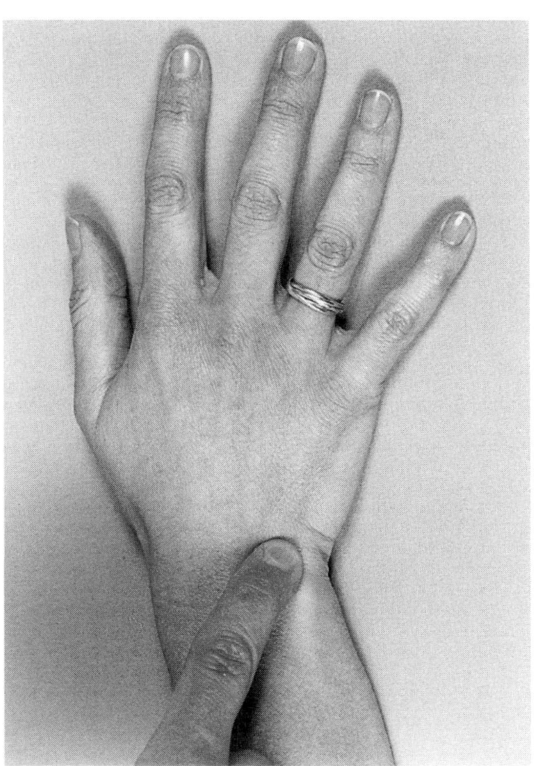

FIGURE 2–5. The triquetrum. The dorsal and ulnar surface of the triquetrum is felt just distal to the ulnar head and styloid.

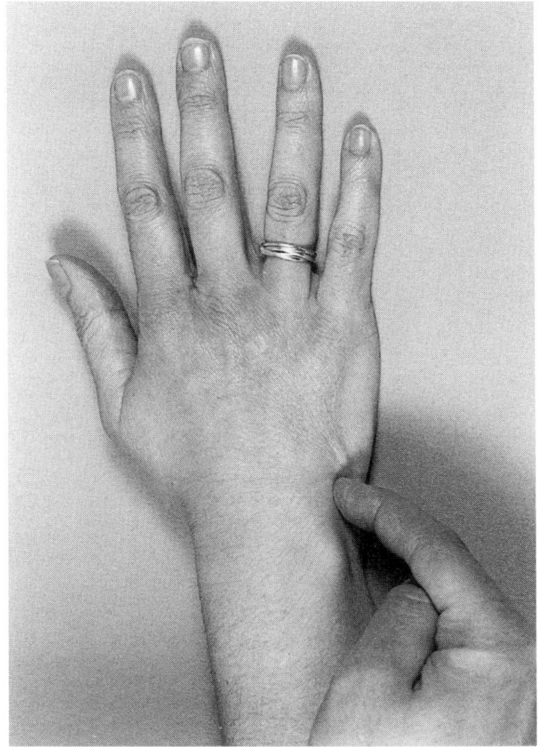

FIGURE 2–7. The triquetrohamate joint. A prominent notch can be felt between the triquetrum and the hamate on the ulnar border of the wrist just distal to the ulnar styloid. Radial deviation of the wrist facilitates palpation of this joint.

ulnar palpation will identify the capitate, which is deep proximally but comes into much more prominence distally until it articulates with the long finger metacarpal (Fig. 2–8). More ulnarly the hamate can be palpated at the base of the ring and small finger metacarpals, as can the capitohamate joint, a ridge between these two carpal bones.

Carpometacarpal Joints

The thumb carpometacarpal joint is easily identified, as previously described, by motion of the thumb. This is a common site of degenerative arthritis, especially in women. The index and long finger carpometacarpal joints are essentially nonmobile; however, the bases of these metacarpals are often quite prominent because the wrist extensor tendons attach to these bones. Tenderness at these sites may indicate a fracture-subluxation of these joints or a painful carpal boss. Rarely does osteoarthritis involve these articulations, probably because of their limited motion. The articulation of the ring and small finger metacarpals with the hamate should be palpated while passively flexing and extending these ulnar border metacarpals. The differential motion between the hamate and the metacarpals can be used to define the margins of the joints. Tenderness at this location, especially with a traumatic history, should raise the possibility of a carpometacarpal joint fracture or fracture subluxation, which can be very difficult to diagnose with plain radiographs.

A useful test to differentiate superficial tenderness from that of underlying osseous, joint, and ligamentous structures is to hyperextend the wrist and digits while palpating the wrist, then having the patient relax and *with the same force* continue to palpate the same location. Pain that is worse with relaxation of the extensor tendons suggests an underlying ligamentous, joint, or osseous abnormality as the source of the patient's discomfort. Pain that is similar with and without resisted wrist and digital extension suggests a soft-tissue source of pain.

The Ventral Aspect

Tendons and Other Soft-Tissue Structures

Beginning radially, the tendons of the first extensor compartment can be identified ventrally. Hyperextension of the thumb facilitates this identification. Just ulnar to this the radial artery can be identified with its pulsation. Ulnar to the artery is the flexor carpi radialis, which can be brought into prominence by resisted flexion of the wrist (Fig. 2–9). Focal swellings in and about this region are often due to ventral wrist ganglions. Distally the thenar muscles should be palpated for tender areas such as those seen in overuse syndromes. The flexor tendons to the digits as well as the palmaris longus can be felt centrally. Cup-

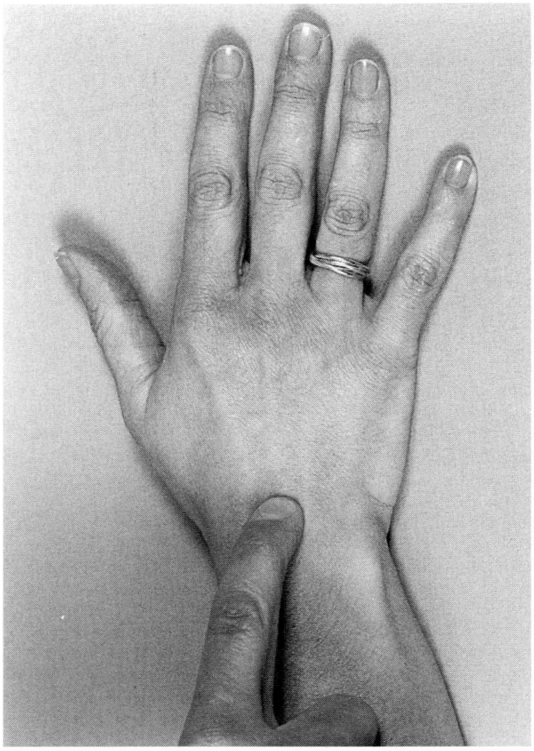

FIGURE 2–8. The capitate. The head of the capitate can be felt as an indentation in the central portion of the wrist deep to the fourth extensor compartment and in line with the long finger metacarpal.

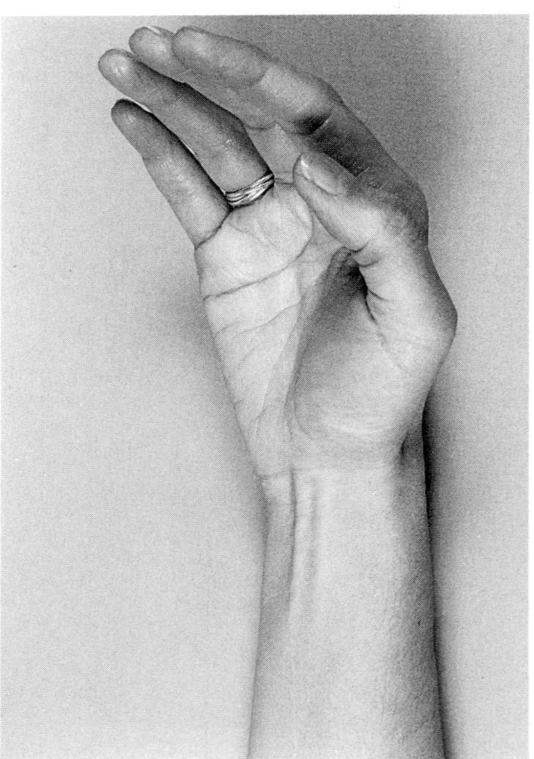

FIGURE 2–9. The ventral aspect of the wrist. Flexion of the wrist and fingers brings the flexor tendons into prominence.

ping the palm brings the palmaris longus into further prominence. Tenderness and crepitus over these tendons with motion may indicate a tendonopathy. Patients with significant flexor tenosynovitis may have swelling in this location as well as a boggy fullness on palpation. The median nerve lies just radial to the palmaris longus. Paresthesias and tenderness over the median nerve may indicate a median neuropathy. The ulnar artery, with the ulnar nerve just ulnar to it, can be palpated just radial to the flexor carpi ulnaris. The flexor carpi ulnaris with the pisiform (a sesamoid bone in the tendon) can be brought into prominence by resisted flexion and ulnar deviation of the wrist.

Distal Radius and Ulna

The articulation of the distal radius with the scaphoid can be palpated just ulnar to the first extensor compartment. This is a common site of tenderness in patients with radioscaphoid arthritis secondary to a scaphoid nonunion. The joint can be best identified by flexion and extension and radial and ulnar deviation of the wrist to identify its articular margin. Articulation of the radius with the lunate and triquetrum is difficult to evaluate ventrally due to intervening soft-tissue structures. The carpus has a convexity based dorsally to allow for passage of the flexor tendons into the wrist beneath the flexor retinaculum. The distance from the skin to the radiolunate and radiotriquetral articulations is large, making these joints difficult to feel from the ventral side. The ventral aspect of the distal radioulnar joint can be felt deep and radial to the flexor carpi ulnaris. Prominence of the distal ulna may indicate ventral subluxation of the DRUJ. Similarly, the ulnar margin of the distal ulna can be palpated just ulnar to the flexor carpi ulnaris.

Proximal Carpal Row

The scaphoid tubercle can be brought into prominence by extension and radial deviation of the wrist. Palpating radially and proximally to this, the entire scaphoid can be palpated from the proximal pole all the way to the scaphotrapezial joint, which can be felt as a prominent structure deep to the thenar musculature. Tenderness over the scaphoid waist from the ventral side, in addition to tenderness in the snuff box, helps confirm the diagnosis of a scaphoid fracture or nonunion. More ulnarly the pisiform can be palpated as it sits within the flexor carpi ulnaris tendon and articulates with the underlying triquetrum. Crepitus and/or pain on moving the pisiform may indicate pisotriquetral arthritis.

Midcarpal Articulation

The midcarpal joints are difficult to palpate ventrally except for the scaphotrapezial joint radially at the distal portion of the scaphoid. Tenderness deep in the hypothenar musculature may indicate an abnormality of the triquetrohamate joint; however, this is usually better appreciated by palpation from the dorsal surface.

Distal Carpal Row

The trapezium and trapezoid are easily felt distal to the scaphoid beneath the thenar musculature. The ridge of the trapezium, the distal and radial attachment of the flexor retinaculum, can usually be felt at this location. More ulnarly the other structures are difficult to identify due to the overlying muscles and tendonous structures. The ulnar margin of the hamate can be felt just distal to the triquetrum. The hook of the hamate can be readily felt if the examiner has an understanding of its normal location. To identify the hook of the hamate the interphalangeal joint of the examiner's thumb is placed on the pisiform and the thumb aimed towards the first web space. Rolling the thumb down into the palm allows one to feel the hook of the hamate deeply as a firmness in the palm (Fig. 2–10). A localized area of tenderness here often signifies a fracture or nonunion of the hook of the hamate.

Carpometacarpal Joints

The carpometacarpal joints are not well identified from the ventral surface except for the basal joint of the thumb. As mentioned with the dorsal examination, circumduction of the thumb can assist the

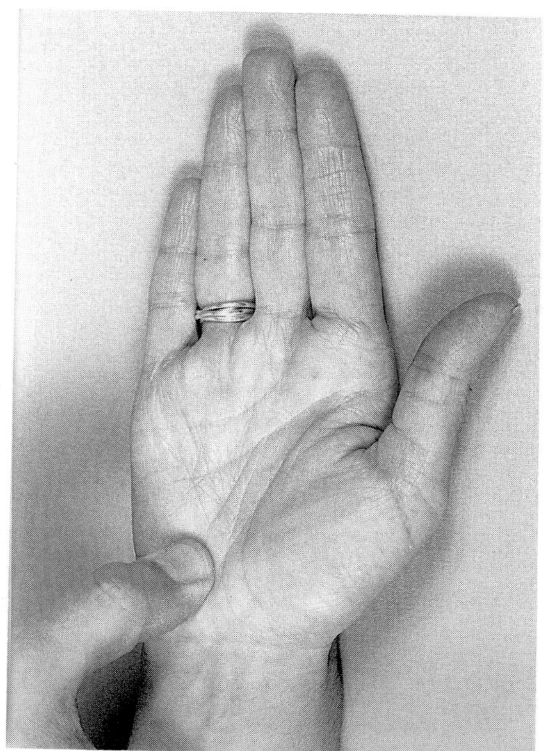

FIGURE 2–10. Hook of the hamate. To identify the hook of the hamate, the interphalangeal joint of the examiner's thumb is placed over the pisiform and aimed toward the first web space. The thumb tip is then rolled into the palm, and the hook of the hamate can be felt as a fullness deep in the palmar tissues.

examiner in identification of this articulation. Tenderness of this joint, both dorsally and ventrally, helps confirm the diagnosis of carpometacarpal joint arthrosis.

MOTION

Pronation and supination should be evaluated with the elbow flexed at 90 degrees and tucked in at the patient's side. Care should be taken to avoid trunk rotation in patients as they try to compensate for a lack of forearm rotation (Fig. 2–11). To avoid measuring radiocarpal supination, rotation should be measured at the level of the DRUJ rather than using objects held in the hand. Normal supination is about 90 degrees while normal pronation is 80 degrees.[3] Wrist extension and flexion and radial and ulnar deviations are checked relative to the long axis of the forearm. Normal wrist flexion is about 80 degrees from neutral while extension reaches about 70 degrees (Fig. 2–12).[3] Ulnar deviation is about 30 degrees and radial deviation 20 degrees (Fig. 2–13).[3] Comparison with the normal side is more accurate than the use of so-called normal values in patients with unilateral disease. Discrepancies between active and passive motion may signify an underlying neurologic abnormality.

The excursion and strength of each of the wrist motors should be evaluated. Resisted wrist flexion and radial deviation tests the flexor carpi radialis while resisted wrist flexion and ulnar deviation primarily tests the flexor carpi ulnaris. Resisted ulnar deviation and extension activates extensor carpi ulnaris and radial deviation and extension activates the extensor carpi radialis longus and brevis. Wrist strength can be quantified using special testing machines to evaluate flexor and extensor function. Grip strength measurement, which is more commonly available, is also a useful method to objectify strength. This measurement is influenced by both wrist and finger flexor and extensor tendon strength. Comparative values from side to side and changes over time make it a useful clinical tool.

PROVOCATIVE TESTS

Phalen's and Tinel's Tests

Hyperflexion of the wrist that reproduces the patient's complaints of numbness in the radial 3.5 digits

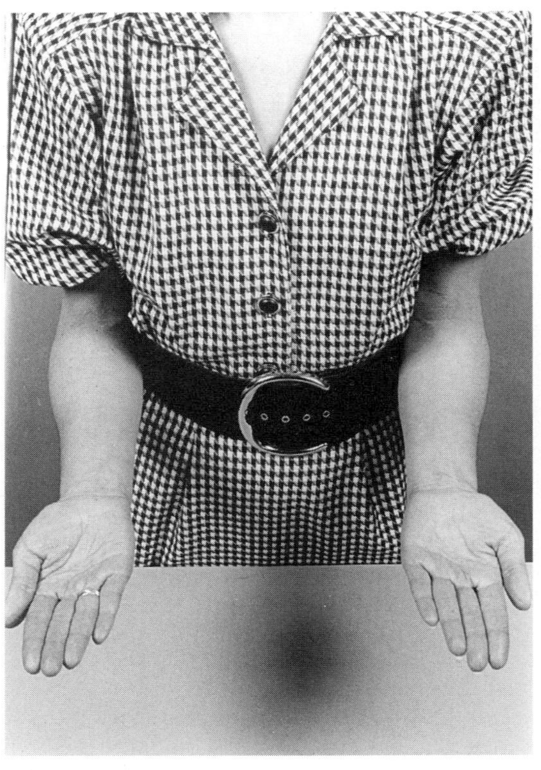

A

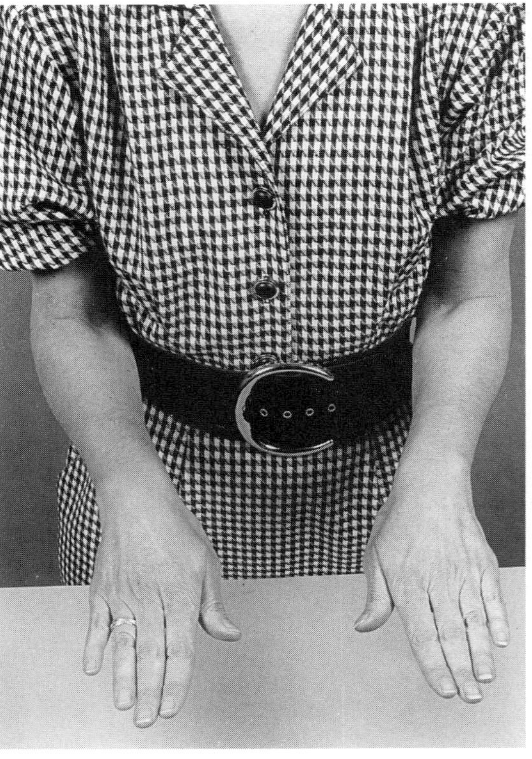

B

FIGURE 2–11. Pronosupination measurement. The elbows should be flexed at the side and the trunk straight with the wrists perpendicular to the floor. Rotation at the level of the distal radioulnar joint should be measured in supination **(A)** and pronation **(B)**.

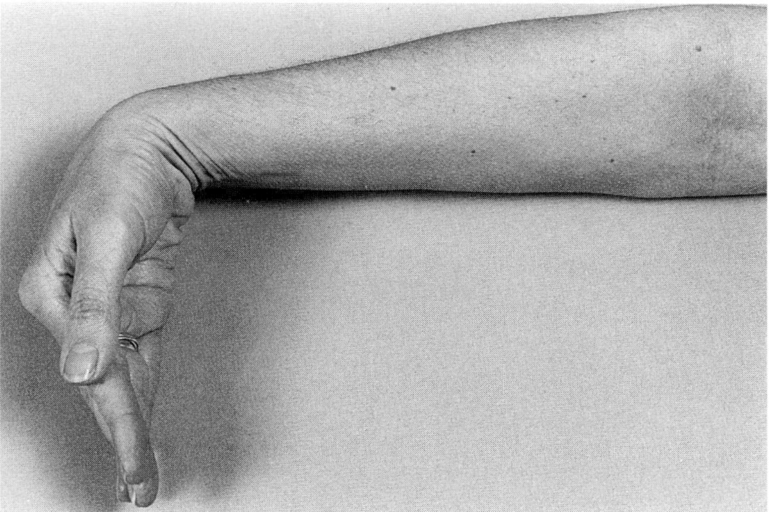

A

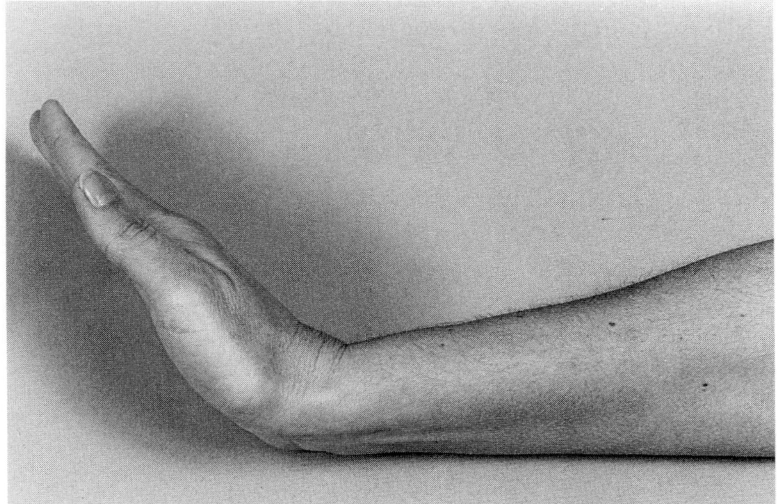

B

FIGURE 2–12. Flexion–extension measurement. Flexion **(A)** and extension **(B)** are best measured from the radial aspect of the wrist.

constitutes a positive Phalen's sign.[4] The addition of pressure over the median nerve can be useful in patients who have a borderline positive or negative Phalen's test (Fig. 2–14). Tapping the median nerve as it passes underneath the flexor retinaculum causes tingling to be referred to the involved digits (Tinel's sign).[5] These findings are usually associated with a diagnosis of carpal tunnel syndrome. In some patients the flexor retinaculum can be palpated at its proximal margin and found to be less compliant (more firm) than normal in patients with carpal tunnel syndrome. A positive Tinel's sign over the ulnar nerve at the wrist and radiating into the ulnar 1.5 digits may indicate entrapment of this nerve in Guyon's canal.

Allen's Test

Allen's test is used to determine the patency of the radial and ulnar arterial supply to the hand.[4,6] After palpation of the radial and ulnar arteries at the level of the wrist the patient is asked to make a tight fist with his or her hand. The examiner then applies firm pressure over both the radial and ulnar artery, and the patient is instructed to open the hand. The examiner then relieves the pressure on the ulnar artery while pressure is maintained over the radial artery. If no filling occurs after 30 seconds, then the pressure is released off the radial artery and radial-artery–dominant circulation to the hand is identified by a red blush filling the hand. This test is then repeated by the patient making a tight fist with pressure again

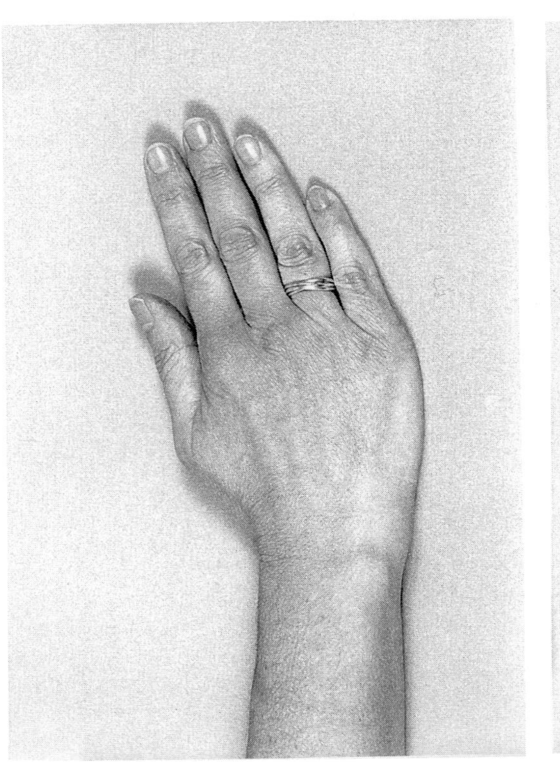

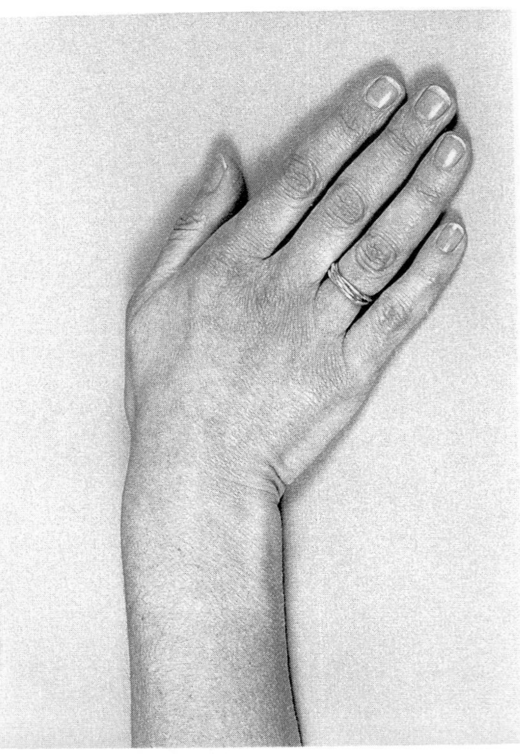

A B

FIGURE 2–13. Radioulnar deviation measurement. These measurements are made relative to the dorsal aspect of the wrist using the long axis of the forearm and the third metacarpal. Radial deviation **(A)** and ulnar deviation **(B)** are measured relative to the neutral position.

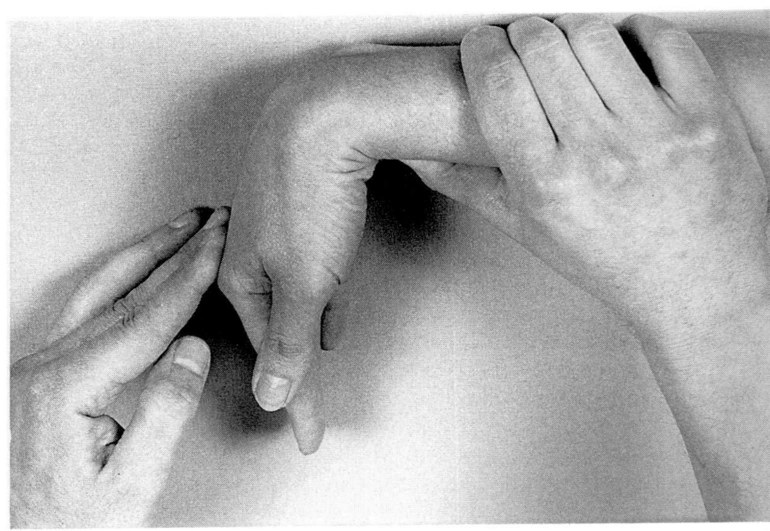

FIGURE 2–14. Phalen's test with provocation. Hyperflexion of the wrist that reproduces complaints of numbness in the radial 3.5 digits constitutes a positive Phalen's test. Concomitant pressure over the median nerve with the thumb accentuates the response.

applied over both vessels. The examiner then releases the pressure over the radial artery, this time leaving the pressure over the ulnar artery and checking for filling of the hand through the radial artery (Fig. 2–15). If no filling occurs then the pressure on the ulnar artery is released. Rapid filling then indicates an ulnar-artery–dominant circulation.

Finkelstein's Test

Finkelstein's test is used in the evaluation of patients with first extensor compartment tenosynovitis (DeQuervain's tenosynovitis).[7,8] The patient's thumb is flexed into the palm and the wrist is passively ulnarly deviated by the examiner (Fig. 2–16). This applies tension to the tendons in the first extensor compartment and reproduces the patient's typical pain. Comparison should be made with the opposite side because occasionally patients without significant tendonitis may report some discomfort with this maneuver. It is important to recognize that patients with trapeziometacarpal arthritis can often have a positive Finkelstein's test as well.

Carpometacarpal Grind Test

Patients with osteoarthritis between the thumb metacarpal and the trapezium have pain and palpable crepitus on axially loading and rotating the thumb ray relative to the carpus (Fig. 2–17). The pain is usually somewhat relieved by distracting the joint.

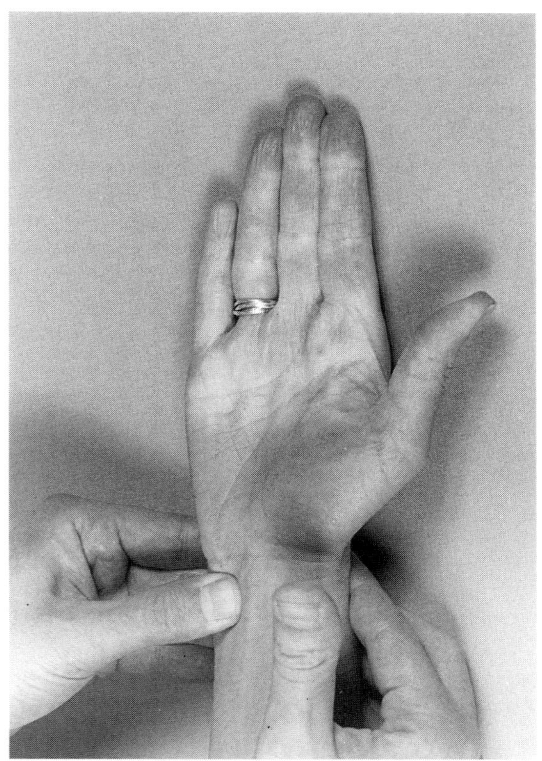

FIGURE 2–15. Allen's test. After exsanguinating the hand using a clenched fist, pressure is applied over the ulnar and radial arteries. A blush consistent with reperfusion can be seen here in the radial four digits after the pressure over the radial artery is released. The rate and extent of hand reperfusion is noted. The test is then repeated by releasing the pressure over the ulnar artery first.

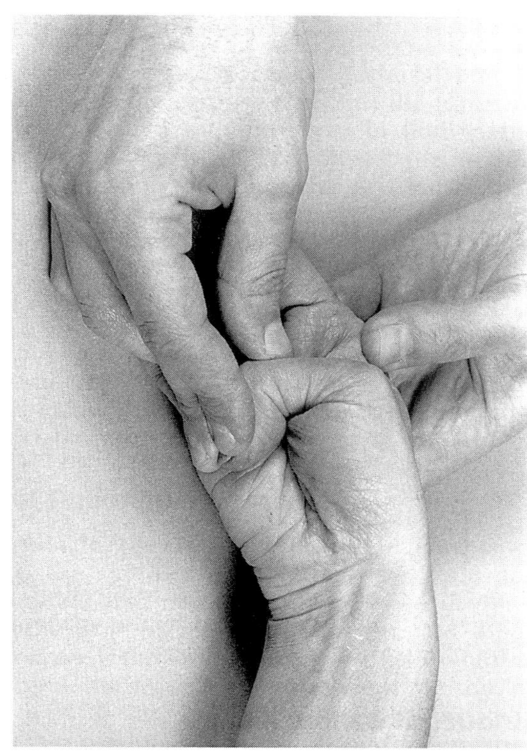

FIGURE 2–16. Finkelstein's test. The patient's thumb is flexed into the palm and the wrist is then forcefully ulnarly deviated by the examiner. This applies tension on the tendons in the first extensor compartment and reproduces the pain experienced in DeQuervain's tenosynovitis.

Scaphoid Shift Test

The scaphoid shift test is used to evaluate patients with dynamic scapholunate instability.[9] The tuberosity of the scaphoid is located on the ventral radial aspect of the wrist by radial deviation and extension of the wrist. Passive radial deviation of the wrist from an ulnarly deviated posture is performed by the examiner while preventing flexion of the scaphoid by firm ventral pressure with the thumb (Fig. 2–18). This loads the scapholunate ligament and reproduces the patient's typical discomfort in patients with a dynamic scapholunate dissociation. A positive test is indicated by a painful clunk that reproduces the patient's typical feeling of wrist instability.

Scapholunate Ballottement

In scapholunate ballottement the index finger is placed on the distal scaphoid tubercle ventrally and the thumb on the dorsal aspect of the proximal pole of the scaphoid just ulnar to the snuff box. The opposite thumb is placed on the dorsum of the lunate. The scaphoid is then translated relative to the

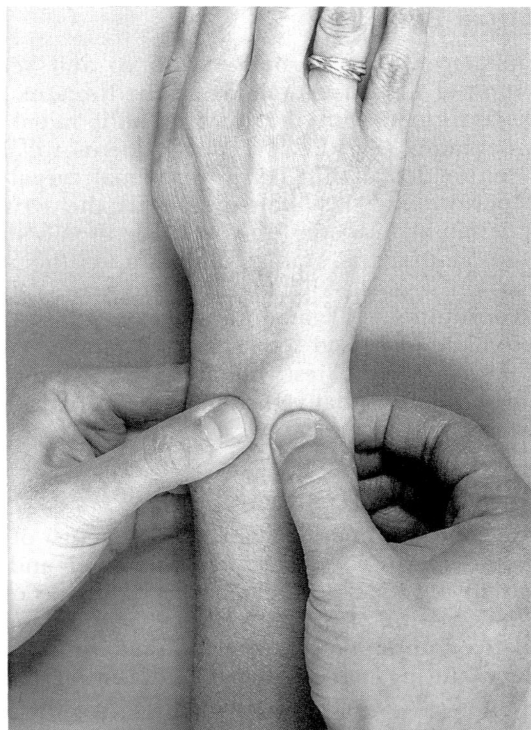

FIGURE 2–22. Distal radioulnar joint ballottement. The translation between the radius and ulna are evaluated with the forearm in supination, neutral, and pronation. Any side-to-side differences are noted.

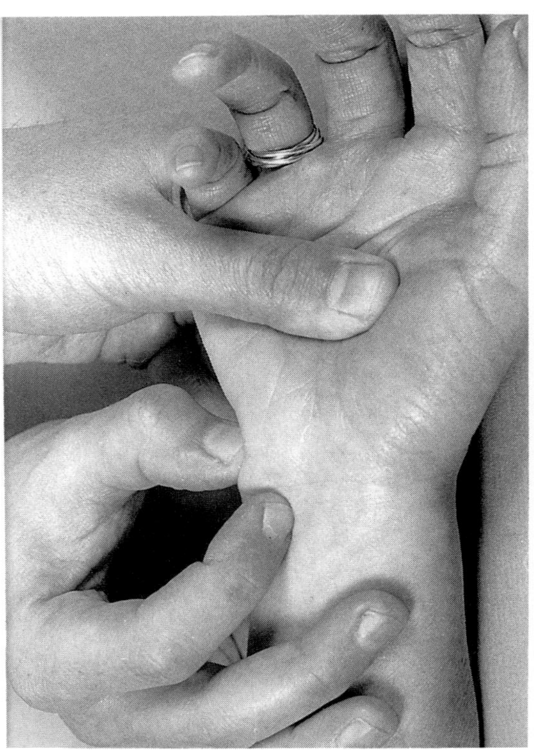

FIGURE 2–23. Pisotriquetral grind test. While applying ventral pressure over the pisiform with the thumb and index finger, the examiner rotates the pisiform on the triquetrum. Painful crepitus suggests pathology of the pisotriquetral joint.

is applied to the pisiform while translating it relative to the triquetrum (Fig. 2–23). Patients with inflammation or articular incongruity of the joint will complain of typical pain and in more advanced cases grinding will be palpated during this maneuver.

LOCAL ANAESTHETIC INJECTIONS

The injection of a local anaesthetic (1% lidocaine hydrochloride, xylocaine) in and about the wrist is a useful method for confirmation of the anatomic source of a patient's discomfort. For example, injections into the carpometacarpal joint of the thumb typically will relieve the majority of the patient's pain if his or her pathology is confined to this articulation. Patients with pantrapezial arthritis often continue to have significant pain after such an injection. Similarly, patients who have the first extensor compartment injected for radial wrist pain usually have near-complete pain relief if their underlying diagnosis is DeQuervain's tenosynovitis. Injections into the pisotriquetral joint are useful in relieving patient's pain from arthrosis of this joint. Intraarticular radiocarpal pathology can be differentiated from soft tissue pain by injection of 5 mL of local anaesthetic into the radiocarpal joint dorsally between the third and fourth extensor compartments. Reduction of the pain and an increase in the functional ability of the patient after such an injection are strong evidence of an intraarticular source of the patient's disability.

SUMMARY

Physical examination of the wrist requires a sound knowledge of the underlying anatomy so that appropriate structures are routinely palpated in the course of the examination. Careful history allows the localization of the areas of the patient's maximal discomfort. The physical examination should be tailored to address the painful site last to avoid losing the confidence of the patient. Whereas the physical examination must be complete, the provocative tests are only applied on an as-needed basis. Appropriate provocative tests are selected based on the patient's history and by localization of the patient's discomfort. Patients with ulnar wrist pain more commonly have tears of the lunotriquetral ligament or triangular fibrocartilage, whereas patients with radial wrist pain most commonly have first extensor compartment tenosynovitis, first carpometacarpal osteoarthritis, occult scaphoid fractures, and/or scapholunate ligament abnormalities. Careful physical examination is essential so that an appropriate provisional diagnosis can be entertained. Appropriate imaging modalities can then be applied in a thoughtful manner with a much greater likelihood of yielding true positive tests that correlate with the patient's underlying pathology.

II. EXAMINATION OF THE HAND AND WRIST

Duffield Ashmead IV and H. Kirk Watson

GENERAL CONSIDERATIONS

Before diagnostic imaging, all patients should undergo a careful interview and physical examination. A detailed history not only defines the hand or wrist problem as the patient sees it, but will enable the clinician to evaluate the hand in its proper context. Pertinent background material will usually include age, hand dominance, and vocational as well as avocational activities. A description of prior or preexisting hand problems will help to establish baseline functional status. The nature of the present problem is explored and recorded, including inciting injury if any, onset and evolution of symptoms, and current functional status, including aggravating and ameliorating factors. With the greater focus afforded by this history, the clinician then proceeds with a thorough examination of the hands.

It is our practice to examine a patient face to face across a narrow table. A pull-out writing slide in a standard desk suits this purpose well. Right and left extremities can be compared side by side; symmetries and asymmetries are readily apparent. The slide itself provides a resting surface for sensory and motor testing as well as a writing surface for note taking.

The examination begins before the patient sits down; however, considerable information can be gleaned from the way the patient approaches the examination room. Is the affected extremity employed, rested, or carefully protected? What is its resting posture? Observation continues as the patient is seated and the extremities placed side by side. Are they developmentally comparable? Are skeletal elements similar in size? A small extremity may be congenitally deficient or may have sustained an early neurologic injury such as an obstetric palsy. Are extension and flexion creases present and normally situated? These creases are a reflection of developmental joint motion and may help distinguish congenital from acquired deficits. Are muscle groups roughly symmetrical? Is there any suggestion of atrophy? Hair and perspiratory distribution are indicators of neurovascular status. Patterns of callous formation, nail length, and soilage will provide insight into how the affected hand or digit is used. Loss of digital pulp bulk, effacement of rugal (fingerprint) pattern, nailfold thinning, and increase in nail curvature are "trophic changes" suggestive of significant neurologic problem, disuse, or reflex sympathetic dystrophy. Are there wounds, swelling, or other signs of acute inflammation or injury?

MOTOR ASSESSMENT

With the patient seated opposite the examiner, active and passive range of motion at the elbow, wrist, and digits are easily demonstrated, assessed for symmetry, and measured with a goniometer. While evaluating active mobility, the examiner may wish to check any limited arcs of motion for passive augmentation. After assessment of the elbow, pronosupination is readily judged with the patient's elbows resting on the table. Left and right wrist motions should mirror each other with the extremities examined side by side. Asymmetries in wrist extension and flexion are highly suggestive of underlying radial or carpal pathology.

Digital ranges of motion may be screened in aggregate, but any suggestion of abnormality should be examined more closely. Is mobility affected by the position of proximal or distal joints? If so, there is a restricting structure bridging multiple articulations. Are there rotational abnormalities such that the digits interfere with each other?

Subjective sensibility is rapidly tested by light touch throughout all cutaneous nerve distributions. This provides a simple screen for neurosensory pathology. More in-depth examination includes static or moving two-point discrimination at all finger pulps. Semmes–Weinstein monofilaments provide an alternative measure of pulp sensibility and are also helpful in areas where two-point discrimination is less well defined and where discriminatory sensibility is less important than protective sensibility. Vibratory threshold testing may also be appropriate.

Motor assessment begins with an examination of specific muscle groups, particularly the intrinsics, for evidence of atrophy. Thereafter individual wrist and digital extensors/flexors are tested against resistance. Total absence of function must be distinguished from weakness; true weakness must be distinguished from volitional or antalgic limitations of patient effort. Presence of a tenodesis effect will reliably distinguish absence of motor function from disruption of a musculotendinous unit. In the context of acute injuries, pain on resisted finger extension or flexion often indicates a partial laceration of the involved tendon.

Certain musculotendinous units will require careful isolation. Whereas only the profundus tendon is capable of flexing the distal interphalangeal (DIP) joint, both sublimis and profundus will flex metacarpophalangeal (MP) and proximal interphalangeal (PIP) joints. Sublimis function must be isolated by holding adjacent digits in hyperextension while asking the patient to flex at the PIP joint. The "commonness" of flexor profundus tendons at the level of the wrist precludes independent excursion of individual slips (quadregia effect). Absence of an independently functioning little finger sublimis is a fairly common variant. A similar isolation of extensor indicis proprius and extensor digiti minimi may be achieved by passive full flexion of the long and ring fingers. Isolated evaluation of communis slips to the index and little fingers is less readily accomplished. Most extensor tendons, however, are readily palpable in the dorsal wrist and hand when wrist and hand extension is resisted. Extensor pollicis longus function should be assessed not by voluntary extension at the thumb interphalangeal (IP) joint, but rather by assessing retroposition of the thumb (extensor pollicis brevis slips will frequently extend to the distal phalanx, as do intrinsic insertions through the extensor hood). Resisted palmar abduction of the thumb provides a measure of opponens and abductor pollicis brevis strength. Resisted abduction and adduction of the fingers tests the interossei. Asking the patient to hold the thumb and index finger tightly side by side while the examiner attempts to separate them will provide a combined measure of the adductor and first dorsal interosseous. More formalized objective measures of grip strength may be appropriate, including the Jamar dynomometer and pinch meter (both key pinch and tripod).

Direct assessment of vascular status may be appropriate even when color, temperature, and capillary refill appear normal. Allen's test provides a visual measure of radial and ulnar perfusion at the level of the wrist. A "digital Allen's test" may be performed to evaluate radial and ulnar proper digital vessels.

MANIPULATIVE ASSESSMENT

Manipulative examination of the hand and upper extremity will serve not only to locate the respective positions of certain bony landmarks, but also to localize areas of tenderness. The medial and lateral epicondyles, radial and ulnar styloids, and extensor and flexor sheaths are all frequent sites of inflammatory change with associated discomfort. Significant pain or paresthesias on gentle compression of the median or ulnar nerves at the elbow, midforearm, or wrist may suggest a compressive neuropathy. Manipulation of individual joints will provide considerable information: Does the patient complain of pain? Is there palpable joint swelling ("synovitis")? Are the articular surfaces smooth and gliding or is there joint noise? Is there any instability?

A thorough manipulative exam is readily integrated with an assessment of passive mobility, and it will include a variety of standard provocative maneuvers. The distal radioulnar joint is assessed from midforearm level, compressing the radius and ulna together. Passive pronosupination, performed from this level, affords clinical access to the distal radioulnar joint, relatively unconfused by adjacent carpal pathology. Although the examiner's hand is quite proximal, the patient will readily localize pathology at the distal level. The radiocarpal and midcarpal joints are examined sequentially, beginning at the radial styloid and adjacent radioscaphoid articulation. Immediately distal to the styloid is the dorsal scaphoid ridge, representing the articular margin of its radial facet. Palpation may be facilitated by passive ulnar deviation of the wrist. Further distal is the dorsal aspect of the scaphotrapeziotrapezoidal (STT) (triscaphe) joint. The scapholunate articulation is readily palpable between the extensor carpi radialis brevis (ECRB) and the extensors of the fourth compartment. The scapholunate joint, triscaphe joint, and the articular/nonarticular margin of the scaphoid are reliable sites of tenderness and occasionally fullness in cases of scaphoid instability (or "rotary subluxation of the scaphoid" [RSS]). A measure of scaphoid stability and surrounding inflammatory change may be gleaned from the *scaphoid shift maneuver.*[10] The examiner places his or her right thumb over the palmar or ventral nose (distal pole) of the patient's right scaphoid with his or her fingers wrapped around the patient's dorsal forearm for counterpressure. As the patient's wrist is brought passively from full ulnar deviation to radial deviation, the examiner's thumb prevents the scaphoid from flexing, driving the proximal pole dorsally. Once the maximum motion position is determined, the scaphoid can be ballotted and its motion evaluated. Significant findings are increased or decreased mobility in comparison with the opposite side, or significant pain usually localized to the dorsal side of the wrist. A final indicator of periscaphoid inflammatory change is the *finger extension test.* With the patient's wrist held passively in flexion, the examiner resists active finger extension. In patients with significant periscaphoid inflammatory change, the combined radiocarpal loading and pressure of extensor tendons will cause considerable discomfort. Currently we believe symptomatic RSS is always associated with a positive finger extension test.

Progressing further ulnarly, the lunotriquetral, triquetrohamate, and pisotriquetral articulations are each examined individually. The adjacent ulnar styloid and extensor carpi ulnaris sheath are also potential sites of pathology.

Throughout the examination it may be necessary to trick a distressed or uncooperative patient. "Substitution maneuvers" and "distraction techniques" are very helpful, and a few examples follow. While appearing to focus on manipulation of one part of the hand, the examiner may simultaneously explore other areas. Concurrent testing of multiple or bilateral muscle groups will often confound a patient with voluntary weakness. Finally, when approaching the patient with multiple complaints, it is frequently helpful to ask the patient to identify the single site of greatest discomfort ("point with one finger . . .") or to identify the solitary symptom he or she finds most distressing ("If I could eliminate a single component of your current problem, what would it be?").

After completion of a thorough physical examination, a single diagnosis or very brief differential is usually apparent. Only infrequently will imaging techniques solve a diagnostic mystery or yield a surprise. These techniques are absolutely essential, however, for precise localization of pathology, estimates of severity, and preinterventional planning.

REFERENCES

1. Paley D, McMurtry RY, Murray JF. Dorsal dislocation of the ulnar styloid and extensor carpi ulnaris tendon into the distal radioulnar joint: The empty sulcus sign. *J Hand Surg* 1987; 12A:1029–1032.
2. Palmer AK, Werner FW. The triangular fibrocartilage complex of the wrist: Anatomy and function. *J Hand Surg* 1981;6:153–162.
3. American Orthopaedic Association. *Manual of orthopaedic surgery.* Chicago: The American Orthopaedic Association, 1979.
4. American Society for Surgery of the Hand. *The hand: Examination and diagnosis.* New York: Churchill Livingstone, 1983.
5. Magee DJ. *Forearm, wrist, and hand: Orthopaedic physical assessment.* Philadelphia: WB Saunders, 1987.
6. Moldaver J. Tinel's sign: Its characteristics and significance. *J Bone Joint Surg* 1978;60A:412–414.
7. Hoppenfeld S. *Physical examination of the spine and extremities.* New York: Appleton-Century-Crofts, 1976.
8. Finkelstein H. Stenosing tendovaginitis at the radial styloid process. *J Bone Joint Surg* 1930;12:509–540.
9. Watson HK, Ryu J, Akelman E. Limited triscaphoid intercarpal arthrodesis for rotatory subluxation of the scaphoid. *J Bone Joint Surg* 1986;68A:345–349.
10. Watson HK, Ashmead D, Makhlouf MV. Examination of the scaphoid. *J Hand Surg* 1988;13A(5):657–660.

CHAPTER 3

PHYSICAL EXAMINATION AND PROVOCATIVE MANEUVERS OF THE WRIST

Richard A. Berger and James H. Dobyns

INTRODUCTION

Injuries of the wrist are often difficult to assess clinically due to the tremendous complexity of carpal anatomy and mechanics. It is not surprising that the clinical examination of the wrist is difficult when one considers that the wrist region contains 15 bones forming 4 major joint regions, which are further divisible into 10 interosseous joints connected by over 20 individual ligaments, all traversed by 23 extrinsic tendons; forms the origins of 8 intrinsic muscles; and transmits 2 major arteries and 6 major nerve branches. Although located in a relatively superficial plane compared with other joint systems, the identification of these structures may be easily confusing, leading to an inaccurate clinical impression. It is therefore of paramount importance that the examiner of the wrist be thoroughly familiar with the underlying anatomy and mechanics of the normal wrist. Once this underlying anatomy is confidently understood, clinical evaluation of the wrist may proceed. We have found that a methodical approach to examination of the wrist is desirable, since critical steps in the examination may be missed if not included in a systematic protocol. This chapter offers a guide to one systematic approach to examination of the wrist. It is often not necessary to complete all testing maneuvers described, and special circumstances may warrant additional tests or maneuvers that may not be listed here.

HISTORY

Common to any complete clinical evaluation will be the accumulation of historical data from the patient or other sources regarding the presenting chief complaint. Of fundamental importance is an absolutely clear understanding of the nature of the chief complaint. Most clinicians have been caught in the dilemma where the most obvious clinical features on examination are not related to the complaint that brought the patient to seek an evaluation in the first place. If we are to expect satisfying results with our patients, we must make every effort to understand why they are seeking help. Additionally, the clinician needs to be wary of descriptive terms such as numbness, pain, and weakness, because these terms may have different meanings to each patient; careful definitions of these symptomatic terms must be mutually agreed on by both the patient and the examiner.

Standard information regarding the circumstances surrounding the onset of the symptoms (trauma, repetitive use, insidious versus sudden onset), the nature of the problem, exacerbating and alleviating factors, severity and constancy of symptoms, and previous treatment efforts should be recorded. The normal use patterns of the hands should be understood, since hand dominance alone will generally not define the use patterns of the hands and wrists. The patient's vocation and avocations should be thoroughly understood, especially when rehabilitation issues emerge. If a puncture, laceration, or other open wound is present, information regarding potential sources and degree of contamination, the time lapsed since the injury occurred, the status of the patient's tetanus prophylaxis, and a drug hypersensitivity profile should be determined, recorded, and appropriately acted on.

CLINICAL ASSESSMENT

General Considerations

Among the first steps in clinical assessment, particularly in a posttraumatic situation, is triage of the entire patient, especially adjacent limb segments. Careful attention should be directed to determining the vascular and neurologic status of the extremity, as well as to obtaining appropriate radiographs of any joint or limb segment suspected of having an injury. The findings of this triage effort should be carefully recorded. If any concern exists regarding an evolving clinical situation, such as a compartment syndrome or progressive neurologic or vascular embarrassment, subsequent examination findings can be easily compared with previous recordings along a time-line, greatly enhancing the understanding of the patient's condition. As noted above, the examiner is always encouraged to compare the extremity under examination with the contralateral extremity, which may often be used as a "control" examination.

Visual Inspection

Visual inspection will give the examiner substantial information regarding probable sources of pathology in a short period of time. Swelling may be evident anywhere on the wrist but the most likely regions are the dorsal, ulnar, and radial. Palmarly, the thick glabrous palmar skin immediately superficial to the thick palmar aponeurosis and flexor retinaculum often obscures swelling; however, swelling proximal to the glabrous skin of the palm may be present through the thin and mobile anterior forearm skin. Discrete swelling, especially near the distal course of the flexor carpi radialis tendon and dorsally or dorsoradially in the wrist region proper, may indicate the presence of a ganglion or cyst. Swelling from the wrist joint proper will most likely be appreciated directly through loss of normal contours, especially in an area of depression such as the anatomic snuff box. The presence of ecchymosis is certainly indicative of vascular trauma or bleeding dyscrasias but generally is not helpful in localizing a specific disorder.

Careful observation of bilateral wrist profiles may reveal asymmetries such as dorsal prominence of the distal ulna, which may result from disruption of the distal radioulnar joint or excessive ulnocarpal supination. Observation of the posture of the fingers should also be made, because flexor tendon lacerations or nerve palsies in the region of the wrist may be clearly reflected in abnormal digital function. Obviously, abnormal dermal perfusion patterns reflected by pallor or venous congestion should be sought and appropriately managed. Finally, much can be gained from casually observing the wrist as the history is taken to determine the degree of spontaneous motion and use of the hand, the presence of guarding or posturing, and to develop an overall sense of the level of discomfort that the patient is experiencing.

Objective Measurement

Range of Motion

One of the first objective measurements to obtain is the active range of motion of the digits, wrist, and forearm. A quick screening test for digital range of motion will determine if active lags are present in the range of extension or flexion. To test for extension lags, the patient is asked to fully extend the fingers, usually with the wrist in a relatively neutral and unconstrained posture. If the finger- or thumbnail touches a straightedge (as a ruler) extending distally from the dorsal plane of the corresponding metacarpal, the patient is said to have no extension lag. Any inability to touch the straightedge is recorded as an *extension lag,* and is quantitatively recorded by measuring the perpendicular distance from the center of the nail to the straightedge. Similarly, full flexion of the digits to the distal palmar flexion crease is considered normal. An inability to fully flex the digits in this manner is recorded as a *flexion lag* and it is quantitated by measuring the perpendicular distance from the center of the pulp of the distal phalanx to the distal palmar flexion crease. If a quantifiable extension or flexion lag is detected, it must be determined if this results from a joint contracture (in which case the lag is not passively correctable) or if the problem rests with tendon excursion. In this instance, care must be taken to rule out tenodesis in the region of the wrist, which may be demonstrated by determining if a change in the lag occurs as a function of wrist position.

Wrist *range of motion* may be recorded in the following way. For palmar flexion, the goniometer is centered over the dorsal surface of the wrist with the edges extending proximally on the dorsal forearm and distally on the dorsal hand, with the wrist maximally actively, and subsequently passively, flexed (Fig. 3–1A). The fingers are allowed to assume an unconstrained posture. Conversely, dorsiflexion is measured actively and passively by placing the goniometer on the palmar surface of the wrist, often with the distal edge extending between the fingers to allow the distal edge to rest on the palm of the hand (Fig. 3–1B). Again, the goniometer is centered on the wrist and the fingers assume an unconstrained posture. Although variability exists, most normal wrists can achieve at least 60 degrees each of palmar-flexion and dorsiflexion. Wrist radial and ulnar deviation are measured by centering the axis of the goniometer on the dorsal surface of the wrist, with the proximal edge centered on the dorsal forearm and the distal edge centered on the third metacarpal. The active and passive ranges of radial and ulnar deviation are recorded, all with the forearm in neutral rotation, if possible. Radial deviation normally exceeds 15 degrees and ulnar deviation usually exceeds 20 degrees.

Forearm rotation is very important to evaluate since the distal radioulnar joint is intimately related to the wrist, both functionally and anatomically. The measurement of forearm pronation and supination can be difficult to quantify, largely due to the lack of uniformly available anatomic benchmarks from which to accurately gauge displacement. One suggested method starts by having the patient rest both humerii comfortably at his or her sides, with the elbows flexed to 90 degrees. It is often easier to evaluate both

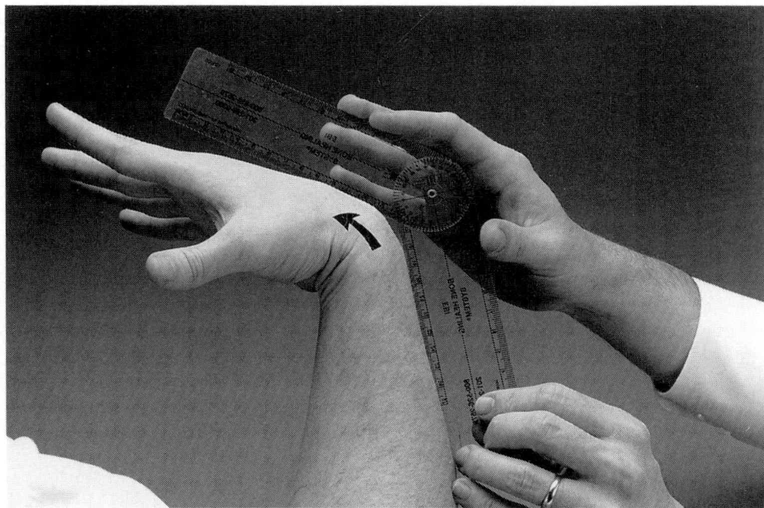

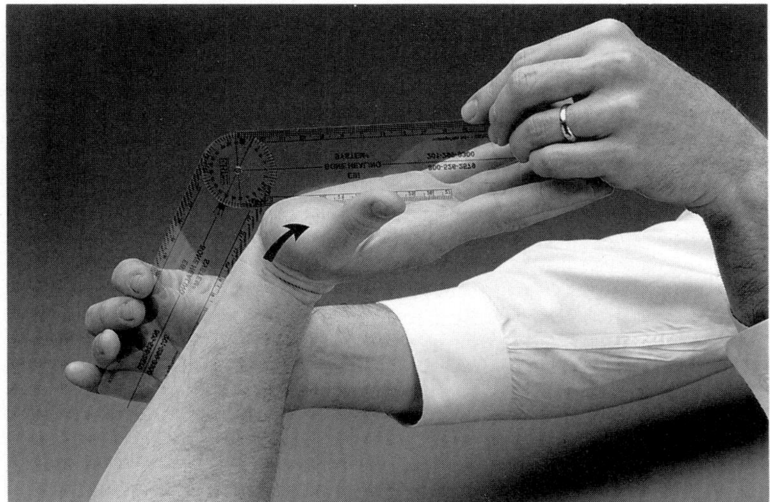

B

FIGURE 3–1. A method to measure wrist range of motion using a standard goniometer. **A:** Measurement of wrist palmar-flexion. **B:** Measurement of wrist dorsiflexion.

forearms simultaneously, because subtle differences will be much more apparent when compared concurrently as opposed to separately. The patient is reminded to keep his or her elbows close to his or her sides. With the humerus used as the reference axis, the goniometer is placed on the anterior surface of the distal forearm for measuring supination and on the dorsal distal forearm surface for measuring pronation. Normal ranges of pronation and supination approach 80 degrees each.

If distal radioulnar joint instability is suspected, the amount of anterior and posterior translation of the radius on the ulna can be *estimated* by placing the forearm in a vertical position with neutral rotation. The examiner gently grasps the distal radius between his or her own thumb and fingers with one hand and the ulna in a similar fashion with the other hand. The bones are passively moved in opposite directions, estimating the linear displacement between the bones. As noted above, it is very important to compare these values with the contralateral extremity. Normally, up to 4 mm of total translation can be passively generated.

Although difficult to quantify, the degree of radiocarpal and midcarpal *passive* pronation and supination should be estimated using a bimanual examination technique with one hand stabilizing the proximal segment (distal forearm or proximal carpal row) and the other hand passively rotating the distal segment (proximal or distal carpal rows, respectively). The range of rotation is then estimated and recorded in degrees. The normal total range of passive radiocarpal/midcarpal rotation is up to 40 degrees.

Carpometacarpal (CMC) motion should be assessed in a complete examination. Thumb CMC motion is measured with a goniometer centered over the first CMC joint and the edges aligned with the first and second metacarpals. Both planar (radial) abduction and palmar abduction should be measured, with 35 to 45 degrees generally being accepted as normal. The second and third CMC motion is normally actively and passively undetectable. Fourth and fifth

CMC motion is primarily flexion–extension and averages 20 and 40 degrees, respectively.

Grip

Grip strength is felt to be one of the most sensitive measures of hand and wrist function. It often proves to be a reliable barometer for progress of convalescence and may be helpful in the detection of malingering.[1] Major limitations to the use of grip measures are the lack of population-wide normal values and the tendency of measuring devices to fall out of calibration and thus reduce the reliability of serial measurements obtained using different devices. These deficiencies can be minimized by comparing values obtained from the symptomatic extremity with those of the contralateral asymptomatic side, recording the serial number of the measuring device to be certain that the same device is used for serial measurements, and having the measuring devices serviced and calibrated in accordance with the manufacturer's suggested schedule.

Overall *hand strength* is best assessed using a dynomometer, with the handle positioned to allow the patient to comfortably hold the device, usually on the third step. We recommend three recordings made by alternating between both hands to allow averaging of efforts and assessment of fatigability. Normally, the dominant extremity should exhibit maximal grip strengths 10% to 20% greater than the nondominant extremity, although patients with ambidexterity, unusual body strength or build, vocations or avocations requiring substantial bilateral hand use, and so on, may confuse this relationship. If any question about patient effort during the testing session occurs, subtle observations such as the degree of digital blanching with grip may help resolve the issue. Additional maneuvers include serially changing the step of the grip handle from the first through the fifth steps, which should normally result in a bell-shaped curve of grip values. A straight-line pattern of maximum grip levels should raise the clinician's suspicions about patient compliance. An additional maneuver is called rapid alternating grip, where the patient rapidly passes the dynamometer between both hands, generating maximum grip with each pass. Substantial differences between single maximum grip and maximum alternating grips should also alert the clinician that an unreliable examination may be in progress. Pinch strength can be quantified in both appositional (key) and oppositional (fingertip) modes. Again, it is suggested that several recordings be made to allow averaging and evaluation of fatiguing. The same relationship between dominant and nondominant hands may be seen as with use of the grip dynamometer; the precautions outlined above should also be employed.

Neurologic Assessment

Neurologic testing in this chapter relates to nerve function in the hand but is based on the integrity of the nerves as they pass through the region of the wrist. Although autonomic functions are transmitted through the wrist, the clinical assessment of the peripheral nerves in this chapter will be limited to assessment of sensory and motor functions.

Sensory function can be assessed through a variety of means with varying sensitivity and specificity. Sensibility of the hand integrates the physiology of sensory input with cognitive use of the hand and may be quickly assessed using the Moberg pick-up test, where the patient is asked to pick up specific small objects, such as a coin, bolt, or pin. Preferential use of ulnar-nerve-innervated fingers may indicate loss of sensibility in the median nerve distribution. Light touch, sharp–dull discrimination, two-point discrimination, and thermesthesia (warm–cold) senses can be reliably assessed in the distributions of the median, dorsal, and palmar sensory branches of the ulnar nerve, the superficial branch of the radial nerve, and terminal branches of the lateral antebrachial cutaneous nerve. Threshold examination, such as vibration and Semmes–Weinstein monofilament testing, are felt to be more sensitive than the aforementioned neurodensity testing but are of limited help in differentiating conditions affecting the wrist per se. Motor examination should include screening of activation and strength of the major motors innervated by the median nerve (abductor and flexor pollicis brevis, opponens pollicis, and the lumbricals to the index and long fingers) and ulnar nerve (abductor, flexor, and opponens digiti minimi, all palmar and dorsal interossei, and the lumbricals to the ring and small fingers). Depending on the level of functional deficit and sparing, lesions of either nerve may be localizable to within the wrist region.

The anterior and posterior interosseous nerves are the principle sources of innervation of the wrist joint capsule, with secondary contributions derived from the median, ulnar, and superficial radial nerves. To date, however, the exact function of these nerves remains unclear. They will probably transmit noxious information, but mechanoreceptor functions such as proprioception and baroreception have not been confirmed. Thus, there are no well-defined clinical examination measures available for the assessment of wrist capsule innervation.

Vascular Assessment

Adequate perfusion of the skin of the hand depends on adequate flow of blood through at least one of the two major arterial systems traversing the wrist, the radial and ulnar arteries. Problems with perfusion most commonly affect the ulnar artery at the level of Guyon's canal, where the artery is susceptible to traumatic compression transmitted through the vessel onto the hamulus of the hamate. If an intravascular thrombus develops, showers of thrombotic emboli may lodge in the arterial tree of the digits, leading to vascular compromise. Signs of such compromise might include focal pallor, necrosis, atrophy, stiffness, and autoamputation. In general, perfusion adequacy can be assessed through observation of skin color, turgor, temperature, and capillary refill response.

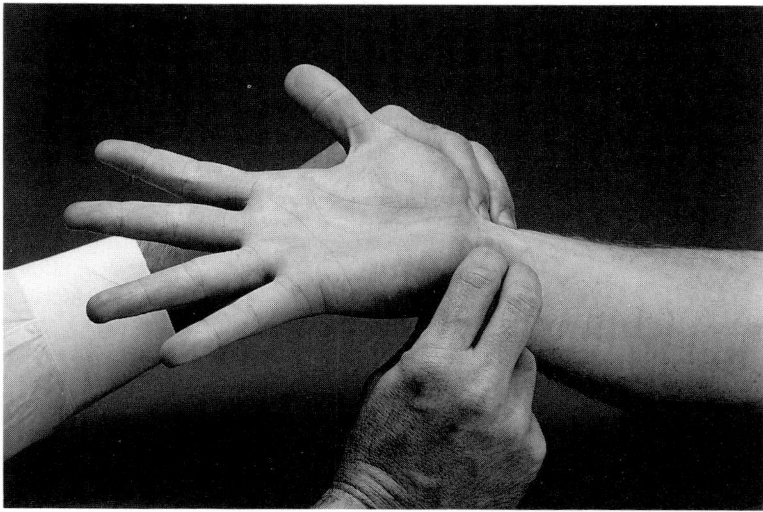

A

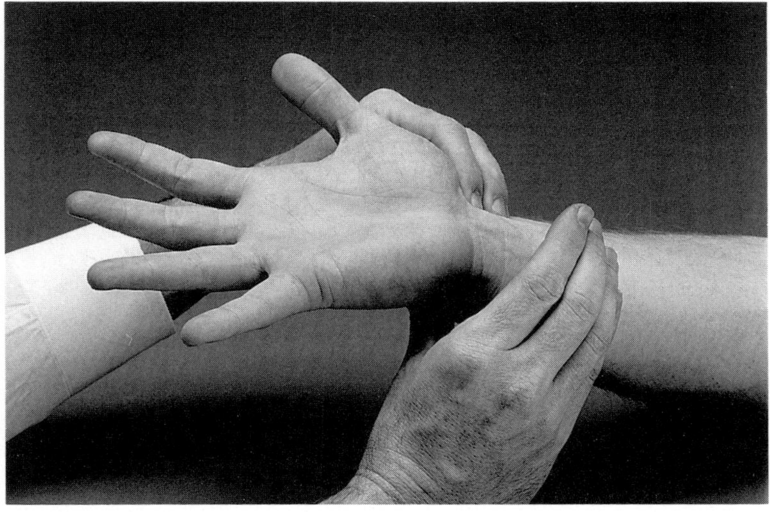

B

FIGURE 3–2. Sequence of application of Allen's test for vascular patency. **A:** With digital pressure applied to temporarily occlude both the radial and ulnar artery, the patient is asked to repetitively make a fist to exsanguinate the hand. **B:** Either the radial or ulnar artery pressure is released while pressure is maintained on the remaining vessel. The time to normal color restoration in the hand is then determined. The test is then repeated, releasing the vessel pressure in the opposite order.

Careful palpation just distal to Guyon's canal and obliquely dorsally and distally through the anatomic snuff box will often reveal distal pulses of the ulnar and radial arteries, respectively.

To assess the functional status of the radial and ulnar arteries, a reliable and simple clinical tool is the *Allen's test* sequence (Figs. 3–2A and 3–2B). The pulses of the radial and ulnar arteries are palpated proximal to the wrist, each found just radial to the flexor carpi radialis and ulnaris tendons, respectively. Gentle occlusive compression is applied simultaneously to the vessels, and the patient is asked to repetitively flex and extend his or her fingers until the digits begin to blanch. The hand is then held in its resting posture as the examiner releases one of the two vessels from compression, timing the capillary refill time to achieve a normal perfusion status of the hand. The test is repeated with the other vessel being released in a similar manner while the first vessel to be released is held occluded. Capillary refill times of more than 5 seconds or unilateral refill times more than 5 seconds slower than the comparison vessel are considered pathologic. Occasionally, use of a portable Doppler signal device may elucidate flow abnormalities such as pseudoaneurysm or arteriovenous malformation or shunting, allow the detection of retrograde flow patterns in cases of proximal occlusion, and possibly detect pulsatile flow not appreciated with palpation. Any substantial questions remaining after such an examination are best addressed using standard arteriographic techniques or magnetic resonance imaging.

Palpation Examination

General Principles

In general, the best palpation examination of the wrist is carried out with the patient relaxed and informed about what is to transpire. Reassuring the patient that no sudden maneuvers will take place and that all reasonable efforts to ensure the least painful examination is often helpful. Additionally, having the patient rest his or her forearm on the examination table, as opposed to suspending it in space, will engender a more reliable examination.

We prefer to progress from the least tender region noted from the patient's history to the most symptomatic region, and progress from light to deep palpation. These methods serve to enhance the patient's trust in the examiner and prevent the patient from unduly guarding during the examination process. As noted above, the contralateral extremity serves as a useful reference, particularly if it is asymptomatic. During the palpation process, be aware of signs other than tenderness, including crepitance, fluctuance, the presence of masses, thrills, and so on.

Attempt to define the location of maximum abnormality and relate it to a specific underlying structure (bone, tendon, joint). This step will rapidly accelerate the definition of further tests or treatment modalities and usually can be accomplished with confidence if sufficient time, effort, and practice are applied.

Finally, it is recommended that the examiner develop a systematic approach and apply it as much as possible. It is through such an approach, especially during the initial evaluation, that the examiner will be certain to evaluate all structures and minimize missed findings.

Regional Examination

Radial Region (Anatomic Snuff Box)

The anatomic snuff box is a triangular region located along the radial margin of the wrist defined by the distal radius proximally, the extensor pollicis longus tendon dorsally, and the extensor pollicis brevis tendon palmarly (Fig. 3–3). The anatomic snuff box ends distally with the convergence of the two thumb extensor tendons, just distal to the first CMC joint. Palpation in the region should readily identify the profile of the radial styloid process. This corresponds with the proximal origin of the radioscaphocapitate ligament. Just distal to the styloid process is the scaphoid, slightly inset from the profile of the radius. Progressing distally, the lateral margin of the scaphotrapezial joint can be palpated, which generally corresponds to the level at which the radial artery can be palpated. Large branches of the superficial radial or lateral antebrachial cutaneous nerves may be palpated in the loose subcutaneous tissue in this region. It is also worthwhile to palpate the subcutaneous courses of the abductor pollicis longus, extensor pollicis brevis, and extensor pollicis longus tendons and to have the patient actively move the thumb to rule out ruptures, cysts, and tenosynovitis. Palpation of the first extensor compartment proximal to the anatomic snuff box may reveal tenderness, swelling, and tendinous nodularity in cases of aseptic tenosynovitis. First extensor compartment tenosynovitis, also referred to as DeQuervain's tendinitis, can be verified clinically by performing *Finkelstein's maneuver.* The examiner places the patient's thumb passively in maximum palmar adduction and flexion and passively ulnarly deviates the patient's wrist. Pain elicited at the first extensor compartment serves as a confirmation of DeQuervain's tendinitis. A stretching sensation or pain at the level of the first metacarpal is not considered a positive sign.

Dorsal-Proximal Region

Palpation of the dorsal-proximal region of the wrist offers the opportunity to examine the radiocarpal joint region (Fig. 3–4). Deep to the extensor tendons is the dorsal rim of the distal radius, which should be palpable in its entirety. Near the midline of the radius, just proximal to the dorsal rim, is a bony prominence referred to as Lister's tubercle, or the dorsal tubercle of the radius. This ubiquitous

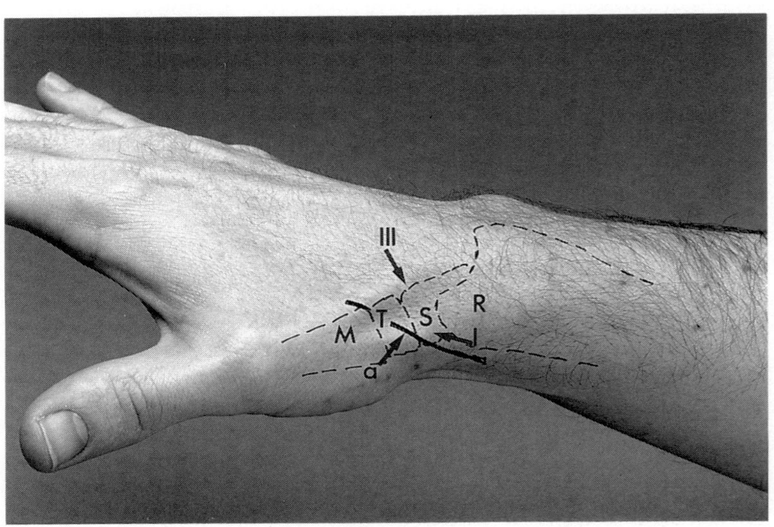

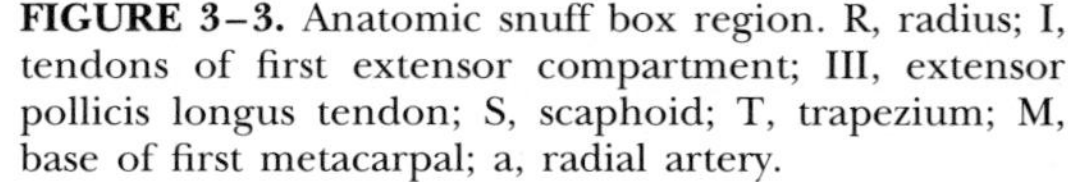
FIGURE 3–3. Anatomic snuff box region. R, radius; I, tendons of first extensor compartment; III, extensor pollicis longus tendon; S, scaphoid; T, trapezium; M, base of first metacarpal; a, radial artery.

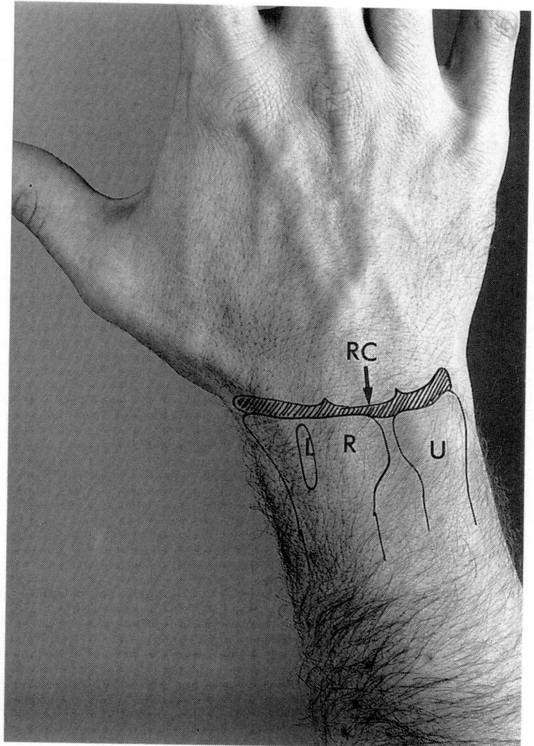

FIGURE 3–4. Dorsoproximal region. R, radius; L, Lister's tubercle; U, ulnar head; RC, radiocarpal joint.

benchmark serves as a guide to several important nearby structures. First, it divides the second and third extensor compartments, with the extensor carpi radialis brevis coursing along its radial side and extensor pollicis longus coursing along the ulnar side. Just distal to the dorsal rim of the distal radius at the level of Lister's tubercle is the scapholunate joint region. Extensor pollicis longus tendinitis, also referred to as Drummer's palsy, is manifested as tenderness in the third extensor compartment, just ulnar to Lister's tubercle. Radially, the intersection syndrome may be detected by identifying tenderness in the bursal region between the abductor pollicis longus and extensor pollicis brevis tendons as they cross over the extensor carpi radialis longus and brevis tendons. The fourth extensor compartment lies centrally over the dorsal-proximal wrist between Lister's tubercle and the head of the ulna. Tenosynovitis of the extensor digitorum communis and extensor indicis proprius tendons is identified by tenderness and swelling in this region.

The distal radioulnar joint lies just ulnar to the fourth extensor compartment; over it courses the extensor digit minimi in the fifth extensor compartment. Swelling and incongruity of the distal radioulnar joint may be detected here. Finally, the head of the ulna may be palpated at the ulnar extreme of the dorsal-proximal wrist region. Substantial ballottement of the head of the ulna indicates dorsal ulnar translation, and distal radioulnar joint stability should be evaluated. The extensor carpi ulnaris tendon traverses this region in the sixth extensor compartment and should be specifically identified as the forearm is rotated through full pronation and supination. Specific findings of extensor carpi ulnaris tendinitis include tenderness and swelling as well as subluxation of the tendon palmarly, particularly in pronation. Ruptures of the extensor carpi ulnaris are not unusual in this region in inflammatory tenopathies found in processes such as rheumatoid arthritis and must be ruled out. Intraarticular synovitis may be substantial enough to allow detection of swelling just distal to the dorsal rim of the radius.

Dorsal-Middle Region

The dorsal-middle region of the wrist corresponds to the midcarpal joint, bounded proximally by the proximal carpal row and distally by the distal carpal row (Fig. 3–5). Just as synovitis of the radiocarpal joint can be detected by dorsal capsular distention, so can the same process be identified in the midcarpal joint. Beginning radially, the scaphoid can be palpated, usually in the interval between the tendons of extensor pollicis longus and extensor carpi radialis longus. Radially and ulnarly deviating the wrist during this palpation maneuver will help to clearly identify the joint line if it initially seems obscure. In line with

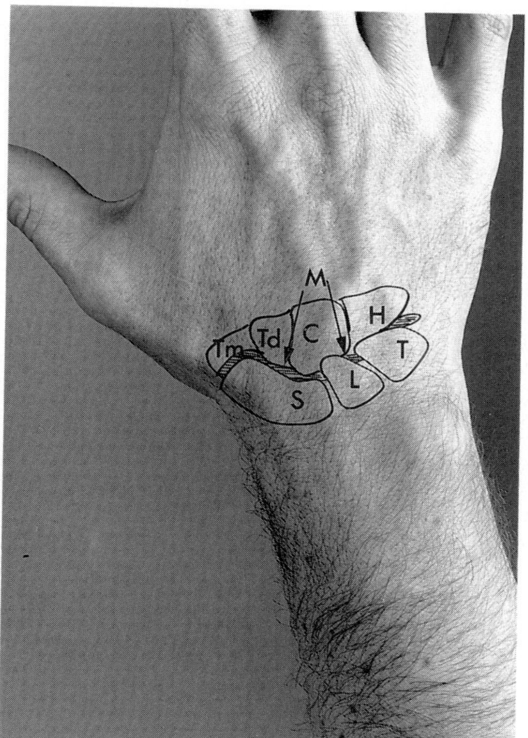

FIGURE 3–5. Dorsal-middle region. S, scaphoid; L, lunate; T, triquetrum; Tm, trapezium; Td, trapezoid; C, capitate; H, hamate; M, midcarpal joint.

Lister's tubercle and just ulnar to the palpable scaphoid is the scapholunate joint. It is common for dorsal carpal ganglia to arise from this region, and tenderness specifically localized to this region may indicate injury to the scapholunate interosseous ligament. Clicks and palpable subluxations emanating from this region should also alert the examiner to the possibility of underlying scapholunate ligament pathology.[2] Progressing ulnarly, the dorsal horn of the lunate is palpable, generally as a region rather than a discrete structure. Tenderness in this region is suggestive of but not specific for underlying pathology of the lunate, such as Kienböck's disease or fracture. Deep pressure is generally required to palpate the lunate with confidence because of the overlying contents of the fourth extensor compartment. A clear deficiency of substrate in this region may indicate a displaced lunate, such as nonreduced perilunate–lunate dislocation. Just ulnar to the lunate is the lunotriquetral joint, again notable in most circumstances as a region rather than a discretely palpable structure. Tenderness in this region is suggestive of lunotriquetral ligament pathology.[3] Finally, the dorsal cortex of the triquetrum is palpable just distal to the ulnar head and deep or just radial to the extensor carpi ulnaris tendon. With the wrist palmarflexed, a substantial palpable exposure of the proximal articulating surface of the triquetrum, and to a lesser extent the lunate, occurs. Tenderness in this proximal region may indicate degenerative changes, including intraosseous ganglia, from ulnar impaction syndrome. Posttraumatic tenderness at the dorsal triquetral cortex may suggest a dorsal cortical fracture or sprain of the common insertions of the dorsal radiocarpal and intercarpal ligaments.

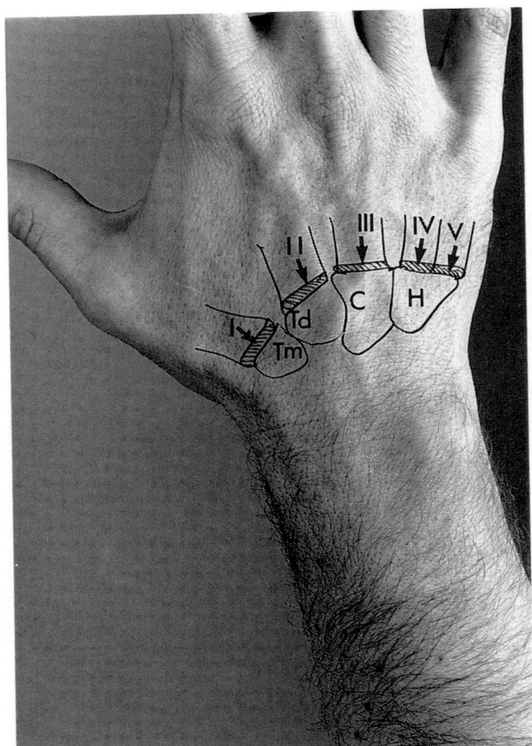

FIGURE 3–6. Dorsal-distal region. Tm, trapezium; Td, trapezoid; C, capitate; H, hamate; I-V, first through fifth CMC joints.

Dorsal-Distal Region

The dorsal-distal region of the carpus (Fig. 3–6) corresponds to the CMC joint region, bounded proximally by the midcarpal joint and the bones of the distal carpal row and distally by the bases of the metacarpals. Rather than having the gently curvilinear contour that the radiocarpal joint enjoys, the midcarpal joint is highly curved, with proximally facing concavity in the radial third and distally, ulnarly facing concavity in the middle third, and nearly linear, obliquely oriented contour in the ulnar third. Effusions in the midcarpal joint may be independent of the radiocarpal joint but will usually directly communicate with the second through fifth CMC joints. Only the thumb (first) CMC joint is normally independent from communication with the midcarpal joint. At this level the extensor tendons, so well encased in the extensor compartments more proximally, are unsheathed and begin to fan out as they approach their insertions. Thus, some of the underlying bones are more readily palpable. Conversely, the interconnections between the bones of the distal carpal row are much more restrictive, thus allowing less motion normally, which diminishes the examiner's ability to define specific joint locations. In distinction are the first, fifth, and fourth CMC joints, which all demonstrate active and passive ranges of motion in decreasing magnitude order. The second and third CMC joints are normally quite immobile due to substantial articular interlocking and ligamentous support.

At the extreme radial margin of the dorsal-distal region, the trapezium can be palpated in the anatomic snuff box. Generally, motion can be detected between the scaphoid and trapezium, thus defining the scaphotrapezial joint. Likewise, motion can be detected between the trapezium and the base of the first metacarpal, thus defining the first CMC joint. Between these two joints, therefore, is the trapezium. Both joints are likely locations for degenerative arthrosis, and it is not unusual to elicit tenderness with this maneuver. As in the anatomic snuff box examination, the radial artery can be palpated crossing the trapezium as its deep branch courses toward the apex of the first web space. Additionally, it may be possible to palpate individual branches of the superficial radial nerve in this region. Progressing ulnarly, the trapezoid is palpated as a prominence dorsal to the plane of the trapezium and is somewhat obscured from direct palpation by the tendon of the extensor carpi radialis longus. The capitate is found just ulnar to the trapezoid, covered in part by the diverging tendons of the fourth extensor compartment. Finally, the hamate is found just ulnar to the region of the capitate and may be directly palpated between the mobile midcarpal joint and the mobile fourth and fifth CMC joints. The hamate will also be palpable through the ulnar snuff box examination. Directly dorsal to the hamate are the tendons of extensor digiti minimi quinti and extensor carpi ulnaris. It may also be possible to palpate distinct branches of the dorsal sensory ulnar nerve.

Ulnar Region (Ulnar Snuff Box)

The ulnar region, or ulnar snuff box, is defined as the interval extending distal to the ulnar head between the flexor and extensor carpi ulnaris tendons and their ligamentous extensions (Fig. 3–7). This region terminates at the base of the fifth metacarpal. Small branches of the dorsal sensory ulnar nerve may be palpated throughout this region.

Proximally, the ulnar head is the most prominent feature in direct continuity with the ulnar shaft. The extensor carpi ulnaris tendon is found in a shallow groove between the prominence of the ulnar head and the ulnar styloid process. When the forearm is in pronation, the most prominent aspect of the distal ulna is its head, with the styloid process difficult to palpate palmarly relative to the radius. In neutral forearm rotation, the ulnar styloid process is palpable directly in the center of the ulnar snuff box. As such, the foveal region, where the triangular fibrocartilage has a substantial insertion, may be palpated. Tenderness in this region may signify a soft-tissue injury to this attachment or surrounding soft-tissue connections. With the forearm in full supination, the ulnar styloid process becomes located dorsally, relative to the radius. Just distal to the ulnar styloid process is the extension of the triangular fibrocartilage complex corresponding to the ulnotriquetral ligament, which may bulge when a substantial radiocarpal joint effusion or synovitis at the prestyloid recess is present. Continuing distally, the examiner encounters the ulnar surface of the triquetrum at the attachment of the ulnotriquetral ligament. Moving slightly palmarly, the pisotriquetral joint is readily palpable. This may be enhanced by grasping the pisiform in one hand while palpating the joint line with the other as the pisiform is translated relative to the triquetrum.

Moving distally, the midcarpal joint is palpated, specifically at the triquetrohamate articulation. Palpating this region while passively moving the wrist through radioulnar deviation clearly demonstrates the complex motion between these two bones. Continuing distally and palmarly, one encounters the hook of the hamate. Tenderness here may be suggestive of a hamulus fracture. Just distal to the body of the hamate is the mobile fifth CMC joint and base of the fifth metacarpal, also approachable from the dorsal-distal region examination.

Throughout this region, the extensor carpi ulnaris tendon is palpable and seems to shift with rotation of the forearm. In reality, it normally stays with the ulnar head, tethered by the sixth extensor compartment. Tenderness in this region and snapping or subluxation of the tendon with forearm rotation may be indicative of extensor carpi ulnaris tendon instability, ulnocarpal subluxation, or distal radioulnar joint instability.[4]

Palmar Region

The palmar region of the wrist has limited palpable landmarks (Fig. 3–8). This is due to the thick glabrous skin of the palm overlying the thick palmar fascia and the flexor retinaculum. However, bony features at the radial and ulnar margins of the palmar wrist region are easily identified.

Proximally, the flat anterior cortex and rim of the distal radius can be palpated. This area serves as the proximal attachment of the palmar radiocarpal ligaments. The flexor carpi radialis tendon is easily

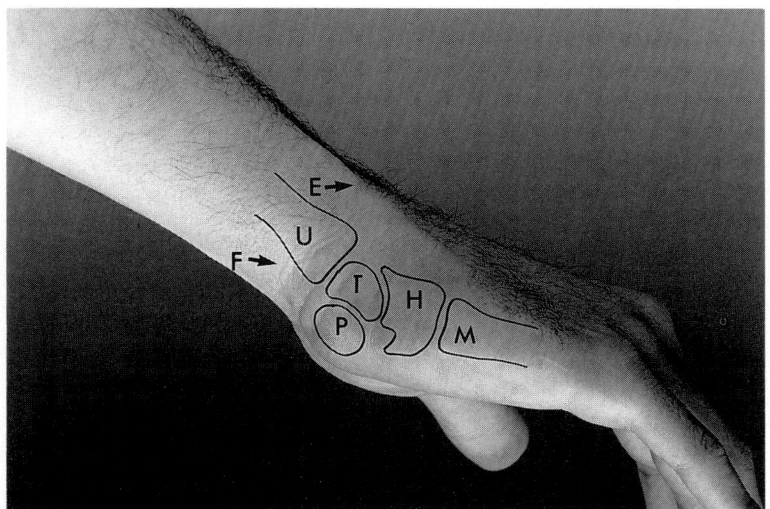

FIGURE 3–7. Ulnar snuff box region. E, tendon of extensor carpi ulnaris; F, tendon of flexor carpi ulnaris; U, ulnar head; T, triquetrum; H, hamate; M, fifth metacarpal base.

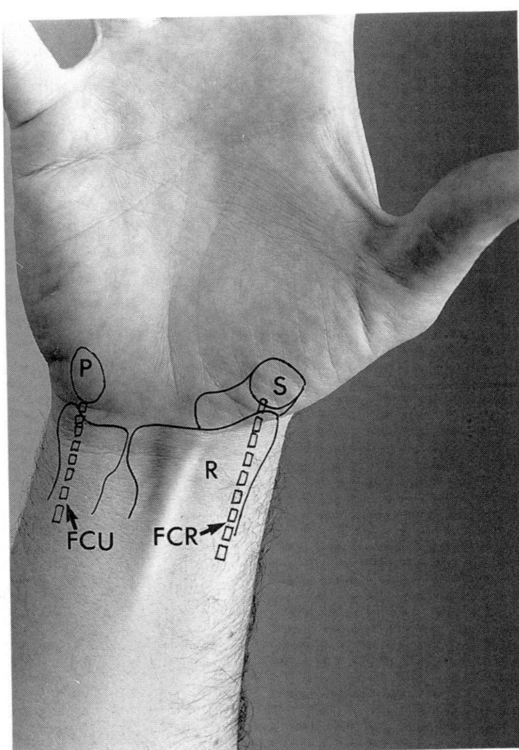

FIGURE 3–8. Palmar region. R, radius; FCR, tendon of flexor carpi radialis; FCU, flexor carpi ulnaris; S, distal pole of scaphoid; P, pisiform.

located near the radial margin of the anterior forearm, and just radial to this is the radial artery. Just distal to the radial styloid process, the artery divides into deep and superficial branches, the former of which is the dominant vessel that deviates dorsally, deep to the tendons of the first extensor compartment. Ulnar to the flexor carpi radialis tendon are the digital flexor tendons and, if present, the tendon of palmaris longus. Swelling in this region is usually associated with flexor tenosynovitis. The ulnar artery pulse can be palpated just ulnar to these tendons and radial to the flexor carpi ulnaris tendon. Following the flexor carpi ulnaris tendon distally leads directly to the pisiform. The other ulnar landmark of the palm is the hook (hamulus) of the hamate, which is located approximately one fingerbreadth distal and radial to the pisiform but may be difficult to palpate with confidence. Tenderness in this region may indicate an underlying fracture of the hamulus.[5]

Radially, following the tendon of flexor carpi radialis will lead directly to the distal pole (tuberosity) of the scaphoid. Verification can be made by radially and ulnarly deviating the wrist while palpating this region. Radial deviation normally will make the tuberosity more palmarly prominent, whereas ulnar deviation creates a recession of the distal pole. Conditions such as scapholunate dissociation may interfere with this normal kinematic behavior. As noted in the dorsal-distal region examination, the trapezium can be palpated just distal to the distal pole of the scaphoid.

PROVOCATIVE MANEUVERS[6]

Introduction

The term provocative maneuver (PM) came into general use in orthopedic sugery in recent years, particularly with regard to clinical stress maneuvers to precipitate symptoms, signs, or other findings that aid in the diagnosis of injury or pain from any cause. In no area has this trend been more evident than the wrist, where the number of categories of problems and specific diagnoses has expanded significantly in the last 3 decades. Examination of the wrist has and continues to be well covered in many texts[3,7–14] and articles.[15–23] The anatomy and biomechanics of the wrist continue to receive much attention. Some of these studies are particularly useful in explaining the genesis of PMs.[24–29] Many clinical descriptions of wrist injury[2–5,19,22,27,28,30–39] and overuse syndromes[16,26,30,40,41] have appeared, as have articles that concentrate on clinical diagnostic features,[1,2,6,20,28,42] radiologic diagnostic features,[13,22,31,34,42] or treatment features.[27,32,33,39] Some of the PMs for the wrist are quite useful in either locating the site of complaint or confirming the diagnosis and will eventually find their way into the general medical lexicon of physical examination. Most will be restricted to specialty usage or even discarded, but they are quite popular at the moment and the list is growing steadily. A PM's value increases if it also can result in a diagnostic imaging finding. This is a clinical chapter, and the PMs described here do not necessarily result in confirmatory imaging findings. It will be interesting to see how many of these maneuvers eventually became part of the imaging techniques to be described. Space does not permit much reference to acute fractures and dislocations although of course there are many useful PMs in that context, also. Our emphasis is on the more subtle PMs that aid in the diagnosis of the painful wrist without a glaringly obvious diagnosis. Even in this context we will not describe the many soft-tissue PMs unless they are pertinent to an underlying bone or joint problem. There are numerous such maneuvers, many of them well known, such as Finkelstein's test for first extensor compartment entrapment, Tinel's and Phalen's tests for carpal tunnel syndrome, Allen's test for arterial patency at the wrist level, Lindberg's test for an anomalous interconnection between the thumb and index flexor tendons, and many others.[13] They are important elements of the wrist examination, since it is often difficult to differentiate core pain from peripheral pain in the snugly packaged wrist mechanism, but they are relatively well described elsewhere, and this chapter is better devoted to those PMs associated with the deep or bone and joint problems of the wrist.

PMs for the wrist may be divided into two groups: general or nonspecific, and site-specific via motion, loading, or combinations of the two.

General Skeletal Provocative Maneuvers[6,13]

The tests are general rather than specific and gross rather than precise. They include the following.

Fist/Grip Compression. This is the gentlest and most controlled of the general maneuvers and can be titrated in degree by the amount of grip pressure generated, as well as by the position of the wrist. However, like most of the general PMs it will aggravate almost any pain-causing mechanism in the wrist; and it may or may not indicate site specificity. Although susceptible to conscious or subconscious control, it is remarkably sensitive to pain or dysfunction at the wrist.[1]

The "Windmill Test." The forearm is grasped and the ballistic hand is whirled rapidly around in widdershins or deasil patterns, perhaps simulating the rotating vanes of a windmill. This is an "all or none" test—lack of resistance or lack of complaint are meaningful, strongly suggesting "no pain foci at the wrist."

The "Shake or Break Test." The forearm is grasped as if it were a fishing pole and the wrist–hand unit is waved vigorously up and down as if it were a fish. This is another "all or none" test.

The "Shuck Test." The wrist is squeezed circumferentially and distraction is applied as the testing hand shucks distally over and off the test hand, similar to shucking corn. This is another "all or none" test.

The "Sitting Hands Test." The patient's hands, either in supination of pronation, are placed on a firm chair or stool seat and the patient sits on them, rocking from one side to the other to induce various combinations of direct pressure, traction, torque, or any of the six motions.

Heavy Traction or Compression Maneuvers. As in "lifting a chair," "hanging from a rod," or doing "push-ups" by a variety of methods, i.e., palm, fist, ulnar border, back of hands, and so on.

Although they are still occasionally useful, most of these similar tests were in vogue when patients were to be seen but not heard, although they often were heard, since moans, screams, or curses were not uncommon.

Many variations of these general tests (the squeeze test, the handshake test, the push tests) are used by some examiners. All use the same principles discussed above.

Provocative Maneuvers That Are Site-Specific via Motion, Loading, Traction, or Combinations of These Maneuvers[2,3,6–15,18–20,22–25,27–29,33,34,36–39,42–46]

Distal Ulna Provocative Maneuvers

The "Piano Key" Test (Fig. 3–9).[17] Simple ventral directed pressure over the dorsum of the dorsally prominent ulna may result in pain, crepitus, snapping, supination, and/or some form of carpal collapse, *but the ulna returns to the start position.* The test means that the distal ulna is unstable and there may be variable degrees of associated adaptive or true carpal instability.

The pisiform boost test (Fig. 3–10).[30] Similar to the "piano key" test, but the translated, supinated carpus is raised and slightly distracted by direct pressure dorsally on the palmar aspect of the pisiform. This test may have the same findings and meanings as the "piano key" test or it may mean damage to the ulnar support system of the carpus.

The Compression–Translation Test (Fig. 3–11).[13] Compression is applied ulnarward to force the ulnar head into the sigmoid fossa. Dorsal and palmar translations are then applied; the test should be performed in various positions of supination and

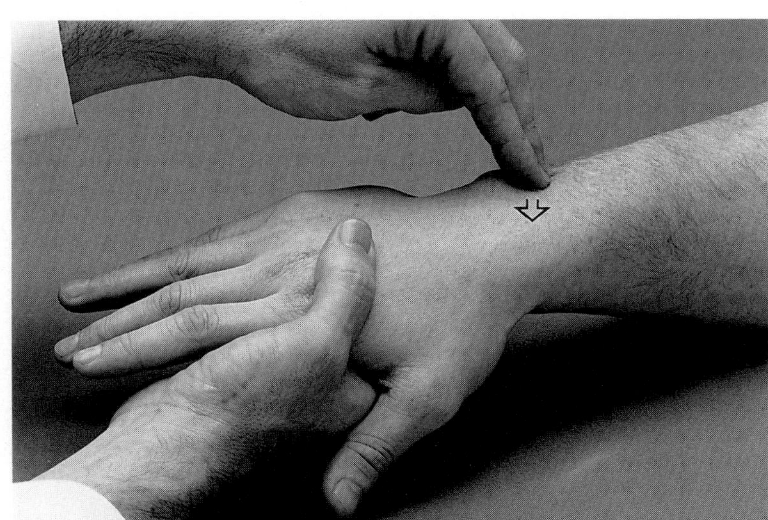

FIGURE 3–9. Piano key test.

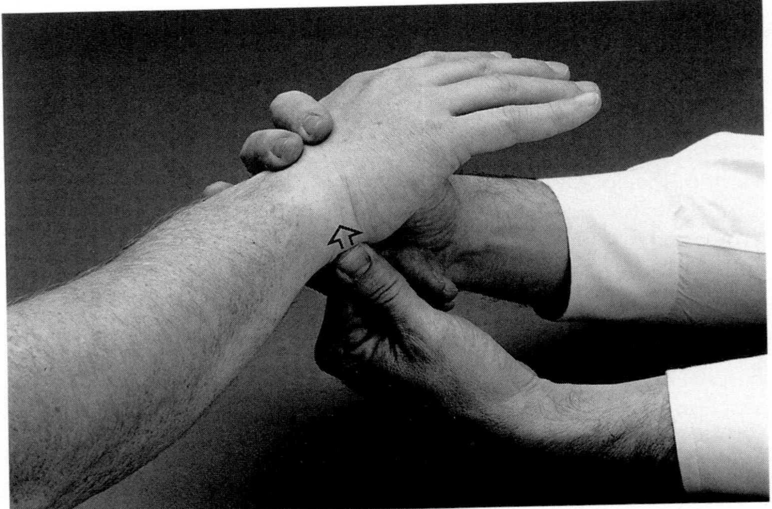

FIGURE 3–10. Pisiform boost test.

pronation. Although principally used to determine the congruity and smoothness of the matching articular surfaces of the distal radioulnar joint, the test also stresses a torn fibrocartilage and may produce pain, entrapment of a flap, and so on. Occasionally the test will reveal such instability that a severe subluxation or dislocation will be produced, or it may reveal a fibrosed or mechanically blocked distal ulna that cannot reproduce a normal range of motion.

The Piston or Screwdriver Test.[6] With grip force maintained (as in gripping a screwdriver) the hand is vigorously pronated and supinated while being advanced and withdrawn (as in driving a screw). This test also checks the congruency and smoothness of the joint and the status of the triangular fibrocartilage.

The Lateral Distraction Test. By either pushing against the radial side of the distal ulna or pulling the ulna ulnarward, a medially unstable ulna may displace away from the radius, either alone or bringing the carpus with it. A positive test can mean either an unstable ulna or an unstable ulna and carpus.

Ulnar Deviation With or Without Grind (compression and dorsipalmar, supination–pronation torque) (Fig. 3–12).[7] Tearing, laxity, or attenuation of the triangular fibrocartilage will cause pain, catching, slipping, crepitus, and sometimes locking of rotation. This test may also be positive for other problems in the ulnocarpal area, e.g., meniscoid tear, chondral flap or other semiloose body, or lunotriquetral ligament tear.

Proximal Carpal Row Provocative Maneuvers

Tests of the bonded or nondissociated proximal carpal row (PCR) include the following.

Ulnar Translation Tests (Fig. 3–13).[37] A carpus, appearing to be aligned, may be unstable enough to be displaced ulnarward by fixing the forearm and applying an ulnar translation force to the hand and carpal unit. There may be crepitus, a sliding or clicking sensation, and pain. If the carpus is already obviously

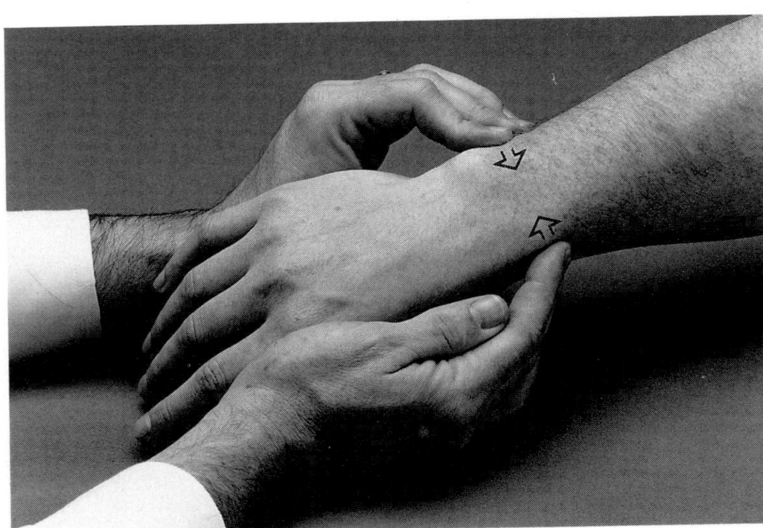

FIGURE 3–11. Ulnar compression–translation test.

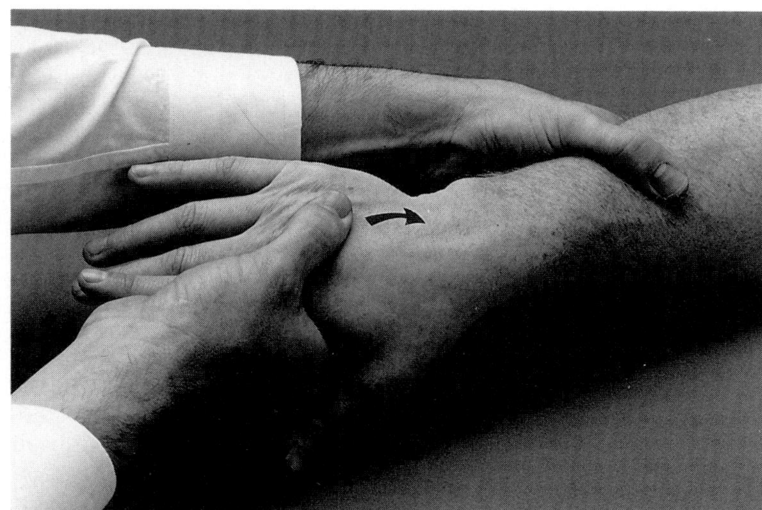

FIGURE 3–12. Ulnar grind test.

displaced ulnarward in relation to the forearm the diagnosis is made, but it is still useful to know whether the subluxation is fixed or still manually correctable. The maneuver is reversed with the hand–wrist unit displaced radially on the fixed forearm. Even if realignment is obtained, malalignment will recur.

Dorsal Translation Test (Fig. 3–13).[19] With the forearm fixed, the PCR is translated dorsally by dorsally directed pressure at the palmar aspects of the pisiform and the scaphoid tuberosity. It is normal for the PCR to translate somewhat, but excessive translation may occur with pain, crepitus, or slipping and a dorsal prominence of the PCR. This test can be used to grade wrist laxity: the normal wrist is fairly snug when this test is done with the wrist in radial deviation, a little looser in the neutral position, and will translate mildly in ulnar deviation. Any translation dorsally from a radial deviation position, moderate translation from a neutral position, or excessive translation from an ulnar deviation position are suggestive of carpal laxity, not necessarily pathologic. All of the maneuvers just discussed assume that there is *no dissociative* condition in the PCR. In the nondissociated wrist, pressure under the scaphoid tuberosity alone or under the pisiform alone may produce the findings mentioned. This means, of course, that similar tests for scapholunate dissociation (SLD) or triquetrolunate dissociation may appear to be positive, because a shift and pain and crepitus may be produced *but not from a dissociative lesion.* This dorsal translation instability of the entire proximal row can mimic a positive scaphoid shift (Watson's) test.

The Palmar Translation Test (Fig. 3–13).[19] Less frequently, it is possible to obtain a similar positive translation in the opposite direction, i.e., palmarward, by displacing the PCR palmarward on the fixed forearm. For both dorsal and palmar translation testing of the PCR, it is necessary to place the translating

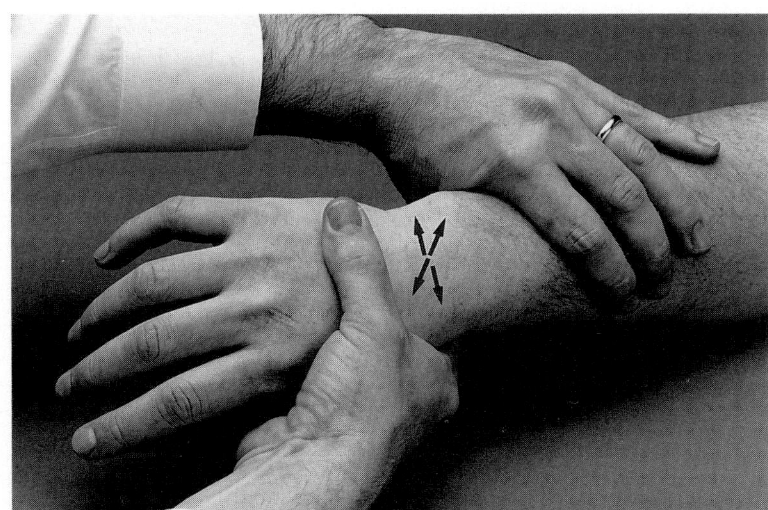

FIGURE 3–13. Ulnar, palmar, and dorsal translation test.

force at the PCR level to avoid testing the midcarpal level at the same time.

The "Catch-up Clunk" Test.[19,24] This test may be positive for either SLD or instability of the entire PCR (commonly referred to in the literature as midcarpal instability, but possible from radiocarpal instability or a combination of the two). The test is done with the wrist moving from a neutral position to a radial deviation and then back to ulnar deviation, or vice versa. In the typical positive test the wrist will clunk, i.e., jump, thud, and hurt, at some point shortly after it passes the midposition and will suddenly be in its standard position for the deviation stance, which is the present. A typical carpal instability nondissociative (CIND) test, as watched on video fluoroscopy, will show the PCR to be flexed over the distal carpal row normally or perhaps slightly to excess in the radial deviation position. As the wrist and hand move toward the midposition and beyond, the PCR remains flexed. As ulnar deviation is increased, the PCR will suddenly shift into extension with the signs noted above. The usual smooth, gradual transition from flexion in radial deviation to extension in ulnar deviation is lost. A positive test indicates instability of the PCR but does not indicate whether the site of the instability is midcarpal, radiocarpal, or both. This same test, carried out in the same manner, will occasionally have similar findings as the unstable scaphoid snaps in and out of near normal and abnormal alignment. There is a subtle difference between the sound and the site of the clunk in SLD, but the best differentiation is to confirm SLD with other clinical testing.

Scaphoid Shift Test (Watson's test) (Figs. 3–14A and 3–14B).[2] This is probably the best-known and most-used test for carpal instability. Watson uses it as one of five confirmatory tests for the diagnosis of SLD or rotary subluxation of the scaphoid, as he prefers to refer to it. The other tests[2] are three areas of tenderness (scapholunate, radial styloscaphoid, and scaphotrapeziotrapezoidal joints) and a stress test (active or slightly resisted finger extension from a flexed wrist position). The scaphoid, trapped between the flexor carpi radialis (FCR) tendon and the extensor tendons, produces pain. The "scaphoid shift test" itself begins with the wrist in neutral extension–flexion and in full ulnar deviation. The examiner stabilizes the patient's forearm–wrist area with his or her fingers dorsally and places the thumb of the same hand palmar to the scaphoid tuberosity, exerting a slight pressure on the scaphoid tuberosity (Fig. 3–14A). The examinee's hand is then brought into radial deviation either actively or passively (Fig. 3–14B). The scaphoid will try to flex further against the examiner's finger and will succeed if scaphoid stability is normal. Mild degrees of SLD will merely be painful at this point, but the more positive test, showing more significant scaphoid instability, will be

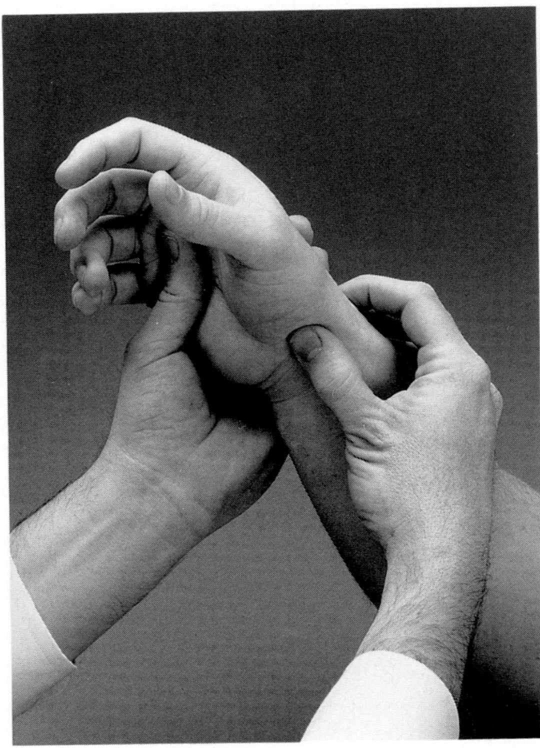

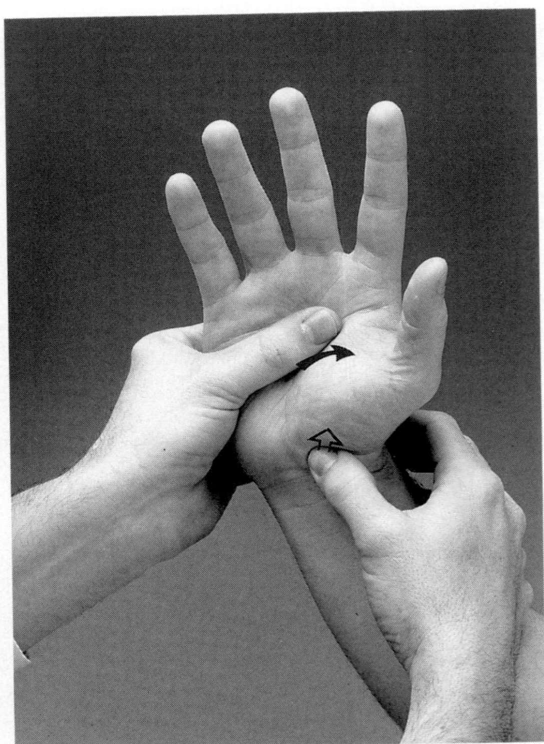

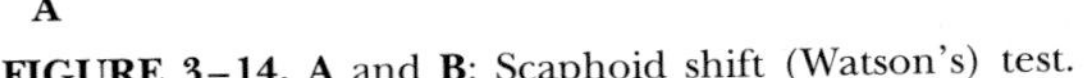

A B

FIGURE 3–14. A and **B**: Scaphoid shift (Watson's) test.

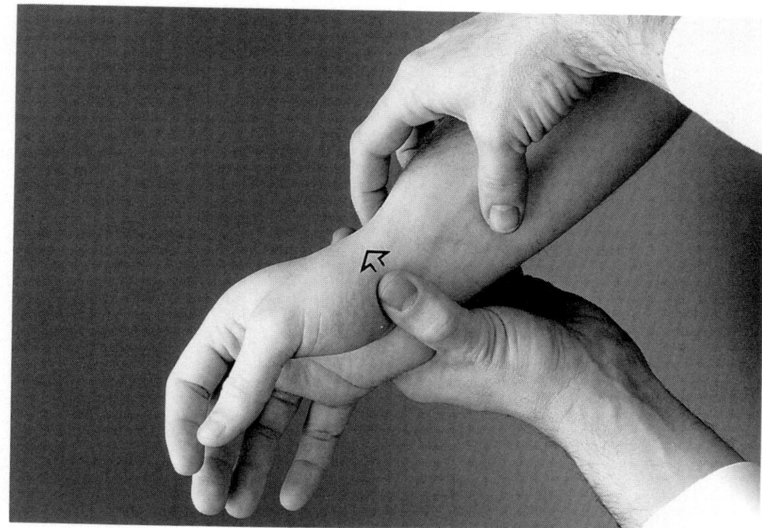

FIGURE 3–15. Scaphoid ballottement test.

indicated by a dorsal shift of the scaphoid as it subluxes dorsally in the scaphoid fossa of the radius, sometimes to the point of dislocation, although usually there is just a subluxation with crepitus and pain. As thumb pressure is relaxed and wrist position returned to neutral, the scaphoid will usually reposition itself with a "clunk." Some examiners use the gradation from pain and tenderness to mild subluxation to greater subluxation to dislocation as a method of quantifying SLD (rotary subluxation of the scaphoid [RSS]). This, of course, can be better appreciated when performed with videofluoroscopy.

Scaphoid Ballottement Test (Fig. 3–15). As suggested in the previous discussion, the scaphoid varies in its degree of instability. Often it is unstable enough that dorsally directed pressure under the scaphoid tuberosity will sublux the scaphoid in the same manner described for Watson's test. As noted previously, it may also sublux the entire PCR if the scaphoid bonding to the lunate is intact but the PCR as a whole is unstable. Dorsal palpation of the proximal pole of scaphoid prominence without associated prominence of the entire PCR is a method of clinically differentiating the two. In fact, the scaphoid ballottement test may be performed from the dorsal aspect if the proximal pole of the scaphoid is prominent even at rest. The scaphoid proximal pole is merely pushed palmarward until it clicks into more normal alignment; release of digit pressure permits it to sublux dorsally again.

Scaphoid Shear Test (Fig. 3–16).[6] When there is significant scaphoid instability the scaphoid can be grasped between the examiner's thumb and fingers, translated dorsally and palmarly, and pushed ulnarward at the same time. Excessive mobility of the

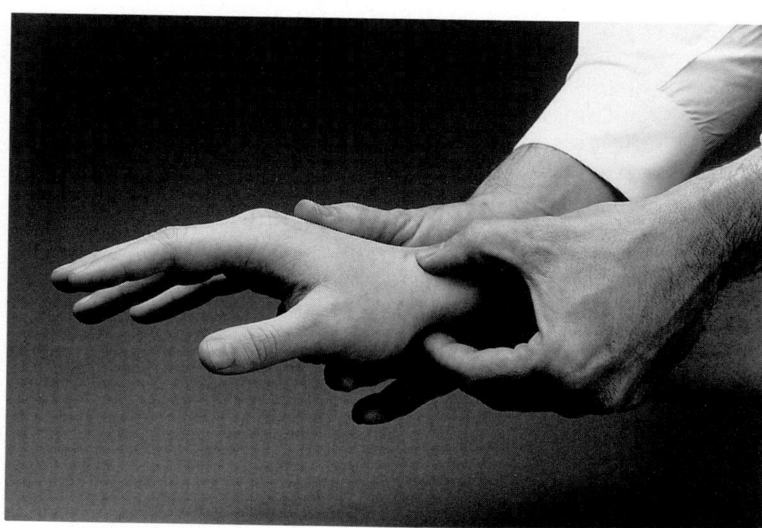

FIGURE 3–16. Scaphoid shear test.

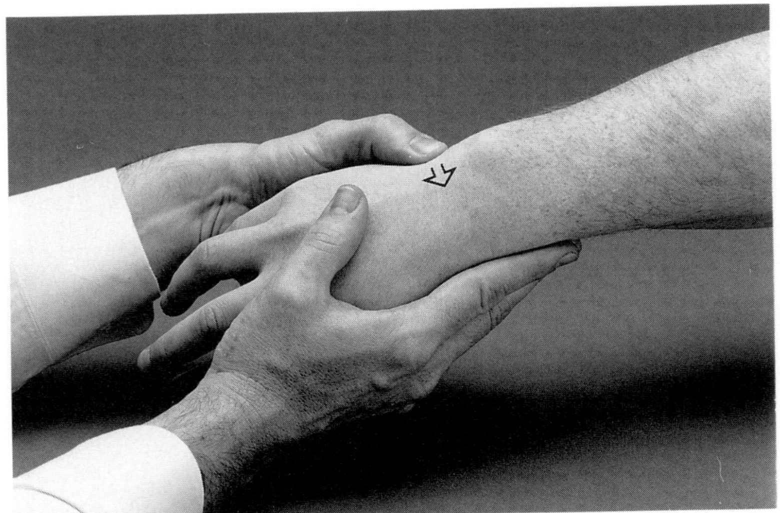

FIGURE 3–17. Lunotriquetral shear (Linscheid's) test.

scaphoid and pain at the scapholunate interval constitute a positive test.

The Lunotriquetral "Shear" (Linscheid's) Test (Fig. 3–17).[13] Simple manual pressure against the medial (ulnar) wall of the triquetrum results in shear stress at the triquetrolunate joint and pain when an established triquetrolunate dissociation is present.

The Lunotriquetral "Shuck" (Kleinman's) Test (Fig. 3–18).[12] This test creates similar shear stress at the lunotriquetral joint (LTJ) by the examiner placing his or her fingers dorsal to the lunate, thumb palmar to the triquetrum just ulnar to the pisotriquetral joint, and applying/releasing translational stress while at the same time radially and ulnarly deviating the wrist.

The Lunotriquetral Ballottement (Reagan's) Test (Fig. 3–19).[3] The lunate is stabilized with one hand, while the other hand grasps the pisiform-triquetrum unit and ballottes it up and down and against the lunate.

The Pisotriquetral Grind Test (Fig. 3–20).[13] Compression and translation in all directions of the pisiform against the triquetrum will produce pain, roughness, and crepitus if arthritis or fracture deformity are present in this joint.

Midcarpal Joint Provocative Tests

The most common test said to be indicative of midcarpal instability is the catch-up clunk test described previously. The authors believe it represents PCR instability, which may come from either the midcarpal area, radiocarpal area, or both.

The Dorsal Translation Test.[19] This test may be done to test the midcarpal joint alone or as a combined test of radiocarpal and midcarpal stability (Louis's test).[34] Louis's test performed according to the author's instructions is quite complex, but in essence it creates a dorsal translational force at both the radiocarpal level and the midcarpal level and there are some people who show instability at both levels. We have already discussed the method of testing the PCR for dorsal translation instability. Using the same method for controlling the PCR with the examiner's fingers lying over it and stabilizing it dorsally, the patient's hand and distal carpal row are translated dorsally by the examiner's other hand. Some laxity is normal, but unusually lax or damaged wrists may sublux the capitate and hamate to the dorsal lips of the PCR or occasionally even dislocate. If there is a variation between the two wrists accompanied by symptoms on one side, this is probably pathologic. If both wrists are equal in instability and symptoms are minimal, such wrists represent another variation of the congenitally lax wrist (see the sections on ulnar deviation and translation testing of the PCR).

The Palmar Translational Test.[19] The test is performed by fixing the forearm (with or without the PCR, depending on whether both the radiocarpal and midcarpal areas are to be tested or only the midcarpal) and applying palmarly-directed force to the hand and distal carpal row. A palmar subluxation is extremely rare, but a collapse into a carpal instability nondissociative ventral (or volar) intercalated segment instability (CIND-VISI) position may be seen in patients with midcarpal instability, although it remains difficult to determine the relative degree of PCR instability from mid- versus radiocarpal joints.

Triquetrohamate Shear Test (Fig. 3–21).[6] The hamate can be grasped between the examiner's thumb and fingers by placing the thumb over the hook and the fingers over the body of the hamate, or vice versa; it can then be translated dorsally and palmarward, stressing the bone itself (all shear and ballottement tests stress the bone(s) that are shifted and specific diagnoses of bony pathology must always be considered in a positive test) and the triquetrohamate joint, the hamate-metacarpal joints, and the hamate-capitate joints. Location of the pain and additional application of site-specific pressure will help to differentiate between these various areas.

Capitate Translational Test.[6] The capitate in various positions can be used to apply pressure to the scaphoid radially, the lunate centrally, the triquetrum ulnarward, or to the entire PCR. The maneuver of capitate positioning and palmarly-directed pressure

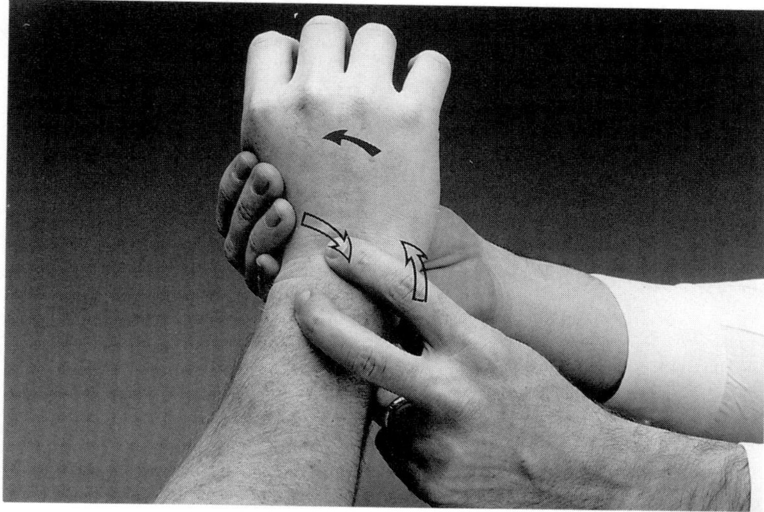

A

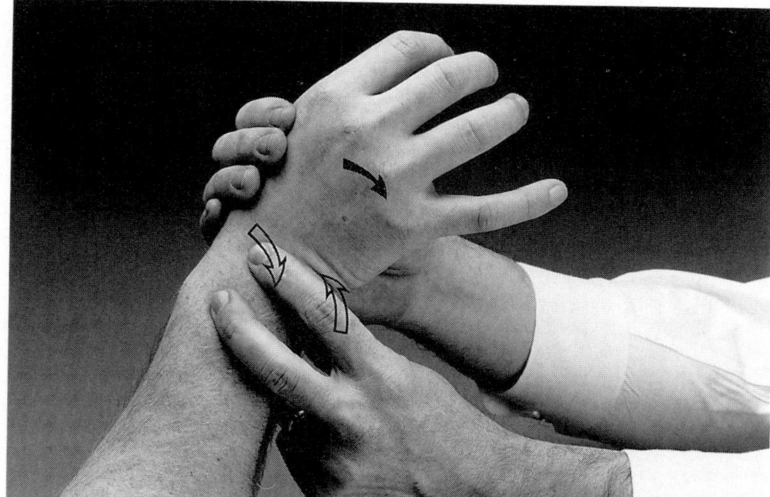

B

FIGURE 3–18. **A** and **B**: Lunotriquetral shuck (Kleinman's) test.

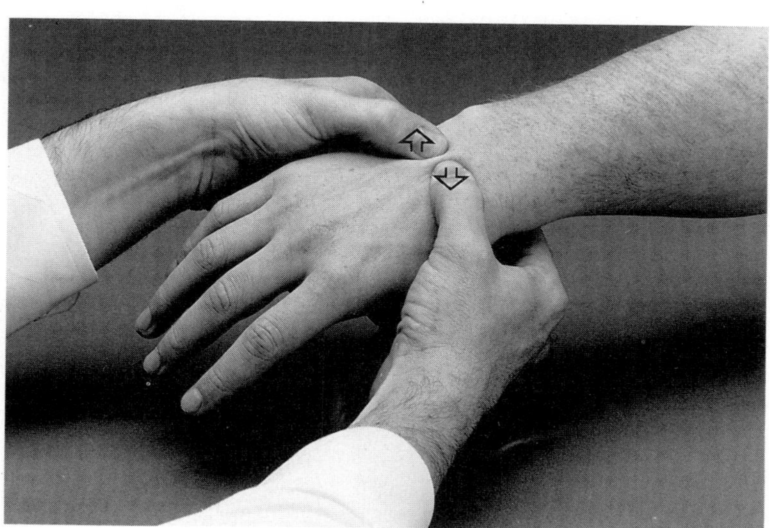

FIGURE 3–19. Lunotriquetral ballottement (Reagan's) test.

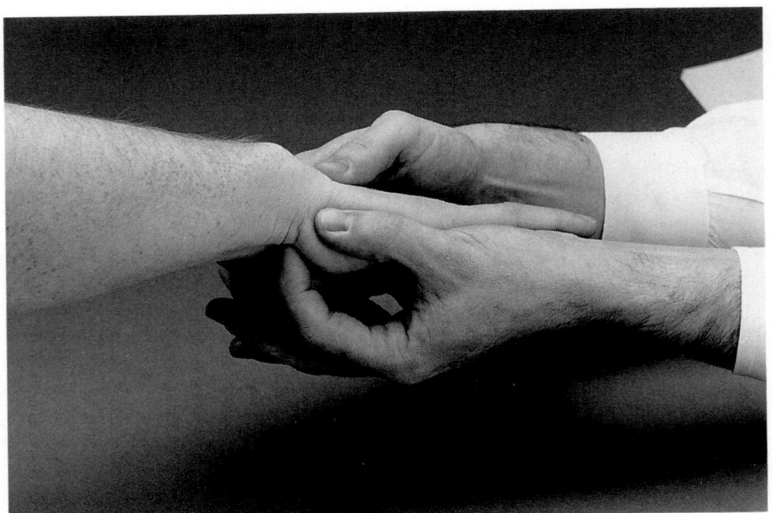
FIGURE 3–20. Pisotriquetral grind test.

over the dorsum of the proximal capitate is usually used to control positioning of the PCR, but can be used for stress testing of the same areas.

Scaphotrapeziotrapezoidal Joint Shear Tests (Fig. 3–22).[30] This joint can be maneuvered between the fingers by grasping the trapezium and trapezoid dorsally and the trapezial ridge palmarly for distal control; and the scaphoid tuberosity palmarly and the dorsal distal scaphoid dorsally for proximal control. Some dorsipalmar translation can be applied or some compression may be applied while the joint is actively moved back and forth from radial to ulnar deviation. The unstable or the arthritic joint will be painful.

CMC Joint Testing

The thumb CMC will be excluded from this discussion since its inclusion in the wrist joint systems may be questioned and PMs at that joint have been known and used clinically for many years. The finger CMC joints are most often tested by the local tenderness, site-specific methods, but they can be tested by motion and stress-loading techniques, also.

Metacarpal Stress Loading.[13] Since the distal carpal row is relatively fixed compared with the PCR or the metacarpals themselves, the simplest way to stress a given finger CMC joint is to passively flex or extend the appropriate metacarpal on its carpal bone. Both ligament stretch and variable articular loading are accomplished with this method and gross instability may be demonstrated.

Translational and Grind Tests (Fig. 3–23).[13] For the mobile fourth and fifth CMC joints translational tests with compression and grind are easily possible by grasping the hamate with one hand and the appropriate metacarpal with the other. The usual findings of pain, crepitus, roughness, subluxation, and/or catching constitute a positive test. The intermetacarpal joints may be the site of symptoms with this test but can be further localized with site-specific pressure testing.

The Metacarpal Squeeze Test (Fig. 3–24).[6] This is similar to but better than the "handshake" test. There is no responding resistance on the part of the examinee and the compressing grasp pressure is

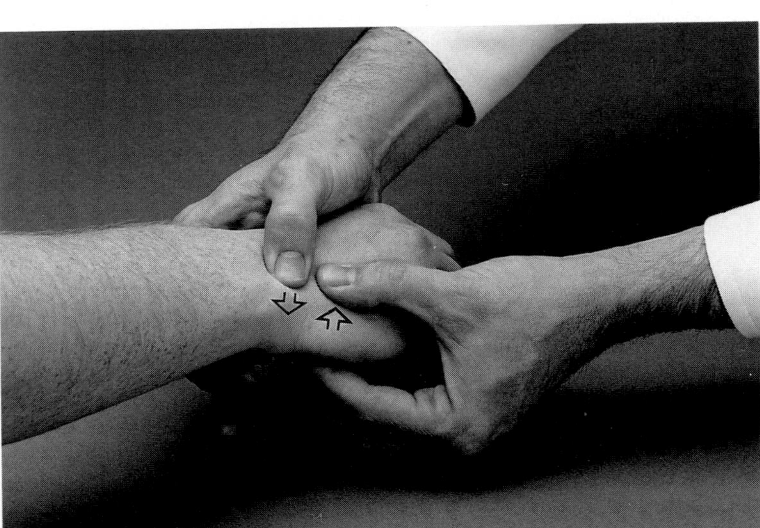
FIGURE 3–21. Triquetrohamate shear test.

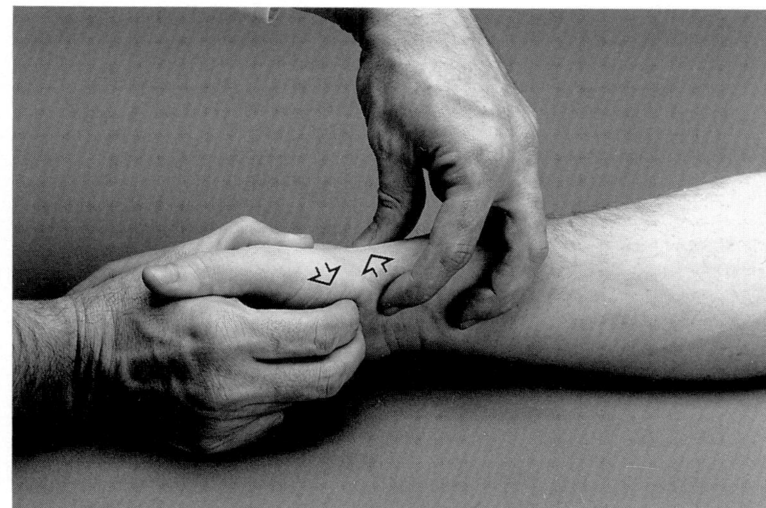

FIGURE 3–22. Scaphotrapeziotrapezoidal shear test.

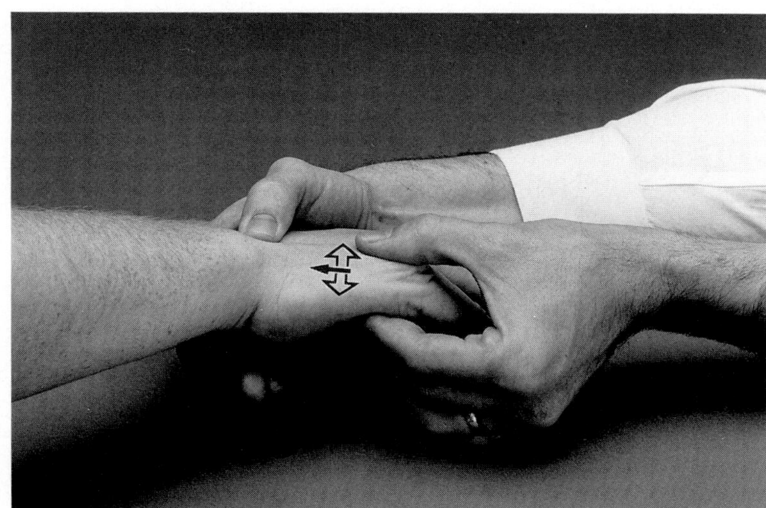

FIGURE 3–23. Metacarpal translation and grind test.

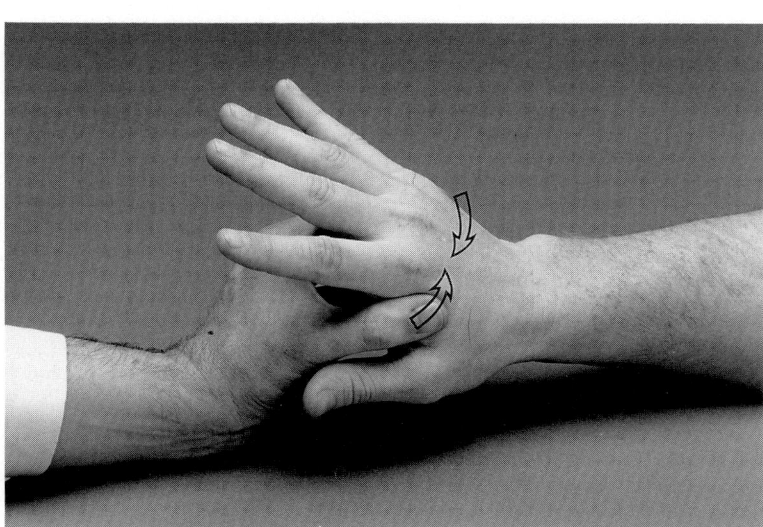

FIGURE 3–24. Metacarpal squeeze test.

applied around the base of the metacarpals. Complaint of pain is considered a positive test, but the pain may not be localizable without further examination.

The tests listed here do not represent a complete listing of all the PMs in clinical use around the world for wrist examination or the many variations that are constantly being developed. In addition, there are as many tests for the soft-tissue structures at the wrist as for the osseous and articular structures. However, the examinations listed here should be sufficient to reveal the principles of provocative testing and to satisfy all but the most adamant curiosity about the techniques in common use for wrist diagnosis.

REFERENCES

1. Czitrom AA, Lister GD. Measurement of grip strength in the diagnosis of wrist pain. *J Hand Surg* 1988;13:16–19.
2. Watson HK, Ashmead D, Makhlouf MV. Examination of the scaphoid. *J Hand Surg* 1988;13(5):657–660.
3. Reagan DS, Linscheid RL, Dobyns JH. Lunotriquetral sprains. *J Hand Surg* 1984;9A:502–514.
4. Burkhart SS, Wood MB, Linscheid RL. Post-traumatic recurrent subluxation of the extensor carpi ulnaris tendon. *J Hand Surg* 1982;7:1–3.
5. Bishop AT, Beckenbaugh RD. Fracture of the hamate hook. *J Hand Surg* 1988;13:135–139.
6. International Wrist Investigator's Workshop. Meeting of 09-28-92, Kansas City, MO; subsequent newsletter/correspondence.
7. Cooney WP, Linscheid RL, Dobyns JH. Fractures and dislocations of the wrist. In: Rockwood CA, Jr, Green DP, Bucholz RW, eds. *Fractures in adults,* vol. I, 3rd ed. Philadelphia: JB Lippincott, 1991:563–678.
8. Dobyns JH, Berger RA. Dislocations of the carpus. In: Chapman MW, Madison M, eds. *Operative orthopedics,* vol. 2, 2nd ed. Philadelphia: JB Lippincott, 1993:1289.
9. Kuhlmann JN. Experimentelle untersuchungen zur stabilitat und instabilitat des Karpus. In: Nigst H, ed. Frakturen, Luxationen und Dissociationen der Karpalknochen: *Bibliothek for Handchirurgie.* Stuttgart: Hippokrates-Verlag, 1982:185.
10. Kuhlmann JN, Fahrer M, Kapandji AI, Tubiana R. Stability of the normal wrist. In: Tubiana R, ed. *The hand,* vol. 2. Philadelphia: WB Saunders, 1985:934–944.
11. Lichtman DM. *The wrist and its disorders.* Philadelphia: WB Saunders, 1988:74–81.
12. Linscheid RL, Dobyns JH. Physical examination of the wrist. In: Post M, ed. *Physical examination of the musculoskeletal system.* Chicago: Year Book Medical Publishers, 1987:80.
13. Schernberg F. Roentgenographic examination of the wrist: A systematic study of the normal, lax and injured wrist. *J Hand Surg* 1990;15B:210–228.
14. Taleisnik J. Wrist anatomy, function and injury. In: *AAOS instructional course lectures,* vol. 27. St. Louis: CV Mosby, 1978:61.
15. Brown DE, Lichtman DM. The evaluation of chronic wrist pain. *Orthop Clin North Am* 1984;15:183–192.
16. Amadio PC, Russotti GM. Evaluation and treatment of hand and wrist disorders in musicians. *Hand Clin* 1990;6(3):405–416.
17. Beckenbaugh RD. Accurate evaluation and management of the painful wrist following injury: An approach to carpal instability. *Orthop Clin North Am* 1984;15:289–306.
18. Cooney WP, Linscheid RL, Dobyns JH. Carpal instability: Pathogenesis, categories and management. In: Eilert RE, ed. *Instructional course lectures,* vol. 41. Park Ridge, IL: AAOS, 1992:33–44.
19. Dobyns JH, Linscheid RL, Chao EYS. Traumatic instability of the wrist. In: *Instructional course lectures, AAOS,* vol. 24. St Louis: CV Mosby, 1975:182–199.
20. Lipschultz T, Osterman AL. New methods in the evaluation of chronic wrist pain. *University of Pennsylvania Orthopedic Journal* 1989;20.
21. McMurtry RY, Youm Y, Flatt AE, et al. Kinematics of the wrist II. *J Bone Joint Surg* 1978;60:955–961.
22. Schernberg F. L'instabilite medio-carpienne. *Ann Chir Main* 1984;3:334.
23. Taleisnik J. *The wrist.* New York: Churchill Livingstone, 1985.
24. Lichtman DM, Schneider JR, Swafford AR, Mack GR. Ulnar midcarpal instability of the wrist: clinical and laboratory analysis. *J Hand Surg* 1981;6:515–523.
25. Linscheid RL, Dobyns JH, Beabout JW. Traumatic instability of the wrist: Diagnosis, classification and pathomechanics. *J Bone Joint Surg* 1972;54:1612–1632.
26. Markison RE. Treatment of musical hands: Redesign of the interface. *Hand Clin* 1990;6(3):525–544.
27. Sutro CJ. Bilateral recurrent intercarpal subluxation. *Am J Surg* 1946;72:110.
28. Vaughan-Jackson OJ. A case of recurrent subluxation of the carpal scaphoid. *J Bone Joint Surg* 1949;31B:532–533.
29. Viegas SF, Patterson R, Peterson PD, et al. The effects of various load paths and different loads on the load transfer characteristics of the wrist. *J Hand Surg* 1989;14A:458–465.
30. Dobyns JH. Sports injuries of the wrist and hand. *J Jpn Soc Surg Hand* 1993;9:831.
31. Gilula LA, Weeks PM. Post traumatic ligamentous instability of the wrist. *Radiology* 1978;129:641–651.
32. Goldner JL. Treatment of carpal instability without joint fusion. *J Hand Surg* 1982;7:325–326.
33. Johnson RP, Carrera GF. Chronic capitolunate instability. *J Bone Joint Surg* 1986;68A:1164–1176.
34. Louis DS, Hankin FM, Greene TL, Braunstein EM, White SJ. Central carpal instability: Capitate lunate instability pattern—diagnosis by dynamic displacement. *Orthopedics* 1984;7:1693–1696.
35. Mouchet A, Belot J. Poignet a ressaut (subluxation medio-carpienne en avant). *Bull Mem Soc Nat Chir* 1934;31:1243.
36. Nigst H. Luxations et subluxations du scaphoide. *Ann Chir* 1973;27:519–525.
37. Rayhack JM, Linscheid RL, Dobyns JH, Smith JH. Posttraumatic ulnar translocation of the carpus. *J Hand Surg* 1987;12A:180–189.
38. Thompson TC, Campbell RD, Arnold WD. Primary and secondary dislocation of the scaphoid bone. *J Bone Joint Surg* 1964;46B:73–82.
39. Watson HK, Ryu J, Akelman E. Limited triscaphoid intercarpal arthrodesis for rotary subluxation of the scaphoid. *J Bone Joint Surg* 1986;68A:345–349.
40. Dobyns JH, Gabel GT. Gymnast's wrist. *Hand Clin* 1990;6:493.
41. Stern PJ. Tendinitis, overuse syndromes and tendon injuries. *Hand Clin* 1990;6(3):467–476.
42. Lichtman DM, Noble WH, Alexander CE. Dynamic triquetrolunate instability: A case report. *J Hand Surg* 1984;9A:185–188.
43. Saffar P. *Carpal injuries: Anatomy, radiology, current treatment.* Paris: Springer-Verlag, 1990.
44. Sennwald G. *The wrist, anatomical and pathophysiological approach to diagnosis and treatment.* Berlin, Heidelberg, New York, London, Paris, Tokyo: Springer-Verlag, 1987.
45. Taleisnik J. Carpal instability: Current concepts review. *J Bone Joint Surg* 1988;70A:1262–1268.
46. Viegas SF, Patterson RM, Peterson PD, et al. Ulnar-sided perilunate instability: An anatomic and biomechanic study. *J Hand Surg* 1990;15A:268–278.

CHAPTER 4

ANATOMY AND FUNCTION OF THE WRIST AND HAND

I. THE WRIST JOINT: ANATOMIC AND FUNCTIONAL CONSIDERATIONS *John M. G. Kauer*

II. ANATOMY AFFECTING THE METACARPAL AND PHALANGEAL BONES OF THE HAND *Bruce A. Kraemer and Louis A. Gilula*

I. THE WRIST JOINT

ANATOMIC AND FUNCTIONAL CONSIDERATIONS

John M. G. Kauer

INTRODUCTION

The wrist links the hand to the forearm. As a region its limits can be set between a horizontal line proximal to the extension of the distal radioulnar joint (DRUJ) space and a distal line through the carpometacarpal (CMC) joints. In the description of the wrist, the distal end of the ulna, as part of the distal radioulnar joint, must be included to represent the functional interactions of the DRUJ and the carpal joint. Understanding the mechanism that underlies carpal function requires detailed insight into carpal bone geometries, ligament behavior, and muscular function. The recognition and analysis of carpal joint disturbances require data concerning bone–ligament interactions that bring about a joint complex with determinate carpal bone-motion patterns.

In the past, different concepts of the mechanism of the carpal joint have been developed. The classical ones emphasize the wrist joint functions with two rigid transverse carpal rows that move toward each other at the midcarpal joint while the proximal carpal row moves toward the radius and the articular disk in the radiocarpal joint.[1–9] The different positions of the hand to the forearm are realized by movements at these two joints of the wrist directed in the same or opposite directions. More detailed x-ray analyses have offered data concerning intercarpal mobility and have thrown light on the mutual displacements of the proximal carpals during flexion and deviation.[10–12]

In this way Destot[13] in particular has offered important contributions to the understanding of the carpal mechanism. He emphasized the interrelationship between carpal bone geometries and the role of specific ligamentous interconnections as a basis for carpal stability and consistent carpal bone mobilities.

In general it can be said that the analysis of clinical material has fundamentally increased understanding of normal wrist function. Classifications of carpal instabilities, although incomplete and often liable to change, have focused on the necessity of having detailed descriptions of the structures involved in the mechanism of the joint and data concerning the kinematics of the carpal joint.[14–19]

SYNOVIAL COMPARTMENTS

Normally the joint space of the wrist is divided into a number of compartments separated by interosseous connections. These compartments develop as separate entities, but in a significant number of cases communications between them are found that are related to aging.[20]

The wrist compartments that can be distinguished are the radiocarpal joint space, the midcarpal joint space, and the pisotriquetral joint space. Adjacent to these cavities are the DRUJ space, the CMC I joint space, and the CMC II–V and intermetacarpal joint spaces.

The *radiocarpal joint space* is bounded by the radius, the radioulnocarpal fibrous complex, and the proximal carpals and their interosseous connections. The extension of the space in the ulnar and distal directions can show interindividual differences. Palmarly to the ulnar styloid process the radiocarpal joint space has an extension known as the prestyloid recess that develops during loss of contact between the ulnar styloid and the triquetrum in later embryonic and early fetal life (Fig. 4–1).[21–23] The prestyloid recess is surrounded by loose and highly vascularized connective tissue[24] that divides the proximal and dis-

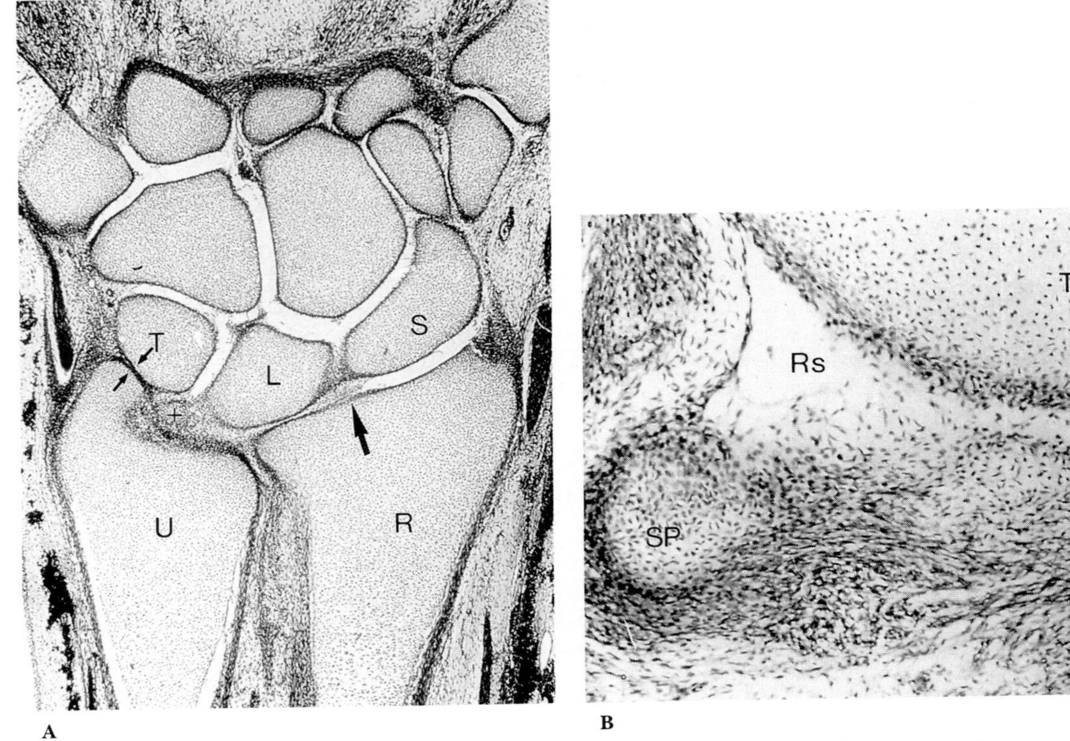

FIGURE 4–1. The early fetal wrist joint. **A:** 10 weeks. Contact between ulnar styloid process and triquetrum (small arrows). Cartilage primordium in disc area (black cross). Large arrow indicates mesodermal barrier in radiocarpal joint space. **B:** 15 weeks. Prestyloid recess lined by synovial tissue. U, ulna; R, radius; T, triquetrum; L, lunate; S, scaphoid; SP, ulnar styloid process; Rs, prestyloid recess.

tal insertions of the ulnar articular disc into the ulnar styloid process.[22]

Sometimes the radiocarpal joint space is divided into a radial and an ulnar part. The division is marked by a loose areolar connective tissue connection between the distal radius and the scapholunate interosseous connection. Normally this separation is incomplete and is formed by the radioscapholunate ligament, which is in fact a vascular pathway to the proximal poles of the scaphoid and lunate at the palmar aspect of the wrist.[25,26] This connection develops from a mesodermal barrier in the joint space present in earlier developmental stages and can remain as a persistent feature. Distally the radiocarpal joint space is bounded by the proximal facets of the proximal carpals and by the scapholunate and lunotriquetral interosseous ligaments that are in line with these facets. Communication through these ligaments becomes a normal feature at advanced ages,[20] as is communication through the articular disc with the DRUJ space at the center of the attachment to the radius.[27] At the palmar aspect of the radius variably sized recesses of the synovial capsule are seen (Fig. 4–2).

The *midcarpal joint space* between the proximal and distal carpal bones follows the irregular line of joint contacts at the midcarpal level. The joint space has extensions into the interfaces of the intercarpal con-

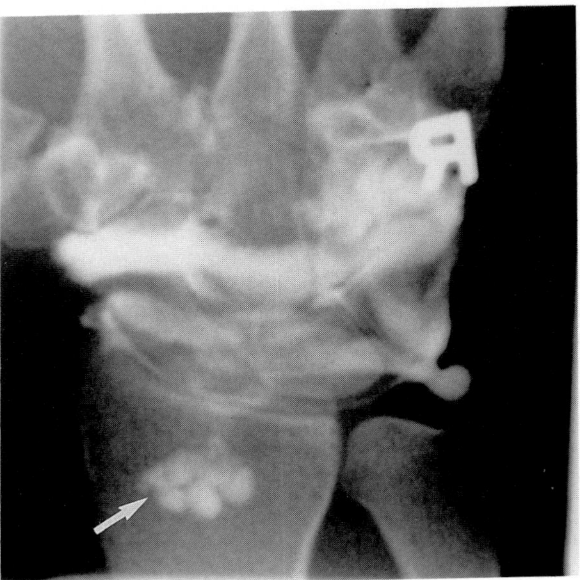

FIGURE 4–2. Large synovial recess (arrow) at the palmar aspect of the radius. (Courtesy of L. A. Gilula, M.D., Mallinckrodt Institute of Radiology, Washington University Medical Center, St. Louis, MO.)

tacts. In the proximal direction the joint space reaches deep into the intercarpal spaces between the proximal carpals, with the interosseous ligament inserted along the borders of the contiguous joint facets. In the distal direction the extensions of the midcarpal joint space can be different interindividually.[28] In most cases there are communications with the CMC joint spaces, most often through the joint between the trapezium and trapezoid and less frequently between the trapezoid and capitate. These communications are the result of an incomplete occlusion of the distal intercarpal joint clefts by the interosseous ligaments. Under normal conditions the joint space of CMC I is separated from the midcarpal joint space and from the CMC II–V and intermetacarpal joint spaces.

The *triquetrum-pisiform (pisotriquetral) joint space* is normally a separate entity. The joint space is situated between the palmar extension of the extensor retinaculum that is attached to the pisiform and the palmar border of the radioulnocarpal complex that is inserted into the triquetrum. Actually, at the ulnar aspect of the ulnocarpal transitional area, the antebrachial fascia divides into a superficial and a deep layer, with the superficial layer forming loops at the dorsal aspect of the wrist around the dorsal tendons, with the exception of the extensor carpi ulnaris tendon. The deep layer of the antebrachial fascia that sheaths the extensor carpi ulnaris muscle at the dorsal aspect of the ulna to the base of metacarpal V is separated from the superficial layer by loose areolar tissue (Fig. 4–3). This situation is functionally related to the mobility of the distal ulna to the carpal joint in pronation–supination of the hand. The pisotriquetral joint space extending proximally as a recess is situated in this loose areolar layer. Serial sections of the wrist in advanced fetal stages show the total separation of this joint space from the carpal joint spaces. However, in at least 40% of the cases a communication is found with the radiocarpal joint space, and this situation is appreciated as a normal feature.[29]

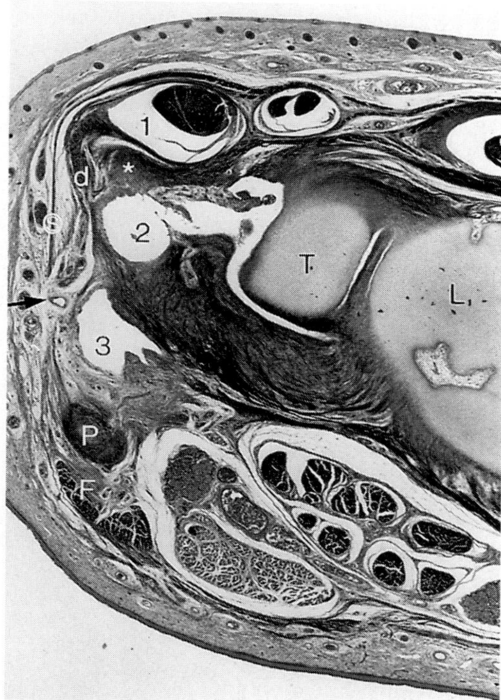

FIGURE 4–3. Transverse section through the late fetal wrist, just distal to the tip of the ulnar styloid (white asterisk). Deep layer (d) of the antebrachial fascia sheaths the tendon of the extensor carpi ulnaris (1). Prestyloid recess (2) and pisotriquetral joint space (3) are separated. Superficial (s) layer (extensor retinaculum) inserts into pisiform (P). Arrow indicates vascular bundle to prestyloid recess surrounding. T, triquetrum; L, lunate; F, flexor carpi ulnaris.

OSSEOUS ANATOMY OF THE WRIST

Seven bones bridge the distance between the bones of the forearm and the midhand. The carpal bones can be grouped into two transverse rows: a proximal one consisting of scaphoid, lunate, triquetrum, and pisiform and a distal row of trapezium, trapezoid, capitate, and hamate (Fig. 4–4). The pisiform does not take part in the wrist joint, being only the sesamoid bone for the tendon of the flexor carpi ulnaris muscle and its extension by the pisiform-metacarpal ligament to metacarpal V. All together the carpals are arranged in a complex of joints, with each carpal bone having several joint contacts with neighboring bones. The very specific geometries of the carpal bones and their joint contacts in association with

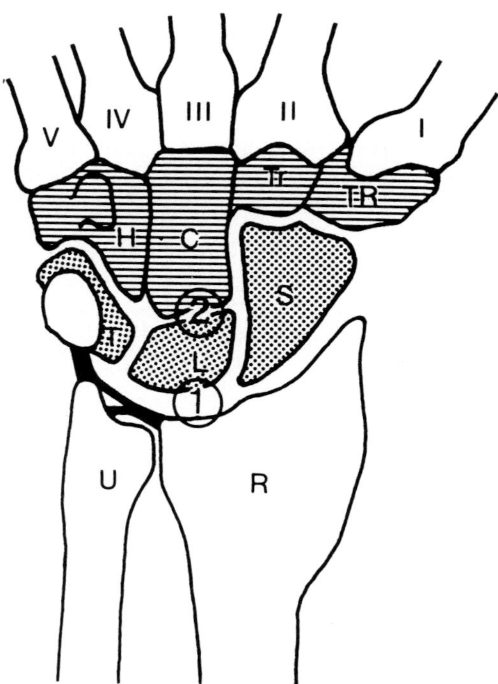

FIGURE 4–4. Carpal bones grouped into two transverse rows and two joints (1, radiocarpal; 2, midcarpal). S, scaphoid; L, lunate; T, triquetrum; TR, trapezium; Tr, trapezoid; C, capitate; H, hamate; I–V, metacarpals.

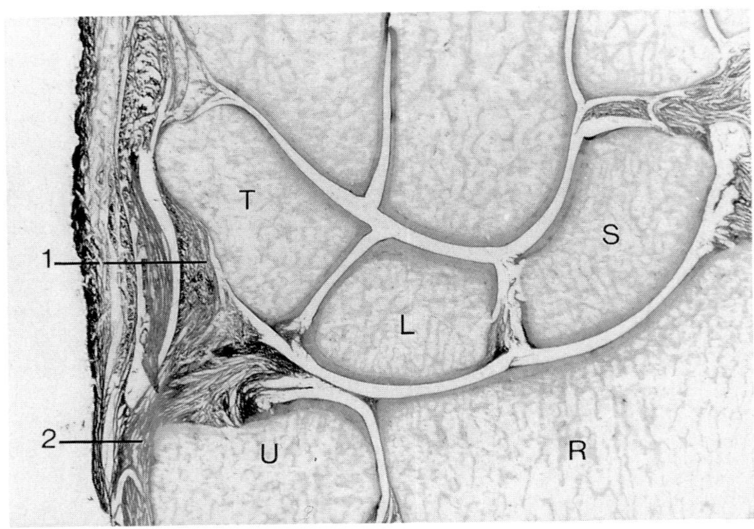

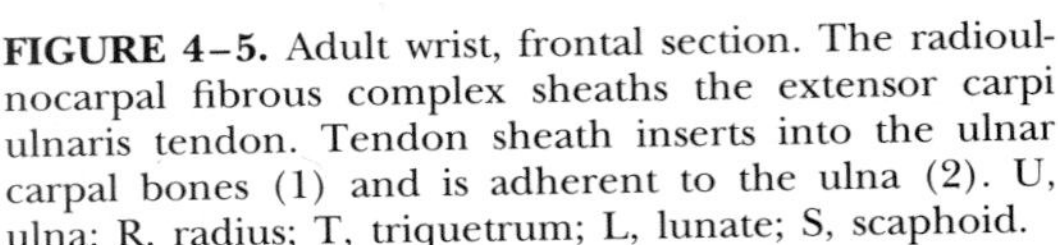
FIGURE 4–5. Adult wrist, frontal section. The radioulnocarpal fibrous complex sheaths the extensor carpi ulnaris tendon. Tendon sheath inserts into the ulnar carpal bones (1) and is adherent to the ulna (2). U, ulna; R, radius; T, triquetrum; L, lunate; S, scaphoid.

their ligamentous interconnections offer the base for the functional behavior of the carpal joint as a defined system.

Of the two forearm bones only the radius contacts the carpal complex. The scaphoid and the lunate contact two facets on the distal radius separated by a dorsopalmar running ridge. In the ulnar direction the facet for the lunate is elongated by a fibrous cartilage that inserts into the base and tip of the ulnar styloid process (Figs. 4–3 and 4–5). This structure, the articular disc, separates the distal ulna from the carpal complex. The articular disc is part of the fibrous complex running along the ulnar side of the carpus.[21–23]

The scaphoid and lunate contact the distal radius in two separate joints. The facets of these joints are irregularly curved, with sharper curvatures in the dorsopalmar direction and more gradual curvatures in the radioulnar direction. The proximal facets of the scaphoid and lunate show the same directional pattern of curvatures. The proximal facet of the scaphoid is curved more sharply than the proximal facet of the lunate, whereas the curvatures of the proximal lunate and triquetral facets are nearly equal (Fig. 4–6).

Intercarpally the proximal row bones are divided by nearly plane joints. The scaphoid and lunate facets in contact with each other are semicircular and reach from the proximal facets to the distal facets for the head of the capitate. The lunotriquetral interface is composed of two flat facets that are directed obliquely from proximal and ulnar to distal and radial. As will be seen, the interosseous ligaments, in combination with the proximal intercarpal joint facets, generate a specific proximal intercarpal mobility.

At the midcarpal level the proximal carpals contact the distal carpals in a series of irregularly shaped joints (Fig. 4–7). The surfaces of the scaphotrapezio-

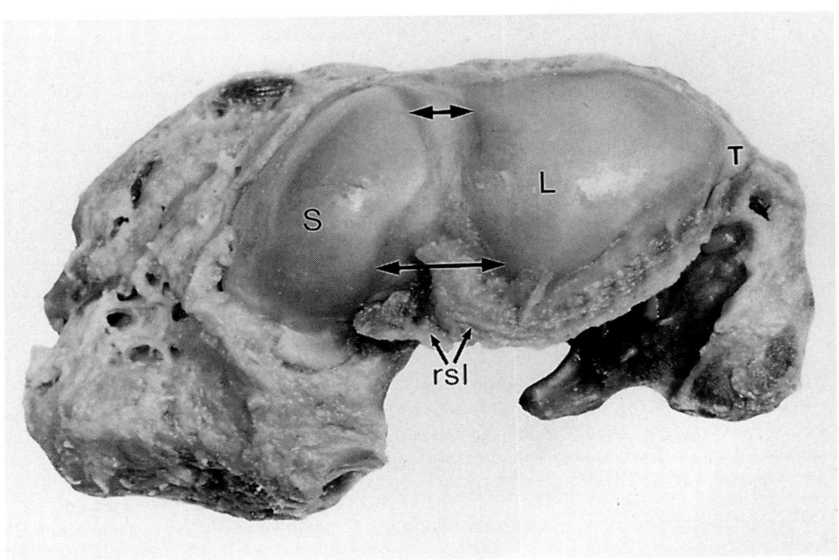

FIGURE 4–6. Proximal joint facets of scaphoid (S) and lunate (L). The proximal triquetral facet (T) is very small. Different lengths of palmar and dorsal parts of interosseous ligament are indicated by the arrows (dorsal is to the top of the figure). rsl, radioscapholunate ligament.

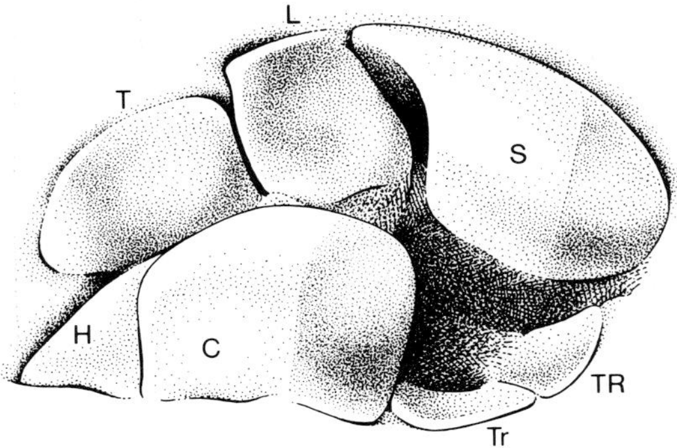

FIGURE 4–7. Wrist joint opened dorsally at the midcarpal joint and flexed. Joint contacts are irregularly curved and close fitting. Labels as in Fig. 4-4. (Reprinted with permission from Kauer JMG, Lange A de. The carpal joint: Anatomy and function. *Hand Clin* 1987;3(1):23–29.)

trapezoidal joint are only slightly curved in both the anteroposterior (AP) and lateral directions, sloping from dorsal and proximal to palmar and distal. The joint cleft between the trapezium and trapezoid corresponds to a ridge on the distal scaphoid facet. A second contact of the scaphoid with the distal carpal row is in the scaphocapitate joint. The facets of this joint show sharp curvatures in the AP direction and less sharp curvature in the proximal-distal direction. The lunocapitate joint has been described as being cylindrical. However, the facet on the capitate head has different and irregular curvatures in the AP direction, the direction of the sharpest curvature. Because the curvatures at the radial border of the capitate facet are less sharp than at the ulnar border of the facet, the facet has a twisted appearance. As a result the palmar part of the facet has an entirely different slope in comparison with its dorsal aspect. In this way the facet gives the impression that the lunate will not move on the capitate in a pure dorsopalmar direction, but with a swerving component in this motion.

The midcarpal contacts at the ulnar side of the carpus show individual variations. In most cases the hamate contacts the triquetrum in an irregularly curved, saddle-shaped joint. The articular facet on the hamate has a dorsopalmar groove that is shaped in a spiral fashion, with the ulnar part of the triquetral facet being more concave and the radial part more convex. This description of Johnston[30] has been elaborated further by MacConaill,[31] who stated that the articular surfaces of the hamate and capitate together form a screw, with the hamate surface being the male part of the screw (Fig. 4–8). The female part is formed by the corresponding facets on the triquetrum and lunate, respectively. In most cases the hamate contacts the lunate on a separate facet at the distal aspect of the lunate. In anatomic textbooks that deal with the osteology of the carpus in more detail this contact is described as the normal situation. In the fetal wrist joint this contact is always present (Fig. 4–9).[23] According to Viegas et al[32] the extent of the

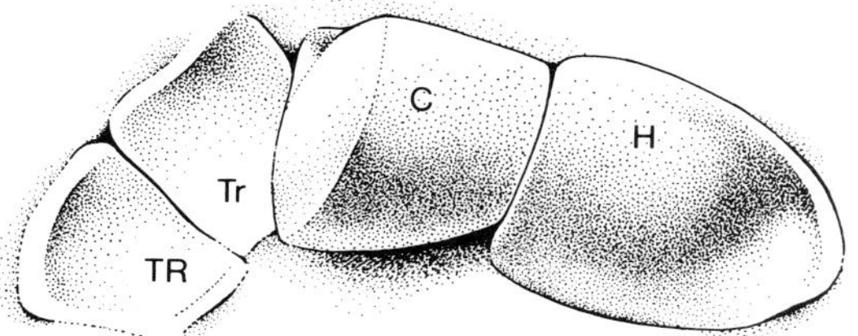

FIGURE 4–8. Proximal joint facets of the distal carpal bones. Curvatures of the facets converge palmarly. (Dorsal is to the top of the figure.) TR, trapezium; Tr, trapezoid. (Reprinted with permission from Kauer JMG. The mechanism of the carpal joint. *Clin Orthop* 1986;202:16–26.)

contact can range from 1 to 6 mm. At the same time the contact from dorsal to palmar differs in extent. In cases of only a small contact, identification by radiograph can be difficult.[32] Of the distal carpals, the trapezoid, capitate, and hamate are in contact with each other by irregularly shaped joint facets, with the bones connected by strong palmar and dorsal ligaments and interosseous ligaments. The trapezium is in contact with the trapezoid by slightly concave–convex facets and with lesser ligamentous constraint than the other distal carpal bones. When the hand moves with respect to the forearm, the distal carpal row can be viewed as a solid whole moving with the hand.

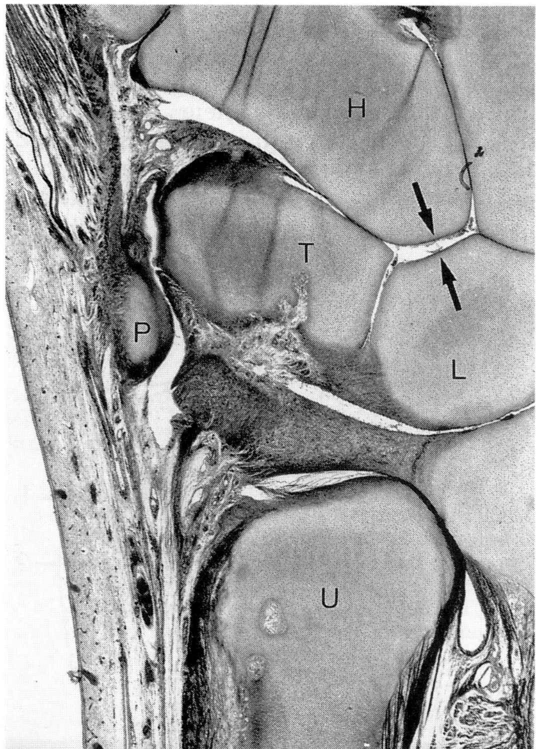

FIGURE 4–9. Late fetal wrist joint, oblique frontal section. Arrows indicate hamate (H)–lunate (L) contact. A proximal joint facet of the triquetrum (T) is absent. P, pisiform; U, ulna.

Radiocarpal and Midcarpal Interdependency

Flexion and deviation movements of the hand lead to angulation at the radiocarpal and midcarpal joint levels. This implies movement of the proximal carpal bones with respect to the radius and movement of the proximal and distal carpal bones with respect to each other. The angulations of the three longitudinal chains are different.[47]

First, the inequality of the joints of the scaphoid and lunate with the radius and the relative shifts between proximal carpal bones during dorsopalmar rotation generate midcarpal displacements. Second, the proximal and distal carpal bones articulate with each other in specifically shaped joints with a different kinematical outcome. These two phenomena are interdependent because if the joints of the proximal carpals moved in equally curved articulations, the distal and proximal carpal bones would move with relation to the radius as a whole. As can be seen in Fig. 4–16, the wedge shape of the proximal carpal bones would position these bones into an end-position to the distal carpal bones without any possibility of changing this position. Therefore the wedge shape of the proximal carpal bones, associated with the tendency of these bones to rotate dorsally, is a third element in this mechanism.

The interdependent displacements of the proximal carpal bones at the radiocarpal and midcarpal levels include displacements in the same and opposite directions at these levels. For the central chain, palmarflexion of the hand results in palmar rotation of the lunate to the radius, while the capitate rotates palmarly with respect to the lunate. Viewed in the sagittal plane, at the radiocarpal level the palmar-flexion end-position resembles the end-position of radial deviation, and at the midcarpal level resembles the end-position of ulnar deviation. In opposite directions the same can be applied to the relative positions in dorsiflexion of the hand (Fig. 4–17). It will be obvious that these rotations in the same and opposite directions can be observed in the radial (scaphoid) and ulnar (triquetrum) chains as well.

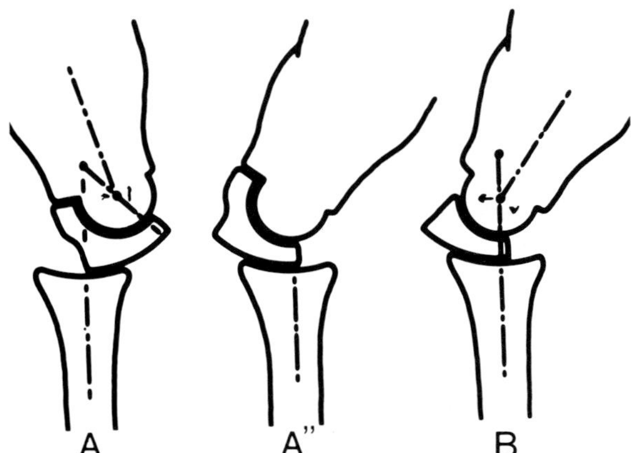

FIGURE 4–16. Scaphoid (A) and lunate (B) modeled as wedge-shaped bones with equally curved proximal facets. Midcarpally both bones will stay in the dorsally rotated end-position.

As stated previously, the proximal carpal bones move in relation to the distal carpal bones through very irregularly curved joint contacts. The shape of the joint facets at the midcarpal level cause an out-of-plane movement of the proximal carpal bones while rotating in either the palmar or dorsal direction with respect to the distal carpal bones. The direction of the midcarpal shift of the proximal carpal bones determines the direction of the out-of-plane motion of the proximal carpal bones. As a result, the direction of the out-of-plane movement of palmarly rotated proximal carpal bones in palmar-flexion and radial deviation will be in opposite directions because the midcarpal shifts are in opposite directions. Dorsal rotation of the proximal carpal row to the radius in dorsiflexion and ulnar deviation will show these phenomena as well. The out-of-plane motions can be described as pronatory and supinatory movements associated with the dorsopalmar rotations of the proximal carpal bones. Therefore specific positions of the proximal carpal bones can be observed for every position of the hand to the forearm, the specificity being the result of a determined mechanism.

Ligament Function

The ligaments of the carpal joints passively restrict mutual movements of the carpal bones and movements of the carpal complex to the radius and ulna.[51] The short CMC and distal intercarpal ligaments join the distal carpals to each other functionally and to the metacarpus as a solid block with the exception of the trapezium, which is mobile to a small extent with respect to the trapezoid. The short (intrinsic) interosseous ligaments of the proximal row, viz. the scapholunate and lunotriquetral interosseous ligaments, allow specific intercarpal mobility between the connected bones. These intrinsic ligaments serve as a control in the linkage of the movements of the proximal carpal bones to one another, a role that is consistent with specific geometries of these bones. The scapholunate and lunotriquetral interactions are primarily based on the integrity of these interosseous connections, since ruptures immediately cause abnormal motion patterns of the proximal carpal bones, with each of them moving into a direction according to their tendency to move. With scapholunate dissociation the scaphoid is palmarly rotated and in the posteroanterior view is foreshortened, while at the same time the lunate and triquetrum are dorsally rotated. When the lunate and triquetrum are dissociated, the lunate moves with the scaphoid into a palmarly rotated position while the triquetrum rotates dorsally. A side effect of both types of dissociation is an ulnar migration of both the lunate and scaphoid in scapholunate dissociation, and of the triquetrum alone in lunotriquetral dissociation. This migration is most probably the result of dorsal rotation of the triquetrum with a shift in the irregular, saddle-shaped triquetrohamate joint. Palmar displacement of the triquetrum on the hamate screws the triquetrum ulnarly; dorsal displacement of the triquetrum moves

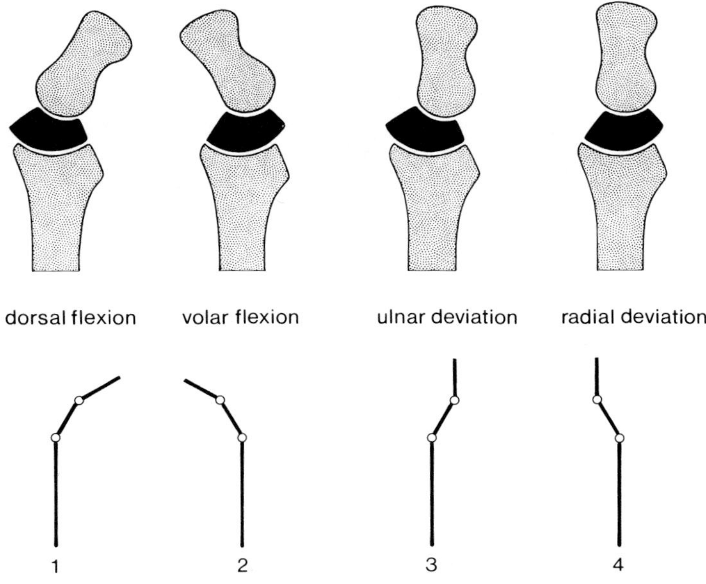

FIGURE 4–17. The different positions of the lunate to the radius and the capitate. The lunate shifts radiocarpally and midcarpally in the same direction in dorsiflexion and ulnar deviation, and in the opposite direction in palmarflexion and radial deviation. (Reprinted with permission from Kauer JMG. The mechanism of the carpal joint. *Clin Orthop* 1986; 202:16–26.)

the triquetrum radially. With scapholunate dissociation the lunate will follow the triquetrum in this ulnar migration.

The longer radiocarpal and ulnocarpal ligaments counteract longitudinal rotation of the carpal complex with respect to the radius. At the same time, because these ligaments have fiber bundles that are intermingled with the short intrinsic ligaments, the stability of the carpal complex depends on the integrity of the ligamentous system as a whole.

To assess the role of the ligaments in maintaining carpal stability, knowledge about the mechanical properties of ligaments and the forces generated in these ligaments is indispensable. Recently data on ligament length changes and force–elongation relationships have been collected.[34,35] From these data it can be suggested that at least in normal loaded movements of the hand the loading of the ligaments is relatively low, with some ligaments becoming strained only at the end-positions of flexion and deviation of the hand. Determining the consistency of these experimental data with ligament behavior in the complex carpal situation requires further investigation. In addition, the proprioceptive function of these structures must be considered.

Ulnocarpal Fibrous Complex

Tendons that cross the carpal joint are an essential part of the stabilizing system of the wrist.[23,42] Tendons play this role by keeping joint facets in close contact. In addition, tendon sheaths at the dorsal aspect of the wrist are connected with the ligamentous system of the carpal joint. This particularly concerns the tendon sheath of the extensor carpi ulnaris tendon at the ulnar aspect of the wrist (Fig. 4–5). In fact the sheath of the extensor carpi ulnaris tendon is part of the ligamentous system of the carpus. For reasons of stability, longitudinal rotation of the hand is excluded from the carpus and is provided by the proximal and the distal radioulnar joints. Movements at the radioulnar and carpal joints are independent. Therefore the spatial organization of the structures in the distal radioulnar and ulnocarpal regions allows a rather free rotational mobility of the distal ulna to the radius and the carpal joint.

An important feature of this mobility at the transitional area of the DRUJ and the carpal joint is the stratification of the antebrachial fascia.[23] At the dorsal aspect of the distal radius the extensor retinaculum forms five extensor tendon compartments, with the retinaculum attached to the distal radius and more distally to the dorsal carpal ligaments. At the dorsal and ulnar aspects of the ulna, the antebrachial fascia is divided into a superficial and a deep layer. Between these layers loose areolar tissue or bursalike structures are found. The extensor retinaculum can be identified with the superficial layer, whereas the deep layer bordering the ulnocarpal fibrous complex, including the articular disc, forms a sheath for the tendon of the extensor carpi ulnaris (Figs. 4–3 and 4–5). Therefore the first five dorsal tendon compartments are radius associated whereas the sixth dorsal tendon compartment is ulna associated. At the palmar side the pisiform serves as an anchor for the superficial layer and encloses the tendon of the flexor carpi ulnaris as a fascial sheath. The deep layer bordering the ulnocarpal fibrous complex has an attachment into the triquetrum (Figs. 4–3 and 4–9). The position of the pisotriquetral joint is just between the superficial and deep layers of the antebrachial fascia. Therefore the pisiform can move with the triquetrum when the hand pronates or supinates.

Within the ulnocarpal fibrous complex is the prestyloid recess (Fig. 4–3) at the palmar aspect of the ulnar styloid process. This diverticulum of the radiocarpal joint space is separated from the pisotriquetral joint. However, in adult hands a communication between the prestyloid recess and the pisotriquetral joint can be found as a normal situation.

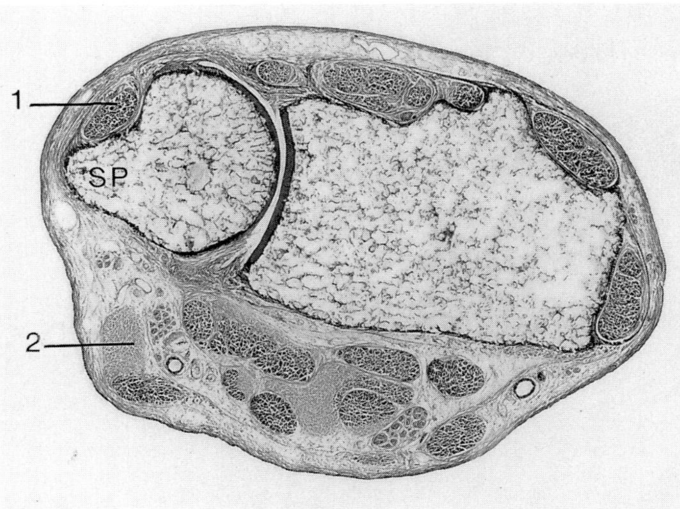

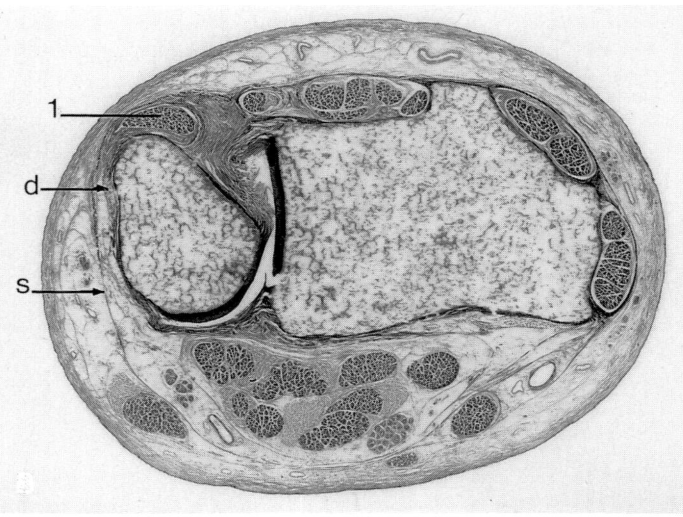

A B

FIGURE 4–18. Transverse sections through the DRUJ. **A:** Pronated hand. **B:** Supinated hand. The tendon of the extensor carpi ulnaris (1) follows the excursion of the ulnar styloid process (SP). In supination the tendon moves ulnarly. The movement is counteracted by the strong ulnar insertion of the deep antebrachial fascial layer (d). s, superficial layer; 2, tendon of flexor carpi ulnaris. Dorsal is to the top of both figures.

It is accepted that the carpal joint has a range of wrist motion that excludes collateral ligaments. Experimental data show that muscles act as "dynamic collaterals;" the extensor carpi ulnaris acts as such at the ulnar side of the carpal joint, and the extensor pollicis brevis and abductor pollicis longus tendons do so at the radial side.[42] In addition, a true ulnar collateral ligament would also affect the range of movement in pronation and supination when the ulna and carpus rotate on each other.

FIGURE 4–19. Tracing of superimposed x-rays of the hand in pronation and supination. The radius (R) is fixed and the ulna (U) rotated. The ulnar styloid process swings from palmar (pronation) to dorsal (supination). The extensor carpi ulnaris tendon marked with metal thread moves with the ulna to the other dorsal (radius-associated) tendons.

To execute the collateral ligament function the extensor carpi ulnaris (ECU) has to follow the ulna as the ECU tendon moves during pronation and supination (Figs. 4–18 and 4–19). The position of the tendon sheath at the dorsal aspect of the ulna supports this view. The layering of the antebrachial fascia with the deeper position of the ECU sheath with respect to the sheaths of the other radius-associated tendons enhances the free mobility of the ulna. Disruption of the ECU tendon sheath followed by a luxation of the tendon seriously affects the stability at the ulnar side of the wrist.

SUMMARY

Analysis of carpal bone motion patterns in flexion and deviation of the hand and the interrelationship between carpal bone geometries and ligamentous interconnections supports the notion that the function of interdependent longitudinal articulation chains is essential in the carpal mechanism. The interdependency includes mutually related movements at the radiocarpal and midcarpal levels. At the same time, there is a linkage of the chains in the transverse direction. With this approach, discussion about the functional grouping of carpal bones in a longitudinal or transverse direction is irrelevant. The proximal carpal bones play the role of intercalated bones, but do so differently based on specific geometries. A normal motion pattern of the carpal bones depends on the linkage of the proximal carpal bones by ligaments, giving a different scapholunate and lunotriquetral intercarpal mobility. In this context the work of Navarro[43] is important. He emphasized the function of the ulnar chain in hand rotation, the central chain as the "flexion–extension column," and the radial chain as the "lateral mobile column" in which the scaphoid plays a stabilizing role. In this concept, later modified by Taleisnik,[19] the differential role of the three intercalated proximal carpal bones is indicated. Both the scaphoid and the triquetrum have a stabilizing function, but under different conditions. The scaphoid is positioned between the trapezium and trapezoid and radius and between the capitate and radius and shows an antagonism in its tendency to move. The triquetrum is the movable anchoring site for the long radiocarpal and ulnocarpal ligaments, including the ulnocarpal fibrous complex. In this concept the shape of the triquetrohamate joint must be acknowledged. The stabilizing function of the ulnar articular chain must compromise with rotational movements around the ulna in the DRUJ during pronation and supination of the hand.

II. ANATOMY AFFECTING THE METACARPAL AND PHALANGEAL BONES OF THE HAND*

Bruce A. Kraemer and Louis A. Gilula

NORMAL OSSEOUS ANATOMY

General Information

The hand, excluding the wrist, contains 19 major bones: 14 phalanges and 5 metacarpals (Fig. 4–20). It also contains a varying number of sesamoid (accessory) bones. Two sesamoids are present in the thumb metacarpophalangeal (MCP) joint palmar plate. Other sesamoids, when present, are usually at the MCP joints of the other digits, most commonly at the little finger. Sesamoids may also be present at the thumb interphalangeal (IP) joint.

Osseous vascular channels pierce the distal third of the proximal phalangeal shafts and characteristically appear as thin, radiolucent lines with faint sclerotic edges, which may be misinterpreted as fractures. These vascular channels usually run obliquely from the external proximal surface to enter the medullary canal more distally.[52] In the middle phalanx, the vascular grooves or foramina may appear as small, round radiolucencies and should not be confused with cyst-like lesions of the bone.[52] Vascular channels

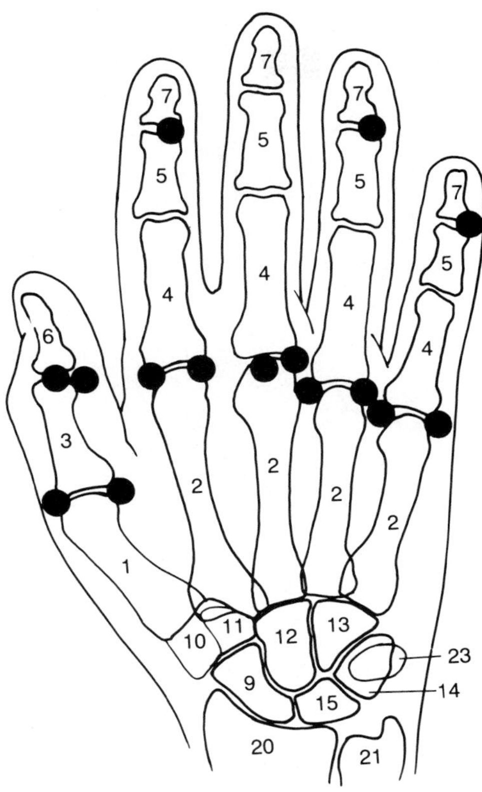

FIGURE 4–20. The major bones of the hand with the most frequent sites of sesamoid bones (found on the palmar joint surfaces) noted by black circles. 1—Thumb metacarpal; 2—finger metacarpals; 3—thumb proximal phalanx; 4—finger proximal phalanges; 5—finger middle phalanges; 6—thumb distal phalanx; 7—finger distal phalanges; 8—sesamoid; 9—scaphoid; 10—trapezium; 11—trapezoid; 12—capitate; 13—hamate; 14—triquetrum; 15—lunate; 20—radius; 21—ulna; 23—pisiform.

are usually best seen on posteroanterior (PA) or anteroposterior (AP) views.

Normal Resting Position

In the normal resting position of the hand, the fingers are flexed, the distal phalanges point toward the scaphoid tubercle without any overlap (Fig. 4–21), and there is a progressive increase in flexion of the digits from the index toward the little finger. The normal position of rest for the thumb is out of the plane of the fingers (Fig. 4–22). The thumb is rotated toward the fingers and angled up and palmarly, taking it out of the plane of the other digits. The distal phalanx of the thumb is flexed slightly in an ulnar direction and is directed toward the palm in opposition.

The tendency toward an ulnar inclination of the fingers is a result of the following:

1. The MCP joint anatomy. The radial-sided prominence of the metacarpal heads and the collateral ligament orientation contribute to ulnar orientation of fingers.
2. The flexor and extensor tendons. The digital flexor and the extensor tendon of each finger

* *Printed material and art reprinted with permission from Gilula LA.* The traumatized hand and wrist: Radiographic and anatomic correlation. *Philadelphia: WB Saunders, 1992:65–104.*

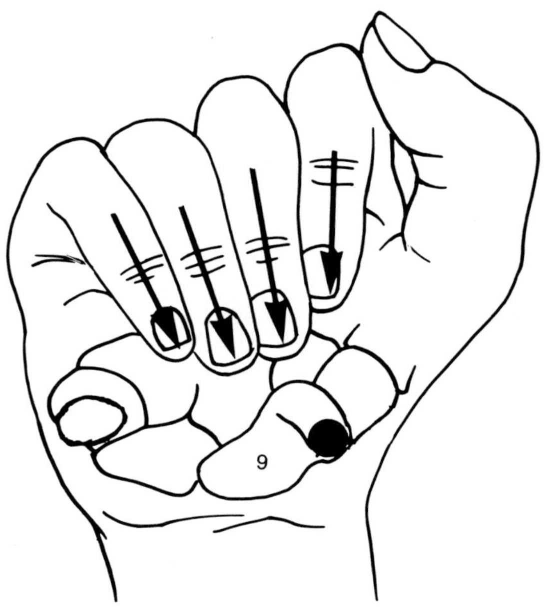

FIGURE 4–21. In the resting hand, the fingers assume a flexed position. In this position, the fingertips point toward the distal pole of the scaphoid (9) (black circle).

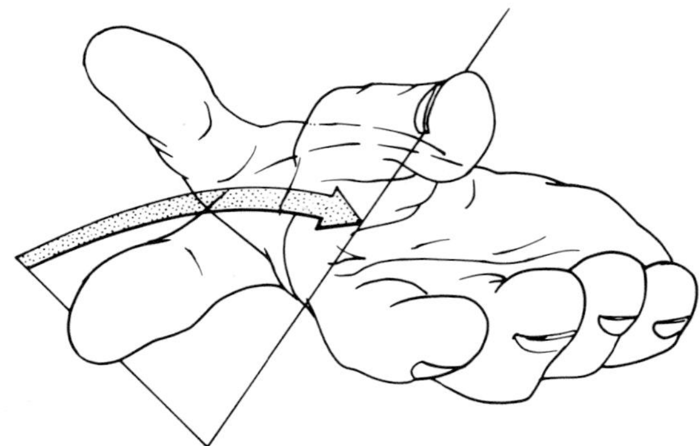

FIGURE 4–22. Thumb motion is out of the plane of the fingers.

cross the hand on the ulnar side of the longitudinal axis of the digits. The pull of these tendons is in a proximal ulnar direction.

3. The muscles. The ulnarly inclined intrinsic muscles predominate over the radial muscles. The insertions of the ulnar intrinsic muscles are more distal than those of the radial intrinsic muscles. The hypothenar muscles pull in an ulnar direction on the little finger.
4. The position of the fourth and fifth metacarpals. The position of the two ulnar metacarpal heads, proximal to the long and index metacarpal heads, pulls their extensor tendons in an ulnar direction. This ulnarward pull is transferred to all of the fingers' junctura tendinae, which interconnect all of the extensor tendons.[54]
5. The physiologic action of the thumb in pinch or key grip is to push the fingers in an ulnar direction.

METACARPALS

General Information

The finger metacarpal axes are roughly parallel to each other, with the heads forming a mobile transverse arch (Fig. 4–23). The thumb metacarpal axis is approximately 45 degrees radial to the index finger metacarpal. The thumb metacarpal is shorter and wider than the finger metacarpals (Fig. 4–20).[55]

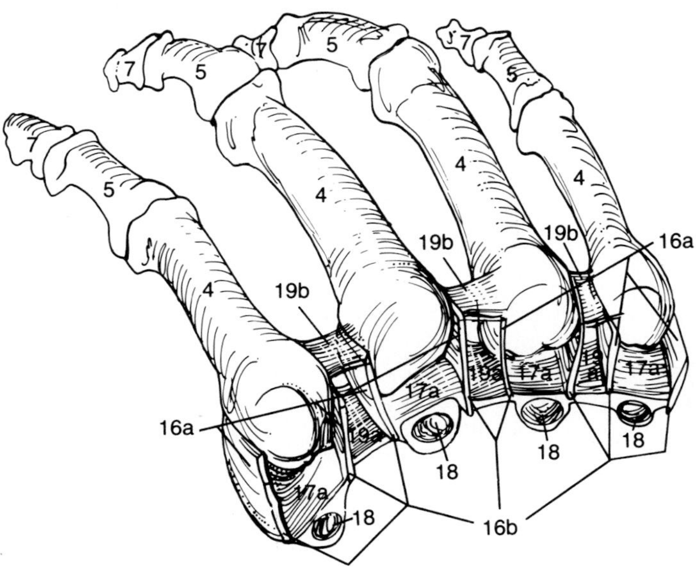

FIGURE 4–23. Cross-section through the finger MCP joints showing the ligamentous joint structures and the longitudinal orientation of the phalanges, as well as their transverse and longitudinal arches. 4—Finger proximal phalanges; 5—finger middle phalanges; 7—finger distal phalanges; 16a—MCP proper collateral ligaments; 16b—MCP accessory (metacarpoglenoid) collateral ligaments; 17a—MCP volar (palmar) plates; 18—finger fibroosseous tunnels; 19a—finger MCP joint volar (palmar) intermetacarpal ligaments; 19b—finger MCP joint dorsal intermetacarpal ligaments.

Metacarpal of the Thumb (Fig. 4–24)

Articular Surface—Base

The proximal end of the thumb metacarpal is concave in the dorsopalmar (posteroanterior) direction and convex in the transverse (mediolateral) direction.[55,56] It has no lateral facets to articulate with adjacent metacarpals (as are found on the finger metacarpals) but has a medial facet to articulate with the trapezoid and the radial edge of the second metacarpal base.[55–57]

Shaft

The diaphysis is narrower than either end of the bone.[55] The shaft is flattened and broad over its dorsal surface.[57]

Articular Surface—Head

The distal end of the first metacarpal is unicondylar and may be flat or rounded, unlike the finger metacarpals, which are round and slightly larger dorsally than palmarly. The metacarpal head presents the same articular surface area in flexion and extension, unlike the finger metacarpals, which present a greater articular surface in flexion.[58] A slight depression is found on the palmar surface of the head on either side of the midline. These surfaces articulate with the thumb sesamoids.[55]

Metacarpals of the Fingers (Figs. 4–23 and 4–24)

Articular Surfaces—Base

These are cuboidal in shape and broader dorsally than palmarly to provide a stable surface for articulation with the carpals.[57,59] The articular surface of the fifth metacarpal has both concave and convex curves, allowing 15 to 30 degrees of flexion. The dorsal and palmar surfaces of the index, long, and little finger metacarpal bases are rough for the attachment of tendons and ligaments.[57]

Shaft

The metacarpals, in cross-section, are oval to triangular in shape, with two lateral surfaces and one dorsal surface.[60] The medial and lateral surfaces are separated from each other by a prominent palmar ridge and are concave for attachment of the interosseous muscles. The diaphysis is narrower centrally than at either end.[60] The palmar cortex is 20% thicker than the dorsal cortex.[60] The weakest point of the metacarpal is just proximal to its head.[61,62]

Articular Surface—Head

There is significant variation in the configurations of the metacarpal heads of the index, long, ring, and little fingers.[58] The distal articular surface is rounded but not spherical, since it is flattened transversely and wider palmarly than dorsally.[63] The radius of the metacarpal head is longer palmarly than dorsally, with a resultant moving axis of rotation as the phalanx is flexed, forming a spiral curve or a cam-shaft effect (Fig. 4–43).[63] The articular head cross-sectional palmar width is nearly twice as wide as the dorsal width, providing more contact surface in flexion than in extension. This allows for more joint mobility in extension while providing more joint stability in flexion. On both the radial and ulnar sides of the metacarpal head are tubercles for attachment of the radial and ulnar MCP collateral ligaments.[57]

Characteristics of the Individual Metacarpals

Index Finger Metacarpal

This is the longest of the metacarpals and its base is larger than those of the other four finger metacarpals.[55,57–59] The base has four articular surfaces for articulation with the trapezium, trapezoid, capitate, and the styloid process of the base of the long finger metacarpal.[55] The palmar radial prominence of the finger metacarpal head is largest on the index metacarpal head and becomes less prominent as one progresses to the little finger.

Six muscles attach to the index metacarpal (Fig. 4–28):

1. The extensor carpi radialis longus.
2. The flexor carpi radialis.
3. The oblique head of the adductor policis.
4. The first and second dorsal interosseous muscles.
5. The first palmar interosseous muscle.

Long Finger Metacarpal[57]

This is usually slightly shorter than the index metacarpal.[55] The base has one articular surface each for the index metacarpal base and capitate and two articular surfaces for the ring metacarpal base. This metacarpal has a roughened dorsal radial prominence that extends proximally and dorsally to the capitate for the attachment of the extensor carpi radialis brevis tendon. The shaft has a palmar longitudinal crest for origin of the adductor pollicis.[59]

Five muscles attach to the long finger metacarpal (Fig. 4–28):

1. The extensor carpi radialis brevis.
2. The flexor carpi radialis.
3. The adductor pollicis oblique and transverse heads.
4. The second dorsal interossei muscle.
5. The third dorsal interossei muscle.

Ring Finger Metacarpal[57]

The base has five articular facets: one each for the capitate, hamate, and little finger metacarpal base and two surfaces for the long finger metacarpal base.

Text continued on page 60

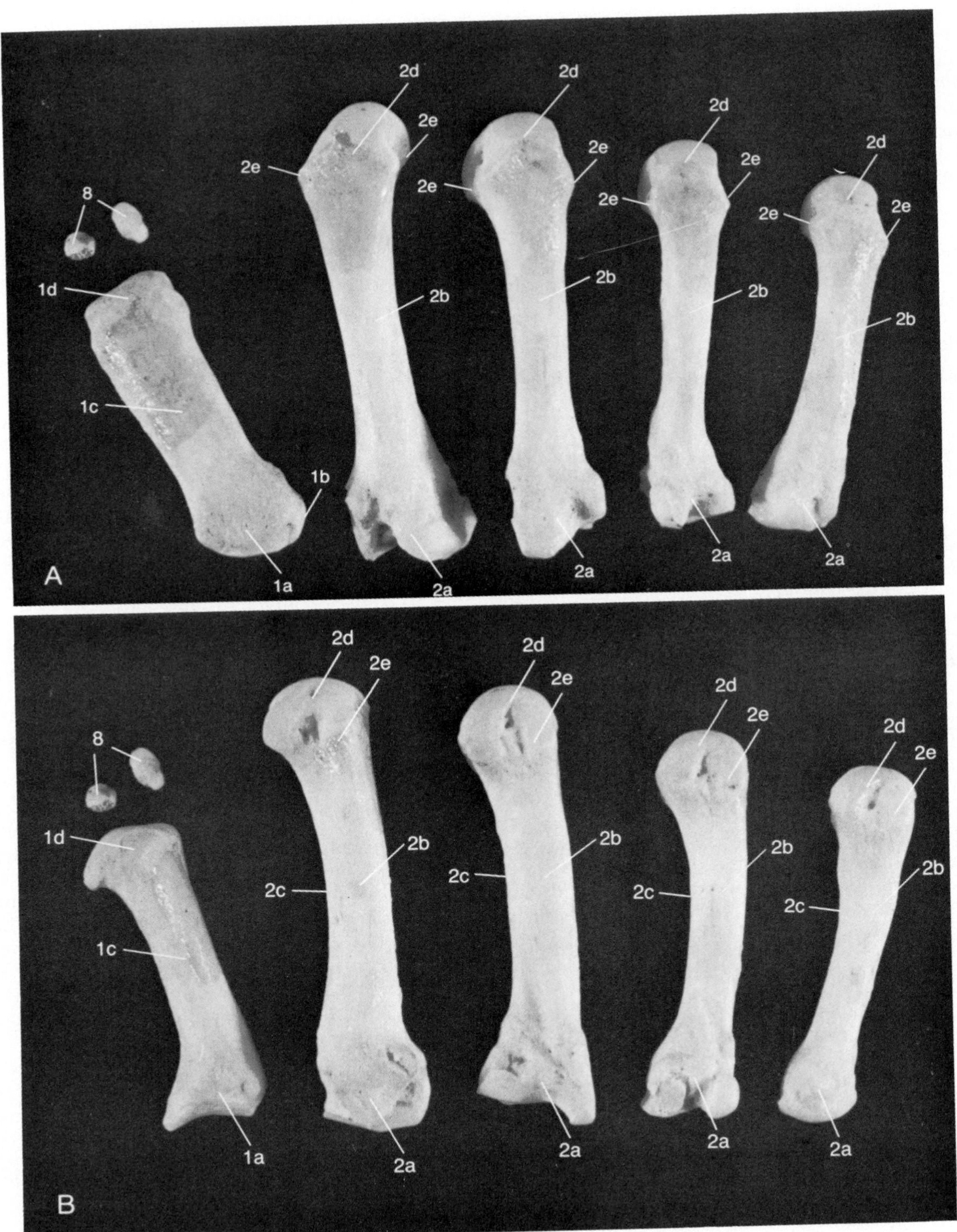

FIGURE 4–24. (panels **A** and **B**) *See legend on opposite page*

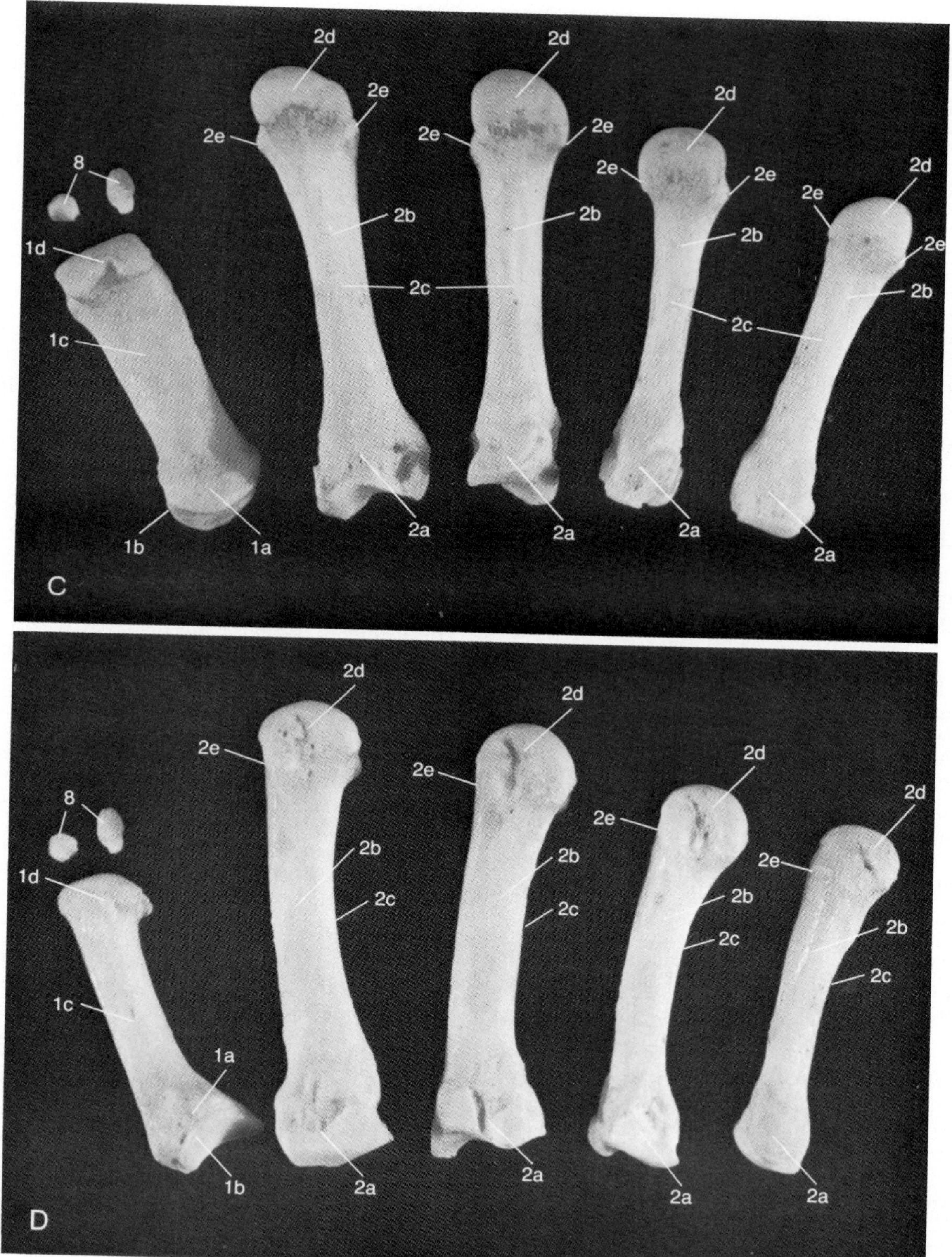

FIGURE 4–24. Dorsal **(A)**, radial **(B)**, palmar **(C)**, and ulnar **(D)**, views of the right thumb and finger metacarpals. The thumb metacarpal is smaller and stouter than the finger metacarpals and usually has two associated sesamoid bones, as shown. 1a—Thumb metacarpal base; 1b—thumb metacarpal base medial facet; 1c—thumb metacarpal shaft; 1d—thumb distal articular head; 2a—finger metacarpal base; 2b—finger metacarpal shaft; 2c—finger metacarpal shaft palmar ridge; 2d—finger metacarpal articular head; 2e—finger metacarpal articular head collateral tubercles; 8—sesamoid bones.

Three muscles attach to the ring finger metacarpal (Fig. 4–28):

1. The third dorsal interosseous.
2. The fourth dorsal interosseous.
3. The second palmar interosseous.

Little Finger Metacarpal[57]

The little finger metacarpal is the shortest metacarpal. The base has two articular surfaces: one for the hamate and one for the fourth metacarpal base. The ulnar side has a prominent tubercle for the attachment of the extensor carpi ulnaris. Five muscles attach to this bone:

1. The extensor carpi ulnaris.
2. The flexor carpi ulnaris.
3. The flexor digiti minimi.
4. The fourth dorsal interosseous.
5. The third palmar interosseous (Fig. 4–28).

PHALANGES

General Information (Figs. 4–25 through 4–27)

Proximal Phalanges

The proximal phalanx of the long finger is the longest. The proximal phalanges of the index and ring fingers are approximately equal in size. The proximal phalanx of the little finger is the smallest.[55]

Middle and Distal Phalanges

The middle phalanges have the same approximate length relationships as the proximal phalanges.[55] The distal phalanx of the long finger is 1 to 2 mm longer than the distal phalanges of the other fingers.[55]

Proximal Phalanx of the Thumb

Articular Surface—Base[58]

The proximal phalangeal base has a broad concave surface that accommodates the thumb metacarpal head (Fig. 4–25). The palmar plate inserts on the broad prominent palmar ridge. The abductor pollicis brevis tendon attaches to the lateral tubercle.

Shaft

The external surface of the palmar cortex is always concave transversely.[64] The external surface of the dorsal cortex is either straight or slightly convex with a larger arch dorsally than palmarly.[64] The annular pulleys attach to the longitudinal palmar crests, which run along the radial and ulnar margins of this bone.[64] The medullary cavity of the diaphysis is narrower in the center than it is at either end.[64]

Articular Surface—Head

The articular surface of the head is formed by a pair of concentric condyles with an intercondylar notch oriented in the anteroposterior direction. The ulnar condyle is usually larger, thus contributing to the rotation, which occurs at the thumb IP joint as it flexes.[58,65]

Proximal Phalanges of the Fingers (Fig. 4–25)

Articular Surface—Base[57]

The concave base provides for joint mobility between flexion and extension. The articular base of a given proximal phalanx is larger than its distal articular head. There are three tubercles at the proximal phalangeal base:

1. A radial tubercle for collateral ligament attachment.[66]
2. An ulnar tubercle for collateral ligament attachment.[66]
3. A dorsal tubercle for insertion of a medial portion of the extensor tendon.[66]

Shaft

The external palmar longitudinal surface is always concave,[64] whereas the external dorsal longitudinal surface is either straight or slightly convex (i.e., a larger arch dorsally than palmarly).[64] Longitudinal palmar crests for the attachments of the annular pulleys are on the radial and ulnar diaphyseal margins.[64] The medullary cavity of the diaphysis is narrower in the center than it is at either end.[64] The proximal and distal metaphyses are equal in length.[64]

Articular Surface—Head

The distal articular surface is composed of two asymmetric condyles separated by a central cleft. The index finger ulnar condyle projects more distally than its radial condyle, and the radial condyles of the long, ring, and little finger project more distally than their ulnar condyles.[63,67] The articular surface extends further palmarly than dorsally.[68] The transverse dimension is almost double the anteroposterior dimension, thus providing greater stability during lateral and oblique stress.[68,69] The central cleft, which provides an effective tracking mechanism for the central projection of the middle phalangeal base, helps resist shearing and rotary stresses.[69] The index finger cleft is inclined in an ulnar direction, whereas the little finger cleft is inclined in a radial direction.[67]

Middle Phalanx

Articular Surface—Base

The base of the middle phalanx (Fig. 4–26) has two complementary concave surfaces that accommodate the two asymmetric condyles of the head of the proximal phalanx. There is a central ridge between the two concave surfaces that is convex in the coronal plane and concave in the sagittal plane.[58] The transverse diameter of the base of the middle phalanx is approximately 10% greater than the bicondylar diameter of its adjacent proximal phalangeal head.[69,70]

There are three tubercles at the middle phalangeal base:

1. A radial tubercle for collateral ligament attachment.
2. An ulnar tubercle for collateral ligament attachment.
3. A dorsal tubercle for insertion of the extensor tendon.[66]

Shaft

The middle phalangeal shaft is similar to the proximal phalanx except that it has less palmar surface concavity and less pronounced marginal longitudinal crests.[64]

The distal metaphysis is longer than the proximal metaphysis.[64]

Articular Surface—Head

This surface is bicondylar but less prominent than that of the head of the proximal phalanx. A shallow cleft separates the two condyles. The transverse dimension is almost double the anteroposterior dimension, thus providing greater stability to lateral and oblique stress.[68,69] The articular surface presents the same surface area to the base of the distal phalanx in flexion and extension but extends farther palmarly than dorsally.[58,68] The central cleft provides an effective tracking mechanism for the central projection of the distal phalangeal base that helps resist shearing and rotary stresses.[69]

Distal Phalanx of the Thumb

Articular Surface

The base of the distal phalanx (Fig. 4–27) has two complementary concave surfaces that accommodate the two condyles of the head of the proximal phalanx of the thumb. The palmar surface of the distal phalangeal base has prominent tubercles on its radial and ulnar edges for the attachments of the radial and ulnar collateral ligaments.[58] The degree of dorsal and palmar lipping of the distal phalangeal base varies.[58]

Shaft and Tuft

The distal phalanx is one-third larger in length and width than the finger distal phalanges.[71] The bone is convex dorsally and flat palmarly.

Distal Phalanges of the Fingers

Articular Surface

The base of the distal phalanx (Fig. 4–27) has two complementary concave surfaces that accommodate the two condyles of the head of the middle phalanx of the same finger. The articular surface is concave in the sagittal and coronal planes and overall is less prominent than the middle phalangeal base. The transverse diameter of the distal phalangeal base is approximately 10% greater than the bicondylar diameter of its adjacent middle phalanx.[69]

Shaft and Tuft

The medullary canal length is two-fifths of the external bone length.[64] There are no palmar longitudinal crests, as are found on the more proximal phalanges and the distal phalanx of the thumb.[64] Fibrous septa radiating out from the distal phalanx to the skin form a dense meshwork that helps to stabilize fractures of the distal phalanx.[61] Vascular grooves or foramina may appear as small, round radiolucencies and should not be confused with cystic lesions of the bone.[52]

The size of the tufts is extremely variable;[52] men have larger tufts than women, and those doing heavy manual labor have heavier tufts than those who do not use their hands as vigorously. Small, palmar, proximally directed projections may be noted on each side of the tuft. These are more commonly seen in the elderly.[52]

One should be aware of a possible Kirner deformity of the little finger in children ages 9 through 12 and not confuse it with a fracture.[52] On radiographic examination the Kirner deformity resembles a transverse fracture of the distal phalanx, with the fingertip bent in a palmar direction.

There is also a growth plate abnormality of the little finger that resembles a mallet finger deformity. Bilateral changes are frequent, and the deformity may be familial. This deformity may represent a stress fracture of the distal phalanx caused by the flexor tendon's insertion into the distal phalanx.

SESAMOID BONES

General Information

Sesamoid bones may be found adjacent to many of the joints of the hand, usually in the volar (palmar) plates of the joints. They are formed early in fetal development but do not ossify until later in life.[52,72] Sesamoids are variable in number and appearance.[52] Small sesamoids may occasionally appear so dense that when projected over a bone, they appear as bone islands. Larger ones are usually well defined and trabeculated. They may be double (bipartite) or multiple (multipartite). Fractured sesamoids are usually differentiated from nonfractured sesamoids by evidence of cortication on all edges of the nonfractured sesamoid and by the fact that fractured sesamoid fragments seem to "fit together," whereas multipartite sesamoids do not.

Text continued on page 67

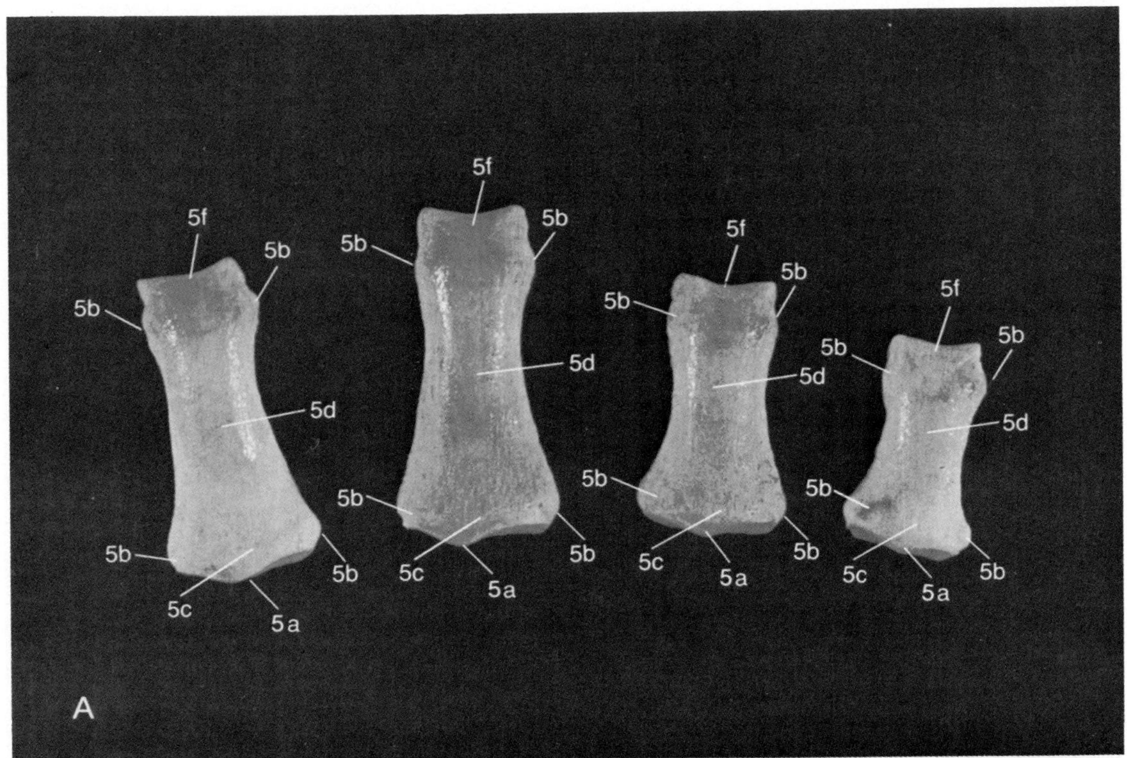

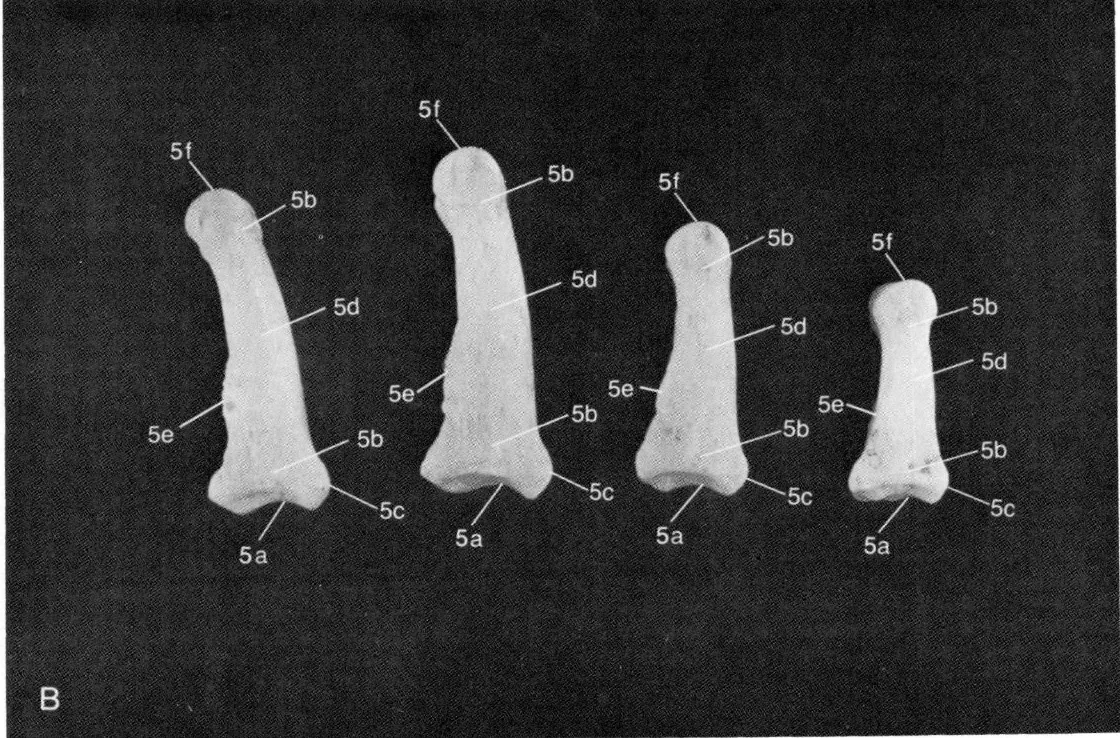

FIGURE 4–26. (panels **A** and **B**) *See legend on opposite page*

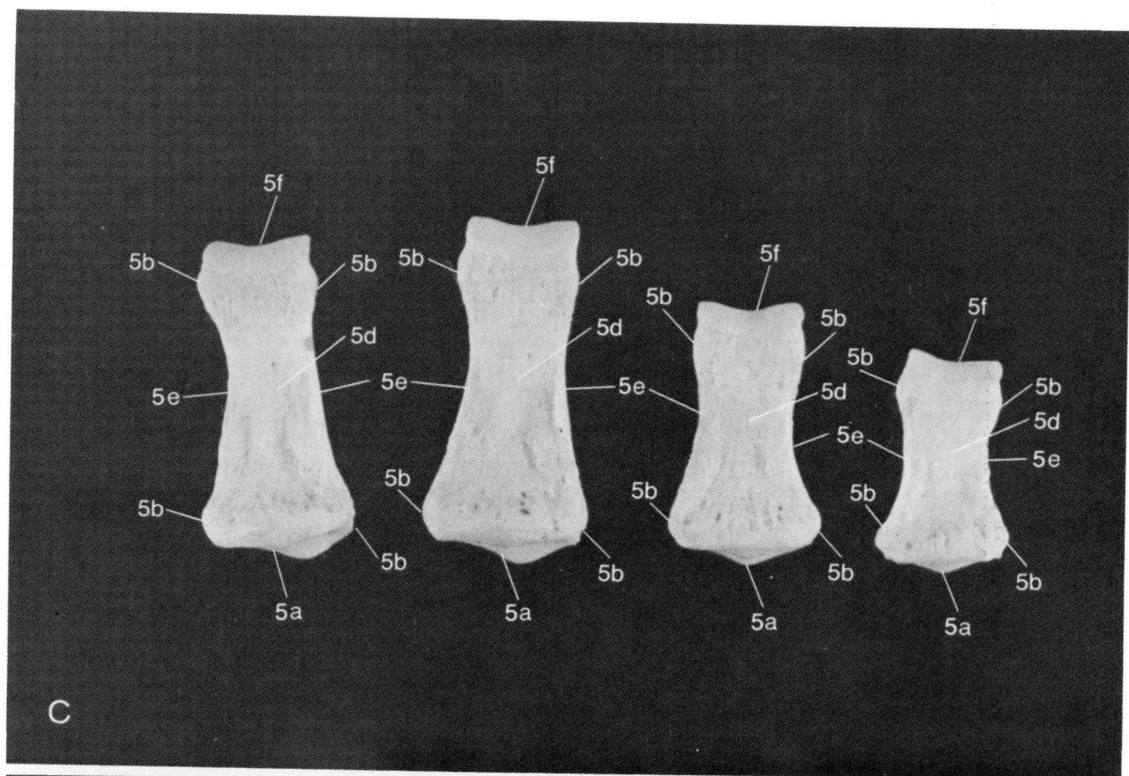

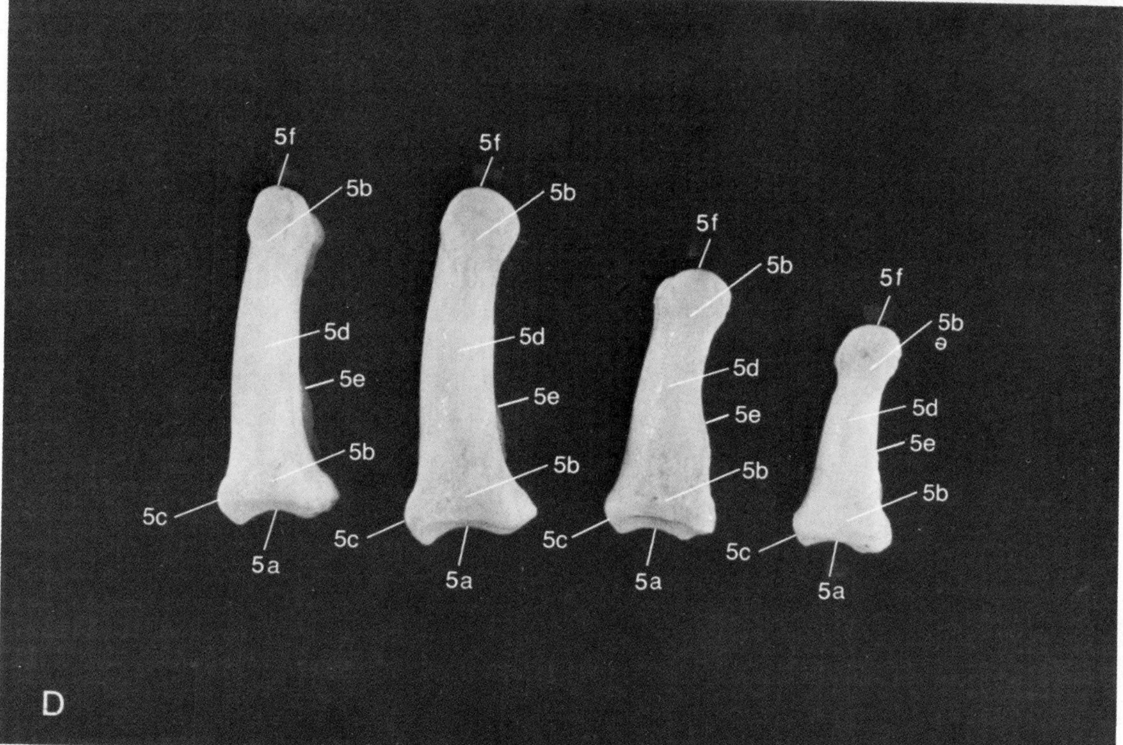

FIGURE 4–26. Dorsal **(A)**, radial **(B)**, palmar **(C)**, and ulnar **(D)**, views of the right index, long, ring, and little finger middle phalanges (left to right), showing fewer variations than the proximal phalanges. 5a—Finger middle phalangeal bases; 5b—finger middle phalangeal collateral tubercles; 5c—finger middle phalangeal dorsal tubercles; 5d—finger middle phalangeal shafts; 5e—finger middle phalangeal longitudinal palmar crests; 5f—finger middle phalangeal articular heads.

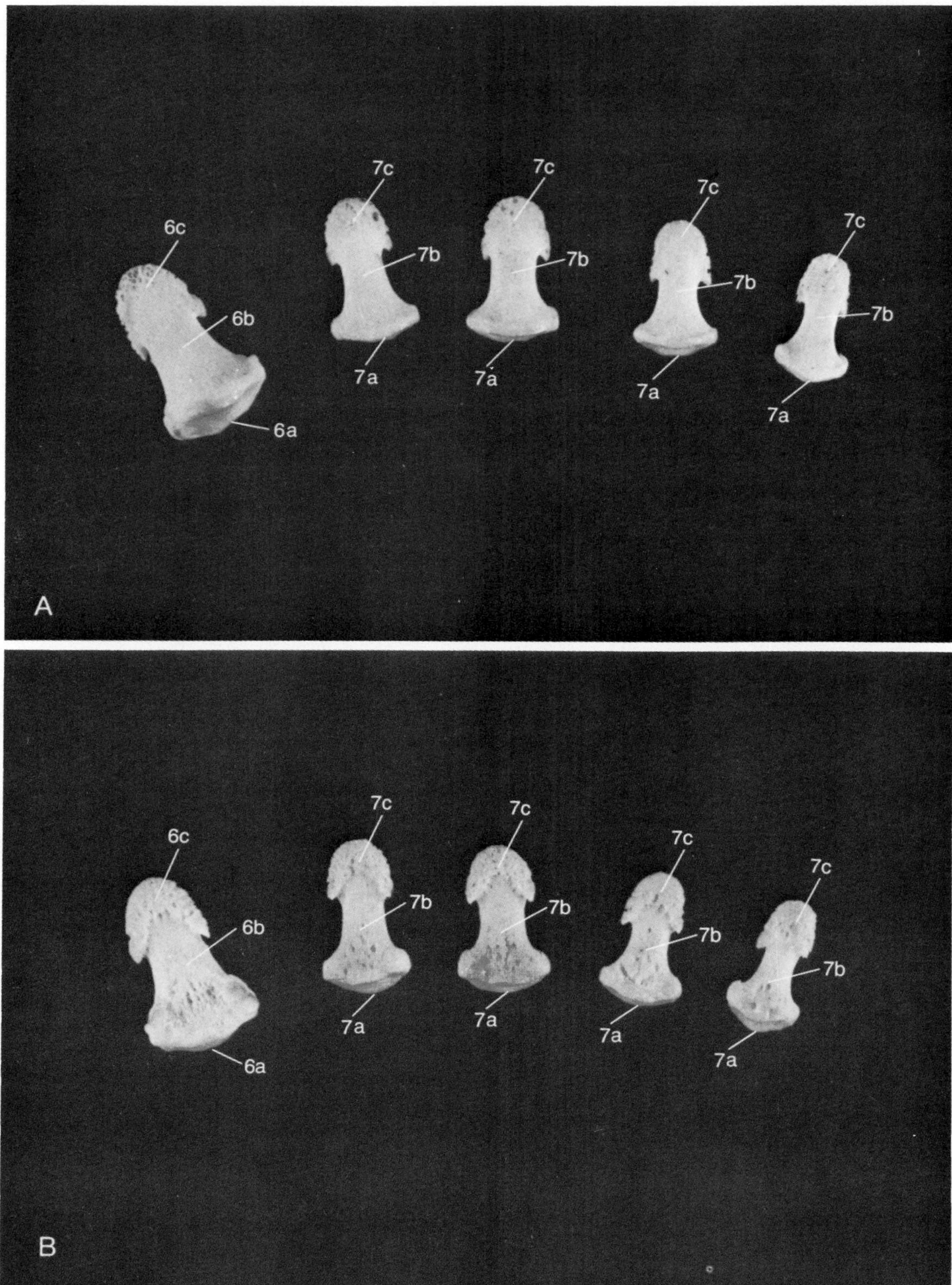

FIGURE 4–27. Dorsal **(A)**, and palmar **(B)**, views of the distal phalanges of the right thumb, index, long, ring, and little fingers (left to right) have a remarkable similarity. 6a—Thumb distal phalangeal base; 6b—thumb distal phalangeal shaft; 6c—Thumb distal phalangeal tuft; 7a—finger distal phalangeal bases; 7b—finger distal phalangeal shafts; 7c—finger distal phalangeal tufts.

Occurrence

Sesamoid Bones of the Thumb[52]

The thumb MCP joint sesamoids are present in virtually all patients,[72,73] whereas sesamoid bones of the thumb IP joint are present in 22% to 73% of patients.[72]

Sesamoid Bones of the Fingers

Finger MCP sesamoids are present in the little finger in 44.6% to 82.5% of patients, the index finger in 47.8% to 64.2% of patients, the ring finger in 0% to 7% of patients, and the long finger in 0% to 5.3% of patients.[72]

Sesamoids are less commonly found at the flexor digitorum at the distal interphalangeal (DIP) joints of the index, ring, and little fingers.

Anatomy

Thumb MCP Sesamoid Bones

The radial and ulnar sesamoids are firmly encased in the MCP joint palmar plate. The medial (ulnar) sesamoid is usually the smaller and rounder of the two sesamoids. The lateral (radial) sesamoid may have a well-defined facet that articulates with the thumb metacarpal head.[74] These sesamoids may be bipartite in 1% to 6% of cases.[72]

Finger Sesamoid Bones

These are also contained within the joint palmar plates. They are usually smaller and are bipartite less often than the thumb sesamoids.

MUSCLES AND TENDONS

Flexor Carpi Radialis

Origin

The flexor carpi radialis (Figs. 4–28, 4–29, and 4–36)[55,57] arises from the medial epicondyle of the humerus lateral to the pronator teres and medial to the palmaris longus and from the epicondylar forearm flexor muscle tendinous origin of the medial humeral epicondyle and the forearm fascia.

Anatomic Course

The flexor carpi radialis descends in the midportion of the forearm, where it becomes tendinous. It traverses the wrist in a special canal under the crest of the trapezium. It is the most superficial muscle of the forearm.

Insertion

The flexor carpi radialis inserts onto the proximal palmar base of the index finger metacarpal. It sends strong, oblique, tendinous slips to the proximal palmar base of the long finger metacarpal. There may be additional tendinous slips to the ring finger metacarpal, the trapezium, and the scaphoid.[55]

Function

The flexor carpi radialis muscle serves to flex the wrist as well as to assist with forearm flexion. It also assists with pronating and abducting the hand.

Flexor Carpi Ulnaris[55,57]

Origin

The flexor carpi ulnaris (Figs. 4–28, 4–29, and 4–36) arises from two heads: a humeral and an ulnar head. The humeral head of the flexor carpi ulnaris arises from the medial epicondyle medial to the palmaris longus and anterolateral to the origin of the flexor digitorum superficialis. The ulnar head arises from the medial border of the olecranon and the upper portion of the dorsal border of the ulna. A tendinous arch unites the two heads of the muscle, beneath which passes the ulnar nerve.

Anatomic Course

The flexor carpi ulnaris descends in the medial aspect of the forearm, becoming tendinous in the middle third of the forearm. Fibers on the ulnar side continue down almost to its distal insertion.

Insertion

The flexor carpi ulnaris tendon inserts onto the pisiform with distal tendinous insertions onto the fibers of the abductor digiti minimi, the proximal palmar base of the little finger metacarpal, and possibly the proximal palmar base of the ring finger metacarpal. A few fibers may wrap around the dorsum of the wrist to insert onto the dorsal transverse carpal ligament.[55]

Function

The flexor carpi ulnaris muscle flexes the wrist, assists with forearm flexion, and assists with adduction of the hand.

Extensor Carpi Radialis Longus

Origin

The extensor carpi radialis longus muscle[55,57] (Figs. 4–28, 4–30, 4–31, and 4–33) arises from the lower third of the lateral epicondylar ridge, as well as the epicondyle of the humerus, along with the other extensor muscles. It also arises from the lateral intermuscular septum.

Anatomic Course

The extensor carpi radialis longus muscle becomes tendinous in the proximal portion of the middle third of the forearm. The tendon then runs along with and radial to the extensor carpi radialis brevis down to the wrist. The tendons are crossed by the

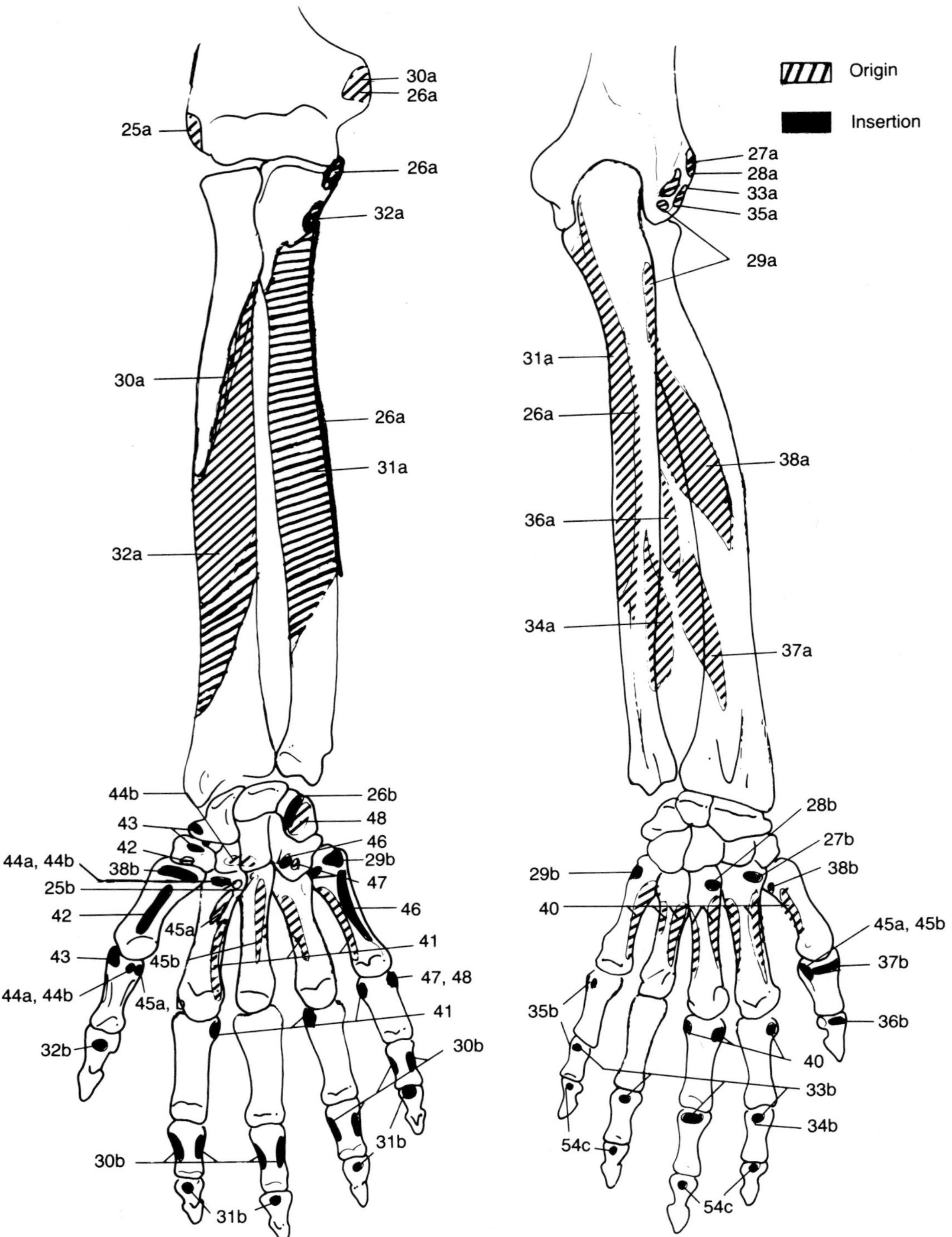

FIGURE 4–28. Palmar (left) and dorsal (right) origins and insertions of the muscles and tendons of the forearm and hand. The sites of origin are indicated by a diagonal pattern, and the sites of insertion are shown in solid black. 25a—Flexor carpi radialis muscle; 25b—flexor carpi radialis tendon; 26a—flexor carpi ulnaris muscle; 26b—flexor carpi ulnaris tendon; 27a—extensor carpi radialis longus muscle; 27b—extensor carpi radialis longus tendon; 28a—extensor carpi radialis brevis muscle; 28b—extensor carpi radialis brevis tendon; 29a—extensor carpi ulnaris muscle; 29b—extensor carpi ulnaris tendon; 30a—flexor digitorum superficialis muscle; 30b—flexor digitorum superficialis tendon; 31a—flexor digitorum profundus muscle; 31b—flexor digitorum profundus tendon; 32a—flexor pollicis longus muscle; 32b—flexor pollicis longus tendon; 33a—extensor digitorum communis muscle; 33b—extensor digitorum communis tendon; 34a—extensor indicis proprius muscle; 34b—extensor indicis proprius tendon; 35a—extensor digiti minimi muscle; 35b—extensor digiti minimi tendon; 36a—extensor pollicis longus muscle; 36b—extensor pollicis longus tendon; 37a—extensor pollicis brevis muscle; 37b—extensor pollicis brevis tendon; 38a—abductor pollicis longus muscle; 38b—abductor pollicis longus tendon; 40—dorsal interosseous muscle; 41—palmar interosseous muscle; 42—opponens pollicis; 43—abductor pollicis brevis; 44a—flexor pollicis brevis superficial head; 45a—adductor pollicis oblique head; 45b—adductor pollicis transverse head; 46—opponens digiti minimi; 47—flexor digiti minimi brevis; 48—abductor digiti minimi; 54c—terminal extensor tendon.

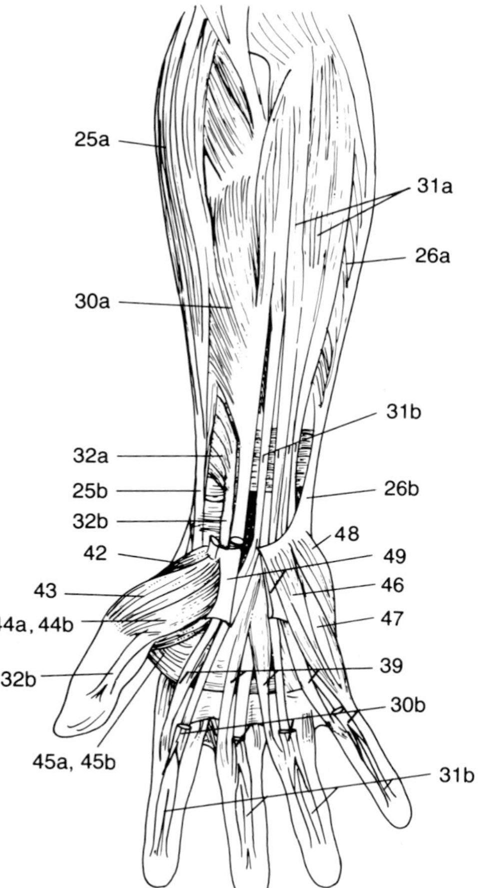

FIGURE 4–29. Palmar surface of the forearm and hand showing the forearm muscles as well as the intrinsic muscles of the hand. The palmar fascia as well as the midportion of the superficialis tendons have been divided. 25a—Flexor carpi radialis muscle; 25b—flexor carpi radialis tendon; 26a—flexor carpi ulnaris muscle; 26b—flexor carpi ulnaris tendon; 30a—flexor digitorum superficialis muscle; 30b—flexor digitorum superficialis tendon (cut); 31a—flexor digitorum profundus muscle; 31b—flexor digitorum profundus tendon; 32a—flexor pollicis longus muscle; 32b—flexor pollicis longus tendon; 39—lumbrical muscles; 42—opponens pollicis; 43—abductor pollicis brevis; 44a—flexor pollicis brevis superficial head; 44b—flexor pollicis brevis deep head; 45a—adductor pollicis oblique head; 45b—adductor pollicis transverse head; 46—opponens digiti minimi; 47—flexor digiti minimi brevis; 48—abductor digiti minimi; 49—palmar transverse carpal ligament.

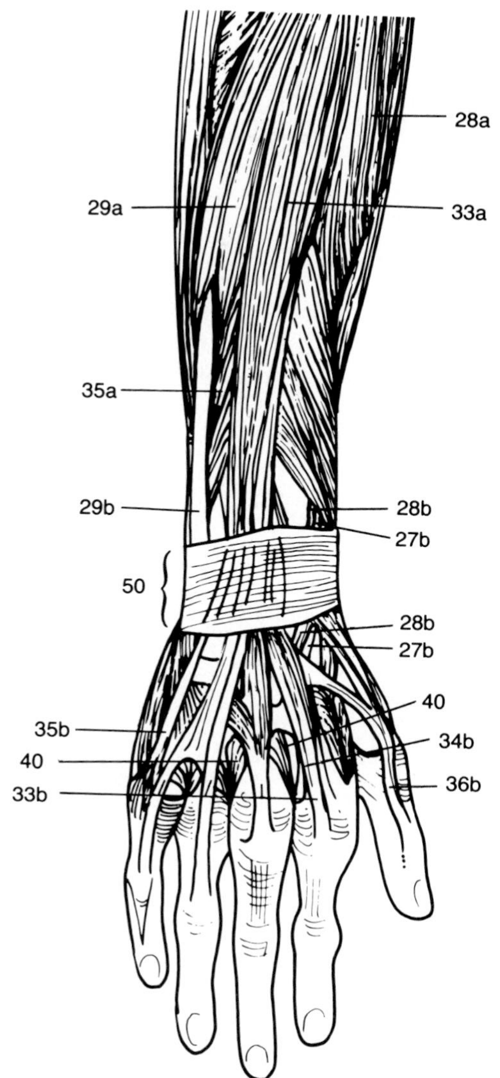

FIGURE 4–30. Dorsal surface of the forearm and hand showing the forearm muscles and tendons traversing the extensor retinaculum. 27b—Extensor carpi radialis longus tendon; 28a—extensor carpi radialis brevis muscle; 28b—extensor carpi radialis brevis tendon; 29a—extensor carpi ulnaris muscle; 29b—extensor carpi ulnaris tendon; 33a—extensor communis digitorum muscle; 33b—extensor communis digitorum tendons; 34b—extensor indicis proprius tendon; 35a—extensor digiti minimi muscle; 35b—extensor digiti minimi tendon; 36b—extensor pollicis longus tendon; 40—dorsal interosseous muscles; 50—extensor retinaculum.

abductor pollicis longus and extensor pollicis brevis in the distal third of the forearm. The tendon then passes through the wrist in the second dorsal extensor compartment.

Insertion

The extensor carpi radialis longus inserts onto the proximal dorsal base of the index finger metacarpal. It may have a tendinous insertion onto the proximal dorsal base of the long finger metacarpal.[55]

Function

The extensor carpi radialis longus muscle extends the wrist and abducts the hand.

Extensor Carpi Radialis Brevis[55,57] (Figs. 4–28, 4–30, 4–31, and 4–33)

Origin

The extensor carpi radialis brevis muscle originates from the common extensor tendon, which arises from the lateral epicondyle of the humerus. It also arises from the radial collateral ligament of the elbow and the proximal ulnar aspect of the intermuscular septum.

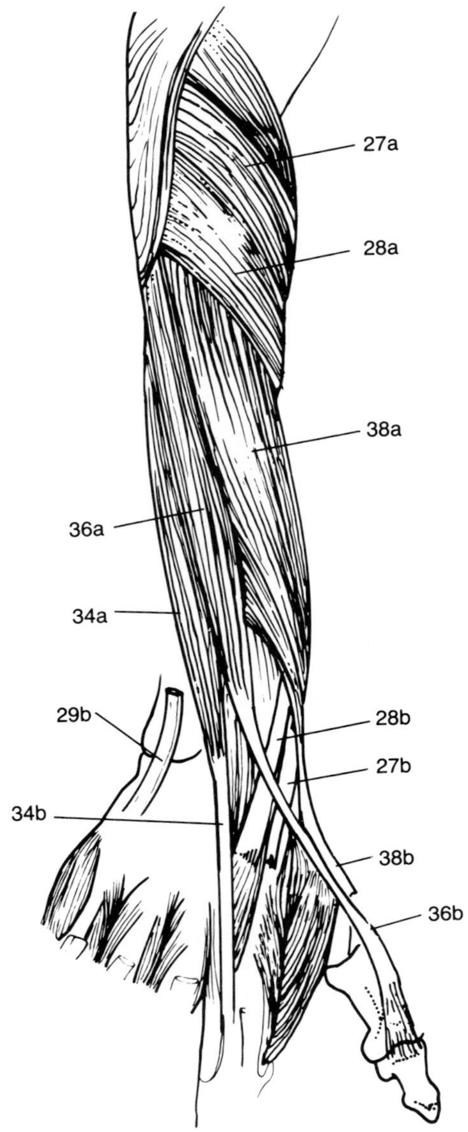

FIGURE 4–31. Deep muscles of the dorsal surface of the forearm. 27a—Extensor carpi radialis longus muscle; 27b—extensor carpi radialis longus tendon; 28a—extensor carpi radialis brevis muscle; 28b—extensor carpi radialis brevis tendon; 29b—extensor carpi ulnaris tendon; 34a—extensor indicis proprius muscle; 34b—extensor indicis proprius tendon; 36a—extensor pollicis longus muscle; 36b—extensor pollicis longus tendon; 38a—abductor pollicis longus muscle; 38b—abductor pollicis longus tendon.

Anatomic Course

The extensor carpi radialis brevis muscle becomes tendinous in the midportion of the forearm. The tendon then runs along with and ulnar to the extensor carpi radialis longus tendon down to the wrist. The tendons are crossed by the abductor pollicis longus and the extensor pollicis brevis in the distal third of the forearm. The extensor carpi radialis brevis passes through the wrist in the second dorsal extensor compartment.

Insertion

The extensor carpi radialis brevis muscle inserts onto the proximal dorsal base of the long finger metacarpal. It may also insert on the proximal dorsal base of the index or ring finger metacarpal.[55]

Function

The extensor carpi radialis brevis muscle extends the wrist and abducts the hand.

Extensor Carpi Ulnaris

Origin

The extensor carpi ulnaris[55,57] (Figs. 4–28, 4–30, 4–31, and 4–33) arises from the dorsal aspect of the lateral humeral epicondyle, the dorsal common extensor tendon of the lateral epicondyle of the humerus, and the dorsal radial border of the ulna.

Anatomic Course

The extensor carpi ulnaris muscle travels down the dorsoulnar aspect of the forearm with its tendon beginning in the mid-forearm. It traverses the wrist in the sixth dorsal extensor compartment.

Insertion

The extensor carpi ulnaris inserts primarily onto the ulnar tubercle of the dorsal proximal base of the metacarpal of the little finger. It may also insert onto the dorsal carpal ligament or the extensor tendons of the little finger.[55]

Function

The extensor carpi ulnaris muscle extends the wrist and adducts the hand.

Flexor Digitorum Superficialis

Origin

The flexor digitorum superficialis (Figs. 4–28, 4–29, 4–32, 4–36, and 4–37) arises from three heads:

1. A humeral head: from the medial epicondyle of the humerus via the common forearm flexor tendon.
2. An ulnar head: from the coronoid process of the ulna.
3. A radial head: from the thin, oblique, muscular line of the radius, which lies on the lateral border of the radius between the bicipital tuberosity and the insertion of the pronator teres.

The flexor digitorum superficialis is the largest muscle of the superficial flexor muscle group and externally covers the flexor digitorum profundus muscle.[55,57]

Anatomic Course

The flexor digitorum superficialis muscle becomes tendinous in the midforearm. At the wrist, the ten-

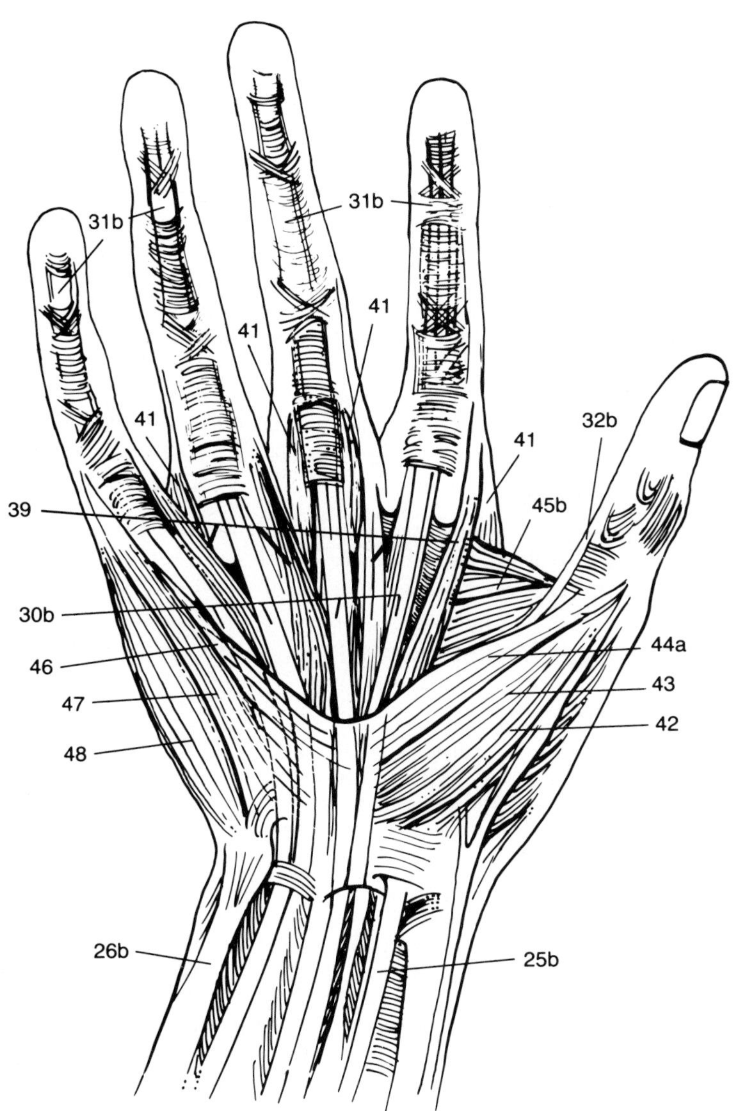

FIGURE 4–32. Intrinsic muscles and tendons of the palmar surface of the hand. 25b—Flexor carpi radialis tendon; 26b—flexor carpi ulnaris tendon; 30b—flexor digitorum superficialis tendon; 31b—flexor digitorum profundus tendon; 32b—flexor pollicis longus tendon; 39—lumbrical muscles; 41—palmar interosseous muscle; 42—opponens pollicis; 43—abductor pollicis brevis; 44a—flexor pollicis brevis superficial head; 45b—adductor pollicis transverse head; 46—opponens digiti minimi; 47—flexor digiti minimi brevis; 48—abductor digiti minimi.

dons pass dorsal to the flexor retinaculum (anterior annular ligament) and palmar (superficial) to the flexor profundus tendons. The flexor retinaculum is a strong, fibrous band that spans the palmar surface of the carpal bones and is a continuation of the forearm fascia. The retinaculum attaches on the radial side to the tuberosity of the scaphoid and the inner (ulnar) part of the anterior surface of the trapezium and on the ulnar side to the pisiform and the hook of the hamate.[57]

At the wrist, the tendons of the index and little fingers lie dorsal to the tendons of the long and ring fingers.

In their anatomic course toward the digital fibroosseous tunnel, the tendons pass through the palm and enter the fibroosseous canal palmar to the profundus tendons. Beyond the first (A1) pulley of the fibroosseous tunnel, at the base of the proximal phalanx, the tendon splits, with each half rolling outward 180 degrees as it passes laterally and then dorsally to the profundus tendon. Once dorsal to the profundus tendon, these two bands rejoin and then decussate again as they insert on the midportion of the middle phalangeal diaphysis. This portion of the tendon, which splits and then rejoins, is referred to as Camper's tendinous chiasm (Fig. 4–37).

Insertion

The flexor digitorum superficialis tendon inserts along margins of the palmar surface of the midportion of the middle phalanges of the index, long, ring, and little fingers. It inserts from a point just distal to the flare of the base of the middle phalanx to only a few millimeters proximal to the neck.[61] This broad area of insertion provides great leverage for powerful proximal interphalangeal (PIP) joint flexion.[70] A deep bundle of fibers of the flexor digitorum superficialis may join the muscle belly in the forearm or the tendon of the flexor digitorum profundus in the hand.[75,76]

Function

The flexor digitorum superficialis muscle flexes the proximal and middle phalanges of the index, long, ring, and little fingers and also assists with wrist flexion.

Flexor Digitorum Profundus

Origin

The flexor digitorum profundus (Figs. 4–28, 4–29, 4–32, 4–36, and 4–37) is located on the ulnar side of the forearm immediately beneath the superficial flexor muscle group.[57]

The flexor digitorum profundus arises from the (1) proximal two-thirds of the ulna's palmar and medial surfaces to the medial side of the coronoid process; (2) the posterior border of the ulna via an aponeurosis (the intermuscular septum between the flexor and extensor carpi ulnaris); (3) the ulnar half of the interosseous membrane; and (4) on occasion, the medial edge of the radius.[55]

Anatomic Course

The flexor digitorum profundus muscle gives rise to 7 to 12 or more tendons, which are held together by a paratenon. The paratenon is a continuation of the fascia of the muscle that extends distally to invest the tendons. Proximal to the flexor retinaculum, the specific tendons to a specific finger are less well defined than they are distally. The radial component to the index finger is the most independent, whereas the fibers to the little finger may arise from the muscle to the long or ring finger.[76]

At the level of the carpal canal, the tendons of the flexor digitorum profundus and superficialis are surrounded by a common synovial sheath (Fig. 4–36). This synovial sheath is attached to the dorsal wall of the carpal canal by a mesotendon, a thin fascial condensation that supports the flexor tendons.

Distal to the flexor retinaculum, the 7 to 12 tendons group themselves into four distinct profundus tendons serving the index, long, ring, and little fingers.

In the palm, interdigital tendinous slips often pass between the profundus flexor tendons leading to the long, ring, and little fingers.

The lumbricals arise from the profundus tendons within the palm.

The proximal region of the fibroosseous tunnel, which contains both the superficialis and the profundus flexor tendons, has been termed "no-man's land" because of the difficulty in obtaining good results with flexor tendon repairs in this region. The zone extends from the metacarpal head to the middle phalangeal level of the finger.[58]

Two tendinous connections, termed vincula, pass to the profundus tendon while it runs with the superficialis tendon.

The profundus tendon lies dorsal to the superficialis tendon until it passes through Camper's chiasm at the proximal phalangeal level. Distally, it continues alone in the digital sheath toward the distal phalanx.

Insertion

The flexor digitorum profundus tendon inserts into the proximal half of the palmar surface of the distal phalanges of the four fingers. A distal vincular connection connects the profundus tendon to the middle phalanx before it inserts into the distal phalanx (Fig. 4–37). The tendon is also intimately associated with the capsule of the DIP, with some fibers inserting onto the palmar plate of this DIP joint.[77] There may be interdigital slips that connect this tendon to the thumb flexor pollicis longus.[75,78]

Function

The flexor digitorum profundus muscle serves to flex the terminal phalanges of the index, long, ring, and little fingers and also assists with wrist flexion.

Flexor Pollicis Longus

Origin

The flexor pollicis longus muscle (Figs. 4–28, 4–29, 4–32, and 4–36) usually arises from the entire middle third of the palmar surface of the radius proximal to the supinator muscle and the radial side of the middle third of the forearm interosseous membrane.

The muscle may also originate from the inner border of the coronoid process or the inner condyle of the humerus, in which case it is often referred to as the accessory muscle of Gantzer.[55,57] The flexor pollicis longus originates in common with the flexor digitorum superficialis. This accessory muscle may have its own tendon, which runs along with the tendon of the flexor pollicis longus.[55]

Anatomic Course

The flexor pollicis longus tendon enters the palm via the radial side of the carpal canal and runs between the two heads of the flexor pollicis brevis. It enters the fibroosseous tunnel via the annular ligament and passes down the tunnel as a flattened tendon running between the flexor pollicis brevis and the oblique head of the adductor pollicis.

Insertion

The flexor pollicis longus muscle inserts onto the palmar base of the distal phalanx of the thumb. The tendon is supported by tendinous vinculae before its insertion. There may be interdigital slips that connect this tendon to the index finger flexor digitorum profundus tendon.[75,78]

Function

The flexor pollicis longus muscle causes the thumb to flex at the IP joint. When the thumb is fixed, the flexor pollicis longus helps to flex the wrist.[57]

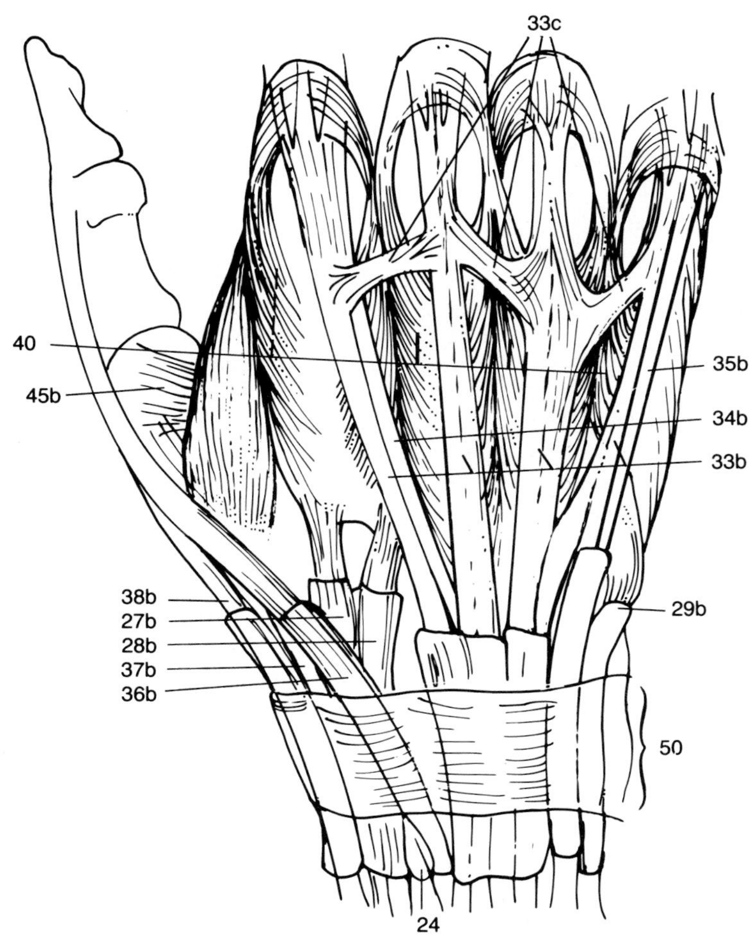

FIGURE 4–33. Intrinsic muscles and tendons of the dorsal surface of the hand. 24—Lister's tubercle; 27b—extensor carpi radialis longus tendon; 28b—extensor carpi radialis brevis tendon; 29b—extensor carpi ulnaris tendon; 33b—extensor digitorum communis tendons; 33c—juncturae tendinae; 34b—extensor indicis proprius tendon; 35b—extensor digiti minimi tendon; 36b—extensor pollicis longus tendon; 37b—extensor pollicis brevis tendon; 38b—abductor pollicis longus tendon; 40—dorsal interosseous muscles; 45b—adductor pollicis muscle, transverse head; 50—extensor retinaculum.

Extensor Digitorum Communis

Origin

The extensor digitorum communis (Figs. 4–28, 4–30, 4–33, and 4–34) arises from the lateral epicondyle of the humerus by a common extensor tendon and the antebrachial fascia (which covers the extensor muscles) and from a small area posterior to the radial notch of the ulna.[55] It is the central extensor muscle of the superficial extensor muscle group and the most superficial forearm extensor muscle.[55,57]

Anatomic Course

The extensor digitorum communis muscle splits into four tendons in the distal third of the forearm. The tendons enter the dorsum of the hand under the extensor retinaculum via the fourth wrist dorsal compartment, which lies between Lister's tubercle and the shallow groove for the extensor digiti minimi. The juncturae tendinae are the intertendinous connections over the dorsum of the hand that unite the index, long, ring, and little fingers in extension. The extensor tendons do not have any vinculae or mesentery supporting them, but they are covered by a synovial bursa while passing under the dorsal carpal ligament. The tendon of the small finger may be absent or very attenuated, and there may be a double or triple tendon to the long finger.[55]

Insertion

The extensor digitorum communis inserts onto the radial, ulnar, and dorsal surfaces of the four middle phalanges via the extensor mechanism detailed below. A slip of the tendon inserts on the dorsal lip of the base of the proximal phalanx or the dorsal capsule of the MCP joint. In some people it is well developed and in others it is a loosely arranged band of deep fibers.[58,62,79–81]

Function

The extensor digitorum communis muscle extends the index, long, ring, and little fingers, primarily at the MCP joint, and assists with wrist extension.

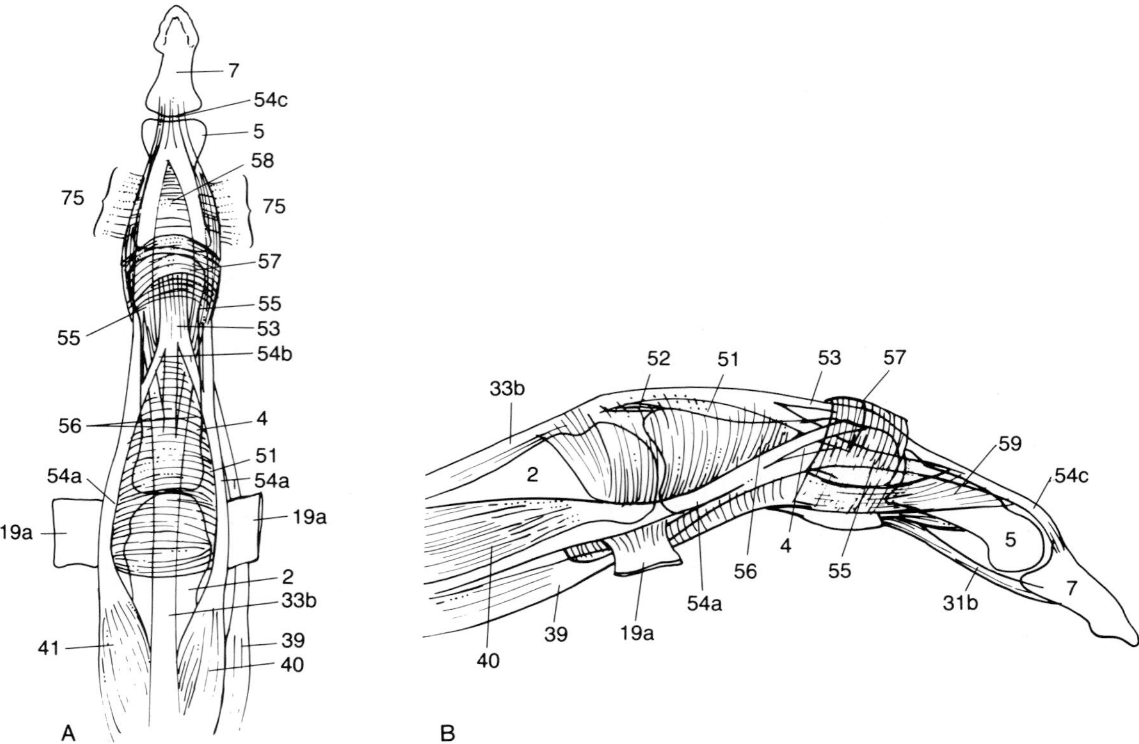

FIGURE 4–34. Dorsal (**A**) and lateral (**B**) views of the digital extensor mechanism. The individual variations of the intrinsic muscle insertions are explained in the text. 2—Finger metacarpal; 4—finger proximal phalanx; 5—finger middle phalanx; 7—finger distal phalanx; 19a—finger MCP joint palmar intermetacarpal ligaments; 31b—flexor digitorum profundus tendon; 33b—extensor digitorum communis tendon; 39—lumbricals; 40—dorsal interosseous muscle; 41—palmar interosseous muscle; 51—sagittal bands; 52—proximal slip of the extensor digitorum communis; 53—central slip of the extensor digitorum longus; 54a—lateral bands; 54b—lateral slips of the finger extensor mechanism; 54c—terminal extensor tendon; 55—conjoined tendon; 56—oblique arcuate fibers; 57—transverse retinacular ligament (of Landsmeer); 58—triangular ligament; 59—oblique retinacular ligament; 75—Cleland's ligament.

Extensor Indicis Proprius

Origin

The extensor indicis proprius muscle (Figs. 4–28, 4–30, 4–31, and 4–33) originates from the posterior surface of the distal third of the ulna below the origin of the extensor pollicis longus and the distal third of the forearm interosseous membrane.[57] The muscle lies on the medial side of the extensor pollicis longus.[57]

Anatomic Course

The extensor indicis proprius tendon enters the dorsum of the hand with the extensor digitorum communis via the fourth dorsal compartment.[57] The extensor indicis proprius tendon is smaller than the extensor digitorum communis tendon and lies on its ulnar side.[57] The tendon may be absent, small in size, or doubled, with both tendons going to the index finger or one each to the index and long fingers.[55]

Insertion

The extensor indicis proprius joins with the index extensor digitorum communis at the level of the distal metacarpal.[57] The extensor indicis inserts onto the proximal ulnar dorsum of the middle phalanx of the index finger.

Function

The extensor indicis proprius extends the proximal phalanx of the index finger and helps to extend the wrist.

Extensor Digiti Minimi

Origin

The extensor digiti minimi muscle (Figs. 4–28, 4–30, and 4–33) arises from a common tendon from the lateral humeral epicondyle and the intermuscular septum between it and the adjacent muscles.[57] It lies on the medial (ulnar) side of the extensor digitorum communis.[57]

Anatomic Course

The extensor digiti minimi tendon enters the dorsum of the hand via a shallow canal on the radius under the dorsal carpal ligament in the fifth dorsal wrist compartment. The tendon of the extensor digiti minimi is larger than the extensor communis tendon of the little finger. It divides into two as it crosses over the dorsum of the hand.[55,57] The outermost portion of the extensor digiti minimi tendon is joined by slips from the innermost portion of the common extensor tendon of the little finger. The two slips spread out to form a broad aponeurosis, which then receives slips from the abductor digiti minimi.

Insertion

The extensor digiti minimi muscle inserts onto the proximal portions of the proximal and middle phalanges of the dorsum of the little finger.[57] The tendon is situated superficial and ulnar to the common digital extensor tendon.[57]

Function

The extensor digiti minimi muscle extends the little finger and assists with wrist extension.[57]

Extensor Pollicis Longus

Origin

The extensor pollicis longus (Figs. 4–28, 4–30, 4–31, 4–33, and 4–35) arises from the middle third of the posterior surface of the ulna and the interosseous membrane. Its origin is distal to the origin of the abductor pollicis longus.

Anatomic Course

The extensor pollicis longus enters the dorsum of the hand through the third dorsal compartment of the wrist. It obliquely crosses the extensor carpi radialis longus and brevis tendons over the dorsum of the hand. It provides the ulnar margin of the anatomic snuffbox of the dorsum of the hand.

Insertion

The extensor pollicis longus inserts onto the distal phalanx of the thumb. There is a dorsal fibrous expansion associated with the extensor pollicis longus tendon that is intimately connected with the thumb IP joint capsule. It receives contributions from the abductor pollicis longus and the adductor pollicis.

Function

The extensor pollicis longus muscle extends the distal phalanx of the thumb and helps to extend and abduct the wrist.

Extensor Pollicis Brevis

Origin

The extensor pollicis brevis muscle (Figs. 4–28, 4–33, and 4–35) originates from the dorsal surface of

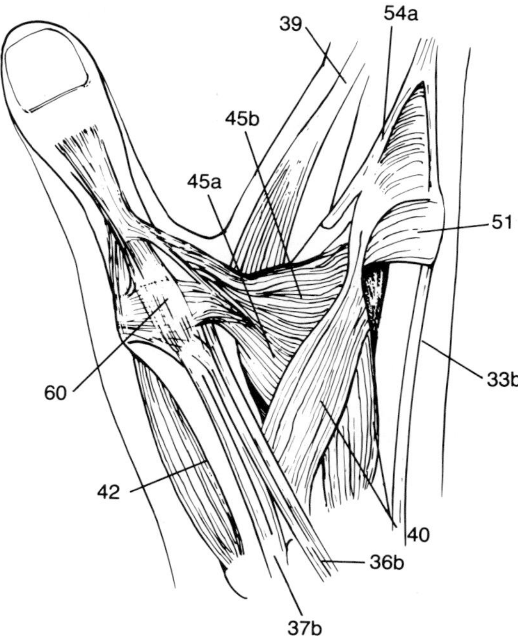

FIGURE 4–35. Extensor mechanism of the thumb. 33b—Extensor digitorum communis tendon; 36b—extensor pollicis longus tendon; 37b—extensor pollicis brevis tendon; 39—lumbrical muscle; 40—dorsal interosseous muscle; 42—opponens pollicis; 45a—adductor pollicis oblique head; 45b—adductor pollicis transverse head; 51—sagittal bands; 54a—lateral bands; 60—dorsal fibrous expansion of the thumb.

the middle third of the radius, the interosseous membrane, and a small area of the ulna distal to the extensor pollicis longus.[55] It is the smallest muscle of the deep extensor muscle group.[57]

Anatomic Course

From its origin, the extensor pollicis brevis runs obliquely in a distal lateral direction toward the radial side of the wrist. With the abductor pollicis longus, it crosses the two radial wrist extensor tendons in the distal forearm. It enters the dorsum of the hand along with the abductor pollicis longus tendon through a groove on the radial side of the styloid process of the radius in the first dorsal compartment.

Insertion

The extensor pollicis brevis inserts into the dorsal base of the proximal phalanx of the thumb.[58,75] The extensor pollicis brevis also sends a tendinous slip that continues with the extensor pollicis longus and inserts onto the distal phalanx.

Function

The extensor pollicis brevis muscle extends the proximal phalanx of the thumb and helps to extend and abduct the wrist.

Abductor Pollicis Longus

Origin

The abductor pollicis longus muscle (Figs. 4–28, 4–31, and 4–33) arises from the posterolateral surface of the shaft of the ulna, the middle third of the posterior shaft of the radius, and the interosseous membrane. It is the most external and the largest of the deep extensor muscles. It may occasionally be absent and be replaced by the extensor pollicis brevis.[75]

Anatomic Course

From its origin, the abductor pollicis longus runs obliquely in a distal lateral direction toward the radial side of the wrist. Along with the extensor pollicis brevis, it crosses the extensor carpi radialis longus and brevis tendons in the distal forearm. It enters the dorsum of the hand along with the extensor pollicis brevis through a groove on the radial side of the styloid process of the radius in the first dorsal compartment.

Insertion

The abductor pollicis longus inserts onto the base of the thumb metacarpal. It may give off two additional tendinous slips at its insertion: (1) one slip to the trapezium and (2) another that blends with the origin of the abductor pollicis brevis.

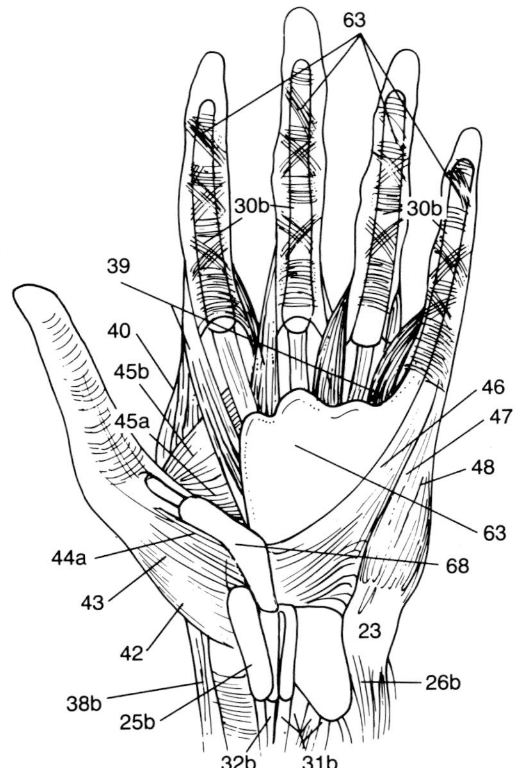

FIGURE 4–36. The tendon sheaths of the flexor tendons are shown. The sheath of the little finger extends down into the palmar bursa. 23—Pisiform; 25b—flexor carpi radialis tendon; 26b—flexor carpi ulnaris tendon; 30b—flexor digitorum superficialis tendon; 31b—flexor digitorum profundus tendons; 32b—flexor pollicis longus tendon; 38b—abductor pollicis longus tendon; 39—lumbrical muscles; 40—dorsal interosseous muscle—index finger; 42—opponens pollicis; 43—abductor pollicis brevis; 44a—flexor pollicis brevis superficial head; 45a—adductor pollicis oblique head; 45b—adductor pollicis transverse head; 46—opponens digiti minimi; 47—flexor digiti minimi brevis; 48—abductor digiti minimi; 63—finger flexor tendon synovial sheaths; 68—thumb synovial sheath.

Function

The chief action of the abductor pollicis longus muscle is to pull the thumb metacarpal dorsally and radially with respect to the palm. It also helps to extend and abduct the wrist.

Lumbrical Muscles

Origin

The lumbricals (Figs. 4–29, 4–32, 4–34, and 4–36) arise from the radiopalmar surface of the flexor tendons at the level of the wrist and proximal palm and, as such, have a moving origin. When the fingers are extended, the proximal muscle end is at the level of the pisiform. When the fingers are flexed, the proximal end of the lumbricals is pulled into the carpal canal and may reach the level of the distal radius.

The first and second lumbricals originate from the radial aspects of the profundus tendons to the index and long fingers, respectively. They are fusiform in shape.[82] The third and fourth lumbricals are bipennate and arise from the adjacent sides of the long and ring finger and the ring and little finger tendons, respectively.[57,82,83] The third lumbrical is occasionally absent.[83] The lumbricals may be completely absent, partially absent, or increased in number.[75] They are the only skeletal muscles that have no direct bone attachments.[82]

Anatomic Course

The lumbricals are separated from the interosseous muscles by a deep transverse intermetacarpal ligament. They lie palmar to this ligament. The muscles pass to the radial side of the corresponding finger MCP joint and then insert into the digital extensor mechanism.

Insertion

The lumbricals insert into the radial aspect of the extensor expansion of the finger, distal to both the insertion of the interossei and the MCP joint.

There may be variations of the insertion of the lumbricals. A lumbrical may also insert into the ulnar side of the adjacent digital extensor mechanism. On occasion, a lumbrical may insert on both sides of the adjacent digital extensor mechanisms.

Function

The lumbricals facilitate IP extension. By pulling the profundus tendon distally at the palmar level, they help take tension off the profundus tendon insertion, thus allowing IP joint extension irrespective of the MCP joint position.[82,84]

Although it has been shown that the lumbricals do not contract during flexion of the MCP joint alone, some researchers believe that they do contribute to coordinated finger flexion when the IP joints are held in extension.[62,82–85] The lumbricals may also contribute to radial deviation and abduction of the digits; however, some researchers debate this point.[82,84]

INTEROSSEOUS MUSCLES

Dorsal Interossei

Origin

There are four dorsal interosseous muscles (Figs. 4–28, 4–33 to 4–35); they are numbered sequentially in a radial to ulnar direction. Each dorsal interosseous muscle arises as two heads from adjacent metacarpals in the proximal four intermetacarpal spaces.[82,83]

The first dorsal interosseous muscle is the largest interosseous muscle and usually is the most distal muscle in the hand innervated by the ulnar nerve. It consists of a deep part that arises from the index metacarpal and a superficial part that arises from both the thumb and the index metacarpals. Each part has a separate tendon that contributes to the index extensor mechanism.[66]

Insertion

The first (most radial) interosseous muscle inserts nearly entirely onto the proximal phalanx and the PIP palmar plate of the index finger.[70] The second interosseous muscle inserts onto the radial side of the proximal phalanx (60%) and the extensor mechanism of the long finger (40%).[62,70] The third interosseous muscle inserts onto the ulnar side of the proximal phalanx of the long finger.[70] The fourth (most ulnar) interosseous muscle inserts onto the ulnar side of the proximal phalanx (40%) as well as the extensor apparatus of the ring finger (60%).[70]

There are tendinous slips that also attach the interossei into the digital extensor hood mechanism.[62] The first dorsal interosseous muscle does not contribute to the index extensor mechanism. Roughly 40% of the second dorsal interosseous muscle inserts into the extensor mechanism and 60% inserts onto the proximal phalanx of the long finger. Roughly 60% of the third and fourth dorsal interosseous muscles inserts into the extensor mechanism and 40% inserts onto the proximal phalanx of the long and ring fingers, respectively.

Function

The dorsal interossei serve to abduct the index, long, and ring fingers from the midline.[82,83] In the act of finger extension, they contribute to the smooth extension of the finger joints.[79,82] Depending on their site of insertion, they help provide lateral stability to the MCP joint.[86] There is no dorsal interosseous muscle of the little finger.

Palmar Interossei

Origin

There are three palmar interossei (Figs. 4–28 and 4–34); they are sequentially numbered in a radial to ulnar direction. The palmar interossei arise from (1) the ulnar side of the base of the index finger metacarpal, (2) the base of the radial sides of the ring and little finger metacarpals, and (3) the adjacent carpal ligaments.[83]

Insertion

The palmar interosseous tendons run dorsal to the transverse intermetacarpal ligaments but palmar to the axis of the MCP joint.[83] They insert onto (1) the lateral band of the extensor aponeurosis[83], (2) the ulnar side of the index proximal phalanx[70], (3) the radial side of the ring and little finger proximal phalanges[70], and (4) the MCP joint capsules of the index, ring, and little fingers (as a minor insertion).[83]

Function

The palmar interossei adduct the index, ring, and little fingers toward the long finger.[82] In the act of finger extension, they contribute to the smooth extension of the finger joints.[79,82,83] They help provide medial or lateral stability on the side of the MCP joint to which they insert.[86] There is no palmar interosseous muscle attaching to the long finger.

THENAR MUSCLES

Opponens Pollicis

Origin

The opponens pollicis muscle (Figs. 4–28, 4–29, 4–32, 4–35, and 4–36)[57,87] arises from (1) the palmar transverse carpal ligament, (2) the palmar ridge of the trapezium, and (3) the palmar capsule of the thumb carpometacarpal joint.

Insertion

The opponens pollicis inserts into (1) the anterior and radial side of the thumb metacarpal distally and (2) the palmar aspect of the thumb MCP joint.

Function

The opponens pollicis muscle causes the thumb to oppose the other digits by bringing the thumb metacarpal forward and medial.

Abductor Pollicis Brevis

Origin

The abductor pollicis brevis muscle (Figs. 4–28, 4–29, 4–32, 4–36, and 4–42)[57,58,87,88] arises from the radial half and distal border of the palmar transverse carpal ligament and the palmar surface of the trapezium. Some believe that the abductor pollicis brevis also arises from the scaphoid, but others refute this.[55]

A tendinous slip from the abductor pollicis longus may join with the abductor pollicis brevis.

Insertion

The abductor pollicis brevis inserts onto (1) the radial side of the thumb proximal phalangeal base, (2) the dorsal aponeurosis, and (3) the lateral aspect of the joint capsule.

Function

The abductor pollicis brevis muscle abducts the thumb and draws it into a right angle to the palm. It is the most superficial of the thenar muscles.

Flexor Pollicis Brevis

Origin

The flexor pollicis brevis muscle (Figs. 4–28, 4–29, 4–32, 4–36, 4–39, and 4–42)[55,57,58,87] arises as two heads.

1. The superficial head arises from the distal lateral border of the palmar transverse carpal ligament and the tunnel of the flexor carpi radialis at the index metacarpal base and the palmar surface of the crest of the trapezium.
2. The deep head arises from the anterior surface of the trapezoid, the ulnar side of the tunnel of the flexor carpi radialis, and the capitate.

Insertion

The flexor pollicis brevis inserts onto the radial (lateral) sesamoid of the palmar plate and the lateral tubercle of the thumb proximal phalangeal base.

Function

The flexor pollicis brevis muscle flexes the proximal phalanx of the thumb and rotates it, turning the thumb pulp toward the pulp of the other fingers and toward the termination of the motion of flexion.[55] It also forms a muscular groove for the flexor pollicis longus tendon.[87]

Adductor Pollicis

Origin

The adductor pollicis muscle (Figs. 4–28, 4–29, 4–32, 4–33, 4–35, 4–39, and 4–42)[57,87,88] arises as two heads.

1. The oblique head arises from the dorsal carpal ligaments over the trapezium, trapezoid, and capitate; the tunnel of the flexor carpi radialis tendon; and the palmar base of the index and long finger metacarpals.[55,57,87]
2. The transverse head arises from the palmar crest of the long finger metacarpal shaft.[87]

Insertion

Both heads of the adductor pollicis muscle converge and insert onto the ulnar tubercle of the thumb proximal phalangeal base, the ulnar (medial) sesamoid of the palmar plate, and the ulnar expansion of the dorsal aponeurosis.[61,87] It is the deepest thenar muscle.

Function

The adductor pollicis muscle adducts the thumb and aids in thumb opposition. It is the most powerful thenar muscle.[87]

HYPOTHENAR MUSCLES

Opponens Digiti Minimi

Origin

The opponens digiti minimi muscle (Figs. 4–28, 4–29, 4–32, and 4–36)[57,88,89] arises from the hook of the hamate and the pisohamate ligament (flexor retinaculum).[89]

Insertion

It inserts on the midshaft ulnar margin of the little finger metacarpal.

Function

The muscle deepens the hollow of the hand and draws the little finger toward the thumb so that the finger pulps oppose each other.

Flexor Digiti Minimi Brevis

Origin

The flexor digiti minimi brevis muscle (see Figs. 4–28, 4–29, 4–32, and 4–36)[57,88,89] arises from the palmar transverse carpal ligament, the hook of the hamate, and the pisohamate ligament.

Insertion

It inserts onto the ulnar side of the base of the little finger proximal phalanx and the palmar plate of the little finger PIP joint.[62]

Function

The flexor digiti minimi brevis muscle flexes the proximal phalanx of the little finger, slightly adducts the little finger, and slightly flexes the little finger metacarpal.[55] It may be absent in up to 40% of patients.[89]

Abductor Digiti Minimi

Origin

The abductor digiti minimi muscle (Figs. 4–28, 4–29, 4–32, and 4–36)[57,89] arises from the distal palmar

mar surface of the pisiform, the tendon of the flexor carpi ulnaris, and the pisohamate ligament. The muscle often may have two bellies, may have a single belly, or may be totally absent. It also may be fused with the flexor digiti minimi brevis.[55]

Insertion

The abductor digiti minimi muscle inserts onto the ulnar edge of the little finger proximal phalangeal base, the little finger MCP joint palmar plate, and the aponeurosis of the extensor digiti minimi.[62,70]

Function

The abductor digiti minimi muscle abducts the little finger from the ring finger, slightly flexes the little finger, and extends the PIP and DIP joints. It functionally acts as a "fifth dorsal interosseous" muscle.[55,62]

DIGITAL EXTENSOR HOOD MECHANISM

Digital Extension: General Information

Digital extension is the result of the complex interaction of the extensor tendons combined with the actions of the intrinsic muscles of the hand. The extensor digitorum communis tendon provides the major force for digital extension. Hyperextension of the MCP joint from hyperactive extensor tendons is restrained because of resistance of the intrinsic muscles.

The digital extensor hood, as defined subsequently, is the fibrous ligamentous expansion over the dorsum of the finger that balances the various extensor forces acting on the phalanges. Although its component parts are described as discrete entities, at the PIP joint level the tendons form a unique pattern of crisscrossing fibers.[90] The outer layer is formed from the extensor digitorum communis, whereas the inner layer is formed by the intrinsic muscles.[90] The exact location of the various components of the extensor mechanism is dependent on the degree of digital flexion–extension.[91,92]

The digital extensor hood is composed of the following:

1. Extrinsic long digital extensor (extensor digitorum communis) tendon.
2. Extensor hood proper.
3. Insertions of the lumbricals and the dorsal and palmar interossei muscles.

Extrinsic and Intrinsic Digital Extensor Mechanism

Extrinsic Digital Extensor Mechanism

The extrinsic long extensor (extensor digitorum communis) tendon (Fig. 4–34) is composed of four components:[93,94]

1. *The sagittal bands, shroud ligaments, or laminae transversae.*[81,95,96] The sagittal bands encircle the metacarpal head and proximal phalangeal base and stabilize the extensor communis over the MCP joint.[81] With MCP joint flexion, the sagittal bands slide distally and apply an extensor force via the central slip, which helps extend the middle phalanx. Hyperextension of the MCP joint from hyperactive extensor tendons is restrained by these ligaments, which limit the proximal excursion of the extensor tendons by virtue of their attachments to the palmar plate.[81,86] These bands (or ligaments) provide some medial and lateral joint stability in extension when the collateral ligaments are relatively lax.[86] Sagittal bands also form "tunnels" for passage of the interosseous tendons.[81]
2. *The proximal slip.* The proximal slip originates from the extensor digitorum communis tendon, inserts onto the base of the proximal phalanx dorsally, and extends the proximal phalanx.
3. *The central slip.* The central slip is actually the distal extent of the extensor digitorum communis tendon, inserts into the dorsal base of the middle phalanx at the central tubercle, and extends the PIP joint.
4. *The lateral bands or slips.* The lateral bands split near the MCP joint, sending a medial portion to the lateral tubercle of the proximal phalanx, which helps abduct or adduct the MCP joint; one insertion to the central slip at the middle phalanx; and one slip to the distal phalanx, which contributes to the conjoined tendon or conjoined lateral band.

The conjoined tendon or conjoined lateral band is composed of a tendinous slip from the lateral band, an extension of the extensor digitorum communis tendon, and the tendinous insertions of the intrinsic muscles, with the palmar and dorsal interossei inserting both radially and ulnarly and the lumbrical inserting radially. The conjoined lateral bands pass dorsal to the axis of rotation of the PIP joint and insert over the entire dorsum of the proximal third of the distal phalanx.

With flexion of the PIP joint, the lateral bands slide palmar to the axis of rotation of the PIP joint and thus relax the extensor forces at the DIP joint and allow it to flex.[79]

Intrinsic Digital Extensor Mechanism

The intrinsic digital extensor hood proper is composed of the following:

1. *Oblique arcuate fibers,* which crisscross between the central slip of the digital extensor tendon and the lateral bands and assist the central slip of the digital extensor tendon to extend the middle phalanx.
2. *The transverse retinacular ligament or lamina (Landsmeer's lamina)*[95,96] traverses the dorsum of the PIP joint from the lateral aspect of the

flexor tendon sheath, joins the lateral bands, and continues dorsally to the central extensor tendon, with some fibers actually crossing over the dorsum of the extensor tendon.[85,96] This ligament helps to hold the extensor mechanism centrally over the PIP joint,[92,97] helps prevent dorsal dislocation and bowstringing of the conjoined lateral bands when the PIP joint is extended,[91,97] and helps prevent hyperextension of the PIP joint.[92] Landsmeer's lamina becomes taut when the finger is flexed, but if contracted, can inhibit PIP joint contraction.[80]

3. *The triangular ligament.* This ligament extends dorsally between the insertions of the radial and ulnar lateral bands at the distal portion of the middle phalanx and prevents the excessive palmar subluxation of the conjoined lateral bands that could occur with middle phalanx flexion.
4. *The oblique retinacular ligament or link ligament (Landsmeer's ligament).* This ligament arises from the flexor tendon sheath of the distal one fourth of the proximal phalanx, passes under the transverse retinacular ligament, and inserts dorsally onto the distal or middle phalanx.[95,96] The link ligament is relaxed when the PIP joint is flexed and taut when the PIP joint is extended.[95,96] It does this by linking the terminal extensor tendon and the lateral slips dorsally over the distal aspect of the middle phalanx and holding them dorsal to the axis of rotation of the DIP joint, thus helping it coordinate flexion and extension at the PIP and DIP joints.

The dynamic action of this tendon is debated, because careful anatomic dissections show that the tendon is present in only 50% of fingers.[98] It is present in 90% of the ulnar side of the ring finger.[98] Its absence or its division does not produce obvious alterations in coordinated finger motion.[98]

INTRINSIC MUSCLE INSERTIONS (Figs. 4–28 and 4–34)

Interosseous Muscles

The interosseous muscles insert via ulnar and radial slips to help form the conjoined lateral band at the level of the PIP joint (see previous discussion). The isolated action of the interossei is to abduct and adduct the digits.

Lumbrical Muscles

The lumbricals insert via the radial lateral slips into the conjoined lateral band at the level of the PIP joint (see previous discussion). The isolated action of the lumbricals is to help initiate MCP flexion (debated) and to assist with IP joint extension.

EXTENSOR MECHANISM OF THE THUMB

Extrinsic Portion of the Thumb Extensor Mechanism (Figs. 4–28 and 4–35)

Extensor Pollicis Longus

The tendon of the extensor pollicis longus runs along the dorsoulnar side of the thumb MCP joint. It inserts onto the base of the distal phalanx of the thumb.

Extensor Pollicis Brevis

The extensor pollicis brevis tendon runs along the middle of the dorsum of the thumb MCP joint. It inserts on the proximal phalanx of the thumb.

Intrinsic Portion of the Thumb Extensor Mechanism (Figs. 4–28, 4–32, 4–35, and 4–36)

Muscles

The abductor pollicis brevis sends tendinous slips to insert on the radial palmar side of the proximal phalanx of the thumb and over the MCP joint to the tendons of the extensor pollicis longus and brevis.

The adductor pollicis sends tendinous slips to insert on the ulnar side of the proximal phalanx of the thumb and over the MCP joint to the tendons of the extensor pollicis longus and brevis.

Dorsal Fibrous Expansion

At the IP joint, the fibers that spread out from the abductor pollicis brevis and the adductor pollicis (see previous discussion) form the thumb equivalent to the digital extensor hood. The dorsal fibrous expansion spreads over the entire width of the distal phalanx and is intimately connected with the thumb IP joint capsule.

DIGITAL FLEXOR TENDON SHEATH

Synovial Flexor Sheath of the Finger

The Flexor Tendon Sheath

The digital flexor tendon sheath (Fig. 4–36) is a double-walled, hollow synovial tube sealed at both ends. The flexor tendon sheath is so tightly restrained that the double-layered synovium assumes a single-layer appearance. The sheath begins proximally at the distal palmar crease, at the level of the metacarpal neck, and continues to the distal insertion of the flexor digitorum profundus tendon. It is traversed by the supporting vinculae longus and brevis to the flexor tendons. These are dorsal synovial condensations at the PIP joint level that not only support the tendons but also carry nutrient blood vessels to them (Fig. 4–37).

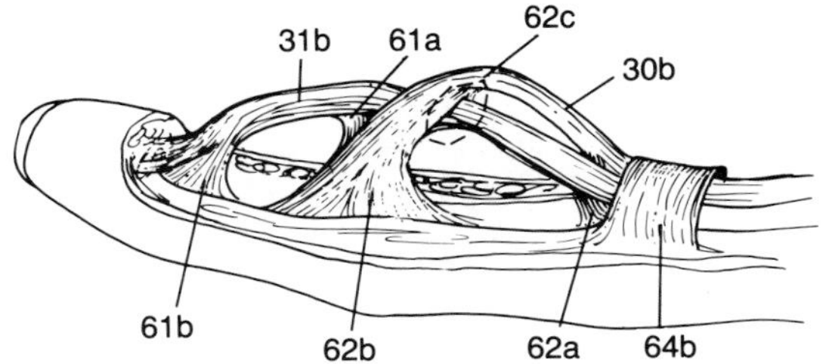

FIGURE 4–37. Distal insertion of the superficialis and profundus tendons plus their vincular attachments to the fibroosseous tunnel. 30b—Flexor digitorum superficialis tendon; 31b—flexor digitorum profundus tendon; 61a—flexor digitorum profundus vinculum longus; 61b—flexor digitorum profundus vinculum brevis; 62a—flexor digitorum superficialis vinculum longus; 62b—flexor digitorum superficialis vinculum brevis; 62c—Camper's chiasm; 64b—finger fibroosseous tunnel A2 annular pulley.

Individual Digital Flexor Tendon Sheaths

The index, long, and ring flexor tendon sheaths are separate, whereas the flexor tendon sheath of the little finger extends proximally to form an ulnar bursa.

Fibroosseous Tunnel of the Finger

General Information

The fibroosseous tunnel (Fig. 4–38)[99,100] is a closely applied, semirigid tunnel through which the flexor tendons pass. Classically, the fibrous portion of the fibroosseous tunnel is described as being composed of (1) five annular pulleys—dense condensations of transversely oriented fibrous bands, (2) three cruciate pulleys, and (3) a floor that is the palmar periosteal surface of the phalanges and the joint palmar plates.

Annular Pulleys

1. The A1 pulley is located at the level of the MCP joint. It attaches to the junction of the palmar plate, the deep transverse intermetacarpal ligament, and the proximal portion of the proximal phalanx. It is the second longest annular pulley.
2. The A2 pulley attaches firmly to the palmar medial and lateral ridges of the proximal half of the proximal phalanx. It lies 1 to 3 mm distal to the A1 pulley and is a critical pulley for maintaining maximal finger flexion. It is the longest of the annular pulleys.
3. The A3 pulley attaches to the palmar plate of the PIP joint and is frequently indistinct.
4. The A4 pulley attaches firmly to the palmar medial and lateral ridges at the middle third of the middle phalanx and is considered a critical pulley for maximal finger flexion.
5. The A5 pulley arises from the palmar aspect of the DIP joint and the proximal palmar base of

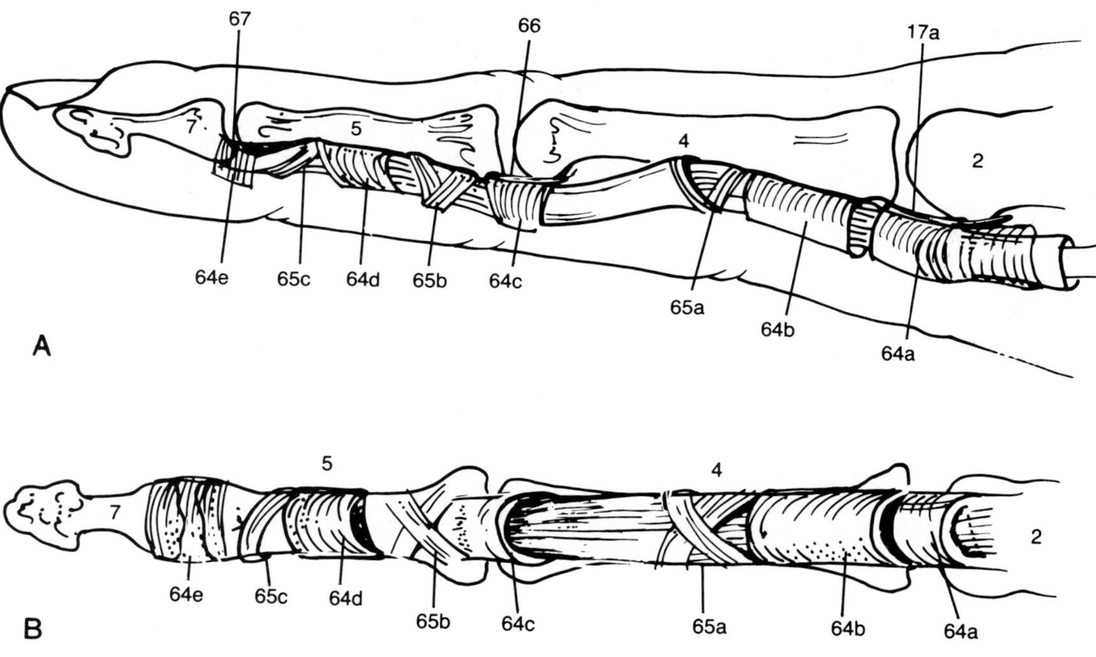

FIGURE 4–38. Lateral **(A)** and palmar **(B)** views of the finger fibroosseous flexor tendon sheath. 2—Finger metacarpal; 4—finger proximal phalanx; 5—finger middle phalanx; 7—finger distal phalanx; 17a—finger MCP joint palmar plate; 64a—finger fibroosseous tunnel A1 annular pulley; 64b—finger fibroosseous tunnel A2 annular pulley; 64c—finger fibroosseous tunnel A3 annular pulley; 64d—finger fibroosseous tunnel A4 annular pulley; 64e—finger fibroosseous tunnel A5 annular pulley; 65a—finger fibroosseous tunnel C1 cruciate pulley; 65b—finger fibroosseous tunnel C2 cruciate pulley; 65c—finger fibroosseous tunnel C3 cruciate pulley; 66—finger PIP joint palmar plate; 67—finger DIP joint palmar plate.

the distal phalanx. It is frequently indistinct as a separate entity.

Cruciate Pulleys

1. The C1 pulley is located at the distal end of the A2 pulley and may partially overlap the distal end of the A2 pulley.
2. The C2 pulley is located beyond the A3 pulley.
3. The C3 pulley is located distal to the A4 pulley.

"Floor" of the Fibroosseous Canal

The floor of the fibroosseous canal is formed by the palmar aspect of the phalanges and the palmar plates of the MCP and proximal IP joints. Fractures of the phalanges often disrupt the periosteum and thus rupture the floor of the superficial and profundus flexor tendons' fibroosseous canal.

Fibroosseous Tunnel of the Thumb (Figs. 4–36 and 4–39)[55,57]

Synovial Sheath of the Thumb

The synovial sheath of the thumb begins in the wrist and extends out to the distal insertion of the flexor pollicis longus. It is also termed the radial bursa because of its proximal extent into the forearm. It supports the flexor pollicis tendon by a mesotendon from the dorsal sheath surface, which forms the vinculum brevis and the vinculum longum. The synovial sheath has an outer parietal (fibrous) and an inner visceral (synovial) layer similar to that of the fingers.

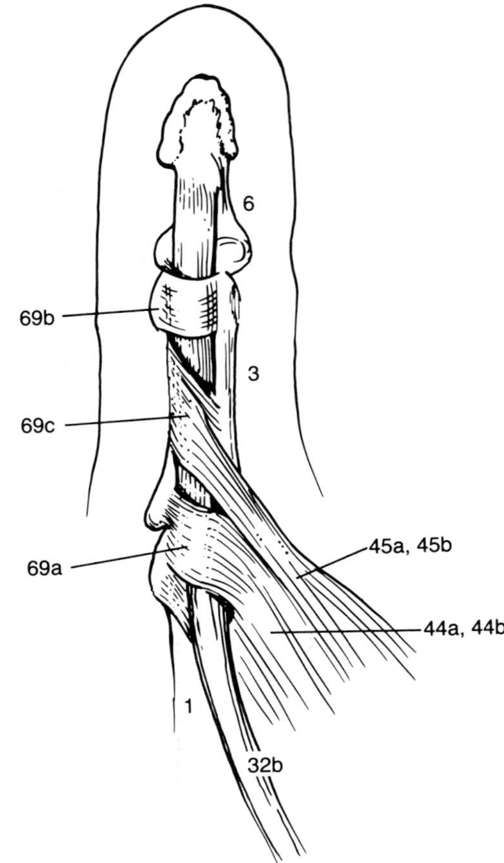

FIGURE 4–39. Palmar view of the flexor tendon sheath of the left thumb. 1—Thumb metacarpal; 3—thumb proximal phalanx; 6—thumb distal phalanx; 32b—flexor pollicis longus tendon; 44a, 44b—flexor pollicis brevis—superficial and deep heads; 45a, 45b—adductor pollicis—oblique and transverse heads; 69a—thumb fibroosseous tunnel A1 annular pulley; 69b—thumb fibroosseous tunnel A2 annular pulley; 69c—thumb fibroosseous tunnel oblique pulley.

Pulleys of the Thumb

The Annular A1 Pulley

This most proximal pulley is over the palmar plate of the MCP joint. Nearly normal thumb flexion is possible if this pulley alone is present.

The Oblique Pulley

This middle pulley is over the palmar surface of the proximal phalanx. The adductor pollicis muscle inserts on the ulnar side.

The Annular A2 Pulley

This distal pulley is over the IP joint of the thumb. It is not essential for thumb flexion. It can be divided, and the thumb retains its normal range of flexion.

JOINT ANATOMY

Carpometacarpal Joint

Carpometacarpal Joint of the Thumb (Fig. 4–40)

General Information[101,102]

The joint between the thumb metacarpal and the trapezium is the first carpometacarpal (CMC) joint, or the trapeziometacarpal joint. It is often described as a saddle-shaped joint, but is more aptly described as being formed by two opposing saddles whose longitudinal axes are perpendicular to each other.[61,70,103,104] In the radioulnar dimension the joint surfaces are fairly congruous, whereas in the dorsopalmar dimension there is disparity among the articular surfaces.[105,106] There are wide variations in the bony configurations of this joint, from saddle shaped to ovoid.[104]

The joint that has great mobility but little bony stability allows 60 degrees of abduction–adduction,[106] 60 degrees of flexion–extension, and 10 degrees of longitudinal axis rotation.

The stability of the thumb CMC joint is provided by the joint capsule, the collateral ligaments, and the elasticity of the articular cartilage. In the midposition, all of the joint ligaments are lax.[105,106] Pieron has described in great detail the variations of the CMC joint ligaments.[102]

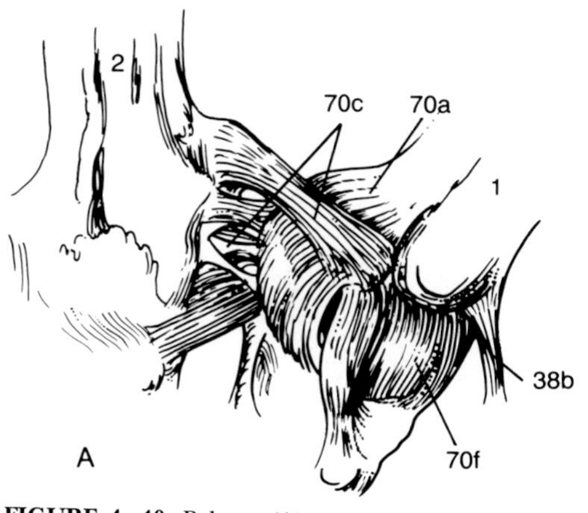

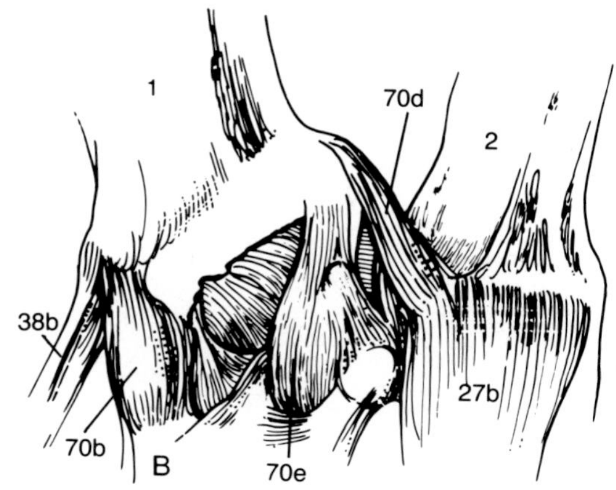

FIGURE 4–40. Palmar **(A)** and dorsal **(B)** views of the right thumb showing the complex ligamentous support of the CMC joint. 1—Thumb metacarpal; 2—finger metacarpal; 27b—extensor carpi radialis longus tendon; 38b—abductor pollicis longus tendon; 70a—thumb CMC ulnar collateral ligament; 70b—thumb CMC radial collateral ligament; 70c—thumb CMC anterior intermetacarpal ligament; 70d—thumb CMC posterior intermetacarpal ligament; 70e—thumb CMC posterior oblique carpometacarpal ligament; 70f—thumb CMC joint capsule.

Ligaments and Joint Capsule[58]

The ulnar collateral ligament is also termed the volar, palmar, or anterior oblique CMC ligament. It firmly holds the palmar lip of the thumb metacarpal base to the tubercle of the trapezium and provides the major resistance to hyperextension and radial subluxation of the joint. It is the strongest ligament of the joint and blends into the joint capsule.[103]

The radial collateral ligament is also termed the dorsal or dorsoradial ligament.[107,108] It is triangular in shape, located along the radial aspect of the joint, and blends with the joint capsule.[108] It attaches the thumb metacarpal to the dorsoradial tubercle of the trapezium[107] and is partially covered by the abductor pollicis longus tendon, which inserts just distal to the ligament.

The anterior and posterior intermetacarpal ligaments connect the dorsal and palmar radial sides of the index metacarpal base to the ulnar side of the thumb metacarpal, often forming a Y configuration.[107] They arise from the dorsoradial aspect of the index metacarpal base near the insertion of the extensor carpi radialis tendon (posterior) and the distal margin of the flexor retinaculum (anterior).[107] They insert as a broad, fan-shaped bundle into the ulnar aspect of the thumb metacarpal base, usually blending with the anterior and posterior oblique ligaments into the palmar-ulnar tubercle of the thumb metacarpal.[61] The posterior intermetacarpal ligament is taut when the joint is flexed and abducted.[105,107]

The posterior oblique CMC ligament is a fan-shaped ligament and is also called the dorsal ligament.[107] It attaches the dorsal surface of the thumb metacarpal base to the trapezium[107] and is covered by the tendon of the extensor pollicis brevis. It is taut with joint flexion and abduction.[105]

The joint capsule is sufficiently lax to allow mobility of the thumb. It does not communicate with the midcarpal joint or other CMC joints, as occurs with some of the finger CMC joints.

Extracapsular Support

Tendons that cross the CMC joint on its palmar and ulnar aspects include (1) the flexor pollicis longus and brevis, (2) the abductor pollicis brevis, and (3) the opponens pollicis.

Tendons that cross the CMC joint on the dorsal and radial aspects include (1) the extensor pollicis longus and brevis, (2) the abductor pollicis longus, and (3) the adductor pollicis.

The adductor pollicis adds support and stability to the joint even though it is slightly removed from the joint. The joint ligaments provide the initial resistance to joint dislocation, whereas the muscles and their tendons provide secondary resistance.

Carpometacarpal Joints of the Fingers (Fig. 4–41)

General Information[58]

1. The index metacarpal articulates primarily with the trapezoid, with minor articulations with the trapezium and the capitate. There is no motion of this joint.[70,109]
2. The long finger metacarpal articulates primarily with the capitate and may articulate with the trapezoid.[109]
3. The ring finger metacarpal articulates with both the capitate and the hamate, whereas the little finger metacarpal articulates exclusively with the hamate.
4. The trapezoid has a consistent articular facet for the index metacarpal and an inconsistent facet for articulation with the long finger metacarpal.[109]

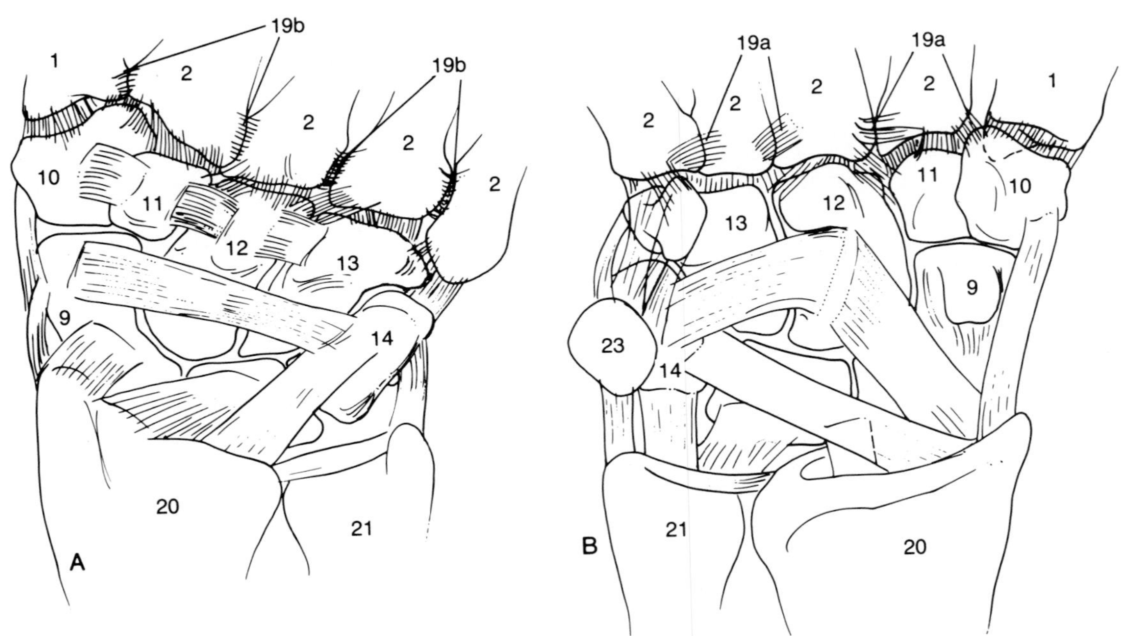

FIGURE 4–41. Dorsal **(A)** and palmar **(B)** views of the finger CMC joints. 1—Thumb metacarpal; 2—finger metacarpals; 9—scaphoid; 10—trapezium; 11—trapezoid; 12—capitate; 13—hamate; 14—triquetrum; 19a—finger MCP joint palmar intermetacarpal ligaments; 19b—finger MCP joint dorsal intermetacarpal ligaments; 20—radius; 21—ulna; 23—pisiform.

5. The capitate articulates mainly with the long metacarpal and, to a lesser extent, with the ring and index finger metacarpals.[109]
6. There is essentially no movement between the long finger metacarpal and the capitate.[70]
7. The CMC joints of the ring and little finger metacarpals are hinge shaped. These joints usually allow 10 to 20 and up to 30 degrees of flexion and extension for the little finger CMC joint and approximately half of this range for the ring finger.[71] They also permit a few degrees of rotation (supination) when attempting opposition with the thumb.[110]
8. The sides of the base of the index through little finger metacarpals articulate with the adjacent metacarpal.[109]

Ligaments and Joint Capsule

The dorsal and palmar proximal intermetacarpal ligaments attach to the bases of each of the finger metacarpals and bind them together. The dorsal ligaments are stronger than the palmar ligaments.[61]

CMC Ligaments. The index finger metacarpal serves for attachment of (1) two dorsal ligaments, one each from the trapezium and the trapezoid and (2) two palmar ligaments, one each from the trapezium and the trapezoid.

The long finger metacarpal serves for attachment of (1) two dorsal ligaments, one each from the trapezoid and the capitate; (2) three palmar ligaments, one each from the trapezoid, the capitate, and the hamate; and (3) an interosseous ligament from the capitate.[57]

The ring finger metacarpal serves for attachment of (1) two dorsal ligaments, one each from the capitate and the hamate; (2) two palmar ligaments, one each from the capitate and the hamate; and (3) an interosseous ligament from the hamate.[57]

The little finger metacarpal serves for attachment of (1) the pisometacarpal ligament, which runs from the proximal carpal row to the palmar and ulnar aspects of the little finger metacarpal; (2) the hamatometacarpal ligament, which extends from the hook of the hamate to the palmar and ulnar aspects of the fifth metacarpal; and (3) a small ligament that extends on the palmar and radial aspects from the hamate to the little finger metacarpal.

Joint Lining. The synovial joint lining is a continuation of the distal carpal row synovium and usually connects to the midcarpal joint.[57] The synovial space of the hamate with the ring and the little metacarpals may be a separate space.[57]

Extracapsular Support

Tendons crossing the finger CMC joint include the following:

1. The digital flexor digitorum superficialis and profundus tendons, which provide weak palmar support.
2. The digital extensor digitorum tendons, which provide some dorsal stability.

3. The flexor and extensor carpi ulnaris tendons, which provide support for the little finger CMC joint.
4. The flexor carpi radialis tendon, which provides support for the index and long finger CMC joints.
5. The extensor carpi radialis longus and brevis tendons, which provide dorsal support for the index and long finger CMC joints.

The oblique head of the adductor pollicis muscle helps to support the long finger CMC joint.

METACARPOPHALANGEAL JOINTS

MCP Joint of the Thumb (Figs. 4–35 and 4–42)

General Information

This condyloid joint allows hyperextension of 20 to 45 degrees and flexion of 5 to 100 degrees in some people. The average range of motion has been estimated to be 75 degrees.[62,70] This wide variation in the range of motion is a result of the round or flat configuration of the metacarpal head. Round heads (more common) allow more flexion, whereas flat heads, present in 10% to 15% of cases, allow little flexion.[62,70] It is also a result of variations of the supporting joint capsular structures.[58]

The MCP joint is condylar, allowing some adduction–abduction. The normal range varies from 0 to 20 degrees, with an average of 10 degrees.[61]

The collateral ligaments and the palmar plate provide great joint stability. They allow more motion on the radial side after an abnormal stretching of the ulnar collateral ligament. Chronic weakness and weakened pinch grip result from weakened collateral ligaments. The collateral ligaments are taut in flexion and more relaxed in extension.[111]

Ligaments and Joint Capsule[58]

Capsular support is provided by the proper radial and ulnar collateral ligaments, which arise from the medial and lateral condyles of the metacarpal head, respectively, then pass obliquely and palmarly to insert on the distal medial or lateral aspect of the palmar plate and the palmar third of the proximal phalanx. These are broad, thick ligaments that are 4 to 8 mm wide and have an average length of 12 to 14 mm.[111] The ulnar ligament is stronger than the radial ligament.[74]

The radial and ulnar metacarpoglenoid ligaments arise superficial and palmar to the proper collateral ligaments.[105] They are thinner than the proper collateral ligaments, attach to the palmar plate, insert onto the palmar plate and its sesamoid, and attach to the proper collateral ligament.[74]

Volar (Palmar) Plate

The palmar plate (anterior or glenoid ligament) arises proximally from two asymmetrical checkrein ligaments from the palmar distal thumb metacarpal. The radial checkrein ligament is short and weak, whereas the ulnar checkrein ligament is longer and stronger.[112]

The palmar plate inserts on the palmar edge of the proximal phalanx and has no flexor tendon palmar to it, as is found in the other digits. It has two sesamoid bones in its center, one radial and one ulnar, which are present in all patients and serve as sites for attachment of the thenar muscles.[58,61,74] It has a thicker fibrocartilage portion distal to the sesamoid bones and a thinner, more pliable portion proximal to the sesamoids.

The palmar plate receives reinforcement from the adductor pollicis, which inserts onto the ulnar sesamoid of the palmar plate, and the flexor pollicis brevis tendon and the abductor pollicis brevis, which insert onto the radial sesamoid.

The joint capsule is thick palmarly (palmar plate) and thin dorsally,[74] and is reinforced dorsally by a slip of the extensor pollicis brevis tendon. It arises proximally near the articular margin of the metacarpal head and attaches distally near the base of the proximal phalanx.[113] The joint capsule usually

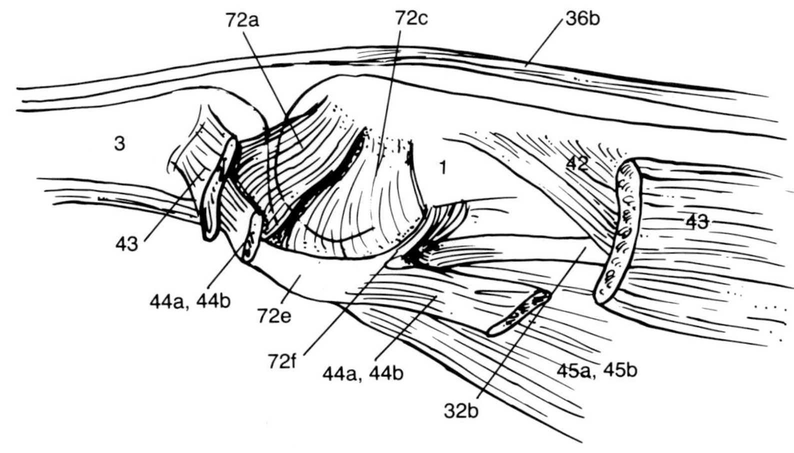

FIGURE 4–42. Radial side view of the thumb MCP joint showing the insertions of the thenar muscles. 1—Thumb metacarpal; 3—thumb proximal phalanx; 32b—flexor pollicis longus tendon; 36b—extensor pollicis longus tendon; 42—opponens pollicis; 43—abductor pollicis brevis (cut); 44a, 44b—flexor pollicis brevis—superficial and deep heads (cut); 45a, 45b—adductor pollicis—oblique and transverse heads; 72a—thumb MCP joint proper radial collateral ligament; 72c—thumb MCP joint radial metacarpoglenoid ligament; 72e—thumb MCP joint palmar plate; 72f—thumb MCP joint palmar plate checkrein ligament.

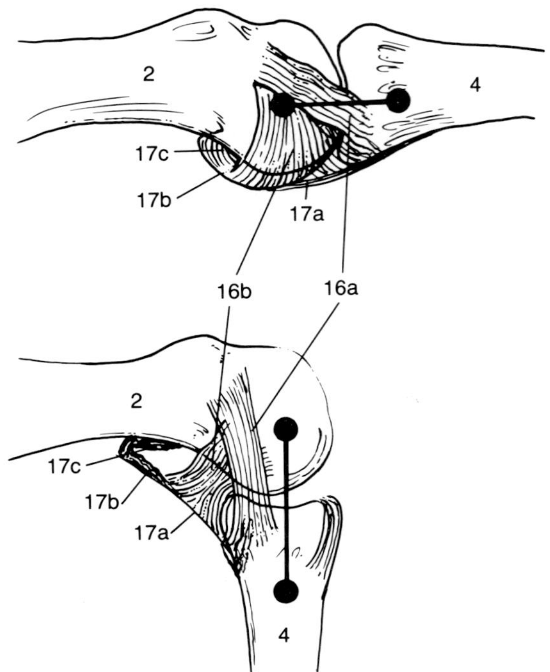

FIGURE 4–43. Lateral view of the finger MCP joint. When flexed (lower), the line connecting the axes of rotation of the two bones at this position is longer, thus demonstrating that the collateral ligaments at this joint are more taut in flexion than in extension. 2—Finger metacarpal; 4—finger proximal phalanx; 16a—finger MCP joint proper collateral ligament; 16b—finger MCP joint accessory (metacarpoglenoid) collateral ligament; 17a—finger MCP joint palmar plate; 17b—finger MCP joint palmar plate checkrein ligament; 17c—finger MCP joint synovial capsule.

consists of a larger proximal palmar recess and a smaller distal dorsal recess.[113]

Extracapsular Support

Tendons that provide extracapsular support include the flexor pollicis longus tendon and the extensor pollicis longus tendon.[70] Muscles that provide extracapsular support via insertions into the extensor mechanism and provide a supportive muscle sling include the adductor pollicis, the flexor pollicis brevis, and the abductor pollicis brevis.[70]

MCP Joints of the Fingers (Figs. 4–23, 4–34, and 4–43)

General Information

In addition to flexion–extension movement, the diarthrodial finger MCP joint allows rotation and abduction from the midline. The range of flexion–extension of the normal joint ranges from 15 to 25 (up to 45 or more) degrees of dorsal extension to 90 degrees of flexion, for a total active flexion of 100 degrees or more.[70,113] In the extended position there is as much as 60 degrees of radioulnar deviation,[97,113] and there may be up to 15 to 20 degrees of rotation.[113]

The border digits, the index fingers and the little fingers, have greater rotation than the long and ring fingers.

Joint stability is very dependent on ligamentous stability; more stability exists in flexion than in extension. This results from[59] (1) palmar flaring of the metacarpal head, which provides more articular surface contact in flexion, and (2) the oblique orientation of the insertion of the collateral ligaments, which are taut in flexion and more lax in extension, thus allowing lateral joint mobility.[70]

The radial collateral ligaments are usually stronger than the ulnar collateral ligaments. This is especially true for the index and long fingers.

Ligaments and Joint Capsule

The thick radial MCP collateral ligament arises from the radial tuberosity on the dorsolateral surface of the metacarpal head dorsal to the axis of rotation.[66,69] The ulnar collateral MCP ligament arises similarly on the ulnar tuberosity on the metacarpal dorsomedial surface. The ligaments, which are triangular in shape, may be up to 3 mm thick and 8 mm wide.[59] The ligaments course obliquely in a dorsal to palmar direction and insert onto the distal-lateral aspect of the palmar plate and the proximal phalanx near the MCP joint.[62,66,86]

The radial collateral ligament inserts more distally on the midradial aspect of the proximal phalangeal base than does the ulnar collateral ligament.[66] The ligaments are more taut in flexion and relaxed in extension.[62,70]

The collateral ligaments are attached further back from the joint on the metacarpal head side than on the proximal phalangeal base side.[114] The radial collateral ligaments of the index and long fingers are more developed than the ulnar collateral ligaments.[66]

The thinner radial and ulnar metacarpoglenoid ligaments (accessory collateral ligaments)[61] arise laterally from the radial and ulnar sides of the metacarpal head, insert onto either side of the palmar plate, and blend into the intermetacarpal ligament.[62] These ligaments are less rigid than the proper collateral ligaments so they can fold on themselves when the joint flexes. They prevent palmar displacement of the proximal phalanx and provide additional joint stability.[59,70]

The strong palmar plate (anterior ligament) has a thin, areolar, and more flexible proximal portion at its proximal attachment to the palmar aspect of the metacarpal neck.[86] This proximal palmar plate attachment is membranous and unlike the more rigid palmar plate attachments of the IP joints (see subsequent discussion).[69] This looseness of the proximal palmar plate attachment allows hyperextension and dorsolateral motion of the MCP joints.[69,70]

The palmar plate has (1) a triangular and thicker (up to 3 to 4 mm thick) distal central portion[114], (2) strong insertion along the narrow palmar border of the articular cartilage of the proximal phalangeal base[77,115], (3) radial and ulnar collateral ligament reinforcement laterally, (4) transverse deep (palmar) intermetacarpal ligament insertion medially and laterally, and (5) a palmar groove for the flexor tendons.[57]

The deep transverse intermetacarpal ligaments (volar, palmar, or transverse interglenoid ligaments)[86] strongly bind together the four finger metacarpal heads via attachments to the palmar plates.[59,115] They arise and insert on the medial and lateral aspects of the palmar plates of each of the finger MCP joints (except radially on the index finger and ulnarly on the little finger where there are no adjacent fingers). They allow dorsal and palmar mobility as well as limited rotation but limit medial and lateral mobility.[110] Dubousset[86] prefers the name transverse interglenoid ligament because the ligament actually runs between the MCP joints and not the metacarpals.

A deep dorsal aponeurosis inserts on the dorsum of the four finger metacarpals and forms a true posterior (dorsal) intermetacarpal ligament.[115] In addition, the joint capsule extends from the metacarpal neck to the base of the proximal phalanx. Dorsally, the capsule is areolar, with a large proximal bursa.[86] Palmarly, it is composed of the thickened palmar plate. Distally, it attaches to a narrow rim along the border of the articular cartilage of the proximal phalangeal base.[77] There is also a proximal palmar synovial recess.[77,86]

Extracapsular Support

Support of the finger MCP joint is provided by the following:[70]

1. The flexor superficialis and profundus tendons, which pass over the palmar surface of the joint.
2. The extensor tendons, which pass over the dorsal surface of the joint.
3. The dorsal and palmar interosseous muscles, which pass lateral to the joint as the sagittal bands.
4. The lumbricals, which pass on the radial side of the digit to insert into the radial aspect of the extensor mechanism.
5. The abductor digiti minimi and flexor digiti minimi muscles.

A slip of the extensor digitorum communis tendon inserts on the dorsal rim of the base of the proximal phalanx and also provides some support. The proximal position of the joint within the webspace also tends to protect it from the extremes of stress.[103]

INTERPHALANGEAL JOINTS

IP JOINT OF THE THUMB

General Information

The interphalangeal (IP) joint of the thumb (Fig. 4–44) is a bicondylar joint permitting flexion–extension, with only a slight degree of rotation in pronation as the joint flexes.[65] The strength of the collateral ligaments of the thumb is equal to the strength of the digital DIP joint collateral ligaments.[58]

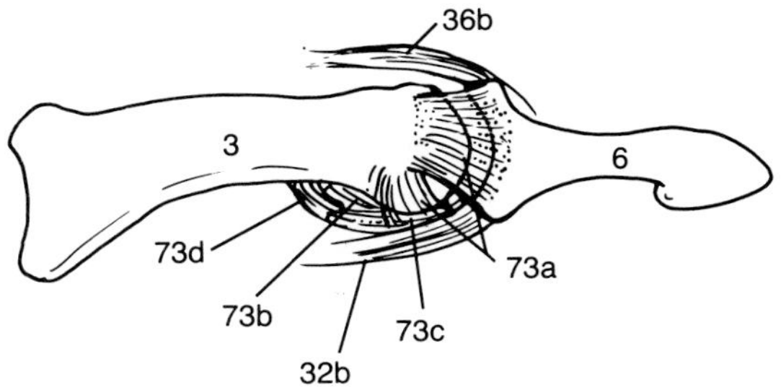

FIGURE 4–44. The lateral view of the IP joint of the thumb is very much like that of the DIP joint of the fingers (see Fig. 4–47). 3—Thumb proximal phalanx; 6—thumb distal phalanx; 32b—flexor pollicis longus tendon; 36b—extensor pollicis longus tendon; 73a—thumb IP joint radial or ulnar collateral ligament; 73b—thumb IP joint capsule and synovial lining; 73c—thumb IP joint palmar plate; 73d—thumb IP palmar plate checkrein ligament.

Ligaments and Joint Capsule

The capsular support is composed of the following:

1. The radial collateral ligament, which has fibers that arise from the lateral (radial) condyle of the proximal phalanx of the thumb and run slightly obliquely across the joint to insert into the lateral (radial) side of the distal phalanx. Additional fibers run vertically to insert into the lateral (radial) side of the palmar plate.[70]
2. The ulnar collateral ligament, which has fibers that arise from the medial (ulnar) condyle of the proximal phalanx of the thumb and run slightly obliquely across the joint to insert into the medial (ulnar) side of the distal phalanx. Additional fibers run vertically to insert into the medial (ulnar) side of the palmar plate.[70]
3. The palmar plate, which has a proximal attachment consisting of two thin, lateral parts and a thinner central (axial) portion and a distal attachment, consisting of a narrow brim along the border of the articular cartilage at the distal phalangeal base.[77]

The synovial lining of the IP thumb joint extends from the proximal edge of the palmar plate to the distal articular surface of the distal phalanx. It also extends dorsally between the distal edge of the articular cartilage of the distal phalanx and the proximal edge of the proximal phalangeal head articular cartilage.[116]

Extracapsular Support

Support is provided by tendons of the flexor pollicis longus, which runs over the palmar surface of the joint to insert broadly on the palmar lip of the distal phalanx, and the extensor pollicis longus, which runs over the dorsal surface of the joint to insert broadly on the dorsal lip of the distal phalanx.[58,70]

Additional joint support is also provided by the snug skin envelope around the joint.[58] Cleland's ligaments reinforce the collateral ligaments and provide additional lateral support.[69]

PROXIMAL INTERPHALANGEAL JOINT

General Information

The proximal interphalangeal (PIP) joint (Figs. 4–34, 4–37, 4–45, and 4–46) is a hinge joint that permits only flexion and extension in the sagittal plane.[117–120] Approximately 100 to 120 degrees of flexion and 5 degrees of extension are allowed, with an average of 105 degrees of motion.[70] Only a minority of whites can hyperextend their joints, but natives of Southeast Asia have a remarkable ability to hyperextend their joints, at times with their fingers extended 90 degrees to the plane of the palm (the position of the "open lotus flower").[117,118] The maximal radial deviation for the index, long, and ring fingers is 5 degrees and for the little finger is 10 degrees.[110]

The bicondylar head of the proximal phalanx articulates with the two reciprocal concave surfaces of the middle phalanx.[69]

The PIP joint has a great deal of stability through its range of motion but is most stable in full extension because of the contour of the joint surfaces. In full flexion, joint stability is dependent on ligamentous strength.[121]

All of the collateral ligament fibers are believed to be taut in 15 to 20 degrees of flexion, whereas in extension only the palmar portion and the palmar plate are stretched (which forms the basis for recommending 15 to 20 degrees of flexion as the preferred position for PIP joint immobilization).[70,92,121]

Because of the multiple structures traversing the PIP joint, Cozzi[122] has described what he terms a lateral fibrous chiasm, one of which lies both medially and laterally. This is composed of a superficial portion, which includes the intermediate bundle of Cleland's ligament, the oblique and transverse retinacular ligaments, and the middle cruciform flexor sheath annular ligament, and a deeper portion, including the collateral ligaments, the palmar plate, and the joint capsule.

Ligaments and Joint Capsule

Lateral capsular support is provided by the tripartite collateral ligament,[58] which is composed of (1) a triangular ligamentous band that extends from the medial or lateral tubercle of the proximal phalangeal head to the lateral margin of the base of the middle phalanx; (2) a proper collateral ligament that extends from a recess palmar to the medial or lateral tubercle of the proximal phalangeal head to the lateral and lateropalmar margin of the base of the middle phalanx; and (3) a fan-shaped ligament or accessory ligament that arises from the lateral or medial tubercle of the proximal phalangeal head and inserts onto the palmar plate. The ligament is 2 to 3 mm thick.[69,103]

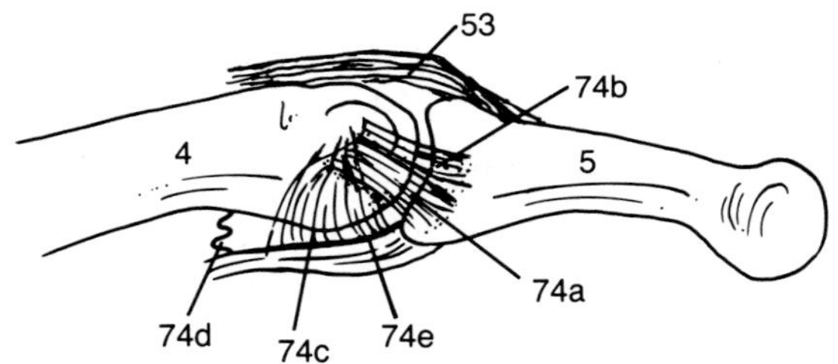

FIGURE 4–45. Lateral view of a finger PIP joint. 4—Finger proximal phalanx; 5—finger middle phalanx; 53—central slip of the extensor digitorum communis; 74a—finger PIP joint radial or ulnar proper collateral ligament; 74b—finger PIP joint radial or ulnar triangular ligamentous band; 74c—finger PIP joint radial or ulnar accessory collateral ligament; 74d—finger PIP joint capsule and synovial lining; 74e—finger PIP palmar plate.

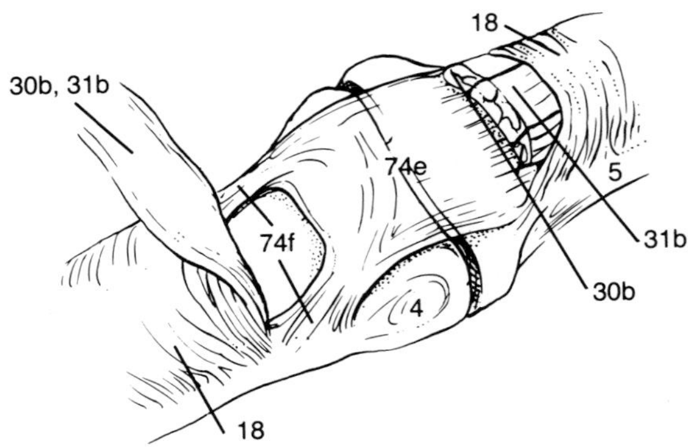

FIGURE 4–46. Palmar view of a finger PIP joint showing that the palmar plate is more fibrous distally and is proximally connected by radial and ulnar checkrein ligaments to the proximal phalanx. 4—Finger proximal phalanx; 5—finger middle phalanx; 18—finger fibroosseous tunnel; 30b—flexor digitorum superficialis tendon (cut); 31b—flexor digitorum profundus tendon (cut); 74e—finger PIP palmar plate; 74f—finger PIP palmar plate checkrein ligaments.

Anatomic Course

The radial and ulnar proper collateral ligaments arise from a concave fossa on the radial and ulnar aspects, respectively, of each condyle of the proximal phalanx. They pass distally in an oblique, palmar direction and insert onto the palmar proximal third of the middle phalanx and the distal medial and lateral margins of the PIP palmar plate.[103]

The fan-shaped portion of the ligament inserts on the palmar tubercle of the middle phalangeal base.[58,70] The collateral ligaments are attached further back from the joint on the proximal phalangeal side.[114] The width of the ligament at its origin and insertion is approximately half of its length.[69]

The oblique orientation of the true collateral ligament fibers is such that they maintain fairly constant tension throughout the range of joint motion.[97,114] The dorsal fibers are more taut in flexion, whereas the palmar fibers are more taut in extension.[97] Palmar capsule support is provided by the strong palmar plate.

Proximal attachment consists of two thick lateral parts (radial and ulnar palmar checkrein ligaments) and a thinner central areolar portion.[68,70,103,123,124] The checkrein ligaments are formed by the confluence of reflected fibers of the dorsal portion of the digital flexor sheath, the accessory ligament insertion, and the lateral (radial and ulnar) margins of the palmar plate.[69,70,124] The central space between the palmar checkrein ligaments allows branches of the digital vessels to run to the flexor tendons as well as protrusion of the palmar synovial pouch.[69,70,123] The blood vessels to the flexor tendons are carried by the vinculum brevis (to the flexor digitorum superficialis) and the vinculum longus (to the flexor digitorum profundus tendon).

Distal attachment consists of a dense fibrous tissue rim along the border of the articular cartilage at the middle phalangeal base that blends with the palmar periosteum.[58,77,123] It is supported medially and laterally by the collateral ligaments. Disruption of the palmar plate usually occurs at the distal attachment into the middle phalanx.[124] The bursting strength of the palmar plate of the PIP joint is 19 kg, compared with 6 kg for the MCP joint.[58,124]

Dorsal capsule support is provided by the central insertion of the extensor tendon onto the dorsal tubercle on the base of the middle phalanx.

The synovial joint enclosure extends from the proximal edge of the palmar plate to the distal edge of the articular surface of the middle phalangeal base. In flexion, the palmar synovial pouch expands around the free proximal edge of the palmar plate.[58] The vinculum brevis helps pull the synovial pouch proximally to prevent it from becoming entrapped in the PIP joint when it is extended. There is also a dorsal proximal extension of the joint synovium.[86,116]

Extracapsular Support

Extracapsular support is provided by the extensor hood, the oblique retinacular ligament, the flexor profundus and superficialis tendons, and the lumbrical and the interosseous muscle tendon combination.

Cleland's ligament extends from the lateral (radial and ulnar) edge of the osseous reflection of the flexor tendon sheath to the overlying skin.

DISTAL INTERPHALANGEAL JOINT

General Information

The distal interphalangeal (DIP) joint (Figs. 4–47 and 4–48) is a hinge joint that permits only flexion and extension in the sagittal plane.[58,117,118,125] It allows 20 to 30 degrees of extension and up to 80 to 90 degrees of flexion.[70] The structure of the DIP joint is much like that of the PIP joint, but the DIP joint palmar plate lacks the strong checkrein ligaments found at the PIP joint; thus the DIP joint has more hyperextension.[58,62,70] The strong ligamentous support and extracapsular support as well as the short lever arm of the distal phalanx are believed to be responsible for the low incidence of DIP joint dislocations.[69]

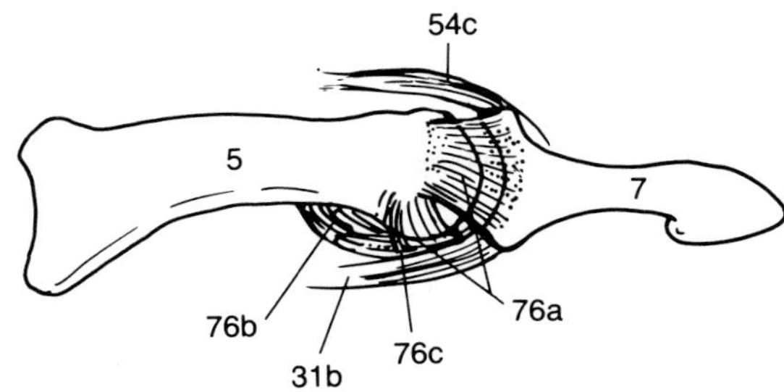

FIGURE 4–47. Lateral view of a finger DIP joint. 5—Finger middle phalanx; 7—finger distal phalanx; 31b—flexor digitorum profundus tendon; 54c—terminal extensor tendon; 76a—finger DIP joint ulnar or radial collateral ligament; 76b—finger DIP joint capsule and synovial lining; 76c—finger DIP joint palmar plate.

Ligaments and Joint Capsule

Capsular support is provided by the following:

1. The collateral ligaments. These short, thick ligaments extend obliquely across the axis of rotation of the DIP joint.[58] They arise from a depression on the lateral (radial and ulnar) side of the head of the middle phalanx.[58] They insert into a prominent midlateral (radial and ulnar) tubercle of the distal phalanx, and the more palmar portion of the ligament inserts onto the lateral (radial and ulnar) edge of the palmar plate.[58] The collateral ligaments are attached further back from the joint on the middle phalangeal side.
2. The palmar plate with its proximal attachment by two thin lateral (radial and ulnar) pillars, which attach to the distal aspect of the middle phalanx as well as merge into the fibroosseous tunnel of the flexor tendons;[126] its thinner central (axial) portion; and its distal attachment by a narrow brim along the width of the palmar articular cartilage border of the distal phalangeal base.[58,77]

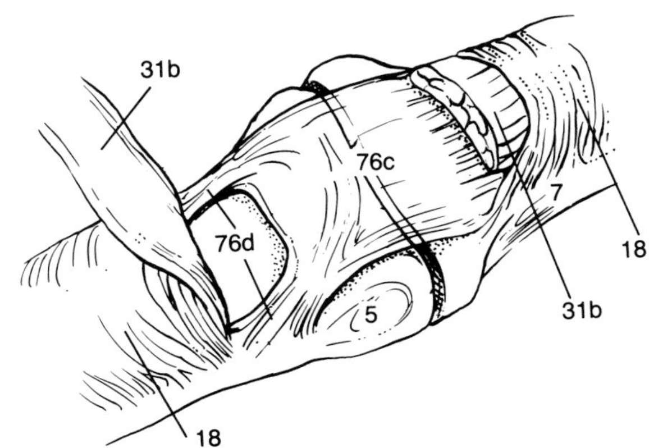

FIGURE 4–48. Palmar view of a finger DIP joint showing the palmar plate is more fibrous distally and is proximally connected by a radial and ulnar checkrein ligament to the middle phalanx. 5—Finger middle phalanx; 7—finger distal phalanx; 18—finger fibrooseous tunnel; 31b—flexor digitorum profundus tendon (cut); 76c—finger DIP palmar plate; 76d—finger DIP palmar plate checkrein ligaments.

Dorsal and palmar synovial pouches extend proximally from the joint capsule.[58,86,116]

Extracapsular Support

Support of the finger DIP joint is provided by the following:

1. The snug skin envelope.[58]
2. The terminal extensions of the flexor profundus tendon, which insert onto the distal phalanx just distal to the insertion of the palmar plate.[58]
3. A few fibers of the flexor profundus tendon, which insert onto the palmar plate.[77]

REFERENCES

1. Bonin von G. A note on the kinematics of the wrist joint. *J Anat* 1929;63:259–262.
2. Cyriax EF. On the rotary movements of the wrist. *J Anat* 1926;60:199–201.
3. Fick R. Handbuch der Anatomie und Mechanik der Gelenke. In: von Bardeleben K, ed. *Handbuch der Anatomie des Menschen: III. Spezielle Gelenk- und Muskelmechanik.* Jena: Gustav Fischer, 1911.
4. Fischer O. Über Gelenke von zwei Graden der Freiheit. *Arch Anat Entwickelungsgesch Suppl Bd,* 1897:242–272.
5. Fischer O. *Kinematik organischer Gelenke.* Vieweg, Braunschweig: 1907.
6. Günther GB. *Das Handgelenk in mechanischer, anatomischer und chirurgischer Beziehung.* Hamburg: Meissner, 1850.
7. Henke W. Die Bewegungen der Handwurzel. *Z Rat Med* 1859;7:27–42.
8. Strasser H. *Lehrbuch der Muskel- und Gelenkmechanik: IV. Spezieller Teil: Die obere Extremität.* Berlin: Springer, 1917.
9. Wright RD. A detailed study of movement of the wrist joint. *J Anat* 1935;70:137–142.
10. Forssel G. Über die Bewegungen im Handgelenke des Menschen. *Scand Arch Physiol* 1902;12:168–258.
11. Virchow H. Die Weiterdrehung des Naviculare carpi bei Dorsalflexion, und die Beziehungen der Handbänder. *Anat Anz* 1902;21:111–126.
12. Virchow H. Über Einzelmechanismen am Handgelenk. *Anat Anz* 1902;21:369–388.
13. Destot E. Anatomie et physiologie du poignet. In: Destot E, ed. *Traumatismes du poignet et rayons X.* Paris: Masson, 1923.
14. Bellinghausen HW, Gilula LA, Young LV, Weeks PM. Posttraumatic palmar carpal subluxation. *J Bone Joint Surg* 1983; 65A:998–1006.
15. Fisk GR. An overview of injuries of the wrist. *Clin Orthop* 1980;149:137–144.
16. Linscheid RL, Dobyns JH, Beabout JW, Bryan RS. Traumatic instability of the wrist. *J Bone Joint Surg* 1972;54A:1612–1632.
17. Mayfield JK, Johnson RP, Kilcoyne RG. The ligaments of the human wrist and their functional significance. *Anat Rec* 1976;186:417–428.
18. Reicher MA, Kellerhouse LE. Carpal instability. In: Reicher MA, Kellerhouse LE, eds. *MRI of the wrist and hand.* New York: Raven, 1990:69–85.
19. Taleisnik J. *The wrist.* New York: Churchill Livingstone, 1985:229–239.
20. Mikic Z. Age changes in the triangular fibrocartilage of the wrist joint. *J Anat* 1978;126:367–384.
21. Kauer JMG. Note sur le développement du ligament triangulaire chez l'homme. *Bull Assoc Anat* 1975;167:893–898.
22. Kauer JMG. The articular disc of the hand. *Acta Anat* 1975;93:590–605.
23. Kauer JMG. The distal radioulnar joint: Anatomic and functional considerations. *Clin Orthop* 1992;275:37–45.
24. Henle J. Handbuch der Bänderlehre des Menschen: *Handbuch der Systematische Anatomie des Menschen,* vol. 1/2. Vieweg, Braunschweig, 1856.
25. Kauer JMG. The radioscaphoid ligament (RSL). *Acta Anat* 1984;120:36–37.
26. Berger RA, Kauer JMG, Landsmeer JMF. Radioscapholunate ligament: A gross anatomic and histologic study of fetal and adult wrists. *J Hand Surg* 1992;16:350–355.
27. Mikic Z. Detailed anatomy of the articular disc of the distal radioulnar joint. *Clin Orthop* 1989;245:123–132.
28. Lanz T von, Wachsmuth W. *Praktische Anatomie 1/3 Arm.* Berlin: Springer, 1959:228.
29. Obermann WR. *Radiology of carpal instability: A clinical and anatomical study.* Ph.D. thesis, University Leiden, the Netherlands, 1991.
30. Johnston HM. Varying positions of the carpal bones in the different movements at the wrist. *J Anat Phys* 1907;41:109–222; 280–292.
31. MacConaill MA. The mechanical anatomy of the carpus and its bearing on some surgical problems. *J Anat* 1941;75:166–175.
32. Viegas SF, Wagner K, Patterson RM, Peterson P. The medial (hamate) facet of the lunate. *J Hand Surg* 1990;15A:564–571.
33. Taleisnik J. The ligaments of the wrist. *J Hand Surg* 1976; 1A:110–118.
34. Savelberg HHCM, Kooloos JGM, Kauer JMG. Kinematics of the human carpal bone ligament complex. *Ann Soc R Zool Belg* 1989;119:65.
35. Savelberg HHCM, Kooloos JGM, Lange A de, Kauer JMG, Huiskes R. Human carpal ligament recruitment and three-dimensional carpal motion. *J Orthop Res* 1991;9:693–704.
36. Fisk GR. Carpal instability and the fractured scaphoid (Hunterian lecture). *Ann R Coll Surg Engl* 1970;46:63–76.
37. Fisk GR. Malalignment of the scaphoid after lunate dislocation. In: Razemon JP, Fisk GR, eds. *The wrist.* Edinburgh: Churchill Livingstone, 1988:135–137.
38. Gilula LA. Carpal injuries: Analytic approach and case exercises. *Am J Roentgenol* 1979;133:503–517.
39. Gilula LA, Weeks PM. Posttraumatic ligamentous instability of the wrist. *Radiology* 1978;129:641–651.
40. Gilford WW, Bolton RH, Lambrinudi C. The mechanism of the wrist joint with special reference to fractures of the scaphoid. *Guys Hosp Rep* 1943;92:52–59.
41. Kauer JMG. The interdependence of carpal articulation chains. *Acta Anat* 1974;88:481–501.
42. Kauer JMG. Functional anatomy of the wrist. *Clin Orthop* 1980;149:9–20.
43. Navarro A. Luxaciones del carpo. (Cited by Taleisnik J. The bones of the wrist.) In: Taleisnik J, ed. *The wrist.* New York: Churchill Livingstone, 1921:1–12.
44. Kauer JMG. The mechanism of the carpal joint. *Clin Orthop* 1986;202:16–26.
45. Kauer JMG. The longitudinal carpal chain, a model of carpal function. *Ann R Coll Surg Engl* 1988;70:166.
46. Kauer JMG, Lange A de. The carpal joint: Anatomy and function. *Hand Clin* 1987;3(1):23–29.
47. Kauer JMG, Lange A de, Savelberg HHCM, Kooloos JGM. The wrist joint: Functional analysis and experimental approach. In: Nakamura R, Linscheid RL, Miura T, eds. *Wrist disorders.* Tokyo: Springer, 1992:3–12.
48. Smith DK, An KN, Cooney WP, Linscheid RL, Chao EY. Effects of a scaphoid wrist osteotomy on carpal kinematics. *J Orthop Res* 1989;7:590–598.
49. Smith DK, Cooney WP, An KN, Linscheid RL, Chao EYS. The effects of simulated unstable scaphoid fractures on carpal motion. *J Hand Surg* 1989;14A:283–291.
50. Lange A de, Kauer JMG, Huiskes R. Kinematic behavior of the human wrist joint: A roentgen-stereophotogrammetric analysis. *J Orthop Res* 1985;3:56–64.
51. Nowak MD, Logan, SE. Distinguishing biomechanical properties of intrinsic and extrinsic human wrist ligaments. *J Biomech Eng* 1991;113:85–93.
52. Poznanski AK. *The hand in radiologic diagnosis.* Philadelphia: WB Saunders, 1984:1.

53. Hakstian RW, Tubiana R. Ulnar deviation of the fingers: The role of joint structure and function. *J Bone Joint Surg* 1967; 49A:299.
54. Zancolli R. *Structural and dynamic basis of hand surgery.* Philadelphia: JB Lippincott, 1968:1.
55. Kaplan EB. *Functional and surgical anatomy of the hand.* 2nd ed. Philadelphia: JB Lippincott, 1965:1.
56. Kuczynski K. Carpometacarpal joint of the human thumb. *J Anat* 1974;118:119.
57. Pick TP, Howden R, eds. *Gray's anatomy, descriptive and surgical.* New York: Crown Publishers, 1978:1.
58. Weeks PM. *Acute bone and joint injuries of the hand and wrist: A clinical guide to management.* St. Louis: CV Mosby, 1981:1.
59. Smith RJ, Peimer CA. Injuries to the metacarpal bones and joints. *Adv Surg* 1977;2:341.
60. Lazar G, Schulter-Ellis FP. Intramedullary structure of human metacarpals. *J Hand Surg* 1980;5:477.
61. Green DP, Rowland SA. Fractures and dislocations in the hand. In: Rockwood CA, Green DP, eds. *Fractures in adults.* 3rd ed. Philadelphia: JB Lippincott, 1991:313.
62. Sandzen SC Jr. *Atlas of wrist and hand fractures.* Littleton, MA: PGS Publishing, 1979:1.
63. Simmons BP, de la Caffiniere JY. Physiology of flexion of the fingers. In: Tubiana R, ed. *The hand,* Vol. 1. Philadelphia: WB Saunders, 1981:377.
64. Schulter-Ellis FP, Lazar GT. Internal morphology of human phalanges. *J Hand Surg* 1984;9A:490.
65. Kapandji AI. Biomechanics of the interphalangeal joint of the thumb. In: Tubiana R, ed. *The hand,* Vol. 1, Philadelphia: WB Saunders, 1981;188.
66. Landsmeer JMF. Anatomical and functional investigations of the human finger and its functional significance. *Acta Anat* (*suppl.* 24) 1955;25:1.
67. Kuczynski, K. Less-known aspects of the proximal interphalangeal joints of the human hand. *Hand* 1975;7:31.
68. Bowers WH. The anatomy of the interphalangeal joints. In: Bowers WH, ed. *The interphalangeal joints.* Edinburgh: Churchill Livingstone, 1987:2.
69. Eaton RG. *Joint injuries of the hand.* Springfield: Charles C. Thomas, 1971:1.
70. Sandzen SC Jr. *Atlas of wrist and hand fractures.* Littleton, MA: PSG Publishing, 1986:1.
71. O'Brien ET. Fractures of the metacarpals and phalanges. In: Green DP, ed. *Operative hand surgery.* New York: Churchill Livingstone, 1982:583.
72. Hubay CA. Sesamoid bones of the hands and feet. *Am J Roentgen Rad Ther* 1949;61:493.
73. Bizarrio AH. On sesamoid and supernumerary bones of the limbs. *J Anat* 1921;55:256.
74. Aubriot JH. The metacarpophalangeal joint of the thumb. In: Tubiana R, ed. *The hand,* Vol. 1. Philadelphia: WB Saunders, 1981:184.
75. Kaplan EB. Anatomical variations of the forearm and hand. In Tubiana R, ed. *The hand,* Vol. 1. Philadelphia: WB Saunders, 1981:361.
76. Valentin P. Extrinsic muscles of the hand and wrist: An introduction. In Tubiana R, ed. *The hand,* Vol. 1. Philadelphia: WB Saunders, 1981:237.
77. Gad P. The anatomy of the palmar parts of the capsules of the finger joints. *J Bone Joint Surg* 1967;49B:362.
78. Fahrer M. Interdependent and independent actions of the fingers. In: Tubiana R, ed. *The hand,* Vol. 1. Philadelphia: WB Saunders, 1981:399.
79. Haines RW. The extensor apparatus of the finger. *J Anat* 1951;85:251.
80. Littler JW. The finger extensor mechanism. *Surg Clin North Am* 1967;47:415.
81. Tubiana R, Valentin P. The anatomy of the extensor apparatus of the fingers. *Surg Clin North Am* 1964;44:897.
82. Valentin P. The interossei and the lumbricals. In: Tubiana R, ed. *The hand,* Vol. 1. Philadelphia: WB Saunders, 1981:244.
83. Eyler DL, Markee JE. The anatomy and function of the intrinsic musculature of the hand. *J Bone Joint Surg* 1954;36A:1.
84. Backhouse KM, Catton WT. An experimental study of the functions of the lumbrical muscles in the human hand. *J Anat* 1954;88:133.
85. Stack G. Muscle function in the fingers. *J Bone Joint Surg* 1962;44B:899.
86. Dubousset JF. The digital joints. In: Tubiana R, ed. *The hand,* Vol. 1. Philadelphia: WB Saunders, 1981:191.
87. Fahrer M. The thenar eminence: An introduction. In: Tubiana R, ed. *The hand,* Vol. 1. Philadelphia: WB Saunders, 1981:255.
88. Kaplan EB. Anatomy and kinesiology of the hand. In: Flynn JE, ed. *Hand surgery.* 3rd ed. Baltimore: Williams and Wilkins, 1982:33.
89. Fahrer M. The hypothenar eminence. In: Tubiana R, ed. *The hand,* Vol. 1. Philadelphia: WB Saunders, 1981:259.
90. Schultz RJ, Furlong J II, Storace A. Detailed anatomy of the extensor mechanism at the proximal aspect of the finger. *J Hand Surg* 1981;6:493.
91. Landsmeer JMF. The coordination of finger-joint motions. *J Bone Joint Surg* 1963;45A:1654.
92. Valentin P. Physiology of extension of the fingers. In: Tubiana R, ed. *The hand,* Vol. 1. Philadelphia: WB Saunders, 1981:389.
93. Ariyan S. *The hand book.* Baltimore: Williams and Wilkins, 1978:1.
94. Landsmeer JMF. The anatomy of the dorsal aponeurosis of the human finger and its functional significance. *Anat Rec* 1941;104:31.
95. Milford LW. *Retaining ligaments of the digits of the hand: Gross and microscopic anatomic study.* Philadelphia: WB Saunders, 1968:1.
96. Milford LW. The retaining ligaments of the digits of the hand. In: Tubiana R, ed. *The hand,* Vol. 1. Philadelphia: WB Saunders, 1981:232.
97. Flatt AE. Biomechanics of the hand and wrist. In: Evarts CMcC, ed. *Surgery of the musculoskeletal system.* 2nd ed. New York: Churchill Livingstone, 1990:311.
98. Shrewsberry MM, Johnson RK. A systematic study of the oblique retinacular ligament of the human finger: Its structure and function. *J Hand Surg* 1977;2:194.
99. Doyle JR, Blythe WF. Anatomy of the flexor tendon sheath and pulleys of the thumb. *J Hand Surg* 1977;2:149.
100. Strauch B, de Moura W. Digital flexor tendon sheath: An anatomic study. *J Hand Surg,* 1985;10A:785.
101. Kapandji AI. Selective radiology of the first carpometacarpal (or trapeziometacarpal) joint. In: Tubiana R, ed. *The hand,* Vol. 2. Philadelphia: WB Saunders, 1985:635.
102. Pieron AP. The mechanism of the first carpometacarpal (CMC) joint: An anatomical and mechanical analysis. *Acta Orthop Scand Suppl* 1973;148:1.
103. Eaton RG, Dray GJ. Dislocations and ligament injuries in the digits. In: Green DP, ed. *Operative hand surgery,* Vol. 1. New York: Churchill Livingstone, 1982:637.
104. Smith SA, Kuczynski K. Observations of the joints of the hand. *Hand* 1978;10:226.
105. Haines RW. The mechanism of rotation at the first carpometacarpal joint. *J Anat* 1944;78:44.
106. Napier JR. The form and function of the carpometacarpal joint of the thumb. *J Anat* 1955;89:362.
107. Bojsen-Moller FB. Osteoligamentous guidance of the movements of the human thumb. *Am J Anat* 1976;147:71.
108. Pieron AP. The first carpometacarpal joint. In: Tubiana R, ed. *The hand,* Vol. 1. Philadelphia: WB Saunders, 1981:169.
109. El-Bacha A. The carpometacarpal joints (excluding the trapeziometacarpal). In: Tubiana R, ed. *The hand,* Vol. 1. Philadelphia: WB Saunders, 1981:158.
110. Dubousset JF. Finger rotation during prehension. In: Tubiana R, ed. *The hand,* Vol. 1. Philadelphia: WB Saunders, 1981:202.
111. Frank WE, Dobyns J. Surgical pathology of the collateral ligamentous injuries of the thumb. *Clin Orthop* 1972;83:102.
112. Gilbert A, Fachinelli A, Kahlil G, Poitevin L. Lesions of the palmar plates. In: Tubiana R, ed. *The hand,* Vol. 2. Philadelphia: WB Saunders, 1985:909.
113. Weissman BNW, Sledge CB. The hand. In: Weissman BNW,

Sledge CB, eds. *Orthopedic radiology.* Philadelphia: WB Saunders, 1986:71.

114. Barton NJ. Fractures and joint injuries of the hand. In: Wilson JN, ed. *Fractures and joint injuries.* 6th ed. New York: Churchill Livingstone, 1982:739.
115. Tubiana R. Architecture and function of the hand. In: Tubiana R, ed. *The hand,* Vol. 1. Philadelphia: WB Saunders, 1981:19.
116. Gilbert A, Busy F. The contribution of arthrography to the diagnosis of lesions of the digital ligaments. In: Tubiana R, ed. *The hand,* Vol. 2. Philadelphia: WB Saunders, 1985:904.
117. Brand PW. *Clinical mechanics of the hand.* St. Louis: CV Mosby, 1985:1.
118. Brand PW, Thompson DE, Micks JE. The biomechanics of the interphalangeal joints. In: Bowers WH, ed. *The interphalangeal joints.* Edinburgh: Churchill Livingstone, 1987:21.
119. Kuczynski K. The proximal interphalangeal joint: Anatomy and causes of stiffness in the fingers. *J Bone Joint Surg* 1968;50B:656.
120. Vicar AJ. Proximal interphalangeal joint dislocations without fracture. *Hand Clin* 1988;4:5.
121. Sprague BL. Proximal interphalangeal joint injuries and their initial treatment. *J Trauma* 1975;15:380.
122. Cozzi EP. The proximal interphalangeal joints—A study of the para-articular fibrous structures. In: Tubiana R, ed. *The hand,* Vol. 2. Philadelphia: WB Saunders 1985:869.
123. Bowers WH, Wolf JW, Nehil JL, Bittinger S. The proximal interphalangeal joint and palmar plate. I: An anatomic and biomechanical study. *J Hand Surg* 1980;5:79.
124. Nance EP, Kaye JJ, Milek MA. palmar plate fractures. *Radiology* 1979;133:61.
125. Shrewsbury MM, Johnson RK. Ligaments of the distal interphalangeal joint and the mallet position. *J Hand Surg* 1980;5(3):214.
126. Landsmeer JMF. *Atlas of anatomy of the hand.* Edinburgh: Churchill Livingstone, 1976:1.

CHAPTER 5

POSITIONS AND TECHNIQUES

Yuming Yin, Frederick A. Mann, and Louis A. Gilula

INTRODUCTION

Various imaging positions and techniques are important in the diagnosis of wrist disorders. The basic method remains plain or routine radiography, although there are many other techniques, such as tomography, arthrography, angiography, computed tomography, magnetic resonance imaging, ultrasound, and bone scintigraphy. Usually, routine radiography provides basic important information about abnormalities that can direct further investigation. When an imaging examination is considered, plain-film examination should first be obtained and studied carefully; then a decision can be made about whether further imaging investigation is needed. This chapter is designed to present most of the described positions for plain or routine radiography of the hand and wrist.

In literature and everyday use, the terms *posteroanterior* (PA) and *anteroposterior* (AP) are incorrectly used as synonyms. Their standard use, as well as of other terms describing radiographic positions, defines the direction of the radiographic beam. The first word defines the surface of the body part through which the x-ray beam enters. The second word describes the surface of the body part through which the x-ray beam exits. The exiting surface of the body part is typically lying on the x-ray cassette or table. Therefore, in the hand or wrist, a PA view describes the view where the palm of the hand or wrist lies on the x-ray cassette or table, an x-ray beam enters the dorsum of the hand, leaves the palm of the hand, and enters the x-ray film. The AP view and position is just the opposite: the x-ray beam enters the palm of the supinated hand and wrist, exits the dorsum of the hand or wrist to then enter the film cassette or table. This is accepted radiographic terminology and will be used throughout this book. We hope that this usage will soon be routine for all who use radiographs, not just radiologists. Without such standardization of terminology, the literature can be confusing.

The number of radiographic positions needed depends on the clinical information provided and the questions to be answered. For a survey examination to evaluate the traumatized hand, PA, oblique, and lateral views are the recommended minimum radiographic examination. For wrist trauma, we feel that PA, oblique, lateral, and scaphoid views of the wrist are necessary for an adequate survey. To determine bone age, only a PA view of the entire hand and wrist is needed.

Usually, unilateral views of the affected hand or wrist are adequate for single extremity trauma. However, for arthritis or systemic disorders, bilateral hand or wrist views are necessary to determine whether there is systemic or local disease. All images of the hand and wrist must be labeled with left and/or right markers, and all pertinent anatomy should be included on the radiographic views. It is important to put patients in a comfortable position that can be held during exposure.

In this chapter, please note that the boldfaced letters (i.e., **(A)**, **(B)**, **(C)**) that frequently come before sections of text refer to figure parts, which in all cases are positioned to the right of the explanatory material. The lettered parts may also be referred to within the body of a corresponding paragraph.

RADIOGRAPHIC POSITIONS FOR THE HAND

HAND: PA VIEW

Synonym Dorsopalmar view

Major Indications This is the basic survey view for the hand and is excellent to profile the entire hand.

Illustration **(A) Position.** The palm of the pronated hand is placed flat on the cassette with 90-degree abduction of the shoulder and 90-degree flexion of the elbow. The fingers are extended and slightly spread. **Central Beam.** The central beam is perpendicular to the cassette and is centered over the head of the third metacarpal.

(B) Criteria for an Adequate Examination. The PA view of the hand should include the distal 2 to 3 cm of the forearm, the entire carpus, metacarpals, and digits. There should be no obliquity or rotation of the hand, as proved by the observation that the concavities of both sides of shafts of phalanges and metacarpals are symmetric. Metacarpals and phalanges should be separated with no overlapping of the bones or soft tissues of the fingers. Minimal to no overlap of the ulna and the radius at the distal radioulnar joint (DRUJ) indicates lack of obliquity or rotation. Both metacarpophalangeal (MCP) and interphalangeal (IP) joint spaces should be profiled or visible if the hand and fingers are placed flat on the film cassette.

Comments This view is not adequate to measure ulnar variance because the central ray is not centered at the wrist (see Wrist: PA View (Fig. 5–29)).

Although it is not necessary to flex the elbow 90 degrees and abduct the shoulder 90 degrees, the value of routinely flexing the elbow and abducting the shoulder to 90-degree position is to obtain a standardized examination for all patients.

As mentioned in the introduction of the chapter, PA and AP views are different. The PA view is obtained when the x-ray beam passes dorsal to palmar, whereas the AP view is taken by passing the x-ray beam from palmar to dorsal (see Fig. 5–5).

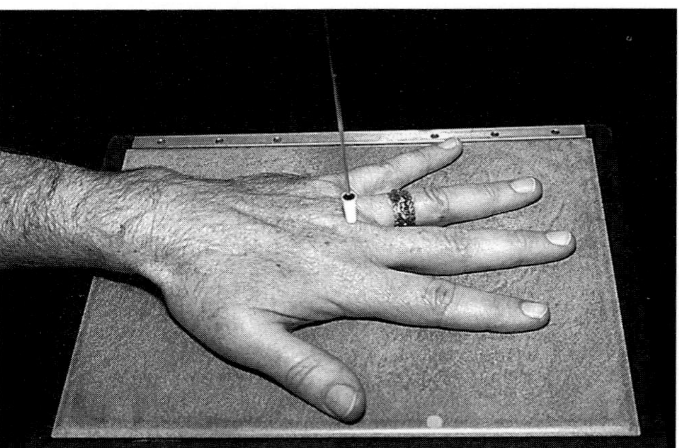

A

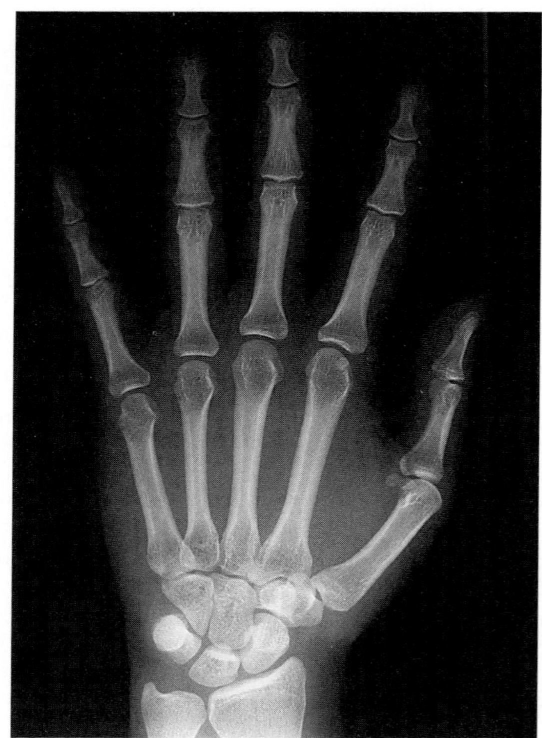

B

FIGURE 5–1. Hand: PA View

HAND: STANDARD PA OBLIQUE VIEW

Synonyms Oblique view, semipronated oblique view

Major Indications This provides a basic survey view of the hand and makes more evident the ventroradial and dorsoulnar sides of the hand and wrist bones. This view is very important for diagnosing metacarpal and phalangeal fractures[1] and can help demonstrate erosions from synovial disease. The space between the first and second metacarpals and the scaphotrapeziotrapezoidal and first carpometacarpal (CMC) joints are displayed. Other features as described for the oblique view of the wrist are also applicable to this view.

Illustration **(A) Position.** The radial side of the hand is elevated 45 degrees from the PA position and the film cassette. The fingers are kept extended to avoid foreshortening of the phalanges and are slightly spread to avoid overlapping. A 45-degree sponge block, especially one with steps, can be used to support this position without motion, especially for the fingers. **Central Beam.** The central beam is perpendicular to the cassette and is centered over the head of the third metacarpal.

(B) Criteria for an Adequate Examination. The examination should include the distal 2 to 3 cm of the distal radius and ulna, the carpus, the metacarpals, and the digits with the fingers well separated. Metacarpals should be imaged with minimal overlapping. If no overlap of metacarpal shafts is present, there is insufficient obliquity of the hand. If overlap exceeds 50% of shaft width, there is too much obliquity of the hand and a lateral view is being approximated. The MCP joint spaces should be open or seen with articular cortices in profile, or parallel, with no overlapping. The dorsal rim of the radius overlaps the ulna at the DRUJ (arrow).

Comments Since metacarpals overlap each other in a true lateral view, this view is important for evaluating metacarpal pathology, especially in trauma.

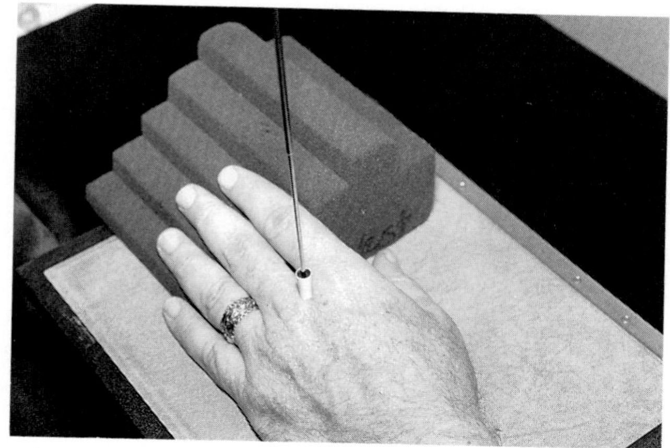

A

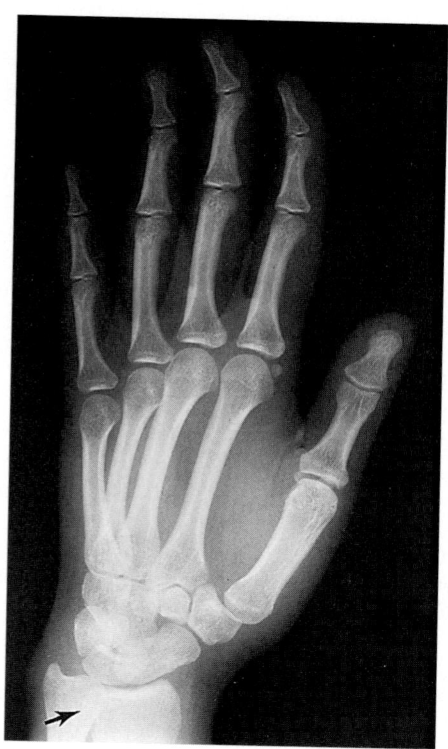

B

FIGURE 5–2. Hand: Standard PA Semipronated Oblique View

HAND: REVERSED PA OBLIQUE VIEW

Synonym Overpronated oblique view

Major Indications This view is used to provide an opposite oblique view when looking for fracture or other bone defects, such as erosions, that do not show on the standard PA oblique view. The dorsoradial and ventroulnar surfaces of the bones of the hand are profiled.[2]

Illustration **(A) Position.** The hand and wrist are overpronated with the radial side of the hand placed on the cassette, while the ulnar side of the hand is elevated 45 degrees off the cassette. The wrist is held straight without flexion or extension. A 45-degree wedge sponge can be placed under the ulnar aspect of the hand and wrist to support the hand. **Central Beam.** The central beam is perpendicular to the cassette and is centered over the head of the third metacarpal.

(B) Criteria for an Adequate Examination. With respect to the amount of hand and wrist inclusion and profile of the joints, the same criteria used for the standard PA oblique view of the hand apply. The pisiform projects more ulnar to the triquetrum (arrow) than the standard PA oblique view or the straight PA view, and the ventral concave surface of the scaphoid faces ulnarly.

Comments This view is usually a supplement to the routine or standard oblique view. When this view is used or when it is unintentionally obtained, as in the difficult-to-position traumatized hand, it is important not to confuse the projectional ulnar positioning of the pisiform for a pisotriquetral dislocation.

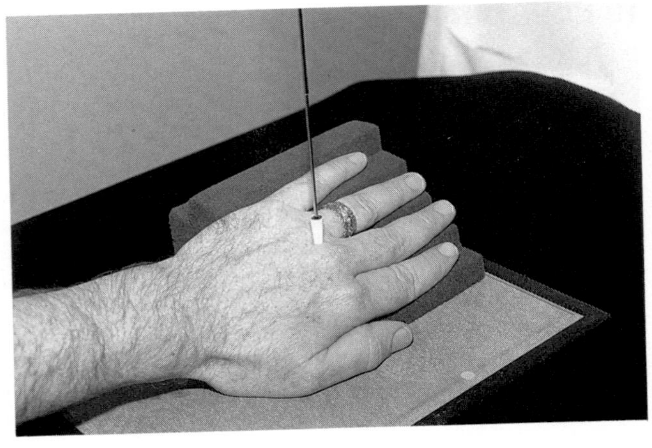

A

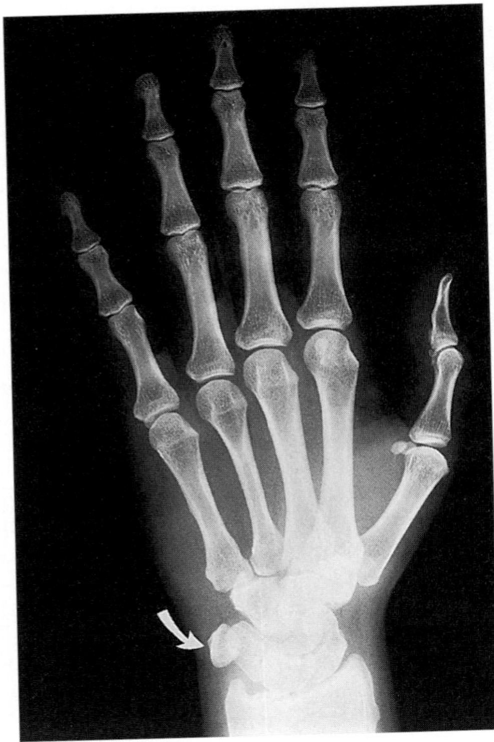

B

FIGURE 5–3. Hand: Reversed (Overpronated) PA Oblique View

HAND: LATERAL VIEW

Synonym Radioulnar view

Major Indications This is one of the basic survey views of the hand. It is excellent to show palmar and dorsal abnormalities of the soft tissues and bones such as palmar (volar) plate avulsions, fractures of the metacarpals and phalanges that may not be evident on the PA or oblique views, ventral and dorsal angulation of fracture fragments, and ventral or dorsal dislocation of the MCP and IP joints. Soft-tissue swelling is easily detected on this view. This view is also necessary to determine the exact location of foreign bodies.

Illustration **(A) Position.** The hand is in neutral position without pronation and supination. No flexion or extension should be present at the wrist. The ulnar side of the hand is in contact with the cassette with the fingers carefully spread to avoid overlap on a step wedge sponge. **Central Beam.** The central beam is perpendicular to the cassette and is centered over the head of the second metacarpal.

(B) Criteria for an Adequate Examination. The true lateral position is recognized with the metacarpals directly superimposed over each other. The distal radius and ulna are superimposed. The dorsum of the metacarpals and the radius and ulna should create a straight line (see "Comments," below).

Comments The hand and wrist should be in neutral position without flexion or extension and without ulnar or radial deviation. Malpositioning may create tilting of the lunate, which may mimic instability. The thumb is in an oblique position in this view. Slight extension at the wrist (undesirable) is present in Fig. 5–4B.

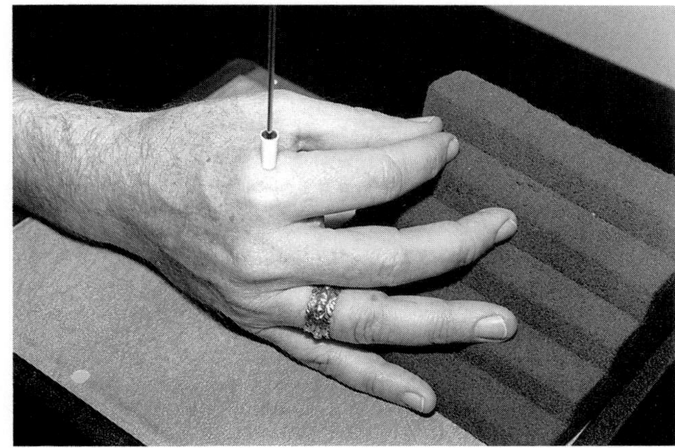

A

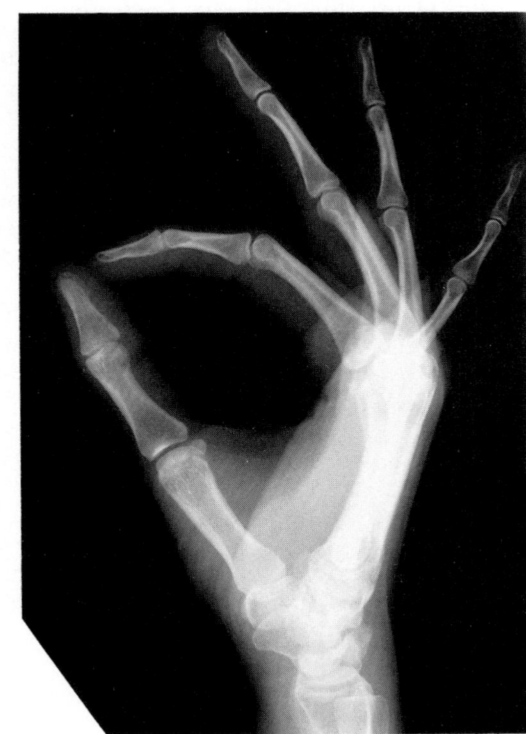

B

FIGURE 5–4. Hand: Lateral View

HAND: AP VIEW

Synonym Palmar dorsal view

Major Indications This view is used when a patient cannot pronate the forearm, such as when it is in a cast.

Illustration **(A) Position.** The dorsal aspect of the hand is placed flat on the cassette in supination. The fingers are extended and slightly spread. **Central Beam.** The central beam is perpendicular to the cassette and is centered over the head of the third metacarpal.

(B) Criteria for an Adequate Examination. The distal 2 to 3 cm of the forearm, the carpus, metacarpals, and digits should be included. The entire hand should be seen without rotation, as evidenced by the observation that the concavities of both sides of the phalangeal and metacarpal shafts are symmetric. This view should profile the CMC, MCP, and IP joint spaces. Metacarpals and phalanges should be profiled without overlapping of the bones or soft tissues of the fingers. The distal radius and ulna should be seen without obliquity or rotation.

Comments This view is not adequate to measure ulnar variance because the central ray is not centered at the wrist (see Wrist: PA View (Fig. 5–29)).

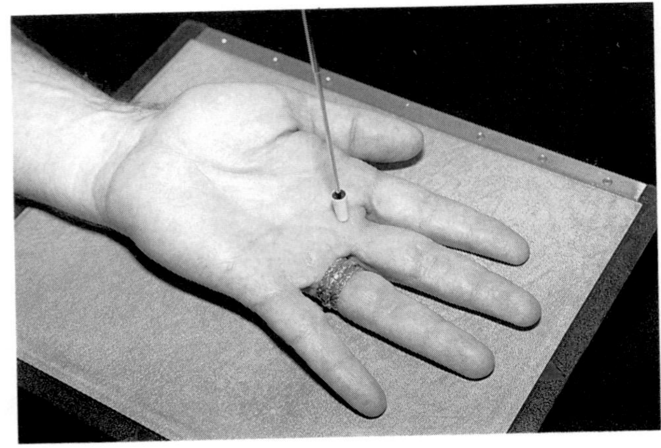

A

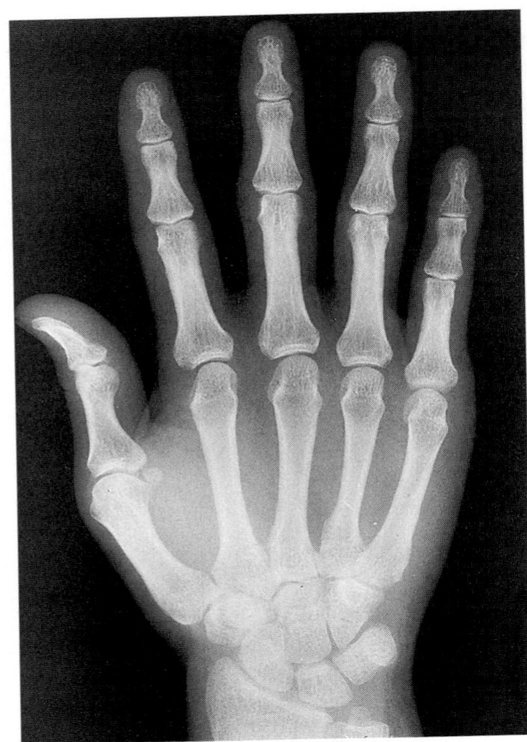

B

FIGURE 5–5. Hand: AP View

HAND: AP OBLIQUE VIEW

Synonym Semisupinated oblique view

Major Indications This view provides an additional oblique view of the hand that better profiles ventroulnar and dorsoradial sides of the phalangeal and metacarpal cortices. This also provides an additional method of performing an oblique view of the hand in the patient who cannot pronate the hand. This view may be of special value when rheumatoid arthritis is suspected.[3]

Illustration **(A) Position.** The hand is placed in 45-degree supination on the cassette. The fingers are fully extended and are slightly spread to avoid overlapping each other. **Central Beam.** The central beam is perpendicular to the cassette and is centered over the third MCP joint.

(B) Criteria for an Adequate Examination. The entire hand and wrist are included. The fingers and metacarpals should not overlap their adjacent rays. The metacarpal shafts should demonstrate more concavity on their ulnar than their radial side. The pisiform is projected ulnarly. This view is similar to the PA overpronated hand view (see Fig. 5–3B). (Reprinted with permission from Totty WG, Gilula LA. Imaging of the hand and wrist. In: Gilula LA, ed. *The traumatized hand and wrist: Radiographic and anatomic correlation.* Philadelphia: WB Saunders, 1992.)

Comments This position may be used when an oblique view is needed and the patient cannot pronate the hand to obtain the PA (semipronated) oblique view. This view is usually used when more than one finger or metacarpal is of concern. When a specific finger or metacarpal is in question, focusing on that ray will provide more structural detail.

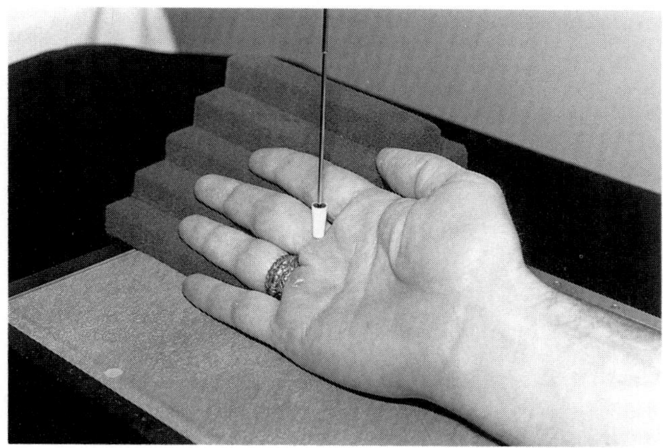

A

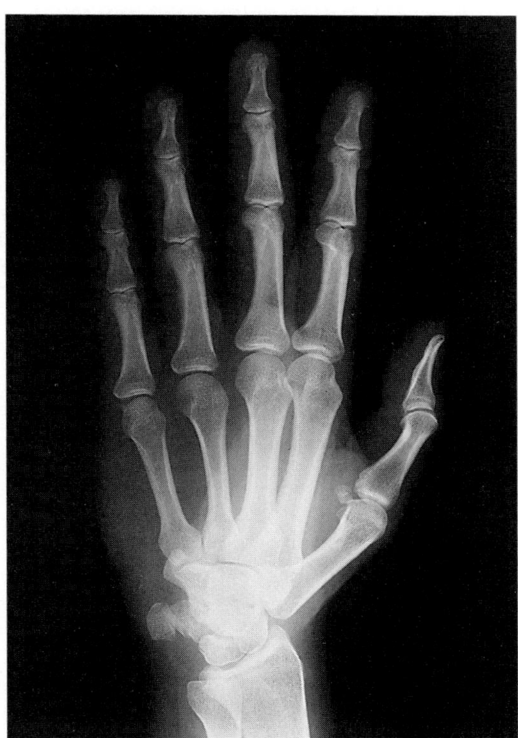

B

FIGURE 5–6. Hand: AP Oblique View

METACARPAL(S): PA VIEW

Synonym Dorsopalmar view

Major Indications This view provides a detailed profile of a specified metacarpal or metacarpals. The PA view is the basic survey examination for this area.

Illustration **(A) Position.** This view has the identical position as the hand PA view, but the field is collimated to the metacarpal(s) of interest. **Central Beam.** The central beam is perpendicular to the cassette and is centered over the midportion of the third metacarpal or over the specific metacarpal(s) of interest. The technique is adjusted to penetrate the metacarpal(s) for better detail than obtained on the hand view. Collimation reduces scatter and improves image detail.

(B) Criteria for an Adequate Examination. Both the metacarpal head and CMC joint should be included in the examination. Lack of rotation can be recognized by the observation of nearly symmetric concavities on both radial and ulnar sides of the metacarpal. Penetration should be adequate to see cortical and medullary detail of the bone.

Comments Usually this view is used when a specific metacarpal bone is strongly suspected to have an abnormality. Commonly, this view is combined with the oblique and lateral positions for a more thorough survey examination of the metacarpal.

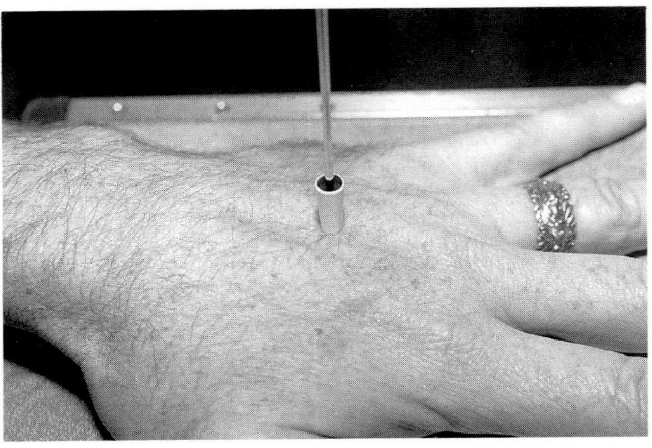

A

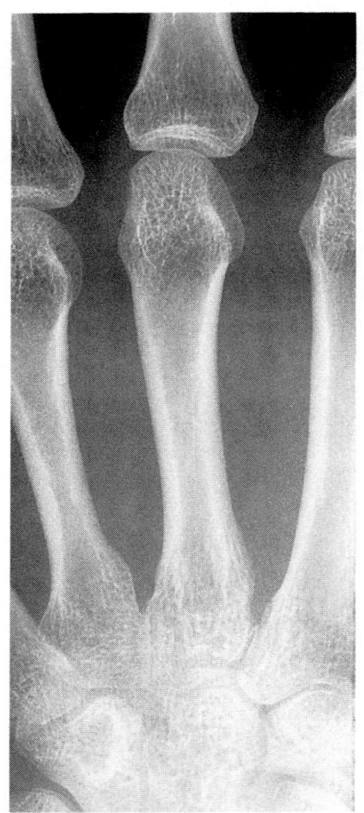

B

FIGURE 5–7. Metacarpal(s): PA View

METACARPAL(S): SEMIPRONATED OBLIQUE VIEW

Synonym Standard metacarpal PA oblique view

Major Indications This view is used when a detailed view of one or more metacarpal bones is desired. Usually this view is combined with the PA and lateral views for a more general survey examination of the metacarpal. The ventroradial and the dorsoulnar surfaces of the metacarpal(s) are demonstrated.

Illustration **(A) Position.** The positioning for this view is the same as for the standard PA oblique view of the hand. **Central Beam.** The central beam is perpendicular to the cassette and is centered over the midportion of the metacarpals between the second and third metacarpals. The technique is adjusted (usually increased) to penetrate the metacarpals for better detail than that obtained on the hand view.

(B) Criteria for an Adequate Examination. The entire metacarpal(s) (both proximal and distal ends), adjacent joints, and the cortical and medullary portions of the bone are clearly demonstrated. The concavities of the ventral surface and the straighter dorsal surface of the metacarpal are evident with minimum overlap of the adjacent metacarpals. See "Criteria for an Adequate Examination" in Hand: Standard PA Oblique View (Fig. 5–2B).

Comments This is an additional view for an individual metacarpal bone. It is usually used when a metacarpal lesion is clinically highly suspect or definite, but in need of more bony detail.

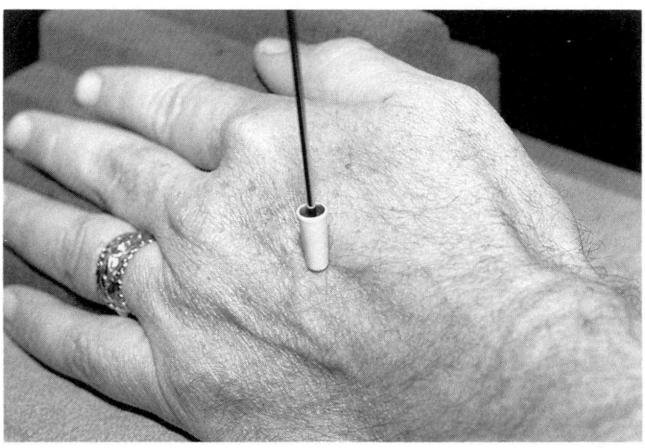

A

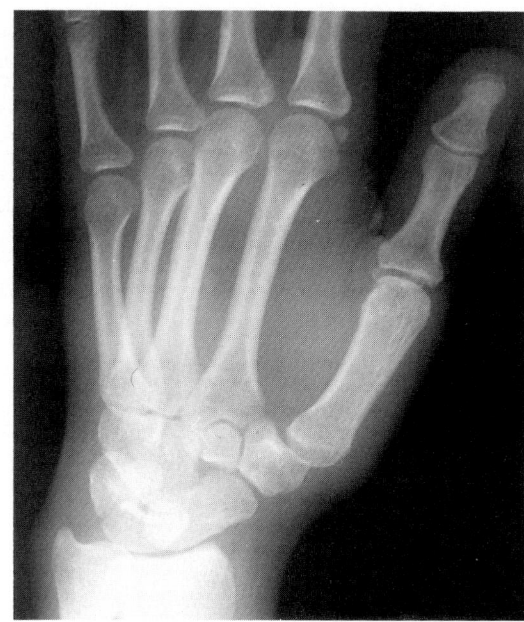

B

FIGURE 5–8. Metacarpal(s): Semipronated Oblique View

METACARPAL(S): REVERSE OBLIQUE PA VIEW

Synonym Overpronated oblique view

Major Indications Indications are the same as for the reverse oblique view of the hand, with collimation to the metacarpal(s) for greater detail.

Illustration **Position.** This position is the same as for the reversed PA oblique view of the hand. The hand and wrist are overpronated, with the radial side of the hand placed on the cassette while the ulnar side of the hand is elevated 45 degrees off the cassette. The wrist is held straight without flexion or extension. A 45-degree wedge sponge can be placed under the ulnar aspect of the hand and wrist to support the hand. **Central Beam.** The central beam is perpendicular to the cassette and is centered over the midportion of the third metacarpal or over the specific metacarpal bone examined.

Criteria for an Adequate Examination. Both the metacarpal head and CMC joint should be included in the examination. The pisiform projects more ulnar to the triquetrum than is seen in a standard PA oblique view, and the palmar concavity of the scaphoid faces ulnarly.

Comments The most common use of this position is as an opposite oblique view to locate fractures or erosions. It can also be used in those patients who cannot supinate their wrists and hands.

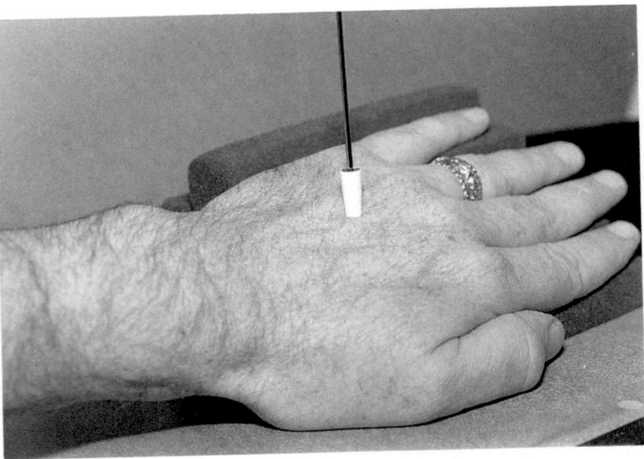

FIGURE 5–9. Metacarpal(s): Reverse Oblique (Overpronated) View

METACARPALS: LATERAL VIEW

Synonym Radioulnar view

Major Indications This view provides a right-angled view to the PA view of the metacarpals and is used when metacarpal detail is desired. Some fractures may be evident only on this view. Accurate evaluation of palmar or dorsal displacement and angulation of metacarpal fractures or other deformities and subluxation/dislocations at the MCP and CMC joints requires this view. This view is excellent for evaluation of focal swelling, especially dorsally, which can be a valuable indicator of underlying bone and/or joint pathology.

Illustration **(A) Position.** The position of the metacarpal is identical to that of the lateral view of the hand. The hand and wrist are aligned with the long axis of the radius in a neutral position without flexion or extension. The ulnar side of the hand lies on the cassette. **Central Beam.** The central beam is perpendicular to the cassette and is centered over the midportion of the second metacarpal.

(B) Criteria for an Adequate Examination. The entire metacarpal(s) should be included with the adjacent MCP and CMC joints. The four ulnar metacarpals are superimposed together. As for the lateral view of the wrist, the palmar surface of the pisiform should project halfway between the palmar surface of the distal pole of the scaphoid and the palmar surface of the head of the capitate. When the ventral surface of the pisiform projects ventral to the distal pole of the scaphoid, or when the pisiform is not seen because it is overlying the carpus, the projection is not a true lateral view.

Comments Usually, this view is combined with the PA and oblique positions for a more thorough survey examination of the metacarpal(s). This view shows overlapping of metacarpal bones but it is the best one for demonstrating palmar or dorsal soft-tissue swelling, especially dorsally. Close evaluation of the overlapping cortices of the metacarpal shaft can demonstrate subtle metacarpal fractures. Some fractures and other abnormalities appear only on the lateral view.

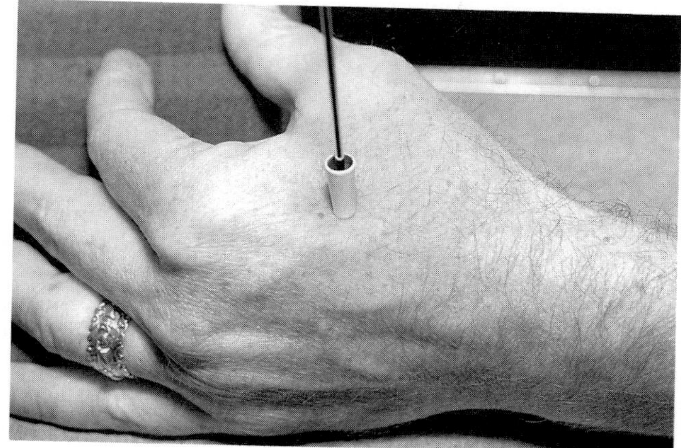

A

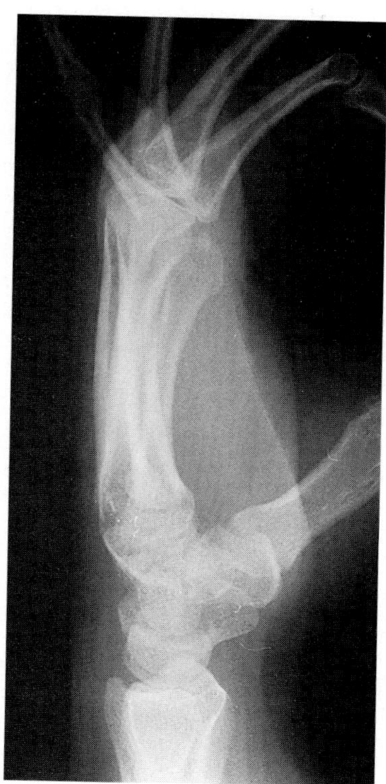

B

FIGURE 5–10. Metacarpal(s): Lateral View

METACARPAL HEADS, SECOND THROUGH FIFTH: BREWERTON'S VIEW

Synonym None

Major Indications This view is designed to demonstrate erosions of the metacarpal heads in the grooved area between the articular cartilage and the bony attachment of the MCP collateral ligaments.[4] Subtle fractures of the metacarpal head that may not be shown on routine views may also be demonstrated.[5] This view also clearly demonstrates the fourth and fifth metacarpals and hook of the hamate.[6]

Illustration **(A) Position.** The dorsum of the fingers are placed flat on the cassette with the MCP joints flexed approximately 45 degrees[7] or 65 degrees.[4,5] **Central Beam.** To prevent the metacarpal head of the index finger from being obscured by the thumb, the central beam is angled 15 to 20 degrees from the ulnar to the radial side of the hand and the thumb is fully extended.[4–6]

(B) Criteria for an Adequate Examination. The second through fifth MCP joints are profiled without any overlapping of adjacent cortical surfaces. Parallel articulating cortices of the MCP joints are clearly seen. Similarly, adjacent metacarpal heads should be separate from each other.

Comment This view is thought to be more sensitive for the demonstration of early erosions of the metacarpal heads in synovial arthritis[4] and occult fractures of the metacarpal heads.[5]

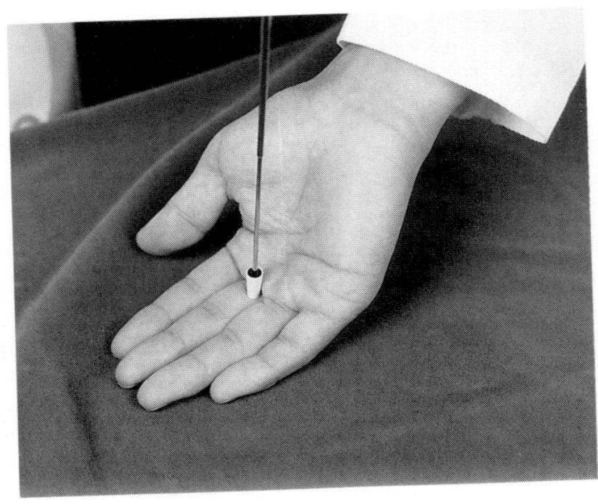

A

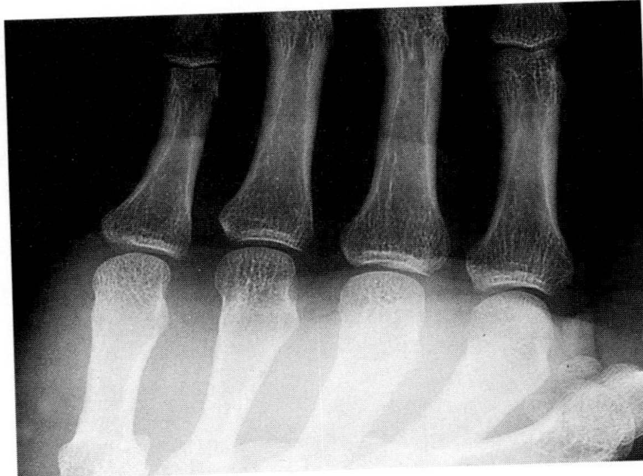

B

FIGURE 5–11. Metacarpal Heads, Second Through Fifth: Brewerton's View

FIRST METACARPAL: PA VIEW

Synonym First metacarpal dorsopalmar view

Major Indications This view provides a detailed survey examination of the first metacarpal bone.

Illustration **Position.** Normally, the transverse axis of the first metacarpal bone is palmarly rotated about 90 degrees with respect to the other metacarpal bones. To obtain a true PA view of the first metacarpal bone, place the thenar eminence on the cassette with abduction of the thumb and let the palm drop off the side of the cassette while closely observing the thumb phalanges to see that they are not rotated. **Central Beam.** The central beam is perpendicular to the cassette and is centered over the midportion of the first metacarpal. The technique is adjusted to penetrate the metacarpal for better detail than that obtained on the hand view.

Criteria for an Adequate Examination. Both the metacarpal head and CMC joint should be included in the examination. Lack of rotation can be recognized by observation of symmetric concavities on both the radial and ulnar sides of the metacarpal. Penetration should be adequate to allow observation of cortical and medullary detail of the bone.

Comment This view is used when first metacarpal pathology is suspected and the other bones are clinically normal.

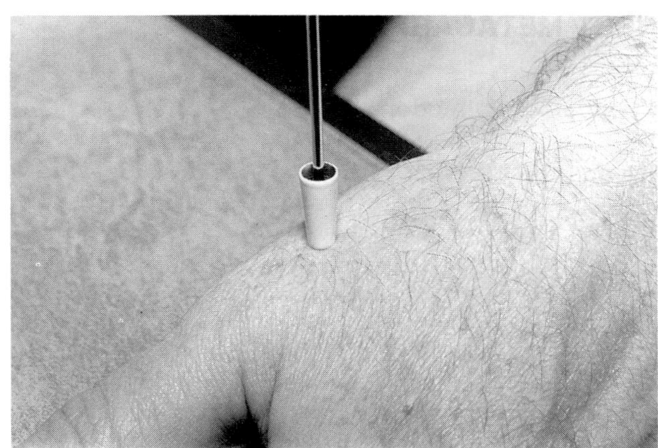

FIGURE 5–12. First Metacarpal: PA View

FINGER(S): PA OBLIQUE VIEW

Synonym Semipronated view of the finger

Major Indications This detailed view of the finger or fingers of interest provides an oblique projection with which to recognize fractures or other pathology. The dorsoulnar and the palmoradial surfaces of the finger(s) are demonstrated.

Illustration **(A) Position.** There are two ways to position the hand for this view. The first is to raise the radial side of the hand 45 degrees from PA view position so that the coronal plane of the hand and finger is positioned to make a 45-degree angle with the cassette. A 45-degree sponge may be used to support the hand and finger. The fingers are fully extended and separated from the affected finger (see Hand: Standard PA Oblique View (Fig. 5–2)). The second is to place the cassette on a 45-degree sponge and put the hand flat on the cassette with the fingers slightly spread. See the correct use of a sponge in Fig. 5–20A. **Central Beam.** The central beam is perpendicular to the cassette in the first position above, is perpendicular to the table in both positions above, and is centered to the PIP joint of the affected finger.

(B) Criteria for an Adequate Examination. The entire finger including the MCP joint, metacarpal head, and fingertip should be clearly demonstrated in the 45-degree oblique position. The IP and MCP joints should be open or visible without foreshortening of the phalanges. Radiographic quality should demonstrate both soft-tissue and bone trabecular detail. Elevating the hand and wrist 45 degrees and resting the fingers on the cassette as in **A** will usually foreshorten the phalanges and prevent obtaining good profile of the IP and MCP joints. Correct use of the 45-degree sponge to support the fingers is shown (of the opposite oblique) in Fig. 5–20.

Comments Street suggests that the internally rotated oblique view is better to show fractures of the phalanges in some instances[2] than is the routine semipronated oblique view (see Finger(s): PA Reverse Oblique View (Figs. 5–20A and 5–20B)).

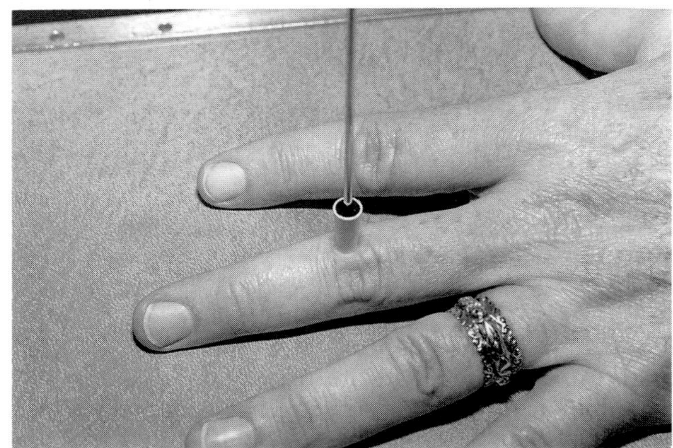

A

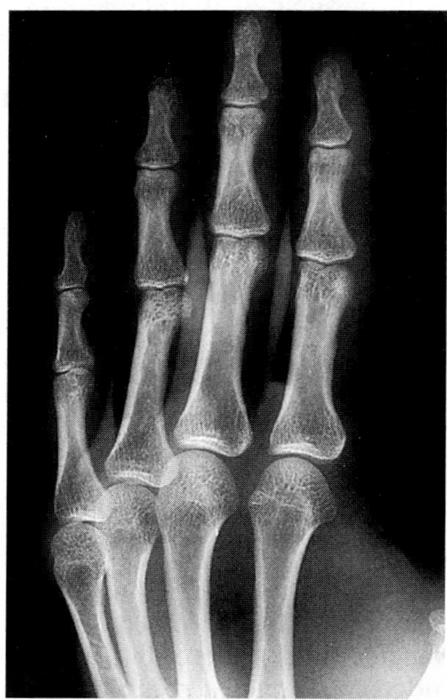

B

FIGURE 5–19. Finger(s): PA Oblique View

FINGER(S): PA REVERSE OBLIQUE VIEW

Synonyms Overpronated PA oblique view, internally rotated oblique projection[2]

Major Indications This view provides additional detail of the phalanges and soft tissues. It demonstrates the palmoulnar and dorsoradial cortices of the phalanges well. It may be used when the AP oblique view of a finger cannot be obtained.

Illustration **(A) Position.** Overpronate the hand 45 degrees from a PA view of the finger, so that the coronal plane of the hand and finger is at a 45-degree angle with the cassette. A 45-degree sponge may be used to support the hand and finger. The fingers are fully extended and separated from the affected finger. **Central Beam.** The central beam is perpendicular to the cassette and is centered at the PIP joint of the affected finger.

(B) Criteria for an Adequate Examination. The entire finger including the MCP joint, metacarpal head, and fingertip should be clearly demonstrated. The IP and MCP joints should be open or visible without foreshortening of the phalanges. This view demonstrates both soft-tissue and bone trabecular detail.

Comment This view may demonstrate some phalangeal fractures better than other finger views.[2]

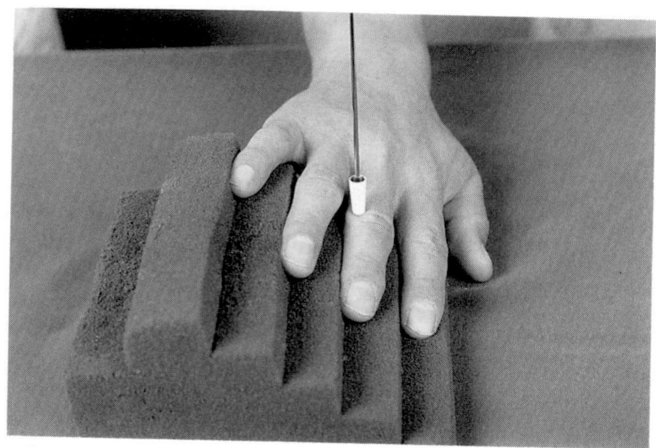

A

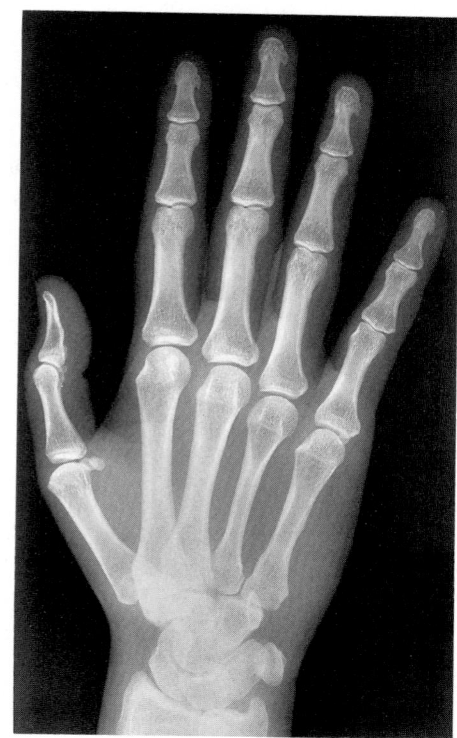

B

FIGURE 5–20. Finger(s): PA Reverse Oblique View

FINGER(S): AP OBLIQUE VIEW

Synonym Semisupinated view

Major Indications This view demonstrates the same structures as does the PA reversed oblique view of the finger(s) and may be of special value when subtle synovial lesions are suspected and when fracture is suspected but not shown on the routine semipronated oblique view. The palmoulnar and the dorsoradial surfaces of the fingers are demonstrated with this position.

Illustration **(A) Position.** The dorsal side of the fingers are placed with 45-degree supination on the cassette. A 45-degree sponge can be used to support the hand. The fingers are fully extended. **Central Beam.** The central beam is perpendicular to the cassette and centered at the PIP joint of the finger of interest.

(B) Criteria for an Adequate Examination. The entire finger(s) should be seen, including the fingertip(s), the MCP joint(s), and the metacarpal head(s). The IP and MCP joints should be profiled and open.

Comment This is an additional view for the fingers. It can be used when the reverse oblique PA view of the fingers cannot be obtained.

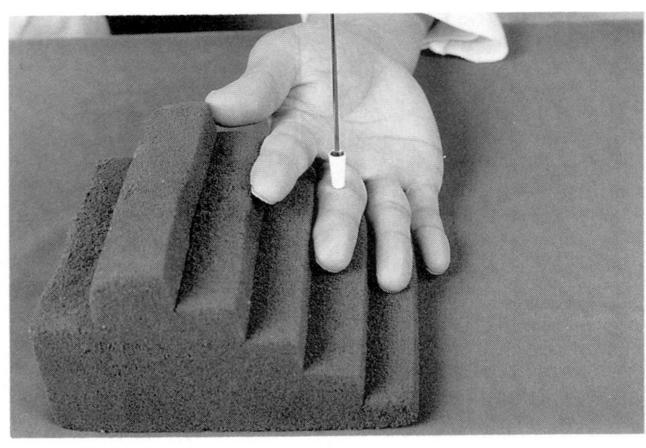

A

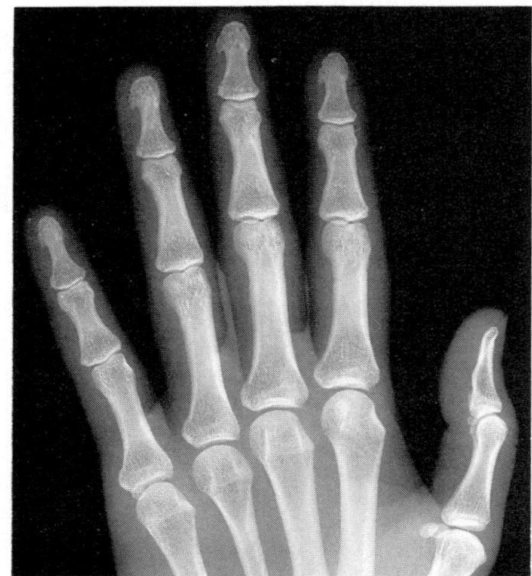

B

FIGURE 5–21. Finger(s): AP Oblique View

FINGER(S): ULNAR AND RADIAL STRESS VIEWS

Synonym None

Major Indications These views are used to demonstrate subluxation, diastasis, or abnormal deviation when MCP or IP joint instability is suspected. With these views, radial or ulnar ligament or capsule abnormality is evaluated.

Illustration **(A) Position.** The finger of interest is held in the PA or AP position by a technologist or a physician with the MCP or IP joint of interest centered on the cassette. With the thumb tip of the person applying the stress placed at the radial side of the joint, radial-directed stress is applied at the ulnar side of the finger distal to the joint of question to test the ulnar collateral ligament. **(B)** To assess the radial collateral ligament, the opposite stress is obtained with the index or long fingertip of the same hand placed at the ulnar side of the joint, and an ulnar-directed stress is applied radially on the digit distal to the joint in question. Some cooperative patients can be instructed to place the described stress on the finger in question with their opposite hand. **Central Beam.** The central beam is perpendicular to the cassette and is centered over the stressed MCP or IP joint. Comparison views of the normal side are recommended.

Criteria for an Adequate Examination. The joint should be carefully profiled and not obscured by the examiner's finger or thumb. Criteria described above to evaluate for rotation and proper positioning on the PA or AP view of the fingers without stress should be used here.

Comments Because commonly there is variation in laxity at the MCP and/or IP joints, it is worthwhile to perform similar stress views of both hands. The stress can be applied by the opposite hand of a cooperative patient, with the maximum stress tolerable applied to the relaxed digit being tested. The plain film without stress should be thoroughly evaluated before applying stress. If a fracture of a phalanx or metacarpal is present, applying stress may displace or flip the bone fragment into the joint. Therefore the presence of an intraarticular fracture is generally a contraindication to applying stress views if stress may be exerted at the joint that has the intraarticular fracture.

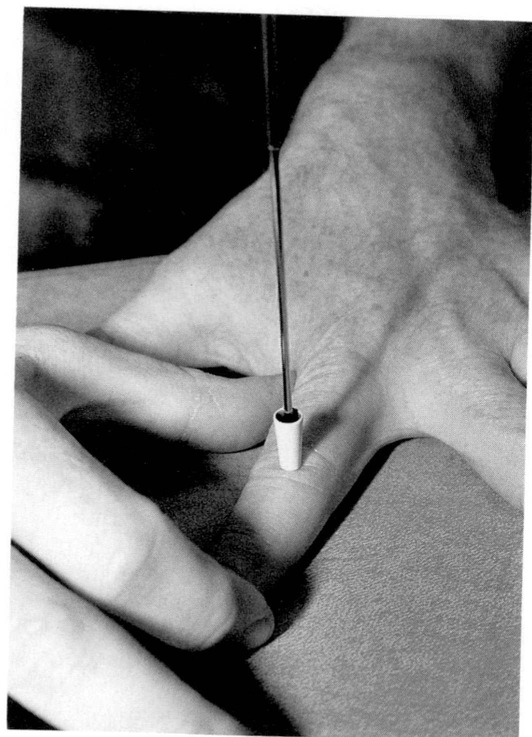

A

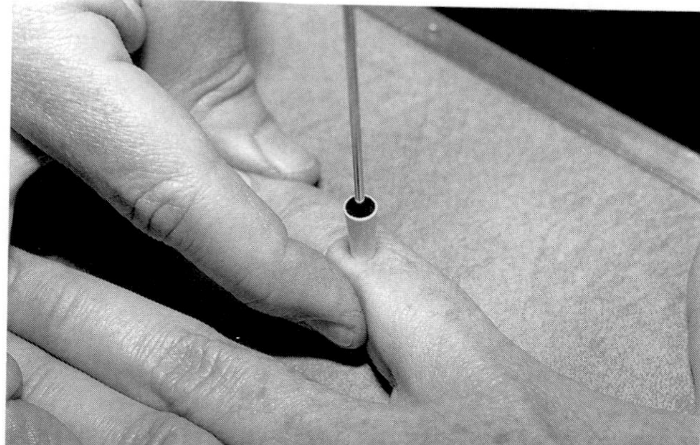

B

FIGURE 5–22. Finger(s): Ulnar and Radial Stress Views

THUMB: AP VIEW (PROFILE OF PHALANGES)

Synonym Palmodorsal view

Major Indications This view provides detailed information of the thumb when pathology is strongly suspected.

Illustration **Position.** Place the thumb in the identical position as for the AP view of the first metacarpal. The forearm is rotated internally nearly 180 degrees so that the dorsal aspect of the thumb is placed on the cassette with fingers extended. **Central Beam.** The central beam is perpendicular to the cassette and is centered on the interphalangeal joint of the thumb.

Criteria for an Adequate Examination. The entire thumb, including soft tissues from the tuft of the distal phalanx to the distal portion of the first metacarpal, should be included without rotation. Lack of rotation is evident by observation of equal concavities of both sides of the phalangeal and metacarpal shafts; the soft tissue should be equal on both sides of the bones. The distal end of the adjacent metacarpal should be seen and the IP and first MCP joints should be profiled and clearly seen.

Comments It is recommended that the technologist demonstrate the desired position with his or her own hand to ensure complete understanding and cooperation so that the patient can maintain this difficult position.[8] The patient can then adjust his or her body position. If the patient cannot tolerate the above position, a PA view can be obtained (see next view).

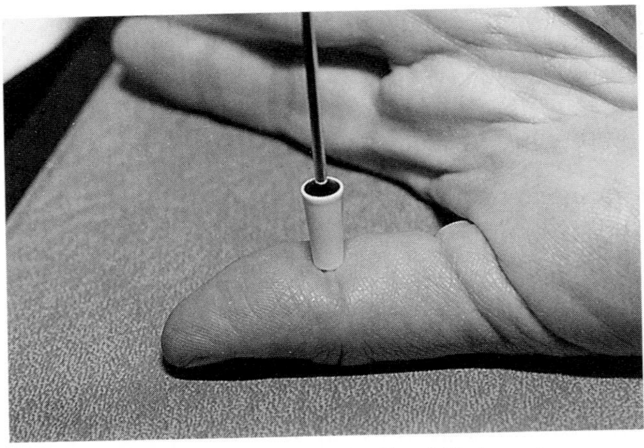

FIGURE 5–23. Thumb: AP View (Profile of Phalanges)

THUMB: PA VIEW (PROFILE OF PHALANGES)

Synonym Dorsopalmar view

Major Indications This view is usually used when the patient cannot tolerate the AP thumb view (see previous view).

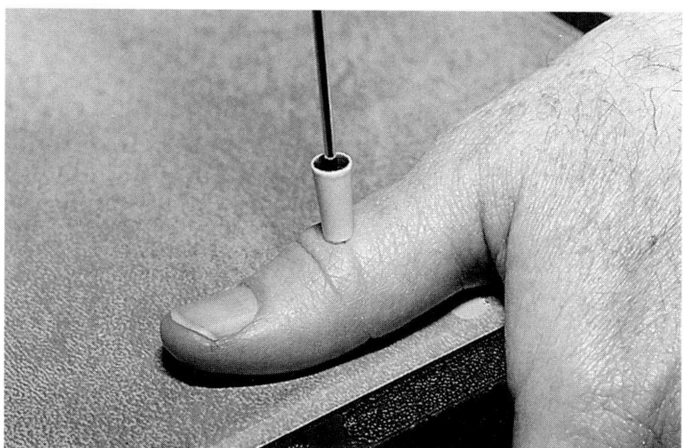

FIGURE 5–24. Thumb: PA View (Profile of Phalanges)

Illustration **Position.** This is identical to the position used for the PA view of the first metacarpal. Place the thenar eminence on the cassette with abduction of the thumb and let the palm drop off the side of the cassette. **Central Beam.** The central beam is perpendicular to the cassette and is centered on the first IP joint.

Criteria for an Adequate Examination. The entire thumb from the distal phalangeal tuft to the scaphotrapezial joint should be seen without rotation. Lack of rotation is recognized by observation of equal concavities of both sides of the phalangeal and metacarpal shafts. Normal soft tissues should be symmetric on both sides of the bones. The articulating cortices of the IP and MCP joints should be clearly profiled and parallel.

Comments In this view, the phalanges will be magnified slightly compared with the AP view because the palmar soft tissues are thicker than those of the dorsum, thus increasing the distance between the phalanges and the x-ray film.

THUMB: LATERAL VIEW

Synonym None

Major Indications This view shows the ventral and dorsal surfaces of the proximal and distal phalanges and first metacarpal bone. It also displays the IP and first MCP and CMC joints.

Illustration **(A) Position.** The forearm is overpronated so that the radial side of the thumb lies on the cassette with the thumb in a true lateral position. **Central Beam.** The central beam is perpendicular to the cassette and is centered on the first IP joint.

(B) Criteria for an Adequate Examination. The entire thumb from the distal phalangeal tuft to the scaphotrapezial joint should be in a true lateral position without rotation. Lack of rotation is recognized by observation of the concavity of ventral surfaces of the phalangeal and first metacarpal shafts with perfect overlapping of the condyles of each phalanx and the first metacarpal. However, due to the diverging x-ray beam when the entire digit is imaged, there may be a slight offset of phalangeal condyles in the proximal distal direction (arrowheads). Both the IP and first MCP joint spaces should be profiled with opposing articulating cortices parallel and not overlapping. Similarly, the radial and ulnar edges of the bases of the proximal and distal phalanges should superimpose each other. (Reprinted with permission from Totty WG, Gilula LA. Imaging of the hand and wrist. In: Gilula LA, ed. *The traumatized hand and wrist: Radiographic and anatomic correlation.* Philadelphia: WB Saunders, 1992.)

Comments The technologist should demonstrate the desired position to the patient to ensure complete understanding and cooperation so that this position can be maintained during exposure.

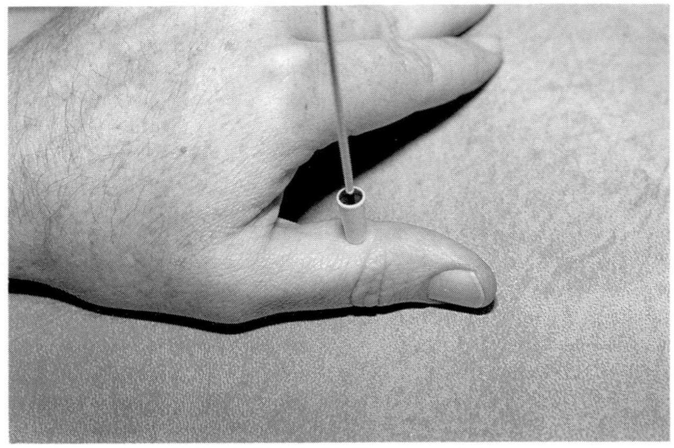

A

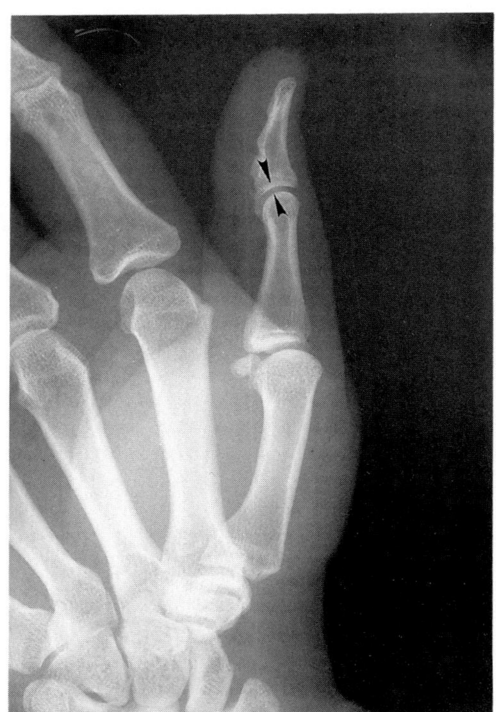

B

FIGURE 5–25. Thumb: Lateral View

THUMB: AP VIEW (PROFILE OF PHALANGES AND METACARPAL)

Synonym None

Major Indications This view may be of special value when subtle synovial lesions and/or fracture are suspected. The AP view is most commonly used when the PA view cannot be obtained. It is a basic survey frontal view of the thumb.

Illustration **Position.** The hand is overpronated with the dorsal surface of the thumb placed on the cassette with fingers extended and the fingers and thumb spread apart as much as possible. **Central Beam.** The central beam is perpendicular to the cassette and is centered on the first MCP joint.

Criteria for an Adequate Examination. The entire thumb should be included from its distal tip to the scaphotrapezial joint. Demonstration of the first MCP joint should be present without overlapping of adjacent cortical surfaces. The trapezium should be well profiled.

Comments Burman described this position for use with the MCP joint and suggested that this be used as a supplemental view when the wrist can be extended.[11]

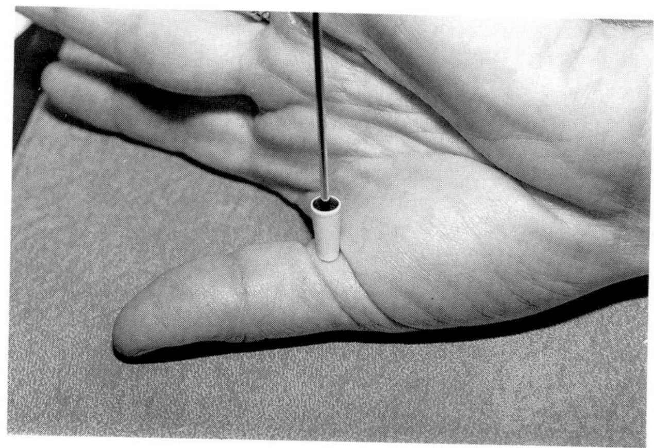

FIGURE 5–26. Thumb: AP View (Profile of Phalanges and Metacarpal)

THUMB: PA VIEW (PROFILE OF PHALANGES AND METACARPAL)

Synonym Dorsopalmar view

Major Indications This view is usually used when the patient cannot tolerate the AP thumb view (see previous view).

Illustration **Position.** The thumb is placed without rotation with the thenar eminence on the side of the cassette. The entire thumb with its first metacarpal should be included on the cassette. **Central Beam.** The central beam is perpendicular to the cassette and is centered on the first MCP joint.

Criteria for an Adequate Examination. The entire thumb from its distal tip to the scaphotrapezial joint should be seen without rotation. Lack of rotation is recognized by observation of equal concavities of both sides of the phalangeal and metacarpal shafts; the soft tissues should be symmetric on both sides of the bones. Articulating cortices of the IP and first MCP joints should be clearly profiled and parallel.

Comments This projection provides an alternative approach to obtain a frontal view of the thumb when an AP view cannot be obtained. A frontal projection should be included as a basic view for evaluation of the thumb.

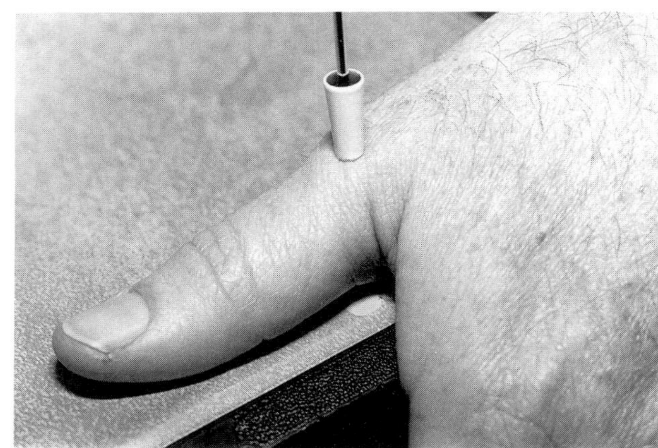

FIGURE 5–27. Thumb: PA View (Profile of Phalanges and Metacarpal)

THUMB: ULNAR AND RADIAL STRESS VIEWS FOR FIRST MCP OR IP JOINT

Synonym None

Major Indications When first MCP or IP joint instability is suspected, stress views are used to demonstrate subluxation, diastasis, or abnormal deviation. Stress views evaluate for radial or ulnar collateral ligament or capsule abnormality.[12]

Illustration **Position.** The thumb is held in the PA or AP position by a technologist or a physician with the MCP joint centered on the cassette. The following descriptions are for AP positions. With PA positions of the thumb, opposite positions of stressing fingers and thumbs would be used. **Stress to test ulnar-sided soft-tissue structures: (A)** With one thumb tip of the person applying the stress placed at the radial side of the MCP or IP joint in question, radial-directed stress is applied distally at the ulnar side of the digit to test the ulnar collateral ligament of the joint in question. Alternatively, this same stress can be applied with one hand by placing the index or long fingertip on the radial side of the joint in question and applying a radially directed stress with the thumb placed distal to the joint to be stressed. **Stress to test radial-sided soft-tissue structures:** The opposite stress is exerted to test the radial collateral ligament. With the thumb tip of the same hand placed at the ulnar side of the first MCP or IP joint, an ulnar-directed stress is applied at the radial side of the thumb distal to the joint to be tested **(B, C)**. **Central Beam.** The central beam is perpendicular to the cassette and is centered over the stressed first MCP or IP joint. Comparison views of the normal side are recommended.

Criteria for an Adequate Examination. The MCP joint should be carefully profiled and not obscured by the examiner's finger or thumb. Criteria described above for evaluation of the AP or PA view of the thumb without stress should be used here.

Comments Because commonly there is variation in laxity at the MCP joint, it is worthwhile to perform similar stress views of both thumbs. The stress can be applied by the opposite hand of a cooperative patient, and the maximum stress tolerable to the cooperative patient should be applied. A routine radiograph without stress should be carefully evaluated before applying stress. If a fracture from a phalanx or metacarpal head is present, applying stress may displace or even flip the bone fragment into the MCP joint and change a nonoperative case into an operative one. The presence of an intraarticular fracture is generally a contraindication to applying stress views at the joint.

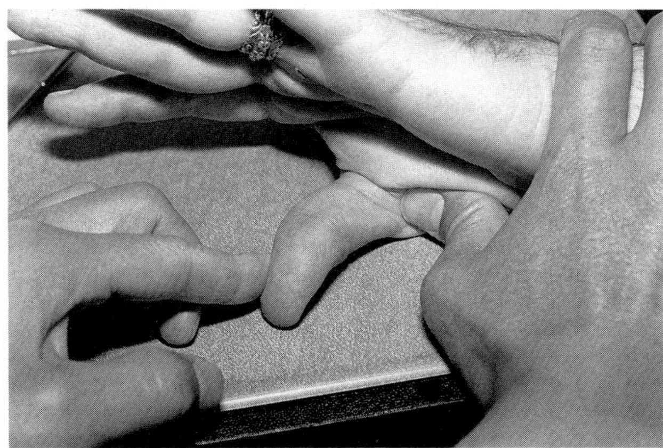

A

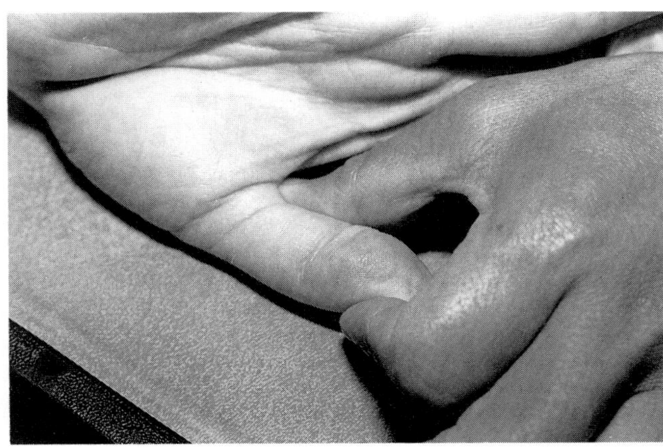

B

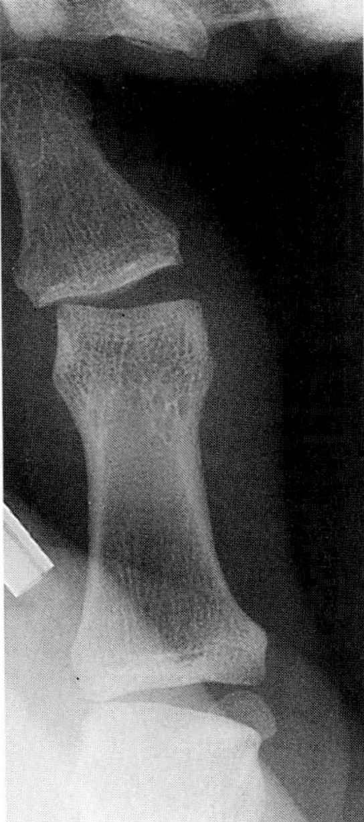

C

FIGURE 5–28. Thumb: Ulnar and Radial Stress Views for First MCP or IP Joint

RADIOGRAPHIC POSITIONS FOR THE WRIST

We suggest that the minimal survey examination for the wrist should include four views: PA, ulnar-deviated PA, semipronated oblique, and lateral views. These four views can be obtained as four exposures on a single film. Many other views for the wrist can be performed, and the following views represent the great majority of the recognized ones. An additional valuable technique not discussed here is the use of fluoroscopic spot views or fluoroscopically directed views. Using the fluoroscope, a specific structure, cortical surface, or fracture line can be more precisely located for fluoroscopic spot views or to position the part in question carefully for overhead views.

WRIST: PA VIEW

Synonym Dorsopalmar view

Major Indications A basic overview of the carpal bones and their connecting bones is best performed with this view. It is used to analyze the three carpal arcs (see Chapter 11) and obtain an overall interpretation of the interrelationship and status of the wrist bones. Ulnar variance is determined on this view. This is one of the four basic survey views for the wrist.

Illustration **(A) Position.** Because the various elbow and shoulder positions affect the relationship between the distal radius and ulna, the standard PA view should be obtained with the elbow flexed 90 degrees and the shoulder abducted 90 degrees. The pronated hand is placed palm flat on the cassette without any flexion, extension, or deviation. The fingers are extended. **Central Beam.** The central beam is perpendicular to the cassette and is centered to the capitate head.

(continued)

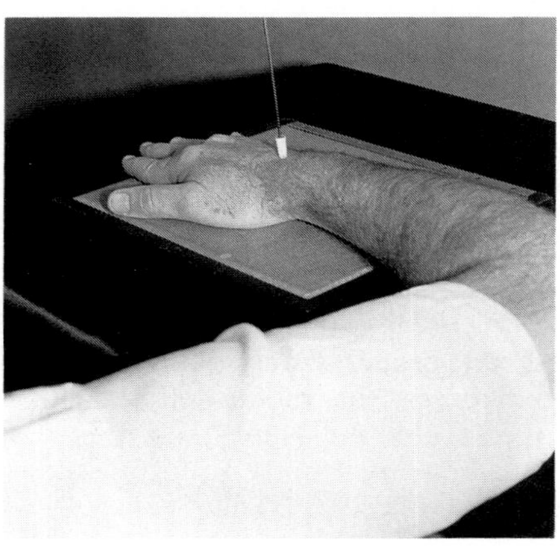

A

FIGURE 5–29. Wrist: PA View

WRIST: PA VIEW (Continued)

(B) Criteria for an Adequate Examination. The standard PA wrist radiograph should include the entire DRUJ with its adjacent radius and ulna, whole carpus, and proximal part of the metacarpals. Metacarpal shafts should be separated without overlap. Lack of rotation is proved by observation of symmetric concavities of both sides of the metacarpal shafts. Collinear alignment of the central axis of the third metacarpal shaft with the mid axis of the radius indicates that there is no radial or ulnar deviation. The second through fifth CMC joints should be evident by recognizing parallel articular cortices at these joints. If profiled, opposing cortices of the scapholunate and lunotriquetral joints should be parallel or demonstrate a clear space; however, commonly one or both of these joints will not be profiled on the routine PA view of the wrist. To recognize the fact that the elbow is at shoulder height, see that the edge (arrowhead **B**) or the entire groove of the extensor carpi ulnaris (ECU) tendon is at or radial to the fovea (white arrow) at the base of the ulnar styloid. See "Comments," below.

Comments This view is from the dorsal direction looking through the hand to the palm. This is not the same as the AP view. Perfect profiling of the scapholunate and/or lunotriquetral joints usually requires fluoroscopic positioning and "spot" radiographs of each joint separately. If the groove of the ECU tendon overlaps the ulnar styloid, this usually means that the elbow is lower than shoulder height; the more the groove overlaps, the lower the elbow will be with respect to shoulder height. We believe that ulnar variance measurements should not be made on a PA view of the wrist unless the ECU groove is in the proper place, since adducting the elbow toward the patient's side will make the ulna become more positive. When treatment decisions are based on the presence of an ulnar-positive or -negative variant, such position variation can potentially change the approach to a wrist problem.

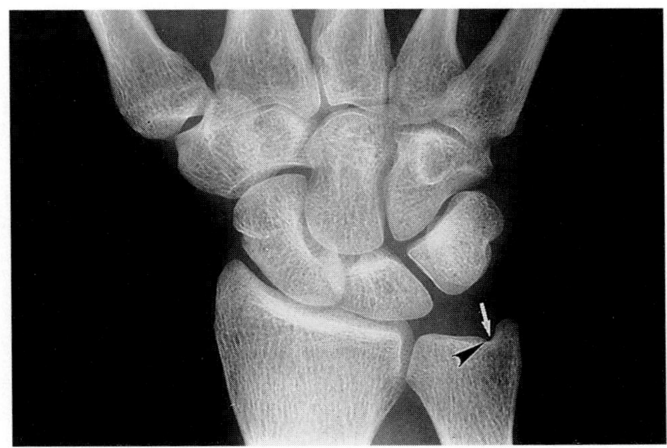

B

FIGURE 5–29. *Continued* Wrist: PA View

WRIST: LATERAL VIEW

Synonyms Neutral lateral view, standard lateral view

Major Indications This is one of the basic wrist views. It is the best view to determine palmar or dorsal displacement and angulation of fracture fragments and dislocations of the distal radius and ulna, some carpal bones, and metacarpal bones. Dorsal and ventral chip fractures or calcifications can often be seen only on this view. The scapholunate, radiolunate, capitolunate, radioscaphoid, and other intercarpal angles are best determined on this neutral lateral view.

Illustration **(A) Position.** At least two methods are available to obtain this view. One is taken with the elbow flexed 90 degrees and adducted against the trunk; a vertical x-ray beam enters radially and exits ulnarly **(A)**. The other has the elbow abducted to the level of the shoulder with a horizontal beam entering radially and exiting ulnarly. When viewed by the technologist from the dorsum of the hand and wrist, the forearm should create a straight line and the long axis of the third metacarpal should be coaxial (parallel) with the long axis of the radius. The ulnar side of the wrist is placed on the cassette with the transverse axis of the carpus perpendicular to the cassette. **Central Beam.** The central beam is perpendicular to the cassette and is centered to the distal pole of the scaphoid. The beam enters radially and exits ulnarly.

(continued)

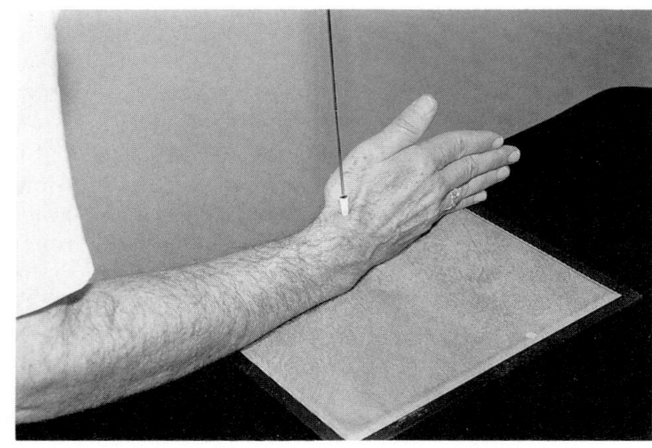

A

FIGURE 5–30. Wrist: Lateral View

WRIST: LATERAL VIEW (Continued)

(B) Criteria for an Adequate Examination. This view should include distal 3 to 5 cm of the radius and ulna, the proximal and distal rows of carpal bones, and the proximal one fourth to one half of the metacarpal shafts. A correct position of the examination shows the palmar surface of the pisiform (white arrow) located at the midpoint between the palmar pole of the scaphoid (ventral end of the double-headed black arrow) and palmar surface of the capitate head (dorsal end of double-headed black arrow). The long axis of the third metacarpal should be coaxial (parallel) with the long axis of the radius. The ulnar styloid should project over the ulnar head and should not demonstrate a fovea at its base. If the ulnar styloid has the same relationship with the ulnar head on both the PA and lateral views, the amount of abduction of the hand was not changed between these two views. Thus, one of the two views was performed incorrectly, and true right-angled views of the ulnar head are not present for evaluation.

Comments Given the wide range of dorsal curvature of the distal ulna in normal wrists, evaluation of the position of ulnar head with respect to the dorsal surface of the radius is not an adequate standard to determine if the lateral projection is correctly positioned.[13] Aligning a radial-sided structure, the ventral surface of the distal pole of the scaphoid, to an ulnar-sided structure, the ventral surface of the pisiform, is an easy and more exact way to check alignment than lining up the dorsal surfaces of the radius and ulna. Using two relatively small surfaces of the pisiform and scaphoid for alignment is more effective than using the broad surface of the radius to line up with the ulna. If the pisiform projects ventral to the distal pole of the scaphoid, the wrist is in slight supination and it is not uncommon that the lunate will falsely appear abnormally dorsally tilted. If none of the pisiform is evident on the lateral view, this would indicate at least a subtle pronation position of the wrist.

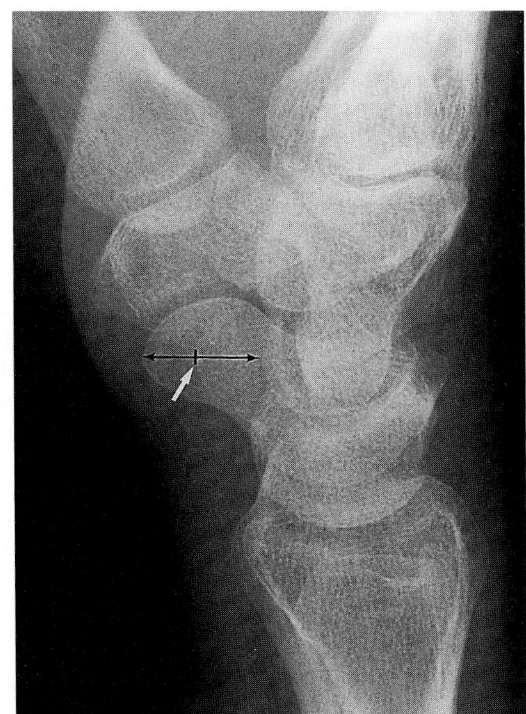

B

FIGURE 5–30. *Continued* Wrist: Lateral View

WRIST: AP VIEW

Synonym Palmodorsal view

Major Indications This view is often obtained in those patients unable to adequately pronate their forearms. The AP view can be used to demonstrate the scapholunate and lunotriquetral carpal interspaces, because these joints are commonly demonstrated in this position (see Fig. 5–33B) better than in the PA position. Other indications mentioned previously for the PA wrist view are also applicable to the AP view of the wrist.

Illustration **(A) Position.** The dorsum of the hand and wrist are flat when contacting the cassette. No extension or flexion of the wrist is present.[10] **Central Beam.** The central beam is perpendicular to the cassette and is centered over the head of the capitate. The beam enters palmarly and exits dorsally.

(B) Criteria for an Adequate Examination. These are the same as with the PA wrist view except that the ulnar styloid projects over the ulnar head. Neither the extensor carpi ulnaris (ECU) groove or the fossa at the base of the ulnar styloid are evident.

Comments Compared with the PA view, on the AP view the apparent spaces between the carpal bones are wider, but this is just because the joints may be much better profiled without overlapping bone structures, rather than true widening of the individual joints. This position is generally easier for the patient with a forearm cast to assume. Recognition of the ulnar styloid position with respect to the ulnar head will usually tell the observer if the wrist image is AP or PA.

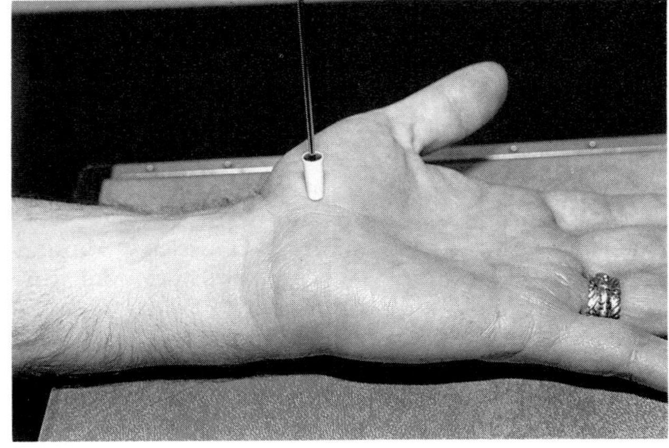

A

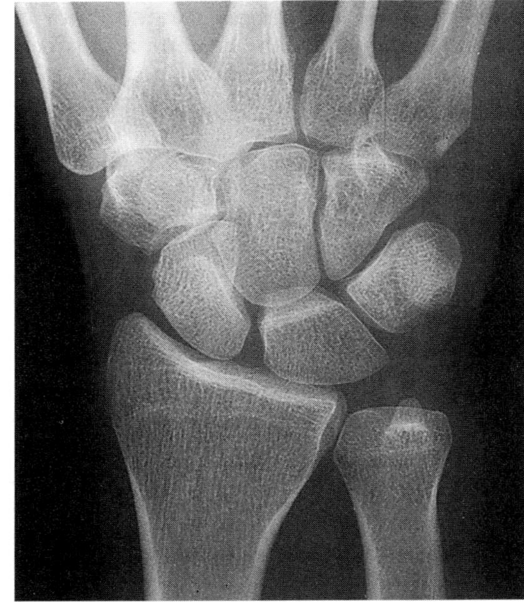

B

FIGURE 5–33. Wrist: AP View

WRIST: LATERAL EXTENSION VIEW

Synonym None

Major Indications In normal wrists, this view demonstrates extension at the radiocarpal and midcarpal joints (see Figure 5–34B). In abnormal wrists, however, abnormal rotation or translation may be evident at either or both the radiocarpal and midcarpal joints. To be more explicit, in the patient with a configuration of dorsiflexion (DISI) or palmar-flexion (VISI) instability pattern, which may be a normal variant or abnormal condition, failure of extension of the capitate (representing the distal carpal row) with respect to the lunate and/or failure of extension of the lunate (representing the proximal carpal row) with respect to the radius (representing the forearm) supports the presence of a true instability and not a normal variant. This view is important when combined with a lateral flexion view, and these two views are an important part of the wrist instability series. See Wrist: Lateral Flexion View, next (Fig. 5–35).

Illustration **(A) Position.** The wrist is placed on the cassette just as it is for the lateral view and then is maximally extended. **Central Beam.** The central beam is perpendicular to the cassette and is centered to the waist of the scaphoid.

(B) Criteria for an Adequate Examination. This view should include the distal radius and ulna, carpus, and proximal portions of the metacarpal shafts. The distal radius and ulna are superimposed as well as the four ulnar-sided metacarpals. Extension of the wrist is recognized by observation of the long axis of the third metacarpal extended dorsally with respect to the long axis of radius and ulna. Just as for the neutral lateral view of the wrist, the ventral surface of the pisiform (arrowheads, **B**) should lie midway between the ventral surface of the head of the capitate (black arrow) and the ventral surface of the distal pole of the scaphoid (white arrow).

Comments In our opinion, this view usually is one of the basic views of the wrist instability series. Unlike the lateral flexion view that follows, the pisiform, which is in the flexor carpi ulnaris tendon, remains closely apposed to the triquetrum and therefore will project over the scaphoid as in the neutral lateral view.

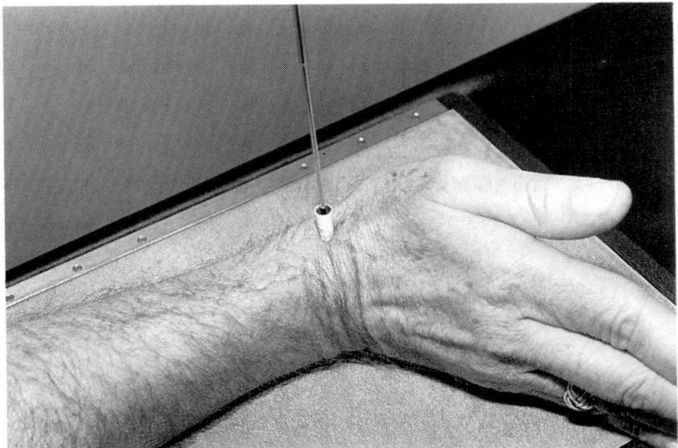

A

B

FIGURE 5–34. Wrist: Lateral Extension View

WRIST: LATERAL FLEXION VIEW

Synonym None

Major Indications The major value of this view is to show flexion of the carpus at the radiocarpal and midcarpal joints to separate the normal configurations of DISI and VISI from true DISI and VISI instability conditions.[16] This view also may show a carpal boss, which when present is a small bony growth occurring dorsally at the third CMC joint.[17] Actually the dorsal or carpal boss view, which is presented later, is a more valuable view to show this bony growth, which is an attached or separate piece of bone.

Illustration **(A) Position.** The wrist is placed on the cassette just as it is in a neutral lateral view and then is maximally flexed. **Central Beam.** The central beam is perpendicular to the cassette and is centered to the scaphoid waist.

(B) Criteria for an Adequate Examination. This view should include the distal radius and ulna, carpus, and the proximal portions of the metacarpal shafts. The distal radius and ulna are superimposed in a similar fashion as in the extension view, as are the four ulnar metacarpals. Since the pisiform is in the flexor carpi ulnaris tendon, which may move away from the triquetrum on flexion, the pisiform (arrow) may normally project anterior to the scaphoid. Flexion of the wrist is recognized by observation of the long axis of the third metacarpal flexed palmarly with respect to the long axis of the radius and ulna.

Comments In our opinion, this view is an important basic view of the instability series. See "Comments" in Wrist: Lateral Extension View (Fig. 5–34); they also apply to the flexion view.

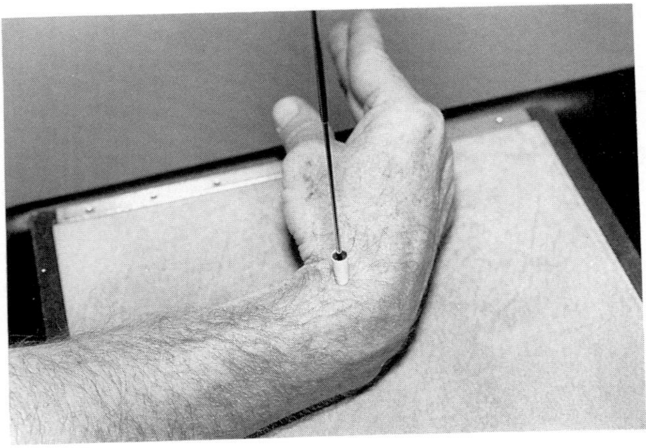

A

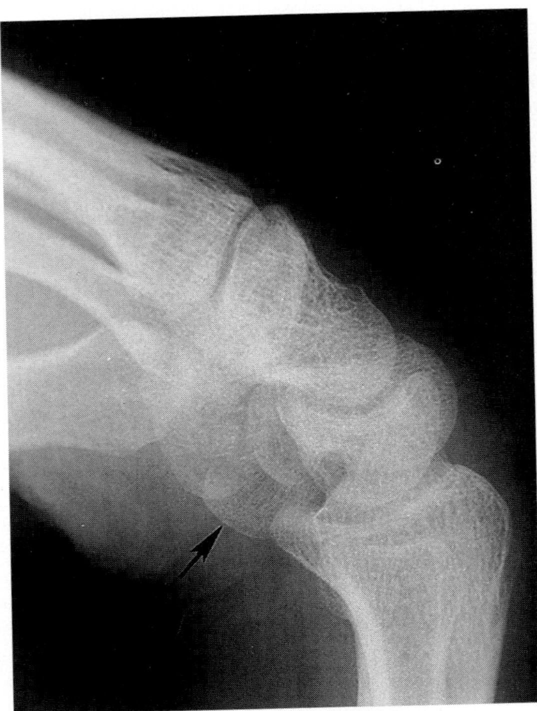

B

FIGURE 5–35. Wrist: Lateral Flexion View

WRIST: PA RADIAL DEVIATION VIEW

Synonym Pronated radial deviation view

Major Indications This view is usually performed as part of a motion study to determine motion between the forearm and the carpus and between the proximal and distal carpal rows. Ulnar-sided carpal interspaces may be better demonstrated in this position (see Fig. 5–36B). An additional view of the carpal bones in the PA position is provided, which may show an abnormality not displayed on the routine PA neutral view.

Illustration **(A) Position.** Place the hand and wrist as described in the standard PA neutral view and then move the wrist and hand into maximal radial deviation. **Central Beam.** The central beam is perpendicular to the cassette and is centered to the capitate head.

(B) Criteria for an Adequate Examination. This view should include the distal radius and ulna, carpus, and proximal part of metacarpal shafts. Radial deviation of the wrist is recognized by observation of the long axis of the third metacarpal deviated radially with respect to the long axes of the radius and ulna. Usually the scaphoid is foreshortened. Lack of rotation is supported by seeing the pisiform remain over the triquetrum and the ventral and dorsal lips of the radius at the DRUJ superimposed or separated by only a few millimeters. Presence of parallel articular cortices at the second through fifth CMC joints indicates that the palm is flat on the cassette or table without wrist extension.

Comments As one basic view of the wrist instability series, motion of the distal carpal row with respect to the proximal row can easily be evaluated by looking at the ulnar edges of the capitate and lunate and comparing these with the alignment of the same two edges on the neutral view. Similarly, motion between the proximal carpal row and radius can be assessed by comparing positions of the ulnar edges of the lunate and radius on this and the neutral PA views.

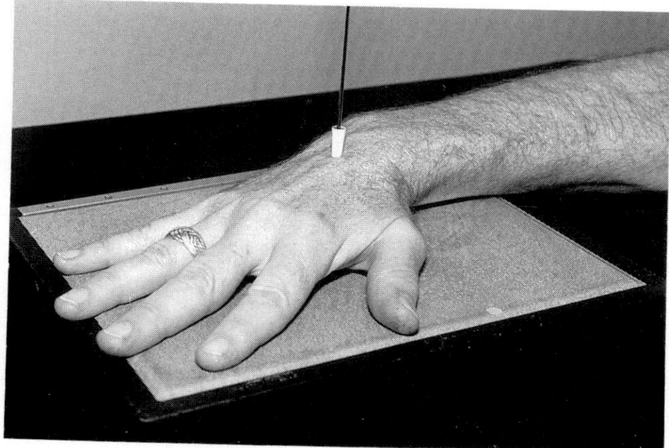

A

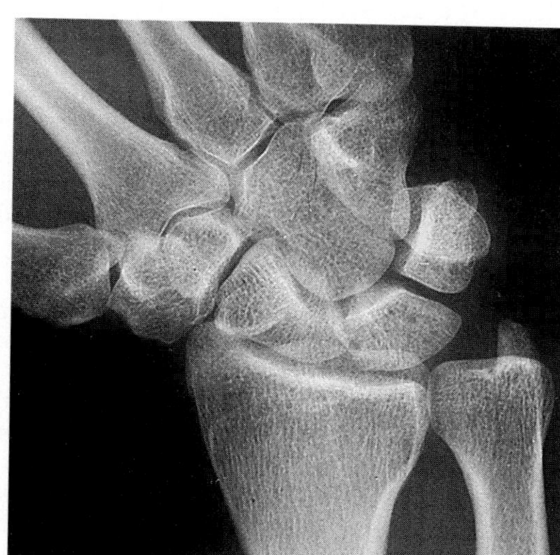

B

FIGURE 5–36. Wrist: PA Radial Deviation View

WRIST: AP RADIAL DEVIATION VIEW

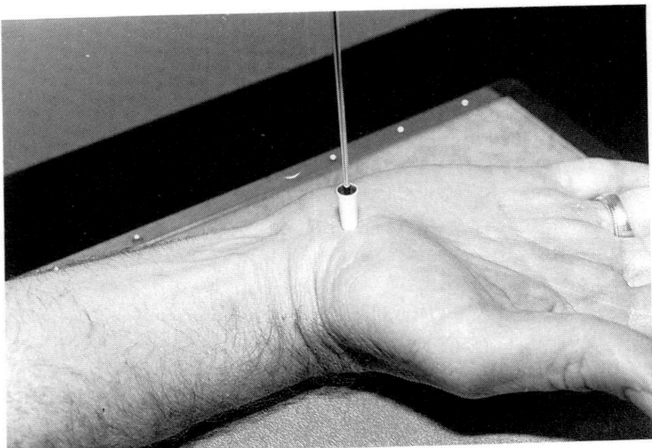

FIGURE 5-37. Wrist: AP Radial Deviation View

Synonym Supinated radial deviation view

Major Indications This view is usually one of the projections in a motion study, or instability study, to determine intercarpal and radiocarpal motion. It may also be used when the patient cannot pronate his or her wrist. The ulnar side of the carpal interspaces may be opened wider and thus better demonstrated in this position.[8]

Illustration **Position.** Place the hand and wrist flat on the cassette as described in the AP wrist view, then deviate the wrist and hand into maximal radial deviation. **Central Beam.** The central beam is perpendicular to the cassette and is centered to the head of the capitate.

Criteria for an Adequate Examination. The distal radius and ulna, entire carpus, and proximal part of metacarpal shafts should be included. Radial deviation of the wrist is recognized by observation of the long axis of the third metacarpal deviated radially with respect to the long axes of the radius and ulna.[8] Lack of rotation is identified by seeing minimal distance (1 to 3 or 4 mm) projected between the dorsal and ventral ulnar edges of the radius.

Comments With any deviation, flexion, or extension view, it usually is not possible to tell if maximal deviation, flexion, or extension was obtained by looking at a radiograph. Only by performing the maneuver is it possible to be certain that maximal motion was obtained. As mentioned previously, radiocarpal motion is recognized by looking at the ulnar edges of the radius and lunate, and midcarpal motion is seen by looking at the ulnar edge of the lunate and capitate while comparing the appearance on this view with that on the neutral or ulnar-deviated view.

WRIST: AP ULNAR DEVIATION VIEW

Synonyms Palmodorsal ulnar-deviated view, supinated ulnar-deviated view

Major Indications This view is usually used for those patients who cannot pronate their forearms. The major value of this view is to see radial/ulnar motion at the midcarpal and radiocarpal joints. In some cases this view will open the radial-sided carpal interspaces. The scaphoid is elongated with ulnar deviation, which allows better evaluation of the waist of the scaphoid for fractures or other pathology.

Illustration **Position.** The dorsal surface of the wrist is placed on the cassette as for an AP wrist view without wrist extension or flexion and then the wrist is placed into maximal ulnar deviation. **Central Beam.** The central beam is perpendicular to the cassette and is centered to the head of capitate.

Criteria for an Adequate Examination. This view should include the distal radius and ulna, the carpus, and proximal part of metacarpals. Ulnar deviation of the wrist is evident by observation of the long axis of the third metacarpal deviated ulnarly with respect to the long axes of the radius and ulna.[8] Lack of or minimal deviation of the wrist is evaluated as mentioned above under "Criteria for an Adequate Examination" in Wrist: AP Radial Deviation View (Fig. 5–37).

Comments This usually is one view of the basic instability series. Elongation of the scaphoid with minimal distortion (foreshortening) and more opening of the radial-sided carpal interspaces[8,14] occurs with this view. There may be better profile of the scapholunate and lunotriquetral joints on the AP rather than the PA view as described for other previous views. With the ulnar-deviated view, prominent widening of the scaphotrapezial joint sometimes takes place; as of yet no significance of this finding is known by these authors.

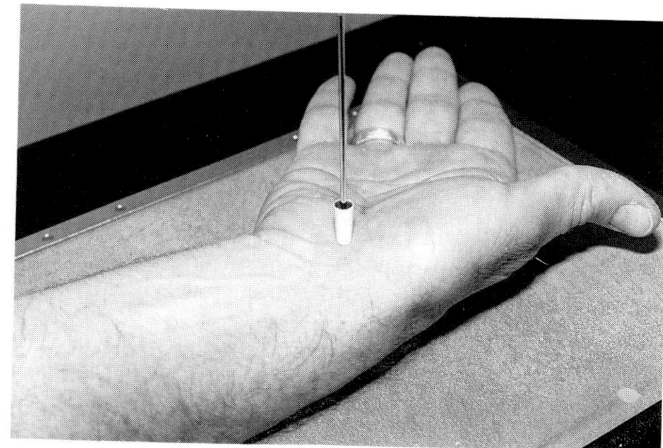

FIGURE 5–38. Wrist: AP Ulnar Deviation View

WRIST: SEMISUPINATED OBLIQUE VIEW

Synonyms Pisiform view, off-lateral view, pisotriquetral joint view

Major Indications This view demonstrates the pisiform, pisotriquetral joint, palmar aspect of the triquetrum, and palmar ulnar surface of the hamate.[19]

Illustration **(A) Position.** The ulnar side of the wrist and hand is placed on the cassette with 30-degree[6] or 45-degree[20] supination from neutral lateral view position. **Central Beam.** The central beam is perpendicular to the cassette and is centered at the level of the capitate head midway between the medial and lateral borders of the wrist.

(B) Criteria for an Adequate Examination. The pisotriquetral joint (between arrows) is clearly profiled without overlapping of the pisiform and triquetrum.[6,20] The distal radius and ulna and bases of the metacarpals are included.

Comments This is the best view to demonstrate the pisiform and pisotriquetral joint in a slightly oblique sagittal plane. A fluoroscopic spot view can more precisely profile this joint.

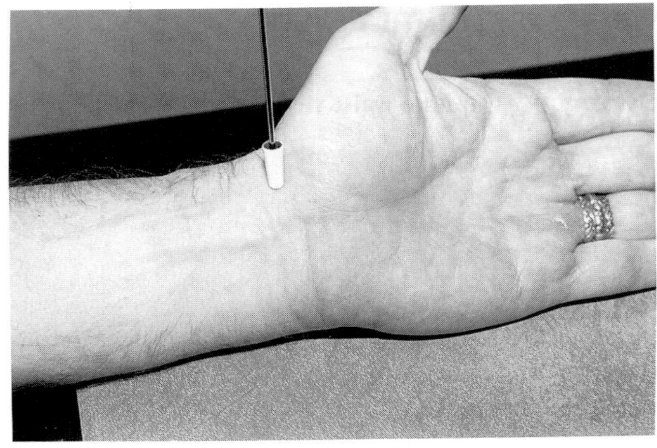

A

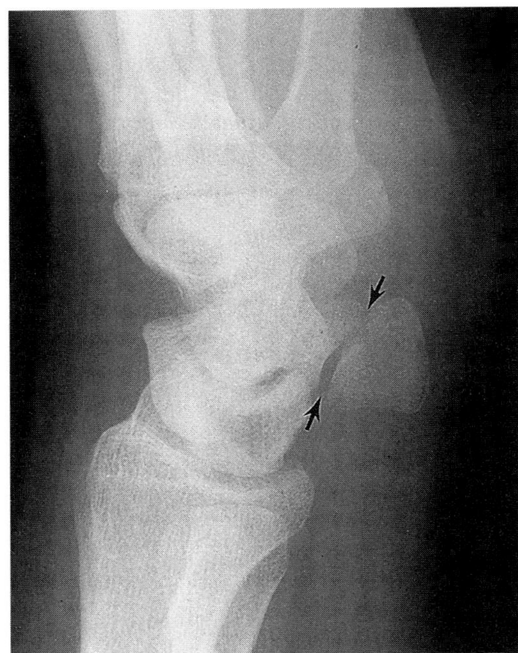

B

FIGURE 5–41. Wrist: Semisupinated Oblique View

WRIST: CLENCHED-FIST VIEW[21]

Synonyms AP fist-compression view, PA fist-compression view

Major Indications This is used to widen the scapholunate joint looking for scapholunate diastasis[21] (see "Comments," below).

Illustration **(A) Position.** For the PA clenched-fist view, the wrist is placed palm flat on the cassette as for a neutral PA view and a tight fist is made. In a similar manner, for the AP clenched-fist view the dorsum of the wrist is placed flat on the cassette and a tight fist is made without extension of the wrist (**B**). **Central Beam.** The central beam is passed through the center of the capitate head.

(C) Criteria for an Adequate Examination. The third metacarpal should be in a straight line with the radius, so that the distal 3 to 5 cm of the radius and ulna and the proximal parts of the metacarpal shafts are included on the film. On the PA view, the CMC joints will not be in profile since the wrist is in extension. However, since the wrist should not be extended on the AP view, the second through fifth metacarpal joints will be in profile.

Comments This is a favorite view of the hand surgeon who wants to investigate for possible scapholunate diastasis. The rationale for this view is that, with a tight fist, the contracting tendons and muscles create a force within the wrist driving the capitate proximally toward the scapholunate joint. In some wrists with a lax scapholunate ligament this maneuver will widen the scapholunate joint. Since the AP view commonly provides a better profile of the scapholunate joint than the PA view without a fluoroscopically controlled profile, the AP fist-compression view may be preferable to use if only the AP or PA view is available. However, since it is uncertain if the scapholunate diastasis will be demonstrated on supination or pronation, it is most desirable to perform both AP and PA fist-compression views. In addition, AP and PA fist-compression views with radial and ulnar deviation positions may show the scapholunate diastasis when it is not evident on neutral AP or PA views. When the CMC joints are not in profile in the PA fist-compression view because of wrist extension, the scapholunate joint may project slightly wider than when no extension is present. This is because the dorsum of the scapholunate joint is in profile with a PA wrist view in extension, and the dorsum of the scapholunate joint is wider than the midportion of the scapholunate joint.[22]

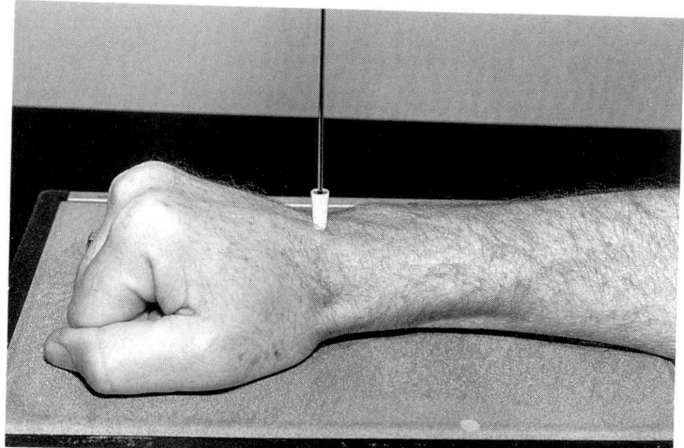

A

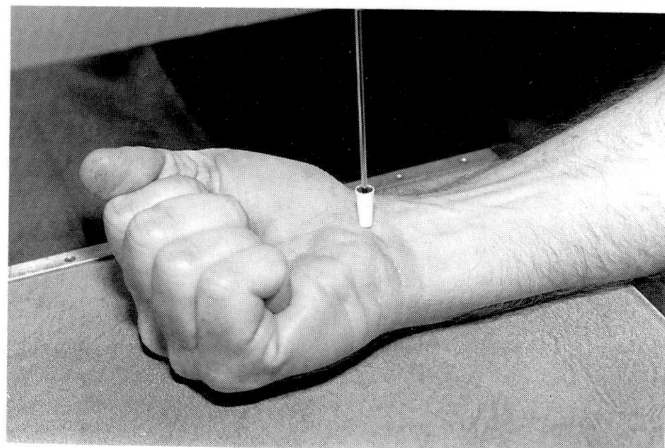

B

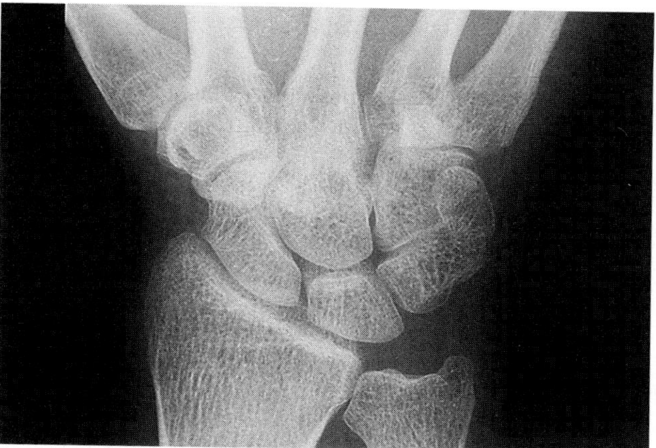

C

FIGURE 5–42. Wrist: Clenched-Fist View

SCAPHOID: SEMIPRONATED OBLIQUE VIEW WITH ULNAR DEVIATION

Synonym Scaphoid oblique ulnar-deviated view[14]

Major Indications This view provides an oblique nonforeshortened view of the scaphoid and shows the scaphotrapeziotrapezoidal articulation.

Illustration **(A) Position.** The wrist is pronated 45 degrees with ulnar deviation. Place the ulnar side of the wrist on the cassette. Pronate the wrist 45 degrees and then maximally ulnarly deviate it. **Central Beam.** The central beam is perpendicular to the cassette and is centered to the waist of the scaphoid.

(B) Criteria for an Adequate Examination. The scaphotrapeziotrapezoidal joint is well profiled, and the scaphoid is elongated. Bases of the metacarpals and the distal ends of the radius and ulna are included. The trapezium is demonstrated free from the other carpal bones.

Comments Ulnar deviation elongates the scaphoid more than occurs with a routine 45-degree semipronated oblique view.

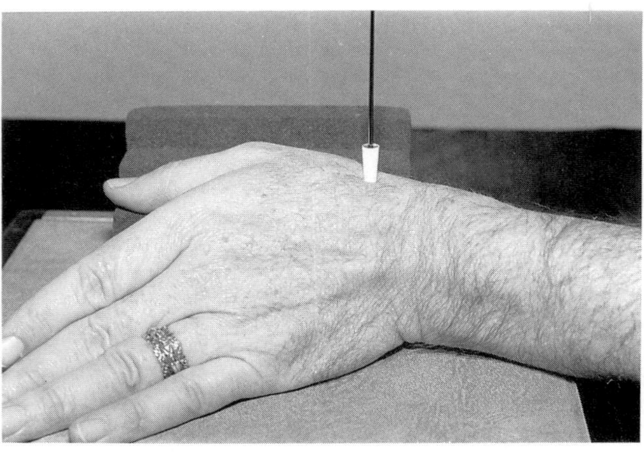

A

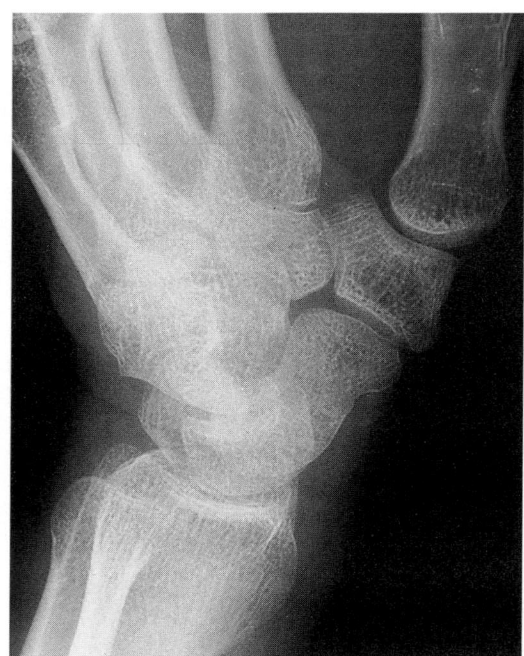

B

FIGURE 5–43. Scaphoid: Semipronated Oblique View with Ulnar Deviation

SCAPHOID: LATERAL SCAPHOID VIEW

Synonym None

Major Indications This position provides a view that elongates and profiles the scaphoid in the sagittal plane.

Illustration **(A) Position.** The ulnar side of the wrist is placed on a cassette with the wrist in extension so that the central axis of the first metacarpal lines up with the long axis of the radius.[12] The fingers are flexed. **Central Beam.** The central beam is perpendicular to the cassette and is centered to the scaphoid waist.

(B) Criteria for an Adequate Examination. The distal pole of the scaphoid projects palmar to the remaining carpal bones. The distal pole of the scaphoid, trapezium, and scaphotrapezial joint are clearly profiled. Central long axes of the radius and scaphoid are collinear.

Comments This provides an additional view for the scaphoid, trapezium, and scaphotrapezial joint. Elongation of the scaphoid occurs in the sagittal plane.

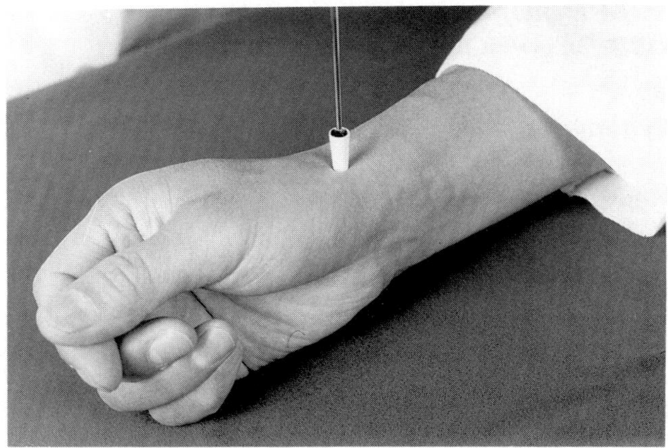

A

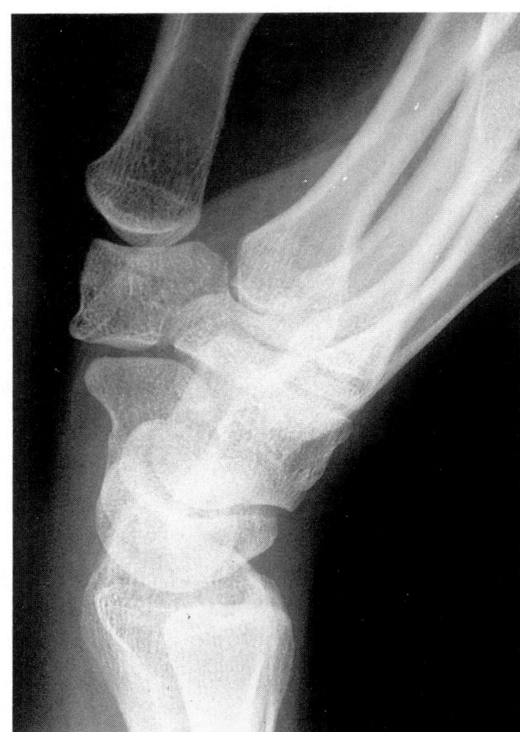

B

FIGURE 5–44. Scaphoid: Lateral Scaphoid View

SCAPHOID: STECHER POSITION FOR SCAPHOID

Synonym None

Major Indications This is a special view to better demonstrate the scaphoid waist.[23]

Illustration **(A) Position.** The film cassette is placed on a 20-degree sponge elevating (extending) the hand with respect to the forearm.[23] The hand is placed on the cassette in a PA position such that the carpus and the distal radius and ulna will be included on the cassette.[24,25] **Central Beam.** The central beam is perpendicular to the table and is centered to the scaphoid waist.

(B) Criteria for an Adequate Examination. The distal radius and ulna, entire carpus, and metacarpal bases are included. Distortion of the ulnar head is present relating to proximal projection of the ulnar styloid process and dorsal surface of the ulnar head from angulation of the central ray with respect to the distal ulna. The scaphoid waist is more in profile, or less foreshortened, and the scaphoid ring sign (due to overlapping of the distal and midportions of the scaphoid) is less evident than on the routine neutral PA position of the same wrist.

(continued)

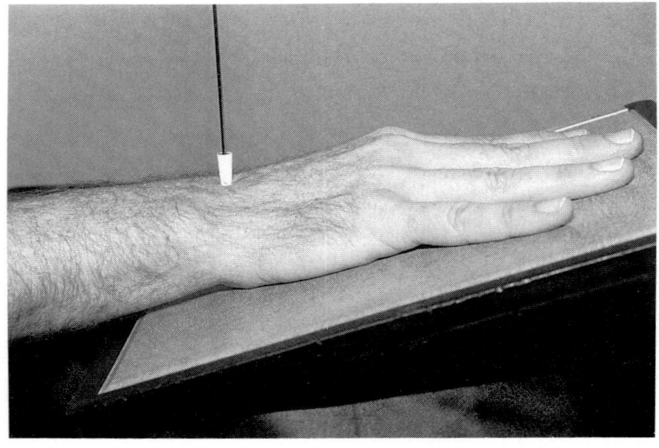

A

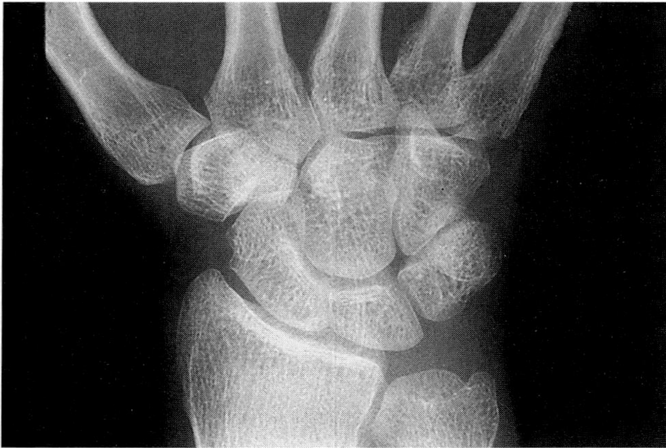

B

FIGURE 5–45. Scaphoid: Stecher Position for Scaphoid

SCAPHOID: STECHER POSITION FOR SCAPHOID (Continued)

Comments

1. Twenty-degree angulation of the wrist places the scaphoid closer to right angles to the central ray so that the scaphoid is projected with less self-superimposition. While some people may prefer this method, Gruber suggested that a similar view can be obtained by placing the hand and wrist in a PA position with the wrist in slight ulnar deviation and the central beam angled 20 degrees toward the elbow.[24] However, since ulnar deviation elongates the scaphoid by decreasing ventral tilting of the scaphoid, addition of 20-degree effective cephalad angulation with respect to the scaphoid will elongate the scaphoid and show the scaphoid waist to better advantage than shown in Fig. 5–45B. Because the long scaphoid axis commonly is angled more than 20 degrees to the long axis of the radius, more effective cephalad angulation (angulation passing toward the elbow) is commonly necessary to pass the central ray exactly perpendicular to the waist or long axis of the scaphoid. A more precise determination of how much cephalad angulation or extension of the wrist is necessary to make the long axis of the scaphoid perpendicular to the central ray can be made by seeing the inclination of the scaphoid on the lateral neutral view of the wrist and passing the beam perpendicular to that inclination.

2. For the purpose of demonstrating a fracture line with superoinferior (proximal-dorsal to distal-ventral) orientation, these positions may be reversed. That is, the wrist is placed with 20 degrees of palmar-flexion or the wrist is placed with neutral position and the central beam is angled toward the fingers.

SCAPHOID: ULNAR OBLIQUE SCAPHOID VIEW

Synonym Ulnar-deviated overpronated scaphoid view

Major Indications This view is one of the common specialty (detailed) films obtained to detect a suspect fracture or lesion of the scaphoid that is not definitely demonstrated on routine views.

Illustration **(A) Position.** The wrist is in slight ulnar deviation, which allows the thumb to align with the forearm with the radial (thumb) side placed on the cassette. Flexion of the fingers will support the wrist position. Alternatively, the fingers and wrist can be supported by a 45-degree sponge placed ulnarly under extended fingers. The thumb is extended.[12] **Central Beam.** The central beam is perpendicular to the cassette and is centered to the scaphoid waist.[12]

(B) Criteria for an Adequate Examination. The scaphoid is overlapped distally by the capitate and proximally by the lunate. Because of the oblique position of the wrist, the scaphoid has more of an oval or kidney bean shape. The radioscaphoid articulation is well profiled and the pisiform (arrow) projects ulnar to the triquetrum. In addition to the carpus, adjacent metacarpals, radius, and ulna are included.

Comments This is an excellent view to show chip fractures of the dorsal aspect of the scaphoid waist.[8] This view should be added to routine wrist or scaphoid views when symptoms suggest a scaphoid fracture and routine views do not show such a fracture. Recognition that the pisiform projects ulnar to the triquetrum, and that the scaphoid has this shape, makes it immediately apparent that the view is a reverse (overpronated) oblique.

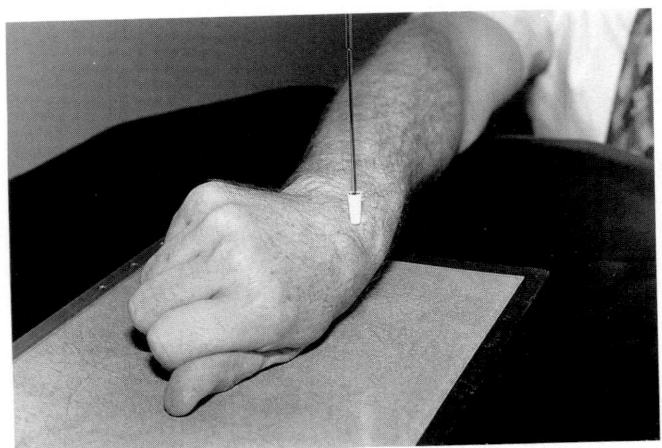

A

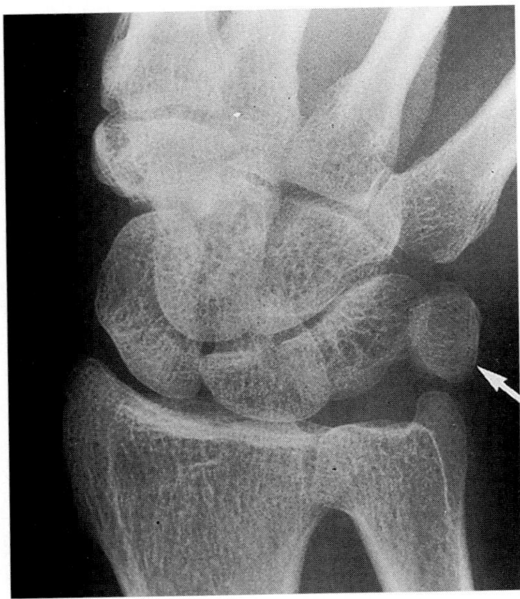

B

FIGURE 5–46. Scaphoid: Ulnar Oblique Scaphoid View

SCAPHOID: THIRTY-DEGREE SEMIPRONATED OBLIQUE PA VIEW

Synonym Modified semipronated oblique PA view[1]

Major Indications This view usually is one of the spot films obtained when a clinically suspected scaphoid fracture or lesion is not definitely shown on routine films. Such a view also shows the scaphotrapezial and may show the trapeziotrapezoidal joints.

Illustration **(A) Position.** The ulnar side of the wrist and hand is placed on the cassette with 30-degree elevation of the radial side of the hand from the cassette. A triangular sponge with or without steps can be placed under the radial side of the hand to support it. **Central Beam.** The central beam is perpendicular to the cassette and is centered to the scaphoid or just ulnar to the scaphoid.

(B) Criteria for an Adequate Examination. This view should include the DRUJ, whole carpus, and the proximal part of the metacarpals. Metacarpal shafts should be separated with no overlapping of the metacarpals distal to their wide bases. This view provides an oblique, less foreshortened view of the scaphoid than seen on the routine PA view and shows the scaphotrapeziotrapezoidal articulation better than on the PA view.

Comments This is a modified view from the routine 45-degree oblique view of the scaphoid. This view should be added to routine views when symptoms suggest a scaphoid fracture and the routine views do not show such a fracture. To obtain slight variations of this view to profile specific cortices, or to look for a fracture line, slight variations of this view may be better obtained under fluoroscopic control.

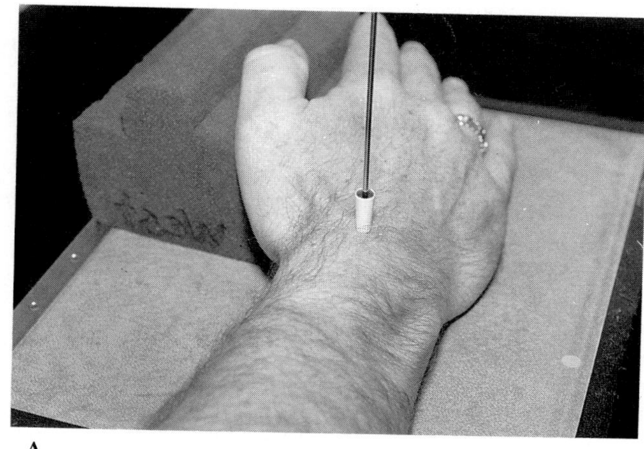

A

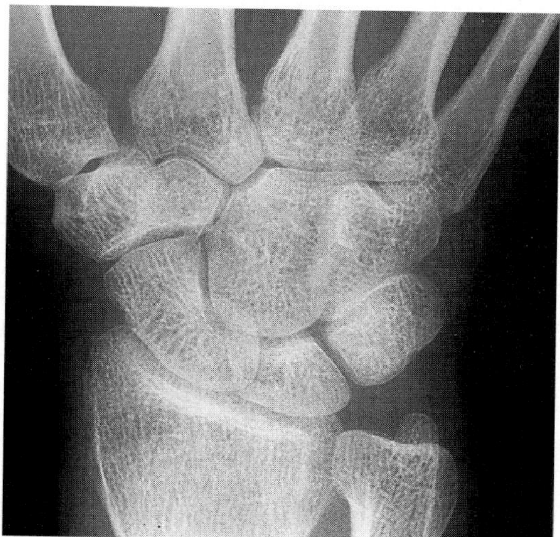

B

FIGURE 5–47. Scaphoid: 30-Degree Semipronated Oblique PA View

SCAPHOID: SIXTY-DEGREE SEMIPRONATED OBLIQUE PA VIEW

Synonym Modified semipronated oblique PA view[1]

Major Indications This view is a good additional specialized spot film obtained when a clinically suspected fracture or lesion of the scaphoid is not definitely shown on routine films. More information about the trapezium and scaphotrapezial and trapeziotrapezoidal joints can be provided by this view.

Illustration **(A) Position.** The ulnar side of the wrist and hand is placed on the cassette with 60-degree elevation of the radial side of the hand from the cassette. A triangular sponge with or without steps can be placed under the radial side of the hand to support it. **Central Beam.** The central beam, perpendicular to the cassette, is centered at the radiocarpal joint distal to Lister's tubercle (**A**). Alternatively, the central ray could be passed through the scaphoid waist or trapezium, whichever is the structure of interest when this view is obtained.

(B) Criteria for an Adequate Examination. This view should demonstrate the distal scaphoid pole and trapezium free from overlapping bone structures. The scaphoid waist, space between the bases of the first and second metacarpals, and scaphotrapezial, trapeziotrapezoidal, and first CMC joints should be evident. The distal radius, ulna, and metacarpal bases should be included.

Comments This is a modified view from the routine 45-degree oblique view of the scaphoid. This view should be added to routine views when symptoms suggest a scaphoid fracture and routine views do not show such a fracture. To clearly profile the scaphoid waist or another specific structure demonstrable with this position, because of variation in carpal bone shapes, this view can be obtained more precisely under fluoroscopic control.

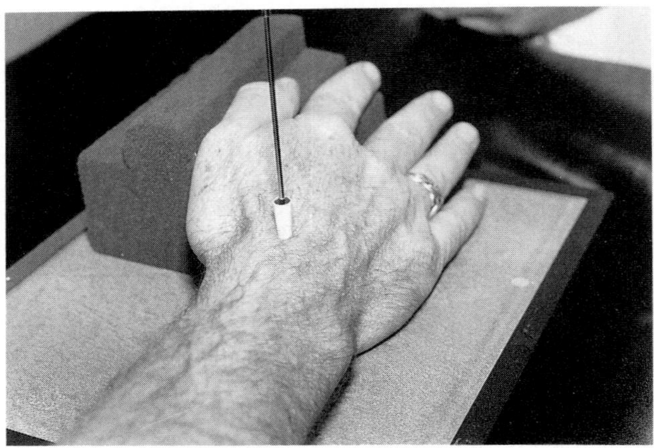

A

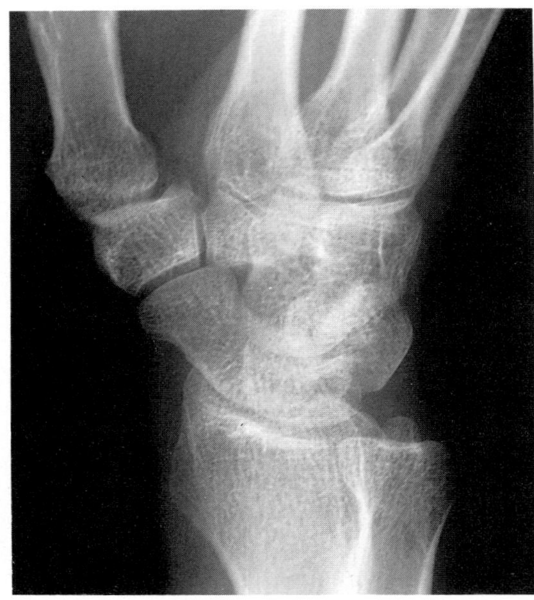

B

FIGURE 5–48. Scaphoid: 60-Degree Semipronated Oblique PA View

SCAPHOID: ELONGATED OBLIQUE VIEW

Synonym None

Major Indications This view is indicated when additional detailed information about the waist of the scaphoid is desired.

Illustration **(A) Position.** Place the hand and wrist as for a PA view position and then raise the radial aspect of the wrist 20 degrees off the cassette.[1] **Central Beam.** With the tube angled 35 degrees toward the elbow, the central beam is centered over the radial styloid and scaphoid waist.[1]

(B) Criteria for an Adequate Examination. The scaphoid is fully elongated and its waist is clearly shown without overlap of adjacent bone structures. Due to angulation of the central beam, the CMC joints are not in profile, the trapezium and trapezoid overlap the distal pole of the scaphoid, and the capitate and hamate overlap the lunate and triquetrum, respectively.

Comments When a fracture or lesion, typically of the scaphoid waist, suspected clinically is not shown on routine films, this specialty view is often diagnostic. This view may be better obtained under fluoroscopic control.

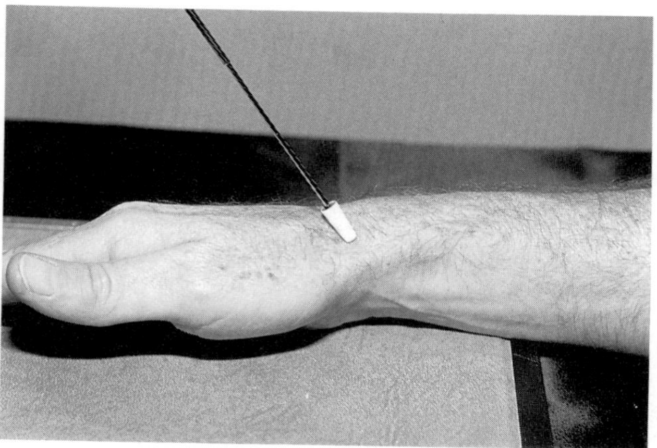

A

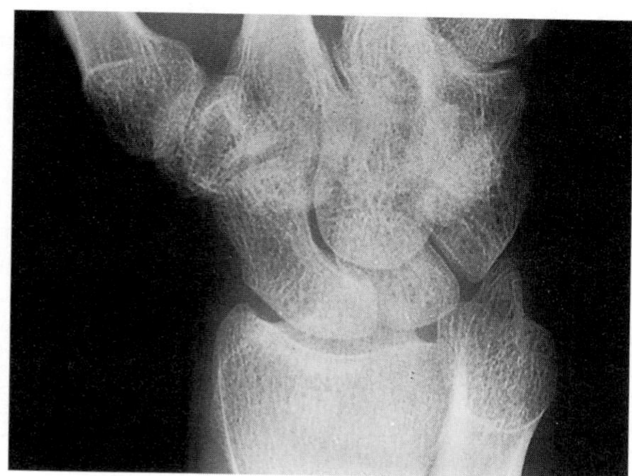

B

FIGURE 5–49. Scaphoid: Elongated Oblique View

CARPAL BRIDGE VIEW

Synonym None

Major Indications This view is recommended to demonstrate dorsal surface fractures of the scaphoid, calcifications and foreign bodies in the dorsal soft tissues of the wrist, and chip fractures of the dorsal aspect of the carpal bones.[26,27] This view provides an additional view of the scaphoid through its long axis. This view can potentially present an additional view of a dorsal boss (carpe bossu).

Illustration **(A) Position.** The dorsum of the forearm is placed on the cassette with the wrist flexed maximally or approximately 90 degrees. **Central Beam.** The central beam is angled 45 degrees proximally and is tangent to the dorsal center of the wrist. However, to be more productive for pathology, the beam should be passed tangent to the precise site of tenderness or interest.

(B) Criteria for an Adequate Examination. This view demonstrates a tangential view of the dorsal aspect of the scaphoid (S), lunate (L), and triquetrum (T).[8,24] An outline of the superimposed capitate (C) should be visible. Correct exposure with adequate penetration without motion shows these structures. Outline of the proximal metacarpals should be faintly visualized through other superimposed structures (radius and ulna).

Comments Fluoroscopic control can be used to better advantage with this view, since the wrist can be positioned under real time to profile more precisely an exact site of interest.

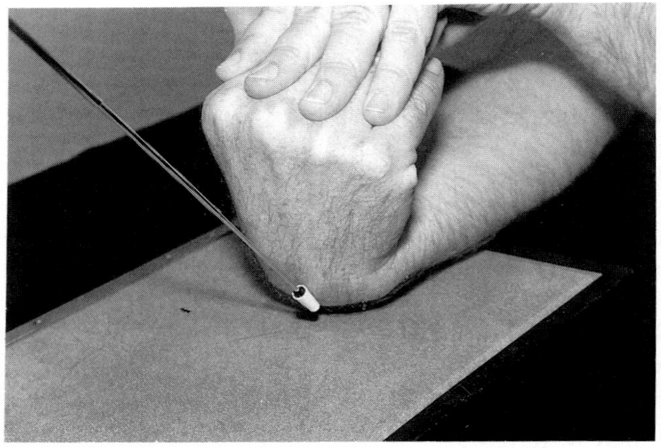

A

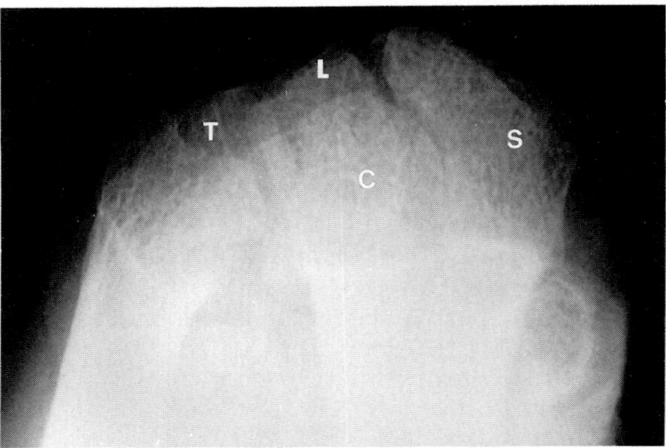

B

FIGURE 5–50. Carpal Bridge View

CARPAL BOSS VIEW

Synonyms Dorsal boss view, carpe bossu view

Major Indications This view is designed to clarify the nature of the bony prominence at the junction of the second and third CMC joints, whether it is an os styloideum, osteophytes, a normal dorsal bony projection attached to the metacarpal base, or a fracture of the dorsal prominence.

Illustration **(A) Position.** The wrist is slightly ulnar-deviated with the ulnar side of the wrist on the cassette. Approximately 30-degree supination of the wrist is performed to place the dorsal prominence at the dorsoradial aspect of the second to third CMC joints tangent to a vertical central ray.[17] **Central Beam.** The central beam is passed through or tangent to the dorsal prominence.

(B) Criteria for an Adequate Examination. The dorsal prominence is clearly profiled to show either a separate bone, osteophytes, or a dorsal exostosis-like projection. (Reprinted with permission from Conway WF, Destouet JM, Gilula LA, Bellinghausen HW, Weeks PM. The carpal boss: An overview of radiographic evaluation. *Radiology* 1985;156:29–31.)

Comments If this view does not show the dorsal bone structure clearly, fluoroscopically directed views can be very effective to profile the bony prominence. This may be especially important to determine if there is a fracture or separate os styloideum at this level. Alternatively, CT performed with thin sections in the direct sagittal or coronal planes could clarify the status of the bone structures in this area, if such detailed plain-film or fluoroscopic spots are unsuccessful. Plain films or fluoroscopy are generally sufficient without the need for CT.

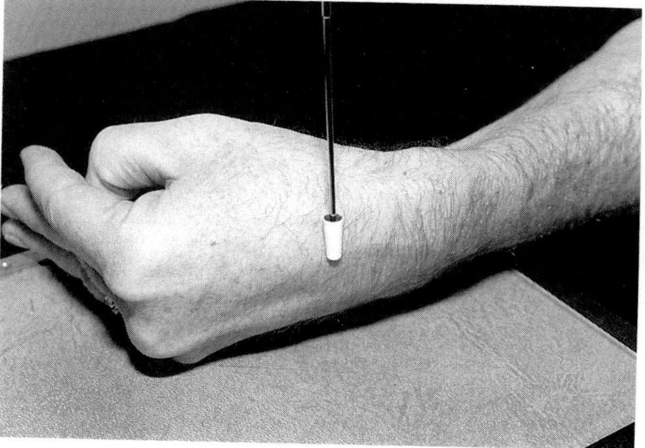

A

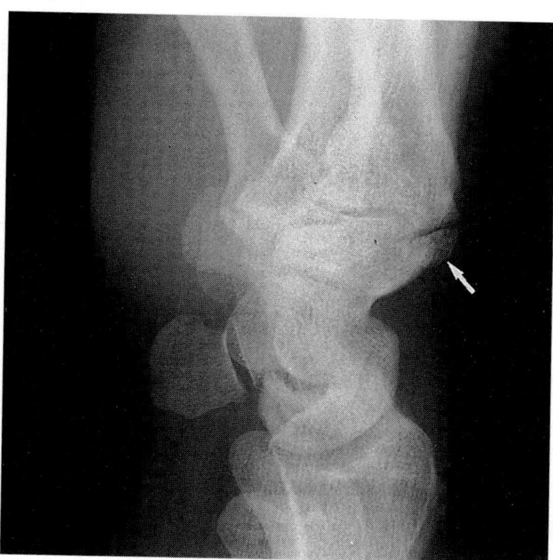

B

FIGURE 5–51. Carpal Boss View

CARPAL TUNNEL: INFEROSUPERIOR VIEW

Synonym Gaynor–Hart position[24,28]

Major Indications This view shows the palmar aspects of the trapezium, the tuberosity of the scaphoid, the trapezoid, the capitate, hamate hook, triquetrum, entire pisiform, the palmar soft-tissue area, and the carpal tunnel between the hook of the hamate and the trapezium.[24,29,30]

Illustration **(A) Position.** The palmar aspect of the wrist is placed on a small sponge centered on the cassette. Maximal dorsiflexion of the wrist joint is maintained by the other hand of the patient or by traction on a bandage placed around the palm of the hand at the MCP joint level. **Central Beam.** The central beam is directed tangent to the center of the palmar aspect of the wrist, 25 to 30 degrees to the long axis of the hand or paralleling the longitudinal axis of the carpal tunnel.[31]

(B) Criteria for an Adequate Examination. This view shows the palmar aspects of the trapezium (Tm), scaphoid tuberosity (S), capitate, hook of the hamate (H), triquetrum, and the entire pisiform (P). The carpus and the carpal tunnel should be demonstrated in a tunnel-like or arch-like arrangement on this view.[28] (Reprinted with permission from Totty WG, Gilula LA. Imaging of the hand and wrist. In: Gilula LA, ed. *The traumatized hand and wrist: Radiographic and anatomic correlation.* Philadelphia: WB Saunders, 1992.)

Comments When the patient cannot tolerate this position, adjust the angle to make the central beam tangent to the palmar aspect of the center of the wrist or parallel with the carpal canal. The carpal canal is easy to palpate on the palmar aspect of the wrist as the concavity between the trapezium, the hamate hook, and pisiform.[18,20]

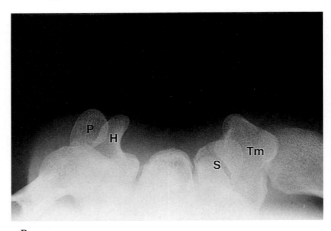

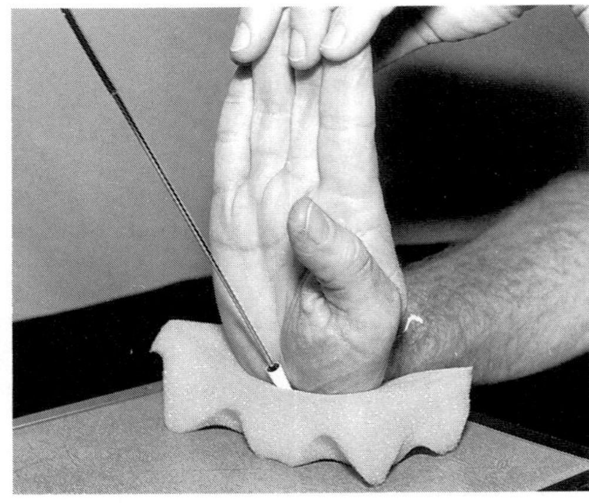

A

P
H
Tm
S

B

FIGURE 5–52. Carpal Tunnel: Inferosuperior View

CARPAL TUNNEL: SUPEROINFERIOR VIEW

Synonym None

Major Indications This view (see Fig. 5–53B) shows the palmar aspects of the trapezium, tuberosity of the scaphoid, the trapezoid, the capitate, the hook of the hamate, the triquetrum, and the entire pisiform.[32]

Illustration **(A) Position.** The hand is placed on the cassette palm down with maximal dorsiflexion of the wrist. **Central Beam.** The central beam is directed tangent to the center of the palmar aspect of the wrist, parallel to the longitudinal axis of the carpal tunnel.

(B) Criteria for an Adequate Examination. This view shows the palmar aspects of the trapezium (Tm), scaphoid tuberosity (S), capitate (C), hamate hook (H), triquetrum (T), and the entire pisiform (P). The carpus should be demonstrated in a tunnel-like or arch-like arrangement on this view.

Comments Sometimes it is necessary to adjust the angle of the tube to make the direction of central ray more parallel with the axis of the carpal tunnel. If the patient cannot perform dorsiflexion of the wrist sufficiently, use the cross-table view (see next view).

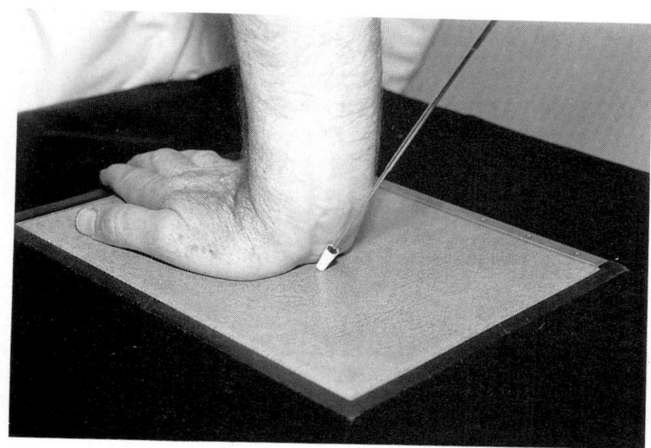

A

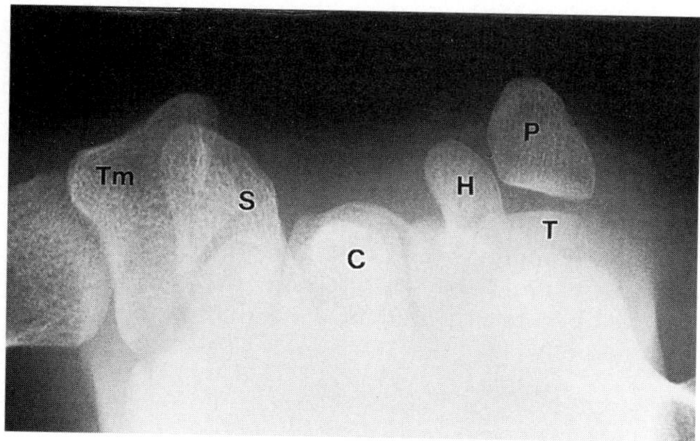

B

FIGURE 5–53. Carpal Tunnel: Superoinferior View

CARPAL TUNNEL: CROSS-TABLE VIEW

Synonym Horizontal beam view

Major Indications This view shows the palmar aspects of the same bone structures as described above in Figs. 5–52 and 5–53 and is designed to show the carpal tunnel when the positions in those figures are not possible.

Illustration **Position.** The cassette is held vertically by the fingers of the wrist to be examined. The maximum possible wrist dorsiflexion is assumed, so that the forearm is not projecting over the carpal tunnel. To assume this position, the hypothenar and thenar eminences usually will not be able to touch the cassette. **Central Beam.** The central beam is directed horizontally, tangent to the center of the palmar aspect of the wrist and parallel to the longitudinal axis of the carpal tunnel.[8]

Criteria for an Adequate Examination. The palmar aspects of the trapezium, scaphoid tuberosity, capitate, hamate hook, triquetrum, and the entire pisiform should be visible and the carpal tunnel should be demonstrated in a tunnel-like or arch-like arrangement.

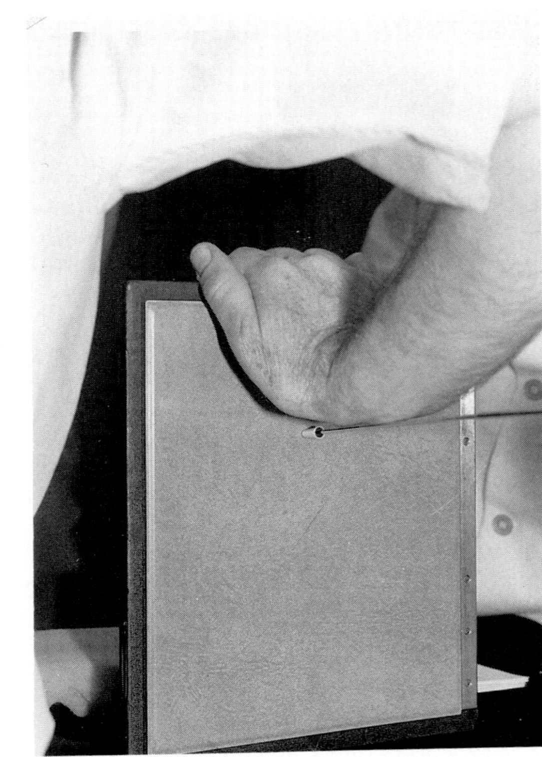

FIGURE 5–54. Carpal Tunnel: Cross-Table View

TRAPEZIUM: PA AXIAL OBLIQUE VIEW

Synonym None

Major Indications This view is used to evaluate the trapezium and its articulation with the scaphoid.

Illustration **(A) Position.** The palmar surface of the hand is placed on a 45-degree sponge with the wrist in a 45-degree oblique position and in ulnar deviation.[27] **Central Beam.** The central beam is perpendicular to the cassette and is centered to the trapezium.

(B) Criteria for an Adequate Examination. This view clearly demonstrates the trapezium free from other carpal bones. The scaphotrapeziotrapezoidal joint is well profiled, and the scaphoid is elongated. Bases of the metacarpals and the distal ends of the radius and ulna are included.

Comments A profile of specific cortices of the trapezium, as for other carpal bones, can be obtained more precisely under fluoroscopic control.

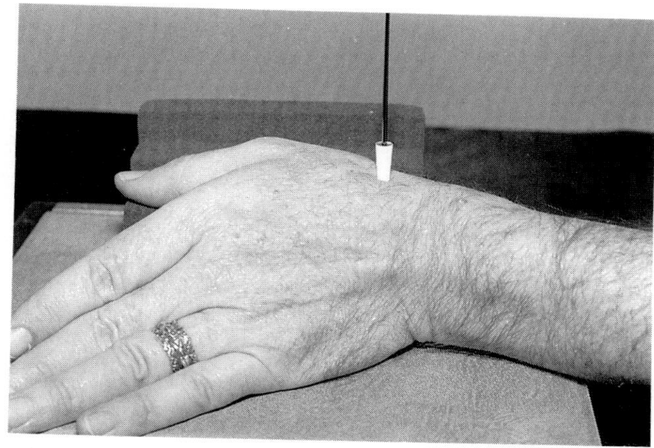

A

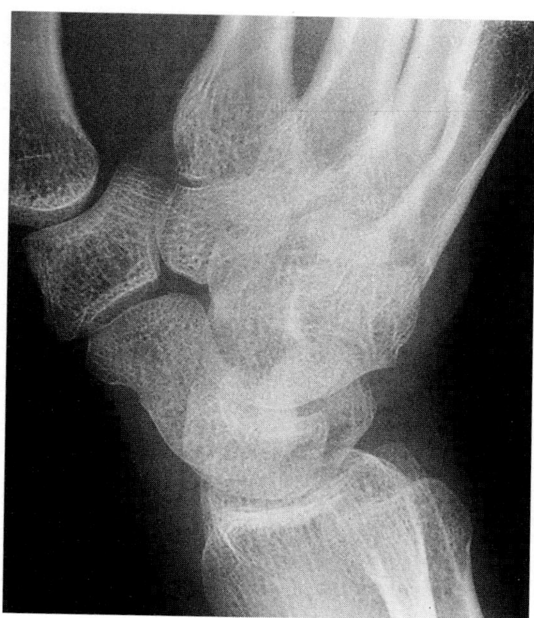

B

FIGURE 5–55. Trapezium: PA Axial Oblique View

HANDS AND WRISTS: BALL-CATCHER'S VIEW

Synonyms Norgaard's view, semisupinated position[7,33,34]

Major Indications The view has been used to look for early erosions in arthritis not seen on routine views, especially on the ventral ulnar sides of bones (see Fig. 5–56B).[14]

Illustration **(A) Position.** The hand or hands are placed palm up, with the thumbs elevated off the film cassette approximately 35 to 45 degrees[7] and the ulnodorsal aspect of the hypothenar eminences flush on the cassette. The interphalangeal joints are slightly flexed. **Central Beam.** The central beam enters the midshaft of the metacarpals of the hand or the space between both hands if both hands are imaged simultaneously.

(B) Criteria for an Adequate Examination. One or both hands must be included from the distal 3 to 5 cm of the forearm to the tips of the fingers. An oblique view is present with the pisiform bone or bones and the pisotriquetral joint(s) evident without overlapping of the second through fifth metacarpal heads.

Comments This view was described by Norgaard[33,34] and was considered useful in detecting early radiographic changes of rheumatoid arthritis. Although the author also stated that a nonscreen technique should be used to obtain high resolution, today's high-resolution film/screen combinations are adequate; however, low kVp (60 to 65) is recommended to obtain optimal contrast.

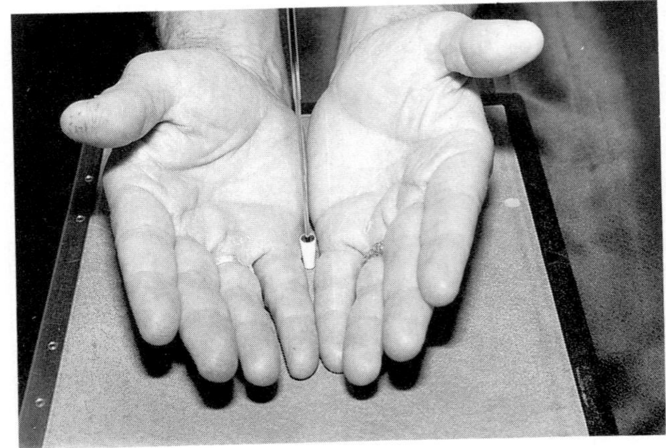

A

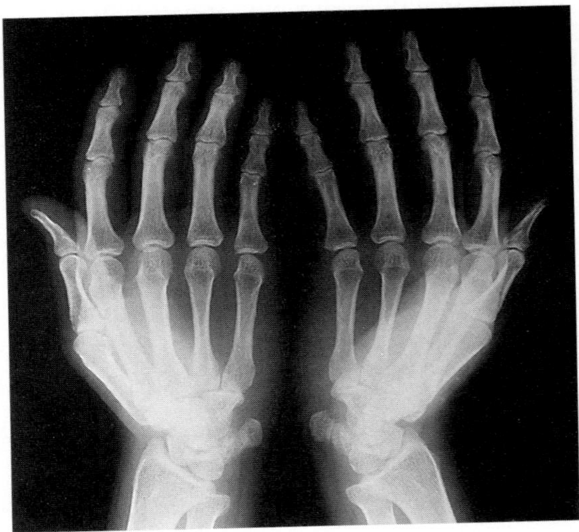

B

FIGURE 5–56. Hands and Wrists: Ball-Catcher's View

STRESS VIEW, WRIST, PRONE: ULNAR AND RADIAL TRANSLATIONS

Synonym None

Major Indications This stress view will display laxity of ligaments in the wrist at the radiocarpal level.[35]

Illustration **(A, C) Position.** With the wrist prone, one of the examiner's hands immobilizes the distal forearm by pushing it firmly onto the table or cassette. The thumb of the opposite hand of the examiner is placed on the base of the patient's thumb and ulnar-directed force is applied for the ulnar translation stress (**A**). For the radial translation stress maneuver, the distal forearm is fixed the same as for ulnar translation stress. The examiner's fingers are placed along the ulnar aspect of the fifth metacarpal and radially directed stress is applied (**C**). **Central Beam.** The central beam should be at the level of the radiolunate joint.

(B, D) Criteria for an Adequate Examination. The radioscaphoid joint should be in profile. Overlap at the DRUJ should be similar between the two views to make comparison between radial and ulnar displacement forces and between both wrists easier to accomplish. Preferably the wrist should not be in radial or ulnar deviation during the examination. **B** shows no radial or ulnar deviation; **D** shows slight ulnar deviation.

Comments The opposite wrist should be examined for comparison, since some people have normal laxity at the radiocarpal level. Fluoroscopy can be readily used rather than overhead views, since fluoroscopy has the advantage of allowing the examiner to watch the wrist to ensure that no rotation of the wrist occurs during application of the maneuvers. Lead gloves should be worn when radiographic exposures are being made. Obscuration of the distal carpus by the lead gloves does not cause problems because attention is directed to the radiocarpal level. As much force as can be placed by the examiner and can be tolerated by the patient should be applied.

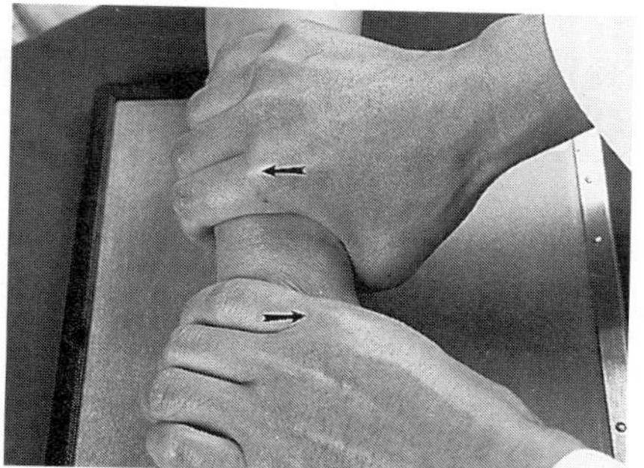

A

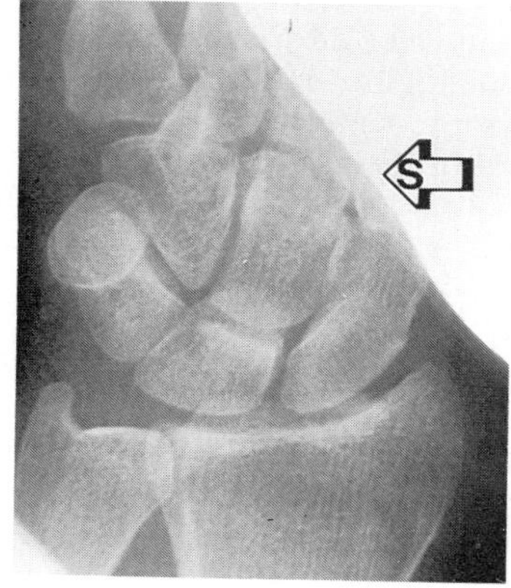

B

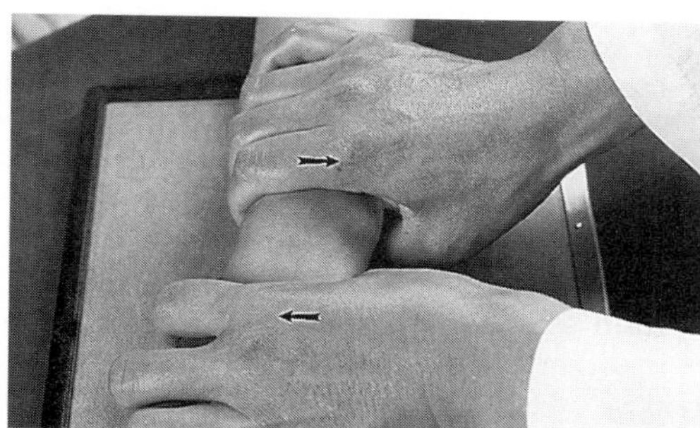

C

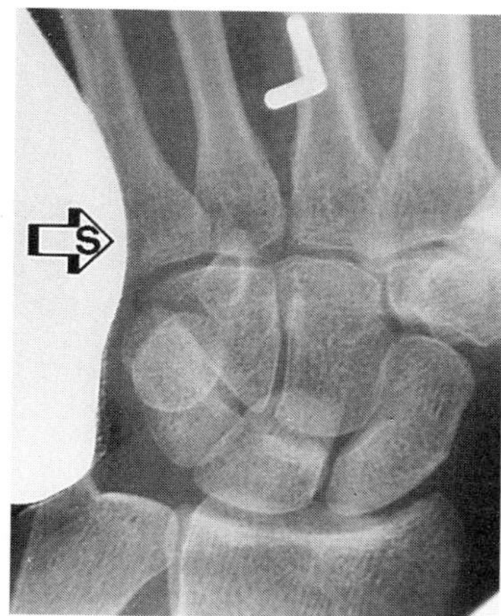

D

FIGURE 5–57. Stress View, Wrist, Prone: Ulnar and Radial Translations

STRESS VIEW, WRIST, LATERAL, CAPITOLUNATE INSTABILITY: VENTRAL AND DORSAL DISPLACEMENTS

Synonym Capitolunate instability pattern (CLIP) wrist maneuvers[35,36]

Major Indications When a patient has pain caused by dorsal (usually) or ventral displacement force, this maneuver can demonstrate how much midcarpal displacement occurs between the capitate (identifying the distal carpal row) and the lunate (identifying the proximal carpal row). More displacement of the capitate out of the lunate on the symptomatic side associated with symptoms, especially when more than one half of the width of the capitate head displaces out of the distal lunate concavity is believed to be positive.[36] This maneuver can also be used to show increased motion at the radiocarpal level.

Illustration **(A, C) Position.** The ulnar side of the patient's hand is placed on the cassette or the table in a true neutral lateral position with slight ulnar deviation at the wrist. A small sponge, sheet, other support, or the examiner's hand can be used to support the distal forearm. One of the examiner's hands holds the distal forearm rigidly to the table (or cassette or support) and the other hand grasps the patient's wrist at the CMC level. The examiner's fingertips placed at the dorsum of the second to fifth CMC joints displace the carpus palmarly for ventral displacing force. To apply the dorsal displacing force, the examiner's thumb is placed at the CMC level at the base of the thumb and the radial aspect of the carpal tunnel at the CMC level. The examiner's hand and thumb should be around the patient's thumb **(A, C)** and not in the web space of the patient's thumb. No flexion or extension of the wrist should be allowed. **Central Beam.** The central beam should pass through the head of the capitate.

(continued)

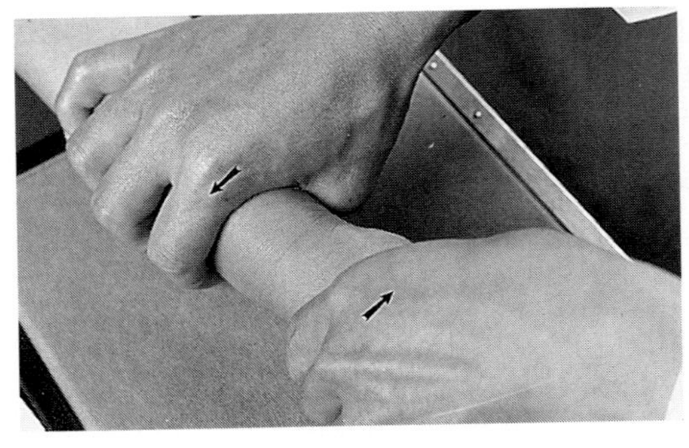

A

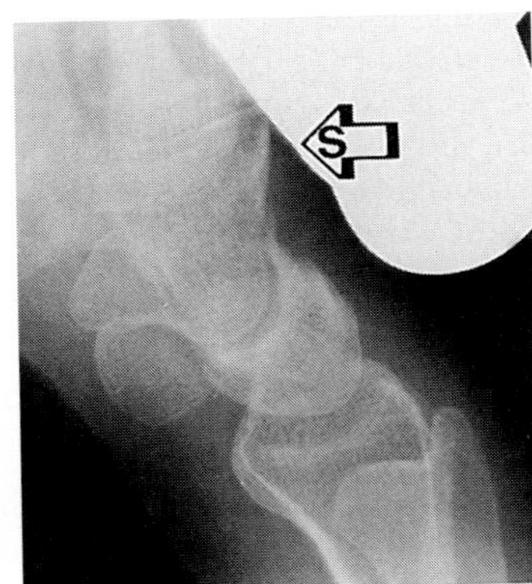

B

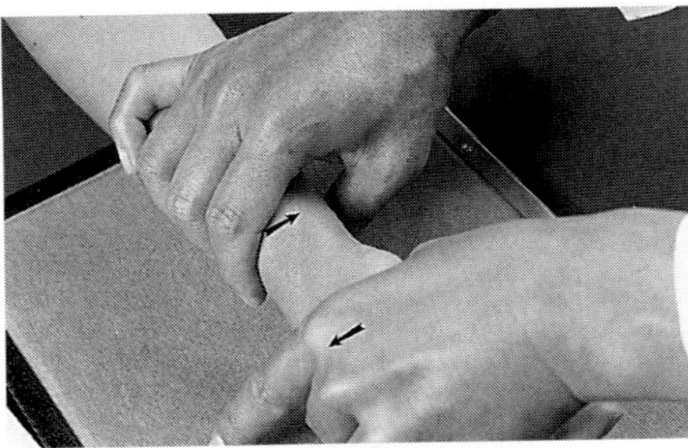

C

FIGURE 5–58. Stress View, Wrist, Lateral, Capitolunate Instability: Ventral and Dorsal Displacements

STRESS VIEW, WRIST, LATERAL, CAPITOLUNATE INSTABILITY: VENTRAL AND DORSAL DISPLACEMENTS (Continued)

(B, D) Criteria for an Adequate Examination. The central axes of the metacarpals and distal radius should be parallel. Pressure should be placed at the CMC level as seen by position of the gloved hands. Lack of rotation of the carpus can be identified by looking at the position of the pisiform with respect to the scaphoid as described above under lateral view of the wrist. Penetration should be adequate to see the capitolunate joint space. With ventral displacing force, the lunate should usually tilt ventrally and often will assume a VISI configuration (**B**). Without such lunate tilting, inadequate stress may be questioned. Some dorsal movement of the capitate out of the distal lunate concavity with dorsal displacing force is expected (**D**), or the question of inadequately applied stress can be raised.

Comments Both sides should be examined to look for differences between sides. Lax wrists will show much more motion than rigid joints. Ulnar deviation tends to loosen the midcarpal joint to enable more displacement with the maneuvers. The significance of these displacing maneuvers is currently in question. Apparently there is no good proof yet as to what this means, although we question if extrinsic ligament stretch or partial injury can account for the pain, when pain occurs in these patients.

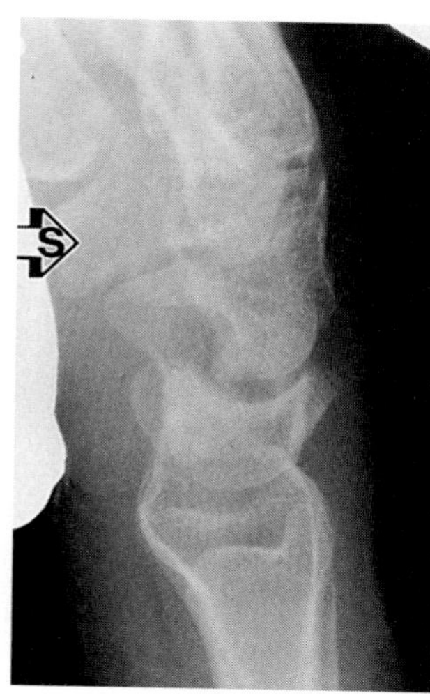

D

FIGURE 5–58. *Continued* Stress View, Wrist, Lateral, Capitolunate Instability: Ventral and Dorsal Displacements

STRESS VIEW, WRIST, LATERAL: ULNAR AND RADIAL DEVIATIONS

Synonym Taleisnik lateral wrist views

Major Indications These maneuvers are designed to show if the lunate moves normally. With ulnar deviation the lunate tilts dorsally and with radial deviation the lunate tilts ventrally. With rotary subluxation of the scaphoid, these views can show if the lunate moves fairly normally, especially when compared with an opposite side that is normal (especially asymptomatic). When the lunate motion is abnormal, the question of more abnormality in the wrist than isolated to the scaphoid is questioned. See "Comments," on the next page, for further discussion.

Illustration **(A, C) Position.** The wrist is placed in a true neutral lateral position on a cassette or table top. Full ulnar deviation is performed followed by full radial deviation. Alternatively, the distal forearm can be supported on a stack of sheets, other object, or by the examiner's lead-gloved hands, so that full ulnar deviation in the lateral position can be obtained easily without hitting the table or cassette. Radial deviation is then performed, maintaining true neutral lateral position. This can all be performed under fluoroscopic control. **Central Beam.** The central beam is directed toward the capitolunate joint or the head of the capitate.

(continued)

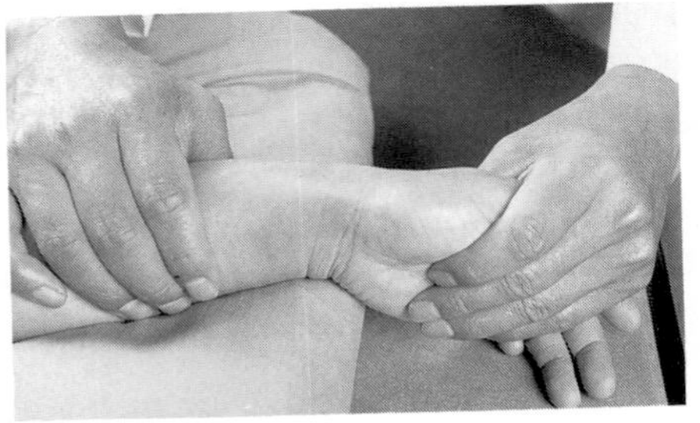

A

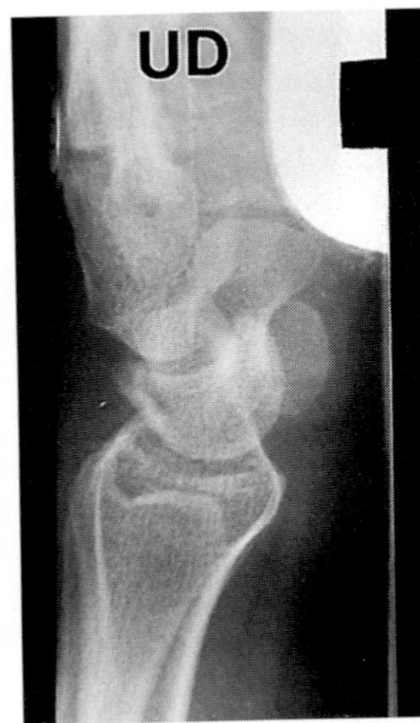

B

FIGURE 5–59. Stress View, Wrist, Lateral: Ulnar and Radial Deviations

STRESS VIEW, WRIST, LATERAL: ULNAR AND RADIAL DEVIATIONS (Continued)

(B, D) Criteria for an Adequate Examination. A true lateral position is identified by positioning the ventral surface of the pisiform between the ventral surfaces of the capitate head and distal pole of the scaphoid (arrows, **B, D**) as mentioned previously under Wrist: Lateral View. If the pisiform projects ventral to the distal pole of the scaphoid, the wrist is in supination and the lunate can normally display dorsiflexion in that position. The dorsum of the metacarpals should line up with the dorsum of the radius to show there is no flexion or extension at the wrist. Ulnar deviation (UD) can be recognized by increased radioscaphoid angle or dorsal tilting of the lunate and the distal pole of the scaphoid. With radial deviation (RD) the scaphoid and the lunate tilt toward the palm, creating a lesser radioscaphoid angle.

Comments The lunate normally tilts dorsally with ulnar deviation in the same direction as the scaphoid. Similar to the scaphoid, with radial deviation the lunate normally tilts toward the palm. The opposite side should be examined in the same manner to recognize differences between sides in motion of the lunate. We believe that this maneuver is valuable to help distinguish rotary subluxation of the scaphoid from DISI. True isolated rotary subluxation of the scaphoid displays abnormal motion of the scaphoid only. When the lunate also has abnormal motion, as can be shown by these maneuvers and by abnormal motion on flexion and/or extension lateral views, more extensive ligament abnormalities especially of the extrinsic ligaments, such as DISI, can be suspected. Fluoroscopy can allow more satisfactory rapid positioning and spot filming to account for variations in individual patient anatomy.

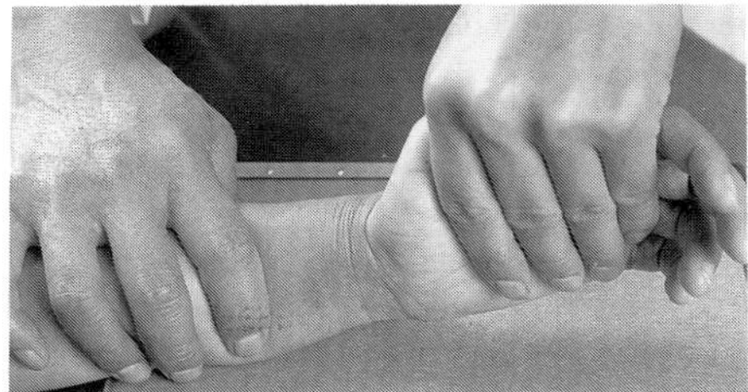

C

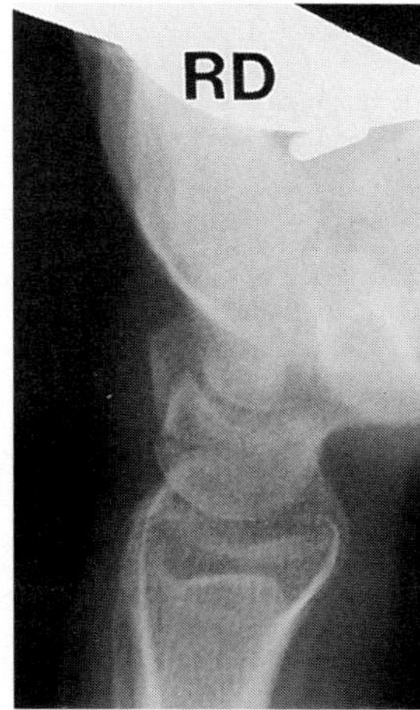

D

FIGURE 5–59. *Continued* Stress View, Wrist, Lateral: Ulnar and Radial Deviations

REFERENCES

1. Kreel L, Paris A. *Clark's positioning in radiography,* Vol. 1. 10th ed. Chicago: William Heinemann, 1979:2–27.
2. Street JM. Radiographs of phalangeal fractures: Importance of the internally rotated oblique projection for diagnosis. *AJR* 1993;160:575–576.
3. Movin A, Karlsson U. *Skeletal projections for diagnostic radiology.* 1st ed. Philadelphia: JB Lippincott, 1975:102–120.
4. Brewerton DA. A tangential radiographic projection for demonstrating involvement of metacarpal heads in rheumatoid arthritis. *Br J Radiol* 1967;40:233–234.
5. Lane CS. Detecting occult fractures of the metacarpal head: The Brewerton view. *J Hand Surg* 1977;2:131–133.
6. Wood MB, Berquist TH. The hand and wrist. In: Berquist TH, ed. *Imaging of orthopedic trauma and surgery.* Philadelphia: WB Saunders, 1986:641–662.
7. Galasko CSB, Isherwood I. *Imaging techniques in orthopaedics.* London: Springer-Verlag, 1989:4–6.
8. Bontrager KL. *Radiographic positioning and related anatomy.* 1st ed. St. Louis: Mosby–Year Book, 1986:111–126.
9. Totty WG, Gilula LA. Imaging of the hand and wrist. In: Gilula LA, ed. *The traumatized hand and wrist: Radiographic and anatomic correlation.* Philadelphia: WB Saunders, 1992:1–12.
10. Eisenberg RL, Dennis CA, May CR. *Radiographic positioning.* 1st ed. Boston: Little, Brown, 1989:42–63.
11. Burman M. Anteroposterior projection of the carpometacarpal joint of the thumb by radial shift of the carpal tunnel view. *J Bone Joint Surg* 1958;40A:1156–1157.
12. Bernau A, Berquist TH. *Orthopaedic positioning in diagnostic radiology.* 1st ed. Baltimore, Munich: Urban & Schwarzenberg, 1983:108–132.
13. Haerr C, Mann FA, Gilula LA. *Anatomic variations of the wrist; selection of landmarks for verifying true frontal and lateral projections.* Abstract presented at RSNA 1993.
14. Ballinger PW. *Merrill's atlas of radiographic positions and radiologic procedures,* Vol. 1. St. Louis: CV Mosby, 1986:50–74.
15. Peh WCG, Gilula LA. Normal disruption of carpal arcs of the wrist. *J Hand Surg (Am)* 1994, submitted.
16. Gilula LA, Weeks PM. Post-traumatic ligamentous instabilities of the wrist. *Radiology* 1978;129:641–651.
17. Conway WF, Destouet JM, Gilula LA, Bellinghausen HW, Weeks PM. The carpal boss: An overview of radiographic evaluation. *Radiology* 1985;156:29–31.
18. Pallardy G, Chevrot A, Galmiche JM, Galmiche B. Radological examination of the hand and wrist. In: Tubiana R, ed. *The hand,* Vol. 1. Philadelphia: WB Saunders, 1981:648–682.
19. Sartoris DJ, Resnick D. Plain film radiography: Routine and specialized techniques and projections. In: Resnick D, Niwayama G, eds. *Diagnosis of bone and joint disorders,* Vol. 1. Philadelphia: WB Saunders, 1988:3–54.
20. Greenfield GB, Cooper SJ. *A manual of radiographic positioning.* Philadelphia: JB Lippincott, 1973:84–109.
21. Jones WA. Beware the sprained wrist: The incidence and diagnosis of scapholunate instability. *J Bone Joint Surg* 1988; 70(B):293–297.
22. Schimmerl SM, Metz VM, Totterman SMS, Mann FA, Gilula LA. Anatomic variation of the scapholunate (SL) joint: Where should the SL joint be measured? *Radiology* 1994, submitted.
23. Stecher WR. Roentgenography of the carpal navicular bone. *AJR* 1937;37:704–705.
24. Gruber L. Practical approaches to obtaining hand radiographs and special techniques in hand radiology. *Hand Clin* 1991;7:1–20.
25. Meschan I. The upper extremity. In: Meschan I, ed. *Radiographic positioning and related anatomy.* 2nd ed. Philadelphia: WB Saunders, 1978:60–68.
26. Lentino W, Lubetsky HW, Jacobson HG, Poppel MH. The carpal-bridge view. *J Bone Joint Surg* 1957;39A:88–90.
27. Swallow RA, Naylor E, Whitley AS, Roebuck EJ. *Clark's positioning in radiography,* Vol. 1. 11th ed. Rockville, MD: Aspen, 1986:35–53.
28. Hart VL, Gaynor V. Radiography of the carpal canal. *Radiogr Clin Photogr* 1942;18:23–24.
29. Wilson JN. Profiles of the carpal canal. *J Bone Joint Surg* 1954;36A:127–132.
30. Hart VL, Gaynor V. Roentgenographic study of the carpal canal. *J Bone Joint Surg* 1941;23:382–383.
31. Cullinan AM. The appendicular skeleton: Upper and lower extremities, shoulder, and pelvic girdles. In: Cullinan A, ed. *Optimizing radiographic positioning.* Philadelphia: JB Lippincott, 1992:53–70.
32. Templeton AW, Zim ID. The carpal tunnel view. *Missouri Med* 1964;61:443–444.
33. Norgaard F. Earliest roentgenological changes in polyarthritis of the rheumatoid type: Rheumatoid arthritis. *Radiology* 1965;85:325–329.
34. Norgaard F. Earliest roentgen changes in polyarthritis of the rheumatoid type. *Radiology* 1969;92:299–303.
35. Schernberg F. Roentgenographic examination of the wrist. A systemic study of the normal, lax and injured wrist. Part 2: The stress views. *J Hand Surg* 1990;15B:220–228.
36. White SJ, Louis DS, Braunstein EM, Hankin FM, Greene TL. Capitate-lunate instability: Recognition by manipulation under fluoroscopy. *AJR* 1984;143:361–364.

Acknowledgments

The authors appreciate the help of Andrew DiCarlo and Dareld LaBeau II, RT (R) with obtaining radiographs and Thomas Murry, photographer, for his help with the photographs of the many positions in this chapter.

CHAPTER 6

RADIOGRAPHY OF SOFT TISSUES IN TRAUMA TO THE HAND AND WRIST*

David J. Curtis

INTRODUCTION

Trauma to the hand and wrist is unique in its soft-tissue expression.[1–3] Swelling is the radiologic hallmark of trauma. It is one of the four signs of injury, which are swelling, pain, redness, and heat. Commonly, trauma with swelling is associated with a fracture in the hand or wrist. The swelling is limited in scope by fascial planes, which are vertically oriented and attach directly into the skin (Fig. 6–1).[4] The limitation of the swelling makes the area of injury predictable. This chapter is intended to describe the areas of limitation and help discern the underlying fracture, sprain, or dislocation.

TECHNICAL METHOD

Soft-tissue or "extremity" cassettes are the preferred means of imaging. These cassettes enhance the soft tissues while maintaining good bony detail. The posteroanterior (PA) and lateral views are the only two views used in the soft-tissue evaluation technique.[3] These two views provide 360 degrees of information and are not confusing when evaluating soft tissues. Additional views may be needed to find a fracture, sprain, or dislocation.

The views added to the soft-tissue evaluation are "stress" views. The clenched-fist view is just as named, i.e., the hand is clenched into a fist to stress the ligaments. It works because both flexors and extensors place full pressure on the collateral ligaments as well as all other ligaments and all the bones within the wrist. The hanging finger-trap view works because of muscle fatigue and the loss of ligamentous integrity.[5] Occasionally an ulnar deviation view will stress the wrist and demonstrate a fracture (Fig. 6–2). Very few fractures are found as a result of these three stress views, but sprains are frequently demonstrated. Patient-induced stress of the thumb is especially helpful.[6] Another "stress" view helpful in the detection of fractures is a delayed image 7 to 10 days after injury. Additional views should be obtained if a fracture, suspected because of swelling, is not demonstrated.

FOREARM

The lateral view of the hand provides unobstructed visualization of soft tissues on the dorsum of the forearm (Fig. 6–3). Small amounts of swelling can be detected and usually signify bony or severe ligamentous injury. The previously described pronator quadratus fat pad (pronator) is also visible in the lateral view on the ventral aspect of the radius and ulna (Figs. 6–3 and 6–4).[7] The pronator fat pad should lie close to the radius and be obvious in a good lateral view. A fracture or dislocation was present in 130 consecutive cases studied at the Children's National Medical Center in which the pronator was disturbed (unpublished study). The pronator fat pad was considered to be disturbed when it was displaced or contrast was lost within the soft tissues, indicating edema within the fat of the pad. The dorsal region of the forearm was considered abnormal when the skin could no longer be distinguished from the subcutaneous fat planes overlying the wrist. The skin is normally 1 mm thick and well distinguished by subcutaneous fat (Fig. 6–5).[8] Because Colles fracture is the most common wrist fracture, usually both the pronator and dorsal wrist fat are disturbed, but on occasion

* *Figures 6–1 through 6–15 reprinted with permission from Curtis DJ, Downey EF Jr. Soft tissue evaluation in trauma. In Gilula LA, ed.* The traumatized hand and wrist: Radiographic and anatomic correlation. *Philadelphia: WB Saunders, 1992.*

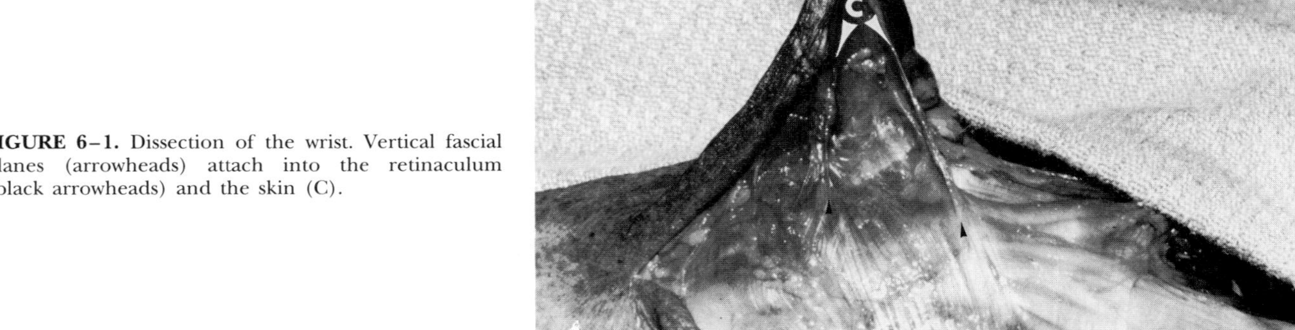

FIGURE 6–1. Dissection of the wrist. Vertical fascial planes (arrowheads) attach into the retinaculum (black arrowheads) and the skin (C).

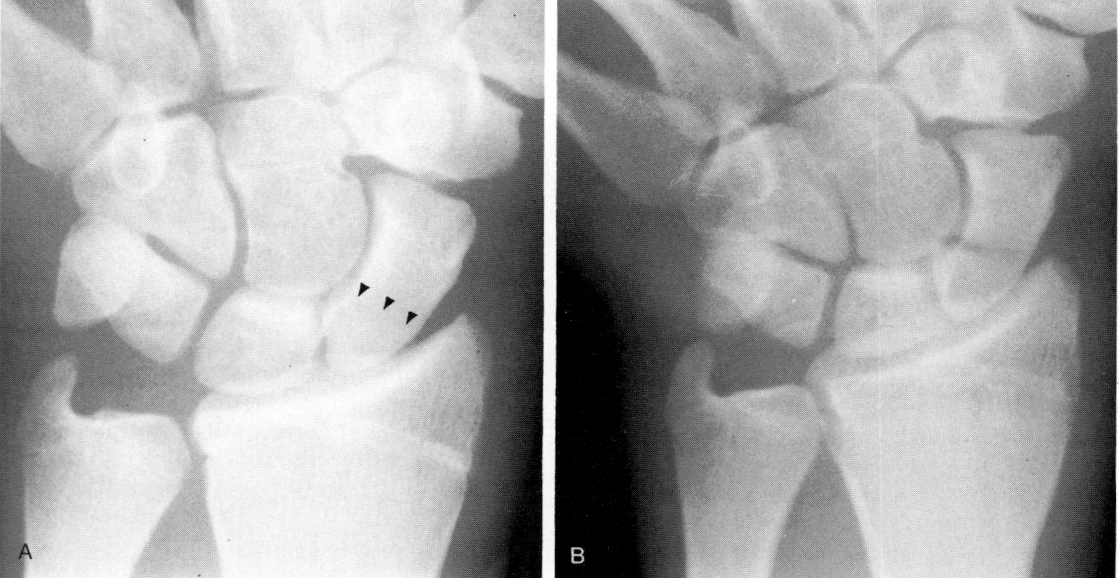

FIGURE 6–2. A: PA view of the wrist. A subtle scaphoid fracture is outlined by arrowheads. **B:** Ulnar deviation stress PA view. The fracture line is distracted.

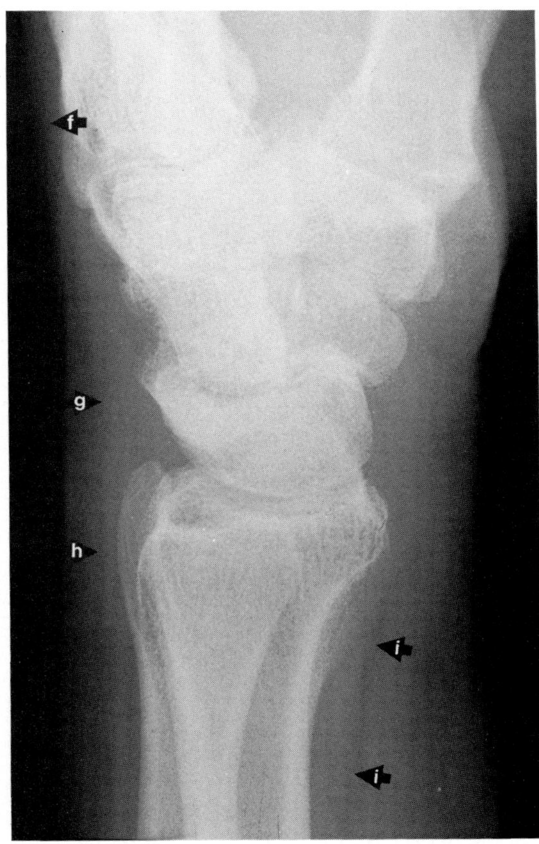

FIGURE 6–3. Lateral view of the wrist. Pronator fat plane ("i" on arrow), dorsal forearm ("h" on arrow), dorsal wrist ("g" on arrow), and dorsal hand ("f" on arrow).

only the pronator fat pad is abnormal when the dorsal bone cortex is intact. Since dorsiflexion is the mechanism of injury most frequently encountered, it is rare that the pronator fat will be undisturbed and the dorsal wrist fat abnormal.

In the PA view of the wrist (Fig. 6–6), the abductor pollicis longus tendon (APLT) is immediately adjacent to the radial styloid process and provides a linear soft-tissue density in contrast to the subcutaneous fat. The skin is well defined as well, and between the two soft-tissue densities the fatty density will become infiltrated if there is an injury to the radius. Infiltration of the fat with edema fluid causes the distinct contrast of the tendon and skin to be lost (Fig. 6–7). The ulna is contained within the subcutaneous fat and will frequently be fractured with the radius. If this happens the styloid process will lose the fatty density adjacent to it (Fig. 6–8). Hence, in many injuries to the wrist both the pararadial and paraulnar regions will show fatty infiltration because of the fractures. Absence of infiltration is strong evidence that no fracture has occurred.

WRIST

The lateral view of the wrist shows an undulating, mixed-density, soft-tissue capsule dorsal to the carpal bones. Ventral to the carpus is a large soft-tissue density that is not as helpful in determining injury. When

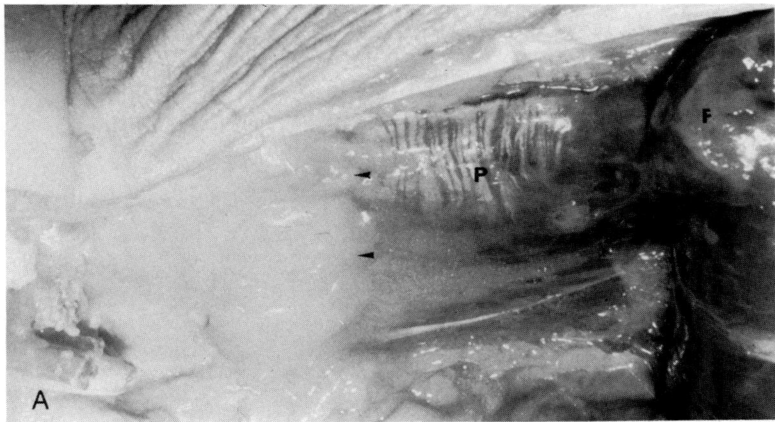

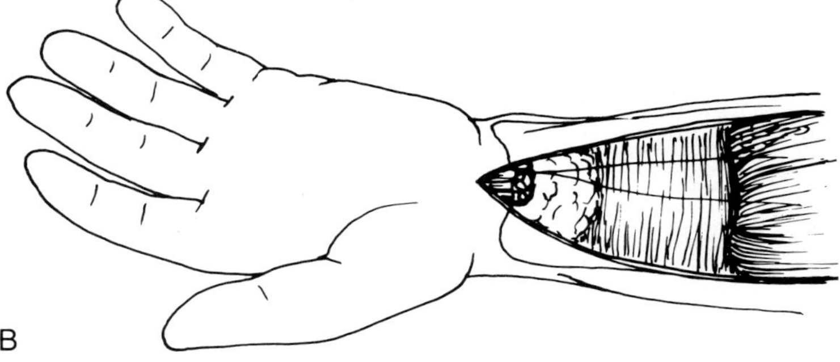

FIGURE 6–4. A: Palmar view of dissected forearm shows the flexor muscle (F). The pronator muscle (P) and its superficial fat plane (arrowheads) are evident. The hand is to the left. **B:** Line drawing corresponding to **A**.

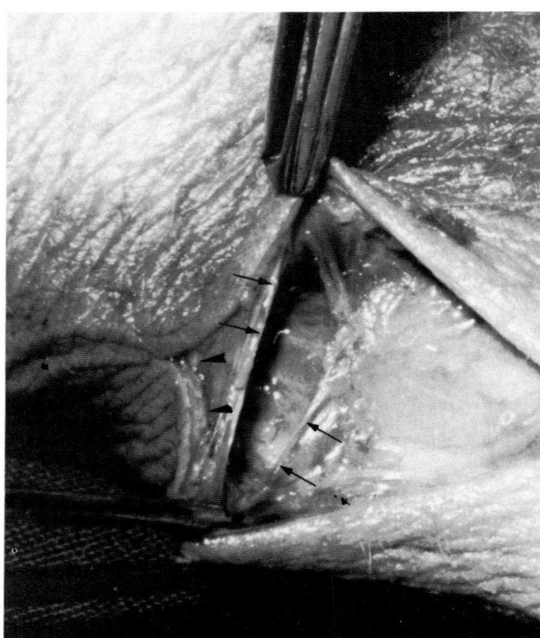

FIGURE 6–5. Lateral (radial) dissection of the skin. Subcutaneous fat (arrowheads) and deeper fascial structures create a space to contain swelling (arrows).

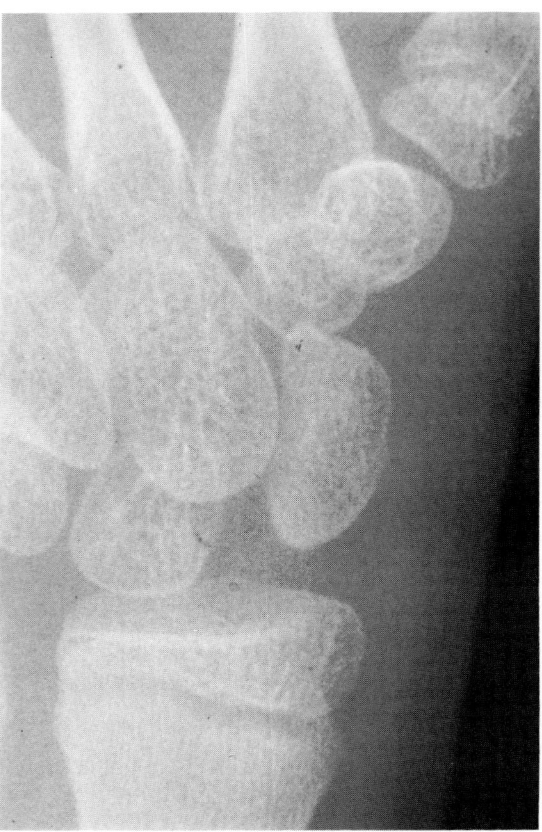

FIGURE 6–7. PA view of the radial side of the wrist in a child. Loss of distinctness of the superficial aspect of the abductor pollicis longus tendon (APLT) radial to the radius indicates an underlying fracture.

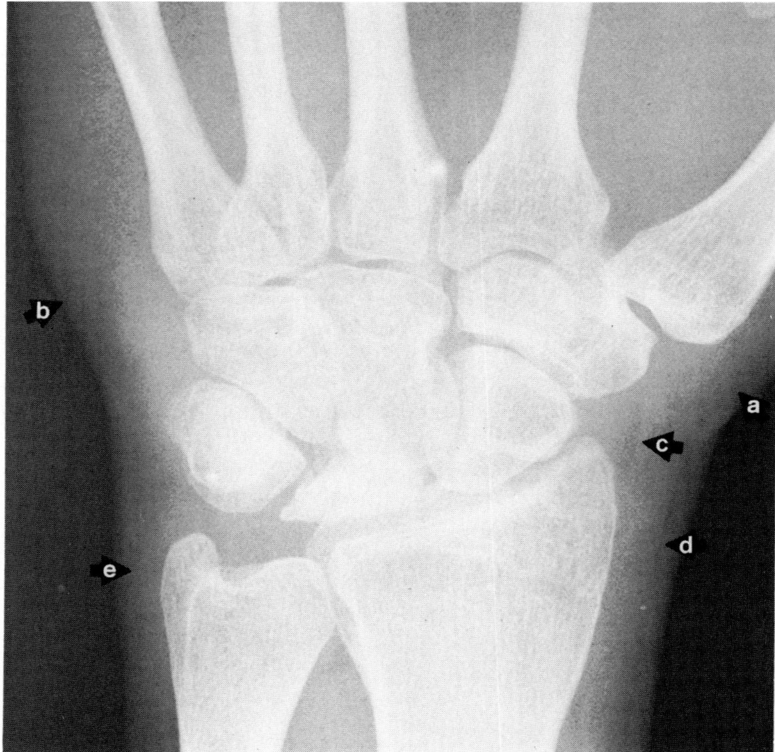

FIGURE 6–6. PA view of the hand in a patient with osteonecrosis of the lunate. The pararadial region and abductor pollicis longus tendon (APLT) (''d'' arrow), the paraulnar subcutaneous region (''e'' arrow), scaphoid fat plane (''c'' arrow), hypothenar region (''b'' arrow), and the subcutaneous fat plane in the thenar region (''a'' arrow) are all evident.

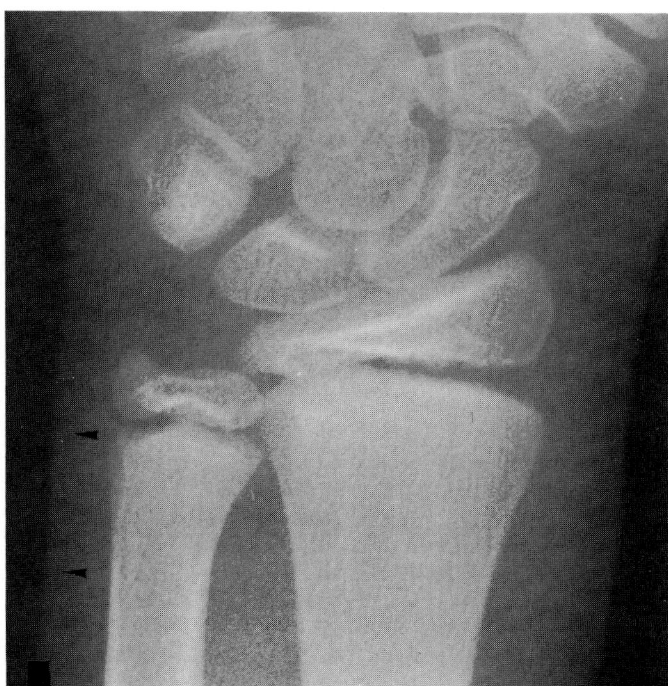

FIGURE 6–8. PA wrist view. Loss of distinctness to the skin–subcutaneous fat interface (arrowheads) strongly suggests an ulnar fracture. An associated fracture of the distal radius (salter II) is present (lateral view is not included).

carpal injury has occurred the undulation becomes smoothed out into a convexity that faces away from the carpals (Fig. 6–9). The mixed density also becomes a more uniform soft-tissue density because of the wrist effusion.[9] These two signs may occur together or separately. Actual fracture lines are usually not visible in the lateral view. The one exception is the dorsal avulsion fracture of the triquetrum. This fracture accounts for approximately half of triquetral fractures. This makes the lateral view essential for eliminating it alone, even if the soft-tissue changes were not present in other trauma.

The PA view of the wrist illustrates useful changes for carpal bones only in the radial aspect. The area of change has been previously described as the navicular (scaphoid) fat plane.[10] The anatomy of the fat plane is of interest because the lateral (radial)-most soft-tissue density that delineates it is the same APLT that makes up the pararadial fat plane. It is the opposite side of the tendon that delineates the fat for the scaphoid fat pad. The medial (ulnar) aspect of the fat pad is the lateral collateral ligament of the wrist, which extends from the radial styloid to the tuberosity of the trapezium (greater multangular). Therefore the fat pad runs from the radial styloid to the trapezium. The fat pad parallels the carpal scaphoid, hence its name. The importance of this fat pad cannot be overemphasized since it reflects injury to the scaphoid, which is the most frequently fractured carpal bone.[9,10] Because of its anatomy this carpal bone is frequently subjected to proximal aseptic necrosis, which leads to a variety of problems, including nonunion, pseudoarthrosis, and fragmentation. The problems become magnified if prompt immobilization is not applied. A missed scaphoid fracture is the most common cause of medicolegal intervention for radiologists in the wrist and hand. We have found that any obliteration of the scaphoid fat plane is indicative of a fracture (Fig. 6–10), especially when the dorsal wrist fat plane is disturbed.[9] This makes the two fat planes in combination extremely sensitive.

If the dorsal wrist fat plane is disturbed but the scaphoid fat plane is normal, injury to the other carpal bones must be suspected. The triquetrum is the next most commonly injured carpal bone and only half of its fractures are of the dorsal avulsion type, which is usually easily seen. The remaining half are subtle linear fractures. The hamate is the next most commonly fractured carpal bone, and may be associated with a metacarpal fracture.

Kienböck's aseptic necrosis of the lunate is a common disorder that must not be mistaken for a fracture. Earlier orthopedic textbooks included it with fractures, resulting in the misstatement that lunate

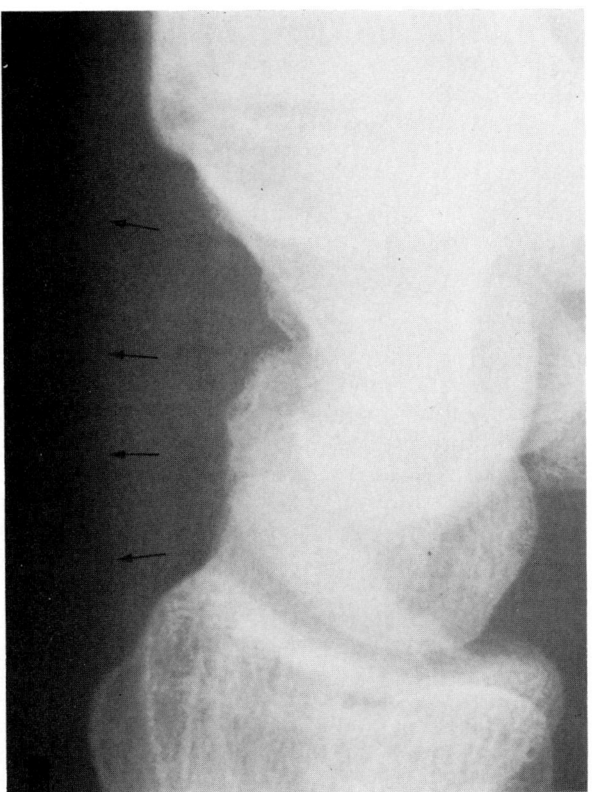

FIGURE 6–9. Lateral view of the wrist. The skin–subcutaneous fat interface (arrows) is lost. An underlying fracture should be suspected.

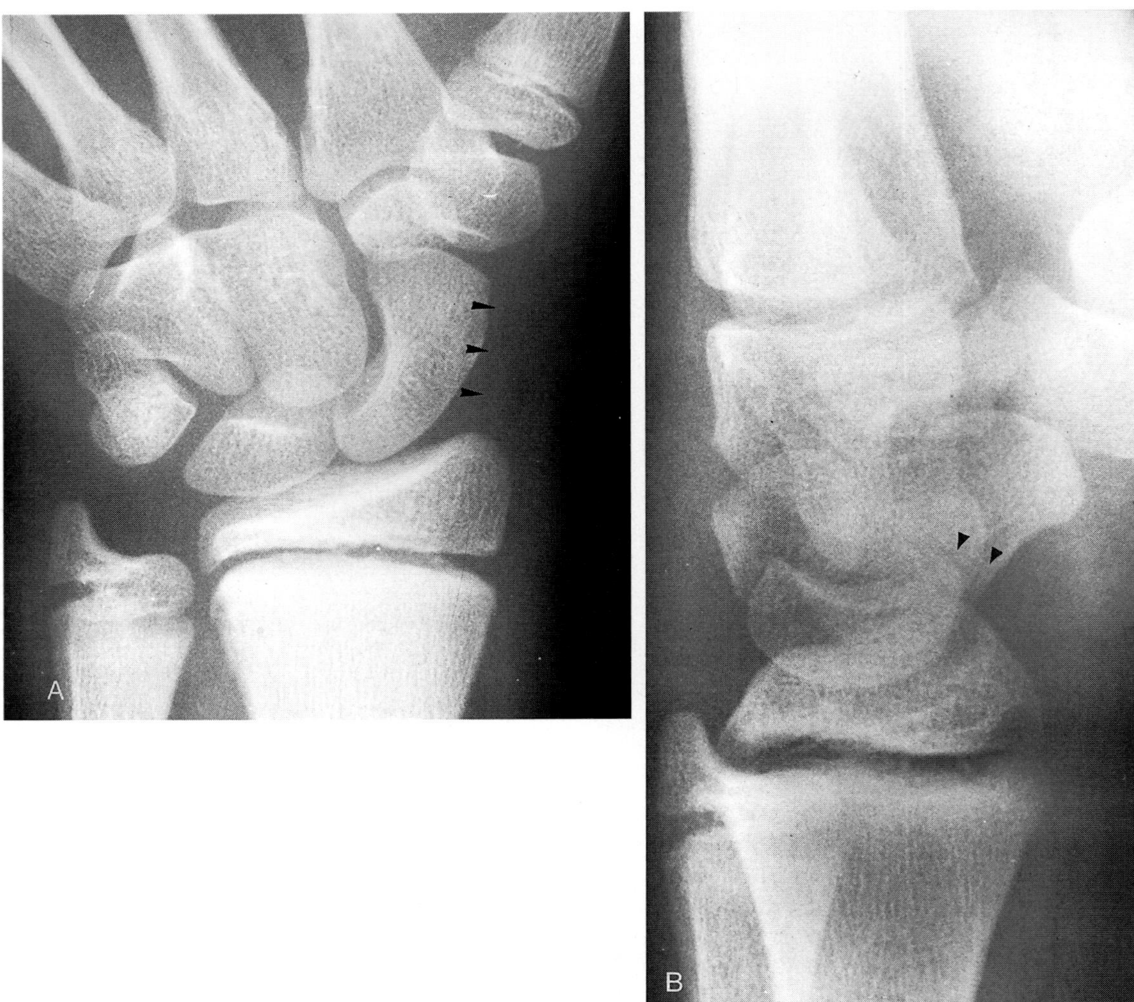

FIGURE 6–10. A: PA mild ulnar deviation view of the wrist. Three-fourths of the fat plane deep to the abductor pollicis longus tendon (APLT) is lost (arrowheads). A scaphoid fracture should be suspected. **B:** Lateral view of the wrist. A scaphoid fracture line is seen (arrowheads).

fractures were more common than scaphoid fractures. Lunate fractures probably are more common than most carpal fractures, except for the three already mentioned (scaphoid, triquetrum, hamate), but they are difficult to detect. The cause of Kienböck's aseptic necrosis has not yet been completely clarified.

In addition to that seen in fractures, soft-tissue swelling may be seen with sprains of the wrist, synovitis, and tenosynovitis. Sprains tend to be more extensive than suspected. They are identified by noting joint spaces that are wider than the uniform 1–2 mm seen throughout the hand and wrist. Besides being wider, the joint spaces may have lost their parallel nature. Loss of parallelism between articulating cortices occurs commonly with osteoarthritis or trauma, and the latter frequently leads to the former. The distinguishing feature between the two entities is the presence of sclerosis deep to the cortical bone in the region of the narrowest joint space, found only in osteoarthritis.[11] Proof of the sprain can be obtained using the clenched-fist or finger-trap hanging-forearm PA view. There may be widening in an acute sprain and no change in most old injuries that have had time to heal. The imaging must include the ulnar-deviated PA projection (see Fig. 6–2) because multiple views may demonstrate laxity that is old; it must not be confused with acute laxity. If traction views are used, however, it may be helpful to perform the traction views on the asymptomatic wrist as well because there can normally be some distraction between carpal bones, especially between the proximal and distal carpal rows. The presence of osteoarthritis does not rule out an acute sprain. In fact, a wrist with osteoarthritis may be more susceptible to a new sprain than a virgin wrist.

Dislocations of the wrist are rare. When they do occur, over 95% of them involve the radiolunocapitate axes and can easily be diagnosed on the lateral view of the wrist. Swelling should be very obvious, and is usually present in the PA view as well as in the pararadial, paraulnar, and scaphoid regions. In the lateral view, swelling may be present in the dorsal forearm, pronator, and dorsal wrist areas. This much swelling should always alert the radiologist to the possibility of a dislocation as well as multiple injuries in both the forearm and wrist compartments. With a dislocation there are usually overlapping bones as well that create an increased density where they overlap. The density of normal bony structures is uniform throughout the hand and wrist, with one area comparable in density to another. The other sign of a dislocation is widened space in the intercarpal or radiocarpal joints. Occasionally there is a widening in the carpometacarpal joints, although this is rare.

HAND

The lateral view of the hand shows swelling dorsally in what is normally a subcutaneous space (Fig. 6–11). If there is enough swelling, it is expressed in the

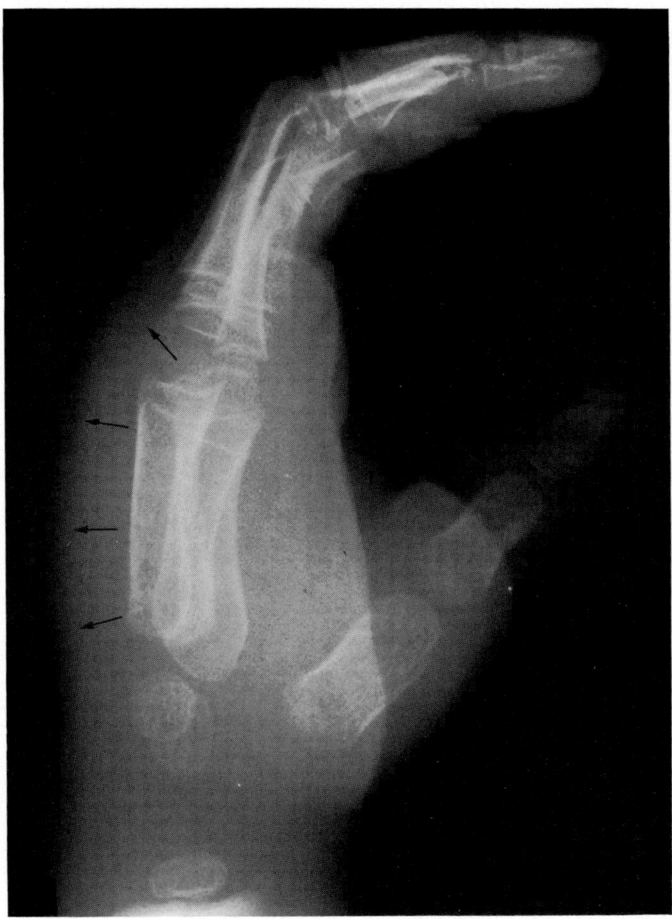

FIGURE 6–11. Lateral view of the hand. Dorsal swelling is seen throughout the hand. Compare with Fig. 6–3. Fractures involve the second and third metacarpal bases (shown on other views).

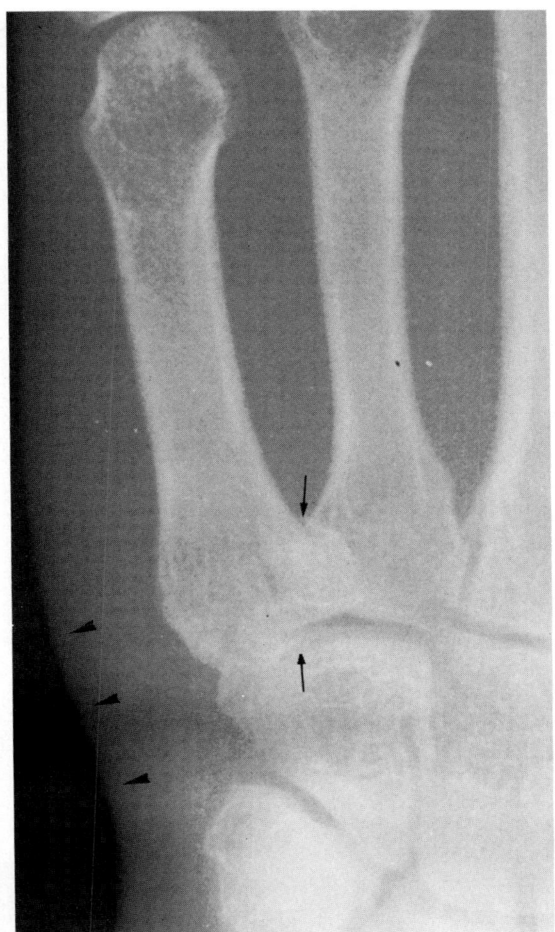

FIGURE 6–12. PA view of the medial (ulnar) side of the hand and wrist. Hypothenar swelling obscures the skin–subcutaneous fat interface (arrowheads). An underlying fracture of the fifth metacarpal is present (arrows).

hypothenar recess in the PA view (Fig. 6–12). The most common expression in the hypothenar space is as an increased density bordering on pure white, whereas in the lateral view the swelling is convex in shape and does not parallel the metacarpals. If the injury is to the metacarpal head rather than to its base or shaft, a convex swelling over the head occurs in the lateral view (Fig. 6–13) and usually there is no swelling seen in the PA view.

DIGITS

The digits have tightly applied skin, which makes swelling almost impossible except over the dorsum of the joints. This is seen in the lateral view as a convex swelling over the joint space (Fig. 6–14). This swelling may be expressed either radially, ulnarly, or both, at the joint level in the PA view. When swelling is present just on the radial or ulnar side of a joint on

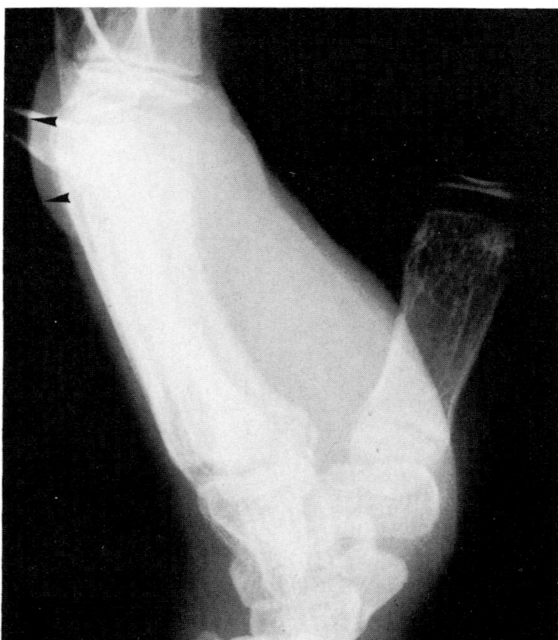

FIGURE 6–13. Lateral view of the hand. Convex swelling is seen distally over the metacarpal heads (arrowheads), indicating a fracture of one or more of them. The base of a proximal phalanx may be fractured instead of or as well as a metacarpal head. In this case a metacarpal head is fractured. From Curtis DJ et al: AJR 142:781, 1984.

the PA view, injury to the radial or ulnar collateral ligament, respectively, should be suspected.

THUMB

The thumb has no region for swelling that can be visualized in the lateral view. In the PA view, swelling is seen at the lateral oblique base of the first metacarpal where the APLT inserts (Fig. 6–15). Injuries as distant as the first metacarpophalangeal joint will cause swelling at this site. This is important because it means that injuries to the thumb can be suspected and imaged when wrist views only are obtained that do not include a PA view of the hand.

SUMMARY

Using radiography that emphasizes the soft-tissue expression of fractures, sprains, and dislocations will increase the accuracy of diagnosis and improve overall treatment of injuries to the hand and the wrist. Absence of any swelling can be taken as assurance that significant acute bony or soft-tissue injury has not occurred.

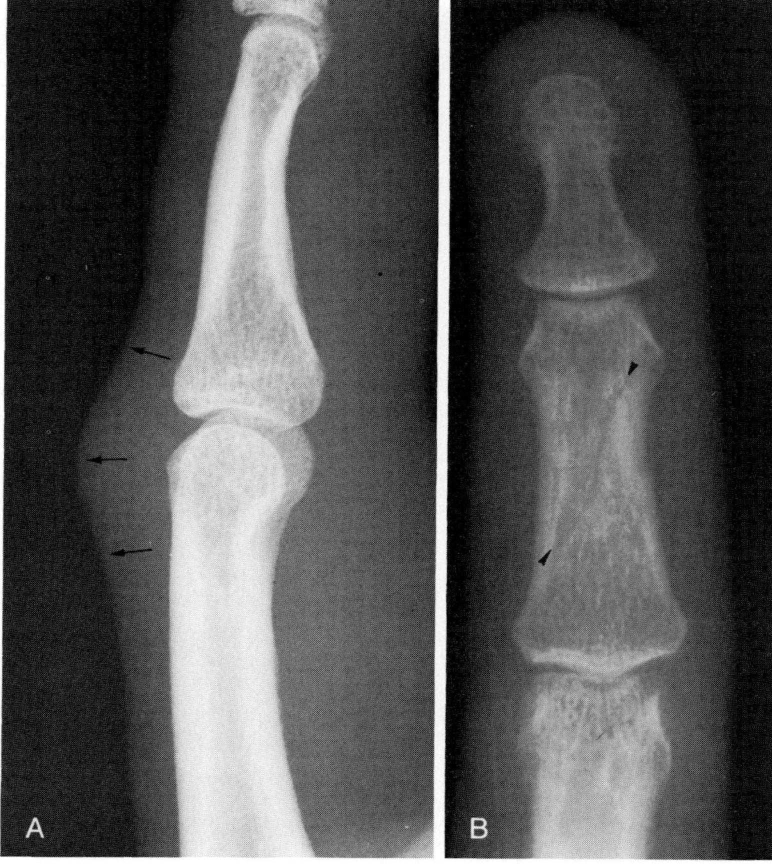

FIGURE 6–14. A: Lateral view of a finger. Swelling is seen over the dorsum of a proximal interphalangeal joint (arrows). **B:** PA view of the middle phalanx of the same digit. An oblique fracture (arrowheads) involves this middle phalanx with minimal swelling present radially and ulnarly to the joint space and middle phalanx.

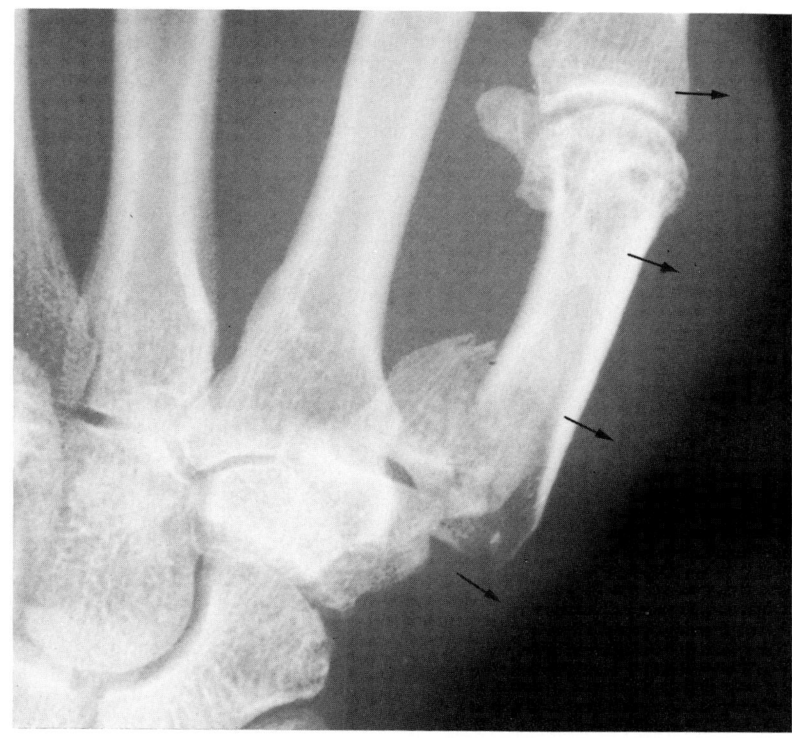

FIGURE 6–15. PA view of the hand. Swelling is seen radially (arrows) with loss of the distinctness of the abductor pollicis longus tendon (APLT) at its attachment with the proximal first metacarpal (proximal arrow). The underlying oblique comminuted fracture of the first metacarpal is seen.

REFERENCES

1. Curtis DJ. Injuries of the wrist: An approach to diagnosis. *Radiol Clin North Am* 1981;19:625–644.
2. Curtis DJ, Downey EF Jr, Brower AC, et al. Importance of soft-tissue evaluation in hand and wrist trauma: Statistical evaluation. *AJR* 1984;142:781–788.
3. Downey EF Jr, Curtis DJ. Soft-tissue radiography of the wrist. In: Lichtman DM, ed. *The wrist and its disorders.* Philadelphia: WB Saunders, 1988:96–107.
4. Curtis DJ, Downey EF Jr, Brahman SL. Letter to the editor. Compartmentalized swelling in hand and wrist trauma. *AJR* 1985;145:195.
5. Yousefzadeh DK. The value of traction during roentgenography of the wrist and metacarpophalangeal joints. *Skeletal Radiol* 1979;4:29–33.
6. Downey EF Jr, Curtis DJ. Patient-induced stress test of the first metacarpophalangeal joint. *Radiology* 1986;158:679–683.
7. MacEwan DW. Changes due to trauma in the fat plane overlying the quadratus muscle: A radiologic sign. *Radiology* 1964;82:879–886.
8. Melson GL, Staple TW, Evens RG. Soft-tissue radiographic technique. *Semin Roentgenol* 1973;8:19–24.
9. Carver RA, Barrington NA. Soft-tissue changes accompanying recent scaphoid injuries. *Clin Radiol* 1985;36:423–425.
10. Terry DW Jr, Ramish JE. The navicular fat stripe: A useful roentgen sign for evaluating wrist trauma. *AJR* 1975;124:25–28.
11. Watson HK, Ryu J. Degenerative disorders of the carpus. *Orthop Clin North Am* 1984;15:337–353.

CHAPTER 7

WRIST INSTABILITY SERIES
An Overview

I. RADIOGRAPHY FOR WRIST INSTABILITIES *F. Schernberg*

II. INDICATIONS FOR WRIST INSTABILITY SERIES AND ITS COST-EFFECTIVENESS *Nhan P. Truong, F. A. Mann, and Louis A. Gilula*

I. RADIOGRAPHY FOR WRIST INSTABILITIES

F. Schernberg

Our classification of injuries limited to ligaments, with no or minimal lesions of the bone or cartilage surface, is a guideline for their diagnoses as well as their treatments. It consists of four main grades. The Grade I injury represents partial disruption of the ligament with the affected joint stable to active or passive stress. This condition may be confused with several other traumatic lesions such as traumatic chondromalacia or occult fractures. The Grade II injury consists of a complete disruption of the involved ligament. The carpals are not displaced and they have normal relationships to each other. Only active movement or passive stress will displace them. The Grade III injury consists of complete disruption of the ligament associated with a permanent displacement of the different carpals with abnormal relationships between them. Because some contact remains between the adjacent articular surfaces, this condition is commonly called subluxation. If no contact exists between adjacent carpal bones, a luxation or Grade IV injury is present.

The Grade I lesion, commonly called a sprain, and the Grade IV lesion are not included in the common concept of wrist instability first introduced by Fisk.[1] Grade II corresponds to dynamic instabilities, and Grade III to a static instability. Displacement can be either a widening of the intercarpal space, angular modifications of the carpals, or even both conditions simultaneously. This classification is the keystone for our therapeutic policy in the case of ligament injuries.

In Grade I and acute Grade II ligament injuries, surgery (i.e., suture) is unnecessary. Healing of the injured ligaments will be achieved by cast immobilization, generally in 3 to 4 weeks in a Grade I lesion and over 6 weeks in a Grade II injury. Only old Grade II ligament injuries (seen later than 6 weeks) and Grade III ligament injuries (acute or old ones) need surgical care; in the former, to repair the retracted stumps of the ligaments, and, in latter, to first reduce the displaced bones as accurately as possible and then to repair the ligament(s).

The imaging techniques available to evaluate injuries of the ligaments must provide three major facts to the surgeon: (1) the precise location of the lesion; (2) the character of the lesion (i.e., tear or an avulsion from its bony insertion) and its severity or extent (i.e., partial or complete lesion); and (3) the significance of that lesion for stability of the joint (i.e., is there evidence of wrist instability?).

The roentgenographic examination was one of the first diagnostic aids for evaluation of the wrist used at the beginning of the twentieth century.[2] In daily practice, it remains a useful and accurate diagnostic tool for evaluating injuries to the wrist ligaments.[3] Currently it is the only diagnostic tool capable of showing the amount of instability resulting from injuries to the wrist ligaments. Radiography provides only indirect information about the ligamentous lesions. Therefore much experience correlating roentgenographic features with information obtained by direct visualization of the lesions is mandatory. In our initial experience this has been obtained mainly during surgery.[4,5] Actually, more direct demonstration of some pathology is possible with the use of arthrography demonstrating abnormal communications between joint compartments.[6–8] Magnetic resonance imaging (MRI)[9–11] is a newer imaging tool that can show the ligamentous structures themselves; however, MRI has many limitations.[11]

Arthroscopy[12,13] is an invasive method associated with iatrogenic complications including infection, anesthesia, dorsal sensory branch of the radial nerve injury, tendon injury, or even further joint damage. It can demonstrate the appearance of the ligaments and the interval between adjacent bones. It also identifies other pathologic conditions such as chondromalacia. At the present time these diagnostic tools appear to be predictable diagnostic aids with a high rate of accuracy for lesions at the level of the first carpal row (i.e., for the scapholunate and lunotriquetral ligaments) as well as for the triangular fibrocartilage. These modalities, however, do not offer a better way to demonstrate injuries to the remaining major wrist ligaments. In our opinion, this results directly from the fact that the first row can be considered as an osteoarticulated meniscus (Fig. 7–1).[14] Because the scapholunate and lunotriquetral ligaments are similar to the triangular fibrocartilage in the coronal plane, they thus can be easily examined by these different direct imaging techniques, similar to the meniscus of the knee. The other ligaments, which are within the capsular tissue in a peripheral plane, are less easily accessible. To be effective, the roengenographic examination must be guided by clinical data and performed with precision, and the analysis of the views must be performed in a stepwise and systematic way in static as well as dynamic conditions.[4,5,14]

Because there is a well-known difficulty of conventional radiology assisting in the diagnosis of injuries to the ligaments at the distal radioulnar joint (DRUJ), we will not address that here. Computed tomography[15,16] and arthrography are currently the most appropriate diagnostic tools in that area. Perhaps in the future MRI may become the tool of choice to evaluate ligamentous abnormalities around the DRUJ. Lesions with advanced collapse and osteoarthritis are also eliminated from discussion here because the management of their imaging is also quite different.

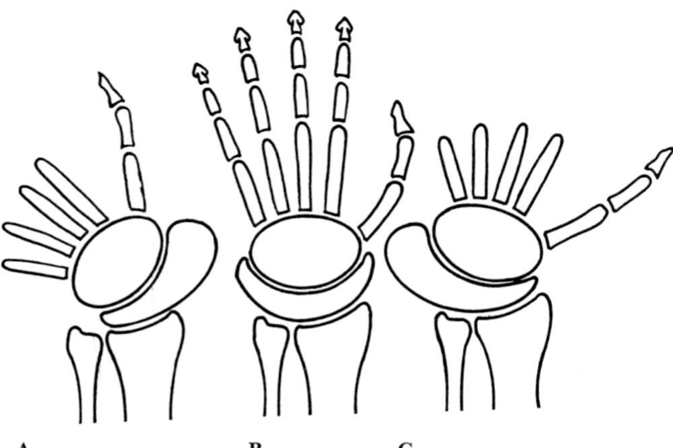

FIGURE 7–1. A schematic drawing of the wrist in the frontal position with the proximal carpal row considered as an osteoarticulated meniscus adapting its shape according to the variation of the interarticular carpal space. **A**: in ulnar deviation; **B**: in standard (neutral) position; **C**: in radial deviation. (Reprinted with permission from Schernberg F. *Le poignet: Anatomie radiologique et chirurgie.* Paris: Masson, 1992.)

THE INITIAL WORKUP

The routine radiographic examination of a painful wrist with suspected injury to the ligaments should include standard posteroanterior (PA), lateral, and oblique views of the wrist. Only standard PA and lateral views are necessary to analyze the relationships between the carpal bones. The oblique views are useful to rule out carpal bone fractures.

The Standard Frontal PA View

The Positioning of the Hand and Its Assessment: The PA View in Neutral Position

It is easy to put the wrist in a neutral position and check that this position is maintained. However, with a vertical beam, the neutral position of the forearm and the hand in position for a PA view can only be achieved if the elbow is in 90 degrees of flexion and the shoulder in 90 degrees of abduction (the elbow is at shoulder height).

The radiographic criteria that confirm neutral rotation of the forearm are demonstrated on both sides of the wrist. Proximally, the ulnar styloid process appears in its most medial (ulnar) position relative to the ulnar shaft. More lateral (radial) position of the ulnar styloid process suggests supination. At the DRUJ there is no overlap of the articular surfaces, and the radioulnar space is clearly seen. The radial styloid is also well outlined without any suggestion of double contour. Distally, the carpometacarpal spaces are well outlined all along the bases of the five metacarpals, and in the hand the metacarpals of the fingers are regularly positioned with equal intervening intermetacarpal spaces.

Analysis of Normal Roentgenographic Aspects of the Wrist

Roentgenographic analysis of the wrist must be carried out in a systematic stepwise manner at three fundamental levels; the first carpal row, the radiocarpal joint, and the midcarpal joint. At each level, the width of the joint spaces and the parallelism between cortices of adjacent articulating bones are analyzed first, followed by analysis of the three arcs of Gilula,[17] and finally the anatomic configuration of the individual carpal bones.

The Spaces Between the Carpal Bones

The spaces between the carpal bones should always be the same and less than 3 mm in width with parallelism between cortices of adjacent articulating bones.[17,18]

The Three Carpal Arcs[17]

The first arc is the convexity formed by proximal articular surfaces of the scaphoid, lunate, and triquetrum. The second arc is the concavity created by the distal articular cortices of these same three bones, scaphoid, lunate, and triquetrum. The third arc is created by the proximal convexities of the capitate and hamate.

The Anatomic Configuration

On frontal views, hand measurements of carpal height or carpal translation[19] are not useful in the field of instabilities. To facilitate the description of anatomic configuration, we will outline normal anatomic aspects in both extreme radial and ulnar deviation positions (Figs. 7–2 and 7–3).

Anatomic Configuration of the First (Proximal) Carpal Row (Fig. 7–2). According to kinematic studies of carpal bone motions during deviation in the frontal position,[20] which clearly showed that ulnar deviation and extension on one hand and radial deviation and flexion on the other hand are linked, the criteria for modification of the appearance of the carpal bones in side-to-side deviation are in fact mainly criteria of flexion and extension.

The Scaphoid.[2,4,5,14,21–24] Radial deviation creates the same configuration as flexion: the scaphoid has a foreshortened appearance with a ring sign. The shape of the scaphoid in neutral deviation is the configuration of neutral position: the scaphoid remains foreshortened but the ring sign is less obvious. Ulnar deviation produces the configuration of extension: the scaphoid is seen in its full length and there is no ring sign.

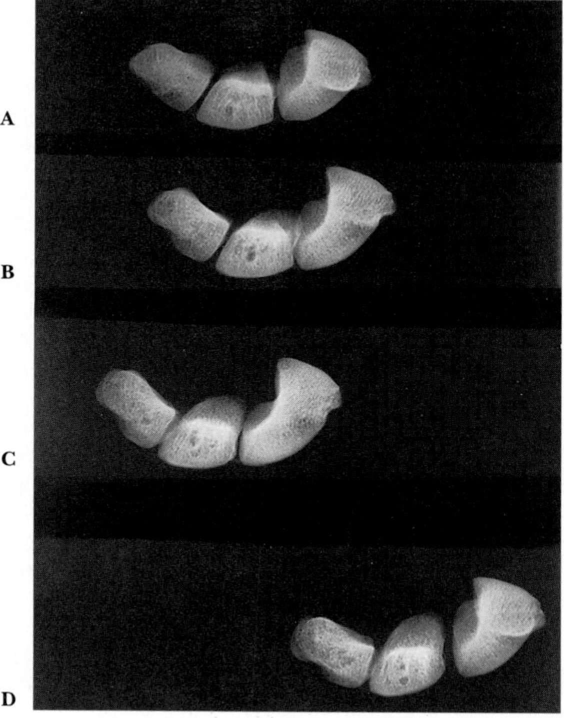

FIGURE 7–2. Normal scapholunotriquetral relationships in different deviations while in the frontal position. **A**: In radial deviation; **B**: in standard neutral position; **C**: in ulnar deviation; **D**: scapholunotriquetral relationship in standard frontal neutral position where the scaphoid shows a configuration of radial deviation or flexion and both the lunate and triquetrum have a configuration of ulnar deviation or extension. Thus the scapholunate dissociation is demonstrated on the AP view by analyzing the roentgenographic shapes of the bones, or it can also be recognized by making careful measurements on the lateral view.

The Lunate.[4,5,14,21–23] In radial deviation the lunate has the configuration of flexion: it appears almost triangular with its small posterior process well outlined. Its shape in neutral deviation is the configuration of neutral position: the lunate has lost its triangular shape and its anterior and posterior processes are superimposed. The shape of the lunate in ulnar deviation is the same as extension and is due to the appearance of the wide anterior process of the lunate, which gives the lunate a trapezoidal-type shape.

The Triquetrum.[4,5,14,22,23] In radial deviation, the triquetrum assumes the configuration of flexion: there is evidence of a tubercle on the radial part of the distal border of the triquetrum. Its shape in neutral deviation is the configuration of neutral position: the tubercle on the lateral (radial) part of the distal border looks smaller. The shape in ulnar deviation is the configuration of extension: the tubercle on the lateral (radial) part of the distal border of the triquetrum has completely disappeared and is now linear.

The Normal Scapholunotriquetral Relationship in Different Deviations in the Frontal Position (Figs. 7–2 and 7–3).[4,5,14,22–26] In radial deviation (Figs. 7–2A and 7–3A) the three bones of the proximal row are in radial deviation showing features of flexion of the proximal carpal row: the scaphoid is foreshortened with a ring sign; the lunate appears almost triangular with its small posterior process well outlined; and there is evidence of a tubercle on the radial part of the distal border of the triquetrum. In neutral hand and wrist position (Figs. 7–2B and 7–3B) the three bones of the proximal row are in neutral position. In neutral position the scaphoid remains forshortened but the ring sign is less obvious; the lunate has lost its triangular shape and its anterior and posterior processes are superimposed; and the tubercle on the lateral part of the distal border of the triquetrum looks smaller. In ulnar deviation (Figs. 7–2C and 7–3C) the three bones of the proximal row are in ulnar position and show a configuration of extension: the scaphoid is seen in its full length and there is no ring sign; because of the appearance of the wide anterior process of the lunate it appears trapezoidal in shape; and the tubercle on the lateral (radial) part of the distal border of the triquetrum has completely disappeared and is now linear.

Anatomic Configuration at the Radiocarpal Level (Fig. 7–3). Radiocarpal rotation is displayed by the relationship of the proximal pole of the lunate to the distal part of the radius and the distal radioulnar space. In radial and neutral deviation (Figs. 7–3A and 7–3B) the proximal surface of the lunate never moves more than half its width off the distal surface of the radius. In ulnar deviation (Fig. 7–3C) most of the proximal surface of the lunate is apposed to the radius, and the lunotriquetral joint is nearly in line with the DRUJ.

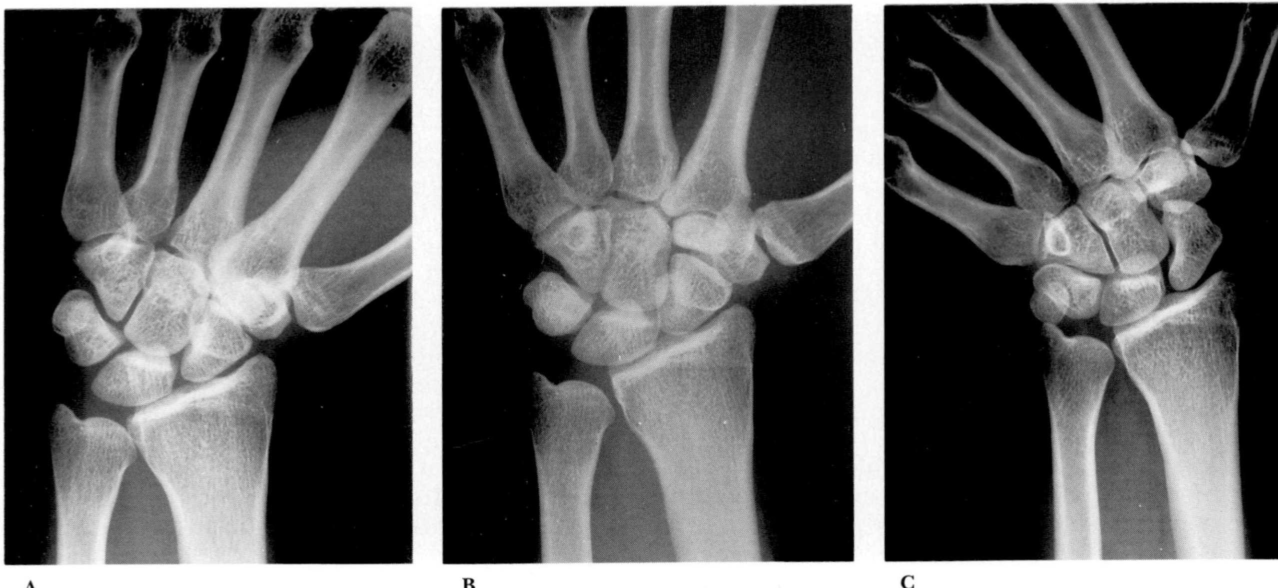

A B C

FIGURE 7–3. Roentgenographic features of a normal wrist on PA views. **A**: In radial deviation; **B**: in standard position; **C**: in ulnar deviation. (Reprinted with permission from Schernberg F. Roentgenographic examination of the wrist: A systematic study of the normal, lax and traumatic wrist. Part one: The standard and the positional views. *J Hand Surg* 1990;15B:210–219.)

Anatomic Configuration at the Midcarpal Level (Fig. 7–3). Midcarpal rotation is assessed by evaluating the relative positions between the triquetrum and the ulnar slope of the hamate[27] and the vertex of the hamate relative to the first carpal row.[14] In radial deviation (Fig. 7–3A) the triquetrum is at a proximal level (''high'') in relation to the hamate, and the vertex of the hamate is articulating with the triquetrum ulnar to the lunotriquetral joint. In the neutral position (Fig. 7–3B) the proximal pole of the hamate is opposite the lunotriquetral joint. In ulnar deviation (Fig. 7–3C) the triquetrum is at its distal level (''low'') in relation to the hamate, and the vertex of the hamate reaches and overlaps the medial (ulnar) and distal part of the lunate.

Normal and Abnormal Configurations

The preceding sections outline the criteria that define the normal carpal bone shapes and interrelationships at the different levels of the wrist that must be systematically checked on the standard PA view.

Normal and Abnormal Features at the First (Proximal) Carpal Row

Normal Features (Figs. 7–2A through 7–2C and 7–3). The proximal row is normal as defined in the preceding section. In addition, interosseous gaps at the scapholunate and lunotriquetral joints are less than 3 mm, and the carpal Arcs I and II as defined by Gilula[17] and the scapholunotriquetral articulation are normal.

Abnormal Conditions.

Scapholunate Lesions.

Scapholunate Dissociation. Scapholunate dissociation shows evidence only of scapholunate space widening with the carpal bones moving into normal flexion and extension positions. On the frontal view (neutral position) the scapholunate space is greater than 3 mm, producing the Terry Thomas sign.[27] On the lateral view the scapholunate angle is normal with normal neutral position of the lunate. It is crucially important not to confuse scapholunate laxity with such a configuration. The scapholunate gap that is well outlined on a standard PA view never exceeds 3 mm. Such an appearance, often encountered in cases of scaphoid fractures (Fig. 7–4A), may be considered abnormal, because usually on the standard PA view the scapholunate space is seldom clearly profiled, its width being less than 2 mm. Scapholunate laxity can easily be confirmed by performing a comparative standard view of the contralateral uninjured wrist or by motion views of the involved wrist (Fig. 7–4B).

Scapholunate Dislocation. Here the major abnormality is the presence of abnormal angular modification of the scaphoid and/or the lunate configurations. The presence of scapholunate diastasis is not constant. Loss of the normal outline of the proximal carpal row on the frontal view (neutral position) consists of the scaphoid displaying an appearance normally seen in radial deviation, while the lunate and triquetrum adopt the appearance seen in ulnar deviation (Fig. 7–2D). On the lateral view the scapholunate angle is increased, reaching about 90

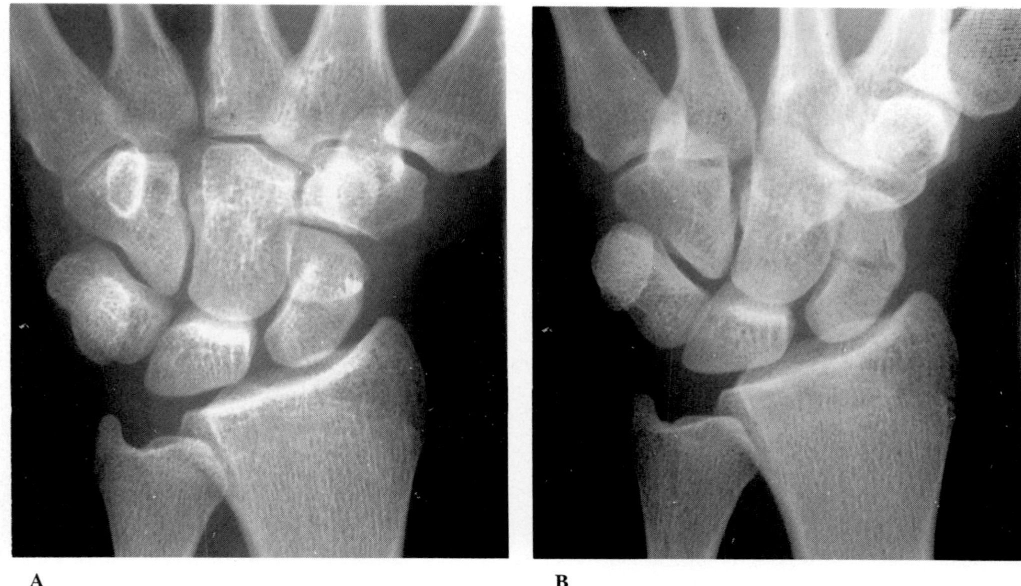

FIGURE 7–4. Appearance of scapholunate (SL) laxity in a case of fractured scaphoid. **A**: In standard PA position, the SL gap is well profiled, seeming enlarged, but it is not abnormal. **B**: The same wrist with a clenched-fist view shows a similar appearance of the SL joint. The space is lax normally. In general, in this chapter laxity is used to denote a normal constitutional condition and not a traumatically induced one.

degrees. The lunate may be normal or dorsiflexed. When the lunate is dorsiflexed, the dorsal intercalated segmental instability (DISI) pattern,[28] associated with a loss of the colinear alignment of the radius and capitate, is realized. In case of any doubt, additional motion views may be helpful (see upcoming sections).

Lunotriquetral Lesions. According to anatomy and biomechanics[29] at this level, isolated abnormalities found on the standard PA view are rather uncommon. They are associated more often with radiocarpal lesions.

Lunotriquetral Dissociation. Dissociation is recognized only by evidence of widening of the lunotriquetral space since the carpal bones are in normal position during flexion and extension. Such a condition has been encountered in our experience only as a residual of perilunate dislocations.

Lunotriquetral Dislocation. In the frontal view there is evidence of disruption of Arcs I and II of Gilula at the lunotriquetral area. The lunotriquetral space may be normal or, if there is a gap greater than 3 mm, it may be abnormal. In our experience this situation is seldom seen as an isolated lesion at the first row. It is mainly encountered as a residual of perilunate dislocations or in association with a radiocarpal lesion such as the ventral intercalated segmental instability (VISI) pattern,[28] where the three carpals of the first row are in a volar-flexed position. With lunotriquetral dislocation, there is loss of the normally congruent movement between the scaphoid, lunate, and triquetrum during the side-to-side (radial-to-ulnar) deviation from neutral position.

Normal and Abnormal Features at the Radiocarpal Level

Normal Features (Fig. 7–3B). The radiocarpal joint is normal when its interosseous gap is less than 3 mm. Simultaneously the scapholunotriquetral relationships must also be normal during side-to-side deviation views (here in neutral position). Radiocarpal rotation must also be normal in the neutral position.

Abnormal Features.

Radiocarpal Laxity.[4,5,14,28] On the frontal view in neutral position the scapholunotriquetral relationship shows features of radial deviation. On the lateral view, as mentioned by Linscheid et al,[28] there is evidence of a VISI pattern with a radiolunate angle of at least − 45 degrees (or higher negative numbers). The most significant radiographic finding to support this as a normal finding is the evidence of the same feature on the opposite side. Additional dorsal stress views also can confirm the laxity (discussed further in the section on lateral stress study).

Ulnar Translocation. The pattern described as ulnar translation by Dobyns et al[30] or ulnar translocation by Taleisnik[31] indicates radiocarpal abnormality. On the standard PA view (Fig. 7–5) in neutral position, the first carpal row is not in its correct position but is in the position normally seen in ulnar deviation. In addition the whole proximal surface of the lunate has moved off the distal end of the radius and the scapholunate joint is opposite the DRUJ. Ulnar translocation with no abnormality seen within the first carpal row (the scapholunotriquetral articulation is normal) is called ulnar translocation Type I. Ulnar transloca-

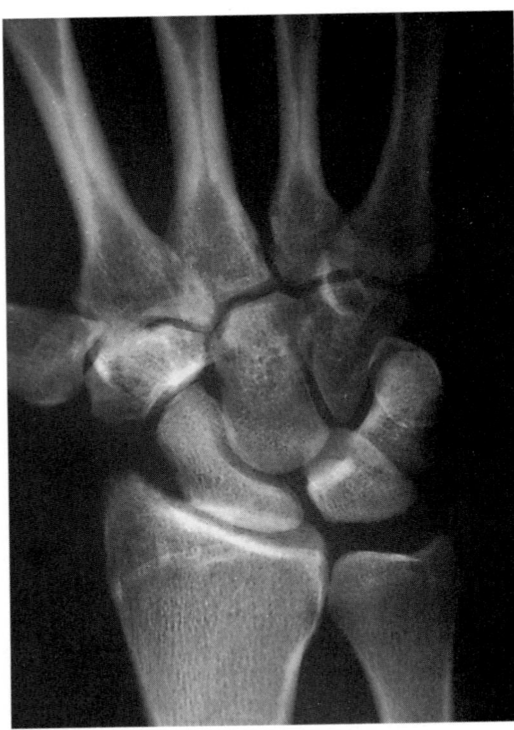

FIGURE 7–5. Type I ulnar translocation in standard PA view. (Reprinted with permission from Schernberg F. Roentgenographic examination of the wrist: A systematic study of the normal, lax and traumatic wrist. Part one: The standard and the positional views. *J Hand Surg* 1990;15B:210–219.)

tion Type II, as described by Taleisnik,[31] is present when the scaphoid is in normal relationship with the radius, with a scapholunate dissociation Grade III, and ulnar position of the lunate as with ulnar translocation Type I. On the lateral view the lunate is dorsiflexed.

Normal and Abnormal Features at the Midcarpal Level

Normal Features (Fig. 7–3B). The normal midcarpal joint has an interosseous gap of less than 3 mm. Scapholunotriquetral relationships must remain normal between side-to-side deviations as well as in the neutral position. Midcarpal rotation in the neutral position is also normal.

Abnormal Features. In our experience any abnormal feature at the midcarpal level is rather rare on the standard frontal view.

The Standard Lateral View (Fig. 7–6)

Positioning of the Hand and Its Assessment: The Lateral View in Neutral Position

It is easy to put the wrist in a neutral position and to ensure that this is maintained. However, with a vertical beam, the neutral position of the forearm with the hand in prone position for a PA view can be achieved only if the elbow is in 90 degrees of flexion with the elbow at shoulder height. For the lateral view, the elbow, which is flexed 90 degrees, is held tightly against the chest in 0 degrees of abduction or anteposition with the x-ray beam applied in the vertical direction.

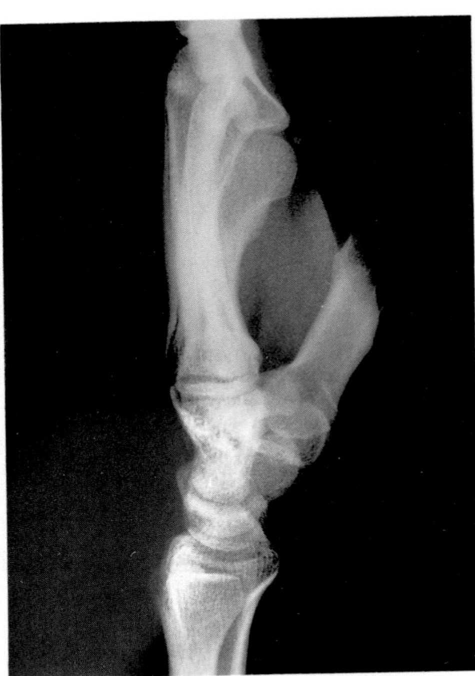

FIGURE 7–6. A standard lateral view of the wrist and metacarpals.

The neutral lateral position is confirmed by superimposition and straight alignment of the convex distal surfaces of the second and third metacarpal heads.[26] The neutral position of flexion and extension is confirmed by parallelism of the axes of the shafts of the radius and the third metacarpal. The radiographic criteria that confirm the neutral rotation of the forearm are demonstrated on both sides of the wrist. Proximally, there is complete overlap of the radius and the ulna. The ulnar styloid is also well outlined at the mid part of the distal border of the ulnar head.[32] Any supination or pronation will bring the styloid more ventral or more dorsal, respectively. Distally, the bases of the metacarpals of the long fingers are superimposed.[33]

Analysis of the Normal Roentgenographic Features of the Wrist

Roentgenographic analysis of the wrist must be carried out in a systematic stepwise manner. One way is to first analyze the width of the joint spaces and the parallelism between cortices of adjacent articulating bones. Next the dorsal part of the wrist is closely scrutinized, followed by examination of the anatomic configuration of the individual carpal bones.

The Joint Spaces

The joint spaces are normal when joint margins are concentric or cortices "fit together" and joints are of similar width.

The Dorsal Part of the Wrist

Instead of studying lines as on frontal views, on the lateral view one considers different structures on the dorsum of the wrist. There is a succession of five main prominences from proximal to distal:[14] dorsal ridge of the distal articular surface of the radius, the posterior border of the lunate, the posterior pole of the triquetrum,[34] and the posterior and distal pole of the hamate and the capitate. The posterior pole of the triquetrum always remains clearly visible in the posterior lunocapitate area defined by the posterior border of the lunate and the capitate.

The Anatomic Configuration

As bones are superimposed, the anatomic alignment of the individual carpal bones is best achieved with their angular measurement.[28] They will be mentioned here and are described in more detail in Chapter 8.

Normal Colinearity of the Radius, Lunate, and Capitate. The normal colinearity of the radius, lunate, and capitate (when the mid axes of these three bones create a single straight line) is present in only 11% of normal wrists.[35] Slight angles between these three axes are common.

Angular Measurements. The *scapholunate angle* has an average value of + 47 degrees, varying from 30 to 60 degrees.[28] The *radiolunate angle* varies from − 25 to + 10 degrees. The *capitolunate angle* varies from − 15 to + 30 degrees.[30] The *triquetrolunate angle* measurement is difficult to determine because the entire triquetrum is often difficult to see on the lateral radiograph. Its average value is + 14 degrees, varying from − 3 to + 31 degrees.[36]

Abnormal Features on the Lateral View

Anatomy on the lateral view can provide a numeric estimation to the features found on frontal views. It is important to recognize that normal measurements on the lateral view may be associated with an abnormal condition on a frontal view, such as joint widenings without any angular modification of the bones (e.g., scapholunate dissociation). Conversely, abnormal measurements on the lateral view do not necessarily indicate a pathologic condition. Such alignment abnormalities may be found in loose-jointed individuals and are especially common in patients with a radiocarpal laxity (as in some VISI configurations).

THE DYNAMIC WORKUP

According to different configurations of the standard views, the dynamic study may become mandatory. The dynamic studies are of the greatest interest in all cases with negative standard views associated with a clinical condition underlying a suspicious lesion. In cases of wrist trauma in which the standard views are suspicious, such additional views can display abnormalities from studies previously labeled normal. Dynamic studies also are useful in cases with abnormal standard views if further specific information is desired.

The Motion Views

Motion views are routine radiographs taken at extremes of motion. They include PA views obtained in maximum radial and ulnar deviation, with clenched fist, and in maximum supination. We rarely perform lateral views in maximum of flexion and extension because they are of less interest to us.

PA Views in Radial and Ulnar Deviation

Normal Radiographic Appearance in Radial Deviation (Fig. 7–3A)

Normalcy at the Proximal Carpal Row Level. The proximal row is normal when there are scapholunate and lunotriquetral interosseous spaces less than 3 mm, normal Arcs I and II as defined by Gilula,[17] and normal scapholunotriquetral articulation. At this level the only condition that must be fulfilled is that these three bones adopt the same position or show the same roentgenographic aspect of positioning; thus normal scapholunotriquetral articulation does not mean a joint. This term is used to indicate that the three proximal carpal row bones adopt the same spatial situation, which may be either in neutral position, flexion, or extension.

Normalcy at the Radiocarpal Level. The radiocarpal joint is normal when three conditions are encountered: the interosseous gap is less than 3 mm, the normal scapholunotriquetral relationship is in a configuration of flexion (or radial deviation), and usually the proximal surface of the lunate does not move more than half its width off the distal surface of the radius.

Normalcy at the Midcarpal Level. The midcarpal joint is normal when the interosseous gap is less than 3 mm, the normal scapholunotriquetral relationship is in the position of flexion or radial deviation, the triquetrum is at a proximal level ("high") in relation to the hamate, and the vertex of the hamate is articulating with the triquetrum ulnar to the lunotriquetral joint.

Normal Radiographic Appearance in Ulnar Deviation (Fig. 7–3C)

Normalcy at the Proximal Carpal Row Level. The proximal row is normal with interosseous gaps at the scapholunate and lunotriquetral spaces of less than 3 mm, normal Arcs I and II as defined by Gilula,[17] and normal scapholunotriquetral articulation. However, proximal-distal motion at the lunotriquetral and scapholunate (SL) joints on radial/ulnar deviation is common. Peh and Gilula reviewed the asymptomatic wrist in 100 patients who had an instability series to determine how much proximal-distal motion can occur at the lunotriquetral and SL joints between radial and ulnar deviation and to determine if the arcs were reliable in a large group of patients in the neutral position. They found that the arcs are intact in the neutral position in 97 of 100 patients in the PA and 98 of 100 patients in the anteroposterior (AP) position, with the exceptions mainly from a break in Arc II due to one case with a Type II lunate (large hamate facet of the lunate) and two cases with slight distal position of the triquetrum. Disrupted arcs on radial or ulnar deviation were found in 95 cases, 74 of which were detected on both PA and AP views, with the other 21 seen on just one view. "On PA radial deviation, at the lunotriquetral (LT) joint, distal triquetral position caused Arc I to be disrupted in 80 and Arc II to be disrupted in 78 cases while at the SL joint, the scaphoid moved distally in 10 cases. Similar findings were detected on AP views. In ulnar deviation, Arc II was disrupted at the SL joint due to proximal scaphoid position in 30 (PA) and 12 (AP) cases, respectively. Arc III was intact in all positions. Between radial and ulnar deviation, the SL joint width increased in 52 cases."[37] This verifies that radiographic carpal arcs normally disrupt with radial and ulnar deviation, and caution should be exercised when interpreting Arcs I and II and SL joint width when the wrist is not strictly neutral in position.[37]

Normalcy at the Radiocarpal Level. The radiocarpal joint is normal when the interosseous gap is less than 3 mm, the scapholunotriquetral relationships are normal in extension (or ulnar deviation), most of the proximal surface of the lunate is apposed to the radius, and the LT joint is nearly in line with the DRUJ.

Normalcy at the Midcarpal Level. The midcarpal joint is normal when the interosseous gap is less than 3 mm, the normal scapholunotriquetral articulation has the configuration of extension or ulnar deviation, the triquetrum is at its distal level ("low") in relation to the hamate, and the vertex of the hamate reaches and overlaps the medial (ulnar) and distal part of the lunate.

Indications and Normal Radiographic Appearance

The PA views in radial and ulnar deviation become helpful in cases of uncertain alignment aspects because they show the two opposite positions of the scapholunotriquetral relationship. The neutral standard position is in fact an incomplete position of radial deviation as mentioned by Fick.[38]

Abnormal Standard PA View

Scapholunate Dissociation. If there is any doubt of the diagnosis of SL dissociation, additional motion views in radial and ulnar deviation may be helpful. This can be monitored best with fluoroscopic spot views when possible. On ulnar deviation, as in the neutral position, the scaphoid shows the appearance seen in radial deviation (foreshortened scaphoid) while the lunate and the triquetrum adopt the appearance they have while in ulnar deviation. On radial deviation the three bones conform to their normal expected position. This confirms that the dissociation is confined to the SL joint.

Static Ulnar Translocation. If there is any question about the presence of ulnar carpal translocation, additional radial and ulnar deviation motion views may be helpful. In radial deviation as well as in the neutral position, the entire proximal carpal row is not in its correct position, but rather is in that position normally seen in radial deviation. In addition, the whole proximal surface of the lunate has moved off the distal end of the radius, and the SL gap is opposite the DRUJ. On ulnar deviation, the carpal bones may or may not return to the normal radiocarpal position.

With a Normal Standard PA View

Dynamic Lunotriquetral Dissociation. Usually there is evidence of abnormality with ulnar deviation as seen by overlap of the lunate and the triquetrum and widening of the LT joint.[36]

Dynamic Ulnar Translocation. The standard PA neutral view is negative (Fig. 7–7B). The frontal views in radial and ulnar deviation show that the three carpals of the proximal row remain in a similar appearance of ulnar deviation. There is no abnormality within the proximal carpal row. The persistent elongation of the scaphoid normally seen in ulnar deviation present here in radial deviation (Fig. 7–7A) demonstrates the radiocarpal abnormality. This is also confirmed by the abnormal ulnar carpal shift on radial deviation, with the lunate lying off the ulnar border of the radius and, in ulnar deviation (Fig. 7–7C), a marked widening of the radioscaphoid joint.

PA View With the Fist Clenched

Description of the Maneuver

Two PA radiographs are taken: one with the hand in the position of fist clenching but without forceful clenching of the fist, and the second one with forceful clenching of the fist.

Normal Radiographic Appearance

Normally there is no widening of the SL gap on either of the two PA views taken with or without tight clenching of the fist.

Indications and Abnormal Radiographic Appearance

This view may be useful to explore the SL area that is normal or of uncertain status. Maintenance of the interosseous space at less than 3 mm confirms its normalcy (Fig. 7–4B). A gap widening of more than 3 mm is usually abnormal (Fig. 7–8).

Active Supination

This represents the AP view. In that view the SL gap is always seen better than in the neutral standard frontal position (PA view), but it never exceeds 3 mm in the normal wrist. Like the clenched-fist view, it is useful in cases where the status of the SL joint is unclear.

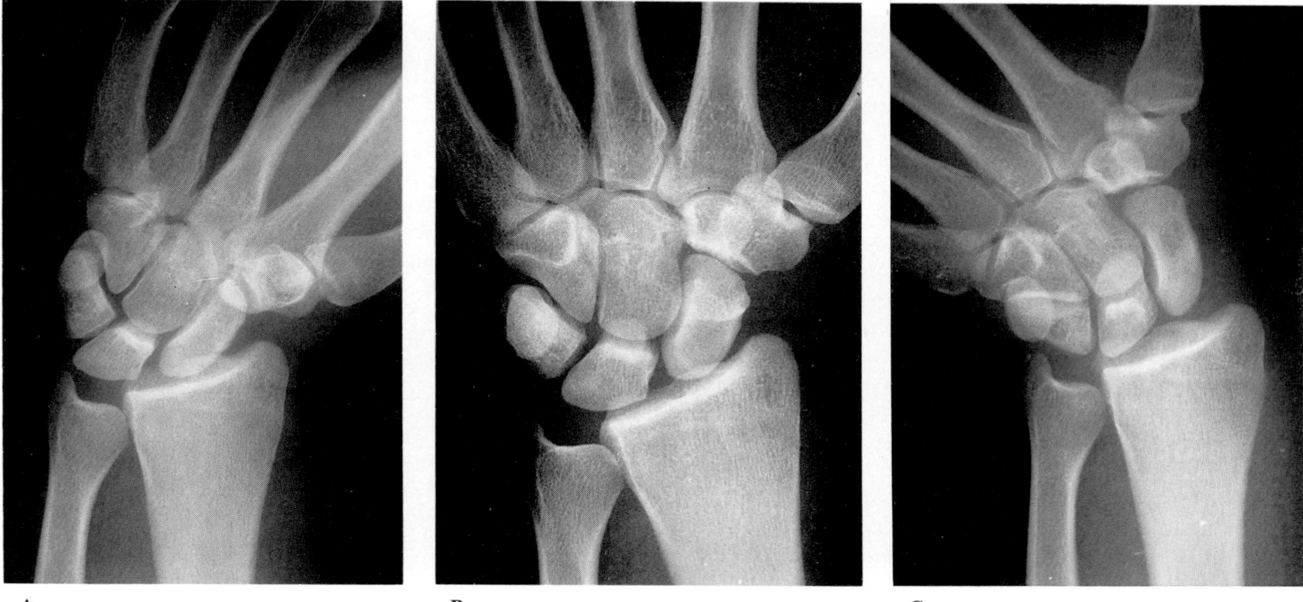

FIGURE 7–7. Dynamic ulnar translocation. **A**: Radial deviation: radioscaphoid joint space widening is present, the scaphoid remains elongated, normal offset of Arcs I and II is present at the lunotriquetral joint, and the entire lunate lies ulnar to the radius. **B**: Neutral position: no abnormality is evident except that the midpoint of the proximal surface of the lunate is on the ulnar edge of the radius, a borderline normal finding. **C**: Ulnar deviation: the radioscaphoid joint is markedly widened and normal offset of Arcs I and II at the scapholunate joint is present. (Reprinted with permission from Schernberg F. Roentgenographic examination of the wrist: A systematic study of the normal, lax and traumatic wrist. Part one: The standard and the positional views. *J Hand Surg* 1990;15B:210–219.)

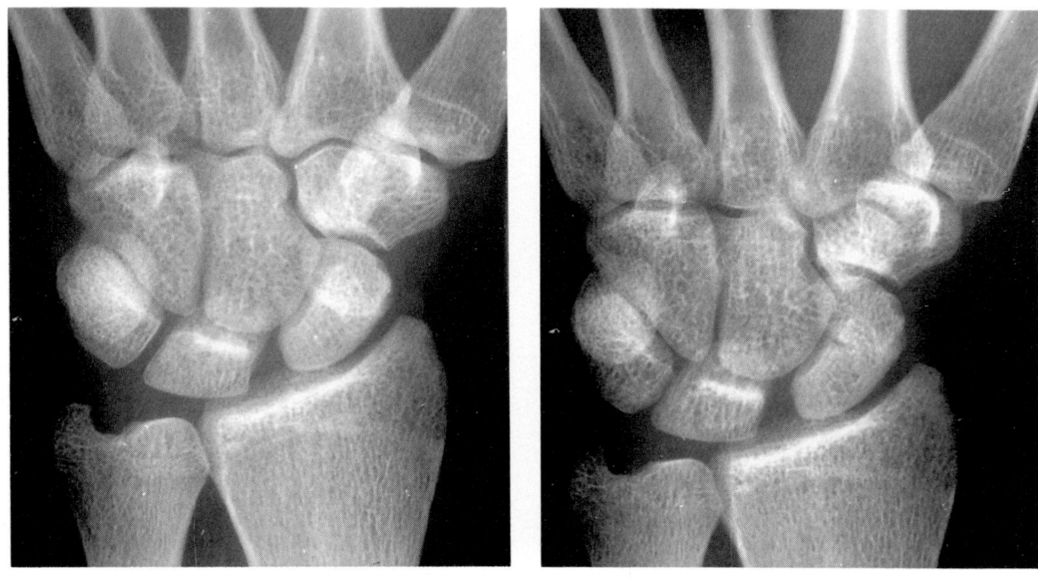

FIGURE 7–8. Clenched-fist view in a case of SL dissociation. **A**: View with the hand in position of fist made but not clenched. Widening of the SL joint is present, but the distal part of this joint is not perfectly profiled. **B**: View with the fist clenched. The SL joint is questionably wider than in **A** but the joint is more perfectly profiled. The slight difference in wrist positioning that can easily occur is evident by looking at the lunotriquetral joint, which is perfectly in profile in **A** and is not in **B**.

The Lateral Views in Flexion and Extension

On lateral views, the angular variations in passive flexion and extension are identical to those reported by Sarrafian, Melamed, and Goshgarian[35] in active movement. We do not use passive flexion and extension views in our normal clinical experience. However, Gilula uses lateral flexion–extension views to see the end-position of the capitate with respect to the lunate and the lunate with respect to the radius in patients with suspected VISI or DISI (see Chapter 8). This is performed with the belief that the VISI or DISI "configuration" (when angles measure VISI or DISI) represents a normal variation when the flexion and extension views are normal; that is, these three bones flex with respect to each other. DISI and VISI "configurations" are believed to be abnormal when any one of the axes does not flex or extend with respect to each other on flexion or extension, respectively, in the patient who does not have marked limitation of motion such as that due to pain.

The Positional Views

Description and Maneuver

We advocate plain-film views in cases of clicks from articular origin rather than conventional cineradiography.[40] It is of crucial importance to clinically eliminate a click of extraarticular origin such as that found in cases of localized tenosynovitis of the fourth extensor compartment. The latter can be confirmed by ultrasound examination.[41] The plain-film positional regimen consists of PA and lateral views with the hand remaining in neutral position between flexion and extension maneuvers and radial and ulnar deviation maneuvers performed in both lateral and frontal positions. The various positions are maintained without any strength. Therefore, the radiographic study is performed as follows. The patient's wrist is placed in the frontal (usually PA) position under the radiographic beam. Then, with the wrist maintained in the neutral position between flexion and extension, the patient is instructed to bring it to the frontal position as near as possible to that in which the click will occur. The first frontal view is taken in that position (PA preclick view). Then the patient moves the wrist slightly into ulnar deviation so that the click occurs. The second frontal view is then taken in that position (PA postclick view).

The same maneuver is performed in the lateral position. First, the patient places his or her wrist in the neutral position between flexion and extension as near as possible to that position at which the click will occur. The first lateral view is then taken in that position (lateral preclick view). Then the patient moves the wrist slightly into ulnar deviation, and the click occurs. The second frontal view is then taken in that position (lateral postclick view).

Thus we get four views, two frontal and two lateral, which allow us to analyze with good detail the modification that happens during the click, i.e., the sudden modification of the position of the proximal carpal row bones that go from a high position of flexion into a full extended position. In normal wrists this modification occurs smoothly and progressively. In unhealthy wrists this phenomenon occurs suddenly near the position of clicking. In case of doubt between a click of articular or abarticular origin (unclear clinical information), if there is no obvious modification between the two preclick and postclick views in the frontal and lateral views, the click is of abarticular origin.

Abnormal Radiographic Appearance: Posteromedial Radiocarpal Instability (Fig. 7–9)[4,5]

Posteromedial radiocarpal instability has also been described as midcarpal instability by Lichtman et al.[42] It is important to remember that such a click can be passively induced by the examiner[14] in a normal wrist by applying a palmarly directed stress in the frontal (prone or supine) position during radial to ulnar deviation. The pathologic condition is defined by the fact that the click occurs in the patient's wrist when the patient actively deviates the symptomatic wrist without any other additional stress. This click will not occur when applying a dorsally directed stress by the examiner's thumb on the ulnar part of the wrist over the palmar surface of the pisiform, counteracted by a force exerted by the index finger on the dorsum of the head of the ulna. Applying force on the pisiform with the thumb and on the ulnar head with the index finger produces a palmar-to-dorsal stress on the pisiform (i.e., on the ulnar part of the proximal carpal row). Just before the click occurs (Figs. 7–9A1 and 7–9B1), even though the hand is in neutral to slightly ulnar deviation on the frontal view, the scapholunotriquetral alignment is in radial deviation or flexion with a radiolunate angle of − 30 degrees on the lateral view. Just after the click occurs (Figs. 7–9A2 and 7–9B2), the three carpal bones of the proximal row are in the alignment of full ulnar deviation on the frontal view with a radiolunate angle of + 30 degrees on the lateral view. These views demonstrate with good detail a loss of normal and smooth reciprocal rotation between the proximal and distal carpal rows with radial and ulnar deviation, as the three carpals move abruptly from flexion to extension. The fact that there is evidence of a marked change in alignment of the proximal carpal row between very slight changes in the amount of ulnar deviation between Figs. 7–9A1 and 7–9A2 supports the presence of a pathologic condition.

The Stress Views

The stress examination consists of applying different stresses on the wrist as the forearm is supported and the hand firmly held. The different stresses we apply to the wrist consist of two main types: normal (i.e., physiologic) and abnormal (i.e., nonphysiologic). The former consist of radial and ulnar deviation on frontal views and flexion and extension positions on

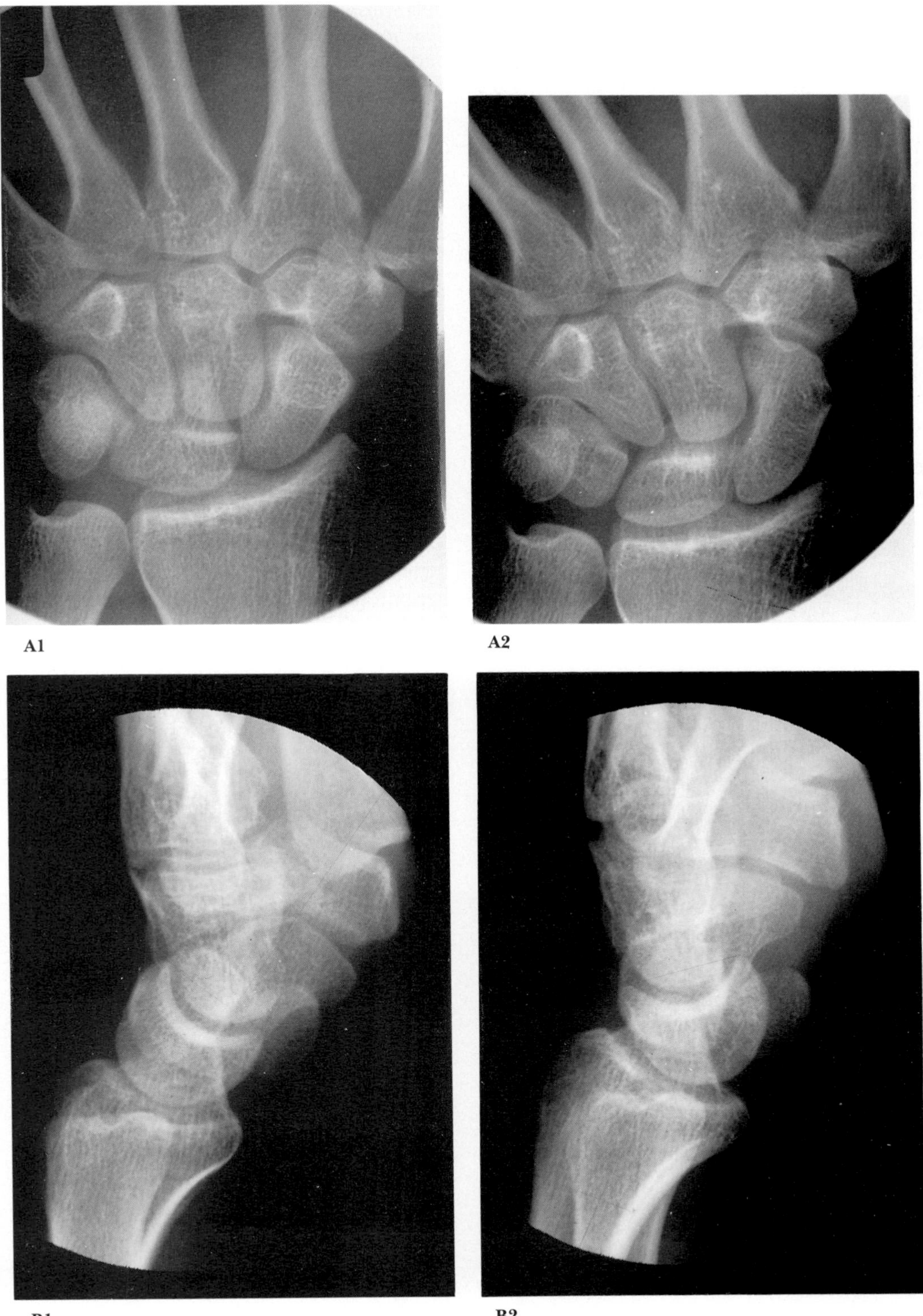

FIGURE 7–9. Posteromedial radiocarpal instability. **A1** and **B1**: Frontal and lateral views just before the click. **A2** and **B2**: Frontal and lateral views just after the click. (See text for details.) (Reprinted with permission from Schernberg F. Roentgenographic examination of the wrist: A systematic study of the normal, lax and traumatic wrist. Part one: The standard and the positional views. *J Hand Surg* 1990;15B:210–219.)

lateral views. The "abnormal" stresses consist of radial and ulnar transposition and passive supination and pronation in the PA view. Palmar and dorsal stress forces are applied in both the frontal and lateral views. Before these forces are applied, the hand is always aligned with the wrist in neutral position in both planes and the forearm is placed in the neutral position midway between pronation and supination. Only one type of stress is applied at a time to easily notice the modifications induced by the stress relative to the standard views described above.

Normal (Physiologic) Stress Views

Description of the Maneuver

The different maneuvers consist of radial and ulnar deviation on frontal views and flexion and extension on lateral views.

Normal Radiographic Appearance

The normal stress views obtained by applying physiologic stresses on the wrist do not demonstrate any significant difference with the motion views.

Indications and Abnormal Radiographic Appearance

According to Ambrose and Posner,[39] motion views in radial deviation are helpful in cases of uncertain findings or occult lesions at the lunotriquetral area. In our experience, when the deviation is performed under stress, more motion at the LT joint in the symptomatic wrist than in the asymptomatic wrist is abnormal (Fig. 7–10); this represents a dynamic LT instability with only minimal ligamentous lesions. Forced ulnar deviation is very useful to disclose a fracture of the scaphoid in the case of an occult fracture or uncertain findings of the scaphoid.[4,5] This position is also the stress view of choice to reveal a Grade II injury to the ligaments at the distal part of the scaphoid (scaphotrapezial ligaments) by a widening of the lateral (radial) aspect of the midcarpal joint (Fig. 7–11). Because widening of the scaphotrapezial joint can occur normally, to call such widening abnormal there should be a history of severe trauma (to rule out any degenerative condition revealed from a minor trauma) and there must be a crucial difference between the traumatic scaphotrapeziotrapezoidal roentgenographic appearance and the appearance of the normal contralateral wrist taken at the same time with the same positioning.

Abnormal (Nonphysiologic) Stress Views

Frontal View

The abnormal stresses consist of transposition and rotation and ventral- and dorsal-directed stresses.

Radial and Ulnar Transposition.

Description of the Maneuver (Fig. 7–12). The patient's hand and forearm are in neutral PA position. To apply ulnar transposition, the examiner's right hand is placed on the ulnar border of the distal

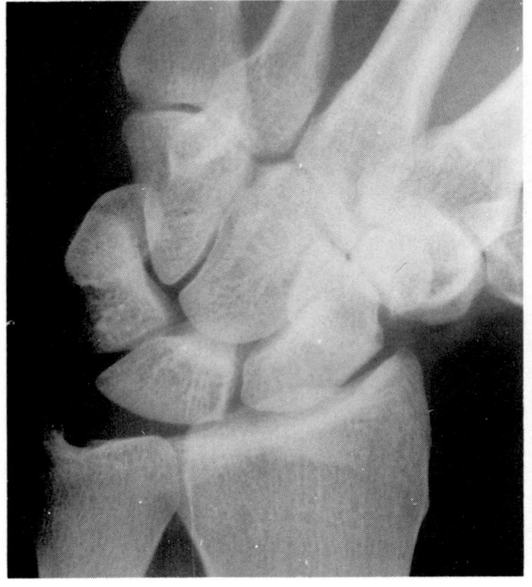

A

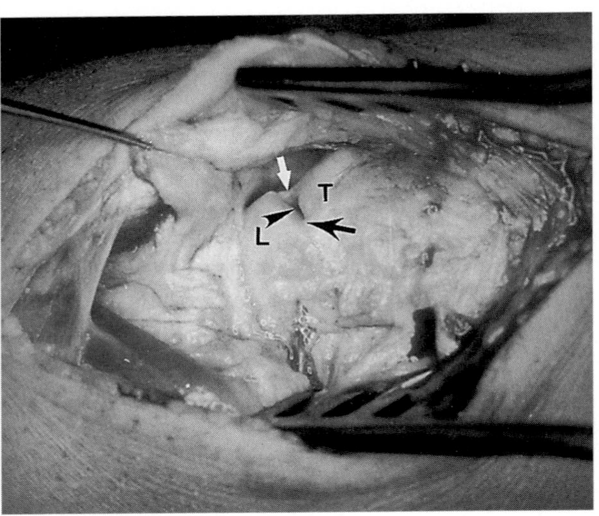

B

FIGURE 7–10. Dynamic lunotriquetral dissociation. **A**: In this case of a dorsoulnar chronic painful wrist, forced radial deviation demonstrates broken arcs I and II at the lunotriquetral joint relative to the lunate. This feature was abnormal relative to the same view taken on the normal uninjured contralateral wrist. **B**: Features of the lesion seen on dorsal exposure of the wrist in radial deviation. The interosseous membrane is torn (black arrowhead). The dorsal (arrow) and palmar (white arrow) lunotriquetral ligaments are not torn but are partially stripped from the triquetrum (T), which is shifted distally relative to the lunate (L).

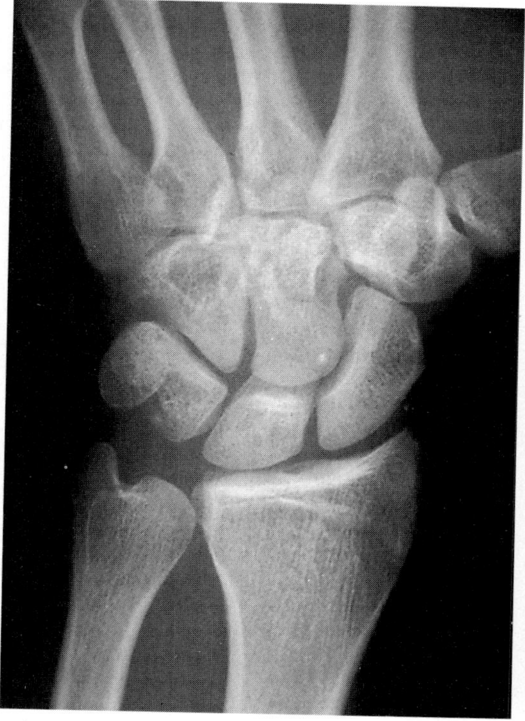

A

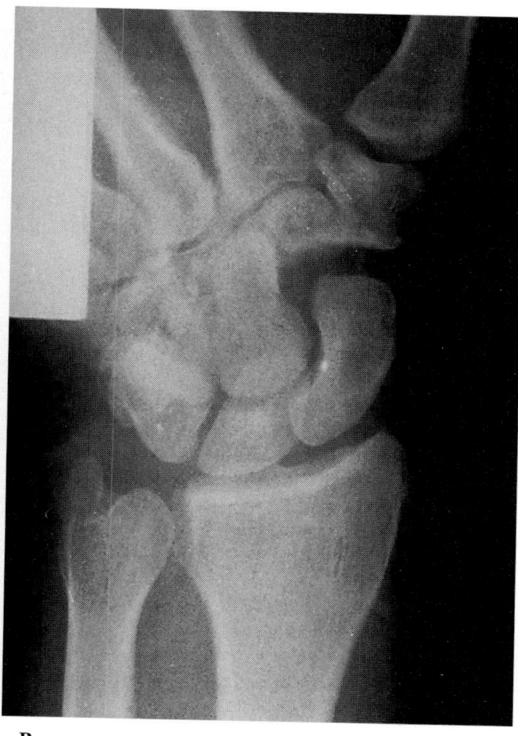

B

FIGURE 7–11. Dynamic scaphotrapeziotrapezoidal instability. **A**: Normal features on frontal standard view; an incidental benign lucent defect involves the hamate. **B**: On forced ulnar deviation, the lateral aspect of the midcarpal joint is widened; a Grade II injury to the lateral (radial) midcarpal ligaments can therefore be assessed. (Reprinted with permission from Schernberg F. *Le poignet: Anatomie radiologique et chirurgie.* Paris: Masson, 1992.)

forearm, firmly holding the forearm proximal to the ulnar styloid. His or her left hand holds the patient's hand firmly distal to the carpometacarpal level within the first web. When applying the ulnar-directed stress, the right hand is a stabilizer and the left one applies the motor power ulnarward without any additional side-to-side rotation. To perform radial transposition the maneuver is applied in the reverse.

Normal Radiographic Appearance. On radial transposition (when displacing the carpus radially), a moderate modification of the features of the three proximal row carpal bones may develop. The joint space between the scaphoid and the lunate may be enlarged, however, it never exceeds 3 mm in a normal wrist. On ulnar transposition, the configuration of the three proximal row carpal bones changes into that of ulnar deviation. The joint space between the scaphoid and radius is now enlarged, and the SL joint is narrowed. The proximal surface of the lunate never displaces more than half its width off the ulnar facet of the radius.

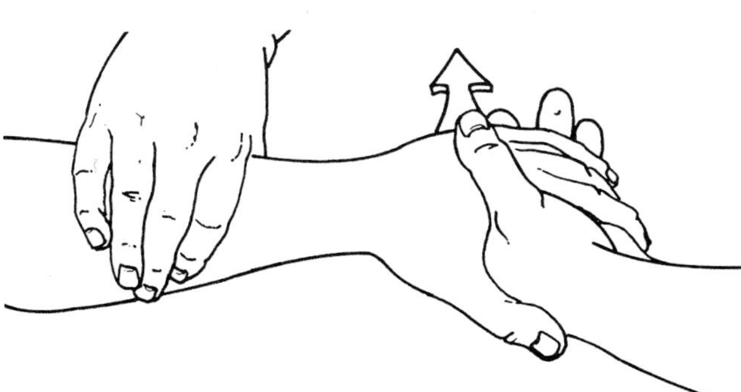

FIGURE 7–12. Drawing of the maneuver of creating radial and ulnar transposition forces. (Reprinted with permission from Schernberg F. *Le poignet: Anatomie radiologique et chirurgie.* Paris: Masson, 1992.)

Indications and Abnormal Radiographic Appearance. These views are of crucial interest to show Grade II injuries located at the SL or radiocarpal area. In the case of Grade II injury to the SL ligament, on PA view with passive radial transposition, diastasis at the SL joint of greater than 3 mm (Fig. 7–13) confirms the Grade II lesion that other views do not disclose.

Pronation and Supination.

Description of the Maneuver. The patient's hand and forearm are in neutral PA position. The examiner's left hand holds the patient's forearm firmly proximal to the ulnar styloid. His or her right hand holds the patient's hand firmly distal to the carpometacarpal level. When applying the pronation–supination stresses, the examiner's left hand is the stabilizer and the right one has the motor power to move the hand into pronation and supination without any additional side-to-side rotation or deviation.

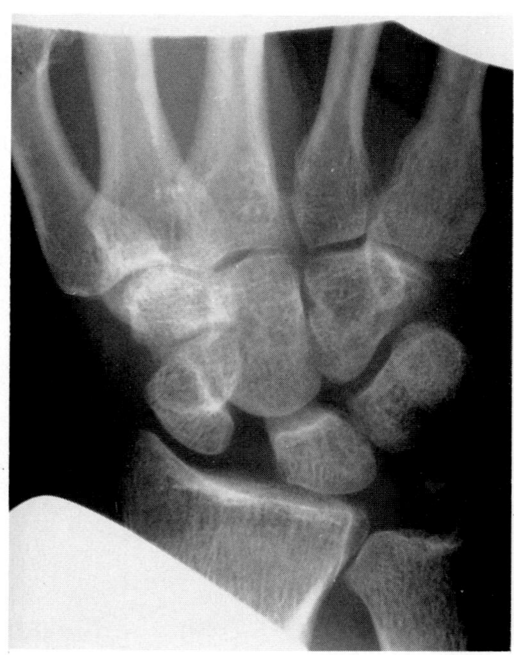
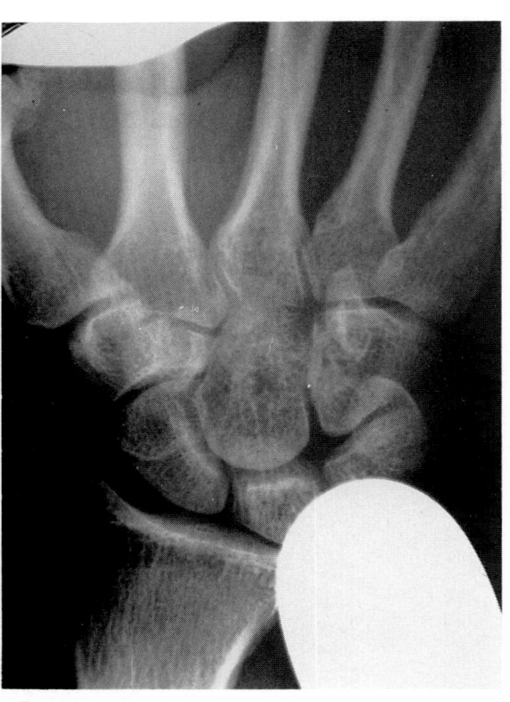

A B

FIGURE 7–13. Dynamic SL dissociation. **A**: On a PA view passive radial transposition demonstrates widening of the SL space; none of the other views showed any abnormality. Grade II injury to the SL ligament can therefore be identified. **B**: PA view on passive ulnar transposition: no SL diastasis is evident. (Reprinted with permission from Schernberg F. Roentgenographic examination of the wrist: A systematic study of the normal, lax and traumatic wrist. Part one: The standard and the positional views. *J Hand Surg* 1990;15B:210–219.)

Radiographic Appearance. Normally, rotational movement within the wrist can only be performed passively except in the case of radioulnar fusion, where it is performed actively.[21] The rotational stresses of passive pronation and supination induce an appearance of increasing pronation or supination of the three proximal row carpal bones. Associated with these appearances, the medial (ulnar) part of the midcarpal space widens in pronation and narrows in supination. In our experience these changes are of lesser utility.

Indications and Normal Radiographic Appearance. We do not use these routinely in our clinical practice. In fact, the application of these maneuvers is the same as that with radial and ulnar transposition forces.

Volar (Palmar) and Dorsal Stress.

Description of the Maneuver. The patient's hand and forearm are in neutral PA position. The examiner's left hand holds the patient's forearm firmly proximal to the ulnar styloid. His or her right hand holds the patient's hand firmly distal to the carpometacarpal level. When applying the stress, the examiner's left hand is a stabilizer, and the right one has the motor power to move the patient's hand from neutral to volar position and from neutral to dorsal position without any additional side-to-side rotation.

Normal Radiographic Appearance. These stresses do not produce any apparent alterations, other than showing coordinated movement of the scaphoid, the lunate, and the triquetrum into the configuration of radial deviation on volar (palmar-directed) stress and into the configuration of ulnar deviation on dorsal-directed stress. These modifications can be confirmed and measured on lateral views.

Indications and Abnormal Radiographic Appearance. They are not routinely used.

Compression and Traction Views.

Description of the Maneuver. The compression and traction views correspond to passive dynamic axial loading forces. The patient's hand and forearm are in neutral PA position. One of the examiner's hands holds the distal part of the patient's forearm firmly just proximal to the ulnar head to maintain the wrist in neutral position. His or her opposite hand holds the patient's hand firmly distal to the carpometacarpal level (at the level of the first web space). When applying stress to the patient's wrist, the examiner's hand on the forearm is a stabilizer, and the opposite one on the patient's hand has the motor power to apply an axial loading force or traction or compression forces without any additional side to side rotation. A *compression force* is defined as a force applied by the examiner's hand on the patient's hand directed from distal to proximal (push). A *traction force* is a force applied by the examiner's hand to the patient's hand directed from proximal to distal (pull). These traction or compression forces are never associated with any kind of radial–ulnar deviation or flexion–extension, since the hand is always maintained in a neutral position.

Normal Radiographic Appearance. The measures of carpal height and carpal translation in the stress views are similar to those defined on standard views by McMurtry et al.[19] Some variation appears with passive compression when the appearance of the three proximal carpal row bones may be slightly modified to represent a configuration of radial deviation. On traction, the bones return to a configuration of neutral position or slight ulnar deviation. Widening at the radiocarpal and midcarpal space can be associated with traction views (where traction is applied longitudinally through the fingers) but it always is identical in both radiocarpal and midcarpal joints. In cases of perilunate laxity, there is evidence of broken Arcs I and II of Gilula[17] at the joints where the ligaments are abnormal. The appearance of the carpus with traction is the same as that seen on frontal views in the case of a fractured distal end of the radius treated by external fixation. At the radiocarpal space, widening limited to the radioscaphoid and ulnotriquetral areas while the radiolunate space remains normal is true in normal and lax patients. In these patients there will be a difference only in the amount of widening, with the widening of lesser importance in normal than in lax patients. The widening of those spaces induces a nonpathologic stepoff at Arcs I and II. In the case of a distal radius fracture treated by an external fixator creating a traction force, this feature is normal; however, some surgeons mention it as an associated pathologic condition. Conversely, if any widening occurs at the radiolunate area, this is diagnostic of an associated ligamentous tear.

Indications and Abnormal Radiographic Appearance. These views are not routinely used.

Lateral Views

Volar (Palmar) and Dorsal Stress.

Description of the Maneuver (Fig. 7–14). The patient's hand and forearm are in the neutral, lateral position. The examiner's left fingers are applied to the dorsal part of the forearm proximal to the distal ulna. The thumb is applied at the palmar (volar) part of the hand distal to the wrist crease. The examiner's right fingers are applied to the dorsal part of the patient's hand distal to the carpometacarpal area, and the right thumb is applied to the volar part just distal to the left thumb. The long fingers of the left hand act as the stabilizer, and both thumbs act as the motor power. Volar stress is obtained with a reverse position.

Comments. These maneuvers are drawer maneuvers that stress the whole wrist as a unit and are not designed to stress the radiocarpal or midcarpal levels specifically. In general, the examiner should not disturb the tested area by applying his or her fingers on the area of interest. Proximally, the fingers must not reach the radiocarpal area, and distally they must be beyond the carpometacarpal area. This is mandatory to avoid superimposition of the examiner's hands on the radiographs and also to avoid disturbing the dynamic effect of the maneuver on the wrist. These maneuvers are different from specific ones such as the specific dorsal stress of the ulnar part of the first row or the maneuver described by Watson, which represents the specific dorsal stress of the radial part of the first row. The dorsal stress described in this paragraph is similar to that described as the capitolunate instability pattern (CLIP) wrist maneuver under fluoroscopy by White et al.[47]

Normal Radiographic Appearance.

Angular Modifications.[4,5,14] On volar- (palmar-) and dorsal-directed stress, Taleisnik[21] has emphasized alterations of the scaphoid and the lunate alignment that take place. We analyzed alterations of alignment, not only for the scaphoid and the lunate, but also for the triquetrum in both lateral and PA views. These observations confirm that the three proximal row carpal bones move as a unit mainly into radial deviation in the frontal view and into flexion in the lateral view with anterior (palmar-directed) stress. Conversely, with dorsal-directed stress, these three bones assume a configuration of ulnar deviation in the frontal view and extension in the lateral view. We also have quantified the angular modification by measuring the variations of the radiolunate angle (Fig. 7–15). On anterior (palmar-directed) stress, the radiolunate angle may decrease as far as −45 degrees, and on dorsal-directed stress it increases, but never to greater than +25 degrees. On standard lateral views, the radiolunate angle ranges from +10 to −25 degrees, as reported by Meyrueis, Cameli, and Jan.[43] On dorsal-directed stress, the angular modifications appear to be less than those obtained on anterior (palmar-directed) stress.

Interarticular Space Modifications.[4,5,14,22,23,25,26] On dorsal-directed stress (Figs. 7–16A and 7–17A), displacement occurs at the lunocapitate joint. The capitate can displace and sublux out of the lunate fossa. In the normal wrist, this displacement of the head of the capitate out from the lunate fossa never exceeds a quarter of the width of the capitate head. The posterior pole of the triquetrum, which remains clearly visible in the posterior lunocapitate area, is a fundamental relationship of the triquetrum for the normality of the wrist in the lateral view. With palmar- (volar-) directed stress, the lunate will commonly tilt or face palmarly but the capitate head does not sublux out of the lunate fossa. Schernberg's unpublished work performing palmar-directed and dorsal-directed stresses on 53 normal wrists showed that with palmar-directed stress the scaphoid and triquetrum also tilt palmarly with the lunate. Similarly, with dorsal-directed stress the scaphoid and triquetrum tilt dorsally with the lunate. This indicates that these three carpal bones move together in the same way in a normal wrist.

Indications and Abnormal Radiographic Appearance. The most useful view in current practice is dorsal-directed stress.

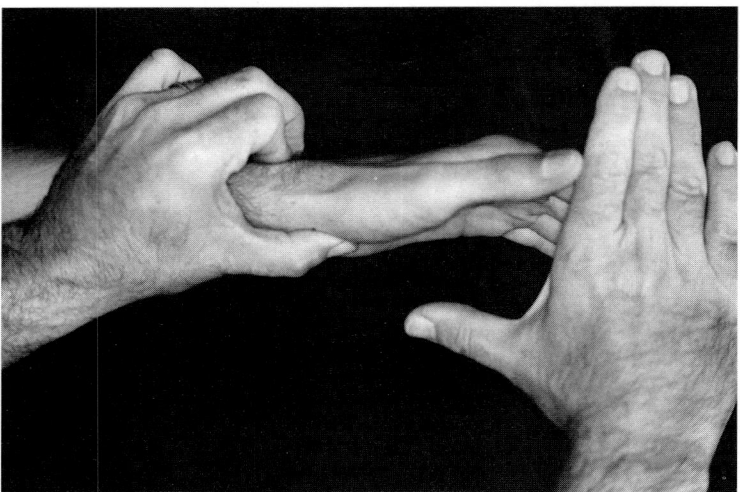

A

FIGURE 7–14. The volar- (palmar-) and dorsal-directed stress maneuvers in the lateral views. **A**: The maneuver with the examiner's right hand removed. **B**: Drawing of the manuever with both hands in place. Dorsal-directed stress is applied by the examiner's right hand while the forearm is stabilized by the examiner's left hand. **C**: Drawing showing the location of both thumbs on the hand, just distal to the wrist crease. (Reprinted with permission from Schernberg F. *Le poignet: Anatomie radiologique et chirurgie.* Paris: Masson, 1992.)

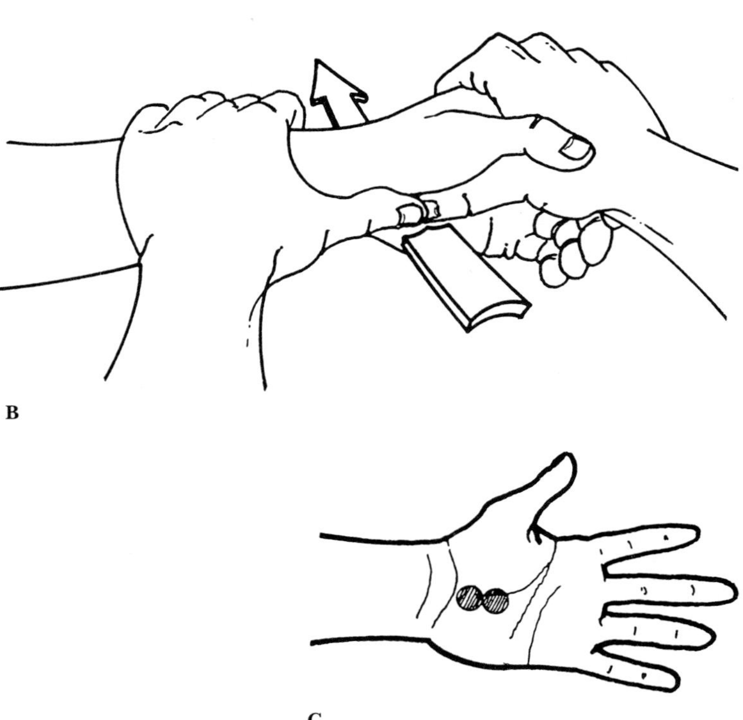

B

C

Laxity.[5] Lax wrists are normally asymptomatic. Here two main types of laxity are considered, the radiocarpal and the perilunate types. In the case of radiocarpal laxity on the frontal view, the scaphoid, lunate, and triquetrum demonstrate a normal scapholunotriquetral articulation with these three bones having the same appearance of positioning in flexion, or an appearance of scapholunotriquetral alignment in radial deviation. Normally on the standard frontal view the scapholunotriquetral alignment should be that of neutral deviation. The radial deviation alignment of these three proximal carpal bones of the lax wrist can be confirmed on a standard lateral view in which the lunate demonstrates a palmarly tilted appearance, e.g., with a radiolunate angle of -45 degrees. Since the plain films of the lax wrist are abnormal relative to normal conditions where the radiolunate angle varies from -25 to $+10$ degrees, a dynamic study is useful to see if this "abnormality" is within normal limits. Examination of the contralateral wrist with standard and dynamic views showing that the abnormality is the same on both sides confirms the diagnosis of constitutional laxity. In the case of the second main type of laxity, the perilunate type, the plain films are normal.

The clinical appearance of the lax wrist is related

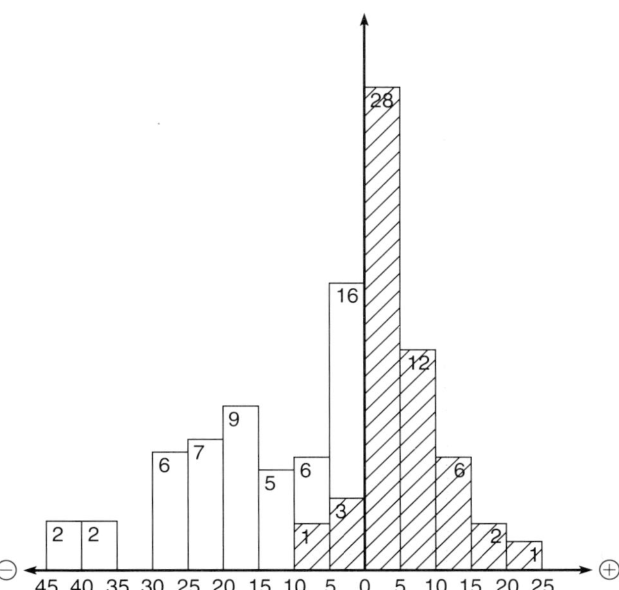

FIGURE 7–15. Histogram showing the radiolunate angle on volar (palmar- or ventral-) and dorsal-directed stress maneuvers in 53 cases of normal wrists. The numbers on the horizontal line are in degrees. (Reprinted with permission from Schernberg F. Roentgenographic examination of the wrist: A systematic study of the normal, lax and traumatic wrist. Part one: The standard and the positional views. *J Hand Surg* 1990;15B:210–219.)

to the level of its activity. Sometimes either after overuse or secondary to trauma, the lax wrist can become symptomatic. In the case of radiocarpal laxity the wrist may become painful with normal standard wrist views. The dorsal stress study demonstrates modification of the proximal row configuration from that of radial deviation (scapholunotriquetral bone mass in volar flexion) into an aspect of neutral position (the scapholunotriquetral bone mass in neutral position). On the lateral view, those modifications can be measured at the radiolunate angle, which increases from − 45 to 0 degrees. In cases of perilunate laxity, the patients complain of dorsal pain and/or either prominent or occult dorsal ganglion cysts.[44–46] The latter can be demonstrated by ultrasonographic examination.[41] The dynamic roentgenographic examination is normal except for traction in the frontal view and dorsal-directed stress in the lateral view on both sides (Figs. 7–16B and 7–17B). The lateral view demonstrates a posterior transposition between the different carpal bones. To locate the abnormality precisely, we must not only pay attention to the capitate and the lunate, but also to the triquetrum. The head of the capitate displaces posteriorly in relation to the distal poles of the lunate and subluxes out of the lunate fossa. In general, dorsal displacement of the capitate reaches, but never exceeds, half the width of its head in relation to the anterior pole of the lunate. In addition to this, the triquetrum usually

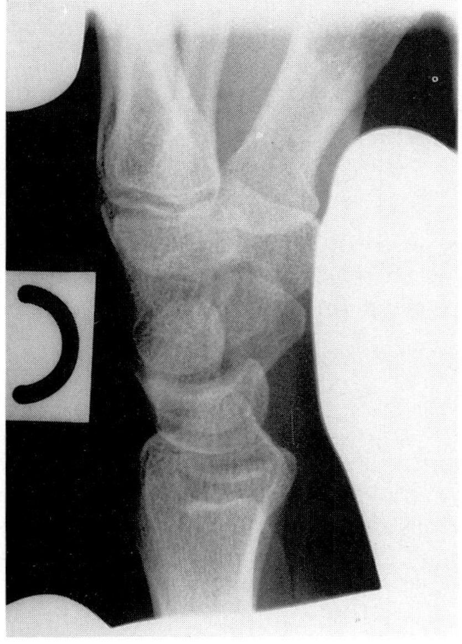
A

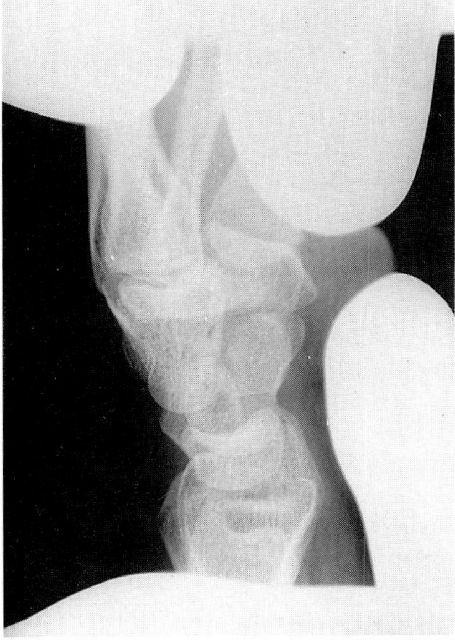
B

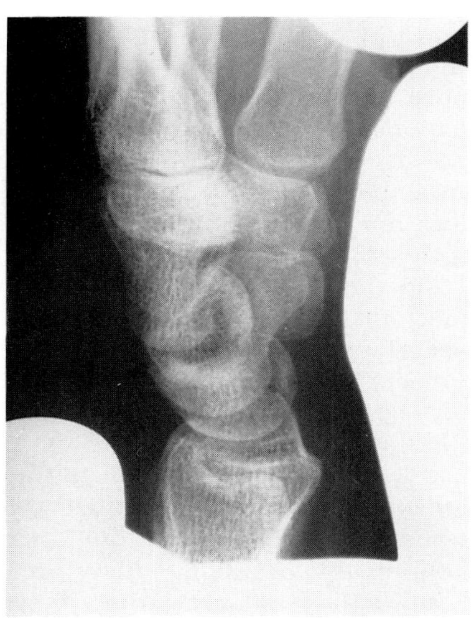
C

FIGURE 7–16. Configurations of the wrist in the lateral view with dorsal-directed stress. **A**: Normal condition: the posterior pole of the triquetrum (arrowhead) always remains clearly visible in the posterior capitolunate area defined by the posterior border of the lunate and the capitate. Less than one fourth of the width of the capitate head displaces out of the distal concavity of the lunate. **B**: Perilunate laxity: more than one fourth of the width of the capitate head displaces dorsal to the dorsal lip of the lunate. In this case, increased widening at the capitolunate joint is also present. **C**: Medioanterior midcarpal instability (MAMI) pattern. See text. (Reprinted with permission from Schernberg F. Roentgenographic examination of the wrist: A systematic study of the normal, lax and traumatic wrist. Part two: Stress views. *J Hand Surg* 1990;15B:220–228.)

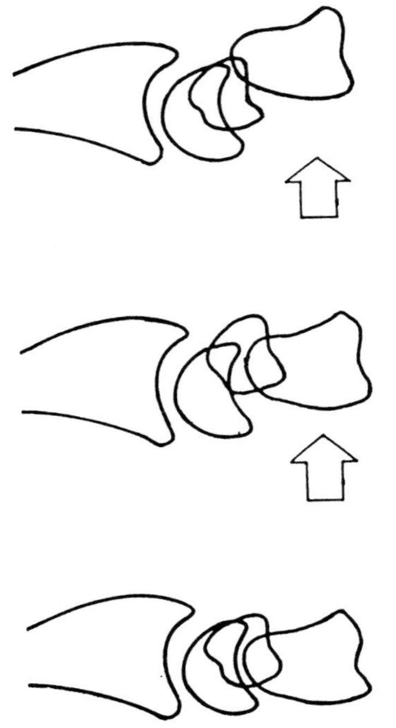

FIGURE 7–17. Drawings of the radiographic aspects of Fig. 7–16. (Reprinted with permission from Schernberg F. *Le poignet: Anatomie radiologique et chirurgie.* Paris: Masson, 1992.)

remains linked to the capitate and moves with it in the same direction.

Capitolunate Translation. The configuration of capitolunate instability or the CLIP wrist described by White et al[47] using fluoroscopy to us appears to be similar to the perilunate lax wrist pattern, whatever more complex maneuvers have been performed to demonstrate it. We are more convinced of this by the fact that only two of the eight reported patients had sustained an injury. In fact, the fluoroscopic study does not give any information about the relationship of the triquetrum.

On the normal standard lateral wrist view, the triquetrum overlaps the lunate and capitate but the posterior surface or pole of the triquetrum normally projects posterior to the capitolunate articulation. With dorsal-directed stress displacing the capitate dorsally, the posterior pole of the triquetrum remains in the same relative position to the capitate. This fact demonstrates that the triquetrum is linked to the capitate. In the case of CLIP wrist, the authors do not mention this problem;[47] therefore, although it is not clear from the literature if the same relationships occur under fluoroscopy, there is no obvious reason why the same relationships cannot be observed with fluoroscopy.

Medioanterior Midcarpal Instability (MAMI Pattern).[4,5,14,26] Standard radiographs show a normal appearance both on PA and lateral views. Dynamic motion views in full ulnar and radial deviation do not demonstrate abnormal findings. Passive traction with a PA view produces an increasing widening of the medial (ulnar) aspect of the midcarpal space, and the lateral view in dorsal stress shows dorsal subluxation of the capitate out of the lunate fossa. The displacement is as far as half of the head of the capitate that was out of the lunate fossa. Obscuring the posterior pole of the triquetrum in the lateral view with dorsal-directed stress is diagnostic of a MAMI pattern, but such a configuration may also be obtained with a lateral view taken with a slight amount of supination, as in Fig. 7–16C. The widening of the medial (ulnar) midcarpal space is more or less obvious on traction views, but it is very demonstrative on AP views taken with passive supination of the distal part of the hand. Operative observations on live patients and experimental findings on cadaveric wrists operated on with dynamic radiographic studies confirmed that the lesion is a tear of the medial (ulnar) sling (limb) of the anterior (palmar) deltoid ligament of the wrist.

A CLINICALLY BASED ALGORITHMIC APPROACH TO WRIST EXAMINATION (FIG. 7–18)

The Basic Initial Workup

The initial workup consists of four basic views: frontal and lateral standard views and two oblique views; in semipronation and in semisupination. In case of an unclear roentgenographic configuration, we routinely perform radial and ulnar motion views to show the extreme end-points of the proximal row carpal bones and/or standard views of the contralateral side. If these radiographs are negative or unclear, a dynamic study is mandatory.

The Secondary Dynamic Workup

Acute Trauma

The examination is performed mostly under anesthesia. It consists of a passive stress study, which will show one of the following findings.

There Is No Evidence of Fracture

If possible, a frontal view with the fist clenched is performed without anesthesia. The passive stress study that we recommend consists of radial and ulnar deviation and also radial and ulnar translocation on frontal views and dorsally directed stress on the lateral view.

There Is Evidence of a Fracture With the Need to Disclose a Possible Associated Ligamentous Injury

Distal Radius Fracture. Only the cases that have been operated on with stabilization of the fractured distal end of the radius will be examined by a dynamic study. It is performed in the operating room, just after stabilization of the fracture. It consists of radial and ulnar translocation on frontal views.

Scaphoid Fracture. In most cases of scaphoid fracture, the problem is not to confuse a configuration of

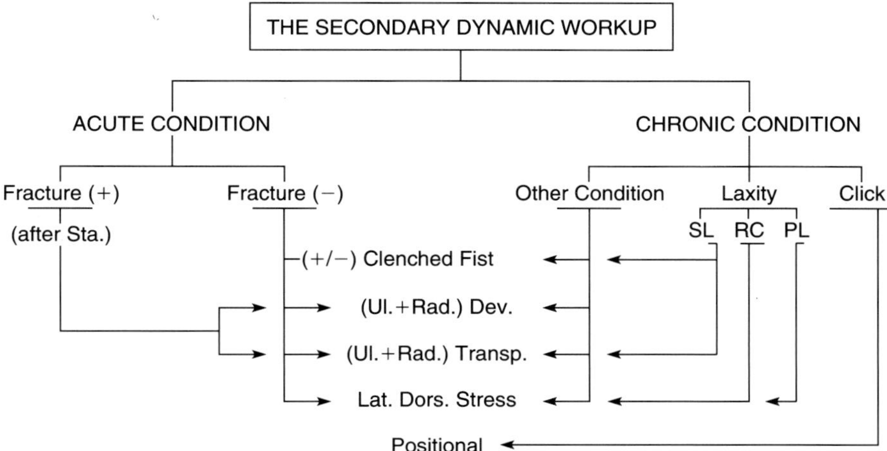

FIGURE 7–18. A clinically based algorithmic approach to wrist examination. SL, Scapholunate laxity; RC, radiocarpal laxity; PL, perilunate laxity; UL, ulnar; rad, radial; lat, lateral view; dors, dorsal; sta, standard view. Fracture (+): in case of fracture (distal radius or carpal). Fracture (−): if there is no evidence of a fracture.

SL laxity with a truly abnormal condition. SL laxity is most easily confirmed by performing a comparative view on the contralateral wrist (Fig. 7–3). With a displaced fracture in which one suspects an associated ligamentous lesion, we recommend performing frontal views in radial and ulnar translocation just after its stabilization by osteosynthesis.

Chronic Conditions

Click, Pop, or Clunk

Positional views with PA and lateral views are taken just before and just after the click.

Lax Wrist

The final study performed is determined by the type of laxity suspected. With SL laxity, in our opinion the frontal view with the fist clenched is the best one. In cases of radiolunate or perilunate laxity, dorsal stress in the lateral view is diagnostic.

In All Other Conditions

In general, if one does not have sufficient clinical information to suspect the location of the injury, we recommend performing a standard regimen accompanied by 1) a frontal view with the fist clenched, 2) passive stress views consisting of radial and ulnar deviation, 3) radial and ulnar translocation on frontal views, and 4) dorsal-directed stress on the lateral view.

If enough clinical information is available to locate the injured ligament, we recommend first performing the specific dynamic view for the ligament in question. For a suspected lesion at the SL joint, the views of choice are frontal views with clenched fist and radial transposition. For a lesion suspected at the lunotriquetral (LT) joint, the views of choice are the frontal motion view in ulnar deviation and the frontal stress view in forced radial deviation. In case of a suspected lesion at the lateral (radial) part of the midcarpal joint, the view of choice is the frontal view in forced ulnar deviation. For a suspected lesion at the medial (ulnar) part of the midcarpal joint, the view of choice is the lateral, dorsal-directed stress view. In our opinion, whatever the information obtained from those specific views, it is also necessary to perform frontal stress views in radial and ulnar translocation and dorsal-directed stress views with a lateral view, if they have not already been done, to avoid overlooking any lesion located at the radiocarpal level.

The Complementary Workup

In Grade II or III ligamentous lesions, in most cases static and dynamic roentgenographic examination of the wrist allows one to make a precise diagnosis. It is crucial not to mistake a configuration of normal laxity for a lesion. Only seldom does one need any additional information. In our experience, radiography is less reliable in Grade II lesions located at the LT area. If one has any doubt about the existence of a lesion at this level, a complementary technique of direct imaging is therefore mandatory. Within the different techniques of direct imaging available (i.e., arthrography, MRI, or arthroscopy), arthrography appears to be the easiest and most accurate diagnostic tool.[48] To this date, in our cases of lesions at other joints, none of the different direct imaging techniques has proven to be more reliable than the above-described roentgenographic examination.

When normal standard and dynamic radiographs are observed in a patient who has already had a painful laxity condition eliminated but who has evidence of a clinically pathologic condition with pain, consistent edema, and motion limitation, some pathologic condition must be considered. This situation represents a confusing condition—it may be a Grade I ligamentous lesion, but it also may be due to an extraarticular or a cartilaginous problem, or even an occult fracture. Because it is also rather difficult to disclose a Grade I ligamentous lesion by direct imaging, such a lesion will be considered only if the other conditions have been eliminated. If an extraarticular condition is ruled out, we manage those cases by informing the patient about the problem and treating the painful wrist with wrist immobilization by a short forearm cast for 3 to 4 weeks. At the end of that treatment period, if the patient is well we consider the diagnosis of Grade I lesion as positive. If the patient is not improved, we must consider another diagnosis. At that point we prefer performing a triple-phase radionuclide bone scan.[49,50] If the bone scan shows changes that favor a fracture, we use computed tomography or trispiral tomography to confirm it, just as we would use tomography immediately in case of an uncertain fracture detected during the stress study. If there is no evidence of a fracture on computed tomography, chondromalacia must be considered as the most reliable diagnosis. When the bone scan shows uptake suggestive of chondromalacia, we do not routinely confirm it by arthroscopy.[51] A final consideration, although uncommon, is that of a "bone bruise" or bone marrow edema. In the case of a very hot bone scan that is unexplained by routine films and tomography, MRI may be of value in showing an abnormal marrow signal, such as that occurring in bone marrow edema or even some subtle fractures that may not show up on computed tomography or polytomography.

II. INDICATIONS FOR WRIST INSTABILITY SERIES AND ITS COST-EFFECTIVENESS

Nhan P. Truong, F. A. Mann, and Louis A. Gilula

WRIST INSTABILITY SERIES

Introduction

Wrist trauma can result in carpal instability or abnormal carpal alignment either early or late.[52,53] All posttraumatic carpal instabilities may not be evident on conventional plain radiographic static views,[53–58] and wrist instability series (WIS) have been designed to search for such dynamic instabilities (Fig. 7–19). The existing literature does not clearly specify when WIS should be performed. As a result, clinical indications and use of WIS varies greatly between different centers and investigators.

Between 1979 and 1990, we routinely performed WIS on all patients with posttraumatic wrist pain referred for wrist arthrography. Despite performing the examination tightly tailored to the patient's clinical symptoms, most of our WIS have been "normal." Since these "normal" WIS represent considerable monetary costs, patient radiation, and physician and patient time without a clear clinical benefit, we believed that there was a need for the development of an inclusion–exclusion filter as a "pre-WIS" screen. To be generally applicable to patients with cryptic wrist pain, an effective filter must substantially improve the number of positive WIS without a clinically significant loss of specificity (i.e., no increase in false negative diagnoses).

Application of the WIS Filter

Survey Radiographs

The four preliminary survey radiographs include posteroanterior (PA), PA 45-degree semisupinated oblique, PA ulnar deviation, and lateral views, and can be analyzed in the following manner. On the PA view, most of the joint spaces should have equal width and be symmetric, especially within a carpal row. The radiocarpal joint can be slightly wider than intercarpal joints, and sometimes the intercarpal joints of the distal carpal row can be slightly narrower than the midcarpal joint. The articular surfaces of the carpal bones should be parallel and carpal Arcs I to III should be smooth (Fig. 7–20A).[59] Abnormal widening or overlapping of normally parallel joint spaces or a disrupted carpal arc strongly suggest ligamentous and/or bone or joint injury (Figs. 7–20B and 7–20C).[60]

On a true lateral view, the ventral border of the pisiform should be centered between the ventral margin of the capitate head and the ventral border of the distal scaphoid pole (Fig. 7–21). Normally, the axes of the capitate, lunate, and radius are nearly parallel on a neutral lateral view. However, true coaxial alignment of the capitate, lunate, and radius axes is observed in only approximately 10% of cases.[61] Abnormal dorsal or ventral tilting of the lunate indicates dorsal intercalated segmented instability (DISI) or volar or ventral intercalated segmental instability (VISI) configurations, respectively. When abnormal carpal alignment is suspected, the scapholunate (SL) and capitolunate (CL) angles, and occasionally lunotriquetral (LT) angles, can be measured to further confirm and subclassify the diagnosis of DISI or VISI configurations, respectively (Fig. 7–22).[52,60,62] We believe that the diagnosis of DISI or VISI configurations

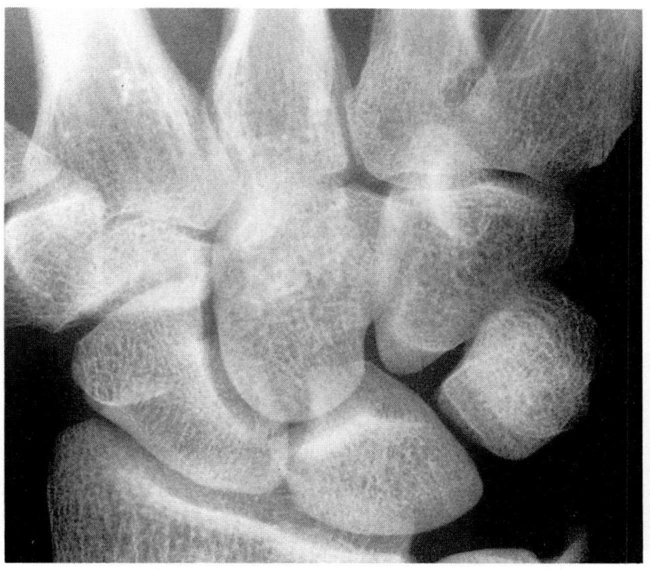

A

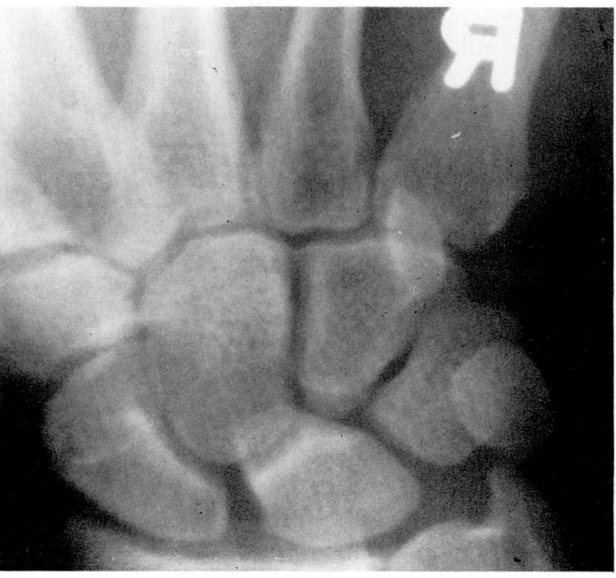

B

FIGURE 7–19. **A**: Static PA view of the right wrist demonstrates no definite abnormal alignment. **B**: Neutral fluoro spot view on instability series with scapholunate joint profiled clearly reveals scapholunate joint space widening evidenced by the fact that the scapholunate joint in its midportion is wider than the capitolunate joint and the third carpometacarpal joint widths.

suggested by abnormal tilting of the lunate is only indicative of abnormal alignment, which in some cases may be a normal variant, and the diagnosis of DISI or VISI instability can be firmly established with imaging only when there is abnormal intercarpal motion demonstrated, as on an instability series (Fig. 7–23). On a normal lateral flexion view, the long axis of the capitate should be in flexion with respect to the lunate axis, which in turn should be flexed with respect to the long axis of the radius. Likewise, on a normal lateral extension view, the long axis of the capitate should be in extension with respect to the lunate axis, which in turn should be extended with respect to the long axis of the radius. Deviation from this normal relationship accompanying a DISI or VISI configuration confirms DISI or VISI instability (Fig. 7–23). The additional semipronated oblique and ulnar deviation PA views will also aid in the routine survey examination for carpus abnormalities.[63]

Directed Physical Examination

Physical examination includes search for the site of maximal point(s) or area(s) of tenderness, capitolunate instability pattern (CLIP) or dorsal pain syndrome, presence of popping, and SL symptomatology. The CLIP wrist maneuver (Figs. 7–24A and 7–24B) is performed with stabilization of the patient's forearm and placing the wrist in slight ulnar deviation. Then first dorsal and subsequently ventral displacing forces are applied at the carpometacarpal joints.[58,64–66] This maneuver is considered positive radiologically when half or more of the head of the capitate displaces out of the lunate fossa[67] (Fig. 7–24C), but especially when pain of the presenting type is elicited.

Positive SL symptomatology is diagnosed when one or more of the five following tests is positive:[68] 1) tenderness in the snuff box (Fig. 7–25A); 2) tenderness over the proximal pole of the scaphoid just dorsal and distal to the radial styloid (Fig. 7–25B); 3) tenderness over the SL joint (Fig. 7–25C); 4) positive Watson's maneuver; and/or 5) positive wrist flexion–finger extension maneuver. The Watson maneuver or scaphoid shift test[69] (Fig. 7–26) is performed with the patient's hand pronated; dorsally directed pressure is applied over the ventral aspect of the distal scaphoid pole. Starting from an ulnar-deviated position, the wrist is moved radially with constant dorsally directed pressure applied to the distal scaphoid pole. The goal of this maneuver is to try to sublux the proximal pole of the scaphoid dorsally out of the scaphoid fossa, which, when present, supports the diagnosis of rotary subluxation of the scaphoid or abnormal laxity of ligaments supporting the scaphoid. The finger extension maneuver (Fig. 7–27) is performed with the elbow on the table, the wrist palmarflexed, and the fingers extended.[68] Downward pressure is then applied by the examiner on the extended fingertips of the patient. The maneuver is considered positive for SL pathology when pain of the presenting type is elicited over the scaphoid. Additional examinations for other sites of symptoms are performed as detailed in Chapters 1 and 2. In general, abnormalities found by various other provocative maneuvers will show nothing using routine imaging

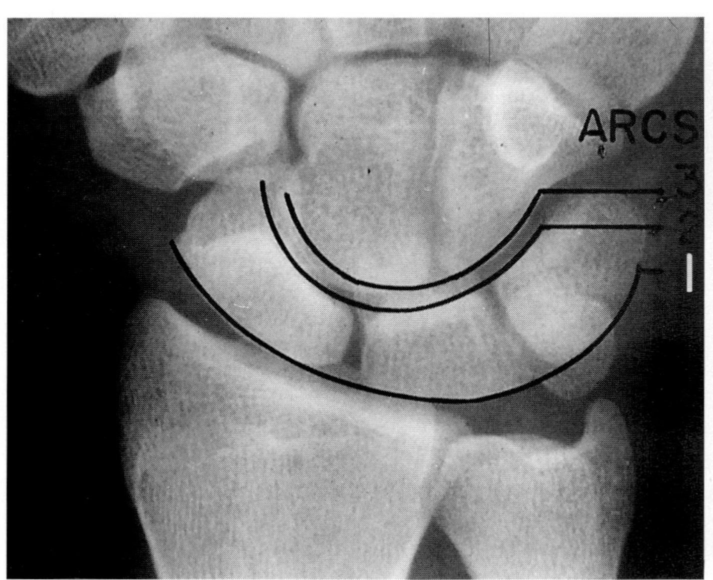

A

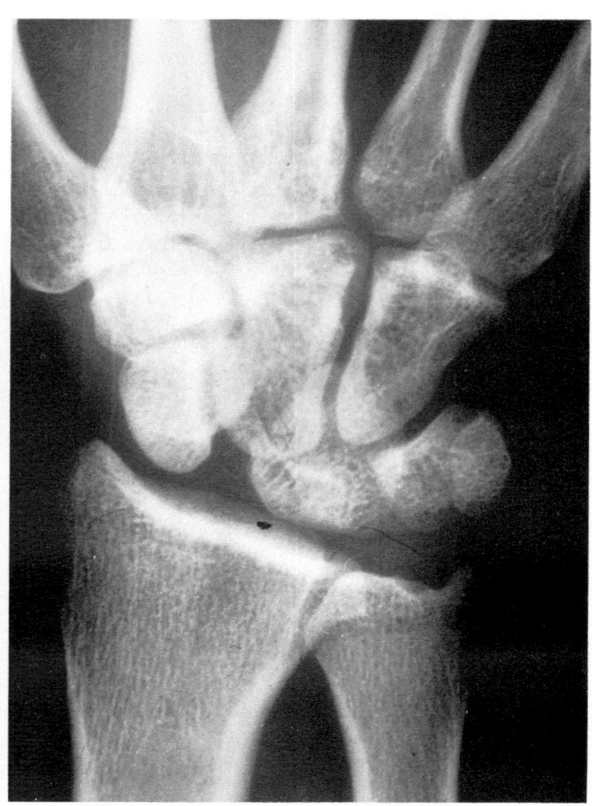

B

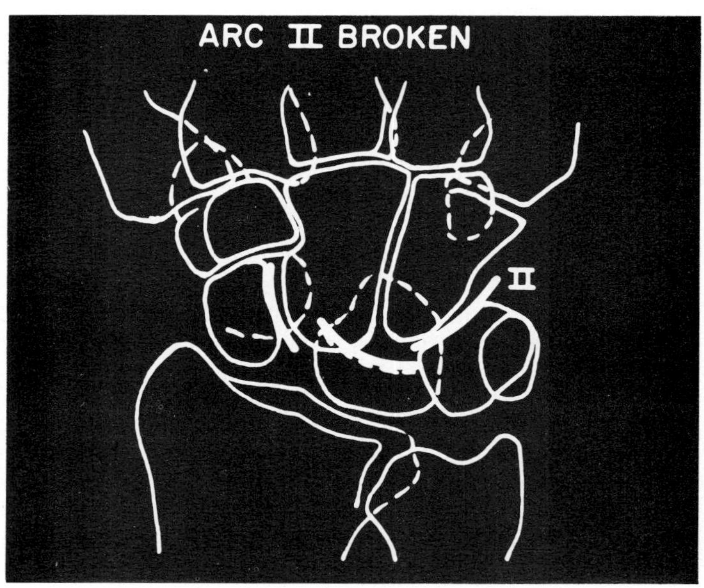

C

FIGURE 7–20. A: On the PA view of a normal wrist, three smooth arcs normally outline proximal and distal cortical margins of the proximal carpal row and proximal cortical surfaces of the capitate and hamate. **B**: Arc II is broken at both the scapholunate and the lunotriquetral joint spaces, indicating abnormal intercarpal relationships at both of these joints. **C**: Diagram of **B**. (Panels A–C reprinted with permission from Gilula LA. Carpal injuries: Analytic approach and case exercises. *AJR* 1979;133:503–517.)

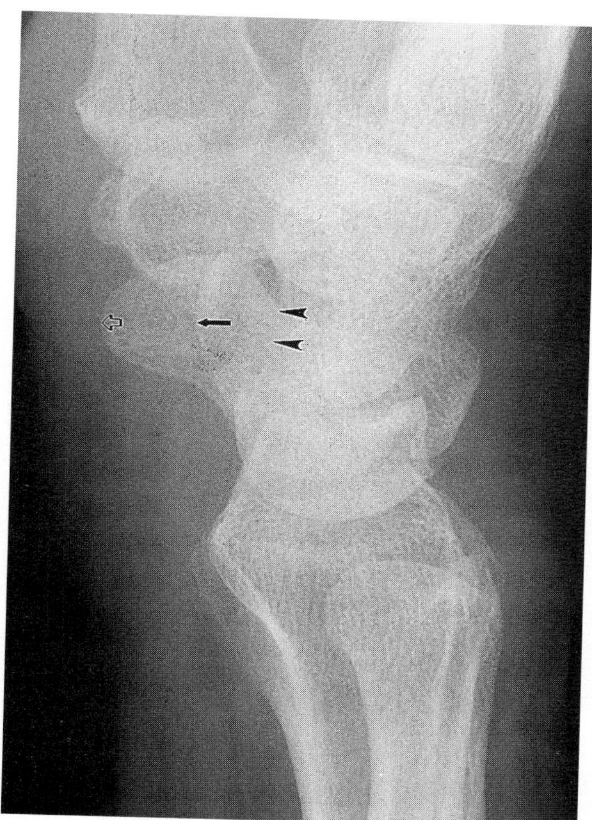

FIGURE 7–21. On a true lateral view, the ventral border of the pisiform (arrow) should lie in the mid third to half of the space between the ventral cortex of the capitate (arrowheads) and distal scaphoid pole (open arrow).

procedures. Examination for popping will be described subsequently.

Wrist Instability Series: Performance and Interpretation

Our full instability series of 17 views is performed under fluoroscopic control and is listed in (Table 7–1):[70] PA in neutral, radial, and ulnar deviation profiling the SL joint; PA with ulnar translocation and radial displacement stresses;[57,58] semisupinated oblique position to profile the scaphotrapeziotrapezoidal joint; true lateral view; lateral views with wrist fully palmar-flexed and fully dorsiflexed; lateral views with the wrist in radial and ulnar deviation to observe lunate motion; the two CLIP wrist views; semisupinated view profiling the pisotriquetral joint; and (AP) anteroposterior views profiling the SL joint with fist clenched in neutral, full ulnar, and full radial deviation positions.

For patients with repetitive painful clunking or popping, fluoroscopic evaluation and, as appropriate, videotape recording is performed in an attempt to identify abnormal bone motion or a soft-tissue cause as the etiology for the popping (Fig. 7–28). If abnormal motion is identified, a full instability series is obtained, mainly to search for other abnormalities.

With normal carpal alignment and positive SL ligament symptomatology, both PA and fist-clenched AP views of the fluoroscopically profiled SL space in neutral, radial, and ulnar deviations of both wrists are performed. In other words, the SL joint should be watched carefully as the wrist is moved slowly between extremes of radial and ulnar deviation in both the supine and prone positions to identify the position in which the SL joint is widest. Additional views between the radial and ulnar deviation positions are obtained if necessary to demonstrate the SL joint space at its widest possible state. If abnormal SL widening is present, a full instability series is then obtained to distinguish rotary subluxation of the scaphoid from DISI or VISI instability. If there is abnormal motion of the lunate in conjunction with DISI or VISI alignment, then the radiographic diagnosis of true DISI or VISI instability is established (Fig. 7–23). With DISI, if the lunate moves normally with respect to the capitate and radius, the abnormality is believed to be centered about the scaphoid (Fig. 7–29) and the condition of rotary subluxation of the scaphoid is supported rather than the diagnosis of DISI.

Development of the Clinicoradiologic Filter

We developed our three-criteria screening filter using an informal, nine-member expert panel under the guidance of Dr. L. A. Gilula.[70] A thorough review of the English-language literature on WIS was performed along with consultations with academic hand surgeons to assemble an "expert" knowledge base. Three criteria were chosen for inclusion in the pre-WIS filter:

1. Radiographically evident static instability—abnormal carpal alignment on routine radiographs such as DISI, VISI, scapholunate diastasis, or lunotriquetral offset;[59]
2. Clinically evident static instability—scapholunate joint or ligament symptomatology;[71] and
3. Clinically evident dynamic instability: a) reproducible painful clicking or popping,[56,71] b) CLIP wrist (positive capitolunate instability pattern)[64] on physical examination.

Validation of and Experience With the WIS Filter

The validity of the screening filter was retrospectively tested in 560 consecutive patients with posttraumatic, cryptic wrist pain referred for wrist arthrography between 1979 and 1990. Plain films, physical examination findings, wrist arthrograms, and WIS on all 560 cases were reviewed. On basis of the review, interpretation of plain radiographs, and the originally recorded physical examination findings, patients who

Text continued on page 194

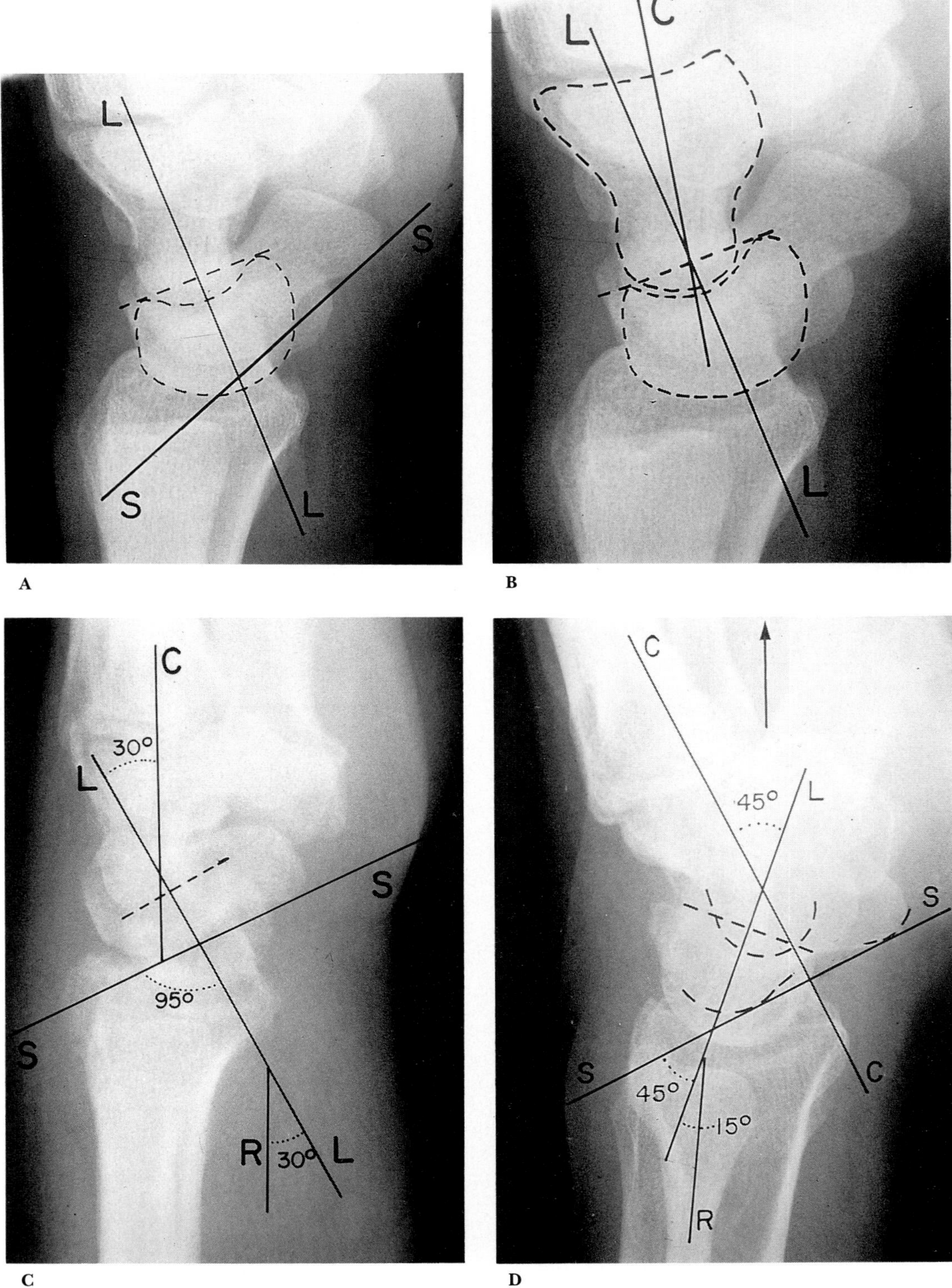

FIGURE 7–22. A, B: The axes of the scaphoid (S), lunate (L), and capitate (C) are represented by the solid straight lines. **C**: DISI configuration is diagnosed when the SLA (scapholunate angle) is 80 degrees or more and/or the CLA (capitolunate angle) is more than 30 degrees. A normal SLA is 30 to 60 degrees, and a normal CLA is less than 30 degrees. **D**: VISI configuration is confirmed when the SLA is less than 30 degrees and/or the CLA is more than 30 degrees. (Panels A–D reprinted with permission from Gilula LA, Weeks PM. Posttraumatic ligamentous instabilities of the wrist. *Radiology* 1978;129:641–651.)

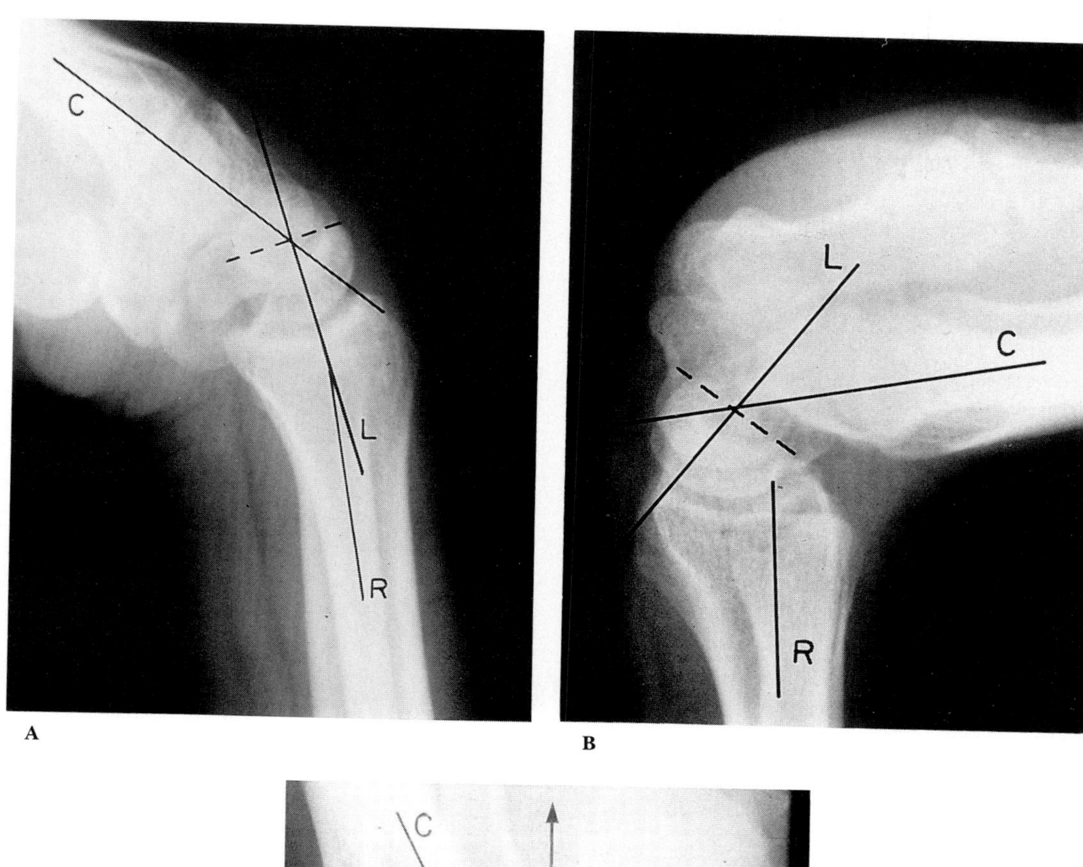

A B

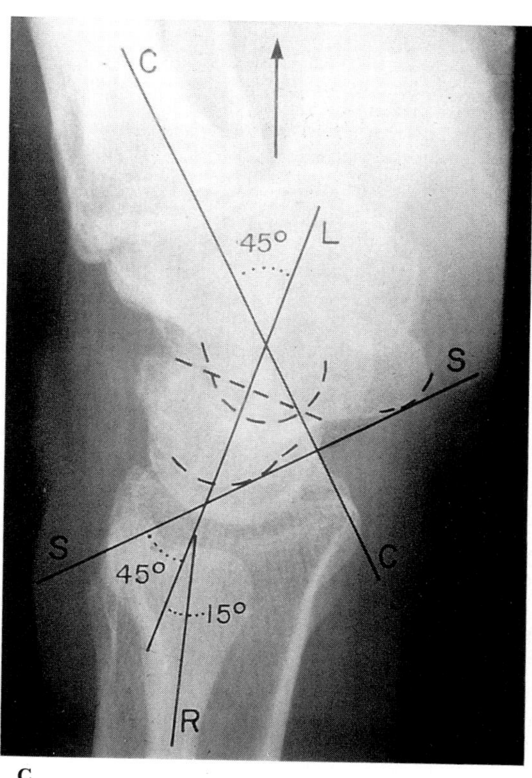

C

FIGURE 7–23. A: Lateral flexion of a normal wrist demonstrates flexion of the capitate axis (C) with respect to the lunate axis (L), which in turn is flexed with respect to the radius axis (R). **B**: Lateral extension (dorsiflexion) of a normal wrist demonstrates extension of the capitate axis (C) with respect to the lunate axis (L), which in turn is extended with respect to the radius axis (R). **C**: VISI configuration is demonstrated with an abnormally increased capitolunate angle of 45 degrees (normal ≤ 30 degrees).

Illustration continued on following page

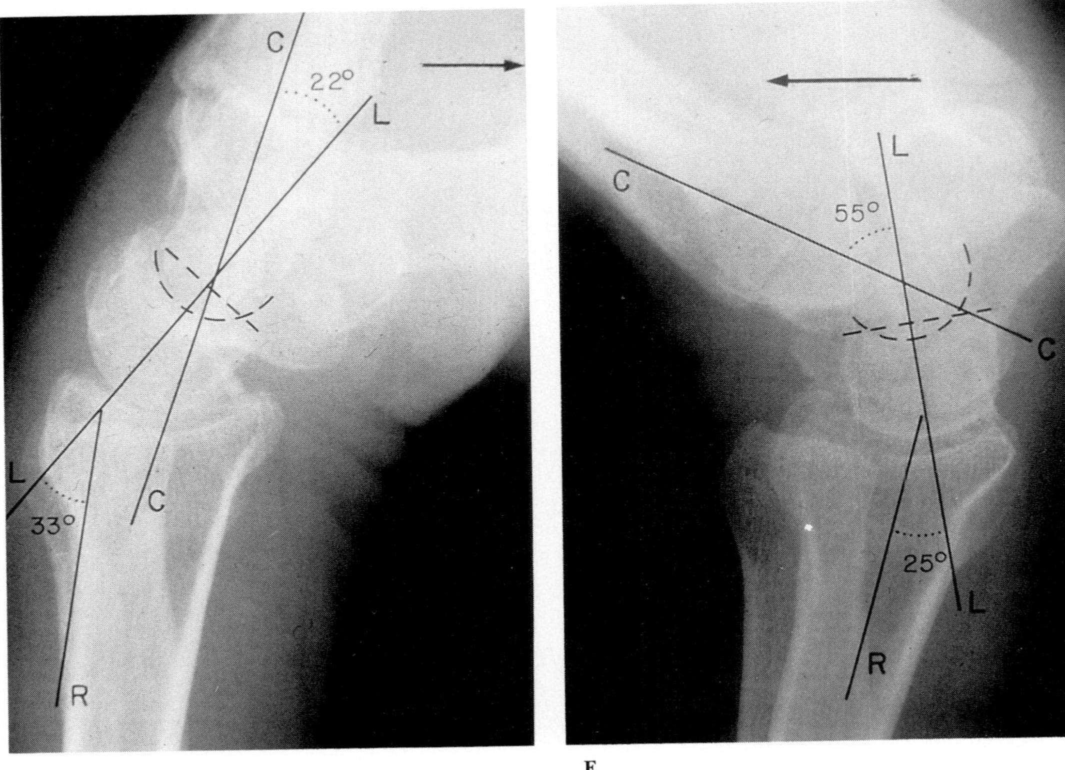

FIGURE 7–23 *Continued* **D**: On lateral view with palmar-flexion, the capitate axis (C) does not flex with respect to the lunate axis (L), indicating abnormal intercarpal motion and supporting the diagnosis of VISI. The lunate axis (L) is flexed with respect to the long axis of the radius (R). **E**: On lateral view obtained in extension, there is normal extension of the capitate axis (C) with respect to the lunate axis (L), which in turn is normally extended with respect to the radius axis (R). (Panels A–E reprinted with permission from Gilula LA, Weeks PM. Posttraumatic ligamentous instabilities of the wrist. *Radiology* 1978;129:641–651.)

had at least one of the screening criteria were assigned to a group with a high probability for wrist instability pattern probable (WIPP). All remaining patients were assigned to a group defined as unlikely (low probability) to have significant wrist instability pattern excluded (WIPE).

Patient Population

Of the 560 patients, 329 were male and 231 female. Patient ages ranged from 11 to 71 years with an average of 35. Wrist trauma in all of these patients was either acute, subacute, or chronic secondary to occupation or avocation. Twenty-five patients with unilateral symptoms but bilateral, symmetrical, abnormal wrist instability series were considered as having hyperlax wrists and were not classified as having posttraumatic wrist instability.[70]

Excluding the 25 "hyperlax" wrists, there were 535 remaining patients. In these 535 patients, 142 had at least one (WIPP) and 393 had none (WIPE) of the three proposed criteria. Of the 142 WIPP patients, 39 had abnormal alignment on plain films, 54 had repetitive clicking or popping, and 35 had scaphoid symptomatology. Five had both abnormal alignment and clicking or popping, seven had both abnormal alignment and scaphoid symptoms, and two patients had both scaphoid symptoms and clicking or popping. Wrist instabilities in these different groups are listed in Table 7–2.

Seventy-eight (15%) of the total 535 patients had an abnormal WIS. In the group of 142 patients who had at least one of the three criteria, 69 patients (45%) had abnormal WIS. Nine patients (2%) of the 408 with none of the three criteria (WIPE) had an abnormal WIS. These nine had dynamic scapholunate diastasis without focal tenderness (condition 2).

Thus the filter produced 69 true positives, 9 false negatives, 384 true negatives, and 73 false positives. The filter's diagnostic performance can be summarized as having a sensitivity of 88.5% and a specificity of 84.0%.

Comment

Application of our three-condition filter identifies almost all the recognized carpal instabilities (69 of 78) in our case series of 535 patients. It appears to systematically overlook those dynamic scapholunate diastases that lack focal scapholunate symptoms (9 of 78). Perhaps this is not surprising, since some radial-

Text continued on page 198

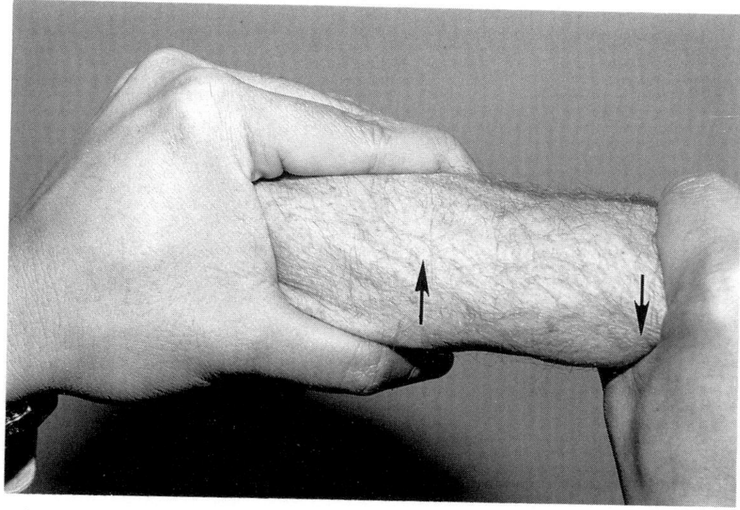

A

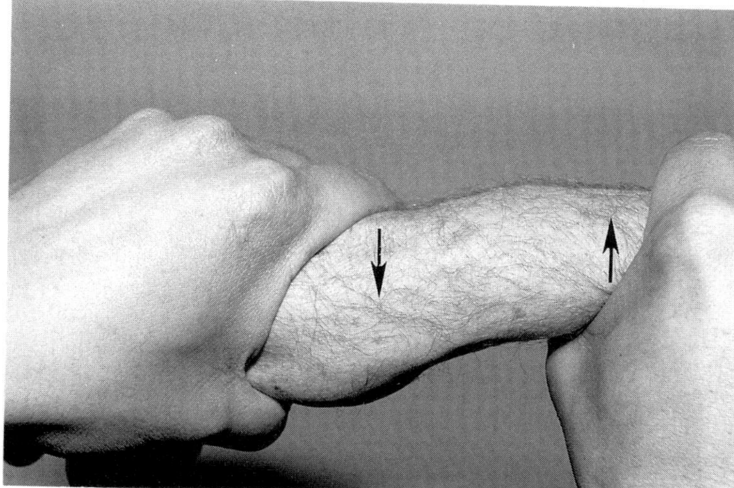

B

FIGURE 7–24. CLIP wrist maneuvers are performed with **A**: dorsal displacing and **B**: ventral displacing forces applied at the level of the carpometacarpal joints. The maneuver is considered positive clinically when pain of the presenting type is elicited, and typically when more than half of the proximal pole of the capitate is displaced outside of the lunate fossa. **C**: Commonly, the capitate will displace dorsally less than half the width of the capitate head. **D**: With palmar-directed force, a VISI configuration can often be transiently created in normal wrists.

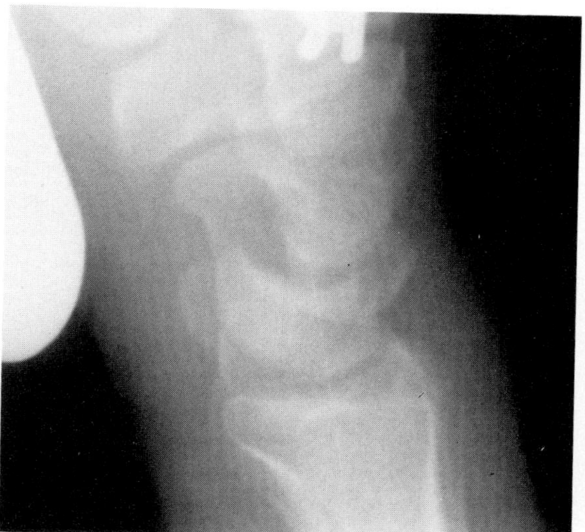

C

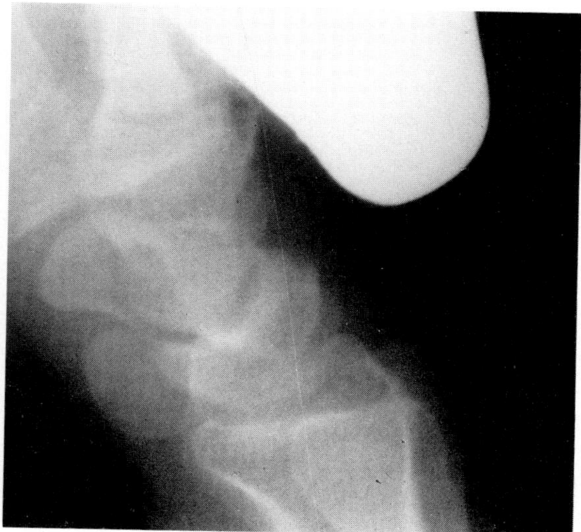

D

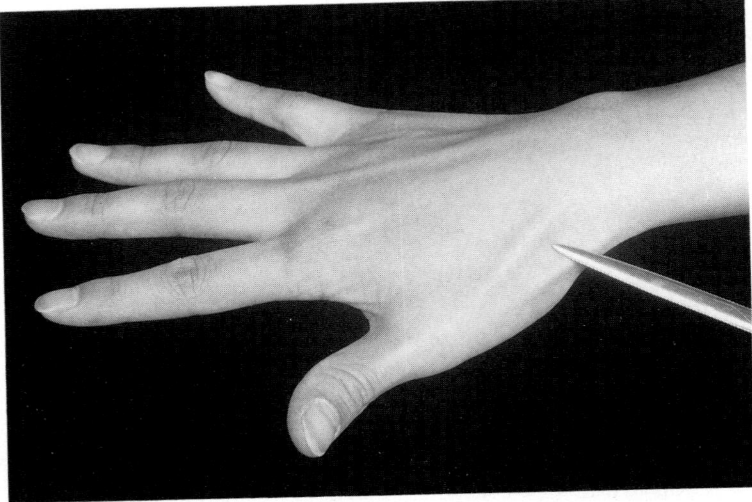

A

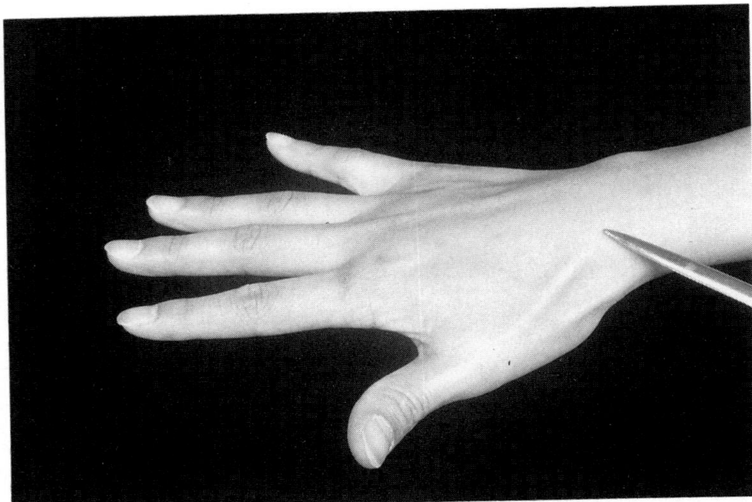

B

FIGURE 7–25. Examination for scaphoid symptomatology includes search for tenderness over **(A)** the snuff box, **(B)** the proximal scaphoid pole just distal to the radial styloid, and **(C)** the scapholunate joint. Flexion of the wrist makes the scapholunate joint more easily palpable, since in this position the dorsal rim of the radius does not cover the scapholunate joint as much as is covered in the neutral nonflexed, or extended position of the wrist.

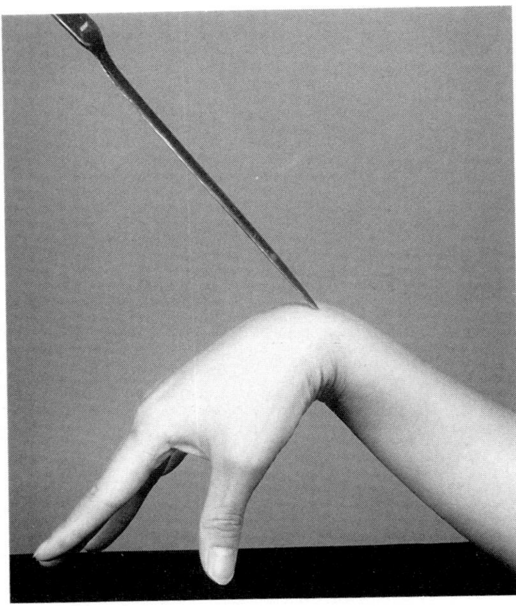

C

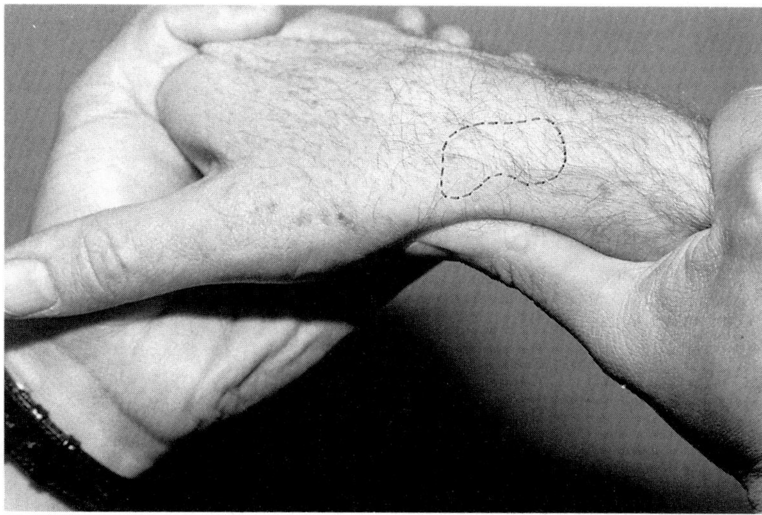

A

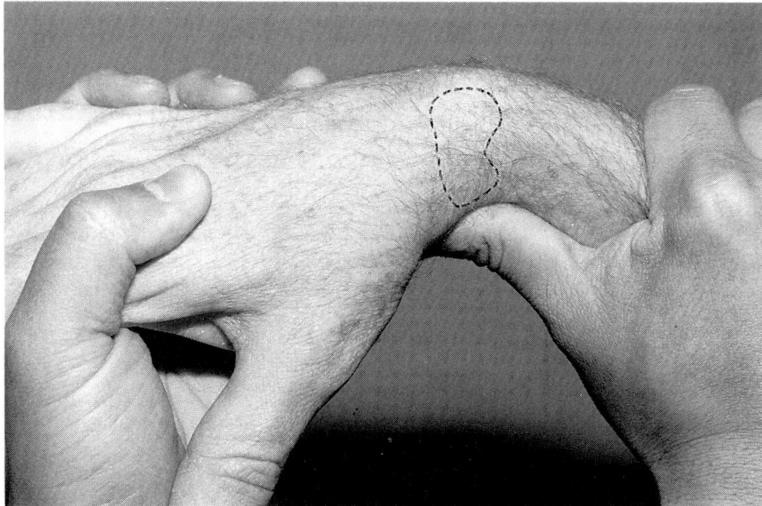

B

FIGURE 7–26. Watson's maneuver or the scaphoid shift test is performed with constant pressure applied to the distal pole of the scaphoid while the wrist is moved from **(A)** ulnar to **(B)** radial deviation in an attempt to sublux the proximal scaphoid pole dorsally out of the scaphoid fossa of the radius. The test is considered positive when pain, especially that of the presenting type, is elicited in the region of the snuff box.

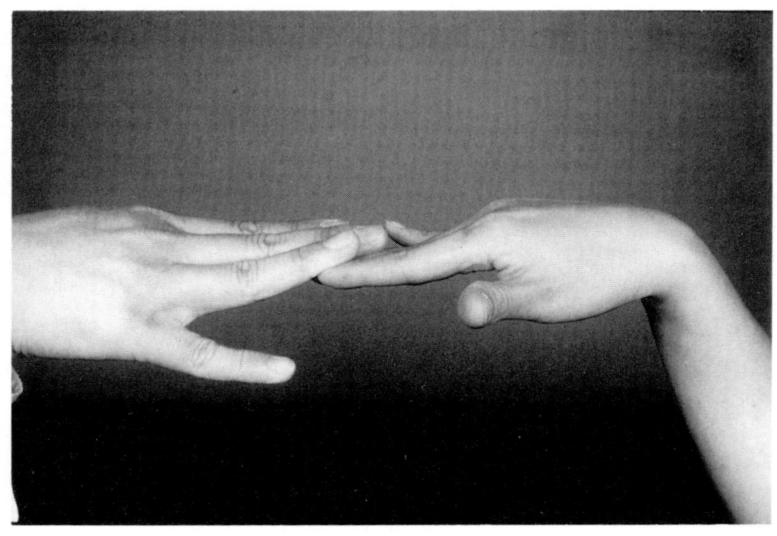

FIGURE 7–27. Finger-extension test is performed with flexion at the wrist joint and downward pressure exerted on the extended fingers. Pain of the presenting type in the region of the snuff box constitutes a positive test.

TABLE 7–1. *Wrist Instability Series*

PA Projections Profiling the Scapholunate Articulation
Neutral
Full ulnar deviation
Full radial deviation
Stress—ulnar translocation (displacement)
Stress—radial translocation (displacement)
Prone Oblique Projection to Profile the Scaphotrapeziotrapezoidal Joint
Lateral Projections
True lateral ("zero neutral")
Fully palmarly flexed
Fully dorsiflexed
Ulnar deviation
Radial deviation
Stress—dorsal CLIP maneuver
Stress—palmar CLIP maneuver
Semisupinated Oblique to Profile the Pisotriquetral Joint
AP Projections With Fist Clenched to Profile the Scapholunate Joint
Neutral
Full ulnar deviation
Full radial deviation

sided pain has a poor correlation with arthrographic findings.[72,73] However, static and dynamic maneuvers producing point-like pain (to be distinguished from more diffuse pain) at the scapholunate articulation (conditions 1 and 2) have not been specifically addressed in the radiology literature. Similarly differentiation of such focal tenderness from more diffuse types of pain or tenderness elsewhere in the wrist and correlated with arthrographic findings has not been reported in the literature. Moreover, some clinicians recommend surgery based on such focal findings.[74]

In any event, our nine "missed" cases required diagnostic information beyond that inherent in WIS and would have necessitated arthrography. Thus, use of this pre-WIS filter led to a diagnostic sequence that identified all carpal instabilities, and did so while using only one fourth of the routine number of WIS. This achieves considerable improvement in diagnostic efficiency while decreasing patient radiation exposure and resource use.

Who should apply the filter? In our opinion, performance of a high-quality physical examination of the wrist should be part of the radiologists' study. Since WIS requires specific dynamic maneuvers, radiologists already perform many tests common to wrist physical examination. However, the filter can be applied by any skilled examiner (e.g., hand surgeon, occupational therapist, radiologist, and so on).

In conclusion, a majority of patients with painful wrists do not need an instability series. Prospectively applying the above three screening criteria will result in a reduction of physician and patient time expenditure, costs, and patient radiation exposure. At the same time, these criteria can enable use of a tailored instability series usually to confirm or exclude the clinical abnormalities in question.

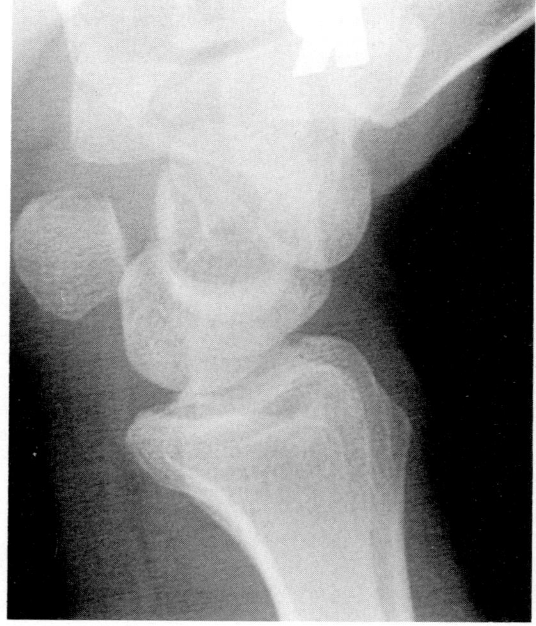

A

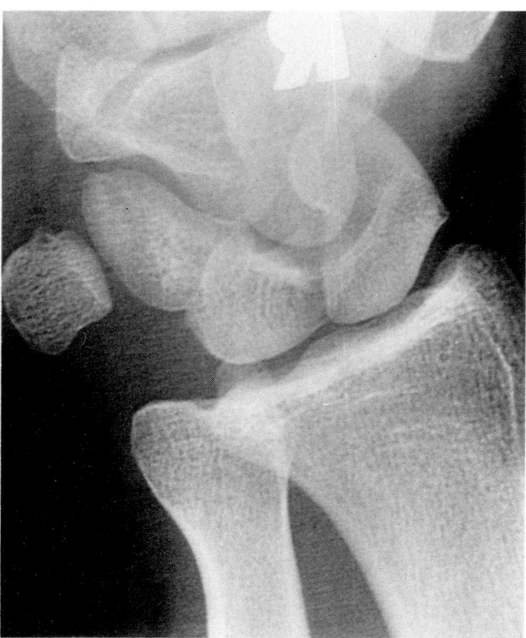

B

FIGURE 7–28. Fluoroscopy demonstrates that reproducible painful popping in this patient is secondary to dorsal dislocation of the capitate with respect to the lunate. Dislocation **(A)** and reduction **(B)** of the capitate were easily performed actively by the patient when he applied a rotary force to his wrist.

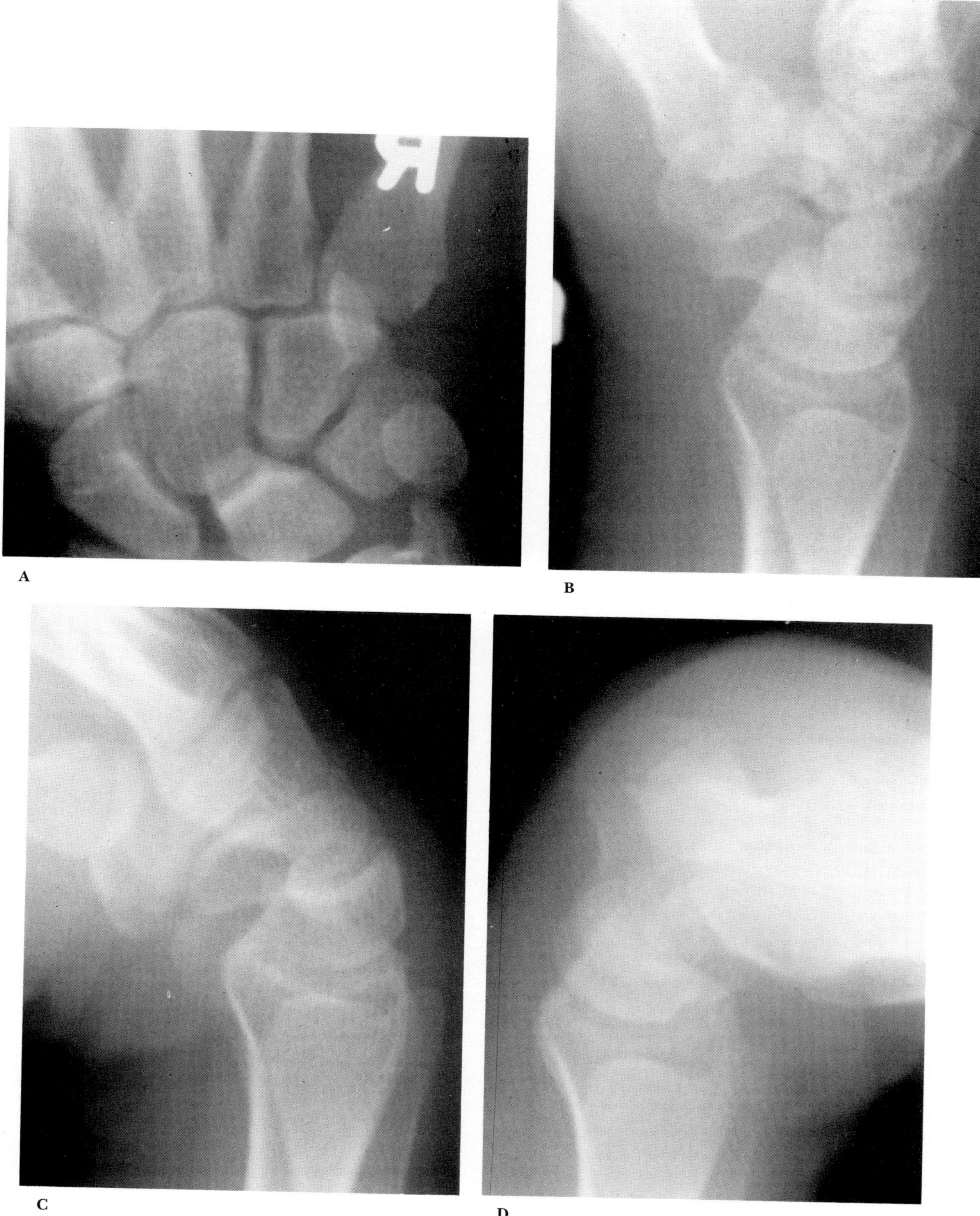

FIGURE 7–29. 105-mm fluoroscopic views of a patient with rotary subluxation of the scaphoid with scapholunate diastasis **(A)**, and ventral scaphoid and slight dorsal lunate tilting **(B)**. Flexion **(C)** and extension **(D)** views demonstrate a normal relationship between the capitate, lunate, and radius axes, confirming scaphoid rotary subluxation and excluding DISI.

TABLE 7–2. *152 Patients With ≥ 1 of the 3 Proposed Criteria*

	Abn. Align.	C/P	Scap. Sxs.	Abn. Align. and C/P	Abn. Align. and Scap. Sxs.	C/P and Scap. Sxs.	Total
All pts.	45	55	37	6	7	2	152
Normal WIS	10*	36	23	2	1	1	73
Abn. bilat. WIS	6	1	2	1			10
Abn. WIS	29	18	12	3	6	1	69
SL widening	10	8	8	1	4		31
DISI	10		1	1			12
VISI	7		1	1			9
CLIP		2					2
Midcar. inst.		2					2
Other	2 (1 LT offset, 1 decr. ROM)	6 (1 VISI conf., 1 bony pop, 1 incr. rad. trans. 1 DRUJ widen., 2 abn. motion)	2 (1 RS and RL widen. with traction, 1 RS widening)		2 (1 RS widen., 1 decr. ROM)	1 (1 incr. rad. and uln. trans.)	13

* *Five with SL widening, 1 VISI configuration, 1 DISI configuration, 1 scapholunate advanced collapse, 2 ulnar impaction. (Reprinted with permission from the Radiological Society of North America from Truong NP, Mann FA, Gilula LA, Kang SW. Clinicoradiologic filter increases yield from wrist instability series.* Radiology *1994;192:481–484.)*

Abn, abnormal; Align, alignment; Bilat, bilateral; C/P, clunk and pop; CLIP, capitolunate instability pattern; Conf, configuration; Decr, decreased; DISI, dorsal intercalated segmental instability; DRUJ, distal radioulnar joint; Incr, increased; Inst, instability; LT, lunotriquetral; Midcar, midcarpal; Rad, radial; ROM, range of motion; RL, radiolunate; RS, radioscaphoid; Scap, Scaphoid; SL, scapholunate; sxs, symptoms; Trans, translation; Uln, ulnar; VISI, ventral intercalated segmental instability; Widen, widening; WIS, wrist instability series.

COST-EFFECTIVENESS OF A PRE-WIS SCREENING FILTER[70]

Since our goals in developing a pre-WIS filter included improved resource management, we wanted to quantify the potential savings in patient radiation exposure, physician and patient time expenditure, and cost related to an inclusion–exclusion-filter-based selection rather than routine performance of WIS.

Patient radiation exposure, time expenditure, and charges related to performance of WIS were retrospectively estimated for the above 560 patients who had WIS and wrist arthrography. The "high probability for instability" criteria group included all patients having at least one of the three proposed criteria (WIPP). Average radiation exposure, times, and charges were calculated per diagnosed instability for the routine and WIPP groups, respectively.

Patient radiation exposure was calculated for 17 digital spot films (8 PA and 9 laterals) and 3 minutes of nonmagnified fluoroscopy per wrist in an adult.[67] The effective doses computed are based on 1) measured entrance exposures during fluoroscopy and spot film imaging of an adult wrist, 2) organ dose values adapted from those specified for the humerus[75] by adjusting for different field sizes, and 3) organ-weighting factors recommended by the International Commission on Radiological Protection.[76]

Cost per WIS was estimated for the amount of fluoroscopic time, spot films taken, and physician interpretation. We also compared our charges to others around the country who performed WIS. None of our 560 patients were charged extra for the WIS, since this study was performed as part of the arthrogram.

Results

Patient Radiation Exposure

The estimated effective doses for PA and lateral digital spots of the wrist at 55 kV are 0.05 mrem/image and 0.07 mrem/image, respectively. Nonmagnified PA and lateral fluoroscopy at 56 kV results in effective doses of 2.1 mrem/min and 3.0 mrem/min, respectively. The average of these two values would be 2.6 mrem/min. As a result, the collective effective dose for a full WIS (including 8 PA/AP and 9 lateral spot images and 3 minutes of fluoroscopy per wrist) is approximately 10 mrem ($2[8 \times 0.05 + 9 \times 0.07 + 3 \times 2.6] = 9.86$ mrem). For perspective, consider that an effective dose of 10 mrem represents approximately 3.3% of the annual effective dose due to naturally occurring radiation sources in the United States (average of 300 mrem per year) or about half of the effective dose attributed to the extra radiation received from one New York-to-Tokyo round trip by commercial aircraft.

The relative difference in patient radiation exposure would be 67 mrem/instability in the routine group (10 mrem $\times$ 560/84 = 66.7 mrem) versus 22 mrem/instability in the criteria-selected group (10 mrem $\times$ 152/69 = 22 mrem).

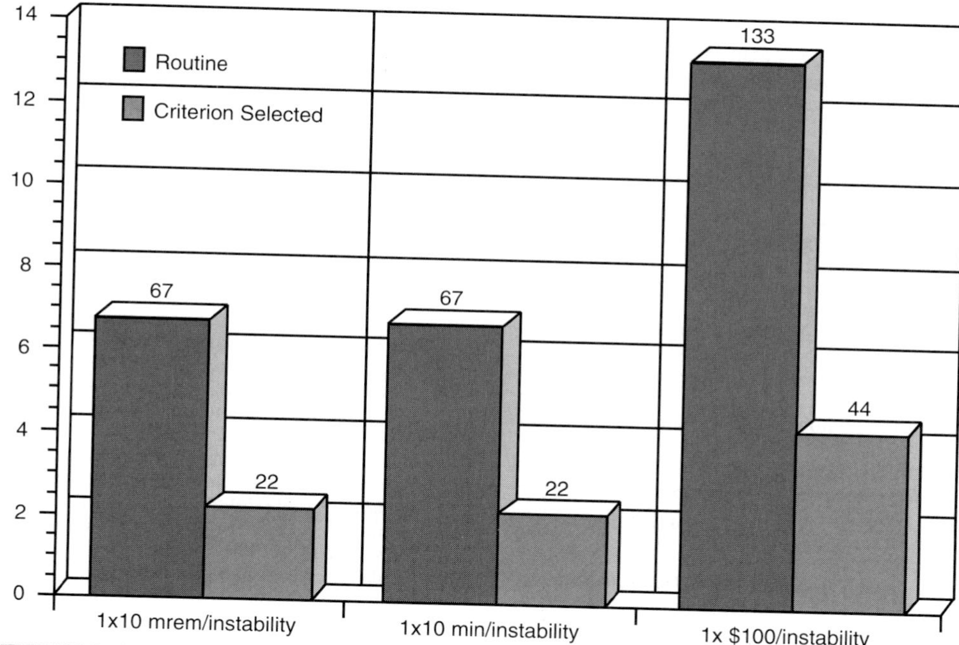

FIGURE 7–30. Bar graph demonstrates the relative reductions in patient radiation exposure, time expenditure, and costs by application of criteria selected versus routine use of WIS.

Physician and Patient Time Expenditure

We estimated a total of 10 minutes for a full WIS (3 minutes of fluoroscopy and 17 spot films per wrist). The relative difference in time expenditure would be 67 min/instability in the routine group versus 22 min/instability in the criteria-selected group.

Total Charges

We estimated a total fee of $200, including both technical and professional costs for each full WIS. The relative difference in costs would be $1330/instability in the routine group versus $440/instability in the criteria-selected group.

Figure 7–30 graphically demonstrates the relative differences in patient radiation exposure, time expenditure, and costs between these two groups.

Conclusion

Prospectively applying the above three screening criteria will result in decreased patient radiation exposure, physician and patient time expenditure, and costs by approximately two thirds for each wrist instability found.

REFERENCES

1. Fisk G. Carpal instability on the fractured scaphoid. *Ann Roy Coll Surg Engl* 1970;46:63–76.
2. Destot E. *Traumatismes du poignet et rayons X.* Paris; Masson, 1923:27–32.
3. Gilula LA, Weeks PM. Ligamentous instability of the wrist. *Radiology* 1978;129:641–651.
4. Schernberg F. Roentgenographic examination of the wrist: A systematic study of the normal, lax and traumatic wrist. Part One: The standard and the positional views. *J Hand Surg* 1990;15B:210–219.
5. Schernberg F. Roentgenographic examination of the wrist: A systematic study of the normal, lax and traumatic wrist. Part Two: Stress views. *J Hand Surg* 1990;15B:220–228.
6. Gilula LA, Hardy DC, Totty WG. Wrist arthrography: An update review. *J Med Imag* 1988;2:251–266.
7. Palmer AK, Levinsohn EM, Kuzma GR. Arthrography of the wrist. *J Hand Surg* 1983;8A:15–23.
8. Zinberg EM, Palmer AK, Coren AB, et al. The triple-injection wrist arthrogram. *J Hand Surg* 1988;13A:803–809.
9. Baker LL, Hajek PC, Bjorkengren A, et al. High resolution magnetic resonance imaging of the wrist: Normal anatomy. *Skeletal Radiol* 1987;16:128–132.
10. Zlatkin MB, Chao PC, Ostermann AL, et al. Chronic wrist pain: Evaluation with high-resolution MR imaging. *Radiology* 1989;173:723–729.
11. Rominger MB, Bernreuter WK, Kenney PJ, et al. MR imaging of anatomy and tears of wrist ligaments. *RadioGraphics* 1993; 13:1233–1246.
12. Roth JM, Haddad RG. Radio-carpal arthroscopy and arthrography in the diagnosis of ulnar wrist pain. *J Arthroscop Rel Surg* 1986;2:234–243.
13. Whipple TL, Marotta J, Powell J. Techniques of wrist arthroscopy. *Arthroscopy* 1986;2:244–252.
14. Schernberg F. *Le poignet: Anatomie radiologique et chirurgie.* Paris: Masson, 1992:37–41.
15. Mino DE, Palmer AK, Levinsohn EM. The role of radiography and computerized tomography in the diagnosis of subluxation and dislocation of the distal radioulnar joint. *J Hand Surg* 1983;8:23–31.
16. Wechsler RJ, Wehbe MA, Rifkin MD, et al. Computed tomography diagnosis of distal radio-ulnar subluxation. *Skeletal Radiol* 1987;16:1–5.
17. Gilula LA. Carpal injuries: Analytic approach and case exercises. *AJR* 1979;133:503–517.
18. Gilula LA, ed. *The traumatized hand and wrist: Radiographic and anatomic correlation.* Philadelphia: WB Saunders, 1992.
19. McMurtry RY, Youm Y, Flatt AE, et al. Kinematics of the wrist. *J Bone Joint Surg* 1978;60A:423–431.

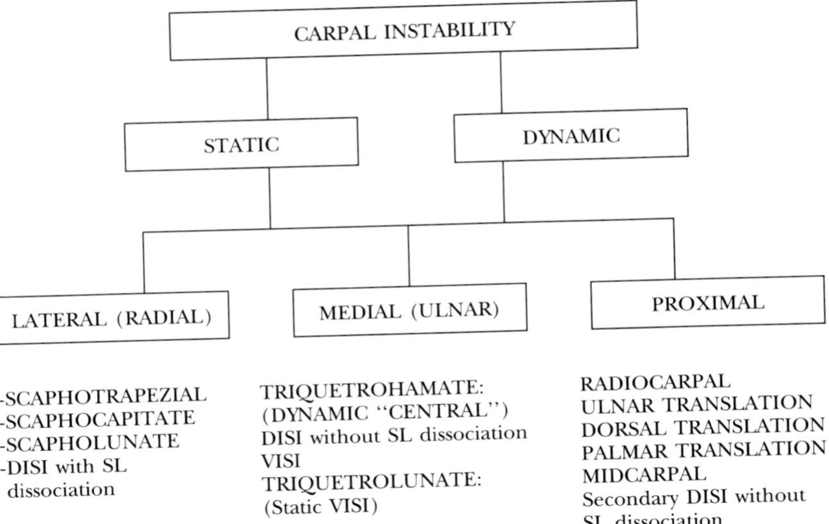

FIGURE 8–1. Classification of carpal instability. SL, scapholunate. (Modified with permission from Taleisnik J. Post-traumatic carpal instability. *Clin Orthop* 1980;149:73–82.)

(scapholunate and lunotriquetral) oriented joints and on those segments of transverse joints that seem to lead intercarpal motion (triquetrohamate, scaphotrapeziotrapezoid, and scaphocapitate). In 1972, Linscheid et al described four carpal instabilities—two each at the radiocarpal (ulnar translation, dorsal subluxation) and midcarpal (dorsiflexion instability, palmar flexion instability) joints.[5] The acronyms DISI (dorsal intercalated segment instability) and VISI (ventral, or volar intercalated segment instability) or PISI (palmar intercalated segment instability), where the lunate is the intercalated segment, are commonly used to describe midcarpal malaligaments. PISI and VISI are synonymous. Further subclassification of DISI and VISI patterns is based on whether there are associated (potentially causal) longitudinal (scapholunate, lunotriquetral) joint dissociations (carpal instability dissociated [CID]) or not (carpal instability nondissociated [CIND], which has normal scapholunate and lunotriquetral alignments and motion).

By convention, the lunate is the keystone landmark for the diagnosis and differential diagnosis of carpal instability, especially in the lateral projection. Abnormal translation (dorsal, palmar, radial, or ulnar) and/or angulation (tilting dorsally or palmarly) implies a certain kind of pathologic condition (Fig. 8–3). As such, the lunate reflects the motion of the intercalated segment (proximal carpal row) within the so-called radiocarpal link, because its orientation is believed to be normally governed by the scaphoid radially and the triquetrum ulnarly.[30,31] When the normal wrist is held in full radial deviation, the proximal carpal row will have translated ulnarly and dorsally and palmar-flexed to allow sufficient radial-sided carpal height shortening necessary to approximate the radial styloid and trapezium.[31] PA radiographs in this position will show scaphoid foreshortening, a triangular-shaped lunate, and the triquetrum in a proximal position in relation to the hamate (Fig. 8–4A). In contrast, for full ulnar deviation, ulnar-sided carpal height shortening is accomplished through radial and palmar translation and dorsiflexion of the proximal carpal row led by the triquetrum as it tracks along the progressively coronal orientation of the semihelicoid triquetrohamate articulations.[30,32] On the PA view, the scaphoid appears elongated and the lunate quadrilateral,[33] and the triquetrum approaches the metacarpal end of its articulation with the hamate (Fig. 8–4B). Thus an intercalated segment itself within the proximal carpal row is led into palmarflexion by the scaphoid in radial deviation and driven into dorsiflexion by the triquetrum in ulnar deviation.

One can extrapolate from these normal, attitude-dependent shapes seen on PA projections. Consider static dorsiflexion instability (DISI) that commonly occurs after a scapholunate dissociation, or a static palmar-flexion instability (PISI) that may complicate a triquetrolunate dislocation.[31,34] On a neutral PA projection, a foreshortened scaphoid (palmar-flexed) with an increased scapholunate gap and a rhomboid-shaped lunate (dorsiflexed) suggest a DISI (CID). Similarly, a foreshortened scaphoid (palmar-flexed) and a triangle-shaped lunate is compatible with a PISI (VISI). Careful attention to the lunotriquetral (LT) articulation on Arcs I and II may help determine whether there is LT dissociation (CID) or not (CIND). Therefore, it is always important to pay attention to the lunate to see if it moves ulnarly, dorsally, or palmarly with or without tilting. Each condition represents different pathologic changes, and important diagnostic "fingerprints" are commonly shown by the conventional radiographic exam.

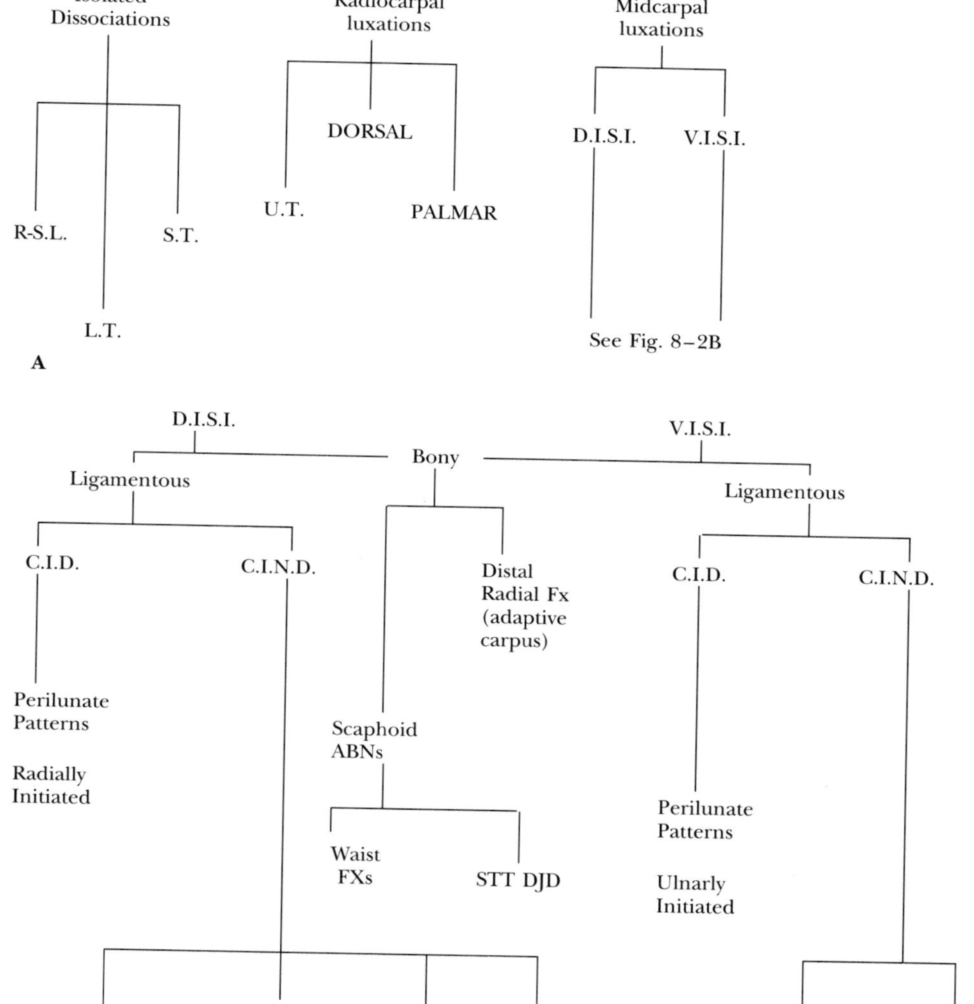

FIGURE 8–2. A: Carpal instabilities. R-SL, rotary scapholunate; ST, scaphotrapezial; LT, lunotriquetral; UT, ulnar translocation; DISI and VISI, dorsal and ventral intercalated segmental instability. **B:** Midcarpal instabilities. C.I.D. and C.I.N.D., carpal instability, dissociated and nondissociated: R.S.C., radioscaphocapitate; TH, triquetrohamate; CT, capitotriquetral; LT, lunotriquetral; CLIP, capitolunate instability pattern ABNs, abnormalities; STT, scaphotrapeziotrapezoid; DJD, degenerative joint disease; Ligs, ligaments. (Reprinted with permission from Wilson AJ, Mann FA, Gilula LA. Imaging the hand and wrist. *J Hand Surg* 1990;15B:153–167.)

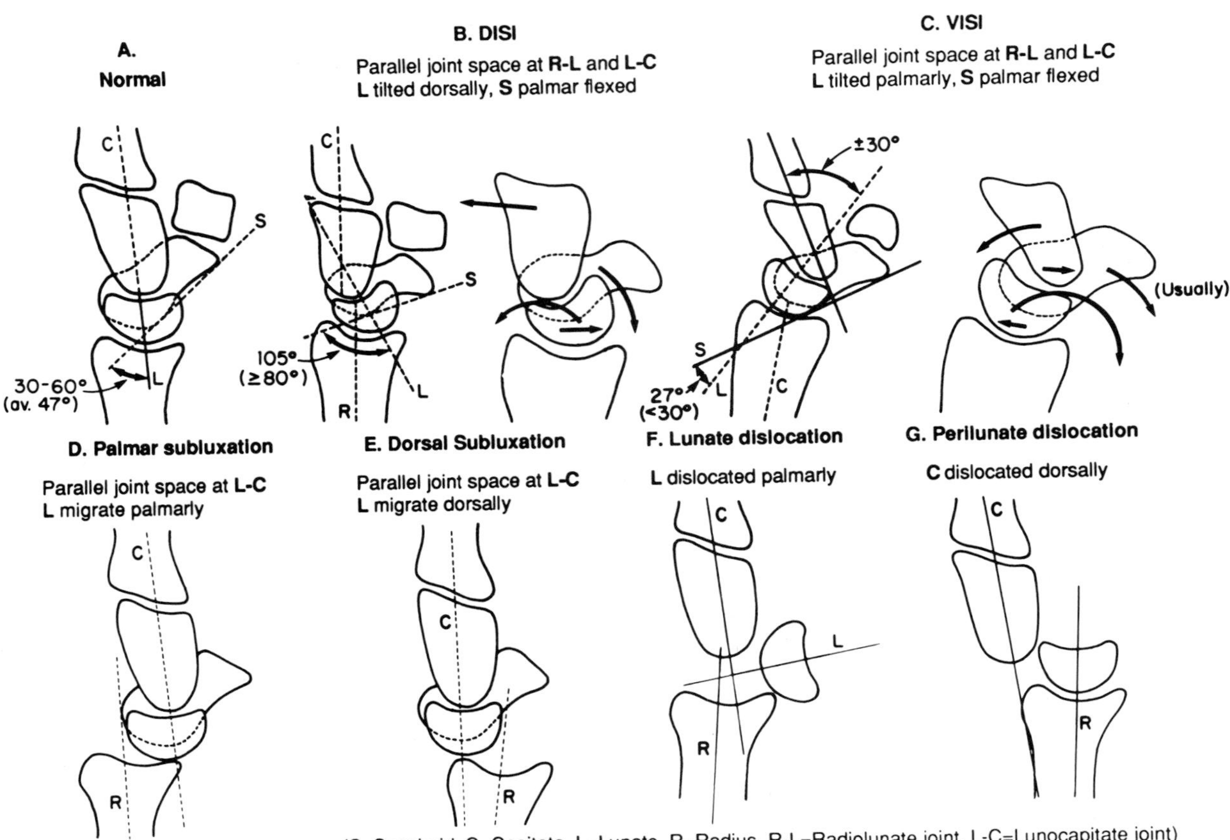

FIGURE 8–3. A line drawing that shows lunate conformational changes in different conditions.

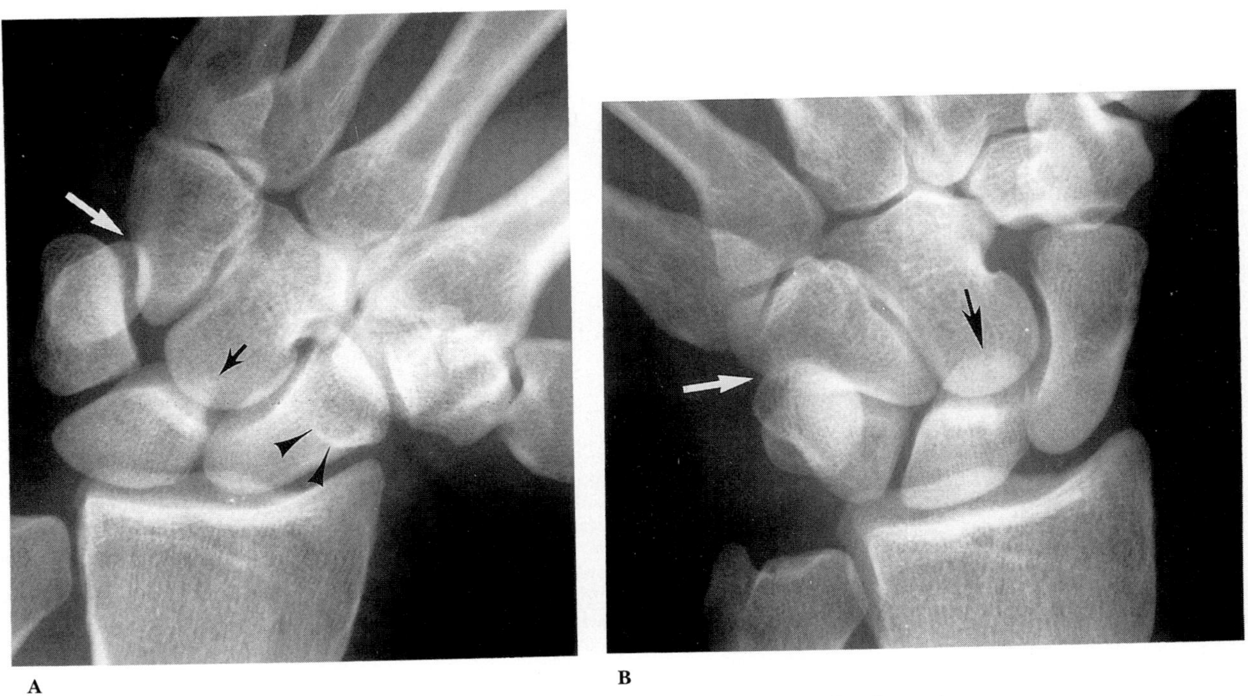

FIGURE 8–4. A: PA view of a normal left wrist in full radial deviation demonstrates foreshortening of the scaphoid creating a "ring sign" (arrowheads), a triangular lunate (black arrow), and the triquetrum in a proximal position in relation to the hamate (white arrow). **B:** PA view of a normal left wrist in full ulnar deviation demonstrates the elongated scaphoid appearance, a somewhat quadrilateral lunate (black arrow), and a triquetrum displaced distally in relation to the hamate (white arrow).

RADIOCARPAL INSTABILITIES: ULNAR, DORSAL, AND PALMAR TRANSLATIONS (TRANSLOCATION)

This group of instabilities is characterized by injuries affecting the integrity and/or course of the extrinsic ligaments, with sparing of the intrinsic (scapholunate and lunotriquetral) ligaments. The resulting displacements are at the radiocarpal joint (radioscaphoid plus radiolunate plus ulnotriquetral joints) such that the carpus translates toward the same-named translocation (ulnar, palmar, and dorsal). Whereas ulnar and palmar translations can complicate either inflammatory (rheumatoid arthritis) or traumatic (fall on outstretched hand with or without fracture) insults, dorsal translocations are seen virtually only with malunions of distal radius fractures where the distal fragment is dorsally angulated.

Ulnar Translocation

Ulnar translocation (UT) is defined as the ulnarward translation of the longitudinal axis of the carpus, represented by the long axes of the capitate and long (third) metacarpal along the distal articular surface of the radius. This is an uncommon traumatic injury,[1,35–38] and is more frequently seen with attenuation of the supporting ligaments caused by chronic synovitis, especially rheumatoid arthritis (Fig. 8–5). With failure or attenuation of the radiocarpal ligaments, the palmar and ulnar "sloping" (inclination) of the distal articular surface of the radius dictates ulnar and anterior translation under ordinary physiologic loading.[22] UT may also be found in some developmental disorders that lead to progressive shortening of the ulna relative to the radius, or in surgical excision of the distal ulna.[23]

The radiographic diagnosis of ulnar carpal translation is based on the neutral PA view.[35–44] Ulnar translation is defined as abnormal translation of the lunate and capitate in an ulnar direction. A key visual measure of ulnar translation is provided by recognizing the position of the lunate in relation to the ulnar edge of the lunate facet of the radius in the neutral PA projection (see Chapter 5). In this position, normally half or more of the articular surface of the lunate should be in contact with the distal radius.[44] Therefore, ulnar translocation is recognized when less than half of the articular surface of the lunate is in contact with the radius in the PA neutral position. Also, widening of the radial styloid scaphoid distance so that this joint space is larger than other intercarpal spaces, especially a normal radiolunate joint width, is supportive of this diagnosis. At least three quantitative methods have been reported for measuring abnormal ulnar migration of the carpus: 1) DiBenedetto's carpal radial distance,[40] 2) McMurtry's carpal ulnar distance ratio,[42] and 3) Chamay's index of carpal translation[39] (Fig. 8–6). Of them, DiBenedetto's carpal radial distance may be both the simplest and most practical measurement to use, since landmarks are uniformly present on standard wrist radiographs. Observation of the lunate's position with respect to the ulnar edge of the lunate fossa, in our experience, remains the easiest way to quickly survey the wrist for ulnar translocation without actually performing a measurement.

Ulnar translocation can be subclassified (Types I and II) on the basis of the position of the scaphoid relative to the radial styloid.[8,23] In Type I, the entire carpus including the scaphoid is translated ulnarly. The distance between the radial styloid and the scaphoid is widened (Fig. 8–7A). In Type II, the relationship and the distance between the scaphoid and the radial styloid remains normal, but the scapholunate space is widened (Fig. 8–7B). In Type II translocations, only the scaphoid remains in its normal position, and the rest of the carpus migrates

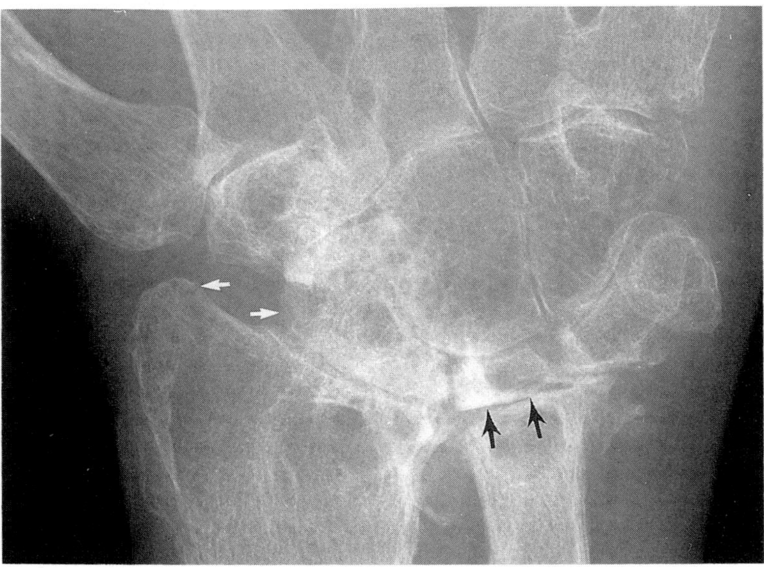

FIGURE 8–5. Rheumatoid arthritis of the right wrist with ulnar translation Type I. PA view of the right wrist demonstrates general osteopenia and narrowing of the joint spaces in the wrist. The whole carpus is migrated to the ulnar side, as evidenced by complete displacement of the lunate from the distal radius fossa toward the distal ulna (black arrows). The distance between the radial styloid and scaphoid is increased (white arrows).

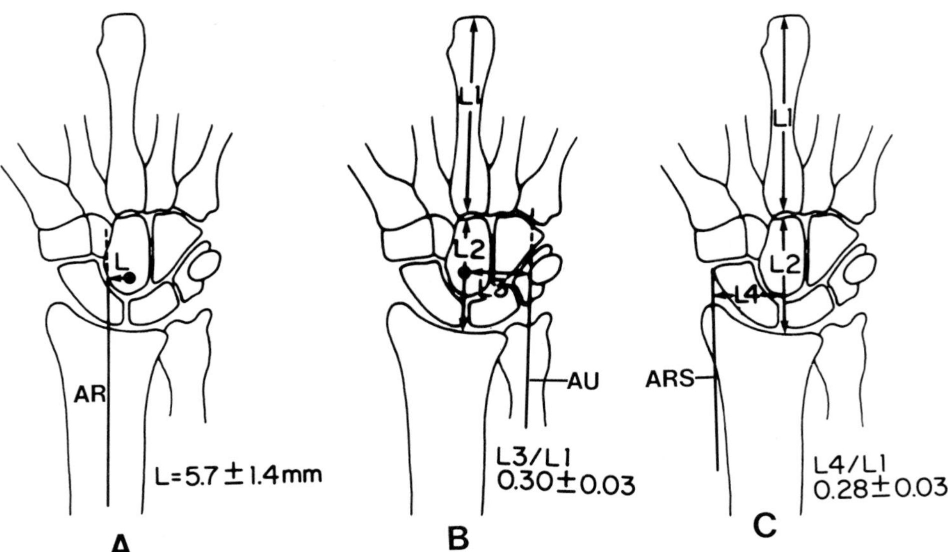

FIGURE 8–6. Three different methods have been described to measure ulnar translation of the carpus. Normal values for each methods are shown. **A:** DiBenedetto's carpal radial distance. This is the simplest measurement method performed by measuring the distance from the center of axis of rotation of the capitate to the longitudinal axis of the radius, which is determined by bisecting two perpendicular lines across the shaft (L = 5.7 ± 1.4mm). **B:** McMurtry's carpal ulnar distance ratio (L3/L1 = 0.3 ± 0.03). **C:** Chamay's index of carpal translation calculates a ratio by using the length of the third metacarpal and the longitudinal axis of the radial styloid as reference point. (L4/L1 = 0.28 ± 0.03. L, carpal radial distance, L1, length of the third metacarpal; L2, carpal height, which is the distance between the distal radial articular surface and the distal point of the capitate drawn along the mid axis of the third metacarpal; L3, carpal ulnar distance (McMurtry); L4, capitate-radial styloid distance (Chamay); AU, axis of ulna; ARS, axis of radial styloid; AR, axis of radius.)

ulnarly. While the distinction between the two types of ulnar translation has little clinical importance, it is vital to ensure that a Type II translocation, with its wide scapholunate gap, is not misdiagnosed as an isolated scapholunate dissociation. When such misdiagnoses occur, any effort to stabilize the scaphoid and lunate will probably fail, and the underlying ulnar carpal translocation will not be corrected. Ulnar translocation Types I and II can coexist, in which case the whole carpus migrates ulnarly with scapholunate space widening (Fig. 8–7C). A case of UT accompanied with palmar translation has recently been reported;[43] however, both of the cases of palmar subluxation described by Bellinghausen et al[45] showed ulnar translocation with their palmar carpal subluxation. Therefore, since all three reported cases show the same associated findings, this implies that palmar subluxation will probably always be associated with some degree of ulnar translocation.

Radial Translocation

Radial translocation is theoretically just the opposite of ulnar translocation; however, no such static instability has been reported except as accompanying a radial styloid fracture–dislocation. However, in our practice, using dynamically applied radially directed stress (see Chapter 7), we have had occasional cases in which the whole carpus can be displaced radially during the fluoroscopic study (Fig. 8–8). Presumably this indicates normal ligament laxity (if bilaterally symmetric and asymptomatic) or torn extrinsic ligaments (if painful and if different from opposite wrist).

Palmar (Ventral) Translocation

Palmar (ventral) translocation or translation (subluxation) (VT) refers to abnormal palmar migration of the entire carpus in relation to the long axis of the radius.[44,45] Clinically, a reversed silver-fork deformity is present with palmar displacement of the proximal carpal row (Fig. 8–9), presumably due to dorsal extrinsic ligament injuries at the radiocarpal level. Other carpal instabilities may also be present, such as DISI, VISI, or ulnar translation. On the PA wrist view, there is overlap of the normally opposing articular surfaces of the distal radius and proximal carpal row. The relationship among carpal bones remains normal and the three carpal arcs are intact. On the lateral view, the lunate, representing the position of the proximal carpal row, is translated palmarly with resultant loss of the normal parallel articular surfaces at the radiocarpal joint (Fig. 8–9). The capitate and lunate may be normally aligned. Comparison views of the opposite (normal) side in a neutral lateral projection should help establish this relationship more precisely, if clinically indicated.

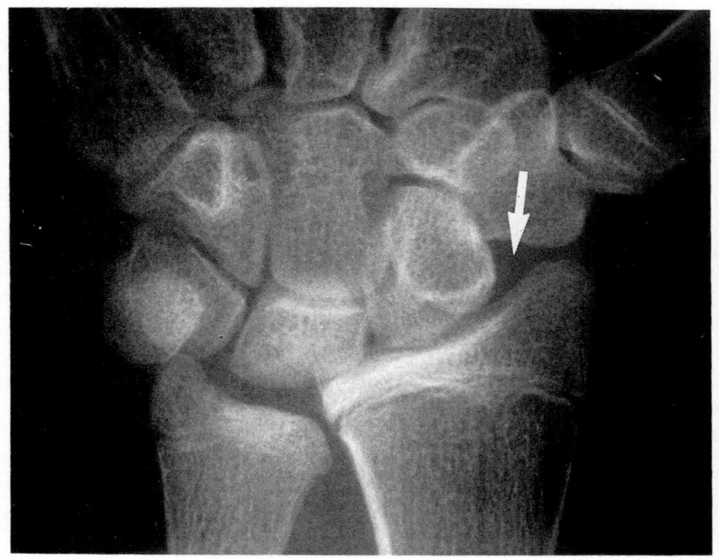

A

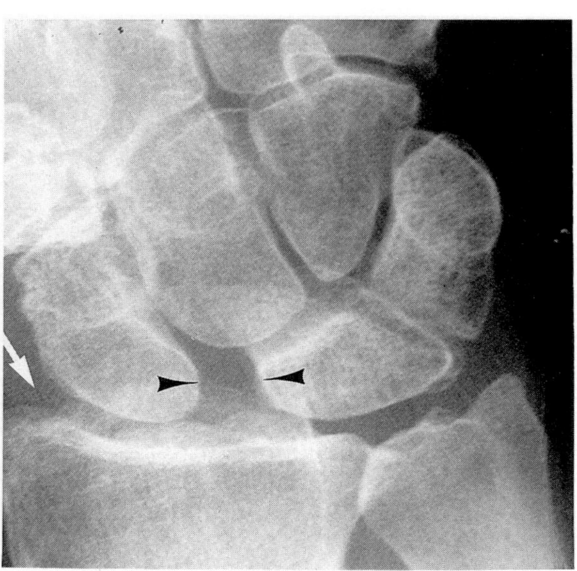

B

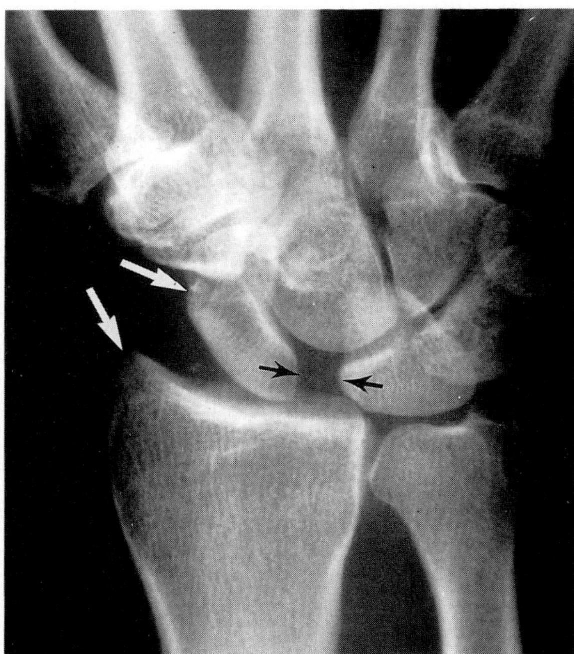

C

FIGURE 8–7. Ulnar translation. **A:** Ulnar translation Type I. PA view of left wrist demonstrates that the lunate along with all other carpal bones has migrated ulnarly. Less than half of the lunate contacts the distal radius. The radial styloid-scaphoid distance is increased (arrow). The relationship between carpal bones is normal. Arcs II and III are intact. Arc I is slightly offset at the scapholunate area due to some flattening and irregularity of the scaphoid and lunate at this joint, presumably due to cartilage loss and subchondral bone alterations between the radius and carpus in the lunate fossa. **B:** Ulnar translation Type II. PA view of right wrist demonstrates the lunate, along with the other carpal bones except for the scaphoid, has migrated ulnarly. The scapholunate joint space is widened (between arrowheads). The distance between the radial styloid and scaphoid is normal (white arrow). **C:** Ulnar translation Types I and II. PA view of right wrist demonstrates scapholunate joint space widening (between black arrows). The lunate has translated ulnarly and more than half of the lunate has moved out of the distal radius fossa. The distance between radial styloid and scaphoid is increased (between white arrows).

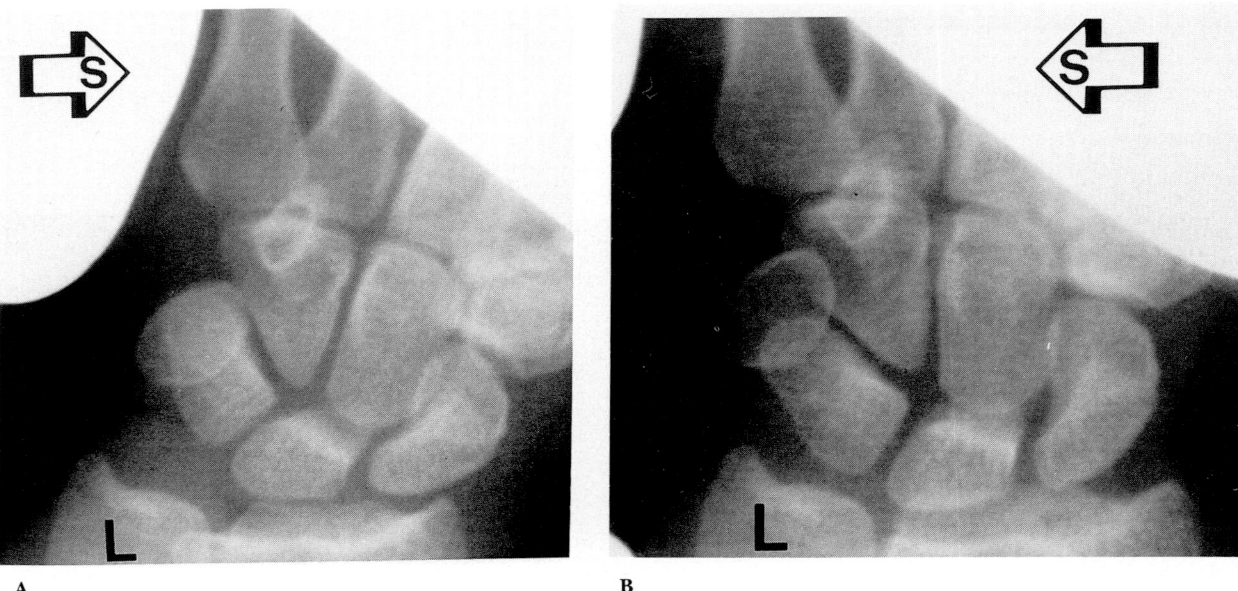

FIGURE 8–8. Radial translation. **A:** PA view of left wrist demonstrates the whole carpus migrated radially under ulnar side stress directed radially. **B:** More normal relationship between the carpus and radius is retained under ulnarly directed stress; however, radiocarpal widening is evident. s = stress applied.

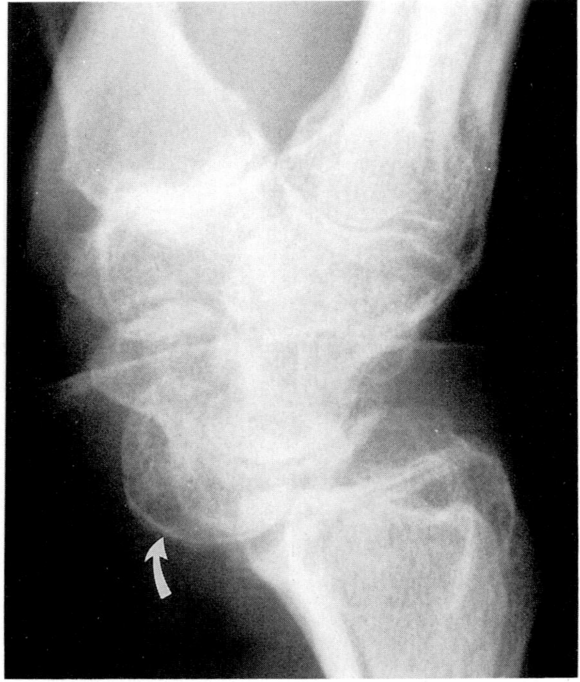

FIGURE 8–9. Palmar carpal translation. Lateral view of the right wrist demonstrates the lunate along with the other carpal bones are displaced out of the distal radial fossa and moved anterior to the distal radius (arrow). Alignment between the lunate and capitate and between the lunate and scaphoid remains intact, although there are increased capitolunate and scapholunate angles. (Reprinted with permission from Bellinghausen HW, Gilula LA, Young LV, Weeks PM. Post-traumatic palmar carpal subluxation: Report of two cases. *J Bone Joint Surg* 1983;65A:998–1006.)

A second and much more common type of palmar carpal subluxation accompanies intraarticular fractures of the distal articular surface of the radius (Barton's fracture, see Chapter 9). This type results in palmar displacement of a major articular fragment(s) of the radius with the carpus still aligned with the fragment(s) (Fig. 8–10).[22] A pure type of palmar subluxation is very rare.[43,45]

Dorsal Translocation

Dorsal translocation (DT) or *dorsal subluxation*[5,25,44] refers to abnormal dorsal migration of the intact carpus with respect to the long axis of the radius. Clinically, isolated dorsal dislocation of the radiocarpal joint is very rare.[46] It is usually associated with acute or remote fractures of the distal radius with uncorrected dorsal angulation of the distal fragment.

On the neutral PA projection, the radiologic findings are very similar, but reversed to those found in palmar translocation. Findings on the neutral lateral view are distinctive:[7,47] the proximal carpal row, as reflected by the lunate, is subluxed or dislocated dorsally and maintains collinearity with the long axis of the capitate and distal radius (Fig. 8–11). It is possible that an adaptive DISI configuration of the carpus could be seen in the situation where the distal articular surface of the radius is dorsally inclined; as the carpus subluxes dorsally the lunate remains dorsally tilted and the capitate palmar-flexes to restore the carpus to more of a functional position ("adaptive carpus" as described by Saffar, Paris, France in a personal communication). Comparison neutral lateral views of the opposite (normal) wrist should help establish this radiocarpal relationship more precisely if there is any question; however, observation that there

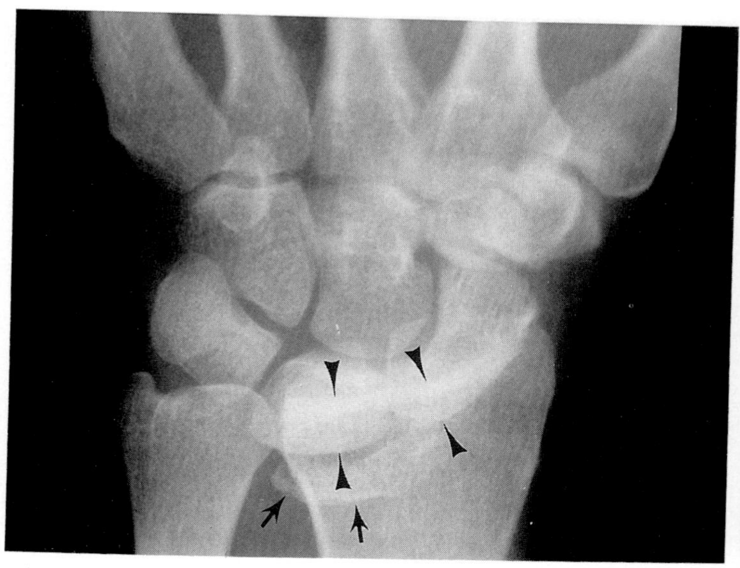
A

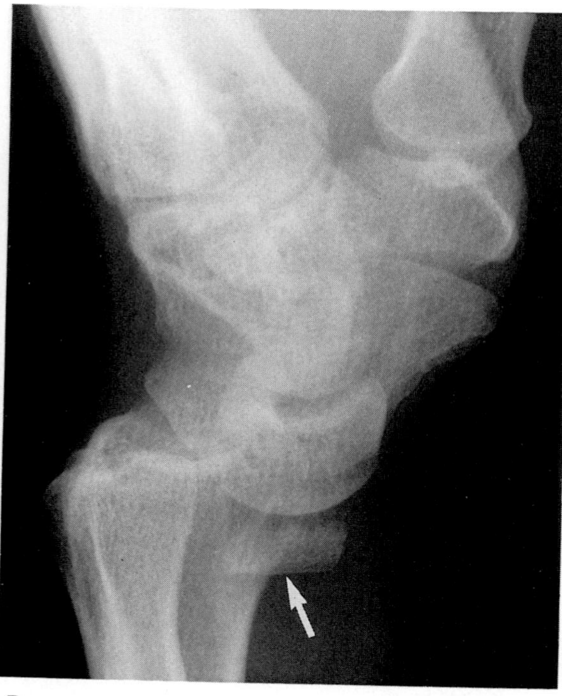
B

FIGURE 8–10. Palmar translation with distal radius fracture. **A:** PA view of the left wrist demonstrates overlapping of the distal radius and proximal carpal row (between arrowheads). The three carpal arcs and the relationships within the carpus are normal except for offset at the lunotriquetral joint, which is apparently due to pressure on the triquetrum as this bone is supported on the ulnar head. A long fracture fragment is attached proximal to the lunate and scaphoid (arrows). The entire carpus has migrated proximally. **B:** Lateral view demonstrates the lunate and other carpal bones displaced palmarly and proximally. The capitolunate relationship is normal. Again a fracture fragment lies proximal to the lunate and anterior to the distal radius (arrow).

is loss of parallelism between articular surfaces of the distal radius and proximal lunate should make recognition of this malalignment easy.

Rotary Subluxation of the Scaphoid

Rotary (rotatory) subluxation of the scaphoid (RSS) is the most common type of wrist instability,[48–53] if instabilities associated with rheumatoid arthritis are ignored. It has also been called scapholunate dissociation (SLD) among other terms by many authors.[54–56] Confusion remains concerning the terms RSS and SLD. Some authors[57,58] believe that RSS is an advanced stage of SLD because it involves more ligaments. Other authors use these two terms interchangeably. We believe that RSS describes a condition in which the scaphoid is unable to maintain its normal position with respect to the radius, and that SLD is a condition in which the scapholunate relationship is abnormal. SLD may occur with or without DISI. RSS may be an isolated instability, or be seen in association with more extensive injury or disease. Primary (isolated) RSS occurs when the scaphoid malrotation is the only end result of wrist damage.[5,59–61] Secondary (associated) RSS is one of the residual abnormalities of reduced major carpal injuries, such as perilunate and lunate dislocation,[55,56,62,63] secondary to chronic synovitis (rheumatoid arthritis),[64–66] or associated with a distal radius fracture.[67]

Scaphoid subluxation refers to displacement of the scaphoid bone, mainly as rotation around its transverse axis; however, the scaphoid can be displaced in two additional methods. With rotation around its transverse axis, the distal pole of the scaphoid is palmar-flexed. When the scapholunate ligamentous connections are loose or disrupted, the proximal pole of the scaphoid may translate dorsally with congruent rotation and translation of the lunate.[68,69] It may be a dynamic or static subluxation. For a second method of rotation, the scaphoid may rotate around its longitudinal axis. This may be not recognizable on radiographs, but can be seen at surgery. Diastasis of the scapholunate joint with movement of the proximal scaphoid pole away from the lunate constitutes a third way the scaphoid may move from the lunate and its normal position in the scaphoid fossa. There could also be combinations of these types of displacements.

Based on their clinical experiences, Watson et al[47,70] have suggested a classification for RSS (Table 8–1). In types 2 to 4, the diagnosis of scapholunate dissociation is confirmed by radiographic examination.[53,70] Radiographic features include foreshortening of the scaphoid, creating a "signet ring" sign;

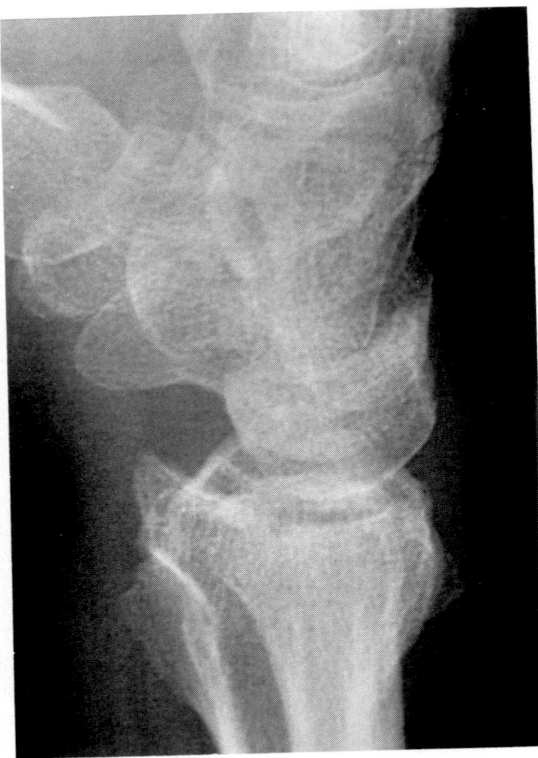

FIGURE 8-11. Distal radius fracture malunion with dorsal translation of the carpus. Lateral view of the right wrist demonstrates the lunate and other carpal bones migrated dorsally. The distal radius malunion results in dorsal tilting of the articular surface. The axes between the lunate, capitate, and scaphoid are normal.

TABLE 8-1. *Classification of Rotary Subluxation of Scaphoid*

Type 1: Dynamic	RSS with no radiographic evidence of abnormality.
Type 2: Static	RSS with radiographic findings of SLD, foreshortening of the scaphoid, a wide scapholunate joint, a ring sign, overlapping of the scaphoid and capitate, and an increased scapholunate angle.
Type 3: Degenerative	Type 1 or Type 2 with concomitant degenerative arthritic changes.
Type 4: Secondary	RSS secondary to Kienbock's disease, scaphoid nonunion, or other causes.

RSS: rotary subluxation of scaphoid
SLD: scapholunate dissociation

scapholunate space widening; an abnormal radioscaphoid angle; and malalignment of the scaphocapitate joint (see below). The other carpal bones may be in normal alignment and position.

In the neutral PA projection, abnormal scapholunate diastasis (the Terry Thomas or David Letterman sign—the name refers to the space between the two front teeth of these people) without evidence of Type II ulnar translocation[8] (Fig. 8-12A) reflects an abnormal scaphoid position. At least three standards have been suggested to differentiate between normal and abnormal (SLD) scapholunate gap: 1) the abnormal scapholunate joint width at its midportion is more than twice that of the normal capitolunate joint (Gilula, personal communication); 2) A normal scapholunate gap measures 2 mm or less at its mid portion,[71] and a scapholunate gap greater than 2 mm should raise suspicions of a dissociation.[5] SLD can be

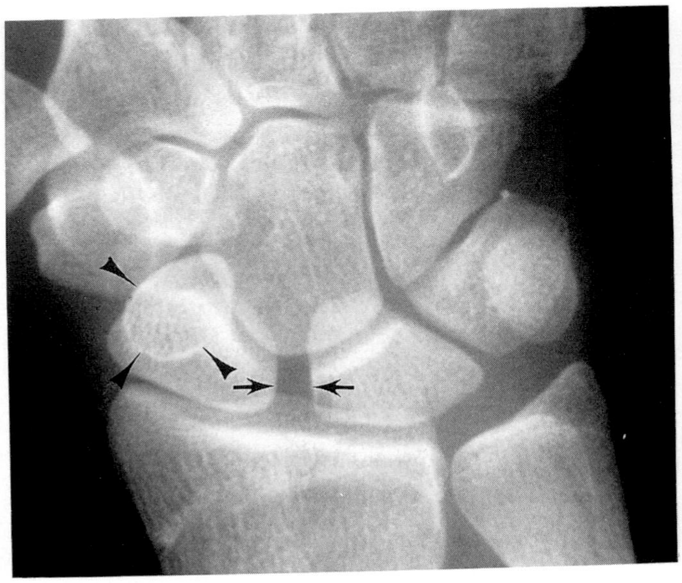

A

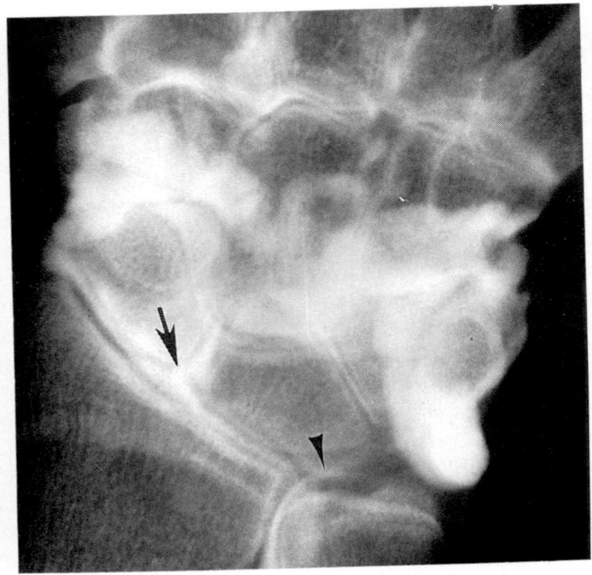

B

FIGURE 8-12. Rotary subluxation of the scaphoid. **A:** PA view of the right wrist demonstrates scapholunate joint space widening (Terry Thomas or David Letterman sign) (arrows) and ring sign (arrowheads). **B:** Wrist arthrogram demonstrates communicating defects in the scapholunate ligament (arrow) and also in the triangular fibrocartilage (TFC) (arrowhead).

considered definite when the scapholunate gap at the midpoint of this joint is greater than 4 mm. 3) The scapholunate gap is abnormal if it is wider than the scapholunate space on the asymptomatic (other) wrist.[8]

Some special radiographic projections were designed to profile the scapholunate joint.[72–75] Generally, the scapholunate joint can be better profiled on an anteroposterior (AP) view than on a PA view.[63] For accurate assessment, it is paramount to profile the "widened" gap by placing the x-ray beam parallel to the opposing surfaces of the scapholunate joint.[75] Additional PA views in ulnar deviation and radial deviation, and longitudinal compression-load views created by having the patient make a tight fist, may also assist in imaging the abnormally wide scapholunate gap.[76]

With abnormal palmar-flexion of the scaphoid on the neutral PA view, the scaphoid is seen end-on as its long axis becomes more vertical. Because of this, RSS may be associated with the "cortical ring" sign on the PA view. This projectional phenomenon is due to palmar-flexion of the scaphoid (Fig. 8–12A), such that the cortices of the distal pole are projected as a circle over the mid body of the foreshortened scaphoid.[50,76] The foreshortened scaphoid is evidenced by a decrease in the minimal distance between the "ring" and the proximal pole of the scaphoid to less than 7 mm, or 4 mm shorter than the normal (contralateral) wrist.[25,54] Reliable use of these findings requires neutral PA positioning views (see Chapter 5), since both the foreshortened appearance and "ring" sign of the scaphoid can appear in a normal wrist positioned in radial deviation.[28,44,77]

In the neutral lateral projection, RSS may show loss of the normal parallelism at the radioscaphoid joint and dorsal displacement of the proximal scaphoid pole. Abnormal palmar rotation of the scaphoid is confirmed by scapholunate angles greater than 70 degrees.[25] Normally this angle is 30 to 60 degrees.[7,25] This is distinct from DISI, as evidenced by the normal lunate alignment with the radius and capitate in RSS. Mayfield et al[6,19,20] believe that RSS is the first stage of a perilunate, scapholunate instability with disruptions of the scapholunate interosseous and palmar radioscaphocapitate ligaments. Specifically, SLD can exist as an isolated injury in the absence of midcarpal disruption.[6] However, RSS can accompany DISI, and the involvement of the remainder of the midcarpal joint is consistent with an injury of greater magnitude.

LUNOTRIQUETRAL (TRIQUETROLUNATE) INSTABILITY

Lunotriquetral (triquetrolunate) instability (LTI) exists when ligament(s) disruption or damage results in abnormal laxity between the lunate and triquetrum (which may be manifested as translational incongruity parallel to the long axis of the radius or abnormally large rotation at the LT joint resulting in an increased LT angle).[8,23,24,31,78–83] Reagan, Linscheid, and Dobyns divided LTI into two groups according to the degree of injured ligament,[31] referring to LT sprains as incomplete tears of the LT interosseous ligament and LT dissociation as complete tears of the LT ligament. Others believe these two stages represent progression of perilunate instability, one without clinical or radiographic evidence of VISI, and the other associated with VISI.[84] The position of the lunate is the key to differentiating these two types. When associated with VISI deformity, the injury is considered severe and the prognosis poor.[47] Viegas et al[84] prefer to call this spectrum ulnar perilunate instability rather than LTI. They have suggested a more complete staging system as follows.

Stage I: Partial or complete disruption of the LT interosseous ligament; *no* clinical and/or radiographic evidence of *dynamic or static* VISI deformity.

Stage II: Complete disruption of the LT interosseous ligament and disruption of the palmar LT ligament; clinical and/or radiographic evidence of *dynamic* VISI deformity.

Stage III: Complete disruption of the LT interosseous ligament and disruption of the palmar LT ligament; attenuation or disruption of the scaphoid and lunate portions of the dorsal radiocarpal ligament; clinical and/or radiographic evidence of *static* VISI deformity with dissociation at the LT joint.[84]

In LTI Stages I and II, neutral PA views may show breaks in carpal Arcs I and II at the LT articulation. The projected shape of the lunate is its normal trapezoidal. In Stage II, provocative maneuvers (ulnar deviation, AP clenched-fist view, and so on) may show rotary dissociation of the lunate and triquetrum to suggest a dynamic VISI. On neutral PA views, Stage III LTI shows palmar-flexion of both the scaphoid and lunate with the foreshortened scaphoid creating a ring sign. The lunate becomes triangular in configuration (Fig. 8–13). The dissociated triquetrum shifts proximal to the scaphoid and lunate and closer to the ulnar head. Arc I is interrupted by an offset between the lunate and triquetrum, leading to disruption of the normal smooth convexity of the proximal carpal row (Arc I).[31] The disruption of Arc I is more prominent in ulnar deviation, producing an overlap of the lunate and triquetrum.[3,31] Because of proximal-distal displacement between and overlap of these two bones on the PA view, the distance between normally articulating surfaces of the lunate and triquetrum may be increased.[43] There is uniform loss of carpal height. In contrast to RSS and DISI, the lunate is flexed palmarly with the scaphoid to become triangular in configuration, and the scapholunate relationship and angle may or may not be normal, depending on whether there is associated abnormality at the scapholunate joint.

On the lateral radiograph, the lunate is palmar-flexed with the scaphoid, and its long axis is perpen-

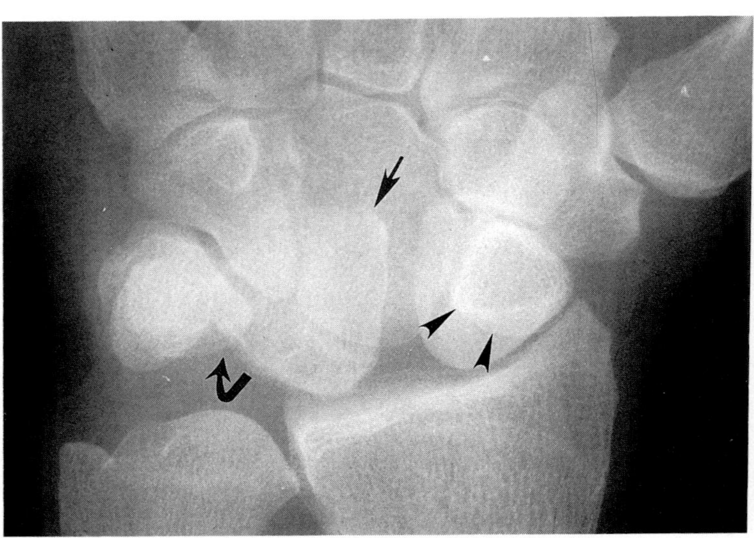

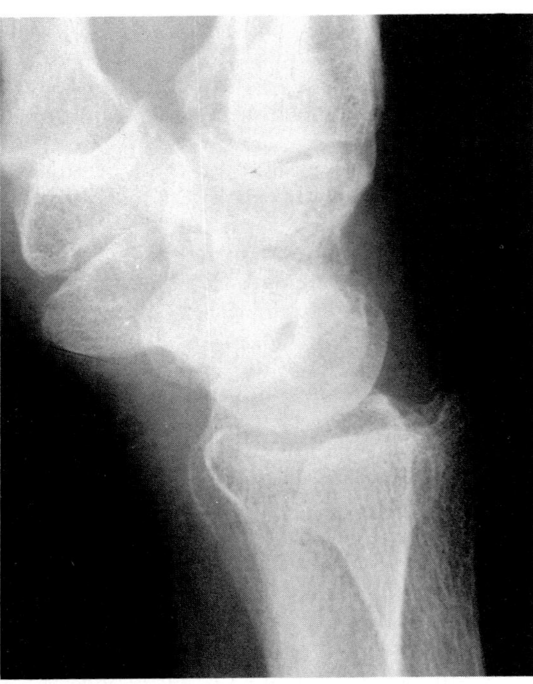

A B

FIGURE 8–13. VISI with lunotriquetral dissociation and scapholunate widening. **A:** PA view of the left wrist demonstrates foreshortening of the scaphoid, creating a ring sign (arrowheads). The lunate is triangular in shape (arrow). Arc I is broken at the lunotriquetral joint (curved arrow). The triquetrum is migrated distally with respect to the hamate; it abnormally overlaps the lunate, and the distal pole of the triquetrum profiles the palmar tubercle and the adjacent sulcus along its radial margin. **B:** Lateral view demonstrates palmar tilt of the lunate and scaphoid and palmar migration of the capitate, all consistent with VISI.

dicular to that of the radius. The LT angle may be neutral or even positive.[2] Specifically, the LT angle is abnormal in "stress" radiographs of Stage II LTI and in neutral lateral radiographs of Stage III LTI. Although it is perceptually more difficult to delineate the triquetral than the lunate outline, the average normal LT angle is reported to be 14 degrees.[31] In contrast, the LT angle is less than 0 degrees with an average of −16 degrees in LT dissociation (LTI) (Fig. 8–14).[31,84] Remembering minus and plus numbers may be a memory problem for some people; if that is the case, remembering that an angle of greater than 14 to 16 degrees in either direction should be abnormal in general should suffice to help the examiner recognize an abnormality. The same comment will subsequently be made about remembering minus and plus numbers for the scapholunate and capitolunate angles in DISI and VISI.

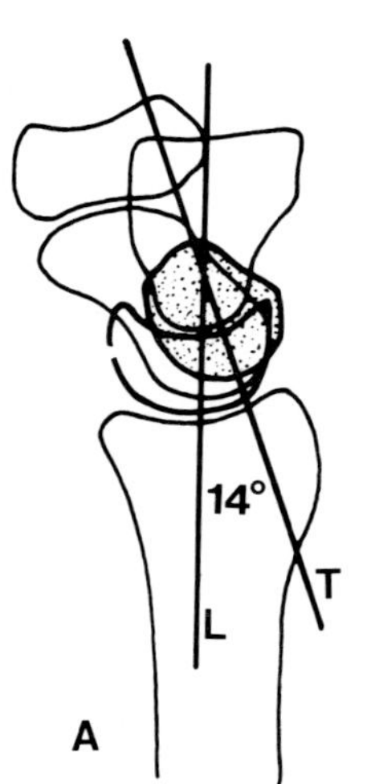

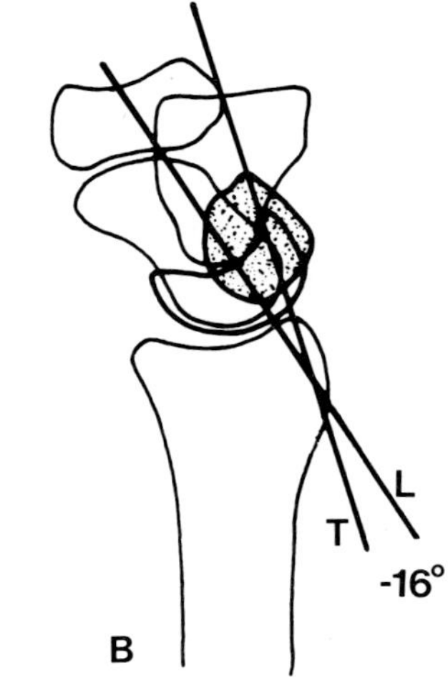

FIGURE 8–14. The lunotriquetral angle. **A:** The normal lunotriquetral angle is about 14 degrees with the triquetral axis palmar to the central lunate axis. **B:** In lunotriquetral dissociation the lunotriquetral angle is decreased or even minus; less than −16 degrees (or greater than 14 to 16 degrees, see text) of dorsiflexion relative to the lunate has been reported by Reagan, Linscheid, and Dobyns. L, lunate axis; T, triquetral axis. (Reprinted with permission from Reagan DS, Linscheid RL, Dobyns JH. Lunotriquetral sprains. *J Hand Surg* 1989;9A:502–514.)

When the triquetral outline cannot be precisely outlined on lateral radiographs, Kleinman[85] has described an indirect sign of triquetral dorsiflexion seen on the PA view: the palmar tubercle (adjacent to the distal margin of the pisotriquetral joint) projects as a convexity from the distal edge of the triquetrum (Fig. 8–13A). Furthermore, when fully dorsiflexed (one can remember this by thinking "distal equals dorsal") the triquetrum approaches the fifth metacarpal base.[85] In contrast, the palmar-flexed (similarly, this can be remembered by thinking "proximal equals palmar") triquetrum approaches the proximal pole of the hamate, reflecting the semihelicoid conformation of the triquetral articular surface of the hamate. Because LT instability is usually a dynamic instability, both neutral PA and lateral views may be normal,

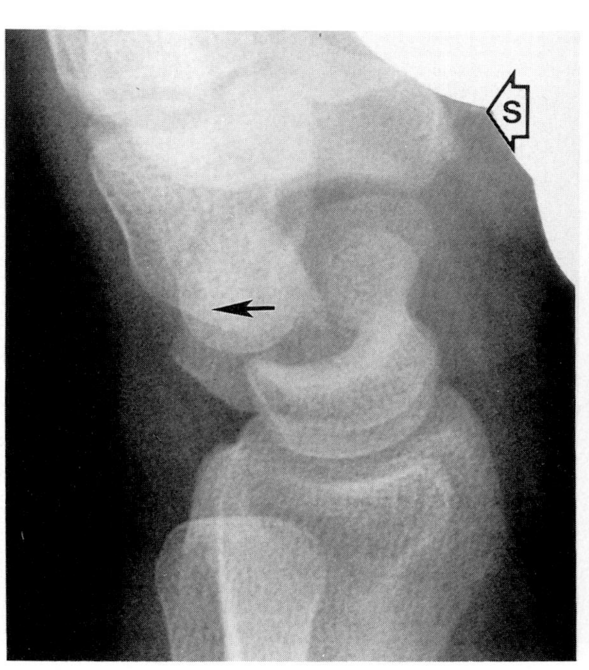

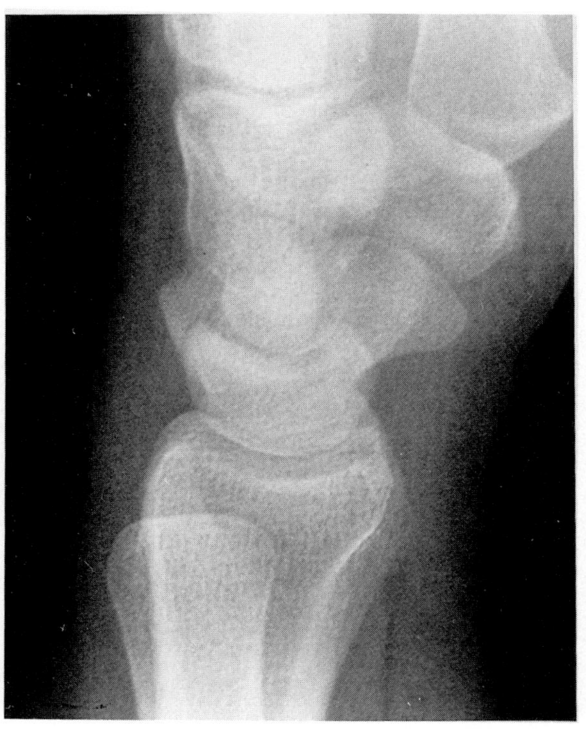

A B

FIGURE 8–15. CLIP wrist. **A:** Lateral view of a left wrist demonstrates the capitate subluxed dorsally (black arrow) from the lunate fossa on stress view under fluoroscopic control. S, direction of applied stress. **B:** The normal alignment is retained in the neutral unstressed position. Often in persons with lax wrists, ventrally directed stress will produce a VISI configuration from palmar tilting of the lunate and scaphoid.

and compression or stress views may be needed to demonstrate the abnormality.[87]

Green suggested that the diagnosis of LTI can be confirmed on neutrally positioned radiographs if the scaphoid and lunate are palmar-flexed and *either* the triquetrum is distally migrated on its hamate articular surface *or* its palmar tubercle is seen.[39]

CAPITOLUNATE INSTABILITY PATTERN

Louis et al and White et al[88,89] described a novel dynamic midcarpal instability centered on the lunocapitate joint, which they named capitolunate instability pattern (CLIP). Clinically, these patients have painful midcarpal clicking or snapping, and positional instability. Tight grasping, especially in the supinated position, tends to precipitate symptoms. The diagnosis rests on the manual displacement of the capitate (and the distal carpal row) from the lunate without an underlying DISI or VISI.[90]

Radiographic confirmation is facilitated by fluoroscopically controlled spot filming during performance of the "CLIP maneuver:" longitudinal traction and dorsal displacement affected by pressing on the scaphoid tubercle in a palmar–dorsal direction. This maneuver is performed in the lateral position usually with the wrist in ulnar deviation (see Chapter 5). In affected patients, there is radiocarpal as well as midcarpal displacement, most evident as the capitate subluxing out of the lunate fossa, especially dorsally (Fig. 8–15).

DORSAL INTERCALATED SEGMENTAL INSTABILITY

In this common midcarpal instability, also known as "dorsiflexion instability," (DISI) the lunate is characteristically more dorsiflexed than normal, and usually the capitolunate angle is greater than 30 degrees (normal is ± 10 degrees[5,24,37,80,83] or 0 to 30 degrees[5] (see Chapter 9). This reflects the underlying abnormal palmar translation of the lunate and the apparent adaptive dorsal translation of the capitate (Fig. 8–16). When associated with scapholunate dissociation, the scaphoid will be in palmar-flexion and the scapholunate angle will be conclusively abnormal (greater than 80 degrees). When angles are mentioned for DISI and subsequently for VISI, the angles may be measured for positive values when in dorsiflexion, or negative values when in palmar-flexion. However, ignoring negative or positive values will not be a problem if one just remembers that a capitolunate angle of greater than 30 degrees and/or a scapholunate angle greater than 80 degrees or less than 30 degrees should be considered as an abnormal configuration. A scapholunate angle of 60 to 80 degrees is borderline. Either or both of the scapholunate and capitolunate angles will be abnormal on the lateral

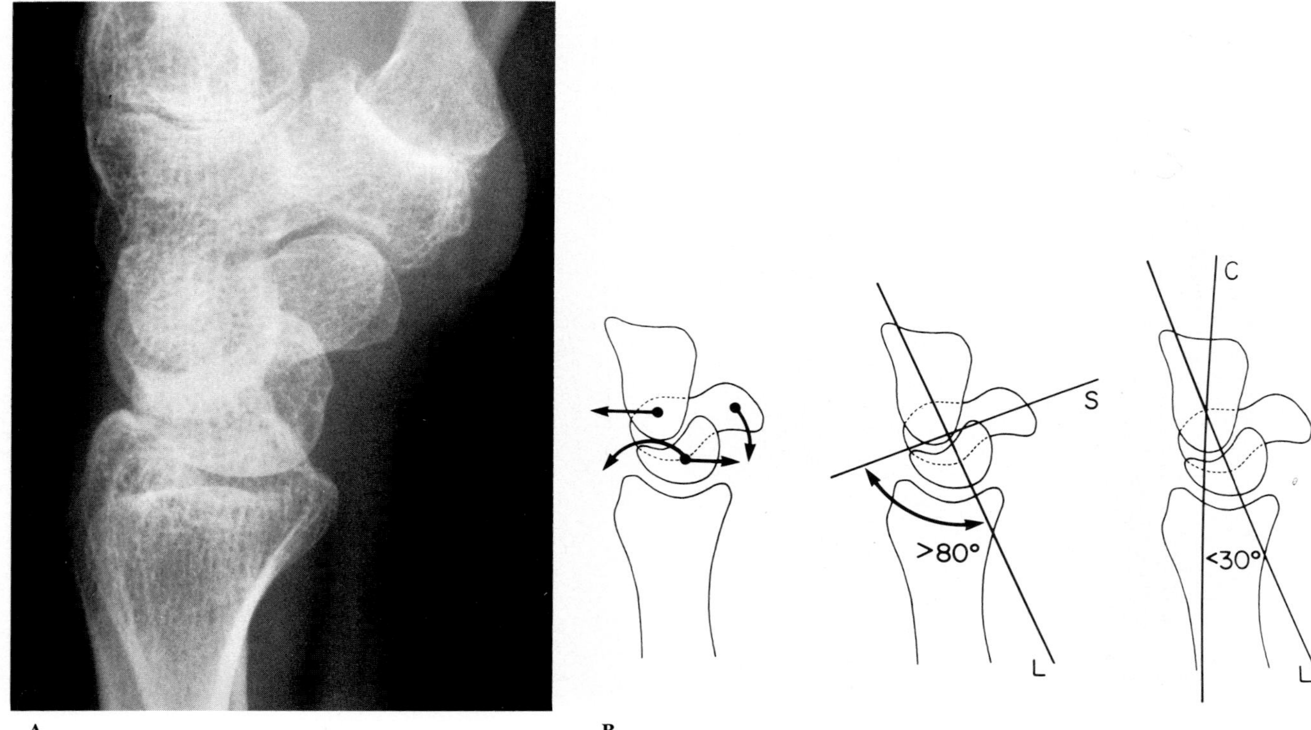

FIGURE 8–16. Dorsiflexion instability (DISI). **A:** Lateral view of a left wrist demonstrates the lunate is tilted dorsally and subluxed palmarly, creating a scapholunate angle of greater than 80 degrees. The capitate is translated dorsally, creating a capitolunate angle more than 30 degrees. **B:** A drawing shows the abnormal change in alignment and position of carpal bones (scaphoid, lunate, and capitate) in DISI. The scapholunate angle is greater than 80 degrees (middle), and the capitolunate angle greater than 30 degrees (right). S, scaphoid axis; L, lunate axis; C, capitate axis.

neutral view in DISI (or VISI). The correlates depicted on the PA view include the cortical ring sign caused by scaphoid foreshortening and triangularly shaped SL diastasis.

In the carpus, static *malalignment* (e.g., DISI *configuration*) is not always associated with *instability* (e.g., DISI pattern). The word "configuration" can be used to refer to the alignment that may measure abnormal on a neutral lateral view but proves to be a normal variant. Instability "pattern" can be used to refer to the malalignment that is abnormal. In our experience, abnormal intercarpal motion is the sine qua non of carpal instability, and the fluoroscopically controlled wrist motion study is the most reliable method to diagnose a DISI pattern. Normally, wrist flexion produces palmar-flexion at the radiolunate and lunocapitate joints. Similarly, wrist extension produces dorsiflexion at both the radiolunate and lunocapitate joints. In other words, "everything should flex on flexion" and "everything should extend on extension" with respect to the radiolunocapitate joints. In DISI pattern or true instability of DISI type, the lunate fails to normally palmar-flex with respect to the radius in wrist flexion and/or the capitate fails to flex with respect to the lunate. DISI pattern patients may also have incomplete capitolunate joint dorsiflexion and/or radiolunate dorsiflexion with wrist extension, and there may be a failure of the radiolunate joint to normally palmar-flex with wrist radial deviation. These relationships are most easily appreciated on lateral radiography. DISI may exist as an isolated abnormality or without dissociation between bones within the proximal carpal row, which is called DISI nondissociated (CIND-DISI, where CIND refers to "carpal instability nondissociated"). The appearance of the PA wrist view may be normal or may show an overlap between the lunate and capitate. A lateral view demonstrates dorsiflexion of the lunate.[37,91] DISI patterns are usually associated with RSS and/or LTD.[37] This is called DISI dissociated (CID-DISI, where CID refers to "carpal instability dissociated") when dissociation is present at the scapholunate or LT joints. We will further address these conditions later. Another condition in which a DISI pattern develops is where there is prominent osteoarthritis at the scaphotrapezial joint, and the entire proximal carpal row tilts dorsally, producing an abnormal capitolunate angle.

VENTRAL INTERCALATED SEGMENT INSTABILITY

Ventral intercalated segment instability (VISI), also known as palmar intercalated segment instability (PISI), is defined by pathologic palmar-flexion at the

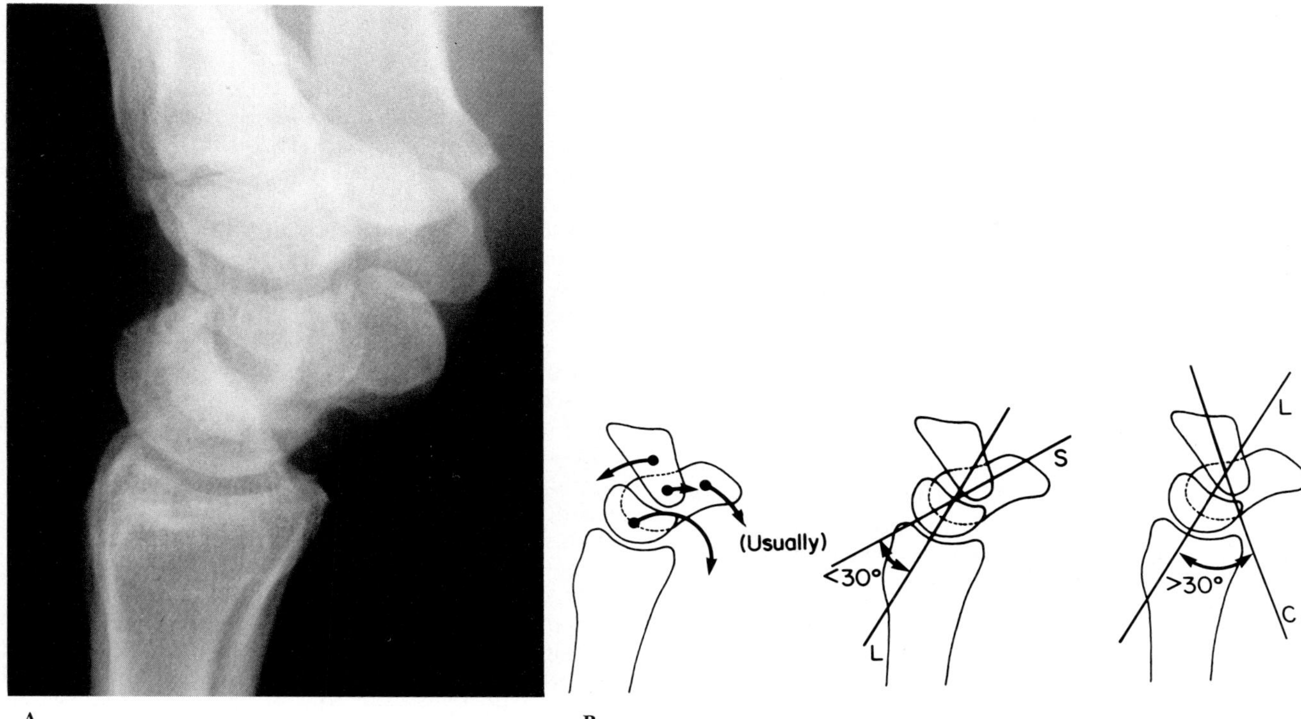

FIGURE 8–17. Palmar-flexion instability or VISI. **A:** Lateral view of the left wrist demonstrates palmar tilting of both the lunate and scaphoid, creating a scapholunate angle of less than 30 degrees. The capitate is subluxed palmarly, creating a capitolunate angle greater than 30 degrees. **B:** Drawings show the abnormal intercarpal bone changes (scaphoid, lunate, and capitate) in VISI. The scapholunate angle is less than 30 degrees (abnormal) (middle), and the capitolunate angle is more than 30 degrees (abnormal) (right). (It is more correct to speak of minus and plus measurements; however, it is much easier to remember that a capitolunate angle greater than 30 degrees and/or a scapholunate angle less than 30 degrees is abnormal, regardless of the direction of the angle, see text.)

radiolunate joint accompanied by pathologic extension at the lunocapitate joint while the wrist is in neutral position.[5,7,22,24,37] The radiographic diagnosis of VISI configuration is based on the neutral lateral radiograph (Fig. 8–17). The characteristic "zig-zag" malalignment is comprised of palmar-flexion at the radiocarpal joint and dorsiflexion at the midcarpal joint when the wrist is in a "zero" neutral lateral position. To distinguish from the normal physiologic laxity common to some asymptomatic young women (this also occurs in men, although apparently in a lesser incidence), alignment is considered abnormal when the radiolunate angle is greater than 10 degrees (of palmar-flexion) and the capitolunate angle is more dorsiflexed than 30 degrees. The scapholunate angle may be less than 30 degrees (normal is 30 to 60 degrees). Again, as mentioned above, it may be easier to remember to consider a capitolunate angle of greater than 30 degrees and a scapholunate angle of less than 30 degrees abnormal and to ignore minus numbers, which are used to indicate the direction of angulation of bones. A VISI pattern is confirmed by an abnormal carpal motion study. Specifically, failure of coordinated palmar- or dorsiflexion at the radiolunate and capitolunate articulations with wrist flexion and extension, respectively, is confirmation of this pattern. The most common cause of VISI-CID (CID refers to the presence of dissociation within the proximal carpal row, at either the scapholunate or lunotriquetral joints) is lunotriquetral laxity.[1,3,22,25,31,91–94] Viegas et al believe that ulnar-sided perilunate instability is a preferred descriptor[84] for VISI with CID at the LT joint.

CARPAL INSTABILITIES: NONDISSOCIATIVE AND DISSOCIATIVE

Radiocarpal and midcarpal (transverse) instabilities may occur with (dissociative, or CID) or without associated dissociation (nondissociative or CIND) within the proximal carpal row (i.e., SLD or lunotriquetral dissociation [LTD]) or very rarely within the distal carpal row. The occurrence of midcarpal (DISI, VISI) or radiocarpal (ulnar translocation) instabilities with SLD or LTD may be coincidental (i.e., not causally related). However, certain patterns are so common that causality or codependence is fairly common (e.g., DISI with SLD, VISI with LTD, SLD with Type II ulnar translocation). In its original and most common use CID/CIND subclassifies instabilities of VISI or DISI into types; 1) ulnar-sided perilunate instability,[84] or 2) without codependent or causally related proximal carpal row interosseous dissociations (i.e., SLD or LTD)[25]. The CIND concept has various names: nondissociative instability of the proximal carpal row,[95] triquetrolunate instability,[92] and dynamic midcarpal instability.[79]

Imaging supplements the clinical assessment of carpal instabilities. Normal carpal alignment (e.g., Gilula's carpal Arcs I and II), intercarpal motion (wrist instability series), and interosseous ligaments (wrist arthrography) confirm a nondissociative type of carpal instability. Allowing for the caveat that "pinhole" communications demonstrated by arthrography may have neither mechanical nor kinematic effect, abnormal proximal carpal row alignment, motion, or interjoint communication(s) may define a midcarpal or radiocarpal instability as a CID. However, it is becoming increasingly recognized through arthrography and arthroscopy that perforations even larger than the pinhole type through the scapholunate and/or LT ligaments may not be associated with abnormal motion at those joints. Therefore, mere presence of a communication through an intrinsic ligament does not mandate a functional dissociation.

There have been no recognized dissociations between the distal carpal row bones without associated metacarpal dissociations. Therefore, CID related to distal carpal row should always be axial carpal dissociations.

Dorsiflexion Instability With Scapholunate Dissociation

Dorsiflexion instability with scapholunate dissociation, also called *carpal instability dissociative dorsal intercalated segment instability (CID-DISI) or DISI with dissociation at the scapholunate joint,* was first described by Linscheid[96] and is a relatively common injury. The distal articular surface of the lunate is tilted dorsally and the scaphoid is rotated palmarly and may be abnormally separated from the lunate. The radiographic features include both DISI and SLD.

On the PA view, the scapholunate joint is widened, with some tilting of the lunate (slight triangular shape) as well as foreshortening (cortical ring sign) of the scaphoid. The articulations of the lunate with the triquetrum, hamate, and capitate are normal. A smooth carpal Arc I is maintained between the lunate and the triquetrum but may be broken at the scapholunate joint. On the lateral view, the most characteristic feature is more dorsal tilting of the distal articular surface of the lunate than normal. The scaphoid is rotated palmarly so that its axis is more perpendicular to the radius than usual. With these abnormal displacements, the scapholunate angle will exceed 80 degrees, the capitolunate angle exceeds 30 degrees, and the capitate subluxes dorsally to adapt to the tendency of the lunate to sublux palmarly (Fig. 8–18).

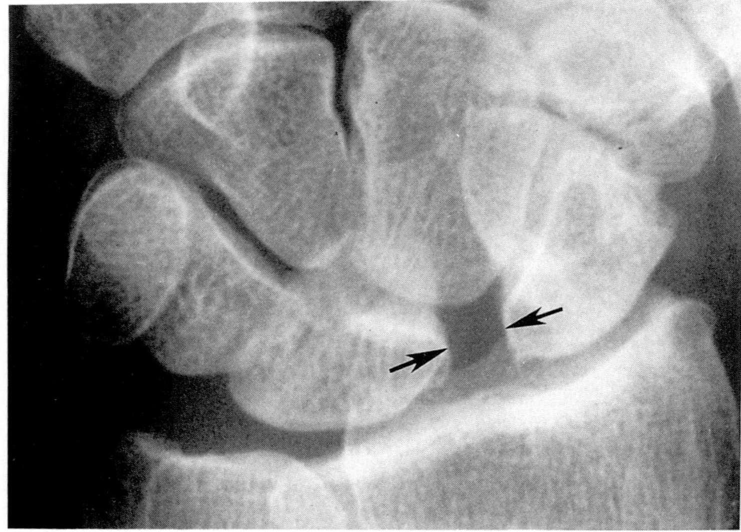

A

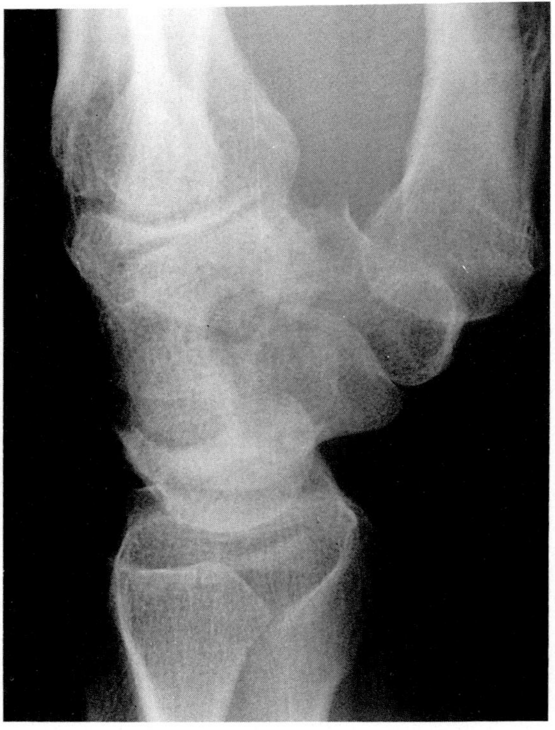

B

FIGURE 8–18. Dorsiflexion instability with scapholunate dissociation (CID–DISI). **A:** PA view of the left wrist demonstrates foreshortening of the scaphoid and scapholunate joint space widening (between arrows). The lunate is triangular in shape. **B:** The lateral view demonstrates lunate tilting dorsally, slight dorsal subluxation of the capitate, and a scapholunate angle greater than 80 degrees.

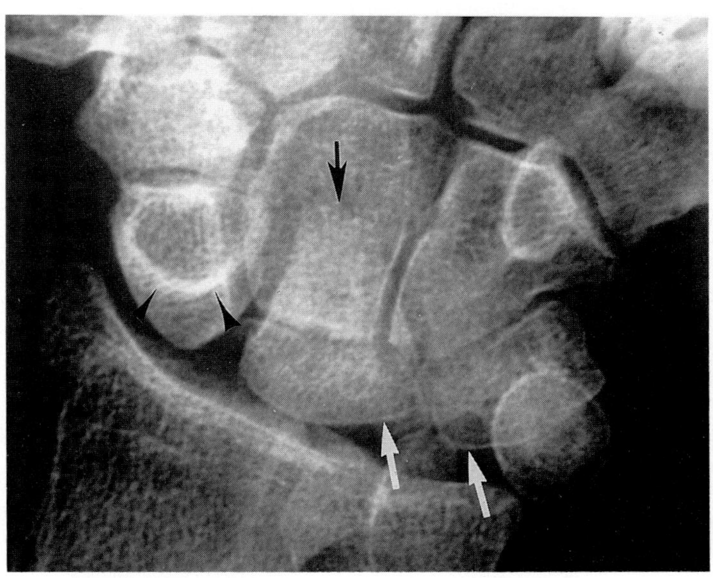
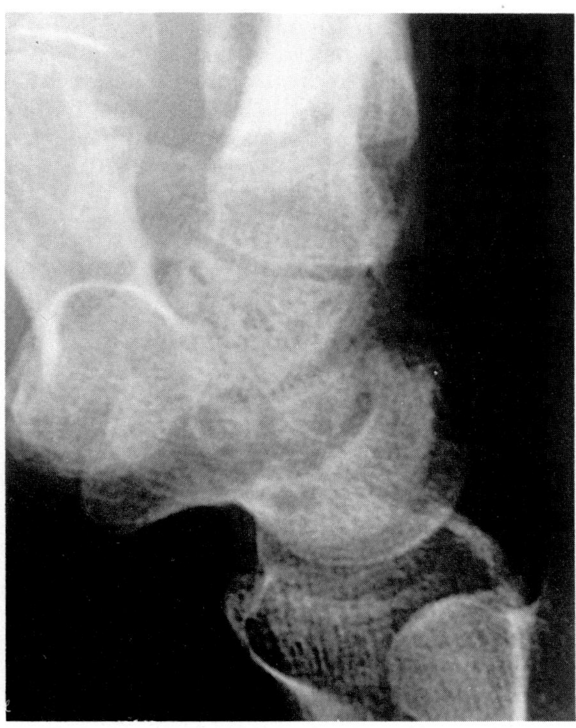

A B

FIGURE 8–19. CID-VISI. **A:** PA view of the right wrist demonstrates that Arc I is broken at the lunotriquetral joint (white arrows). The scaphoid is foreshortened with a ring sign (arrowheads) and the lunate is triangular in shape (black arrow). **B:** The lateral view demonstrates palmar-flexion of the lunate and scaphoid, the long axis of the scaphoid is perpendicular to that of the radius, and the capitolunate and scapholunate angles are abnormal (see text).

Carpal Instability Dissociative–Ventral Intercalated Segment Instability

Carpal instability dissociative–ventral intercalated segment instability (CID-VISI), also known as *palmar-flexion instability with LT dissociation* is most commonly found with triquetrolunate dissociation (TLD).[31,92,97]

Lichtman et al[79] described this as rotary subluxation of the scaphoid with TLD and Stage IV perilunate instability (PLI). Loss of the dorsal ligamentous attachments to the lunate (dorsal radiocarpal ligament) allows the lunate to rotate palmarly. Normally all three bones of the proximal row are tied to each other by intrinsic ligaments (the lunotriquetral (LT) and scapholunate (SL)). With LT dissociation, the lunate and scaphoid through the intact scapholunate joint tilt palmarly. On the PA view (Fig. 8–19A), the LT joint space width is usually normal, the lunate palmarly tilted (triangularly shaped), and the scaphoid foreshortened from palmar-flexion (cortical ring sign). Carpal Arcs I and II are normal at the scapholunate articulation, but may be "broken" at the LT joint. The triquetrum is distally located along its articulation with the hamate and its palmar tubercle is visible at its distal pole due to its dorsiflexion. On neutral lateral views (Fig. 8–19B), the distal articular surface of the lunate and the long axis of the scaphoid are tilted palmarly more than normal. The capitolunate angle is abnormal (exceeds 30 degrees of dorsiflexion of the capitate with respect to the lunate), while the scapholunate angle is normal or decreased. The capitate adapts to the dorsal lunate translation with a compensatory palmar translation.

Carpal Instability Nondissociative–Ventral Intercalated Segment Instability

Carpal instability nondissociative–ventral intercalated segment instability (CIND-VISI, or CIND-PISI) is defined as carpal derangement characterized by pathologic palmar-flexion of the lunate associated with intact proximal and distal carpal rows. This condition may occur with laxity of the capitotriquetral ligament, leading to triquetrohamate joint dissociation,[93] or triquetrohamate disruption and capitolunate laxity.[94] Hankin et al have reported two cases of CIND-VISI that they believe were caused by scaphotrapezial ligament tear or laxity.[98]

The radiologic criteria are the same as for CIND-DISI except that the presenting deformity is a VISI rather than DISI. On lateral view of the wrist, the lunate is palmar-flexed relative to the longitudinal axis of the radius with adaptive capitate extension evidenced by a capitolunate angle less than − 30 degrees (or "greater" than 30 degrees if one ignores minus numbers as mentioned above), and a radiolunate angle greater than + 35 degrees (or just greater than 30 or 35 degrees for ease of memory). The SL angle should be normal (30–60 degrees) or less than 30 degrees. On the PA view, the scaphoid often appears foreshortened but there is no dissociation of the scapholunate or LT joints.[5]

CARPOMETACARPAL INSTABILITY

Carpometacarpal instability is an abnormal condition occurring between the metacarpal(s) and the distal carpal row that results in the inability to maintain normal anatomic relationship(s), either dynamic or static. It usually refers to subluxation, which must be determined in reference to the normal alignment and range of motion of the joint. Subluxation is loss of contact in any direction between the distal articular surface of the distal row of carpal bone(s) and its (their) respective metacarpal articulation(s) to any degree less than total displacement. Complete loss of contact would be a dislocation. The direction of subluxation is defined by the direction of displacement of the distal segment. The amount of subluxation can be given as a percentage determined by the measured displacement divided by the normal articular dimension in that same plane.

In the neutral PA view of a normal wrist, each metacarpal bone has a distinct cortical rim that, when profiled, should have a parallel opposing carpal bone articular surface also in profile. The joint space should measure between 1 and 2 mm and these joints should form a continuous broad letter "M." The proximal line of the M is formed by the distal articular surfaces of the trapezoid, capitate, and hamate. The distal line of the M is composed of the surfaces of the bases of the second through fifth metacarpals.[99–101] Loss of the parallel relationship and/or overlap between carpal and metacarpal bones, when at least one cortical surface is in profile, should be considered abnormal.

Another radiographic parameter, the metacarpal line, may help assess metacarpal shortening that may represent subluxation or dislocation of the carpometacarpal joint. The metacarpal line is a tangential line drawn across the distal articular surfaces of the heads of the fourth and fifth metacarpals. Normally, this oblique line should pass distal to the head of the third metacarpal (Fig. 8–20). If the distal end of the third metacarpal is on this line, the fourth metacarpal is short and there is a differential for the short fourth metacarpal.[102] This includes old or new trauma, any conditions causing early closure of the growth plate, such as sickle cell disease, pseudo- and pseudopseudohypoparathyroidism, familial, and idiopathic. However, in the face of trauma, observation of the opposite side may be of immediate help when looking for asymmetric length and appearance of these bones. On the lateral view, an offset or loss of smooth alignment of the dorsal cortices at the carpometacarpal joint(s) should be a subluxation or dislocation. Due to superimposition of carpometacarpal joints on true lateral radiographs, a slightly oblique lateral projection may be needed to demonstrate the presence of offset at a specific carpometacarpal joint.[103] In addition, if a subluxation is recognized and the specific joint(s) is (are) not identified, slightly off obliques or fluoroscopic spots can help identify which joint is abnormal. Computed tomography can also be definitive for showing the abnormalities at this level (see Chapter 16).

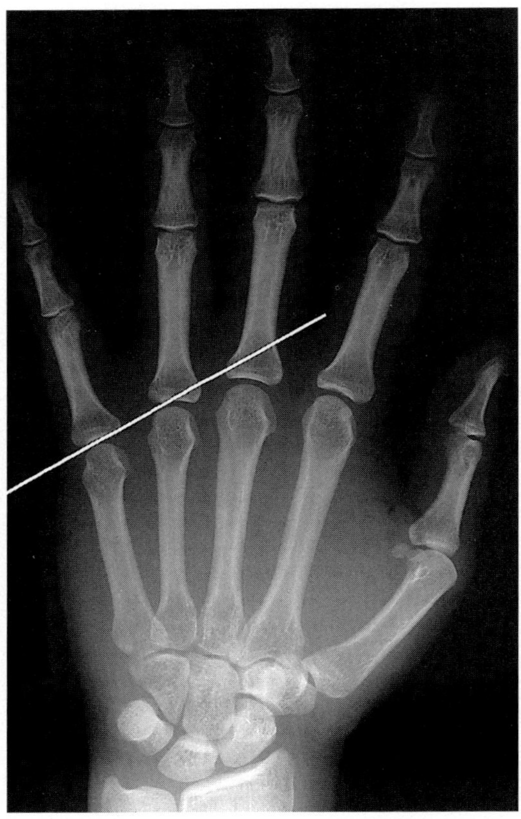

FIGURE 8–20. PA view of a normal left wrist demonstrates the metacarpal line drawn tangentially across the distal articular surfaces of the heads of the fourth and fifth metacarpals. Normally this oblique line should pass distal to the head of the third metacarpal.

A radiographic diagnosis of carpometacarpal instability is made if there is any evidence of subluxation of a carpometacarpal joint as seen either on a static or dynamic (i.e., stress) radiograph.

AXIAL CARPAL SUBLUXATION

Axial carpal or longitudinal subluxation of the carpus is usually caused by a crush or blast mechanism to the wrist. The principal bony injury consists of a longitudinal subluxation of the metacarpal and carpal transverse arches of the hand with partial loss of the normal relationship between the parts into which the carpus has been divided.[104–106]

Radiographic features include abnormal widening of any joint between bones of the distal carpal row and/or a displaced fracture of any distal carpal row bone with diastasis between the bases of two contiguous metacarpals. Usually the proximal carpal row is normal. Diagnostic criteria are met when each of the following are fulfilled: 1) diastasis between the bases of two contiguous metacarpals, and 2) diastasis between any two adjacent bones in the distal carpal row (trapezium, trapezoid, capitate, and hamate) and/or fractures of the distal carpal row with no or little displacement.

Garcia-Elias et al have recognized three groups of axial carpal dislocation.[107] Type AU (axial-ulnar) (Fig. 8–21A), Type AR (axial-radial) (Fig. 8–21B), and Type ARU (axial-radial-ulnar, or combined). The common feature of all these is a longitudinal separation of metacarpals with carpal bone involvement, with or without carpal bone fracture(s). Green prefers to use the terms that indicate the main line of longitudinal separation, such as capitate-hamate diastasis or III to IV dissociation (contrasting to perihamate dissociation).[39]

DISTAL RADIOULNAR INSTABILITY

Distal radioulnar instability is an abnormal alignment or instability between the distal radius and ulnar head that results in the loss of normal joint relationship(s). The causes may be traumatic, degenerative, surgical (iatrogenic), or congenital. It can be either subluxation or dislocation. Dislocation can often be diagnosed on plain films; however, it may be difficult to obtain a true lateral view because of pain or immobility.[108] When it is not possible to obtain a routine lateral view, a cross-table lateral approach may be of value.

The diagnosis of distal radioulnar joint (DRUJ) subluxation usually is difficult to confirm on plain films alone.[109] Partial loss of the normal articular contact between the distal radius and ulna is best defined by comparing symptomatic to asymptomatic wrists imaged by transaxial views of the DRUJ on computed tomography or magnetic resonance imaging scans in at least three positions of forearm rotation (full pronation, full supination, midrotation).[110–114] Supplemental positions that recreate a patient's symptom complex may be necessary to demonstrate loss of congruence not evident on the three standard positions. To save time, one of the above three positions can be replaced by the position that causes the presenting pain, such as overpronation, oversupination, and so on.

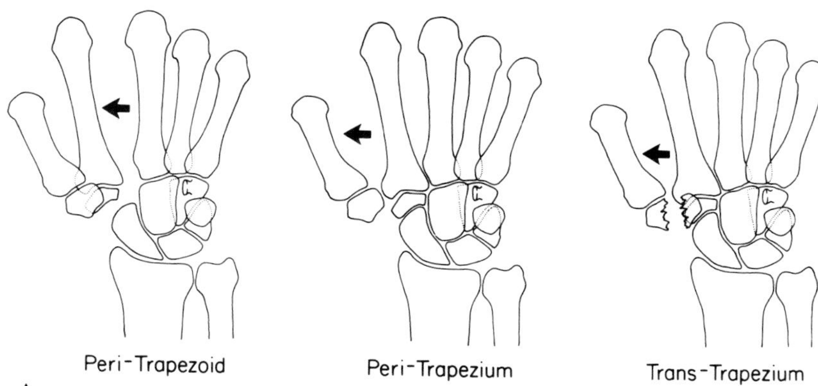

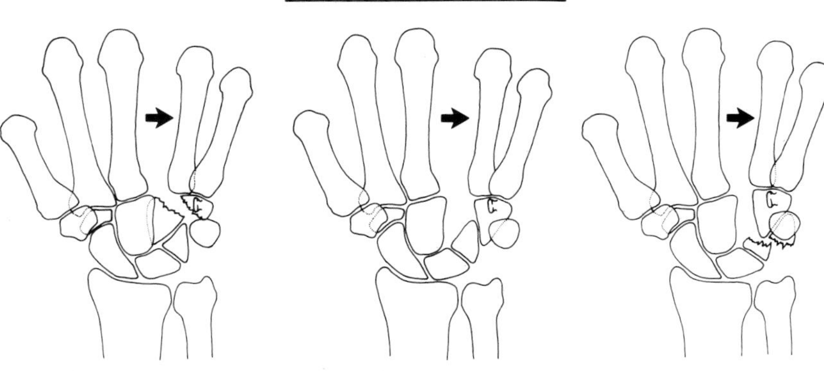

FIGURE 8–21. A drawing of the most common types of axial dislocations of the carpus. **A:** Axial-radial fracture dislocation. **B:** Axial-ulnar fracture dislocation. (Reprinted with permission from Gilula LA, Totty WG. Wrist trauma: Roentgenographic analysis. In: Gilula LA, ed. *The traumatized hand and wrist: Radiographic and anatomic correlation.* Philadelphia: WB Saunders, 1992:221–239.)

107. Garcia-Elias M, Dobyns JH, Cooney WP, Linscheid RL. Traumatic axial dislocations of the carpus. *J Hand Surg* 1989;14A:446–457.
108. Mino DE, Palmer AK, Levinsohn EM. Radiography and computerized tomography in the diagnosis of incongruity of the distal radio-ulnar joint: A prospective study. *J Bone Joint Surg* 1985;67A:247–252.
109. Space TC, Louis DS, Francis I, Braunstein EM. CT findings in distal radioulnar dislocation. *J Comput Assist Tomogr* 1986;10:689–690.
110. King GJ, McMurtry RY, Rubenstein JD, Ogston NG. Computerized tomography of the distal radioulnar joint: Correlation with ligamentous pathology in a cadaveric model. *J Hand Surg* 1986;11A:711–717.
111. Levinsohn EM. Imaging of the wrist. *Radiol Clin North Am* 1990;28:905–921.
112. Pirela-Cruz MA, Goll SR, Klug M, Windler D. Stress computed tomography analysis of the distal radioulnar joint: A diagnostic tool for determining translational motion. *J Hand Surg* 1991;16A:75–82.
113. Magid D, Thompson JS, Fishman EK. Computed tomography of the hand and wrist. *Hand Clin* 1991;7:219–233.
114. Stewart NR, Gilula LA. CT of the wrist: A tailored approach. *Radiology* 1992;183:13–20.

CHAPTER 9

WRIST AND HAND MEASUREMENTS AND CLASSIFICATION SCHEMES

Mark Everett Baratz and Claus Falck Larsen

INTRODUCTION

A variety of measurements and classification schemes have been used to categorize disorders of the wrist and hand. In this chapter we will concentrate on normal measurements and classifications of traumatic, degenerative, and rheumatoid conditions in the adult. Because of space limitations, all measurements and classifications could not be included here, but selected articles are in the list of references at the end of the chapter.[1,2]

A number of measurements are important when evaluating the injured or diseased wrist and hand. Although measurements must be incorporated in the decision-making process, treatment decisions should not be based on measurements alone, but rather on the total clinical evaluation of the patient.[3] Because normal variations and abnormalities may be bilateral, when an abnormality is detected, comparison to the opposite uninjured wrist can be of value.

WRIST AND HAND MEASUREMENTS

MEASUREMENTS

In the last decades several new diagnostic methods for evaluating the wrist have been introduced. However, conventional radiography is still the most important diagnostic procedure for everyday investigation of the injured wrist. Before proceeding to more advanced and often expensive investigation, it is important that the physician is certain that all possible information has been extracted from conventional radiographs. Often ligamentous disruptions demonstrate only subtle or no radiographic changes and are easily missed. Since all information is not obtained from plain films, especially evidence of ligamentous injury and joint instability, it is important to recognize normal carpal relationships on routine radiographs.

Radiographic measurements are useful in the evaluation of alterations in the length of metacarpals and phalanges, in the evaluation of appearance and size of the carpus, and in the evaluation of bone mass. These measurements will not be included in this text,

Standardized Method for Obtaining Wrist Radiographs

A prerequisite for assessing alignment between the carpal bones is to fully understand the importance of a correct lateral and posteroanterior (PA) wrist radiographic projection. A standardized method for obtaining wrist radiographs is necessary to ensure correct positioning and reproducibility.[4,5] The PA position is obtained as described in Chapter 5. The elbow is flexed 90 degrees, and the shoulder is abducted 90 degrees, so that the elbow is at shoulder height (Fig. 9–1A). Lateral wrist radiographs should be obtained in the so-called zero position: the arm is adducted against the trunk, the elbow flexed 90 degrees, the forearm in neutral rotation (no supination or pronation), and the wrist in neutral position (no radial or ulnar deviation and no palmar-flexion or extension) (Fig. 9–1B).[5]

Consistent and comparable right-angled projections can be facilitated using a device to stabilize and control the wrist in the desired position. A device fixing the wrist position in all directions during radiographic examination has been used to measure the radiographic changes in carpal bone angles in various wrist positions (Figs. 9–2A and 9–2B).[6] It proved suitable and accurate for radiographic wrist examinations. However, only mobile, cooperative patients could be examined by using it. Patients in bed,

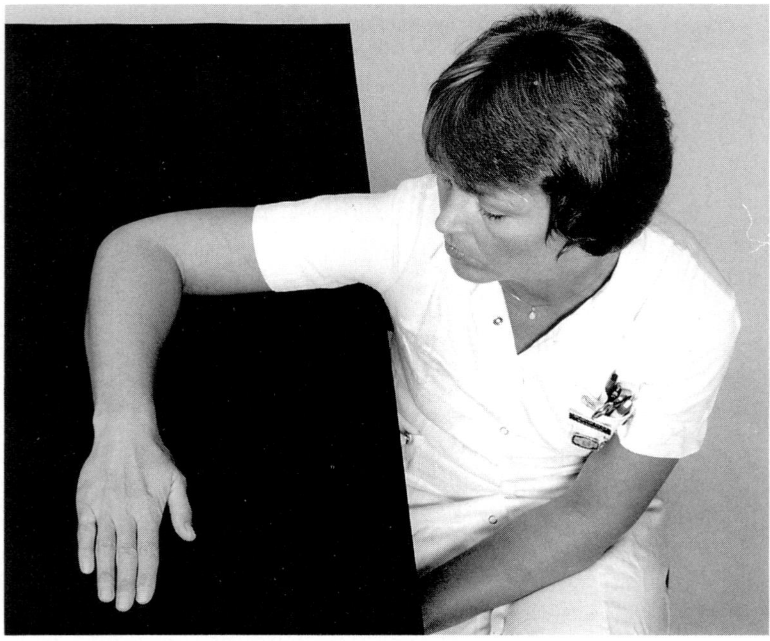

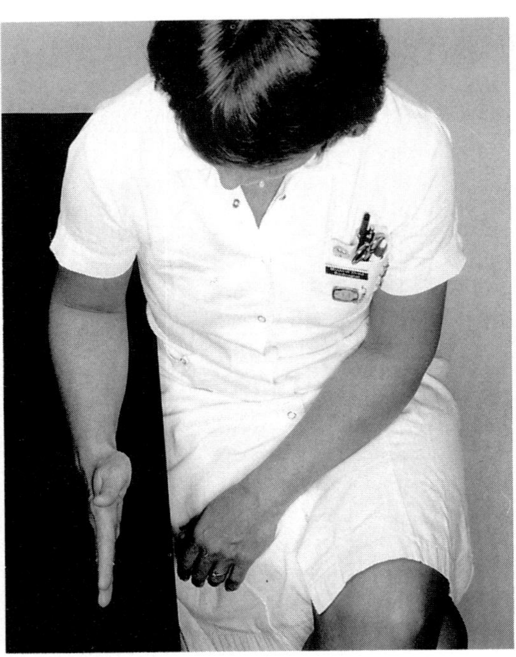

A B

FIGURE 9–1. Radiographs of the normal wrist. **A:** PA projection (zero position). **B:** Lateral projection (zero position). Refer to text.

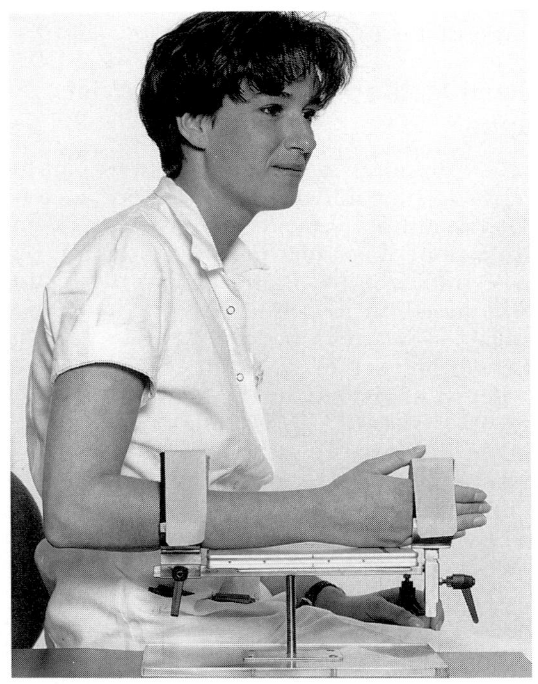

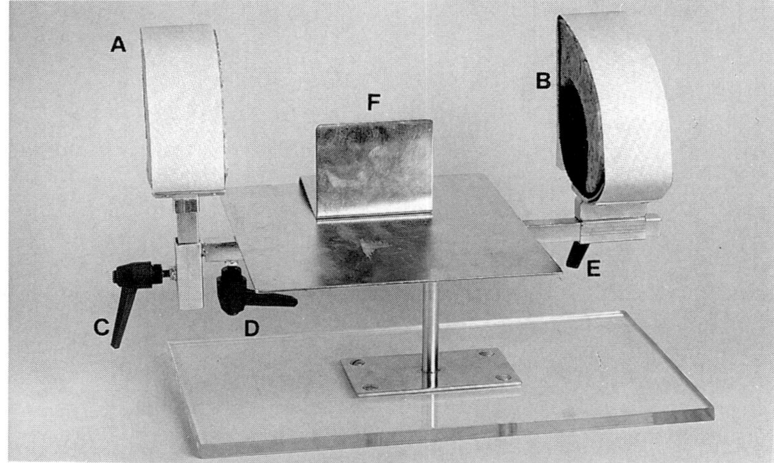

A B

FIGURE 9–2. A: The stabilizing device shown with cassette prepared for lateral projection. **B:** The stabilizing device. A, finger support (changeable foam rubber shell, which can be adjusted to the size of the hand); B, forearm support (changeable foam rubber shell, which can be adjusted to the size of the forearm); C, height-adjustment screw; D, angulation adjustment screw; E, length-adjustment screw; F, cassette support. (Reprinted with permission from Larsen CF, Mathiesen FK, Lindequist S. Measurements of carpal bone angles on lateral wrist radiographs. *J Hand Surg* 1991;16A:888–893.)

as well as those with painful fractures or dislocations, could not be examined by this method. Despite the simplicity of the device, some training is necessary to obtain sufficient radiographs. Radiologic examination using a device is more time-consuming than examination without extra equipment. However, if lateral radiographs are to be used for measurements of carpal bone angles, the wrist must be supported and the position in the remaining planes controlled.

The importance of correct positioning of the wrist for determining carpal bone angles was demonstrated by Larsen et al.[6] Imamura[7] reported similar observations. Varying positions of the carpal bones with different wrist movements have been discussed in detail.[7–11] In neutral position the carpal bones are easy to identify on lateral radiographs, but even 10 degrees of supination or pronation provides a different appearance of the carpal bones, sometimes making it more difficult to identify the recognized shape of the bones, resulting in less accurate tracings for measurement purposes. Criteria for true lateral and PA projections seem to be missing in the literature. When cross-table lateral wrist radiographs are obtained in supination or pronation, the intercarpal angles are significantly changed. However, the error is easily detected as overlapping of the radius and ulna changes and the desired relationship between the scaphoid and pisiform is lost. To recognize a routine lateral view, Gilula (personal communication, 1991 and Chap. 5) has suggested that the palmar cortex of the pisiform should overlie the midportion of the scaphoid between the ventral surface of the distal pole of the scaphoid and the ventral cortex of the capitate head. The significant changes of intercarpal angles during radial and ulnar deviation in the lateral position are also important, because it is often difficult to control radioulnar abduction, such as in the patient with a large hypothenar eminence who in the lateral position is actually radially deviated.

A recent study has demonstrated that landmark-verified standardized position can obtain true right-angled views of the ulna as accurately as positioning in a wrist-holding device. However, the radiologist and treating surgeon must rely on recognition of anatomic landmarks to ensure positioning of sufficient precision to obtain accurate measurements in all cases with or without the use of a positioning device.[12]

Reliability of Measurements

It is important to realize that measurements are subject to significant variation. The reproducibility and variability of the measurements may be caused by biologic or observer variation. One of many factors leading to observer variation is the difference in assessment of radiographic landmarks used for measurements. The "best" method will have low intra- and interobserver variation. A low intraobserver variation is important in cases where the injured or diseased wrist is compared with the normal side by one observer only. In this chapter we have chosen to include information on variation in all cases where such information is available.

Usually measurements are performed using a standard plastic goniometer. Measurements of angles with a goniometer have been accomplished in whole degrees[13,14] and in 2-degree intervals.[15] Measurements can be performed with higher accuracy on digitized enlargements of radiographs.[16] The margin of error in measurements using the digitizer was within 0.4 degrees and 0.1 mm. To precisely measure length, the error due to magnification imposed by divergence of the x-ray beam must be calculated, unless the measurements are used to calculate ratios.

CARPAL COLLAPSE

Carpal collapse occurs in rheumatoid arthritis, Kienböck's disease, scapholunate advanced collapse (SLAC), and other conditions affecting the wrist. Qualification of carpal collapse is performed by measuring the carpal height (Table 9–1).[17,18] *Carpal height* is defined as the distance from the base of the third metacarpal to the distal articular surface of the radius. This is measured along the axis of the third metacarpal on PA radiographs. In the normal hand carpal height remains the same in all positions of radioulnar deviation.

The *carpal height ratio* is defined as the ratio of the carpal height to the length of the third metacarpal (Table 9–1). Carpal collapse will result in a decrease in this ratio. To obtain reproducible values for the carpal height ratio, Stahelin et al defined precise points of measurements (Fig. 9–3).[19] Standardized radiographic technique is required for these measurements (zero position). An alternate carpal height ratio has been proposed in which the carpal height is divided by the capitate length.[20] The capitate length is defined as the longest line between the point at the angular distal cortex of the capitate at the second to third carpometacarpal (CMC) junction to the proximal cortex of the capitate. This would allow quantification of carpal collapse using radiographs obtained without the full length of the third metacarpal (Table 9–1).

The *carpal height index* is determined by dividing the carpal height ratio of the dominant side by that of the nondominant side (Table 9–1).[19,21] The carpal height index has been found to be superior to the carpal height ratio for the evaluation of unilateral disease.[19]

ULNAR TRANSLOCATION OF THE WRIST

Ulnar carpal translocation (Table 9–2) is a complication of rheumatoid arthritis and other synovial arthritides, but is also seen in rare cases of posttraumatic carpal instability with injury and intercarpal arthritis. Ulnar translocation has been divided into two

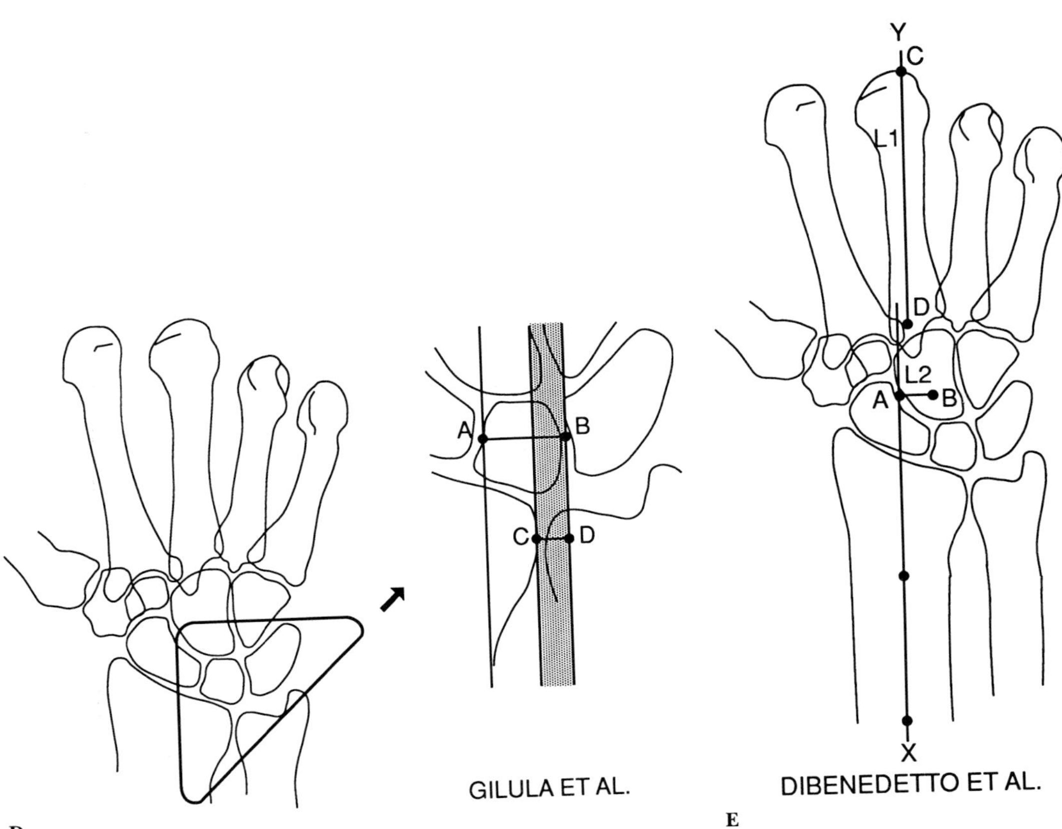

D E

FIGURE 9–4 *Continued* **D:** The method of Gilula and Weeks[23] indicates that ulnar translocation of the carpus is present if more than 50% of the lunate overhang (CD) is ulnar to the lunate fossa. The lunate overhang (CD) is divided by the lunate width (AB) to obtain a quantitative measurement (ratio). The semiquantitative measurement involves visual inspection of the x-ray film and determination of whether the lunate is translated more than 50% ulnarly. The right half of the figure is an enlargement of what is in the triangular area on the left. **E:** The method of DiBenedetto et al[25] uses a perpendicular line measured from the head of the capitate (B) to a reference line based on the radius (X). This line is obtained by bisection of the distal radius 2 and 4 cm proximal to the articular surface of the radius. The distance AB (L2) is the ulnar translation distance and increases as progressive ulnar translation occurs. The normal ratio of radiocapitate distance to the metacarpal length (CD, L1 on line Y) is 0.09 ± 0.02. (Modified with permission from Pirela-Cruz MA, Firoozbakhsh K, Moneim MS. Ulnar translation of the carpus in rheumatoid arthritis: An analysis of five determination methods. *J Hand Surg* 1993;18A:299–306.)

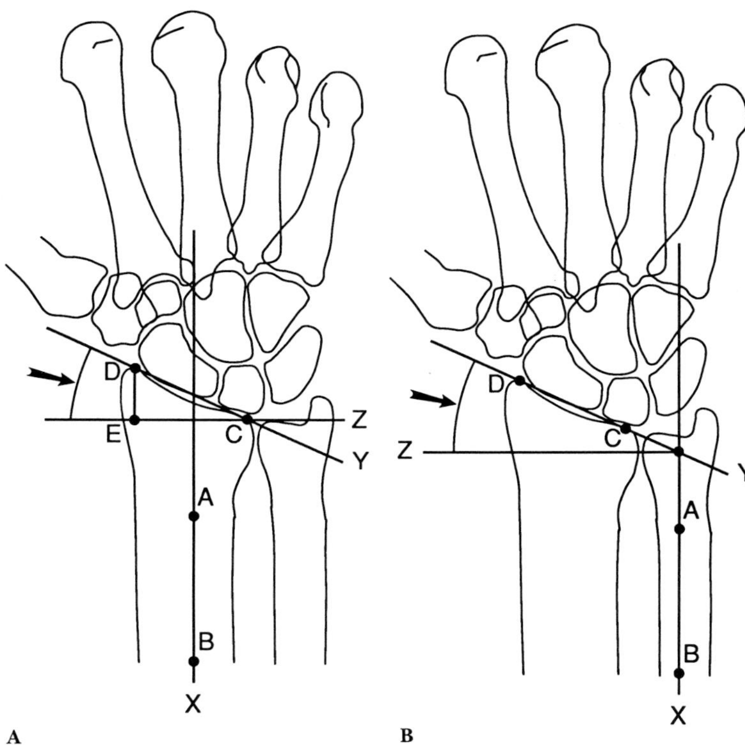

FIGURE 9–5. Radial inclination angle. **A:** The method of DiBenedetto et al. A line is drawn bisecting the distal radial shaft (X), 4 and 8 cm proximal to the radiocarpal joint (AB). The radial inclination angle (arrow) is formed between a line perpendicular to the radial bisection line (Z) and the line (Y) formed between the radial styloid (D) and the distal sigmoid notch (C). The radial height in this case is measured as the distance between the points D and E. (Modified with permission from DiBenedetto MR, Lubbers LM, Ruff ME, Nappi JF, Coleman CR. Quantification of error in measurements of radial inclination and radial-carpal distance. *J Hand Surg* 1991;16A:399–400 and DiBenedetto MR, Lubbers LM, Coleman CR. A standardized measurement of carpal translocation. *J Hand Surg* 1990;15A:1009–1010.) **B:** The method of Matsushita, Firrell, and Tsai. Radial inclination is defined as the angle (arrow) in the PA plane between a line (Y) connecting the radial and ulnar limits of the distal joint surfaces of the radius (DC) and a line (Z) perpendicular to the long axis of the distal ulna (X). The ulnar axis is determined as a line joining the two midpoints of the ulna at 2 cm and 4 to 5 cm (depending on the size of the x-ray film) (AB) proximal from the carpal ulnar joint surface. (Modified with permission from Matsushita K, Firrell JC, Tsai T-M. X-ray evaluation of radial shortening for Kienbock's disease. *J Hand Surg* 1992;17A:450–455.)

measuring angles are minimal.[26] This measure generally can be used with confidence in the description of radiographic findings between physicians. One instance where radial inclination is difficult to determine is in the case of distal radius fracture with intra-articular displacement and comminution.

Radial length, also called radial height and length of radial styloid, is defined as the distance between two lines perpendicular to the long axis of the radius.[31,33] One passes through the distal tip of the radial styloid, and the other passes through the most distal aspect of the ulnar articular surface (Table 9–3).

Palmar tilt, also called dorsal tilt, dorsal angle, volar tilt, volar angle, and palmar slope, is determined by the line drawn across the most distal points of the dorsal and ventral rims of the distal articular surface.[16,29,30,34–40] The degree of palmar tilt is derived by intersection of the line of palmar tilt and a line perpendicular to the long axis of the radius (determined by a line through the center of its medullary space at 2 and 5 cm proximal to the radiocarpal joint) (Fig. 9–6). Mann, Kang, and Gilula reported the results of a series of measurements in 100 normal wrists using specific reproducible criteria for radiographic positioning and measurements, with the radiographs obtained in a standardized fashion.[34] Two methods of measurement were used: 1) measuring the palmar tilt using the more proximal articular margin of the distal radius (method 1); and 2) measuring the more distal articular margin (method 2) (Fig. 9–7). The results of these measurements and other studies are listed in Table 9–3. Specifying the definition of the specific landmarks is recommended when reporting measurements of palmar tilt as well as other measurements in the wrist.

Van der Linden and Ericson[41] reviewed the outcome of treatment for fractures of the distal radius. They observed that only radial shift and palmar tilt of the distal fragment were independent of each other. It was concluded that displacement and anatomic results can be described adequately with only two measurements, one for dorsal angulation and one for radial displacement of the distal fragment. Abbaszadegan, Jonsson, and Sivers[42] followed 267 consecutive Colles fractures to determine prognostic factors for fracture displacement during plaster-cast treatment. They found that *radial axial shortening* (best defined as the distance from the distal-most radial to the distal ulnar articular surfaces)[32] had the greatest prognostic power, followed by Lindstrom class,[43] and the patient's age. A view of the contralateral uninjured wrist is necessary to determine the preexisting ulnar variance before measuring the radial shortening. Residual incongruity of the articular surface of the distal radius has been divided into four grades by Knirk and Jupiter.[44] Grade 0 incongruity was defined as a stepoff of 0 to 1 mm, Grade 1 was 1 to 2 mm, Grade 2 was 2 to 3 mm, and Grade 3 incongruity was 3 mm or more. Radiographic evidence of posttraumatic arthritis and a poor clinical outcome were seen more frequently with wrists having Grades 2 and 3 incongruity. Many studies have focused on the radiologic outcome with little attention paid to the fact

TABLE 9–3. Distal Radius and the DRUJ
The PA and Lateral Radiographs. Normal Data for Radiographic Measurements of the Distal Radius and DRUJ

Parameter/Source	Mean	Median	Range	Normal Limits
Distal Radius				
Radial Inclination (Tilt, Angulation) (degrees)				
Friberg and Lundstrom[28]	25.4 ± 2.2			
Altissimi et al[29]		16–28		
Aro and Koivunen[30]	21.3 ± 3.6			
DiBenedetto et al[26]	22 ± 3			
Schuind et al[16]	23.8	23.8 ± 2.6	12.9–30.3	18.8–29.3
Solgaard[31]	23 ± 3.7		16–35	
Warwick et al[32]	25.5 ± 6.2		15–35	
Radial Length (Length of Radial Styloid) (mm)				
Solgaard[31]	12 ± 2.2		8–17	
Mann et al[33]	13.5 ± 3.8			
Palmar Tilt (Dorsal Tilt, Ventral/Dorsal Tilt) (degrees)				
Gartland and Werley[35]	11		1–21	
DePalma[36]	11		1–23	
Golden[37]	12			
Smaill[38]	13			
Sarmiento et al[39]	11		(−2)–28	
Taleisnik and Watson[40]	11		(−7)–28	
Altissimi et al[29]				0–18
Aro and Koivunen[30]	9.9 ± 4.9			
Schuind et al[16]	12 ± 3.5		4–23	
Mann et al[34] method 1	10.8		3–20	CI95% 10.0–11.6
Mann et al[34] method 2	12.1		2–20	CI95% 11.3–13.0
Lunate Fossa Inclination (degrees)				
Linscheid[47]			0–20	
Carpal Angle (degrees)				
Harper et al[46]	130.88			
DRUJ (refer to text)				
Space (mm)				
Schuind et al[16]	1.6	1.5 ± 0.5	0.7–3.4	0.8–2.9
Length (mm)				
Schuind et al[16]				
(Radial Part)	7.5	7.2 ± 1.5	4.6–11.6	5.1–11.2
(Ulnar Part)	6.2	6.1 ± 1.0	4.0–8.7	4.2–8.3
UI (degrees)				
Tornvall et al[49]			18.6±4.1	11–27
RU (degrees)				
Tornvall et al[49]	100.4 ± 4.5		90–111	

UI, ulnar head inclination; RU, radioulnar angle; CI, confidence index.

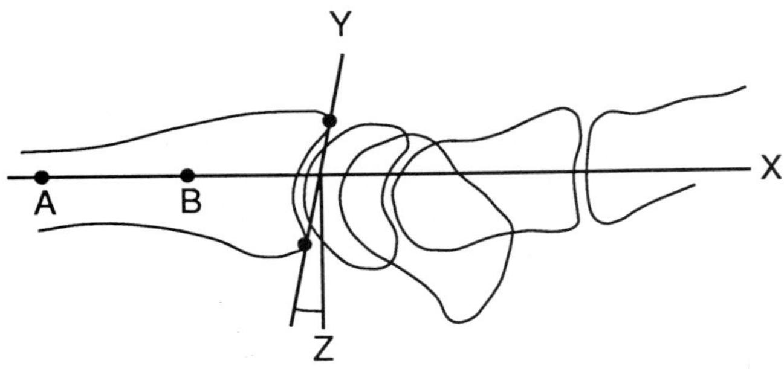

FIGURE 9–6. Palmar tilt is determined by the line (Y) joining the most distal points of the dorsal and ventral rims of the distal articular surface of the radius. The degree of palmar tilt is derived by the intersection of the line of palmar tilt and one perpendicular (Z) to the long axis of the radius (X) determined by a line through the center of its medullary space at 2 and 5 cm (AB) proximal to the radiocarpal joint.

that, regardless of the radiologic appearance, most patients achieve similar levels of activity, pain, and range of motion.[45] An extensive analysis of the correlation between radiographic and functional results after different alternatives of treatment of distal radius fractures was done by Solgaard.[31]

The *carpal angle* is defined as the angle resulting from the intersection of two lines, one tangent to the proximal edges of the lunate and scaphoid and one tangent to the proximal edges of the lunate and triquetrum (Fig. 9–8).[46] A change in the carpal angle can reflect congenital malformations. Significant ethnic differences have been found, however, and the carpal angle is altered by positioning of the wrist.

Lunate fossa inclination has been used to correlate lunate collapse to inclination of the distal radius and to evaluate the effect of radial shortening procedures.

Lunate fossa inclination was measured by Linscheid[47] by using the long axis of the radius for the measurements. Matsushita, Firrell, and Tsai[48] used the long axis of the ulna to describe preoperative and postoperative measurements because of the difficulty in determining the true axis of the radius; however, they did not provide data on normal values (Fig. 9–9 and Table 9–3).

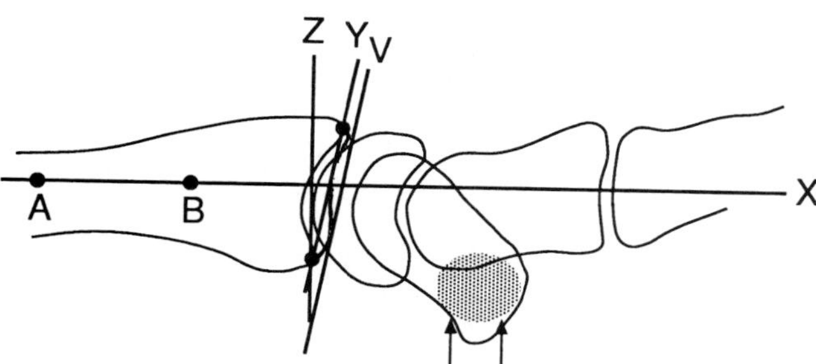

FIGURE 9–7. Zero lateral view of the carpus as judged by relative positions of the pisiform and scaphoid tuberosity. At least 5 cm of the distal radius is included to allow for accurate assessment of the long axis of the radius (A, B, X). Small arrows mark the palmar contour of the pisiform overlapping the distal pole of the scaphoid. Palmar tilt is determined by the line drawn across the most distal part of the dorsal and the volar rims of the distal radial articular surface. The degree of the palmar tilt is derived by an intersection of the line of palmar tilt and one perpendicular to the radial axis (Z). In method 1 the palmar tilt is measured using the more proximal articular margin of the distal radius (Y) and in method 2 it is measured using the distal articular margin (V). (Modified with permission from Mann FA, Kang SW, Gilula LA. Normal palmar tilt: Is dorsal tilting really normal? *J Hand Surg* 1992;17B:315–317.)

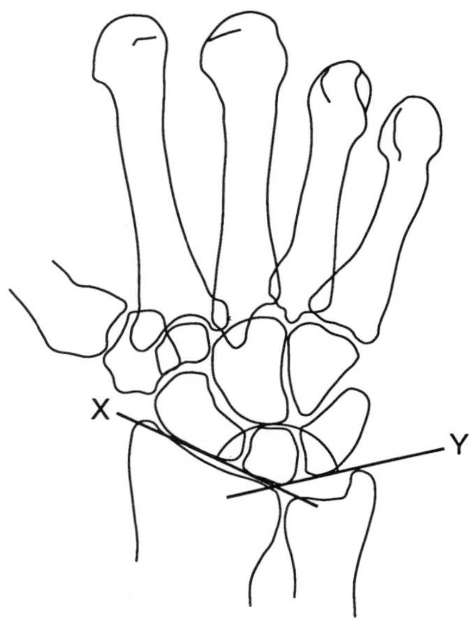

FIGURE 9–8. Carpal angle. The carpal angle was first described by Jercy Kosowicz in 1962. The angle is defined as that resulting from the intersection of two lines, one tangent to the proximal edges of the lunate and the scaphoid (X) and one tangent to the proximal edges of the lunate and the triquetrum (Y). (Modified with permission from Kosowicz J. The carpal sign in gonadal dysgenesis. *J Clin Endocrinol Metab* 1962;22:949; Kosowicz J. The roentgen appearance of the hand and wrist in gonadal dysgenesis. *Am J Roentgenol Rad Ther Nucl Med* 1965;99:354; and Harper HAS, Poznanski AK, Garn SM. The carpal angle in American population. *Invest Radiol* 1974;9:217–221.)

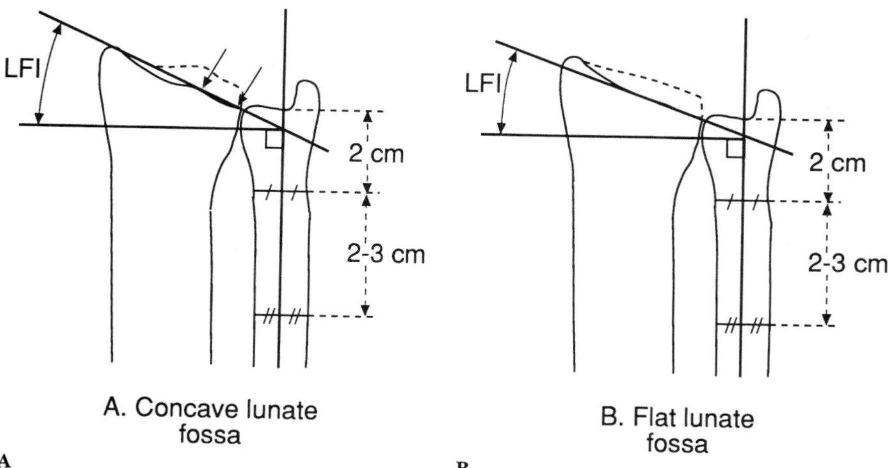

FIGURE 9–9. Lunate fossa inclination (LFI), defined as the angle between the sclerotic line of the lunate fossa of the radius and the line perpendicular to the long axis of the distal ulna. If the sclerotic line of the lunate fossa was concave, a line was drawn between the radial and the ulnar prominances of the lunate fossa **(A).** If the sclerotic line of the lunate fossa was flat, this line was simply extended **(B).** The ulnar axis was found by determining a line joining the two midpoints of the ulna at 2 cm and 4 to 5 cm (depending on the size of the x-ray film) proximal from the carpal ulnar joint surface. (Modified with permission from Matsushita K, Firrell JC, Tsai T-M. X-ray evaluation of radial shortening for Kienbock's disease. *J Hand Surg* 1992;17A:450–455.)

Normal data for the *distal radioulnar joint* (DRUJ) has been reported by Schuind et al (Table 9–3).[16] Tornvall et al[49] introduced *ulnar head inclination* (UI) and the *radioulnar* (RU) *angle* to describe the DRUJ (Fig. 9–10). The UI might be altered by pathologic conditions in the wrist, such as congenital disease. RU angle changes reflect malalignments of the DRUJ in the frontal plane. In cases of wrist injuries, comparing these angles with those of the uninjured wrist is recommended.

ULNAR VARIANCE

The term *ulnar variance,* also called *radioulnar index,* is used to describe the relative positions of the distal articular surfaces of the radius and ulna (Table 9–4).[14,16,28,29,33,50–58] A positive ulnar variance occurs when the distal cortical surface of the ulna projects more distally than the adjacent distal radial articular surface. In negative ulnar variance the distal edge of the ulna is proximal to the distal articular surface of the radius. Three techniques for measurements of ulnar variance have been described (Figs. 9–11A through 9–11C). Standardized radiographic technique is essential.[50,51] Kristensen, Thomassen, and Christensen[52] determined the intra- and interobserver variation when measuring ulnar variance using different methods. A modification of the method described by Palmer et al[51] had the highest reliability expressed in "weighted kappa" values, but both methods were reliable. Steyers and Blair[53] compared three methods of measuring ulnar variance and

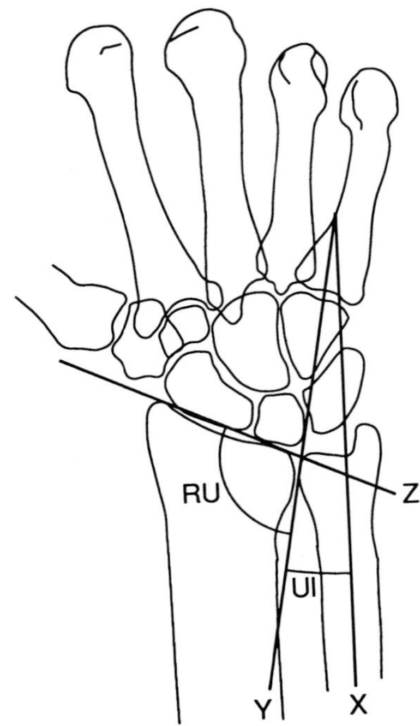

FIGURE 9–10. Ulnar head inclination (UI) and radioulnar (RU) angle. UI was defined as the angle between the long axis of the ulna (X) in a PA x-ray and a line drawn along the articular surface of the ulnar head facing the sigmoid notch (Y). RU angle was defined as an angle between the previous line along the ulnar head surface facing the sigmoid notch and a line drawn between the radial and the ulnar limits of the distal radius joint surface (Z). (Modified with permission from Tornvall AH, af Ekenstan F, Hagert CG, Irstam L. Radiological examination and measurements of the wrist and distal radioulnar joint. *Acta Radiol Diagn* 1986;27:581–588.)

TABLE 9–4. Ulnar Variance
The PA Radiograph. Normal Data for Radiographic Measurements of the Ulnar Variance Using Different Methods (Figs. 9–11 to 9–13)

				Ulnar Variance (mm)			
Source	**No.**	**Gender**	**Age (y)**	*Mean*	*SD*	*Range*	**Ethnic Group**
Chan and Huang[86]	400	NA	NA	+0.69	NA	(−3.0)–5.0	Chinese
Gelberman et al[54]	419	NA	NA	+0.27	1.69	(−6.0)–7.0	US (blacks)‡
Friberg and Lundstrom[28]				+0.70	1.73	(−5.0)–6.0	US (whites)‡
Palmer et al[51]	14	NA	NA	−0.14	NA	NA	Cadaver wrists*
Altissimi et al[29]	233	NA	NA	NA	NA	(−2.5)–3.1	Italian
Kristensen et al[52]	100	NA	NA	−0.60	1.38	(−4.0)–2.0	Scandinavian*
	100	NA	NA	−0.84	1.23	(−4.0)–3.0	Scandinavian†
Czitrom et al[55]	65	NA	NA	−0.38	1.48	(−5.0)–2.0	N. American*
Chen and Shih[56]	1000	527 M	23–69	+0.31	1.27	(−5.0)–5.0	Taiwan*
		473 F					
Nakamura et al[57]	325	203 M	14–79	+0.20	1.39	(−4.0)–5.0	Japanese*
		122 M					
Larsen et al[14]	75	NA	>17	−0.03	1.56	(−5.0)–5.0	Scandinavian†
Schuind et al[16]	120	M	NA	−0.90	1.5	NA	N. American*
	120	F	NA	−0.90	1.4	NA	N. American*
Hafner et al[58]	NA	NA	2–6	2.1	95%CI	0.3–3.88	N. American
	NA	NA	7–13	2.2	95%CI	(−1.1)–6.7	Japanese
	NA	NA	>14	2.3	95%CI	(−2.4)–7.0	Japanese
Mann et al[33]	26	M	NA	−0.46	1.64	NA	N. American§
	10	F	NA	−0.10	2.11	NA	N. American§

* *Measurements done using the method described by Palmer et al.*[51]

† *Measurements done using a modification of the method described by Palmer et al.*[51]

‡ *Measurement done using the method described by Gelberman et al.*[54]

§ *Unpublished data, 1991 (in Mann et al*[33]*).*

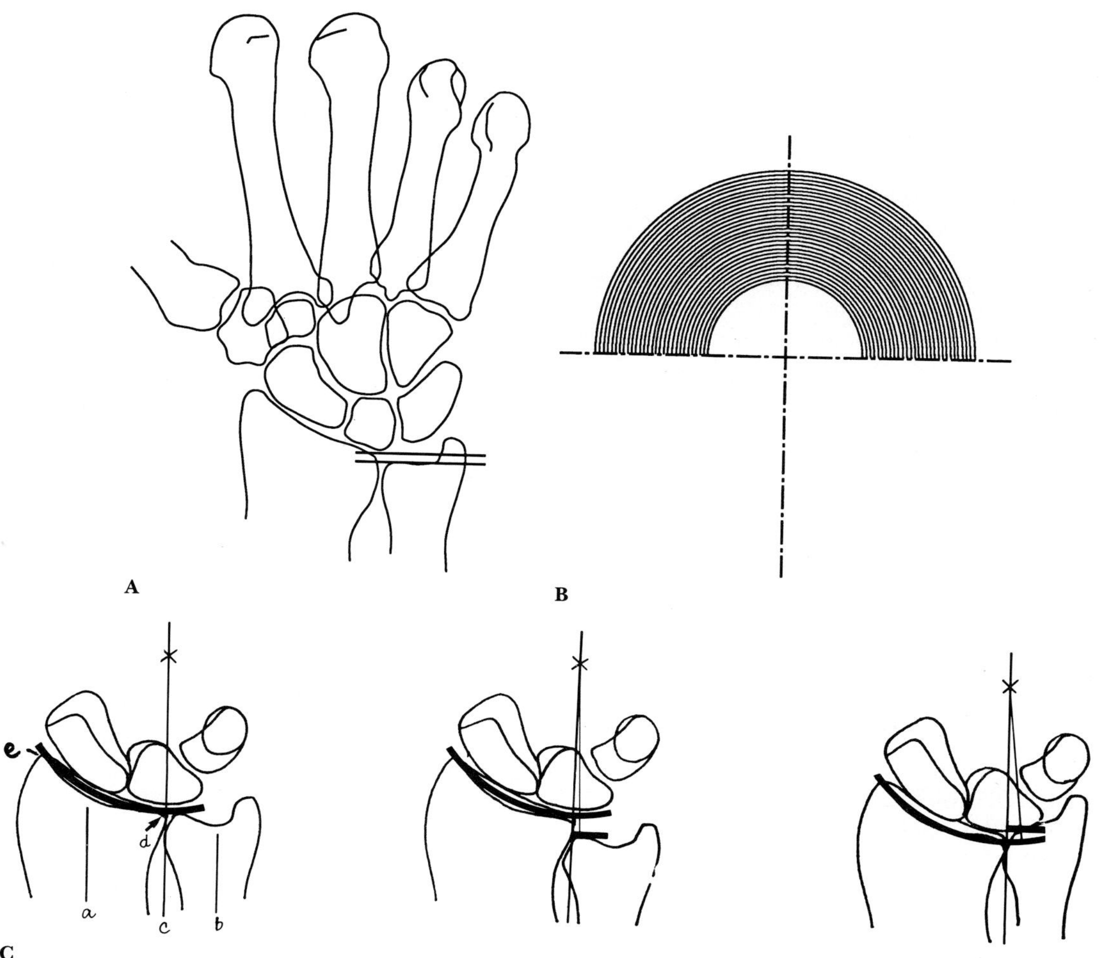

FIGURE 9–11. A: Ulnar variance measured as described by Gelberman et al.[54] The measurement was obtained by projecting a line from the carpal joint surface of the distal end of the radius toward the ulna and measuring the distance in millimeters between this line and the carpal surface of the ulna. **B:** Template of concentric semicircles ranging from 22 to 50 mm were used for measuring ulnar variance. (Modified with permission from Palmer AK, Richard R, Glisson BS, Werner FW. Ulnar variance determination. *J Hand Surg* 1982;7A:376–379.) **C:** A standardized PA x-ray in usual position was used. Ulnar variance determination. In this projection the radius and ulna are parallel. Two parallel lines are outlined (a, b). A new line (c), parallel to a and b, which strikes the ulnar border of the distal subchondral sclerotic radial line (d), is outlined. A semicircle, the radius being the distance between the point D and the styloid process of the radius (e), is drawn. The center of the semicircle lies on line c. This semicircle approximates the distal subchondral sclerotic line of the radius. The ulnar variance is determined as the distance between the most distal part of the ulnar cortical rim and the semicircle (thick black curved line). b: Negative variance. The radial articular surface is projecting more distally than the ulnar articular surface. c: Positive variance. The ulnar articular surface projects more distally than the radial articular surface. (Method described by Kristensen SS, Thomassen E, Christensen F. Ulnar variance determination. *J Hand Surg* 1986;11B:255–257. Modified and redrawn with permission.)

found all to be highly reliable. The authors concluded that the clinician may use whichever technique he or she prefers when measuring ulnar variance.

Several clinical wrist problems are considered directly or indirectly related to relative differences in the lengths of the radius and ulna (e.g., Kienböck's disease and ulnar impaction syndrome). It has been proposed that negative ulnar variance is a predisposing factor to the development of posttraumatic carpal instability.[55,59,60] In a study by Larsen, Lindequist, and Bellstrom[61] no correlation was found between the carpal angles on lateral wrist radiographs and ulnar variance in normal wrist. In the absence of ''preclinical'' carpal instability, it is unclear why there is an apparent increased incidence of posttraumatic carpal instability in individuals with ulnar-minus wrists.

Studies comparing ulnar variance require carefully selected age- and sex-matched controls, since a positive correlation between ulnar variance and both age and sex has been demonstrated.[57] Kristensen and Soballe[62] made the important observation that an apparent pseudolengthening of the distal radius had taken place in several patients with Kienböck's disease as a result of radiocarpal joint arthrosis. This observation suggested that the overrepresentation of ulnar-minus variance among patients with Kienböck's disease was a result of arthrosis, and thereby a consequence of rather than a cause of avascular necrosis of the lunate. There is continued controversy regarding the clinical significance of ulnar variance.

LUNATE DEFORMATION QUOTIENT, LUNATE UNCOVERING RATIO, SCAPHOLUNATE DISTANCE, AND THE LENGTH OF THE SCAPHOID

Several measurements are used to quantify deformation of the lunate and to determine the prognosis and stage of Kienböck's disease. None of these radiographic measurements has proven to be strongly correlated with clinical findings.[63] The *lunate deformation quotient* (LDQ) was described by Stahl (Fig. 9–12).[64] The longitudinal height of the lunate is divided by its greatest dorsopalmar dimension. Mirabello, Rosenthal, and Smith[63] report a ratio of 0.53 in normal wrists.

According to Schuind et al,[16] an index describing uncovering of the lunate by the radius was described by Razemon,[65] but the precise anatomic landmarks used to measure the lunate uncovering-length index still had not been clearly defined. Schuind et al[16] measured the uncovered portion of the lunate on a line perpendicular to the longitudinal axis of the radial side of the DRUJ. The index was calculated by dividing the length of the uncovered lunate by the projection of the entire lunate width on the same line. This is in fact similar to the method for evaluation of ulnar translocation described by Gilula and Weeks (see Fig. 9–4).[23] The average percentage measured in 100 normal wrists was 33% (range 11% to 69%). The PA view of the wrist must be taken in neutral position so that the mid-axis of the third metacarpal is coaxial with the mid-axis of the distal radius. Schuind et al[16] found an association between the lunate uncovering ratio (LUR) and the *carpal ulnar distance ratio.* They suggested that the LUR can be used to quantify ulnar translocation of the carpus.

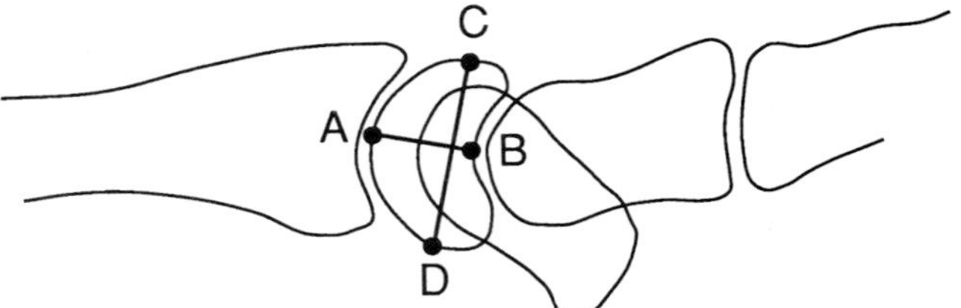

FIGURE 9–12. The lunate deformation quotient (LDQ). The longitudinal height (AB) of the lunate measured on the lateral view is divided by its greatest dorsopalmar dimension (CD). The ratio of these two measurements is considered the LDQ. (Reprinted with permission from Stahl F. On lunatomalacia (Kienbock's disease). *Acta Chir Scand* (suppl) 1947;95:126.)

The *length of the scaphoid* has been measured by Imamura[7] (18 mm ± standard deviation [SD] 0.8), but the measurement will depend on positioning of the wrist.

A widening of the scapholunate joint has been reported as suggestive of scapholunate dissociation in carpal instability. Cautilli and Wehbe[66] measured the *scapholunate distance* in PA radiographs in 100 normal wrists. The mean was 3.7 mm ± SD 0.6 (range, 2.5 to 5.0 mm). Measurements were made from the proximal ulnar corner of the scaphoid to the radial corner of the lunate using a standardized radiographic technique. All radiographs were taken in the zero position. A statistically significant difference was demonstrated with respect to sex. The average scapholunate distance was 4.0 mm in men and 3.6 mm in women. Information on standard deviation was not stated, but there was a significant statistical difference.

This technique does not measure the scapholunate width through the center of the scapholunate joint. Another problem that can occur with this approach is determining, on a curved surface, the exact location of the proximal ulnar corner of the scaphoid and the radial corner of the lunate. On routine frontal wrist views, the scapholunate joint is often not profiled, however. A solution to this problem might be even simpler if anteroposterior (AP) views are taken instead of PA views[22] and if the contralateral wrist is used for reference. The radiographic landmarks used in this method may be difficult to determine on routine radiographs. It is helpful to identify parallel adjacent articular surfaces of the scaphoid and lunate when trying to identify the width of the scapholunate joint. When widening of the scapholunate joint is suspected, a dynamic examination can be performed and the contralateral wrist used as a reference. Obermann[67] used fluoroscopically adjusted PA radiographs to evaluate scapholunate joint width. Similarly, Gilula has used fluoroscopy for years to evaluate scapholunate joint width in prone and supine positions. In a group of 70 patients with different carpal instabilities, the standard PA and lateral radiographs were falsely negative in 25% and falsely positive in 6.5% in the diagnosis of carpal instability. The main reason for this, according to Obermann,[67] is that with standard views the scapholunate joint is not always clearly profiled. The lateral view is not always completely neutral and it is difficult to control the amount of relaxation of the hand and wrist when radiographs are obtained. To profile the scapholunate joint, Kindynis et al[68] suggested the use of a PA radiograph with the tube angled 10 degrees medial (ulnar) to lateral (radial). They believed this allowed a better presentation of the scapholunate joint, making it easier to measure the space through the midportion of the flat medial facet of the scaphoid. Other approaches to profiling the scapholunate joint have also been described in the literature; however, dynamic fluoroscopic evaluation of the scapholunate joint using radial and ulnar deviation in both prone and supine positions provides the only reliable method to show maximum scapholunate widening.

CARPAL ANGLES ON LATERAL RADIOGRAPHS OF THE WRIST

A number of measuring methods have been designed for evaluating carpal bone angles on lateral radiographs (Table 9–5). Nakamura et al[69] stated that a difference of more than 10 degrees between contralateral bone angles only should be considered of diagnostic significance. Their study was based on 25 patients with bilateral wrist measurements and an SD of 5 to 6 degrees. No calculations of a possible statistical difference were reported. Garcia-Elias et al[15] showed that any determination of intercarpal angles using a goniometer has an SD of 5.2 degrees of observer variation. They reported an even higher interobserver variation when the method was used for exact quantification of carpal motion. Larsen, Mathiesen, and Lindequist[13] found that using defined bone axes was associated with the least observer variability. A study by these same authors to determine the differences between carpal bone angles on lateral wrist radiographs showed that the largest difference between the right and left wrists in the same person was 3 degrees.[13] The variance of the radioscaphoid angle and the radiolunate angle measured on radiographs from both wrists was 3.1 degrees and 3.4 degrees, respectively. In a series of 23 normal wrists measured twice by the same observer, the variance for the same two carpal bone angles was 1.57 degrees and 3.65 degrees. Variance-ratio tests showing no significant difference between the variance in the two series of patients shows that any radiologic or anatomic side differences were not clinically significant. Therefore, using defined bone axes, a difference exceeding 5 degrees between the carpal bone angles on lateral radiographs in both wrists of the same person can be considered significant, since they found no significant difference between the angles in the two wrists of the same person.

Several authors have described in detail the normal angular relationships in the wrist.[7,13,23,67,69–75] The range of angles in normal wrists varies considerably in different studies. This variation may be due to the use of different definitions for the angles measured or to statistical variation, since the number of

TABLE 9–5. *The Use of Definitions of the Axes of Carpal Bones in Lateral Radiographs According to Various Authors[13]*

Source	Radius	Scaphoid	Lunate	Capitate	Triquetrum
Linscheid et al[70]	R1	S1	L1	C1	
Sarrafian et al[71]	R1	S1	L1	C1	
Gilula and Weeks[23]	R1	S1/S2	L1	C1	
Reagan et al[72]				T1	
Chaise et al[73]	R1	S1	L1	C1	
Imamura[7]	R2	S1	L1	C2	
Yamada[74]	R2	S2	L1	C2	
Nakamura et al[69]	R2	S1	L1	C2	
Larsen et al[13]	R1	S2	L1	C2	
Obermann[67]	R3	S1/S2	L1	C1	
Belsole et al[75]	D	D	D	D	D

R1: the line through the center of the medulla at 2 and 5 cm proximally to the radiocarpal joint.

R2: the tangent of the dorsal margin of radius more than 3 cm from the distal articular surface.

R3: the line drawn parallel to the borders of the distal radius diaphysis and through the midpoint of the distal articulating surface of the radius (not included in the evaluation of observer variation).

L1: the line perpendicular to the tangent of the two distal poles.

S1: the line through the proximal and distal poles.

S2: the tangent of the volar proximal and distal convexities.

C1: the line through the midpoints of the proximal and distal poles.

C2: the tangent of the dorsal margin of the diaphysis of the third metacarpal bone (substitute axis).

D: using volumetric centroids and principal axes of computed carpal models (digital data from CT scans) to describe the relative position of each carpal bone.

T1: the line passing through the distal angulation and bisecting the sagittal profile proximally.

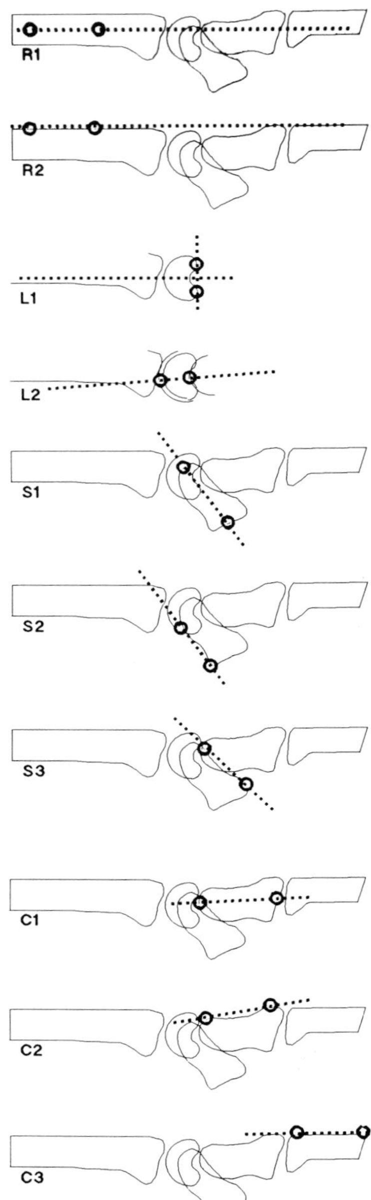

FIGURE 9–13. Frequently referred-to radiologic measures in lateral projections of the wrist assessed using the following definition of axes. *Radius:* R1, the line through the center of medullary canal at 2 and 5 cm proximal to the radiocarpal joint; R2, the tangent of the dorsal margin of the radius more than 3 cm from the distal articular surface. *Lunate:* L1, the line perpendicular to the tangent of the two distal poles; L2, the line through the top points of the proximal convexity and the distal concavity. *Scaphoid:* S1, the line through the proximal and distal poles; S2, the tangent of the palmar proximal and distal margins; S3, the tangent of the dorsal proximal and distal margins. *Capitate;* C1, the line through the proximal and distal poles; C2, the tangent of the dorsal proximal and distal margins; C3, the tangent of the dorsal margins of the diaphysis of the third metacarpal bone (substitute axis). (Reprinted with permission from Larsen CF, Mathiesen FK, Lindequist S. Measurements of carpal bone angles on lateral wrist radiographs. *J Hand Surg* 1991;16A:888–893.)

patients used was small in these studies. A study was performed to establish the most reproducible radiographic measurements for angles between the different wrist bones by calculating the intraobserver and interobserver variabilities using different definitions of the angles.[13] Eleven frequently referred-to radiologic measurements for lateral wrist projections were assessed in 23 wrists using 10 different definitions of axes (Fig. 9–13). The SD of the interobserver variation ranged from 2.60 to 18.15 degrees; and the intraobserver variation ranged from 1.89 to 4.66 degrees depending on the angles measured. The lowest variability is achieved by using four axes for the assessment of carpal alignment (Fig. 9–14).

Precise positioning of the arm and wrist, use of a support, and evaluation using well-defined carpal bone axes are necessary to make accurate wrist measurements. Hardy et al[4] emphasized that radiographic examination of the wrist should be performed with standardized wrist positioning. Several methods of positioning the upper extremity during radiographic examination have been reported.[77–79] Few authors have stated the position of the arm during their examinations.[74,76]

Linscheid et al[70] stated that the scapholunate angle averages 46 degrees (47 degrees is shown in an illustration) and ranges from 30 degrees to 60 degrees in normal wrists (Table 9–6). Gilula and Weeks[23] proposed the same range for the scapholunate angle and added a range of 0 to 30 degrees for the capitolunate angle. However, no description of radiographic technique or material was given. Sarrafian, Melamed, and Goshgarian[71] gave detailed measurements of intercarpal bone angles. Their method controlled flexion and extension of the wrist but not radial or ulnar

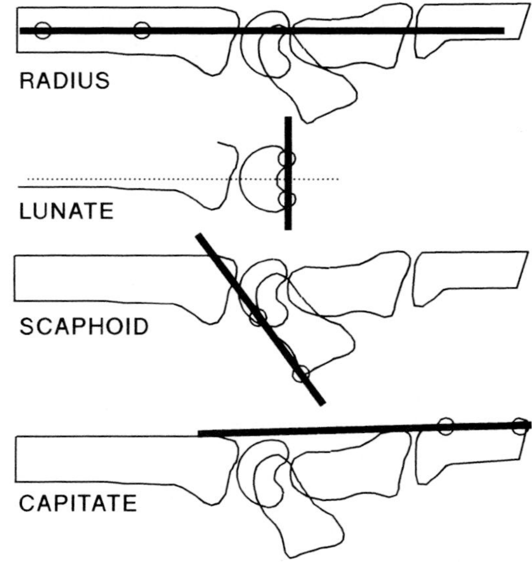

FIGURE 9–14. The four axes providing the least observer variability for assessment of carpal alignment as recommended by Larsen et al.[13] For definition of bone axes, refer to Fig. 9–13. (Reprinted with permission from Larsen CF, Mathiesen FK, Lindequist S. Measurements of carpal bone angles on lateral wrist radiographs. *J Hand Surg* 1991;16A:888–893.)

TABLE 9–6. *Mean, Range, Standard Deviation (SD), and Mean ± 2 SD of Each Carpal Angle According to Various Sources*

Angle Source	No.	Mean	Range	SD	M − 2SD	M + 2SD
RL						
Sarrafian et al[71]	55		(−31)−?			
Chaise et al[73]	50		(−30)−15			
Nishikawa et al[76]	50	10		7.6	− 5.2	25.2
Imamura[7]	40	− 7.4		3.3	−14.2	0.8
Yamada[74]	60	4.5	(−15)−27	9.1	−13.7	22.7
Nakamura et al[69]	84	10	(−22)−6	8	−26	4
Larsen et al[13]	75	− 1.02	(−10)−12	5.3	−11.7	9.65
Belsole et al[75]	22	−13.5				
RS						
Sarrafian et al[71]	55	58	33−73			
Chaise et al[73]	50	50	30−75			
Nishikawa et al[76]	84	66		6.1	53.8	78.2
Imamura[7]	40	66.6		5.1	56.4	76.8
Yamada[74]	60	54.5	37−69	6.6	41.3	67.7
Nakamura et al[69]	84	66	54−78	6	54	78
Larsen et al[13]	75	51.8	35−65	6.4	39	64.6
Obermann[67]	30	53	40−58			
Belsole et al[75]	22	53.7				
RC						
Sarrafian et al[71]	55		(−5)−20			
Chaise et al[73]	50		(−5)−20			
Nishikawa et al[76]	50	2.6		5.9	− 9.2	14.4
Yamada[74]	60					
Belsole et al[75]	22	16.4				
SC						
Sarrafian et al[71]	55	63	41−83			
Chaise et al[73]	50	60	35−85			
Imamura[7]	40	65.8		4.1	57.6	74
Yamada[74]	60					
SL						
Linscheid et al[70]	NS	46	30−60			
Sarrafian et al[71]	55	51	28−101			
Gilula and Weeks[23]	NS		30−60			
Chaise et al[73]	50	50	30−80			
Imamura[7]	40	56		3.5	49	63
Yamada[74]	60	50	30−67	8.2	33.6	66.4
Nakamura et al[69]	84	56	42−70	7	42	70
Larsen et al[13]	75	50.8	36−66	6.7	37.3	64.2
Obermann[67]	14	50	40−60			
CL						
Sarrafian et al[71]	55					
Gilula and Weeks[23]	NS		0−30			
Imamura[7]	40	7.4		3.3	0.8	14
Yamada[74]	60	− 4.5		9.1	−22.7	13.7
Nakamura et al[69]	84	−10		8	−26	4
RT						
Belsole et al[75]	22	−34.5				
LT						
Reagan et al[72]	30	14	(−3)−31			

NS, not stated; RL, radiolunate; RS, radioscaphoid; RC, radiocapitate; SC, scaphocapitate; SL, scapholunate; CL, capitolunate; RT radiotriquetral; LT, lunotriquetral.

deviation or forearm rotation. A series of 50 normal wrists was analyzed by Chaise et al[73] using a method described by Meyrueis, Cameli, and Jan.[77] In this and subsequent studies[7,69,74,76] the position of the wrist was controlled using a device. None of the studies used methods that controlled ulnar or radial deviation. Ulnar or radial deviation cannot be controlled by placing the ulnar border firmly on the table or film cassette, since differences in the hypothenar muscle mass might cause varying degrees of radial deviation. If lateral radiographs are to be used for measurements of intercarpal bone angles, ideally the wrist should be stabilized with a support and the position of the wrist in the two remaining planes controlled. Obermann[67] reported measurements performed with fluoroscopically controlled positioning of the wrist.

Using a device that controlled wrist position in all planes (Fig. 9–2) Larsen et al[6] found wrist measurements were not significantly different from previous studies that used standardized radiographic techniques. They concluded that controlling for ulnar and radial deviation might be of minor importance if the remaining planes are controlled.

Ulnar variance has been mentioned as one of the factors that could have an influence on carpal bone angles.[55,59,60] Ligamentous laxity is another factor that has received very little attention with respect to carpal bone angles. Musculoskeletal problems, injuries, dislocations, and premature development of degenerative joint disease have been related to generalized joint laxity.[79–81] A wide variation in normal joint mobility exists.[80,82] Ethnic differences have been reported, and joint motion varies with age and sex.[80] A correlation between joint laxity and carpal instability is likely, but thus far no studies have focused on this question.

The digital data from computed tomography (CT) of carpal bones can be assembled to three-dimensional (3D) images[83] and used to compute the volumetric centroid and principal axes of each bone.[75] Three-dimensional reconstructions of CT scans of human cadaver carpal bones have been compared with the measured dimensions and volume of the same specimens.[84] Using a novel computer program permitting "boundry tracking," Viegas et al[84] found they could accurately measure volume and dimensions of the carpal bones, as well as minimum intercarpal distance. Despite these advances, there is no direct correlation between the three-plane angles measured from CT and conventional two-plane measurements.[75] When the technique is developed further and made commercially available, it may prove to be a major improvement in the assessment of carpal alignment, since the axes reflect the total geometry of the bones.

Normal mean values and ranges for two-plane radiographic intercarpal bone angles on lateral radiographs may be of assistance in the diagnostic evaluation of ligamentous injury to the wrist, provided a standardized technique is used. In a recent experimental study, however, Meade, Schneider, and Cherry[85] reported that significant ligamentous damage had to be present to change the "normal" intercarpal angles, implying that further studies, such as arthrography or arthroscopy, where clinically indicated, should be performed in patients with normal radiographs.

It is essential to provide a detailed definition of axes used when reporting the results of measurements of carpal bone angles on lateral wrist radiographs. Radiographic examination for classification of abnormal alignments needs to be standardized. Using the same methods for determining carpal bone angles, preferably with the least inter- and intraobserver variation, is an important step. The uninjured wrist in a patient with unilateral wrist trauma can be used as a reference, since no significant difference between the two wrists of the same person has been demonstrated. If the measurements are based on bone axes described by Larsen, Mathiesen, and Lindequist[13] and are compared with a normal contralateral wrist, a difference between the carpal bone angles on lateral radiographs exceeding 5 degrees can be considered significant.

CLASSIFICATION SCHEMES

CLASSIFICATION OF TRAUMATIC CONDITIONS

Distal Phalangeal Fractures

Extraarticular distal phalangeal fractures are common injuries. Most are managed with splinting; therefore the radiographic findings serve to document the injury and further classification is not necessary. Avulsion fractures involving the extensor or flexor apparatus have been classified because different fracture types may be subject to different forms of treatment.

Mallet injuries occur in one of three ways: the extensor tendon can rupture at its attachment on the dorsal cortex; there can be avulsion of a small fragment of the dorsal cortex with the tendon; or there can be avulsion of a larger fragment with ventral subluxation of the distal phalanx (Fig. 9–15). Small avulsion fractures and soft-tissue disruptions are treated with splinting. Some surgeons consider oper-

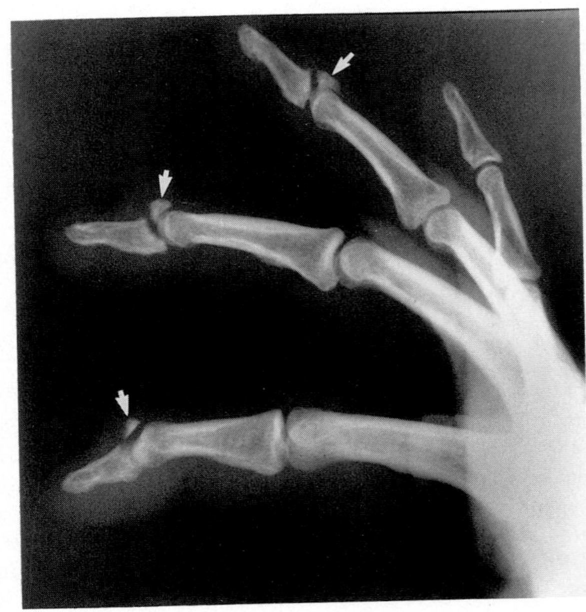

FIGURE 9–15. Multiple mallet fractures (arrows) with and without ventral subluxation of the distal phalanx.

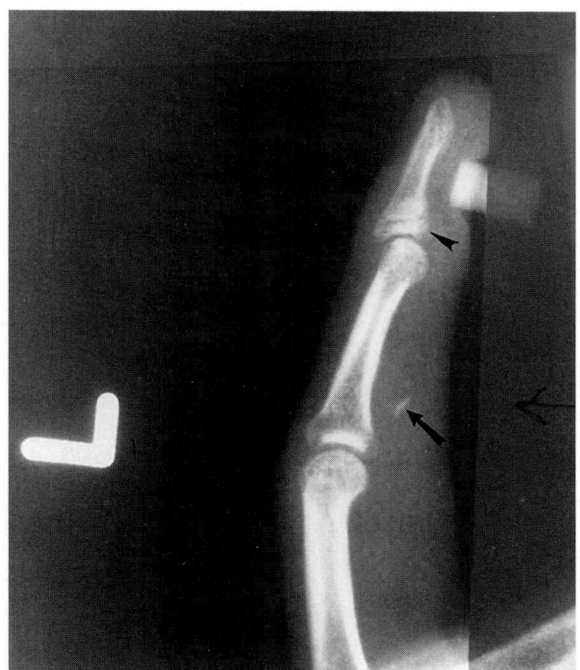

FIGURE 9–16. Type II avulsion of flexor digitorum profundus tendon. A small bone fragment (arrow) is avulsed from the base of the distal phalanx (arrowhead) and is moved proximally. (Courtesy of Glenn A. Buterbaugh, M.D., Pittsburgh, PA.)

ative treatment for mallet fractures with ventral subluxation of the distal phalanx. As a result, it is valuable to document if subluxation is present.

Leddy and Packer[87] describe three types of avulsion injuries involving the flexor digitorum profundus tendon. In the Type I injury, the profundus tendon ruptures at its insertion on the distal phalanx and retracts into the palm. In the Type II injury, a small fleck of bone is avulsed from the distal phalanx. This fragment becomes incarcerated in the flexor apparatus near the proximal interphalangeal joint (Fig. 9–16). In the Type III injury, a larger fragment of bone is avulsed from the distal phalanx. This fragment becomes snared in the flexor apparatus beneath the middle phalanx. Robins and Dobyns[88] describe a fourth type of injury in which there is an avulsion fracture of the distal phalanx combined with an avulsion of the profundus tendon from the avulsed fracture fragment. This classification system has clinical relevance in that Type I avulsions are associated with disruption of blood supply to the tendon and should be repaired within 7 to 10 days.[88]

Fracture-Dislocations of the Proximal Interphalangeal Joint

Three types of proximal interphalangeal (PIP) dislocation or fracture-dislocation were described by Eaton and Littler (Fig. 9–17A).[89] The Type I injury results from hyperextension of the PIP joint. The palmar plate is disrupted and there is a partial longitudinal split in the collateral ligaments. With this injury, the finger assumes a hyperextended position at the PIP joint. In the Type II injury there is a complete longitudinal split between the collateral ligaments. The middle phalanx is dorsally dislocated and assumes a position parallel to that of the proximal phalanx. In the Type III injury there is a fracture-dislocation with avulsion of the palmar lip of the middle phalanx (Figs. 9–17A (part C) and 9–17B). This avulsed fragment can involve varying degrees of the articular surface and may be comminuted. When the fracture involves more than 40 percent of the joint, there is significant associated instability.

The middle phalanx can also be dislocated in either a lateral or a palmar direction. Both are uncommon injuries.

Middle and Proximal Phalangeal Fractures

Fractures of the proximal and middle phalanges commonly involve the shaft and can be subject to rotational and angular deformities. Fractures of the phalangeal head are classified according to displacement, stability, and comminution.[90] Fractures of the base with intraarticular extension have been classified by Steele[91,92] (Figs. 9–18A through 9–18C) as follows:

I. nondisplaced marginal fractures,
II. comminuted, impaction fractures, and
III. displaced with subluxation.

Metacarpophalangeal Joint Dislocations

Dislocations at the metacarpophalangeal (MCP) joint occur most frequently with hyperextension and are rarely associated with a fracture. In a "simple" dorsal dislocation or subluxation, the proximal phalanx assumes a hyperextended position on the metacarpal. With a "complex" dorsal dislocation the base of the proximal phalanx rests on the neck of the metacarpal head creating bayonet apposition of the two bones. In this position the palmar plate becomes interposed between the head of the metacarpal and the base of the proximal phalanx. This is often irreducible without surgery, hence the designation "complex." Depending on the roentgenographic view there may be the appearance of a widened joint space, and there should be a loss of the normal parallelism between adjacent articulating cortices of the MCP joint when these cortices are in profile.

Thumb Metacarpal Fractures and Carpometacarpal Fracture-Dislocations

Fracture-dislocations at the thumb CMC joint have been described as "Bennett's fractures."[93] The fracture occurs through the palmar rim of the thumb metacarpal base and the fragment remains attached to the anterior oblique ligament. Loss of this restraint allows the metacarpal to move dorsal, radial, and proximal to its normal position. This is best visualized on a true lateral projection.[94] Green and O'Brien classified fractures and fracture-dislocations at the

Text continued on page 244

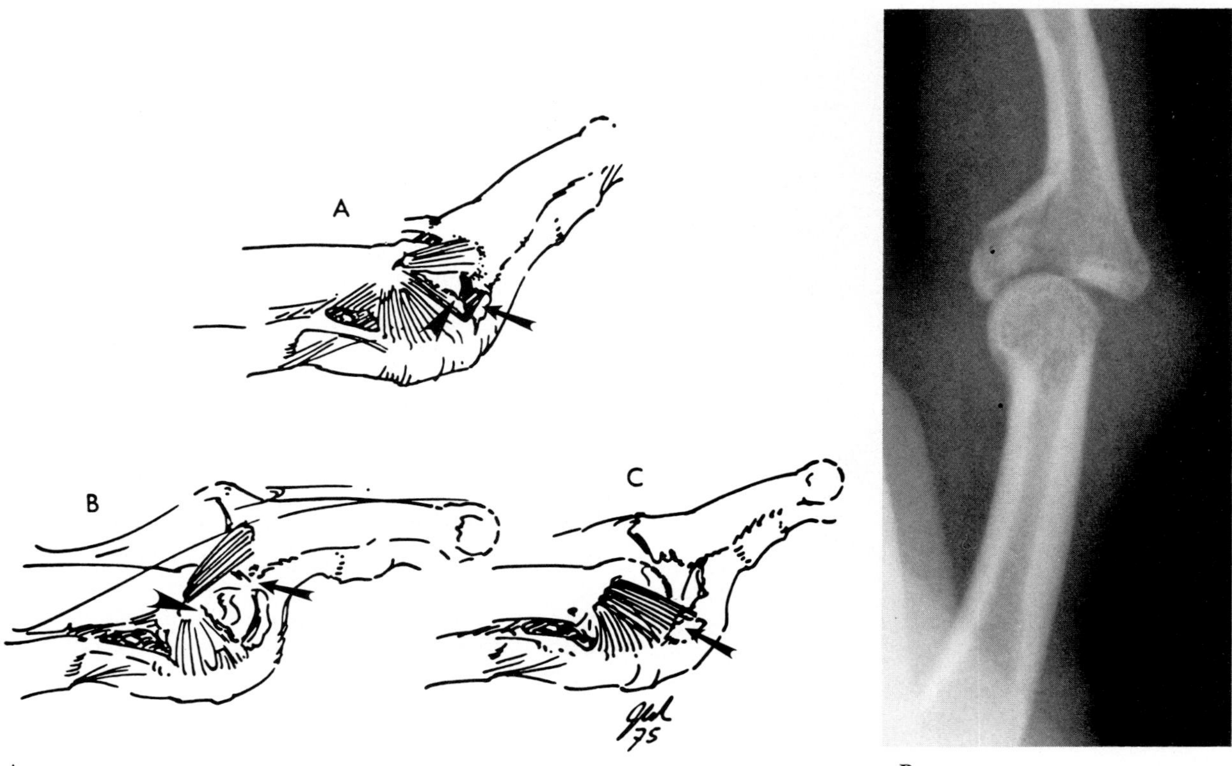

A B

FIGURE 9–17. A: Eaton–Littler classification of proximal interphalangeal joint fracture-dislocations. A: Type I—rupture of palmar plate (arrow) with incomplete split of collateral ligament (arrowhead). B: Hyperextension at the interphalangeal joint is present. Type II—rupture of palmar plate (arrow) with complete split of collateral ligaments (arrowhead) and dorsal dislocation of middle phalanx on proximal phalanx. C: Type III—avulsion fracture (arrow) of the palmar lip of the middle phalanx with dorsal subluxation of the middle phalanx. (Reprinted with permission from Green DP. *Operative hand surgery.* 3rd ed. New York: Churchill Livingstone, 1993.) **B:** Type III fracture—subluxation of the proximal interphalangeal joint (see panel A, part C). Comminution of the ventral half of the middle phalangeal base is associated with dorsal subluxation of the middle phalanx.

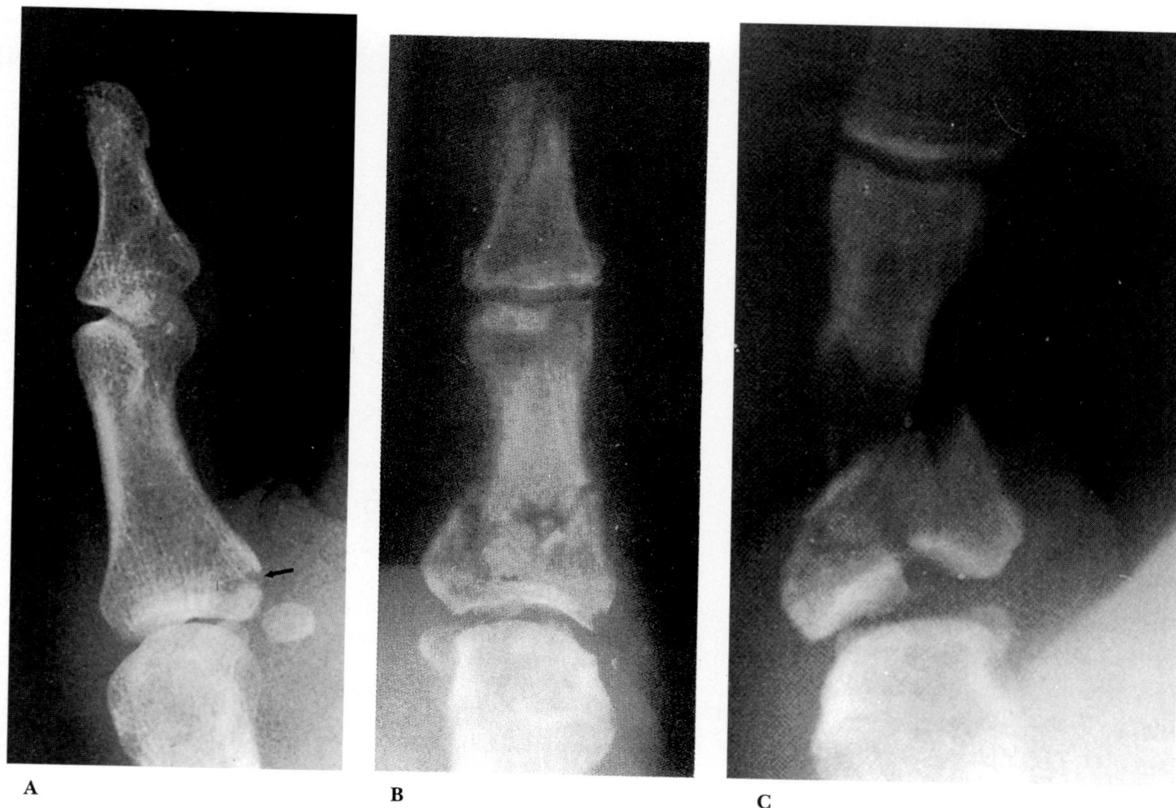

A B C

FIGURE 9–18. A: Steele's classification of intraarticular fractures at the base of the phalanges. Type I: nondisplaced marginal fractures (arrow) at the base of the thumb proximal phalanx. **B:** Steele's classification of intraarticular fractures at the base of the phalanges. Type II: comminuted impaction fracture at the base of the thumb proximal phalanx with intraarticular extension. Minimal displacement of articular fragments is present. **C:** Steele's classification of intraarticular fractures at the base of the phalanges. Type III: displaced intraarticular fracture of the thumb proximal phalanx with subluxation. (Panels A to C reprinted with permission from Gilula LA. *The traumatized hand and wrist: Radiographic and anatomic correlation.* Philadelphia: WB Saunders, 1992.)

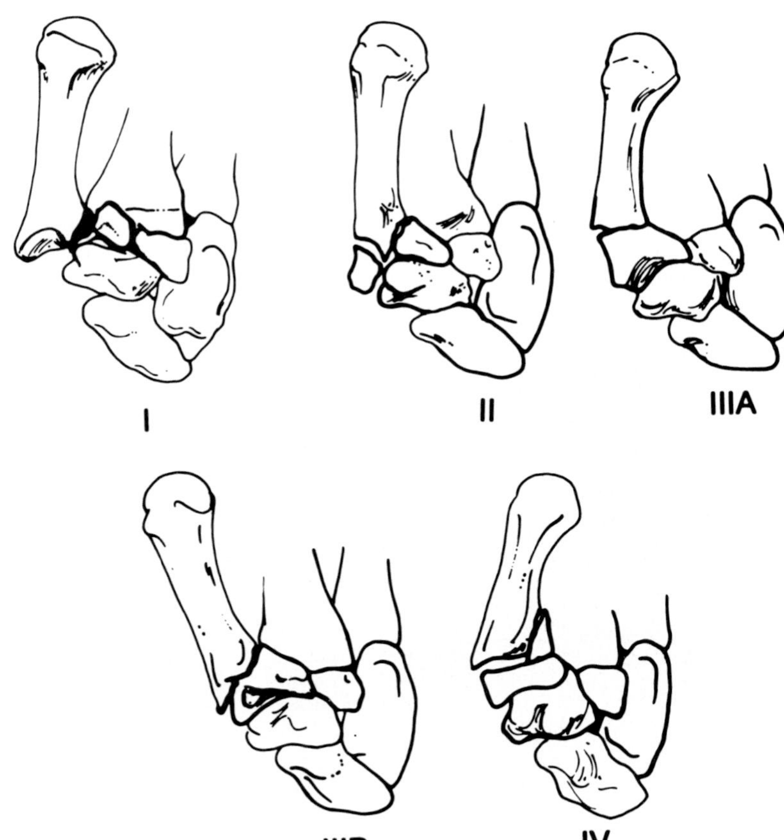

FIGURE 9–19. Greene's classification of fractures at the base of the thumb metacarpal. Type I: intraarticular Bennett's fracture-dislocation. Type II: intraarticular Rolando's fracture or comminuted fracture. Type IIIA: transverse extraarticular fracture. Type IIIB: oblique extraarticular fracture. Type IV: epiphyseal fracture in a child. (Reprinted with permission from Gilula LA. *The traumatized hand and wrist: Radiographic and anatomic correlation.* Philadelphia: WB Saunders, 1992.)

base of the thumb metacarpal as follows (Fig. 9–19):[95]

- I. fracture-dislocation (Bennett's),
- II. y-shaped (Rolando's) or comminuted fracture,
- IIIA. transverse extraarticular fracture,
- IIIB. oblique extraarticular, and
- IV. epiphyseal injury (usually Salter–Harris Type II).

Fractures involving the finger CMC joints occur most commonly at the base of the fifth metacarpal. In the "reverse Bennett's" fracture the radial lip of the fifth metacarpal is avulsed from the metacarpal base. The term *reverse Bennett's* fracture is usually used when there is ulnar subluxation of the fifth metacarpal. An axial load applied to the fifth metacarpal can create a pure dorsal dislocation of the fifth metacarpal or a fracture-dislocation with fracture through the dorsal cortex of the hamate. A loss of the normal joint space or overlapping articular cortices between the hamate and the base of the fourth and fifth metacarpals can be apparent on both plain films and tomograms (Figs. 9–20A and 9–20B). This is most reliably recognized when the other CMC joints (second through fourth) are plainly visible or are in profile. This means that when the CMC joints are clearly seen on the PA or AP view, they are not flexed or extended. In other words, a common cause of failure to see the fifth (or second through fourth) CMC joint(s) can be merely the result of positioning.

Scaphoid Fractures

Russe proposed a classification system of scaphoid fractures based on the direction of the fracture line as it passed through the waist of the scaphoid.[96] The vertical oblique fracture was considered to have greater potential for displacement (Fig. 9–21).[97] Herbert proposed a classification system that subdivided scaphoid fractures into four types:[98]

- A. stable acute fractures,
- B. unstable acute fractures,
- C. delayed unions, and
- D. established nonunions.

Each of these was subsequently subdivided according to fracture location and displacement as well as the type of nonunion in those fractures that had failed to heal (Fig. 9–22). Herbert contended that this classification system had prognostic significance.

Lunate Fractures

Acute fractures of the lunate occur with substantially less frequency than fractures of the scaphoid or triquetrum. Teisen and Hjarbaek[99] proposed a classification that includes five types of acute lunate fractures not due to Kienböck's disease (Fig. 9–23).

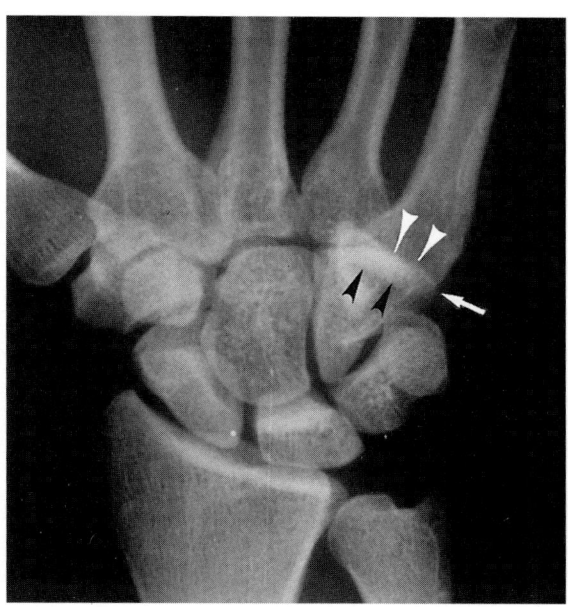

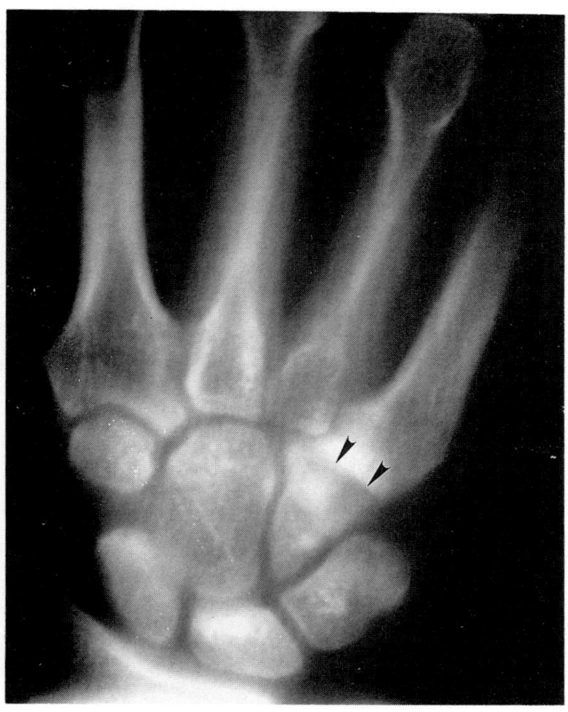

A B

FIGURE 9–20. A: Fracture-dislocation of the small finger CMC joint. Arrow points to loss of fifth CMC joint space and overlapping of cortices of the fifth metacarpal base (black arrowheads) and distal surface of the hamate (white arrowheads). **B:** Tomogram of a fracture-dislocation of the fifth CMC joint shows the fifth metacarpal base cortex (arrowheads) sharply defined without evidence of hamate cortex (when one cortex is seen well the adjacent articulating cortex should be evident). (Reprinted with permission from Gilula LA. *The traumatized hand and wrist: Radiographic and anatomic correlation.* Philadelphia: WB Saunders, 1992.)

Kienböck's Disease

Most authors consider repetitive trauma to be an important component of the cause of Kienböck's disease.[64,100–102] A negative ulnar variance[103] and increased radial inclination[63] are radiographic findings believed to be associated with this disorder. Stahl[64] described four stages of Kienböck's disease. Lichtman et al[101] modified this classification as follows (Fig. 9–24):

Stage I: Lunate is normal or has a small linear compression fracture. A bone scan or magnetic resonance image (MRI) in Stage I will be abnormal.

Stage II: Lunate appears sclerotic; shape is unchanged except for slight collapse.

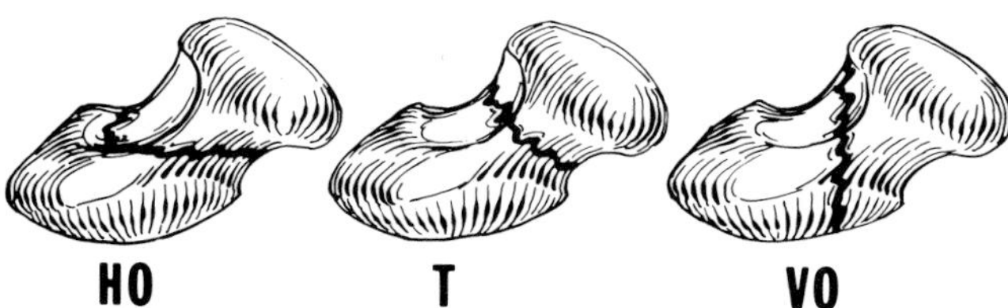

FIGURE 9–21. Russe's classification of scaphoid fractures. HO, horizontal fracture; T, transverse fracture; VO, vertical oblique fracture. (Reprinted with permission from Green DP. *Operative hand surgery.* 3rd ed. New York: Churchill Livingstone, 1993.)

Stage III: Lunate has collapsed.
- A. Normal carpal position,
- B. Rotary subluxation of the scaphoid.

Stage IV: Degenerative changes in the midcarpal, intercarpal, and/or radiocarpal joints.

Hamate Fractures

Fractures of the body of the hamate can occur in association with fracture-dislocations of the fourth and fifth CMC joints. Fractures of the hamate hook may be diagnosed by loss of the normally distinct ring on a PA view. The fracture can be seen on a carpal tunnel view when it is in the ventral half to three quarters of the hamate and the patient's wrist is supple enough to perform an adequate carpal tunnel view (Fig. 9–25A). When the fracture is more dorsal, it may be best seen on a CT scan (Fig. 9–25B) or MRI. Milch classified hamate hook fractures as avulsion fractures of the tip, through the waist, and through the base of the hamate hook.[104]

Fractures of the Trapezium

Fractures of the trapezium have been classified into two categories: ridge avulsions at the insertion of the transverse carpal ligament and fractures through the body of the trapezium.[105] Fractures of the trapezium

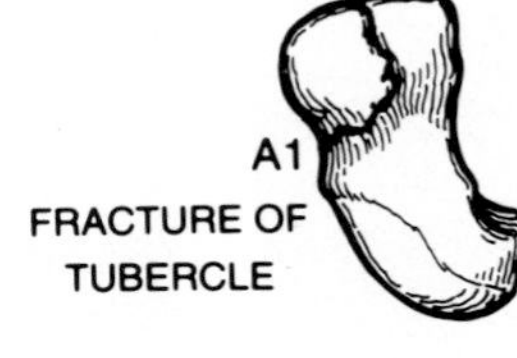

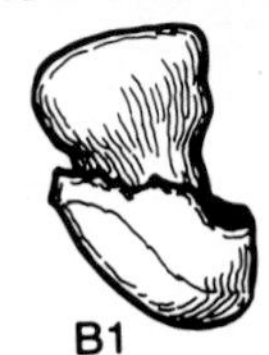
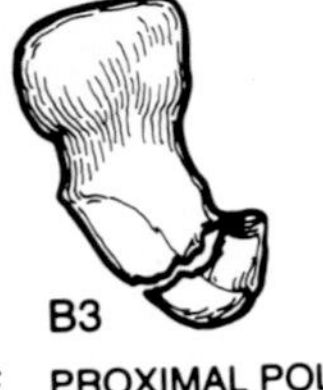

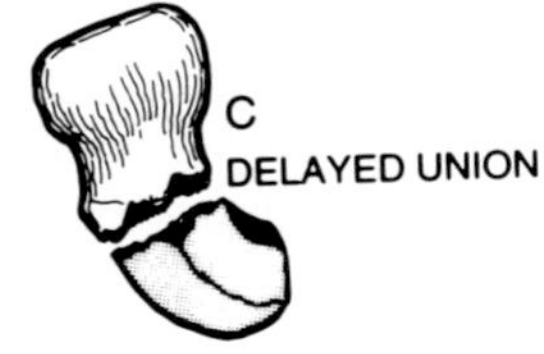

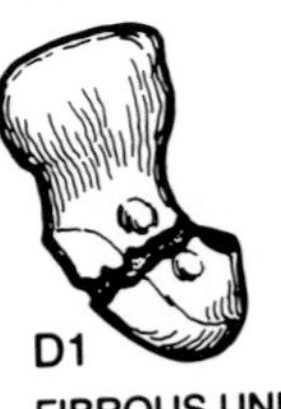
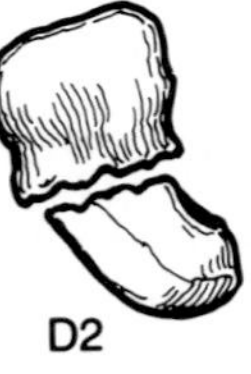

FIGURE 9–22. Herbert's classification of scaphoid fractures. (Reprinted with permission from Green DP. *Operative hand surgery.* 3rd ed. New York: Churchill Livingstone, 1993.)

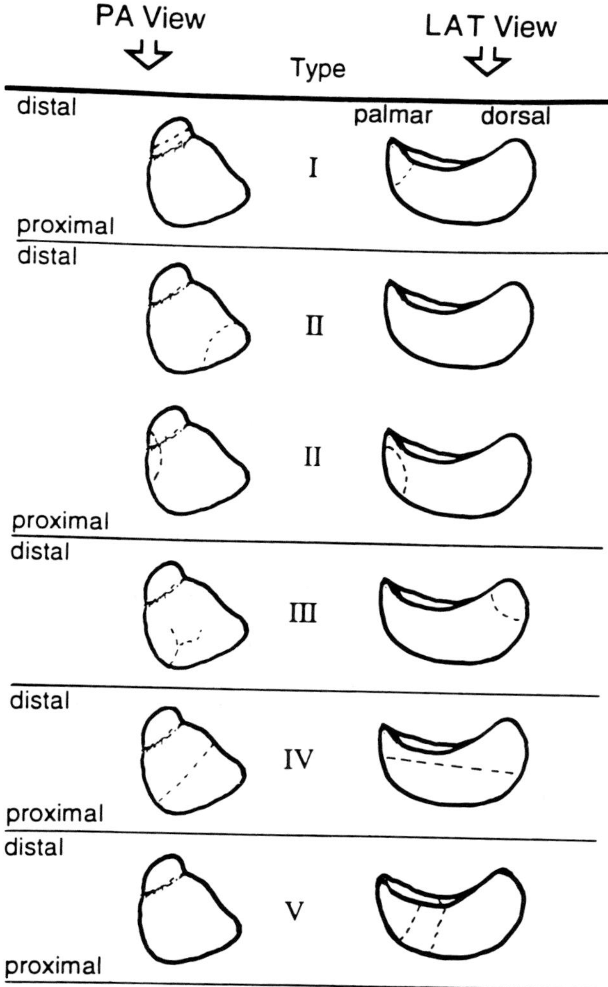

FIGURE 9–23. Classification of acute lunate fractures. I, palmar pole, may involve palmar nutrient artery; II, chip fracture; III, dorsal pole, may involve dorsal nutrient artery; IV, sagittal fracture; V, transverse fracture. (Reprinted with permission from Teisen H, Hjarbaek J. Classification of fresh fractures of the lunate. *J Hand Surg* 1988;13B:458.)

are frequently seen in association with fracture-dislocations of the wrist.

Carpal Dislocations

Based on laboratory simulations of hyperextension injuries to the wrist, Mayfield, Johnson, and Kilcoyne developed the concept of progressive perilunar instability (PPI).[106] With forced hyperextension, they observed a predictable sequence of ligamentous ruptures around the lunate (Fig. 9–26). In Stage I there was disruption of the scapholunate joint (Fig. 9–27). In Stage II the head of the capitate was subluxed on the lunate. With a Stage III injury they observed a perilunate dislocation (Figs. 9–28A and 9–28B) and in Stage IV, a ventral dislocation of the lunate (Fig. 9–29). Johnson[107] observed that dislocations in the carpus can be associated with fractures of the carpus and radial styloid. He described pure ligamentous injuries around the lunate as "lesser arc injuries" and those associated with fractures of the carpal bones adjacent to the lunate as "greater arc injuries." Cooney et al[108] classified these as Mayo Clinic Type I and Type II injuries, respectively. Greater arc injuries can include fractures extending through the radial styloid, scaphoid, capitate, hamate, and triquetrum. An example of a transradialstyloid, transscaphoid, transcapitate, transtriquetral dorsal perilunate fracture subluxation is shown in Figs. 9–30A and 9–30B.

Fractures of the Distal Radius

Classification systems for distal radius fractures usually distinguish between intraarticular and extraarticular fractures. The term *Colles's fracture* has become a colloquialism for any fracture involving the distal radius. In most current classifications it includes extraarticular fractures of the distal radius. Eponyms for intraarticular fractures include Barton's, Smith's, Chauffeur's, and die-punch fractures. Barton's fracture is one in which there is a fracture of the dorsal or ventral lip with associated subluxation of the carpus.[109] Smith's fracture refers to a fracture of the ventral lip or an extraarticular fracture with ventral angulation or ventral displacement of the distal fracture fragment.[110,111] The overlap between the definition of Barton's fracture and Thomas's subclassification of Smith's fracture is illustrated in Fig. 9–31. Chauffer's fracture refers to fractures of the radial styloid,[112] and die-punch fracture refers to those fractures involving the lunate fossa.[113,114] However, a focal depressed fracture fragment of the die-punch type could also involve the scaphoid fossa as well as the lunate fossa. A number of classification systems have been described to group these fracture patterns.[35,43,93,115–120] For brevity, we present a selection of these systems. Frykman[115] developed a classification system of intraarticular and extraarticular distal radial fractures (Fig. 9–32). This classification system, although complete, does not appear to have prognostic significance except for identification of intraarticular involvement and is used less frequently in current orthopaedic literature. In 1951 Gartland and Werley[35] classified fractures according to the degree in which the fracture extended into the articular surface. Melone has stated that most distal radius fractures with intraarticular extension consist of one or more of the following components: the radial shaft, radial styloid, a dorsomedial fragment, and a palmar-medial fragment (Fig. 9–33).[117] Melone classified distal radius fractures as follows:

Type I: Stable, minimally displaced fractures involving the lunate fossa and ulnar styloid.

Type II (die-punch fracture): Displacement of the "medial complex." These are unstable because of comminution of both the dorsal and ventral cortices of the radius, as evidenced by

Text continued on page 253

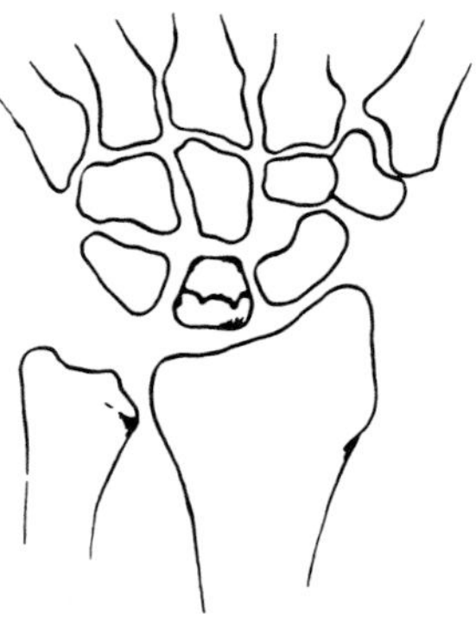

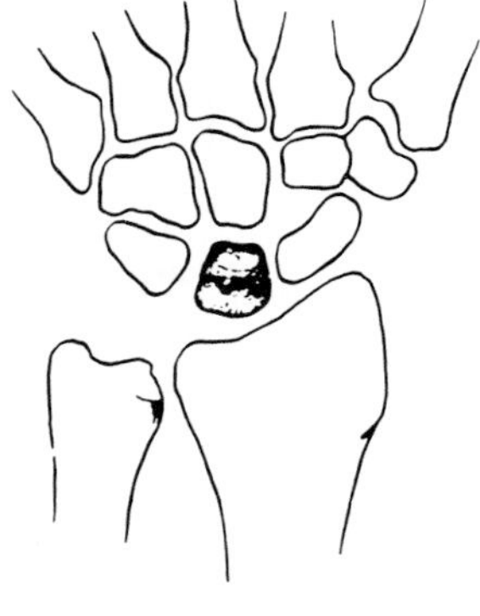

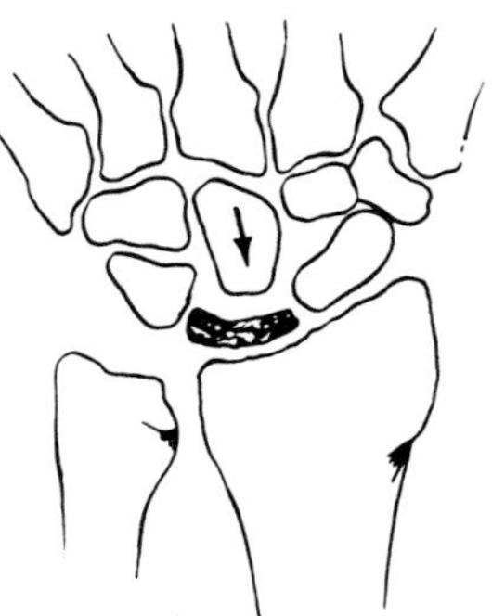

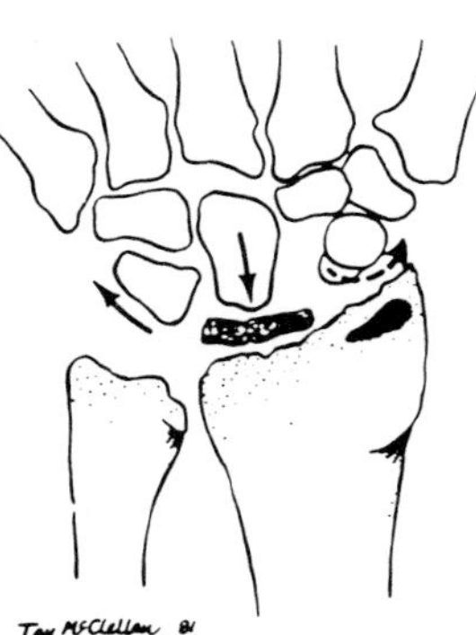

FIGURE 9–24. Schematic and plain radiographic representation of the four stages of Kienböck's disease. See description in text. (Reprinted with permission from Lichtman DM, Alexander AH, Mack GR, Gunther SF. Kienbock's disease: Update on silicone replacement arthroplasty. *J Hand Surg* 1982;7A:343–347.)

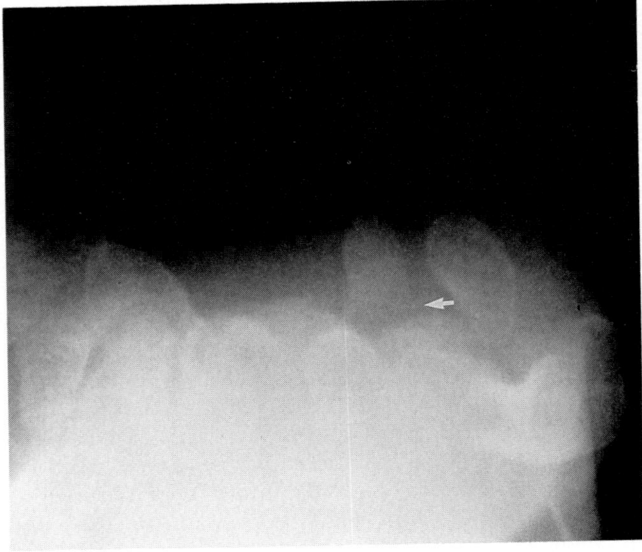

A

FIGURE 9–25. A: Hook of hamate fracture (arrow) seen on carpal tunnel view.

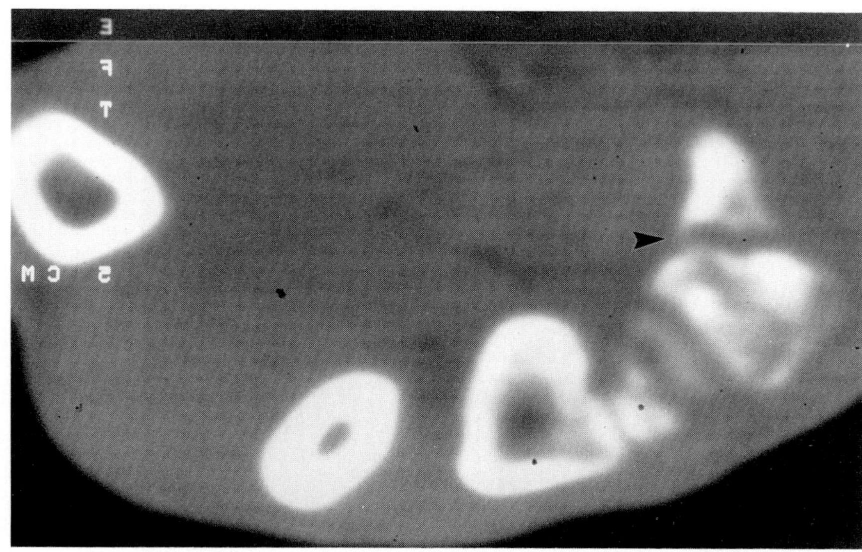

B

FIGURE 9–25 *Continued* **B:** Hook of hamate fracture (arrowhead) demonstrated on CT scan.

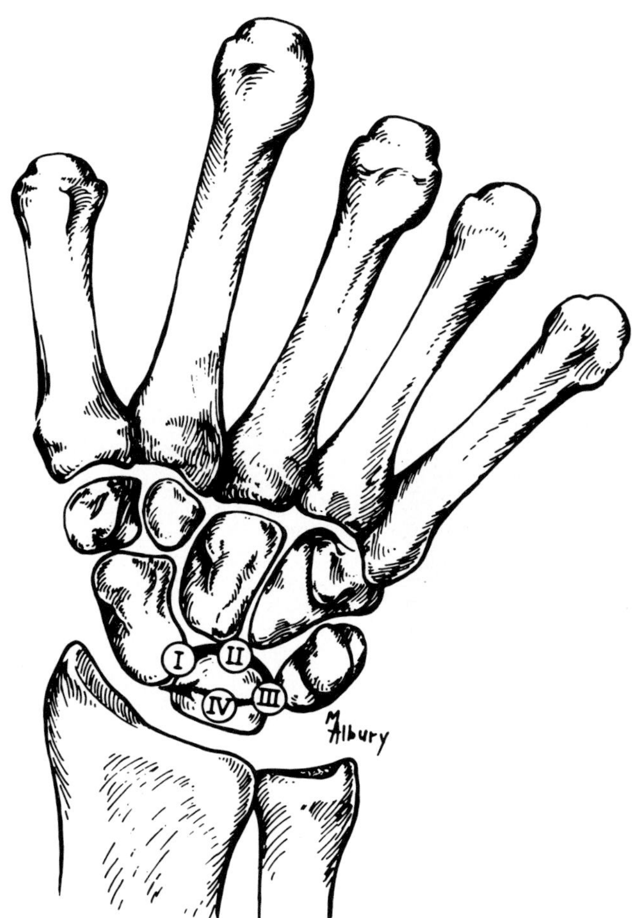

FIGURE 9–26. Mayfield's classification of four stages of PPI. See description in text. (Reprinted with permission from Mayfield JK, Johnson RP, Kilcoyne RK. Carpal dislocations: Pathomechanics and progressive perilunar instability. *J Hand Surg* 1980;5A:226–241.)

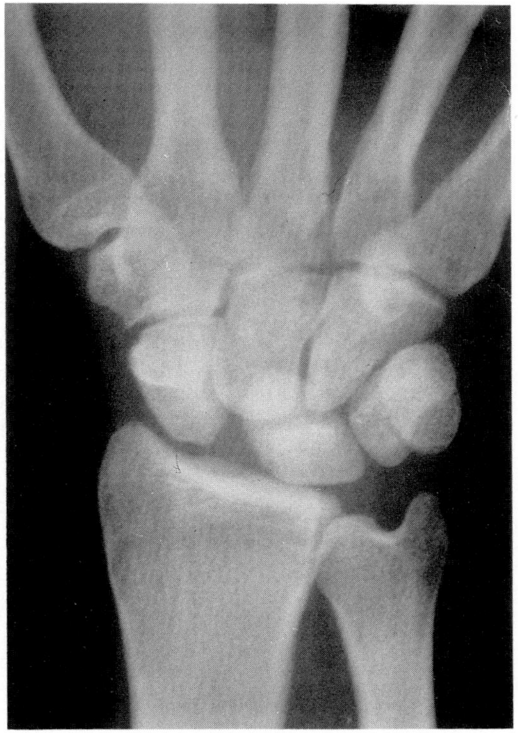

FIGURE 9–27. Mayfield Stage I PPI. Scapholunate dissociation is present.

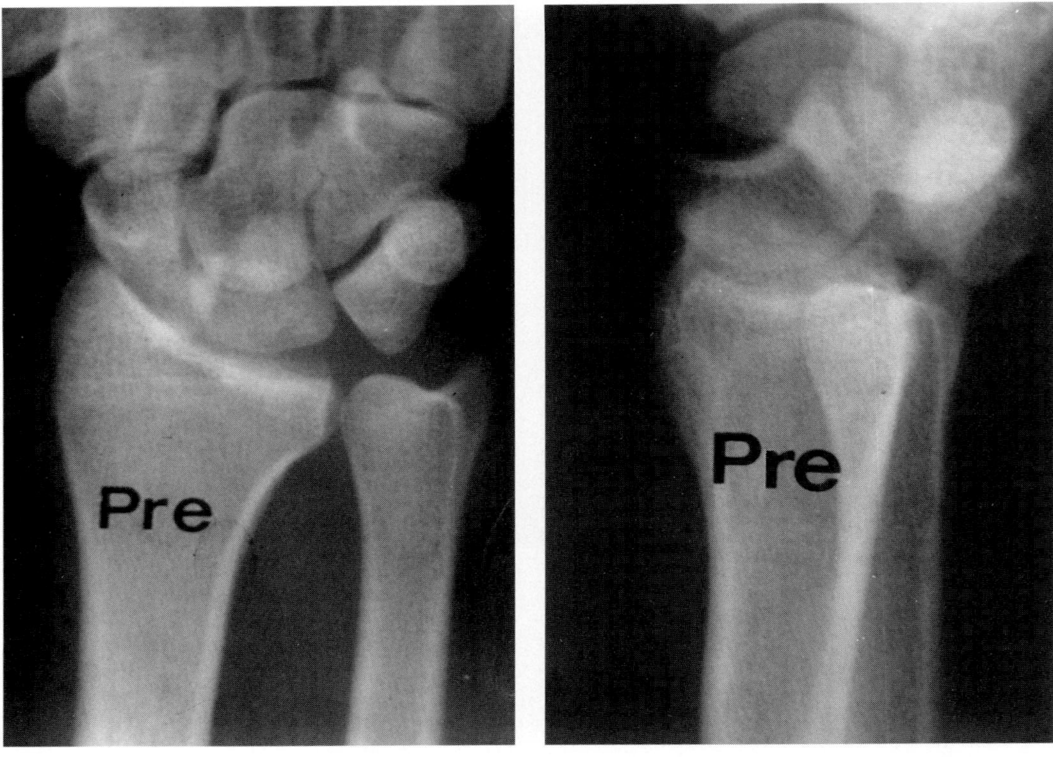

FIGURE 9–28. PA (**A**) and lateral (**B**) radiographs illustrating dorsal perilunate dislocation, Stage III PPI. (Courtesy of R. Daffner, M.D., Pittsburgh, PA.)

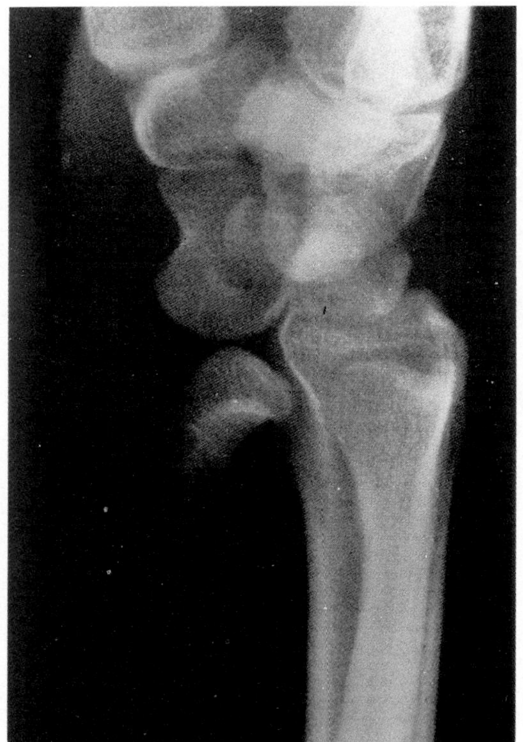

FIGURE 9–29. Stage IV PPI. A lateral radiograph illustrates ventral lunate dislocation, 180-degree ventral flip of the lunate, and ventral dislocation of the proximal pole of the scaphoid.

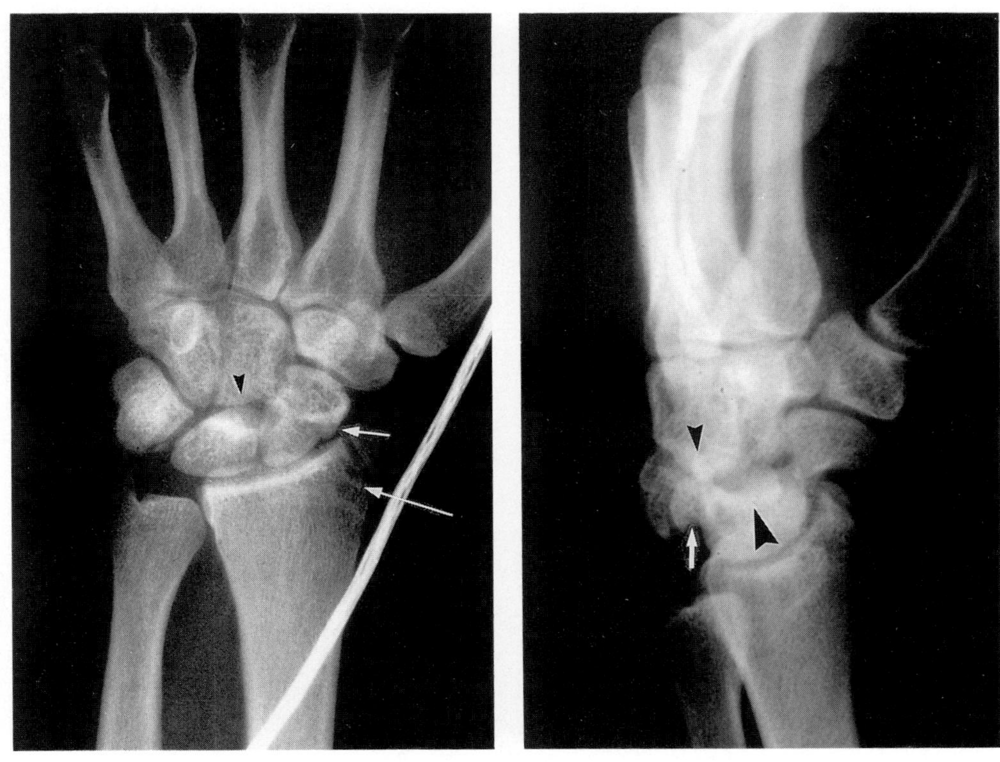

A B

FIGURE 9–30. A: PA radiograph illustrating transradialstyloid, transcapitate, transtriquetral, perilunate fracture subluxation. Long white arrow, radial styloid fracture; short white arrow, scaphoid fracture; black arrowhead, fractured neck of capitate. A small chip fracture is off the proximal radial border of the triquetrum. **B:** Lateral radiograph of case in **A.** Large black arrowhead, longitudinal axis of lunate; small black arrowhead, longitudinal axis of capitate; small white arrow, fractured head of capitate. The scaphoid waist fracture is evident overlying the ventral pole of the lunate. Additional fracture fragments of uncertain origin, but probably from the triquetrum and additional fragments of the capitate head, project dorsal to the lunate. An additional fracture fragment from either the scaphoid waist or the capitate head is at the ventral tip of the large arrowhead.

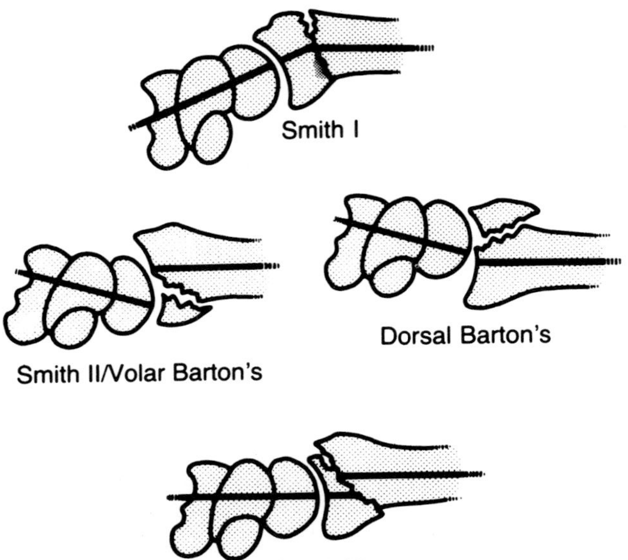

FIGURE 9–31. Thomas's classification of Smith's fractures with consolidation of the two fracture classification systems. Smith's fracture has palmar angulation or palmar displacement of a fracture fragment and Barton's fracture has dorsal or palmar rim fractures with associated subluxation of the carpus. (Reprinted with permission from Green DP. *Operative hand surgery.* 3rd ed. New York: Churchill Livingstone, 1993.)

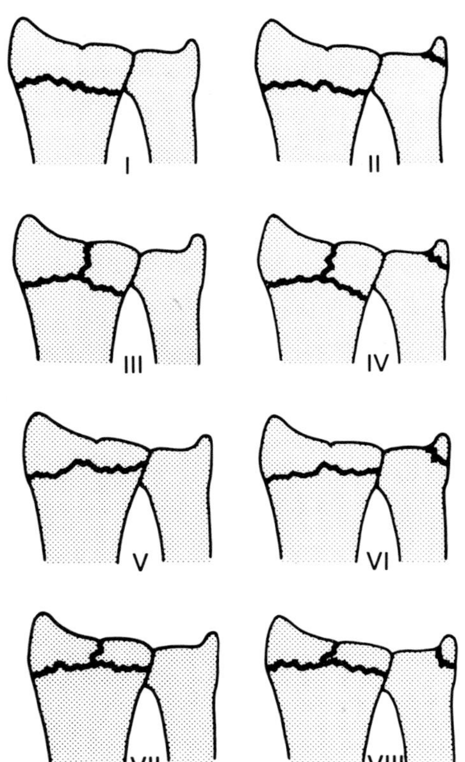

FIGURE 9–32. Frykman's classification of distal radius fractures. I and II are extraarticular fractures; III and IV are intraarticular fractures of the radiocarpal joint; V and VI are intraarticular fractures of the DRUJ; and VII and VIII are intraarticular fractures involving both the radiocarpal joint and DRUJ. Types II, IV, VI, and VIII have associated ulnar styloid fractures. (Reprinted with permission from Green DP. *Operative hand surgery.* 3rd ed. New York: Churchill Livingstone, 1993.)

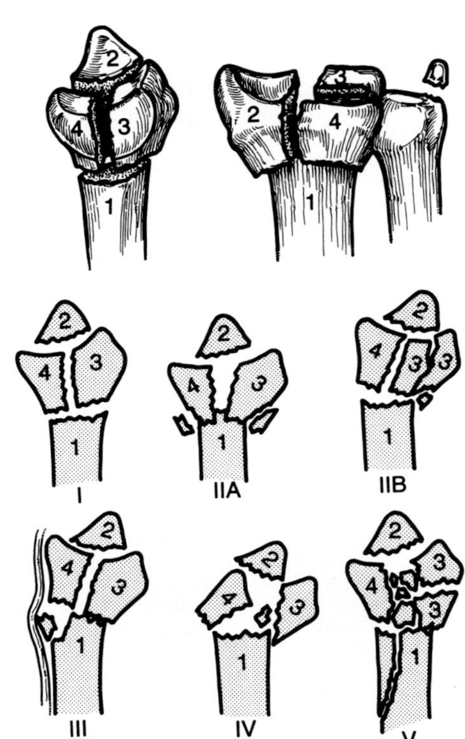

FIGURE 9–33. Melone's classification of distal radius fractures. See description in text. Top two panels: 1, shaft; 2, radial styloid; 3, dorsomedial; 4, ventromedial fragments. Types I to V illustrate the increasing comminution of fragments. (Reprinted with permission from Green DP. *Operative hand surgery.* 3rd ed. New York: Churchill Livingstone, 1993.)

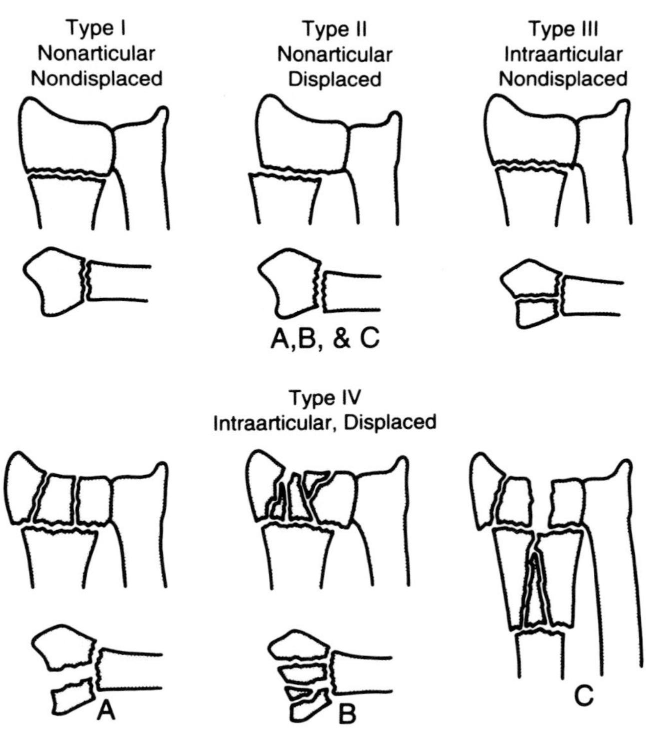

FIGURE 9–34. Rayhack's classification of distal radius fractures. (Reprinted with permission from Green DP. *Operative hand surgery.* 3rd ed. New York: Churchill Livingstone, 1993.)

Mayo Classification

Extraarticular
• Nondisplaced
• Displaced
– Stable
– Unstable

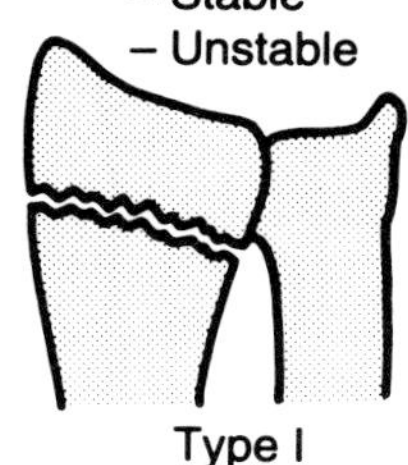

Intraarticular
• Nondisplaced
• Displaced (Reducible)
• Displaced (Unreducible)
• Complex

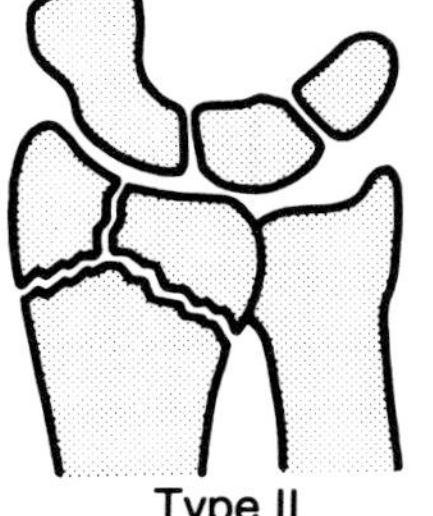

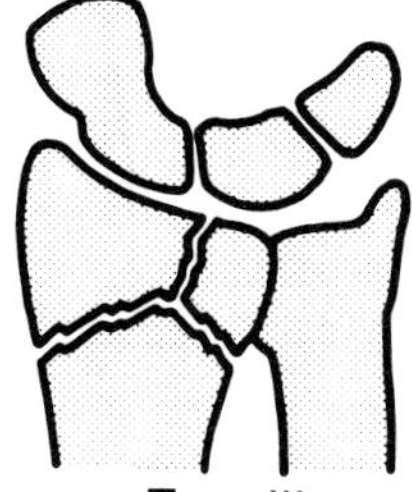

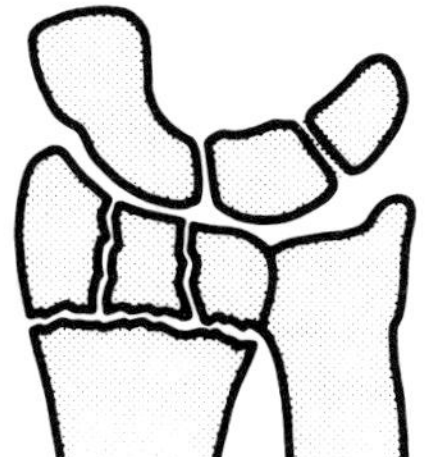

FIGURE 9–35. Mayo classification of distal radius fractures. (Reprinted with permission from Green DP. *Operative hand surgery.* 3rd ed. New York: Churchill Livingstone, 1993.)

1) separation of fracture fragments,
2) radial shortening in excess of 5 mm, and
3) angulation exceeding 20 degrees.

Type III (spike fracture): Displaced lunate fossa with a comminuted radial shaft creating a "spike fragment" that projects into the flexor compartment of the wrist.

Type IV: Split fractures with separation of the dorsal and palmar halves of the lunate fossa.

Rayhack, Langworthy, and Belsole[120] and Bradway, Amadio, and Cooney[121] independently developed classification systems that were based on whether the fracture was intraarticular or extraarticular and if it could be reduced with traction (Figs. 9–34 and 9–35). The Swiss Association for the Study of Internal Fixation (AO) has used a classification system that distinguishes extraarticular, simple intraarticular, and complex fractures.[116,122] The major contribution of this classification system is that it categorizes the locations of the fracture fragments as well as the associated comminution of the subchondral plate and the metaphysis. The ultimate value of any classification system is its ability to predict outcome. Solgaard[131] found that wrist function measured 3.5 years after a fracture of the distal radius correlated with fracture type as defined by Older, Stabler, and Cassebaum (Fig. 9–36).[119]

DEGENERATIVE CONDITIONS

Osteoarthritis

Osteoarthritis (OA) can involve any joint in the hand and wrist. The most common sites for OA are the distal and proximal interphalangeal joints, the thumb CMC joint, and the scaphotrapeziotrapezoidal (STT) joint. Posttraumatic OA in the wrist commonly involves the radioscaphoid and midcarpal joints.

Eaton and Glickel[123] described four stages of degenerative changes about the thumb CMC joint (Fig. 9–37):

Stage I: Joint may appear widened but is otherwise normal.

Stage II: Joint space narrowing and sclerosis; joint debris not greater than 2 mm in diameter.

Stage III: CMC joint obliterated, usually with subluxation of the metacarpal on the trapezium; cystic changes, sclerotic bone and varying degrees of dorsal subluxation. Bone debris greater than 2 mm.

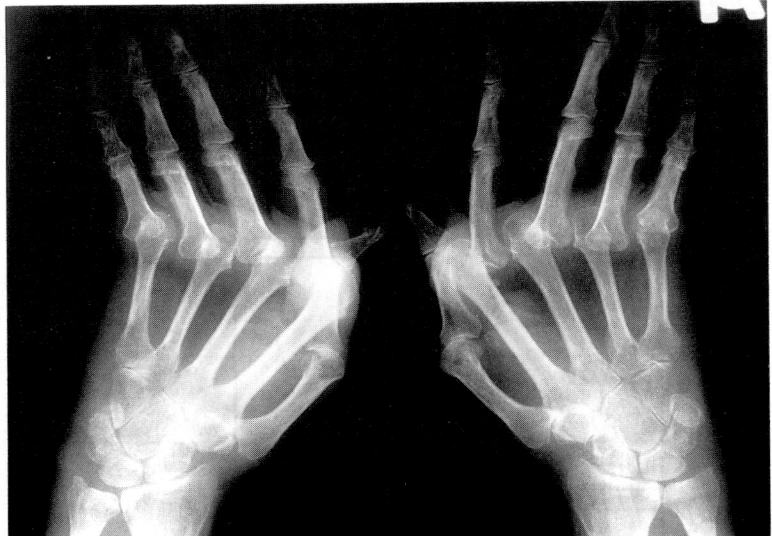

FIGURE 9–40. Ulnar deviation of the phalanges with radial deviation of the metacarpals in rheumatoid arthritis.

and ventrally subluxed in Stage III and there is ulnar deviation that is correctable on physical examination. In Stage IV there is a fixed dislocation of the MCP joint with advanced joint degeneration.

Rheumatoid Arthritis of the Wrist

The radiographic changes in the wrist can vary substantially from one patient to another. The earliest signs of erosion occur in proximity to synovial pouches, such as the ulnar styloid and along the radial aspect of the scaphoid and trapezium.[128,129] Erosion of the normal ligamentous restraints of the carpus can lead to ulnar subluxation or translocation with radial deviation of the metacarpals and ulnar deviation of the fingers, creating the "Z-deformity" (Fig. 9–40). Supination and ventral subluxation of the carpus in conjunction with laxity at the DRUJ conspire to create the caput ulnae syndrome, a dorsal subluxation of the ulnar head.[130] Palmar subluxation of the carpus can progress to radiocarpal dislocation (Fig. 9–41).

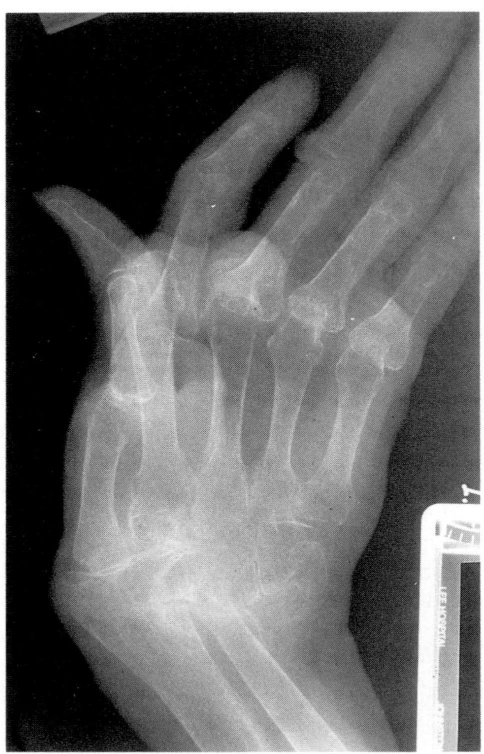

FIGURE 9–41. Ulnar radiocarpal dislocation in rheumatoid arthritis.

REFERENCES

Wrist and Hand Measurements

1. Poznanski AK. *The hand in radiologic diagnosis.* Philadelphia: WB Saunders, 1974.
2. Poznanski AK. Useful measurements in the evaluation of hand radiographs. *Hand Clin* 1991;7:21–35.
3. Cowell HR. Radiographic measurements and clinical decisions (editorial). *J Bone Joint Surg* 1990;72A:319.
4. Hardy DC, Totty WG, Reinus WR, Gilula LA. Posteroanterior wrist radiographs: Importance of arm positioning. *J Hand Surg* 1987;12A:504–508.
5. Taleisnik J. Pain on the ulnar side of the wrist. In: Taleisnik J, ed. *Hand clinics: Management of wrist problems.* Philadelphia: WB Saunders, 1987:51–68.
6. Larsen CF, Stigsby B, Mathiesen FK, Lindequist S. Radiographic examination of the wrist: A new device for standardized radiographs. *Acta Radiol* 1990;31:459–462.
7. Imamura K. Cineradiography. *J Jpn Orthop Assoc* 1987;61:499–510.
8. Johnston HM. Varying positions of the carpal bones in different movements of the wrist: Part I. *J Anat Physiol* 1907; 41:109–122.
9. Kauer JMG. Functional anatomy of the wrist. *Clin Orthop* 1980;149:9–20.
10. Kauer JMG, Landsmeer JMF. Functional anatomy of the wrist. In: Tubiana R, ed. *The hand.* Philadelphia: WB Saunders, 1981:142–157.
11. Kauer JMG. The mechanism of the carpal joint. *Clin Orthop* 1986;202:16–27.

12. Haerr CA, Gilula LA, Mann FA, Larsen CF. *Accurate assessment of the "true" neutral posteroanterior projection of the wrist: Importance of determining ulnar variance.* Presented at RSNA 93, Chicago, IL, 1993.
13. Larsen CF, Mathiesen FK, Lindequist S. Measurements of carpal bone angles on lateral wrist radiographs. *J Hand Surg* 1991;16A:888–893.
14. Larsen CF, Stigby B, Lindequist S, Bellstrom T, Mathiesen FK, Ipsen T. Observer variability in radiographic measurements of carpal bone angles on lateral radiographs of the wrist. *J Hand Surg* 1991;16A:893–898.
15. Garcia-Elias M, Kai-Nan A, Amadio PC, Cooney WP, Linscheid RL. Reliability of carpal angle determinations. *J Hand Surg* 1989;14A:1017–1021.
16. Schuind FA, Linscheid RL, An K-A, Chao EYS. A normal database of posteroanterior measurements of the wrist. *J Bone Joint Surg* 1992;74A:1418–1429.
17. McMurtry RY, Youm Y, Flatt AD, Gillespie TE. Kinematics of the wrist: II. Clinical applications. *J Bone Joint Surg* 1978;60A:955–961.
18. Youm Y, McMurtry RY, Flatt AE, Gillespie TE. Kinematics of the wrist I: An experimental study of radial-ulnar deviation and flexion-extension. *J Bone Joint Surg* 1978;60A:423–431.
19. Stahelin A, Pfeiffer K, Sennwald G, Segmuller G. Determining carpal collapse. *J Bone Joint Surg* 1989;71A:1400–1405.
20. Nattrass GR, McMurtry R, King G. *An alternate method for determination of the carpal height ratio.* Presented at the meeting of the American Society for Surgery of the Hand, Toronto, Canada, September 1990.
21. Kato H, Udui M, Minami A. Long-term results of Kienbock's disease treated by excisional arthroplasty with a silicone implant or coiled palmaris longus tendon. *J Hand Surg* 1986;11A:645–653.
22. Taleisnik J. Current concepts review: Carpal instability. *J Bone Joint Surg* 1988;70A:1262–1268.
23. Gilula LA, Weeks PM. Post-traumatic ligamentous instabilities of the wrist. *Radiology* 1978;129:641–651.
24. Chamay A, Pella Santa D, Vilaseca A. Radiolunate arthrodesis: Factor of stability for the rheumatoid wrist. *Ann Chir Main* 1983;2:5–17.
25. DiBenedetto MR, Lubbers LM, Coleman CR. Relationship between radial inclination and ulnar deviation of the fingers. *J Hand Surg* 1991;16A:36–39.
26. DiBenedetto MR, Lubbers LM, Ruff ME, Nappi JF, Coleman CR. Quantification of error in measurements of radial inclination and radial-carpal distance. *J Hand Surg* 1991;16A:399–400.
27. Pirela-Cruz MA, Firoozbakhsh K, Moneim MS. Ulnar translation of the carpus in rheumatoid arthritis: An analysis of five determination methods. *J Hand Surg* 1993;18A:299–306.
28. Friberg S, Lundstrom B. Radiographic measurements of the radio-carpal joint in normal adults. *Acta Radiol Diagn* Vol. 92, 1976;17:249–256.
29. Altissimi M, Antenucci R, Fiacca C, Mancini GB. Long-term results of conservative treatment of the distal radius. *Clin Orthop* 1986;206:202–210.
30. Aro HT, Koivunen T. Minor axial shortening of the radius affects outcome of Colles' fracture treatment. *J Hand Surg* 1991;16A:82–90.
31. Solgaard S. *Distal radius fracture* (dissertation). Copenhagen, Denmark: University of Copenhagen, 1992:1–16.
32. Warwick D, Prothero D, Field J, Bannister G. Radiological measurements of radial shortening in Colles' fracture. *J Hand Surg* 1993;18B:50–52.
33. Mann FA, Raissdana SS, Wilson AJ, Gilula LA. The influence of age and gender on radial height. *J Hand Surg* 1992;18A:711–713.
34. Mann FA, Kang SW, Gilula LA. Normal palmar tilt: Is dorsal tilting really normal? *J Hand Surg* 1992;17B:315–317.
35. Gartland JJ, Werley CW. Evaluation of healed Colles' fractures. *J Bone Joint Surg* 1951;33A:895–907.
36. DePalma AF. Comminuted fractures of the distal end of radius treated by ulnar pinning. *J Bone Joint Surg* 1952;34A:651–662.
37. Golden GN. Treatment and prognosis of Colles' fracture. *Lancet* 1963;1:511–514.
38. Smaill GB. Long-term follow-up of Colles' fracture. *J Bone Joint Surg* 1965;47B(1):145–148.
39. Sarmiento A, Pratt GW, Berry NC, Sinclair WF. Colles' fractures. *J Bone Joint Surg* 1975;57A:311–317.
40. Taleisnik J, Watson HK. Midcarpal instability caused by malunited fractures of the distal radius. *J Hand Surg* 1984;9A:350–357.
41. Van der Linden W, Ericson R. Colles' fracture: How should its displacement be measured and how should it be immobilized. *J Bone Joint Surg* 1981;63A:1285–1288.
42. Abbaszadegan H, Jonsson U, Sivers K. Prediction of Colles' fractures. *Acta Orthop Scand* 1989;60:646–650.
43. Lindstrom A. Fractures of the distal end of the radius: A clinical and statistical study of end results (dissertation). *Acta Orthop Scand* (suppl) 1959;41.
44. Knirk JL, Jupiter JB. Intra-articular fractures of the distal end of radius in young adults. *J Bone Joint Surg* 1986;68A: 647–659.
45. Rubinovich RM, Rennie WR. Colles' fracture: End results in relation to radiological parameters. *Can J Surg* 1983;26: 361–363.
46. Harper HAS, Poznanski AK, Garn SM. The carpal angle in American populations. *Invest Radiol* 1974;9:217–221.
47. Linscheid RL. Kinematic considerations of the wrist. *Clin Orthop* 1986;202:27–39.
48. Matsushita K, Firrell JC, Tsai T-M. X-ray evaluation of radial shortening for Kienbock's disease. *J Hand Surg* 1992;17A: 450–455.
49. Tornvall AH, af Ekenstam F, Hagert CG, Irstam L. Radiological examination and measurements of the wrist and distal radioulnar joint. *Acta Radiol Diagn* 1986;27:581–588.
50. Epner RA, Bowers WH, Guilford WB. Ulnar variance: The effect of wrist positioning and roentgen filming technique. *J Hand Surg* 1982A;7:298–305.
51. Palmer AK, Richard R, Glisson BS, Werner FW. Ulnar variance determination. *J Hand Surg* 1982;7A:376–379.
52. Kristensen SS, Thomassen E, Christensen F. Ulnar variance determination. *J Hand Surg* 1986;11B:255–257.
53. Steyers CM, Blair WF. Measuring ulnar variance: A comparison of techniques. *J Hand Surg* 1989;14A:607–612.
54. Gelberman RH, Salamon RB, Jurist JM, Posch JL. Ulnar variance in Kienbock's disease. *J Bone Joint Surg* 1975;57A: 674–676.
55. Czitrom AA, Dobyns JH, Linscheid RL. Ulnar variance in carpal instability. *J Hand Surg* 1987;12A:205–212.
56. Chen W-S, Shih C-H. Ulnar variance in Kienbock's disease. *Clin Orthop* 1990;255:124–127.
57. Nakamura R, Tanaka Y, Imaeda T, Miura I. The influence of age and sex on ulnar variance. *J Hand Surg* 1991;16B: 84–88.
58. Hafner R, Poznanski AK, Donovan JM. Ulnar variance in children: Standard measurements for evaluation of ulnar-shortening in juvenile rheumatoid arthritis, hereditary multiple exostosis and other bone or joint disorders in childhood. *Skeletal Radiol* 1989;18:513–516.
59. Voorhees DE, Daffner RH, Nunley JA, Gilula LA. Carpal ligamentous disruptions and negative ulnar variance. *Skeletal Radiol* 1985;13:257–262.
60. Bourne MH, Linscheid RL, Dobyns JH. Concomitant scapholunate dissociation and Kienbock's disease. *J Hand Surg* 1991;16A:460–464.
61. Larsen CF, Lindequist S, Bellstrom T. Lack of correlation between ulnar variance and carpal bone angles on wrist radiographs in normal wrists. *Acta Radiol* 1992;33:275–276.
62. Kristensen SS, Soballe K. Kienbock's disease: The influence of arthrosis on ulnar variance measurements. *J Hand Surg* 1987;12B:301–305.
63. Mirabello SC, Rosenthal DI, Smith RJ. Correlation of clinical and radiographic findings in Kienbock's disease. *J Hand Surg* 1987;12A:1049–1054.
64. Stahl F. On lunatomalacia (Kienbock's disease): Clinical and roentgenological study, especially on its pathogenesis and

late results of immobilization treatment. *Acta Chir Scand* (suppl) 1947;95.

65. Razemon JP. Kienbock's disease: Radiographic and therapeutic study: A review of 22 cases of shortening of the radius. In: Razemon JP, Fisk GF, eds. *The wrist.* Edinburgh: Churchill Livingstone, 1988:188–193.
66. Cautilli GP, Wehbe MA. Scapho-lunate distance and cortical ring sign. *J Hand Surg* 1991;16A:501–503.
67. Obermann WR. *Radiology of carpal instability: A clinical and anatomical study* (dissertation). Leiden, the Netherlands: State University Leiden, 1991.
68. Kindynis P, Resnick D, Kang HS, Haller J, Sartoris DJ. Demonstration of the scapholunate space with radiology. *Radiology* 1990;175:278–280.
69. Nakamura R, Hori M, Imamura T, Horii E, Miura T. Method for measurement and evaluation of carpal bone angles. *J Hand Surg* 1989;14A:412–416.
70. Linscheid RL, Dobyns JH, Beabout JW, Bryan RS. Traumatic carpal instability of the wrist: Diagnosis, classification, and pathomechanics. *J Bone Joint Surg* 1972;54A:1612–1632.
71. Sarrafian SK, Melamed JL, Goshgarian GM. Study of wrist motion in flexion and extension. *Clin Orthop* 1977;126: 153–159.
72. Reagan DS, Linscheid RL, Dobyns JH. Lunotriquetral sprains. *J Hand Surg* 1984;9A:502–513.
73. Chaise F, Rogers B, Witvoet J, Laval-Jeantet M. Analyse de l'incidence radiologique de profil du carpe normal. *Ann Radiol* 1985;28:381–386.
74. Yamada J. A cineradiographic study of normal wrist motion. *J Jpn Orthop Assoc* 1988;62:1043–1054.
75. Belsole RJ, Hilbelink DR, Llewellyn A, Dale M, Ogden JA. Carpal orientation from computed reference axes. *J Hand Surg* 1991;16A:82–90.
76. Nishikawa T, Nakamura R, Kanie J, Hori M, Miura T. Functional radiography of the wrist joint. *J Jpn Hand Assoc* 1985;2:54–57.
77. Meyrueis JP, Cameli M, Jan P. Instabilité du carpe: Diagnostic et formes clinques. *Ann Chir* 1978;32:555–560.
78. Micks JE. A method for evaluating carpal alignment on lateral radiographs. *J Hand Surg* 1985;10A:580–582.
79. Kirk JA, Ansell BM, Bywaters EGL. The hypermobility syndrome: Musculoskeletal complaints associated with generalized joint hypermobility. *Ann Rheum Dis* 1967;26:419–425.
80. Grahame R. Joint hypermobility: Clinical aspects. *Proc R Soc Med* 1971;64:692–694.
81. Scott D, Bird H, Wright V. Joint laxity leading to osteoarthrosis. *Rheumat Rehab* 1979;18:167–169.
82. Bird HA. *Joint hypermobility* (dissertation). Cambridge, UK: The University of Leeds, 1980.
83. Weeks PM, Vannier MW, Stevens WG, Gayou D, Gilula LA. Three dimensional imaging of the wrist. *J Hand Surg* 1985A;10:32–39.
84. Viegas SF, Patterson RM, Todd PD, McCarty P. Measurement of carpal bone geometry by computer analysis of three dimensional CT images. *J Hand Surg* 1993;18A:341–349.
85. Meade TD, Schneider LH, Cherry K. Radiographic analysis of selective ligament sectioning at the carpal scaphoid: A cadaver study. *J Hand Surg* 1990;15A:855–862.
86. Chan KP, Huang P. Anatomic variations in radial and ulnar lengths in the wrists of Chinese. *Clin Orthop* 1971;80:17–20.

Classification Schemes

87. Leddy JP, Packer JW. Avulsion of the profundus tendon insertion in athletes. *J Hand Surg* 1977A;2:66–69.
88. Robins PR, Dobyns JH. Avulsion of the insertion of the flexor digitorum profundus tendon associated with fracture of the distal phalanx: A brief review. In: *AAOS symposium on tendon surgery in the hand.* St. Louis: CV Mosby, 1975:151.
89. Eaton RG, Littler JW. Joint injuries and their sequelae. *Clin Plast Surg* 1976;3:85–98.
90. Barton NJ. Intra-articular fractures and fracture-dislocations. In: Bowers WH, ed. *The interphalangeal joints.* Edinburgh: Churchill Livingstone, 1987:77–93.
91. Steele WM. Articular fractures. In: Barton NJ, ed. *Fractures of the hand and wrist.* Edinburgh: Churchill Livingstone, 1988:55–73.
92. Kraemer BA, Gilula LA. Phalangeal fractures and dislocations. In: Gilula LA, ed. *The traumatized hand and wrist: Radiographic and anatomic correlation.* Philadelphia: WB Saunders, 1992:105–170.
93. Bennett EH. Fractures of the metacarpal bones. *Dublin J Med Sci* 1882;73:72–75.
94. Billing L, Gedda KO. Roentgen examination of Bennett's fracture. *Acta Radiol* 1952;38:471–476.
95. Green DP, O'Brien ET. Fractures of the thumb metacarpal. *South Med J* 1972;42:931.
96. Russe O. Fracture of the carpal navicular: Diagnosis, non-operative treatment and operative treatment. *J Bone Joint Surg* 1960;42A:759–768.
97. Green DP. *Operative hand surgery.* 2nd ed. New York: Churchill Livingstone, 1988:813–873.
98. Herbert TJ. *The fractured scaphoid.* St. Louis: Quality Medical Publishing, 1990:62.
99. Teisen H, Hjarbaek J. Classification of fresh fractures of the lunate. *J Hand Surg* 1988;13B:458–462.
100. Gelberman RH, Bauman TD, Menon J, Akeson WH. The vascularity of the lunate bone and Kienbock's disease. *J Hand Surg* 1980;5:272–278.
101. Lichtman DM, Alexander AH, Mack GR, Gunther SF. Kienbock's disease: Update on silicone replacement arthroplasty. *J Hand Surg* 1982;7A:343–347.
102. Linscheid RL. Kienbock's disease. *J Hand Surg* 1985;10A:1–3.
103. Hulten O. Uber anatomische Variationen der Gelenkknochen. *Acta Radiol Scand* 1928;9:155–168.
104. Milch H. Fracture of the hamate bone. *J Bone Joint Surg* 1934;16:459–462.
105. Palmer AK. Trapezial ridge fractures. *J Hand Surg* 1981; 6:561–567.
106. Mayfield JK, Johnson RP, Kilcoyne RK. Carpal dislocations: Pathomechanics and progressive perilunar instability. *J Hand Surg* 1980;5A:226–241.
107. Johnson RP. The acutely injured wrist and its residuals. *Clin Orthop* 1980;149:33–44.
108. Cooney WP, Bussey R, Dobyns JH, Linscheid RL. Difficult wrist fractures: Perilunate fracture-dislocations of the wrist. *Clin Orthop* 1987;214:136–147.
109. Barton JR. Views and treatment of an important injury to the wrist. *Med Examiner* 1838;1:365.
110. Peltier LF. Eponymic fractures: Robert William Smith and Smith's fracture. *Surgery* 1959;45:1035–1042.
111. Thomas FB. Reduction of Smith's fracture. *J Bone Joint Surg* 1957;39B:463–470.
112. Edwards HC. The mechanism and treatment of backfire fracture. *J Bone Joint Surg* 1926;8:701–711.
113. Cotton FJ. The pathology of fracture of the lower extremity of the radius. *Ann Surg* 1900;32:388–415.
114. Scheck M. Long-term follow-up of treatment of comminuted fractures of the distal end of the radius by transfixation with Kirschner wires and cast. *J Bone Joint Surg* 1962;44A:337–351.
115. Frykman G. Fracture of the distal radius including sequelae: Shoulder-hand-finger syndrome, disturbance in the distal radioulnar joint and impairment of nerve function. *Acta Orthop Scand* (suppl) 1967;108:1–155.
116. Heim U, Pfeiffer KM. *Small fragment set manual.* 2nd ed. New York: Springer-Verlag, 1982:119.
117. Melone CP. Articular fractures of the distal radius. *Orthop Clin North Am* 1984;15:217–236.
118. Nissen-Lie H. Fracture radii "typica." *Norsk Magasin for Laegevidenskapen* 1939;1:293–303.
119. Older TM, Stabler VE, Cassebaum WH. Colles fracture: Evaluation and selection of therapy. *J Trauma* 1965;5:469–476.
120. Rayhack JM, Langworthy JN, Belsole RJ. Transulnar percutaneous pinning of displaced distal radius fractures: A preliminary report. *J Orthop Trauma* 1989;3:107–114.
121. Bradway JK, Amadio PC, Cooney WP. Open reduction and internal fixation of displaced, comminuted intra-articular

fractures of the distal end of the radius. *J Bone Joint Surg* 1989;71A:839–847.

122. Prince H, Worlock P. The small external fixator in the treatment of unstable distal forearm fractures. *J Hand Surg* 1988;13B:294–297.
123. Eaton RG, Glickel SZ. Trapeziometacarpal osteoarthritis: Staging as a rationale for treatment. *Hand Clin* 1987;3:455–471.
124. Larsen A, Dale K, Eek M. Radiographic evaluation of rheumatoid arthritis and related conditions by standard reference films. *Acta Radiol Diagn* 1977;18:481–491.
125. Nalebuff EA. The rheumatoid swan-neck deformity. *Hand Clin* 1989;5:203–214.
126. Nalebuff EA, Millender CH. Surgical treatment of the boutonniere deformity in rheumatoid arthritis. *Orthop Clin North Am* 1975;6:753–763.
127. Wilson RL, Carlblom ER. The rheumatoid metacarpophalangeal joint. *Hand Clin* 1989;5:223–237.
128. Bywaters EGL. The early radiological signs of rheumatoid arthritis. *Bull Rheum Dis* 1960;11:231–234.
129. Martel W, Hayes JT, Duff IF. The pattern of bone erosion in the hand and wrist in rheumatoid arthritis. *Radiology* 1965;84:204–214.
130. Backdahl M. The caput ulnae syndrome in rheumatoid arthritis: A study of the morphology, abnormal anatomy and clinical picture. *Acta Rheumatol Scand* 1963;5:1–75.

CHAPTER 10

NORMAL VARIANTS

Jürgen Freyschmidt and Sylvia Venzke

INTRODUCTION

Compared with other anatomic regions, the hand has a disproportionately large number of small irregular and tubular bones in a very confined space. It is easily understandable that the individual development of all the bones and the coordinated development of the bony structures leads to more disturbances of growth here than in other skeletal regions, along with the consequences of innumerable variants and true malformations. This justifies a special chapter on the variants of normal hand development. The definition of variants as a link between normal and early pathology can be extremely difficult and is based on experience. This experience has been collected for decades in the book by A. Köhler and E. A. Zimmer.* Its 13th German and 4th English editions have been revised and edited by us together with H. Schmidt. The generosity of the publisher, G. Hauff, made it possible for us to borrow a number of figures from this book.

Our definition of a "variant" is an anatomic structure that is (a) not caused by a genetic aberration, (b) usually clinical asymptomatic, and (c) found by chance on radiographs. It could be compared with a large, tiny, or crooked nose. Such a variant only rarely leads to symptomatic disease, such as bursitis or necrosis caused by an accessory bone interfering with normal motion because of its "unphysiologic" location. The main problem with such variants is the possibility of mistaking them for the result of trauma or for changes caused by local infection or generalized inflammatory or metabolic processes. Because the transition between "variant" and true pathologic change can only be understood if one knows the symptomatology of true pathology, this chapter includes a large number of unambiguously pathologic alterations of the hand skeleton.

* *Köhler A and Zimmer EA. Grenzen des Normalen und Anfänge des Pathologischen im Röntgenbild des Skeletts. 13th German ed. 1989;* Borderlands of normal and early pathologic findings in skeletal radiography, *4th English ed. Schmidt H, Freyschmidt J, eds. Stuttgart, New York: Thieme, 1993.*

DEVELOPMENT

The Long Hand Bones

At birth phalangeal and metacarpal diaphyses are ossified. The epiphyses ossify later; those of the distal and middle phalanges ossify between 5 months and 2 years of age and those of the proximal phalanges do so later. Fusion of the epiphyseal plates occurs at ages 15 (metacarpals) to 17 (distal/middle phalanges) to 18 (proximal phalanges). Fusion in females occurs approximately 2 years prior to that in males. The epiphyseal centers of the phalanges are located proximally, as is the ossification center of the first metacarpal. In contrast, the epiphyseal centers of the second through fifth metacarpals are localized distally. Roentgenographic morphology shows the asymmetric (thickened palmar portion, Fig. 10–1) development of the epiphyses of the proximal phalanges. During adolescence the epiphyses can appear relatively broad (Fig. 10–2). The epiphyseal lines of the metacarpal heads in particular show a characteristic course (Fig. 10–3).

The Short Hand Bones

The appearance of the epiphyseal centers of the carpal bones can vary widely, and multiple ossification centers can occur in any of the carpal bones. A wide range of potential pitfalls results from these multiple ossification centers. The first calcified epiphyseal centers are those of the capitate and hamate (before 6 months of age). The triquetrum appears in the second year of life, and doubled epiphyseal centers of the triquetrum are visible regularly. The onset of ossification of the lunate ranges from the second to the fifth year. Rarely, two ossification centers occur. The trapezium, trapezoid, and scaphoid centers are detectable at age 5, and two ossification centers may be visible in the scaphoid. The pisiform ossifies in the ninth to tenth year and shows multiple ossification centers almost regularly. These centers can appear irregular in shape and structure and should not be misinterpreted as an osteochondrosis (Fig. 10–4).

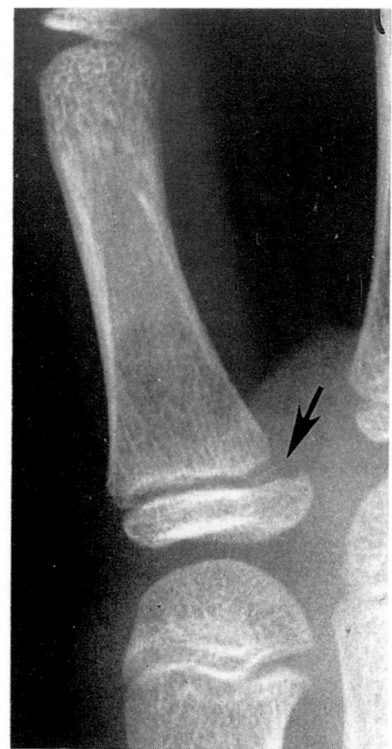

FIGURE 10–1. A "step" (arrow) involves the palmoulnar side.

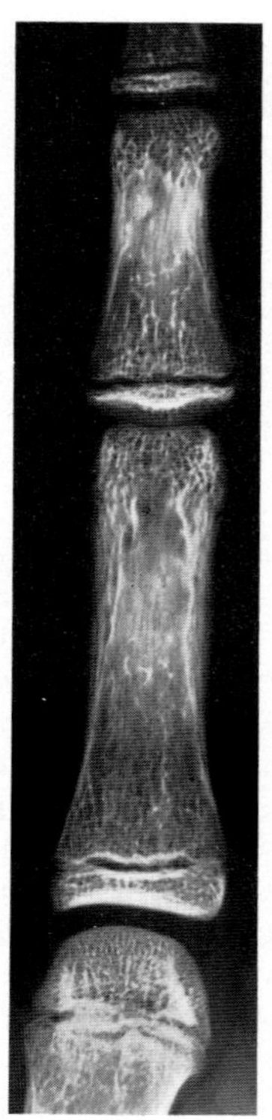

FIGURE 10–2. Broad epiphysis in a 13- to 15-year-old boy. (Reprinted with permission from Schmidt H, Freyschmidt J, eds. *Borderlands of normal and early pathologic findings in skeletal radiology.* 4th English ed. Stuttgart, New York: Thieme, 1993.)

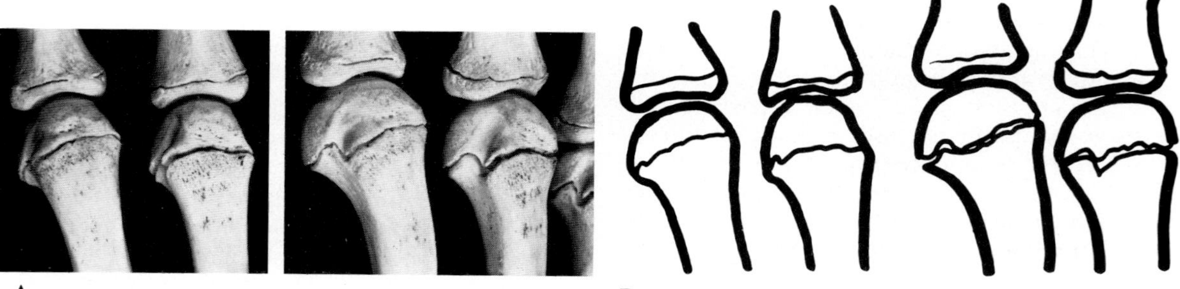

FIGURE 10–3. Epiphyseal lines of the metacarpal heads, shown schematically **(A)** and anatomically **(B)**. (Reprinted with permission from Schmidt H, Freyschmidt J, eds. *Borderlands of normal and early pathologic findings in skeletal radiology.* 4th English ed. Stuttgart, New York: Thieme, 1993.)

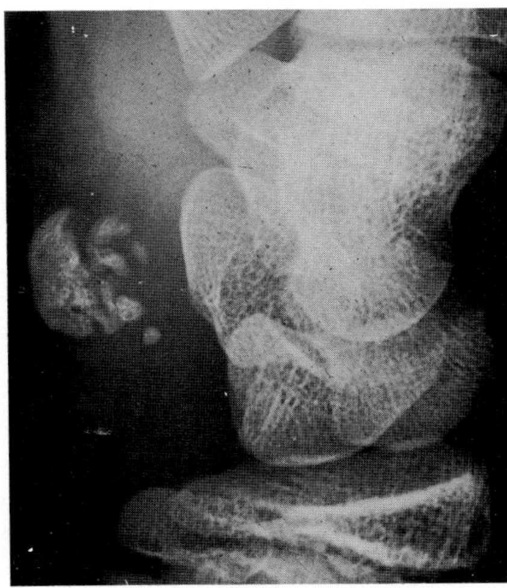

FIGURE 10–4. Multiple ossification centers of the pisiform. Not an osteochondrosis. (Reprinted with permission from Schmidt H, Freyschmidt J, eds. *Borderlands of normal and early pathologic findings in skeletal radiology.* 4th English ed. Stuttgart, New York: Thieme, 1993.)

Figure 10–5A demonstrates the case of unusual ossification of the distal pole of the scaphoid in an otherwise normally developed boy. The irregular structure of the scaphoid could be interpreted as an infectious process involving the cartilaginous structures, but magnetic resonance imaging (MRI) showed an intact cartilage. Follow-up 1 year later (Fig. 10–5B) showed smoothing of the structures secondary to further ossification of the previously invisible distal pole of the scaphoid.

The Distal Forearm

The distal radial epiphysis becomes visible at the age of 8 to 18 months, and the distal ulnar epiphysis usually appears with two ossification centers at the age of 6 years. Between the fifth and tenth years of life, the epiphysis of the distal radius is smaller in size than the metaphysis, especially on the lateral view. The irregular width of the epiphyseal line should not lead to misinterpretation as epiphyseal separation. The epiphysis has its final size at the age of 18 years and shows a typical spur at its radial side before fusion (Fig. 10–6).

VARIANTS AND DEVELOPMENT DISORDERS

The Long Hand Bones

The long hand bones are monoepiphyseal tubular bones. The appearance of multiple ossification centers is a normal finding in epiphyseal growth and should never be misinterpreted as a fragmentation of the epiphysis. Multiple ossification centers are commonly visible at the proximal phalanx of the index and small fingers and are sometimes misinterpreted as Thiemann's disease (congenital acrodysplasia with

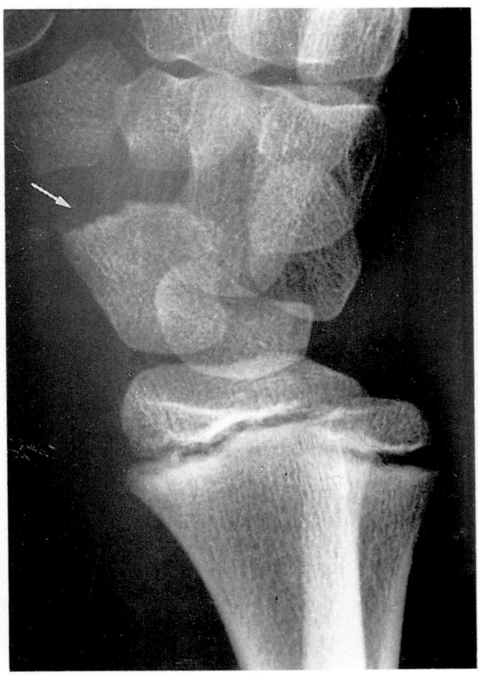

A

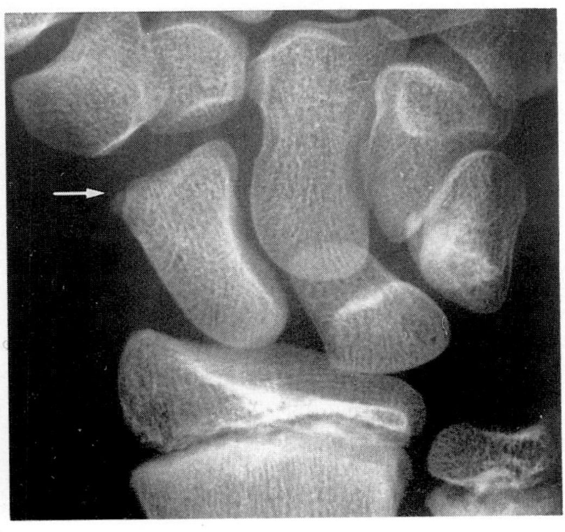

B

FIGURE 10–5. A: Irregular distal pole of the scaphoid (arrow) in a 14- to 16-year-old boy, on a radiograph taken after trauma. No pain in patient's history. **B:** Follow-up after 1 year. Smoothing of the distal pole (arrow). (Reprinted with permission from Schmidt H, Freyschmidt J, eds. *Borderlands of normal and early pathologic findings in skeletal radiology.* 4th English ed. Stuttgart, New York: Thieme, 1993.)

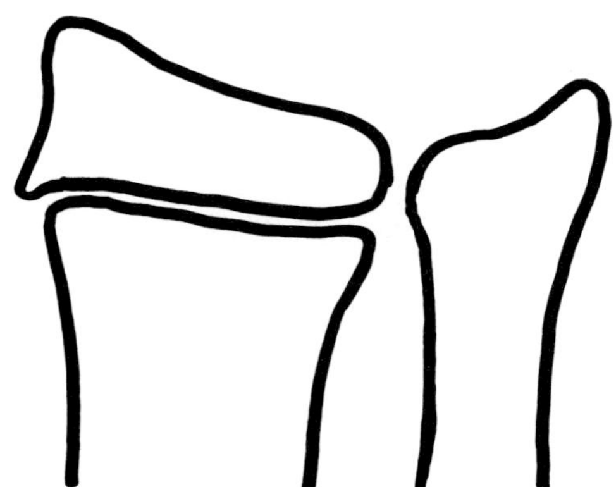

FIGURE 10–6. Schematic illustration of the typical shape of the growth plate. Small spur on the radial side is a normal finding.

aseptic necroses of the phalanges), which is predominately found during puberty. Multiple epiphyseal ossification centers of the first metacarpal have the differential diagnosis of an aseptic epiphyseal necrosis found in Dietrich's disease. Typical findings in epiphyseal necrosis (Fig. 10–7), however, such as joint space widening and a beak-like transformation of the epiphyses, are not visible.

Another entity in the differential diagnosis of Thiemann's disease are the so-called dense or ivory epiphyses, which occur as a normal variant in the distal phalanges and the middle phalanx of the small finger. They are smaller in size than the corresponding epiphyses and may change so as to appear normal during growth and maturation. The higher density on radiographs is based on an inadequate differentiation of the spongiosa. An association of dense or ivory epiphyses with epiphyseal necrosis is reported.[1] Retardation of skeletal development secondary to acquired diseases (i.e., renal osteodystrophy) or congenital disorders (hypothyroidism) may also cause dense epiphyses,[2] but the location and number of these pathologically dense epiphyses distinguish them from transient variants of normal.

Ossification disturbance in rickets is caused by a lack of calcification of the otherwise normal osteoid. Highly specific changes of the epiphyses arise. The first change is a disappearance of the metaphyseal ring (virole) of the distal forearms and metacarpals. Demineralization of the epiphyseal ossification centers with widening of the epimetaphyseal space follows.[3] Figure 10–8 demonstrates cupping of the metaphyses in rickets, which should be easily differentiated from normal epiphyseal regions. It is impossible to determine the etiologic factors of rickets on radiographs, but at least it can be detected early.

The so-called cone epiphyses of the phalanges (Fig. 10–9) are caused by a disturbance of the temporal sequence of growth. The growth of the central region is transiently arrested or blocked while the peripheral regions continue to grow. They occur in otherwise healthy children but also in those with congenital anomalies or endocrine disorders. Giedion classified cone epiphyses and found that some cone epiphyses may be pathognomonic for certain malformations and acquired conditions, such as trauma, infection, or infarction.[4] Cone epiphyses accompanied by brachydactyly of some of the metacarpals and phalanges were found in hyperthyroidism in children, probably secondary to an accelerated skeletal maturation.[5]

Additional epiphyses are a rare finding both in the

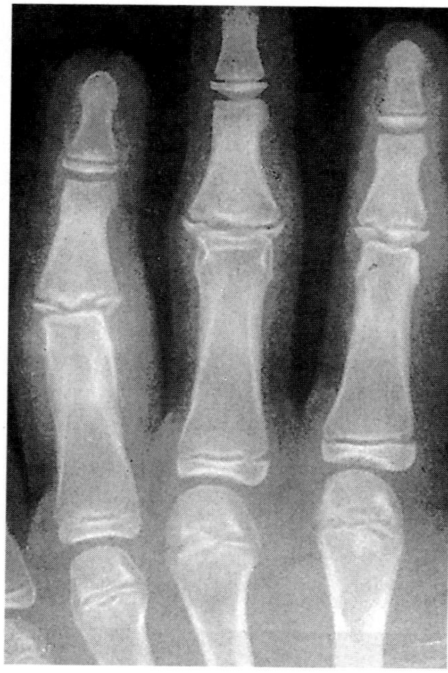

FIGURE 10–7. Thiemann's disease with typical beak-like transformation of the epiphyseal centers. (Reprinted with permission from Schmidt H, Freyschmidt J, eds. *Borderlands of normal and early pathologic findings in skeletal radiology.* 4th English ed. Stuttgart, New York: Thieme, 1993.)

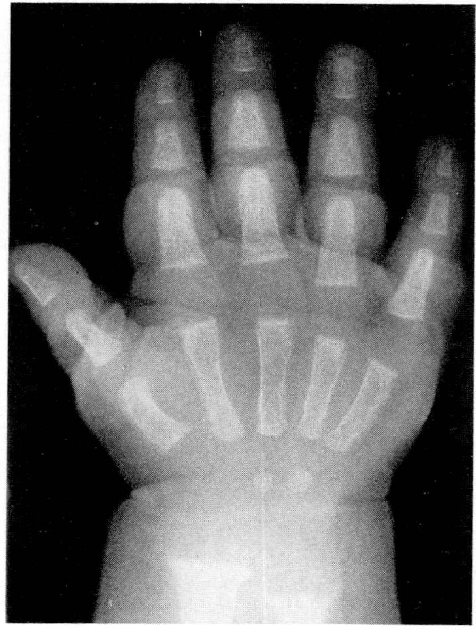

FIGURE 10–8. Rickets in a 1-year-old girl. Typical cupping of the metaphyses.

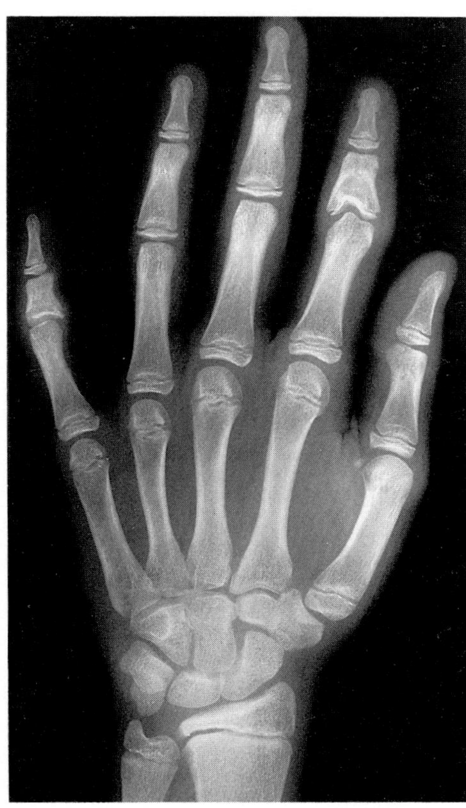

FIGURE 10–9. Cone epiphyses of the middle phalanges of digits 2 to 4 in a 13-year-old girl. Brachymesophalangy D_5; patient's history is unknown. D, digit.

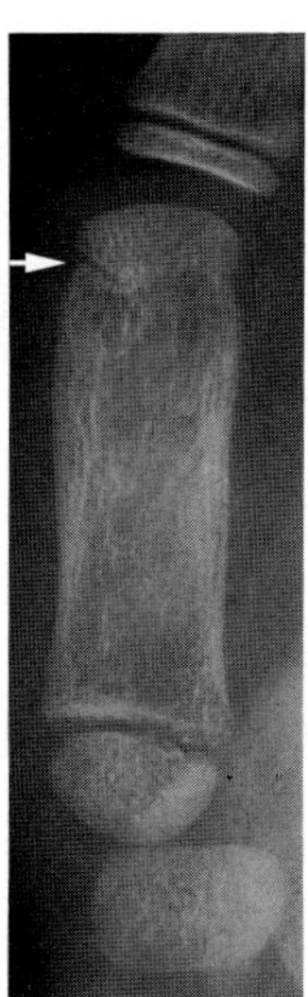

FIGURE 10–10. Additional epiphysis (pseudoepiphysis) in the distal end of the first metacarpal (arrow). (Reprinted with permission from Schmidt H, Freyschmidt J, eds. *Borderlands of normal and early pathologic findings in skeletal radiology.* 4th English ed. Stuttgart, New York: Thieme, 1993.)

normally developed and diseased child. They are erroneously called "pseudoepiphyses." They can be seen particularly in the first metacarpal distally and in the second metacarpal proximally (Fig. 10–10). The additional epiphyses appear earlier, grow more rapidly than the normal epiphyses, and fuse earlier with the diaphyses. (Fig. 10–11). Fusion is often complete before the age of 10 years.[6]

The Short Hand Bones

By a lack of segmentation in development, carpal synostoses may occur as normal variants usually involving the corresponding row.[7] The most common synostoses are the lunotriquetral and the capitohamate coalitions. A possibly compensatory wide scapholunate joint space is seen regularly in lunotriquetral synostosis.[8] Synostoses involving multiple carpal bones or both rows are described in congenital anomalies (Holt–Oram syndrome, oto-palato-digital syndrome, and others).[7] As Taylor et al reported, synostoses in the medial bones of the distal row rather than interrow are synostoses found in Ellis–van Creveld syndrome.[9]

Acquired carpal fusions can result from rheumatoid and other arthritides, posttraumatic conditions, and inflammatory bone lesions, particularly during growth.[6]

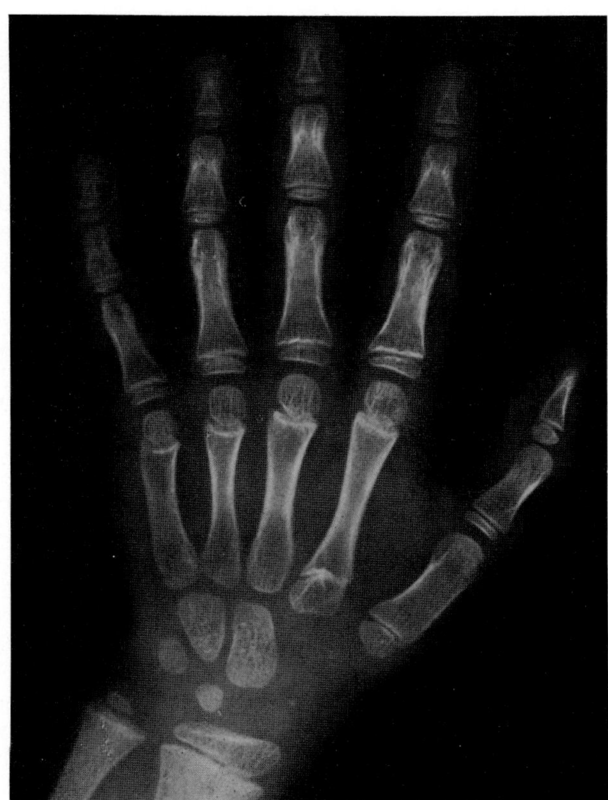

FIGURE 10–11. Premature fusion of an additional epiphysis proximally at the second metacarpal in a 10-year-old boy. (Reprinted with permission from Schmidt H, Freyschmidt J, eds. *Borderlands of normal and early pathologic findings in skeletal radiology.* 4th English ed. Stuttgart, New York: Thieme, 1993.)

Synostoses may be mimicked on radiographs by superimposition of adjacent structures, especially by incorrect projection. Usually the bony structures reveal normally shaped bones after the radiograph is repeated in standard position or if the space between the overlapping structures is profiled, as with fluoroscopy.

THE HAND IN THE ADULT

The Long Hand Bones

The shape of the long hand bones is influenced by sex, constitution, and the type and extent of mechanical stress placed on them. People who do heavy manual labor will often have thick, dense bones with prominent muscle attachments, while slender delicate bones are seen in people who are mainly engaged in nonmanual labor and do not play sports. Pathologic enlargement (i.e., in acromegaly) as well as shortening (i.e., in hypothyroidism) can occur. It may be proportionate or disproportionate, unilateral or symmetric. A *proportionately* short or enlarged hand skeleton usually signifies endocrine disorders. Disproportionate changes in size of the long hand bones indicate congenital anomalies or focal acquired causes, such as early closure of an epiphysis from trauma or sickle cell disease.

In radiologic anthropometry various measurements are described in an attempt to assess supposedly pathologic findings using the length of metacarpals and phalanges. The phalangeal sign according to Kosowicz is useful in the determination of the ratio between phalangeal and metacarpal length. Normally the sum of the length of distal and proximal phalanges should be equal to that of the corresponding metacarpal.[10] Another method—a tangential line drawn from the fifth to the fourth metacarpal head should not intersect the third metacarpal head—developed by Archibald, Finby, and De Vito,[11] was found to be positive in otherwise healthy people,[12] which means that shortened fourth and fifth metacarpals may be normal variants, especially if no other changes exist. Further details are discussed by Poznanski.[7]

Distal Phalanges

Normal Findings and Variants in Shape

The size and form of the distal phalangeal tufts is variable and, as mentioned above, depends on constitutional conditions and muscular stress. The outer contour can appear irregular and spiculated because of variations of small spurs extending from the tufts. With age, the shape of the tuft changes from a nearly conical to a more rounded form, and thorn-like overgrowths, which are most prominent on the palmar side, can appear in the elderly (Fig. 10–12). Such normal findings must be differentiated from cartilaginous exostoses (osteochondromata), which are rare and occur at the bases of the distal phalanges near the former growth plate and not at the tufts. For further details, see Freyschmidt and Ostertag.[13]

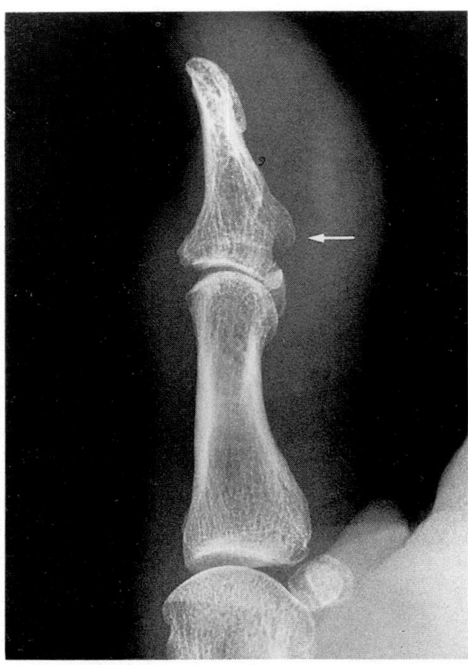

FIGURE 10–12. A typical thorn-like overgrowth (arrow) in an elderly woman, not an exostosis.

Osteophytes combined with juxtaarticular lucent defects (geodes) are typical signs of Heberden osteoarthritis (Fig. 10–13) and should not be mistaken for

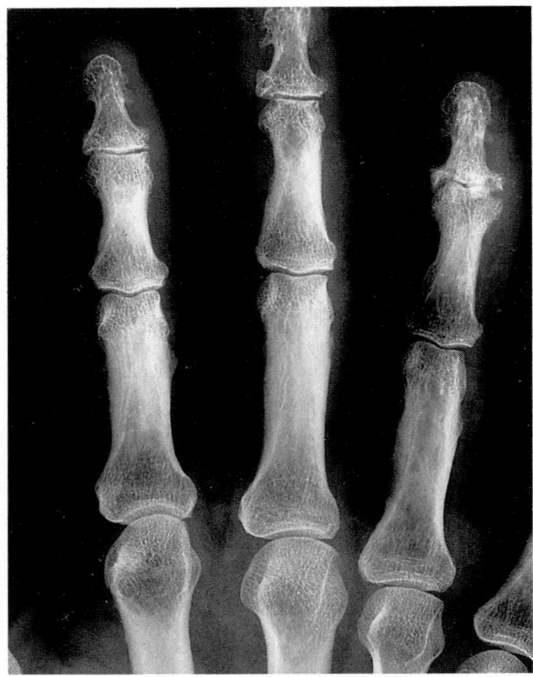

FIGURE 10–13. Heberden's osteoarthritis. Osteophytes are combined with small juxtaarticular lucent defects (geodes), especially in the distal interphalangeal joint of the fourth digit.

normal variants, especially in the elderly. Usually they are asymptomatic. Pain and stiffness occur in the cold and after consumption of alcohol. In many cases it is combined with rhizarthrosis (osteoarthritis of the first carpometacarpal (CMC) joint). One differential diagnostic consideration of Heberden's osteoarthritis is the transverse type of psoriatic osteoarthropathy. Usually pathognomonic protuberances at the bases of the distal phalanges are visible in psoriatic arthropathy (Fig. 10–14).[14]

An enlargement of the distal phalanges may be a sign of acromegaly. Typical anchor deformities of the tufts and pronged protuberances at the bases of the distal phalanges are visible on roentgenograms (Fig. 10–15).[15]

Figure 10–16A shows recalcified deformed tufts after therapy of renal hyperparathyroidism. The previously lytic changes are well calcified, and bowing of the distal phalanges results from the softness of the bone before treatment. In hyperparathyroidism subperiosteal resorptions at the shafts as well as at the tufts cause a spiculated and wooly appearance; moreover, the cortex becomes lamellated. In early stages these changes are extremely subtle.[16] Total radiographic disappearance of the margins of the distal phalanges as a symptom of renal osteopathy is possible, as demonstrated in Fig. 10–16B.

Atrophy of the soft tissues at the fingertips is an early finding in scleroderma. These trophic changes found at the tufts can be measured and calculated by the Yune soft tissue index (Fig. 10–17).[17] Acroosteolysis starts on the palmar side of the tufts (Table 10–1). Later, the distal phalanges may appear chewed. In Gorham's disease (vanishing-bone disease) as well as in Cheney's syndrome, which can occur in any part of the skeleton, disappearance of the distal phalanges is possible.

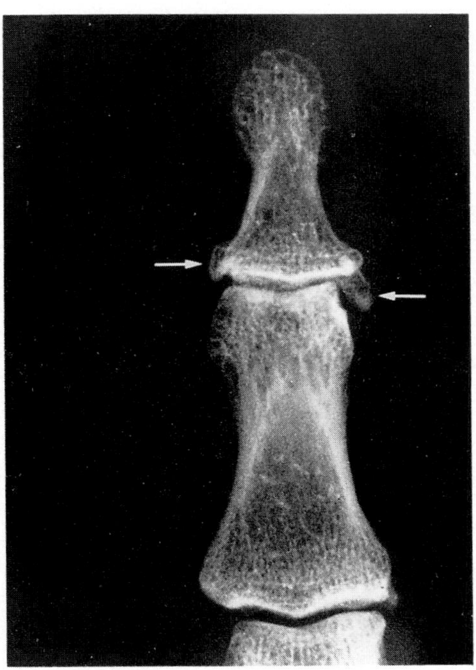

FIGURE 10–14. Transverse type of psoriatic arthropathy. Arrows indicate bone excrescences.

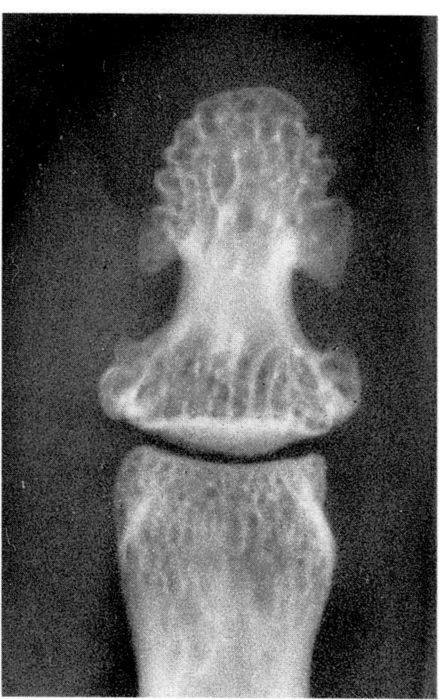

FIGURE 10–15. Findings at the tufts in acromegaly. The tufts have an anchor-like form.

Cortical rarefaction at the lateral margin of the distal phalanges and indistinctness is an early sign in an osseous paronychia. In later stages this may progress to osteolytic changes, as visible in Fig. 10–18.

Clubbing (drumstick fingers), which occurs in some systemic diseases, such as liver cirrhosis, cystic fibrosis, cardiac disease, and paraneoplastic syndromes, among others, is an enlargement of the tufts accompanied by swelling of the soft tissue. Atrophy of the tufts with ragged margins may arise later.

Claw-like bowed distal phalanges of the fifth digits occur in Kirner's deformity (Fig. 10–19). This variant is seen in otherwise healthy people. It is congenital and is passed as an autosomal dominant trait.[6]

Normal Findings and Variants in Structure

In the otherwise normally shaped distal phalanges a well-defined patchy increase in density is possible (Figs. 10–20 and 10–24 and Table 10–2) and is often found in middle-aged women. In contrast to these harmless normal variants, ill-defined sclerotic foci may be seen in sarcoidosis and tuberous sclerosis. In most cases they are combined with coarsening of the trabecular structure and small lucent defects. In some systemic osteopathies (hyperparathyroidism, advanced osteomyelosclerosis) a faint increase in density is observed. For the differential diagnosis of osteomas, see Table 10–2 and Fig. 10–30.

Small round lucencies in the distal phalanges

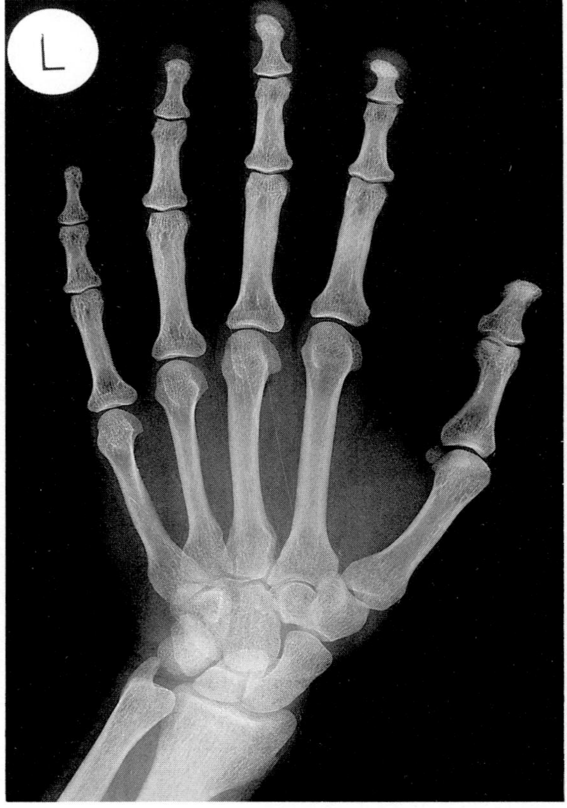

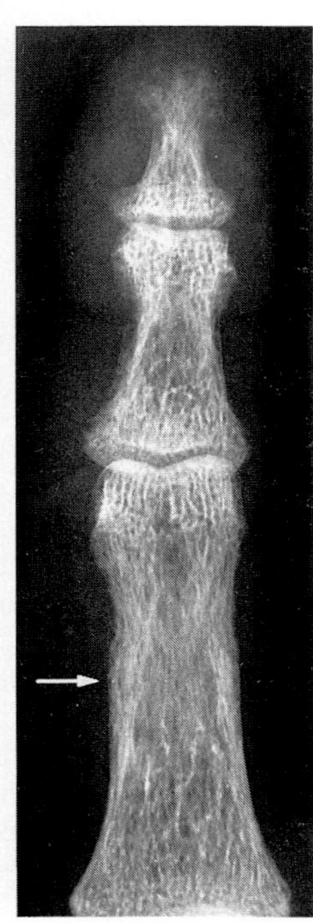

A B

FIGURE 10–16. A: Recalcification and bowing of the tufts as the result of therapy in renal hyperparathyroidism. **B:** Renal hyperparathyroidism. The trabecular structure is coarsened and ill defined. Massive resorption of the tuft and severe subperiosteal resorptions involve the middle phalanx. Lamellated cortex of the proximal phalanx is evident (arrow).

caused by the nutrient canals should not be considered as pathologic cystic lesions. The latter occur in the diseases listed in Table 10–3. Figure 10–21 demonstrates an enchondroma in a distal phalanx. The trabecular bone is destroyed with expansion of almost the entire phalanx. The highly vascularized glomus tumors most commonly arise in the nailbed. They cause erosion of the adjacent bone with a decrease in density in the dorsopalmar projection. Pressure-induced large defects, especially on the dorsal surface of the distal phalanx, can occur in advanced disease.

So-called epithelial cysts or epidermoid inclusion cysts are usually found in the distal phalanx of the

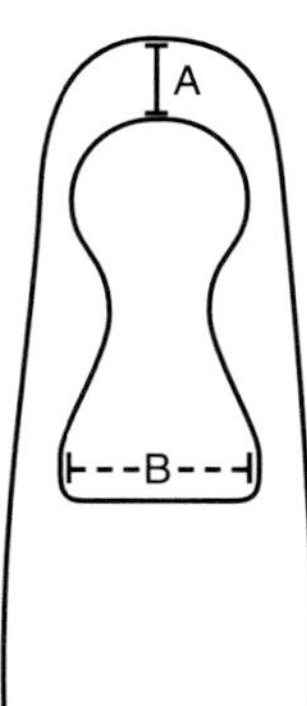

FIGURE 10–17. Calculations of the Yune soft-tissue index. Normal: A ≥ 25% B. pathologic: A ≤ 25% B.

TABLE 10–1. *Differential Diagnosis of Acroosteolysis*[14]

Trophic (vascular/neurogenic/lymphatic)
Raynaud's syndrome
Mixed connective tissue disease
Scleroderma
Epidermolysis bullosa
Chronic acrodermatitis Pick–Herzheimer
Lues nervosa
Syringomyelia
Leprosy
Hyperostosis with pachydermia (Uehlinger's syndrome)
Hypertrophic osteoarthropathy

Traumatic
Frostbite
Burn
Electrical injury
Chronic exposure to ionizing radiation
Chronic mechanical stress (guitar players)

Hormonal
Primary and secondary hyperparathyroidism
Pheochromocytoma

Toxic
Chronic polyvinyl chloride intoxication

Other
Gorham's disease (vanishing-bone disease)
Ainhum syndrome (dactylosis spontanea)
Familial (acro)osteolysis (Cheney's syndrome)
Idiopathic or cryptogenetic acroosteolysis disease
Pycnodysostosis
Inflammatory processes (osseus panaritium or paronychia)
Tumors
Joint diseases (arthritis, arthroses)
Glomus tumor
Epithelial cyst

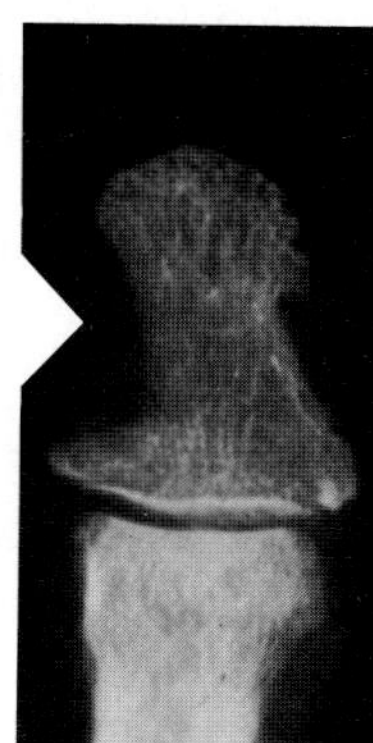

FIGURE 10–18. Osseous paronychia of the distal phalanx. Destruction of the cortex and subcortical bone (arrowhead) is present. (Reprinted with permission from Schmidt H, Freyschmidt J, eds. *Borderlands of normal and early pathologic findings in skeletal radiology.* 4th English ed. Stuttgart, New York: Thieme, 1993.)

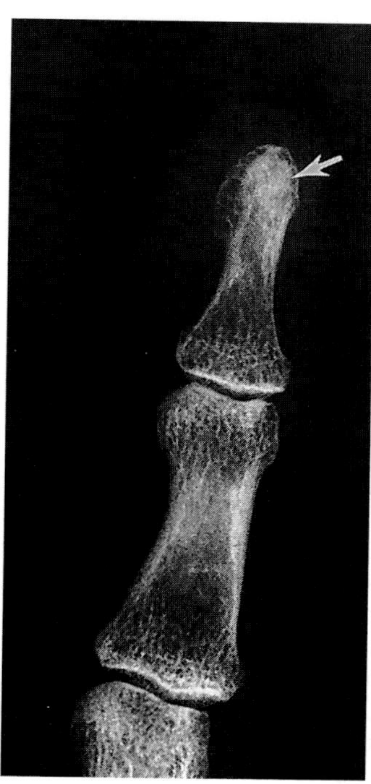

FIGURE 10–20. Dense, osteoma-like structure (arrow) is a normal variant in the distal phalanx of this middle-aged woman.

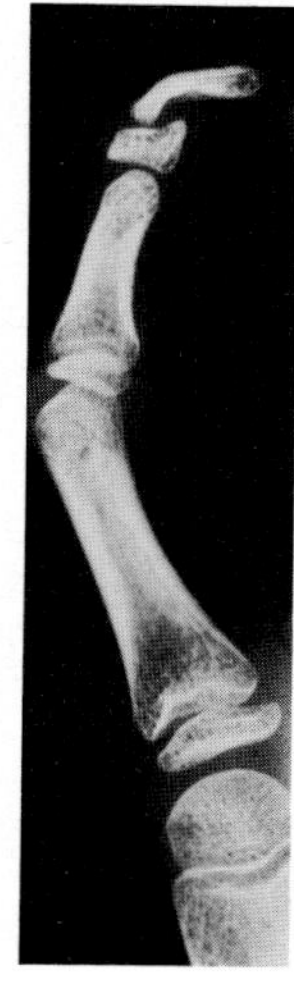

FIGURE 10–19. Kirner deformity with claw-like bowed distal phalanx. (Reprinted with permission from Schmidt H, Freyschmidt J, eds. *Borderlands of normal and early pathologic findings in skeletal radiology.* 4th English ed. Stuttgart, New York: Thieme, 1993.)

TABLE 10–2. ***Differential Diagnoses for Normal Patchy Sclerosis Especially in the Distal Phalanges of Middle-Aged Women***

Oligo- or Multiloculated (Few or Multiple)	Circumscribed (Solitary)
Osteopoikilosis, sarcoidosis, osteomyelosclerosis, toxicity osteopathy, tuberous sclerosis, renal osteopathy	True (en)osteoma (enostosis), osteoid osteoma, infarction, inflammation

Reprinted with permission from Freyschmidt J. *Skeletterkrankunger: Klinisch-radiologische Diagnose und Differentialdiagnose.* Berlin, New York: Springer-Verlag, 1993.

Irregularities in contour at the bases of the proximal phalanges have been described as an early sign of rheumatoid arthritis by Norgaard in 1965.[21] In 1982 Stelling, Keats, and Keats found that these changes can occur in otherwise healthy people and should be considered pathologic processes only if local pain and juxtaarticular decrease in density is found.[22]

In so-called Bouchard's polyarthrosis a heterogeneous occurrence of "cysts" (lucent defects), osteophytes, and erosions at the proximal interphalangeal joints is seen. This disorder is comparable with and often combined with Heberden's polyarthrosis. These changes should not be mistaken for rheumatoid arthritis, given that the proximal interphalangeal joint is one of the preferred regions of rheumatoid arthritis.[6]

Brachymesophalangy, a congenital shortening of the middle phalanx, most commonly of the fifth digit, is seen as a normal variant in the Asian races with a frequency of 20%. In whites these changes are found in 1% of the population. The so-called Bells A3 variant, seen frequently, is shown in Figs. 10–26A and 10–26B. A symmetric brachymesophalangy in both fifth digits combined with a mild clinodactyly is visible in an otherwise healthy young man. Brachymesophalangy accompanied by syndactyly, symphalangism, or severe clinodactyly are visible in a wide variety of syndromes as an expression of congenital anomalies. In trisomy 21, brachymesophalangy is found in about 60% of patients.[7]

Normal Findings and Variants in Structure

The compacta or cortex of the metacarpals and phalanges shows a homogeneous density that changes with resorptive processes. The width of the compacta decreases slowly with age. Women are affected earlier than men. A decreasing density of compacta and trabecular bone is also seen in old age due to a loss of bone mass. These normal findings must be differentiated from resorptive processes in acquired diseases. Because of increased bone turnover in primary and secondary hyperparathyroidism, subperiosteal resorption may be seen on the radial side of middle phalanges of the index and long fingers as one of the early signs. The cortical margin in this area becomes lamellated and destroyed with a brush-like contour in severe cases combined with a coarsened ill-defined trabecular structure (see the section on distal phalanges and Fig. 10–16B).

Linear and small round radiolucencies can have different causes. They may be purely projection related (i.e., Mach effect). In other cases they correspond to linearly configured vascular canals in the proximal phalanges and metacarpals. As demonstrated in Fig. 10–27A, they traverse the cortex and could be mistaken for fracture lines, especially in the oblique projection, when the entrance can be seen in

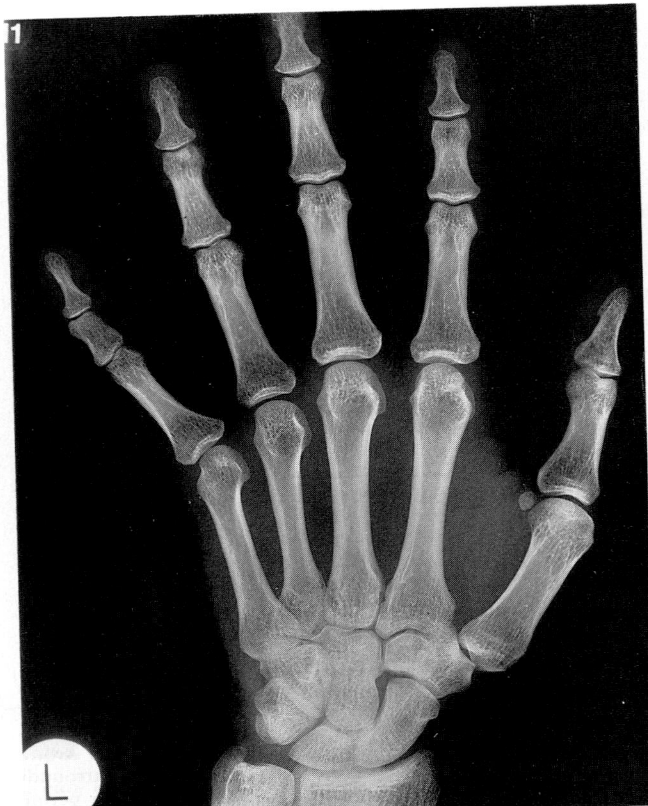

FIGURE 10–26. A: Brachymesophalangy of the fifth digit in an otherwise healthy man. This short middle phalanx is typically combined with a mild clinodactyly. **B:** The same case enlarged.

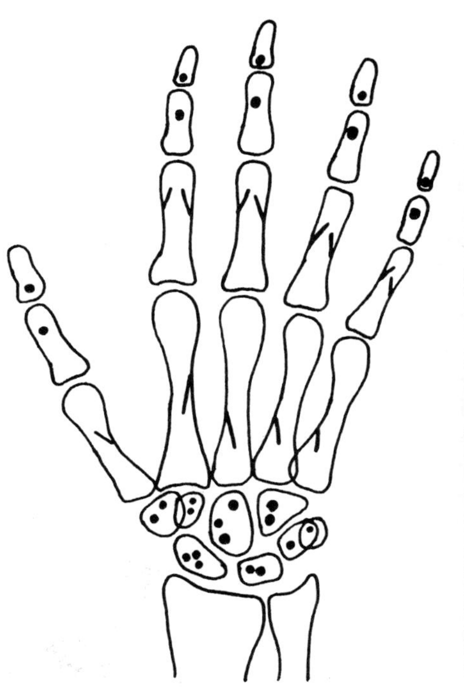

A

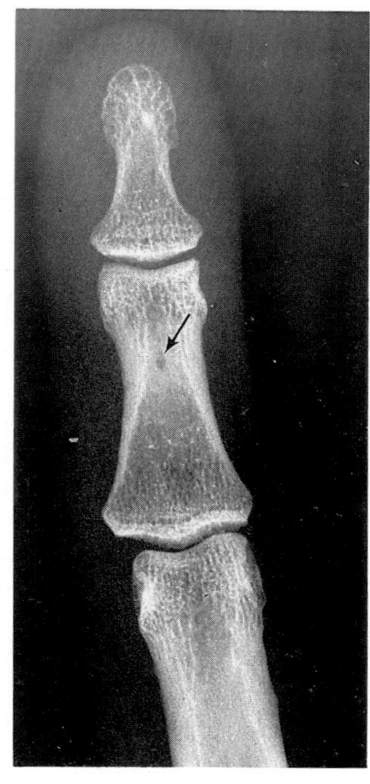

B

FIGURE 10–27. A: Course of nutrient canals. **B:** Nutrient canal (arrow) in the middle phalanx in the dorsopalmar view.

profile. Adjacent osseous ridges could be misinterpreted as callus. A widening of these lines is visible particularly in diseases with marrow hyperplasia (such as anemias). The same implies for small round lucencies created by orthograde projected vascular canals, which are found more frequently in the middle than in the distal phalanges (Fig. 10–27B).[6]

True cysts or cystlike lucencies in the hand skeleton are frequently observed. Figure 10–28 demonstrates typical so-called idiopathic bone cysts of the long as well as the short hand bones. They may be the result of localized osseous resorption with subsequent replacement by connective tissue or fluid. Vascular disturbances with focal necrosis following trauma may be initial etiologic factors. They can also arise secondary to degenerative changes.[23,24] For demonstration of juxtaarticular cyst-like structures, an oblique projection should be performed to determine their intraspongious location and differentiate them from orthograde projected marginal erosions, particularly in the metacarpal heads. The idiopathic bone cysts must be differentiated from symptomatic oligocystic and polycystic changes in acquired diseases, as listed in Table 10–3. A cyst-like change in hyperparathyroidism because of "brown tumor" is shown in Fig. 10–29.

Fluoride abuse or intoxication causes an increased density especially of the proximal phalanges, but also of all other hand bones. Advanced osteomyelosclerosis can also be a cause of increased density of the hand skeleton (Fig. 10–30). Coarsening of the tubular bone structure and bone marrow infarctions may be visible in other chronic hematologic disorders.[6]

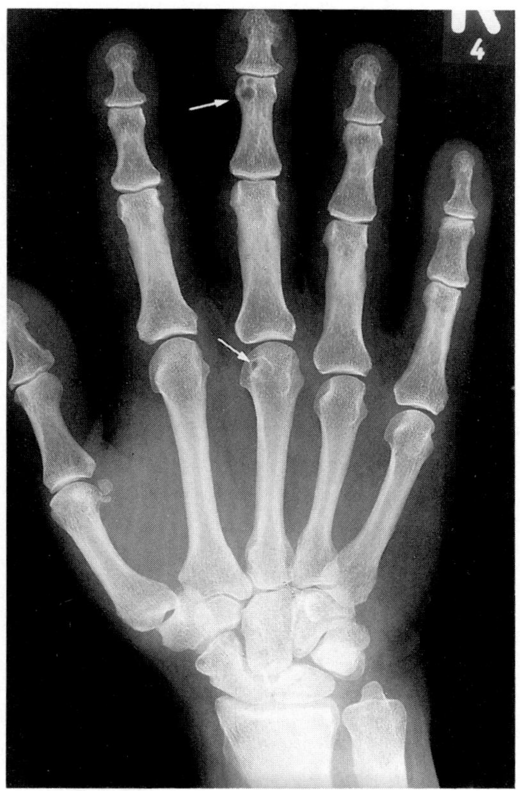

FIGURE 10–28. So-called idiopathic bone cysts or benign, focal, radiolucent defects (arrows) in the hand skeleton without any associated symptoms.

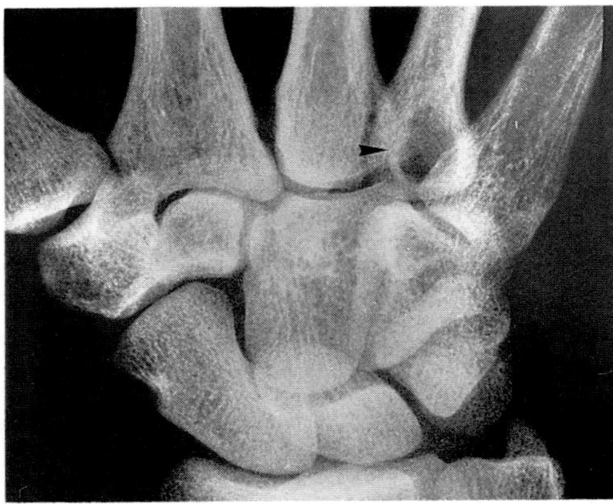

FIGURE 10–29. "Bone cyst" (arrowhead) caused by a brown tumor in hyperparathyroidism.

Leukemia has no pathognomonic signs, but a mixture of different findings with periosteal reaction, metaphyseal lucencies, and often osteolytic processes occur. The hand–foot syndrome in sickle cell anemia can produce similar findings.[6]

A localized homogeneous increase in density in a phalanx usually is caused by an osteoma (Fig. 10–31). The differential diagnosis for the well-known patchy or spotty densities (Fig. 10–20 and Table 10–2) seen especially in the end phalanges of middle-aged women is only of academic interest. Both focal sclerotic entities are asymptomatic. An osteoma may be assumed if the "lesion" in question is relatively large, very dense, and single.[6]

The Metacarpals

Normal Findings and Variants in Shape

The shape of the metacarpal heads and bases is variable. Different features could be mistaken for pathologic findings. Symmetric radial-sided pronounced protuberances in the metaphyseal region can simulate exostoses (Fig. 10–32). Protuberances at the bases of the second to fifth metacarpals are caused by muscle attachments and ligament insertions from the intermetacarpal joints, similar to those of the phalanges. Clefts close to the bases (Fig. 10–32) may be mistaken for fractures. An overlapping of the margins of adjacent bases can cause lines simulating fractures (Mach effects; Fig. 10–32).[6]

The position of the first metacarpal on its articulating surface with the trapezium may easily be misinterpreted as a subluxation. This peculiar joint allows not only flexion and extension but also rotation similar to ball-and-socket joints. In a rotated position of the first metacarpal its radial border overlaps the joint contour of the trapezium, creating the so-called step sign shown in Fig. 10–33.[6]

Normal Findings and Variants in Structure

Dense irregular structures can appear in the juxta-articular region of metacarpals and proximal phalanges because of crossing spongiosa lines, which lead to summation effects.

One or two ivory-like round or oval densities in the metacarpals of an asymptomatic patient usually correspond to simple (en-)osteomas or enostoses. In symptomatic patients an osteoma-like lesion is some-

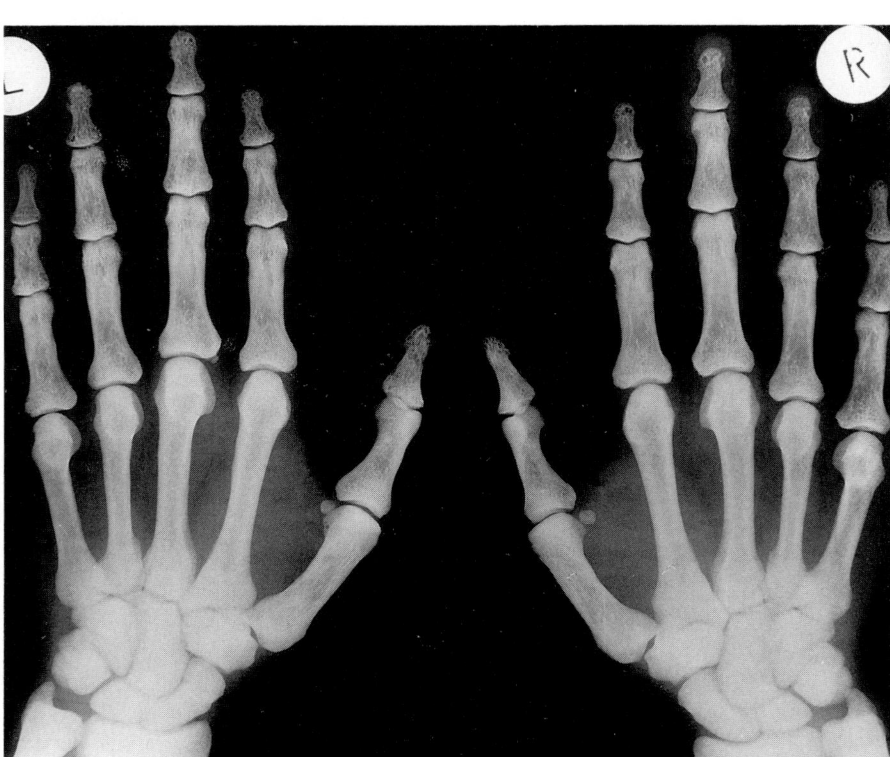

FIGURE 10–30. Generalized increase in density of the hand skeleton in osteomyelosclerosis.

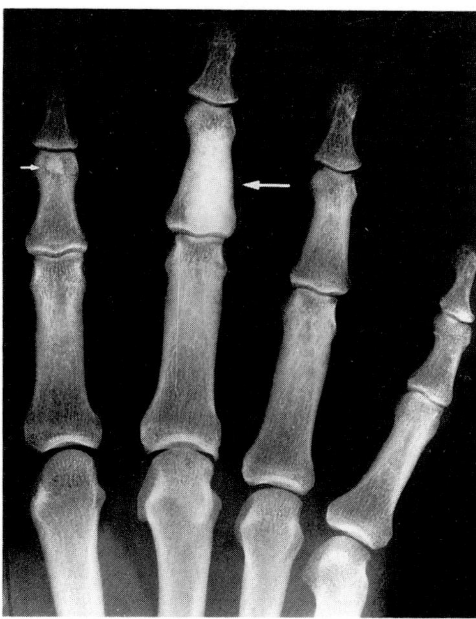

FIGURE 10–31. Large osteoma (large arrow) in the middle phalanx of the third digit and small osteoma (small arrow) in the distal portion of the middle phalanx of the second digit found in an asymptomatic middle-aged male.

times a calcified nidus of an osteoid osteoma (Fig. 10–34A). In contrast to simple enostoses the adjacent trabecular bone is sclerotic, a radiolucent nidus may be visible, and periosteal ossification is possible. Painless osteoid osteomas of the fingers have been de-

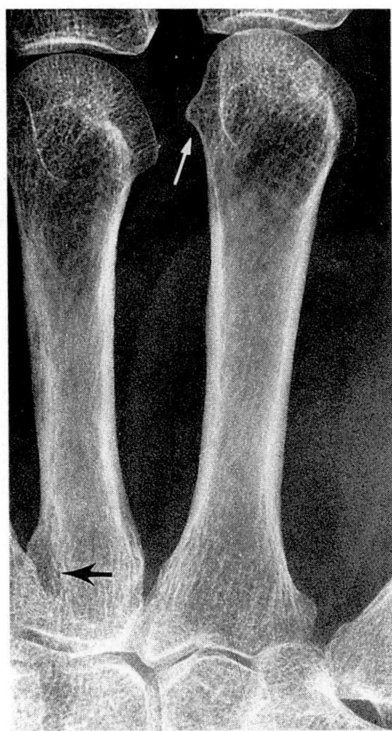

FIGURE 10–32. Exostosis-like shape variants of the second metacarpal head (white arrow), and a cleft at the base of the third metacarpal (black arrow).

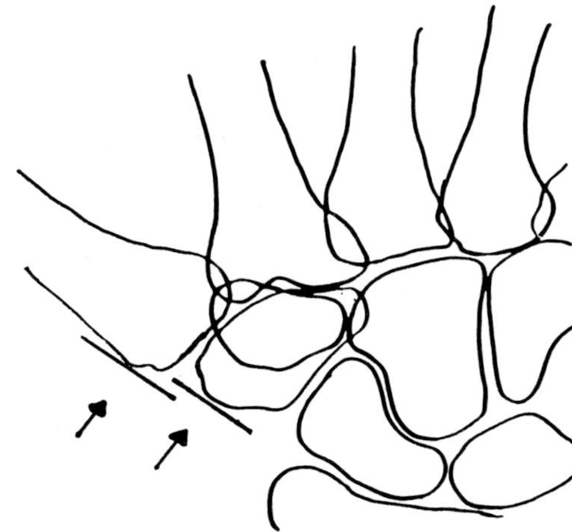

FIGURE 10–33. Schematic showing apparent malalignment of the first metacarpal and the trapezium, the so-called step sign.

scribed, and a lack of pain does not exclude the diagnosis of osteoid osteoma when the typical radiographic appearance is found.[25] Usually a scintigraphic study is negative in enostoses. In an osteoid osteoma the so-called double-density sign (the center is more dense or hot than the periphery) may be found (Fig. 10–34B).[13]

A large number of well-defined sclerotic areas can be found in osteopoikilosis (Fig. 10–35). The "lesions" occur juxtaarticular in the metaphyseal heads but also in other long hand bones, and especially in the carpal bones.

In the healthy adult the Barnett–Nordin index can be taken as an approximate guideline for a normal compacta thickness. A ratio of the cortical width to the total diameter in the middle of the second metacarpal is taken. This index shows a relatively wide range (minimum, 43 to 44%). This method is useful for estimation of the peripheral bone mineralization. An early diagnosis of possible osteoporosis should be made by other methods.

Lucencies caused by thin bony structures on the posteroanterior (PA) or anteroposterior (AP) projection, not to be mistaken for lytic changes, are seen at the base of the fifth metacarpal and the ulnar side of the hamate.

Short Hand Bones

Normal Findings and Variants in Form and Structure

Scaphoid

This carpal bone has a large variability in shape, secondary to projection and form variants (Fig. 10–36). In radial and palmar-flexion the distal pole of the scaphoid turns palmar physiologically. This results in a ring-like appearance of the distal pole.

Occasionally, a radial notch with a sclerotic margin

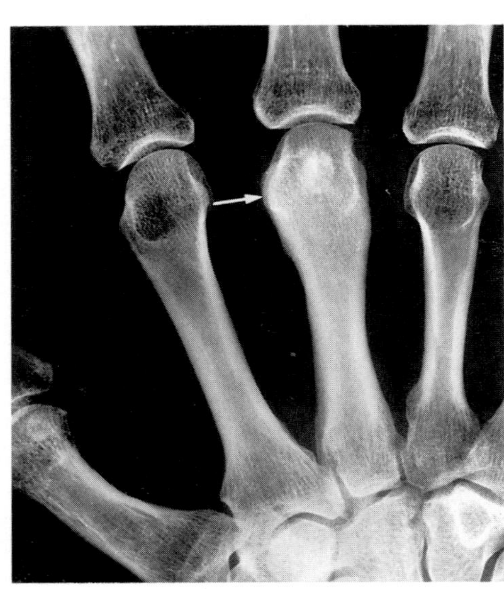

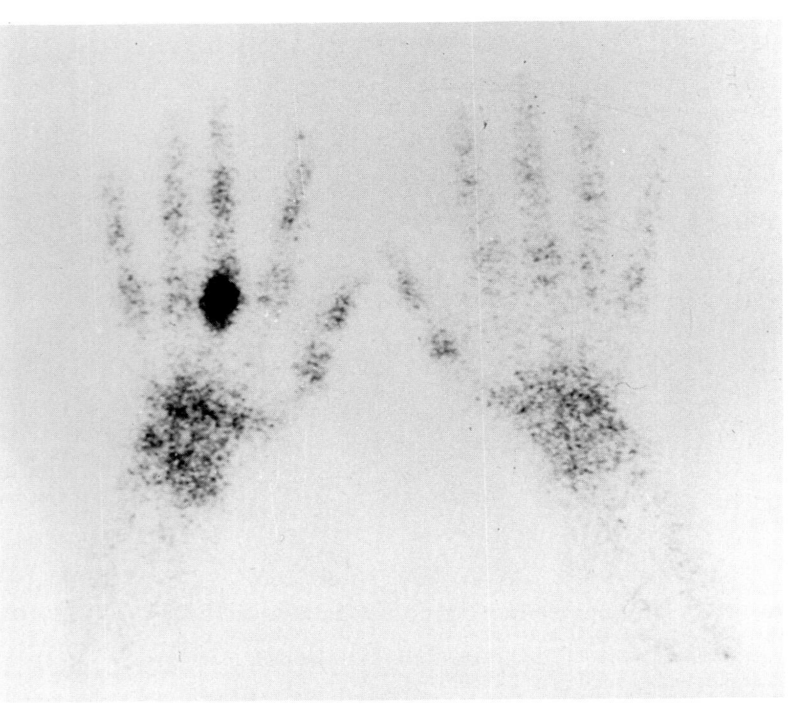

A B

FIGURE 10–34. A: Osteoid osteoma (arrow) in the third metacarpal head. The nidus is calcified with increased volume of the surrounding bony structures: **B:** Double-density sign in osteoid-osteoma of the third metacarpal. The outer edge of increased uptake is not as hot as the center of the increased uptake.

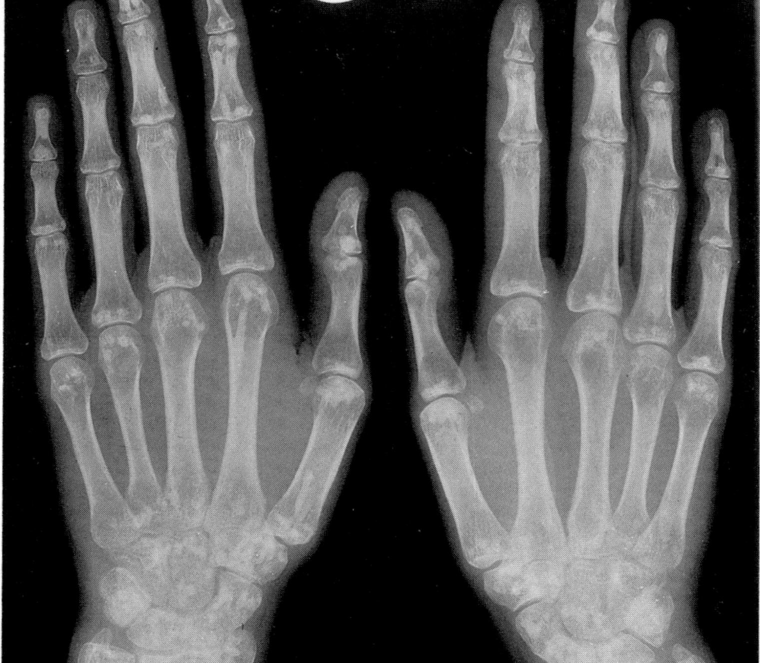

FIGURE 10–35. Osteopoikilosis.

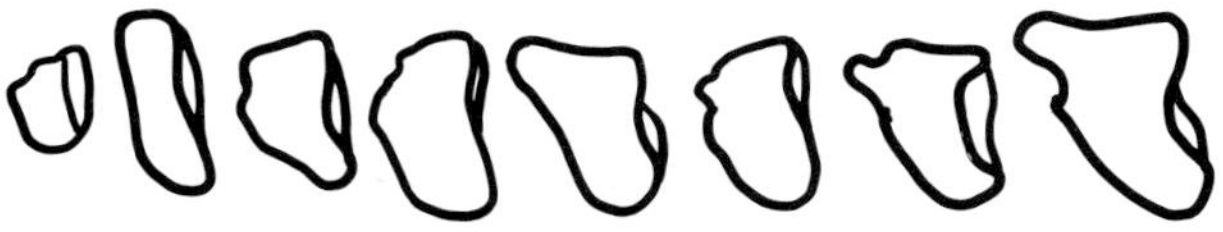

FIGURE 10–36. Variants in shape of the scaphoid. (Reprinted with permission from Schmidt H, Freyschmidt J, eds. *Borderlands of normal and early pathologic findings in skeletal radiology.* 4th English ed. Stuttgart, New York: Thieme, 1993.)

can occur. This should not be mistaken for an erosion in rheumatoid arthritis, particularly if there are no other structural changes.

Protuberances may be idiopathic or seen after complete healing of waist fractures.[24] They are usually visible radiologically in the oblique projection (Fig. 10–37). These protuberances should not be mistaken for the more distal scaphoid tubercle. A fusion of the sometimes separated ossification centers of the tubercle and the scaphoid can cause an exostotic appearance of the tubercle (Fig. 10–38).

A bipartite scaphoid is described by several authors. This may be caused by lack of fusion of two or more ossification centers. Bilateral occurrence is possible. A partial bipartition (Fig. 10–39) on the ulnar side of the scaphoid should not be misinterpreted as a fracture. A conventional tomogram (Fig. 10–40) shows a deep groove in the region of the partial bipartition cleft. The differential diagnosis for a bipartition is a pseudarthrosis or, especially after injury, fracture of the scaphoid.

A bone scan six days after trauma may be helpful if only a small delicate lucency is visible and pain persists. A clinically symptomatic wrist with negative x-ray examination should be considered as an invisible fracture and x-ray examination should be repeated after 10 days. Much literature deals with difficulties in detecting scaphoid fractures and the late complications after overlooked fractures.[26,27]

Rarely, the scaphoid may be absent or hypoplastic

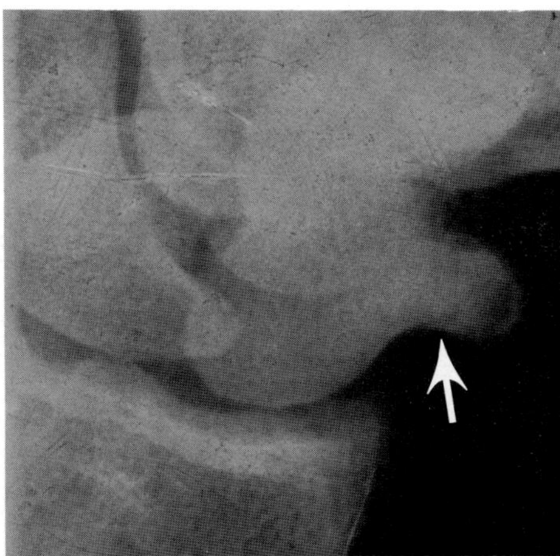

FIGURE 10–37. Genuine exostosis (arrow) of the scaphoid waist. (Reprinted with permission from Schmidt H, Freyschmidt J, eds. *Borderlands of normal and early pathologic findings in skeletal radiology.* 4th English ed. Stuttgart, New York: Thieme, 1993.)

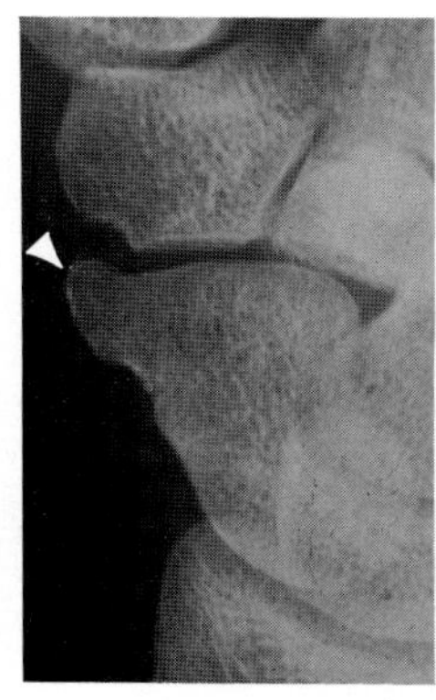

FIGURE 10–38. Protuberance (arrowhead) of the fused separate ossification center of the scaphoid tubercle. (Reprinted with permission from Schmidt H, Freyschmidt J, eds. *Borderlands of normal and early pathologic findings in skeletal radiology.* 4th English ed. Stuttgart, New York: Thieme, 1993.)

as a normal variant. In certain syndromes such as Holt–Oram syndrome, associations with malformations of the radius, thumb, or short hand bones occur.

Lunate

Obvious changes in form and density are visible in acquired disorders (i.e., Kienböck's disease), as discussed in Chapter 20.

On lateral projection cleft-like vertical lines occur as a normal variant (Fig. 10–41). These clefts should not be mistaken for fractures of the lunate, which are extremely rare. The explanation for the clefts, such as nonfusion of multiple ossification centers or some other cause, remains to be found.

Triquetrum

A dorsolateral groove on the lateral view can cause a protuberance at the proximal part of the triquetrum that should not be mistaken for an exostosis (Fig. 10–42). On a PA projection this may be hidden by the overlying pisiform.

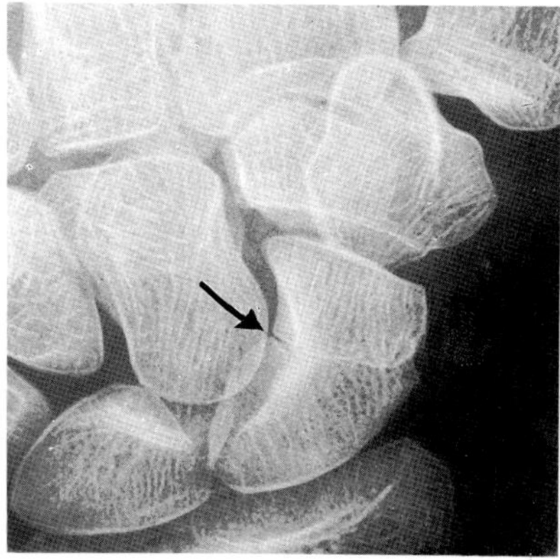

FIGURE 10–39. Partial bipartition of the scaphoid (arrow). (Reprinted with permission from Schmidt H, Freyschmidt J, eds. *Borderlands of normal and early pathologic findings in skeletal radiology.* 4th English ed. Stuttgart, New York: Thieme, 1993.)

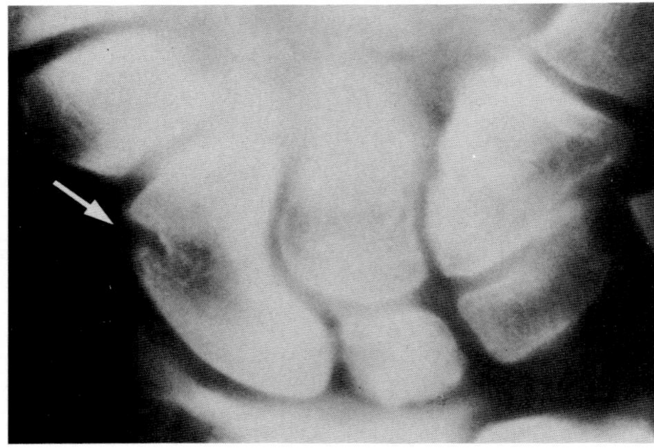

A

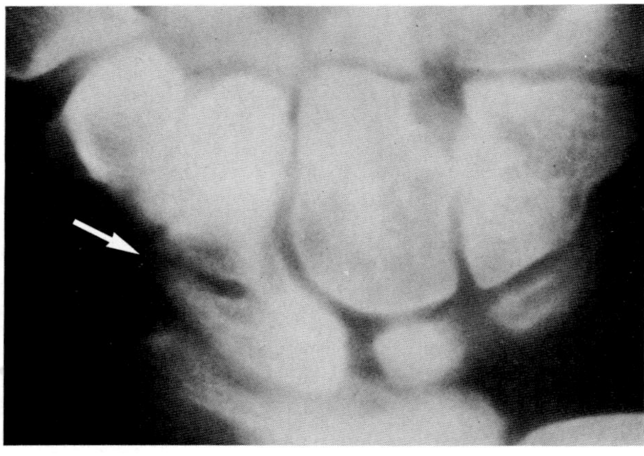

B

FIGURE 10–40. A and **B:** Conventional tomography revealing a deep groove in a partial bipartition of the scaphoid (arrows). (Reprinted with permission from Schmidt H, Freyschmidt J, eds. *Borderlands of normal and early pathologic findings in skeletal radiology.* 4th English ed. Stuttgart, New York: Thieme, 1993.)

Pisiform

Köhler and Zimmer observed irregularities at the distal margin of the pisiform as a normal variant;[6] these should not be misinterpreted as productive processes.

Subchondral sclerosis at the corresponding articulating surfaces of the pisiform and triquetrum is a common site for degenerative changes. An exostosis-like hypertrophy of the distal portion of the pisiform is described as a variant (Fig. 10–43).[6] After trauma, an isolated dislocation of the pisiform is possible.

Trapezium

A normal protuberance, the tuberculum osseous trapezii, is visible at the ventral radial part of the trapezium (Fig. 10–44). A bridging of trapezium, trapezoid, and capitate can be simulated by a projection effect (Fig. 10–45).

Trapezoid

The form and structure of the trapezoid vary less than that of the other short hand bones. The accessory ossicles and other possibilities are discussed later in this chapter. Bipartition of this carpal bone as a normal variant is possible. In the oto-palato-digital syndrome, the trapezoid has a comma-like shape.

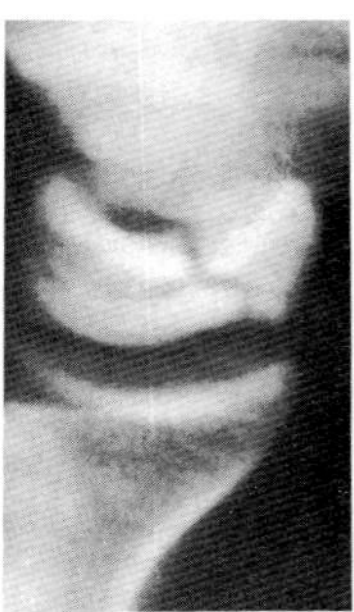

FIGURE 10–41. Vertical cleft in the lunate; no history of trauma. (Reprinted with permission from Schmidt H, Freyschmidt J, eds. *Borderlands of normal and early pathologic findings in skeletal radiology.* 4th English ed. Stuttgart, New York: Thieme, 1993.)

Capitate

This bone has a radially located central indentation. A gap can appear between the capitate, scaphoid, and trapezoid (Fig. 10–46); this has been discussed as a consequence of the os centrale carpi, an accessory ossicle which can fuse with either of the three bones. Frequently a hump-like protuberance may be seen along the ulnar margin, which has a corresponding notch in the hamate (Fig. 10–47). In some cases a narrowing of the joint between the capitate and hamate is visible; this has no pathologic meaning and should not lead to an erroneous interpretation as an arthritic change. Bipartition of the capitate has been described.[6]

Hamate

The radial indentation opposite the capitate is described above. In the dorsopalmar view a ring-like cortical density is caused by the orthograde projection of the hamulus (hook of the hamate) (Fig. 10–48). The absence of this ring structure after hand trauma may signify a fracture of the hamulus with

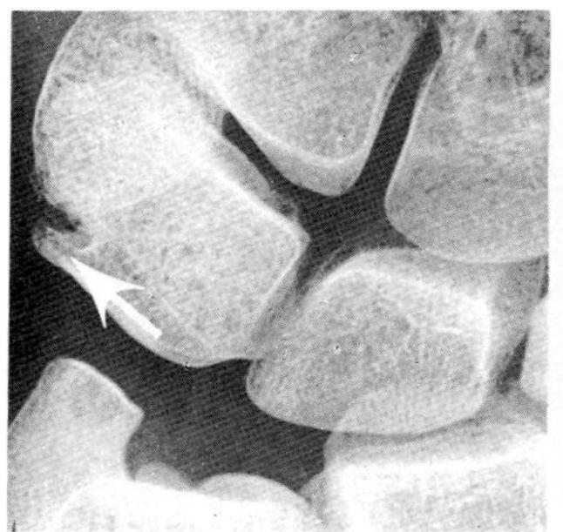

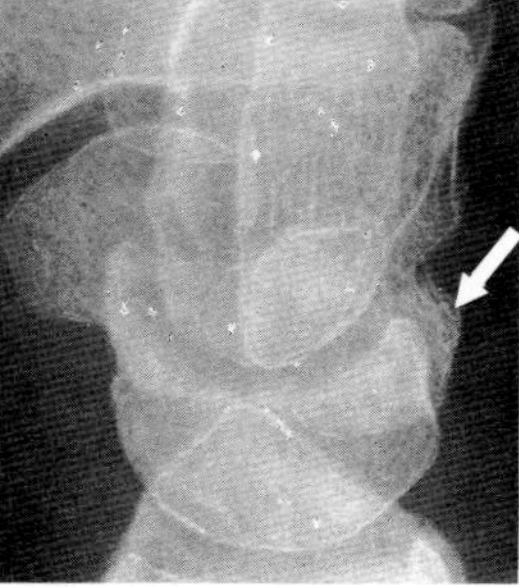

FIGURE 10–42. Groove along the dorsal surface (arrow) that causes an exostosis-like appearance at the triquetrum. (Reprinted with permission from Schmidt H, Freyschmidt J, eds. *Borderlands of normal and early pathologic findings in skeletal radiology.* 4th English ed. Stuttgart, New York: Thieme, 1993.)

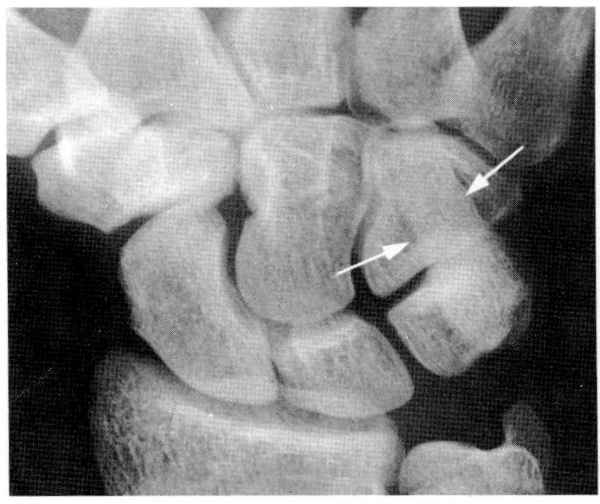
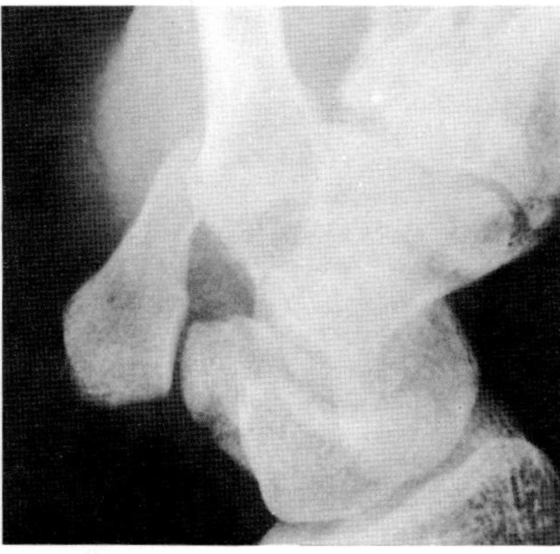

A B

FIGURE 10–43. A and **B:** Hyperplasia of the pisiform with an exostosis-like appearance (between arrows). (Reprinted with permission from Schmidt H, Freyschmidt J, eds. *Borderlands of normal and early pathologic findings in skeletal radiology.* 4th English ed. Stuttgart, New York: Thieme, 1993.)

dislocation.[28] However, its differential diagnosis should include bilateral congenital absence of the hamulus as reported by Seeger, Bassett, and Gold. It may be present in its cartilaginous form, provable with MRI.[29] Bipartition of the hamulus may have clinical relevance by causing pain in the carpal tunnel.

Distal Forearm

A symmetric shortening or lengthening of the ulna in relation to the radius occurs as a frequent normal variant. Posttraumatic radial shortening in the adult, growth disturbances after trauma, and rheumatoid arthritis are acquired causes for ulnar length variations. The distal articulating contours of the radius and ulna are normally aligned. Much has been published about possible disorders in the radiocarpal joint arising from cartilage and ligamentous overstraining by the so-called minus (Fig. 10–49) and plus variants (Fig. 10–50). An association of these ulnar variants with ulnocarpal impaction, radioulnar impingement, acute scapholunate instability, and Kienböck's disease is discussed (Chap. 20).[30]

Small protuberances on the distal radius at the level of the growth plate should not be misinterpreted as exostoses (Fig. 10–51). A thin osseous ridge may be detectable at the ulnar side of the distal radius; this should not be mistaken for a periosteal reaction (Fig. 10–51). Persisting epiphyseal lines in the adult are a normal variant and may mimic a fracture.

Cystic (Lucent Defect) Findings

Cyst-like radiolucencies caused by vascular canals are commonly visible in the capitate, hamate, and lunate. The diameter of such vascular canals ranges from 0.3 to 1 mm[24] and they are well defined, often with a sclerotic rim. Larger lucencies in an asymptomatic patient usually correspond to so-called idiopathic bone cysts, which are visible in carpal bones more often than in the long hand bones. These cyst-like lucent defects have a sclerotic margin and can occasionally reach a size of about 7 to 8 mm (Fig. 10–52). Figures 10–53A and 10–53B show a large round lucency, which had a defect in the radial cortex of the lunate. The patient suffered from a painful reduction of carpal mobility. An intraosseous ganglion was found histologically. For the spectrum of causes for cyst-like lesions in the hand skeleton, see Table 10–3.

Accessory Bones at the Carpus According to Köhler and Zimmer

Radiologists and trauma surgeons should be familiar with accessory bones and the necessity of differentiat-

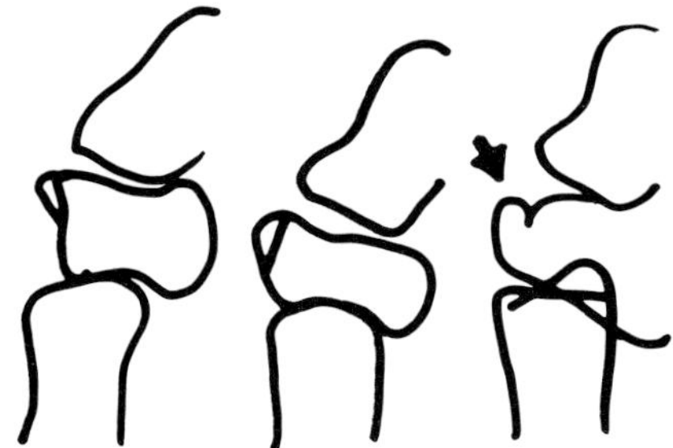

FIGURE 10–44. Tubercle of the trapezium (arrow) shown schematically. (Reprinted with permission from Schmidt H, Freyschmidt J, eds. *Borderlands of normal and early pathologic findings in skeletal radiology.* 4th English ed. Stuttgart, New York: Thieme, 1993.)

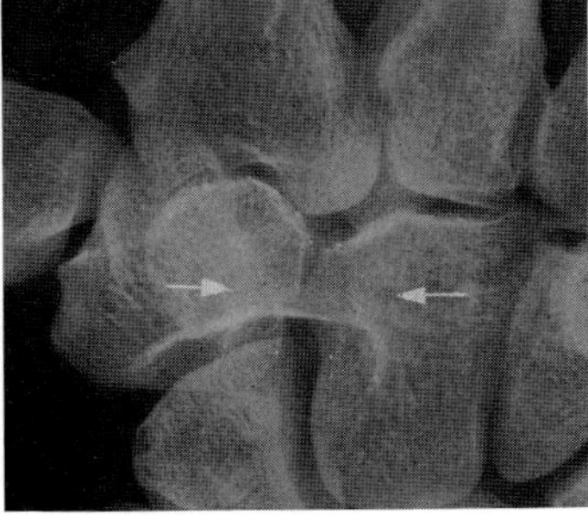

FIGURE 10–45. No synostosis (between arrows), but projection-related effect. (Reprinted with permission from Schmidt H, Freyschmidt J, eds. *Borderlands of normal and early pathologic findings in skeletal radiology.* 4th English ed. Stuttgart, New York: Thieme, 1993.)

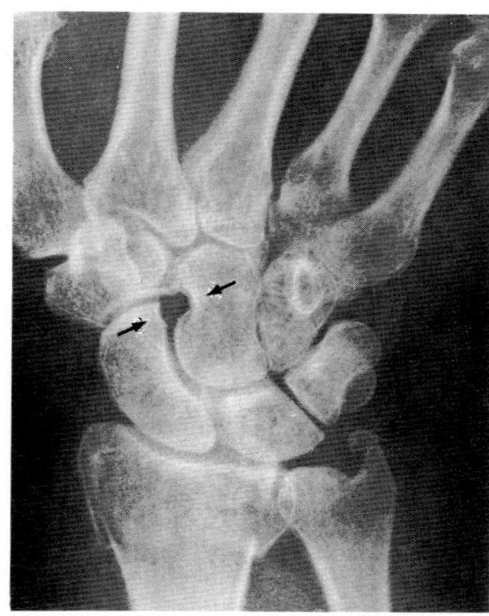

FIGURE 10–46. Typical gap (between arrows) between capitate, scaphoid, and trapezoid. (Reprinted with permission from Schmidt H, Freyschmidt J, eds. *Borderlands of normal and early pathologic findings in skeletal radiology.* 4th English ed. Stuttgart, New York: Thieme, 1993.)

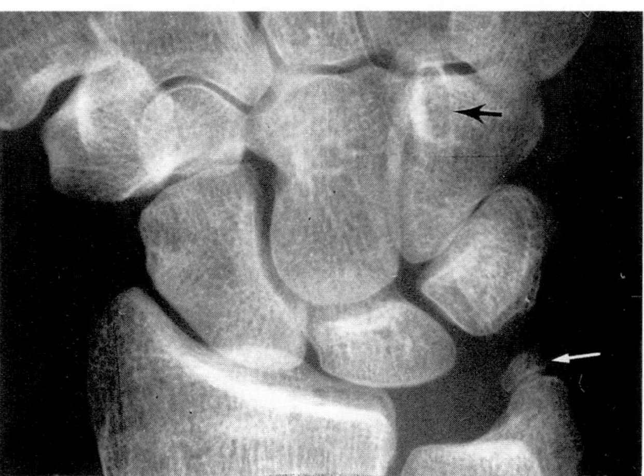

FIGURE 10–48. Normal sclerotic ring in the hamate by orthograde projection of the hamulus (black arrow). Persistent epiphyseal center at the ulnar styloid process (white arrow) has a differential of old fracture, or possibly an os ulnare externum. Patient's history is unknown.

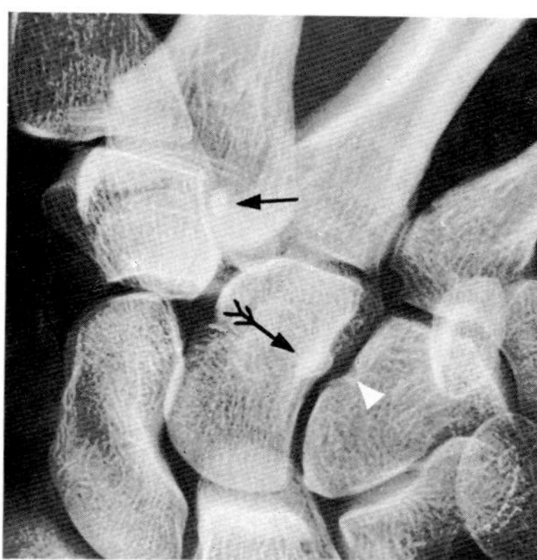

FIGURE 10–47. Protuberance at the capitate (double-tailed arrow) and a notch (arrowhead) at the corresponding side of the hamate. Trapezoides secondarius or bone island (arrow). (Reprinted with permission from Schmidt H, Freyschmidt J, eds. *Borderlands of normal and early pathologic findings in skeletal radiology.* 4th English ed. Stuttgart, New York: Thieme, 1993.)

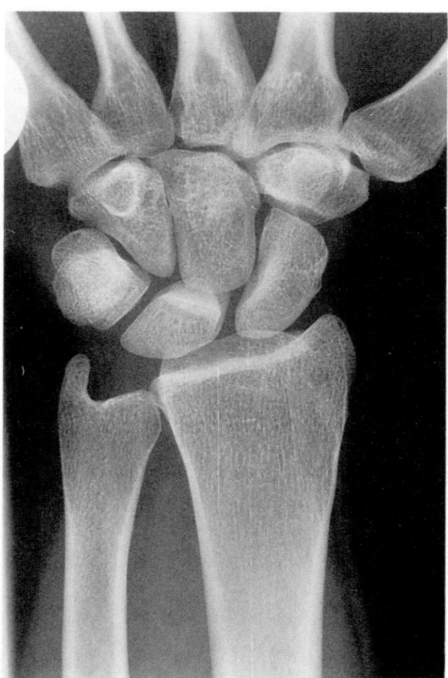

FIGURE 10–49. Ulna minus variant.

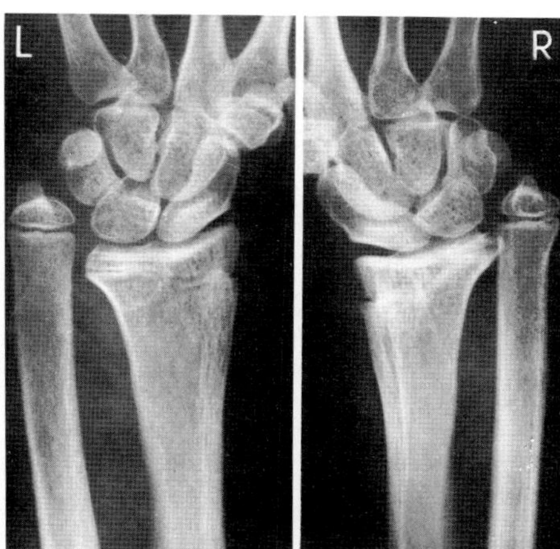

FIGURE 10–50. Ulna-plus variant. The epiphyseal plate of the right radius is closed in some areas, especially centrally. (Reprinted with permission from Schmidt H, Freyschmidt J, eds. *Borderlands of normal and early pathologic findings in skeletal radiology.* 4th English ed. Stuttgart, New York: Thieme, 1993.)

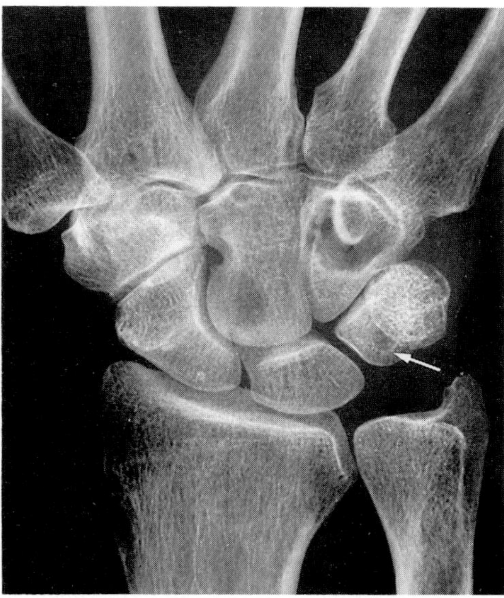

FIGURE 10–52. Large lucent defects compatible with idiopathic bone cysts in the hamate and capitate and a small cyst-like defect (arrow) in the triquetrum of an asymptomatic middle-aged woman.

ing them from fracture fragments to avoid misdiagnoses for their patients. Additional projections are occasionally necessary for a clear interpretation of the extra bones or bone fragments. Depending on the location of the suspicious finding, projections in slight supination or pronation may be helpful. If the bony structures in question are too small for sufficient interpretation, a direct magnification technique or exposure on high-resolution mammography film and interpretation with a magnifying glass may be necessary.

Figure 10–54 gives an overview of the main accessory ossicles of the carpus in the dorsopalmar projection, and Table 10–5 lists the corresponding small hand bone fractures and other lesions. Accessory ossicles usually have a well-defined cortical shell, whereas fresh fragments or avulsions are irregular and lack the cortical shell at the side of the fracture. In contrast to fresh lesions, old partly necrotic fragments are frequently more dense than the adjacent bone. If a diagnostic decision is impossible despite magnification technique and additional projections, a scintigraphic bone scan 6 to 10 days later may clarify the situation. Old fragments usually show normal or only insignificantly increased activity; thus bone scans will be useful when cold, to exclude an acute fracture, and fresh fractures will light up after six days.

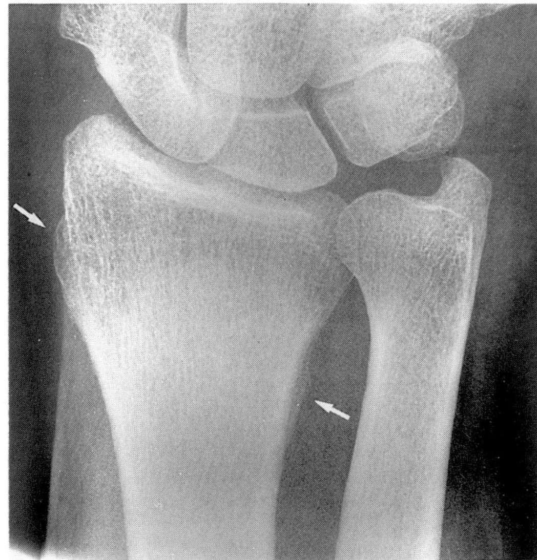

FIGURE 10–51. Normal protuberance at the previous growth plate (arrow, radially), and a normal osseous ridge on the ulnar side of the distal radius (arrow, ulnarly), not a periosteal reaction.

Obvious changes in number and shape of the short hand bones occur with congenital anomalies (i.e., dysostosis multiplex), which must be differentiated from the normal variants we discuss next.

Scaphoid

A bipartition[14] can occur as schematically shown in Fig. 10–54/*9* and mentioned previously. A bipartite scaphoid as well as a hypoplastic scaphoid may be associated with an os centrale carpi (Fig. 10–54/*11*).[4] This accessory ossicle occurs in a gap between the scaphoid, trapezium, and capitate. Pfitzner, who examined 419 wrists in 1894, found an os centrale carpi in 1% of patients.[31] A cartilaginous os centrale carpi has been described during fetal development. The incidence of an os centrale carpi is increased in congenital malformations.[7] Therefore one should look for an associated malformation syndrome when finding an os centrale carpi, sometimes with incomplete expression and only mild clinical findings. An os centrale can be identified and distinguished from an avulsion because of its obvious symmetric occurrence

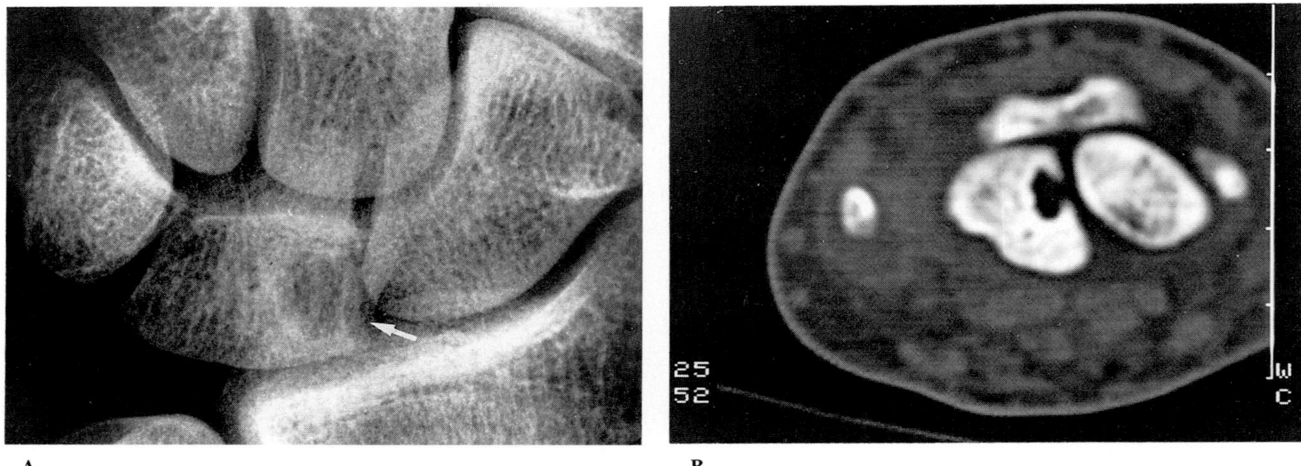

A B

FIGURE 10–53. A: Cyst-like osteolysis in the lunate (arrow), causing pain. **B:** Computed tomography of the lunate shows a defect at its radial margin. An intraosseous ganglion must be considered.

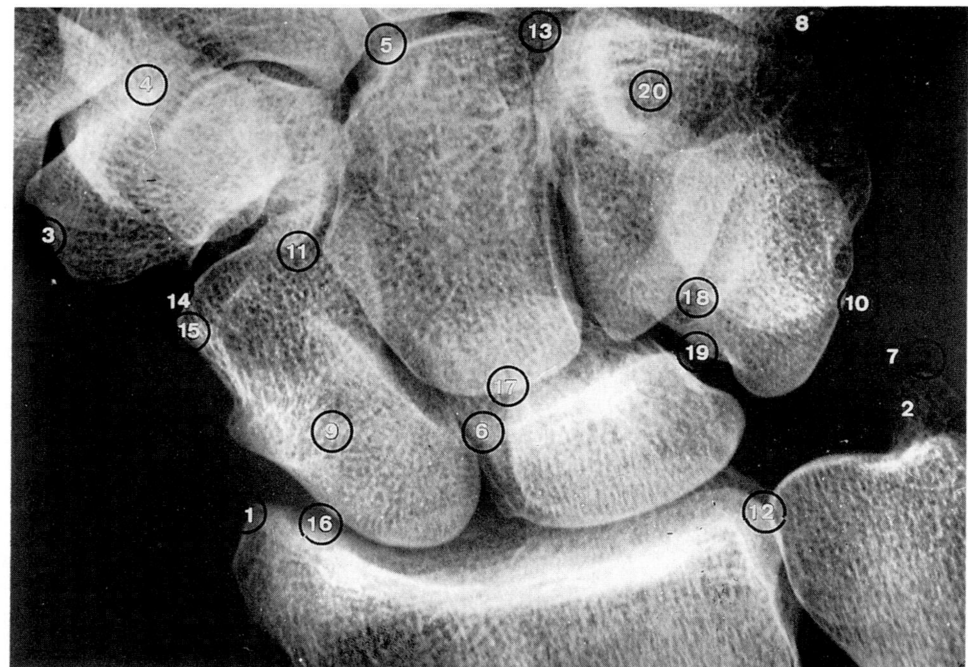

FIGURE 10–54. Schematic overview of some accessory ossicles of the carpus that may simulate disease.[6] 1: persistent ossification center; 2: persistent ossification center/"os triangulare"; 3: paratrapezium; 4: sec. trapezoid/sec. trapezium; 5: os styloideum; 6: epilunate; 7: unnamed ossicles; 8: os vesalianum/os ulnare externum; 9: bi- or multiple partition of the scaphoid; 10: multiple ossification centers; 11: os centrale carpi; 12: ossicles in the distal radioulnar joint; 13: sec. capitate/ossiculum Gruberi; 14: epitrapezium; 15: os radiale externum; 16: os paranaviculare; 17: hypolunate; 18: epitriquetrum; 19: epipyramis; 20: os hamuli proprium. sec, secondary or secondarius.

TABLE 10–5. ***Differential Diagnosis of Accessory Ossicles in the Dorsopalmar View of the Carpus (see Fig. 10–54)***

	Accessory Ossicles	Corresponding Fractures
1	Persistent ossification center	Radial styloid process
2	Persistent ossification center/"os triangulare"	Ulnar styloid process
3	Paratrapezium	Trapezium
4	Sec. trapezoid/sec. trapezium	Trapezoid, trapezium
5	Os styloideum	Base of metacarpal III, capitate, trapezoid
6	Epilunate	Lunate
7	Unnamed ossicles	Triquetrum
8	Os vesalianum/os ulnare externum	Base of metacarpal V, hamulus
9	Bi- or multiple partition of the scaphoid	Scaphoid
10	Multiple ossification centers	Pisiform
11	Os centrale carpi	Capitate
12	Ossicles in the DRUJ	Radius
13	Sec. capitate/ossiculum Gruberi	Capitate, hamate, bases of the III and IV metacarpals
14	Epitrapezium	Tubercle of the scaphoid
15	Os radiale externum	Tubercle of the scaphoid
16	Os paranaviculare	Calcification in chondrocalcinosis
17	Hypolunate	Lunate
18	Epitriquetrum	Triquetrum
19	Epipyramis	Triquetrum
20	Os hamuli proprium	Hamulus

sec, secondary or secondarius; III, IV, V, 3rd, 4th, 5th; DRUJ, distal radioulnar joint.

as shown in Fig. 10–55. In this case an interpretation as a bilateral bipartite scaphoid is also possible.

An os radiale externum (see Fig. 10–54/*15*) is visible in the dorsopalmar projection as well as in the lateral projection, and difficulties could arise in differentiating it from a dislocated flake fragment of the tubercle of the scaphoid. The os radiale externum is highly variable in shape and size. Georgy and Hilger[32] reported an os radiale externum as large as a "cherry." A well-defined accessory bone is shown in Fig. 10–56. In this case it is impossible to differentiate between a large epitrapezium or an os radiale externum. The epitrapezium (Fig. 10–54/*14*) occurs on the radial side between the scaphoid and trapzium. Its differentiation from the os radiale externum is usually academic. A posttraumatic ossification in this region after a fracture of the first metacarpal has been reported by Köhler and Zimmer.[6] Without the history, it could erroneously be diagnosed as an os radiale externum or an epitrapezium (Figs. 10–57A and 10–57B).

The amorphous calcification on the radial side of the scaphoid (Fig. 10–58) is not an accessory ossicle but a calcifying tendinitis. Spontaneous erythema, swelling, and pain was observed clinically.

The os paranaviculare (Fig. 10–54/*16*) in the ra-

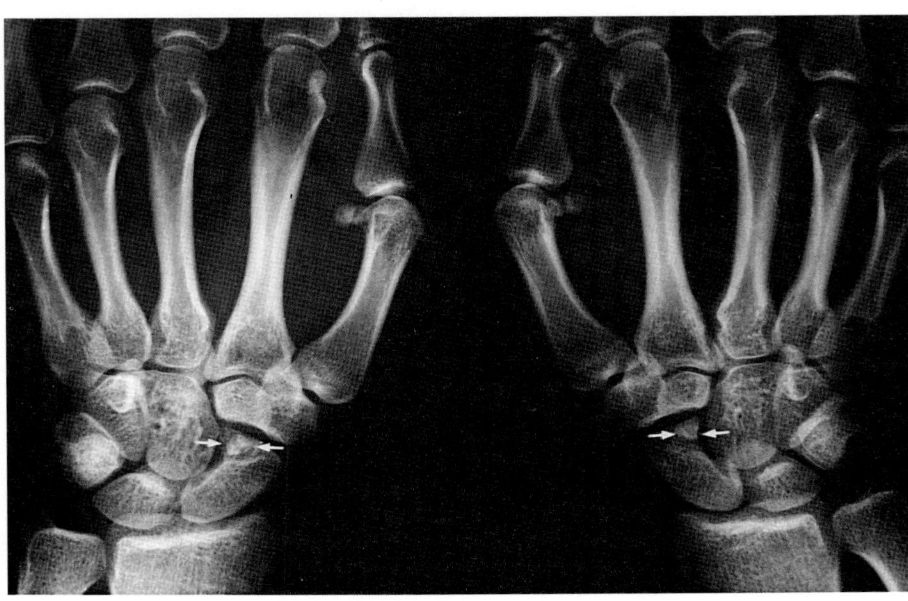

FIGURE 10–55. Bilateral os centrale carpi (arrows). (Reprinted with permission from Schmidt H, Freyschmidt J, eds. *Borderlands of normal and early pathologic findings in skeletal radiology.* 4th English ed. Stuttgart, New York: Thieme, 1993.)

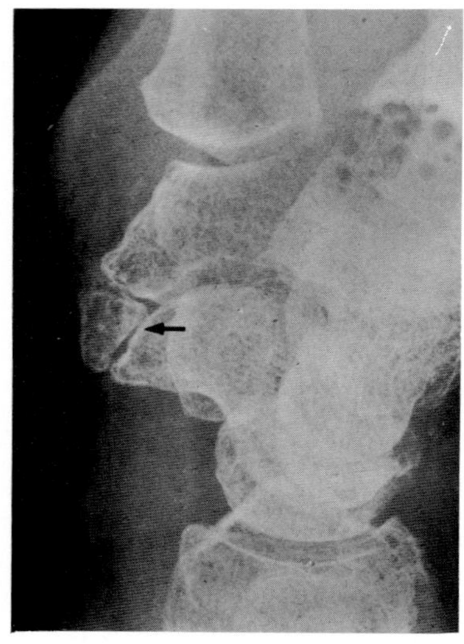

FIGURE 10–56. This may depict an epitrapezium or os radiale externum (arrow). (Reprinted with permission from Schmidt H, Freyschmidt J, eds. *Borderlands of normal and early pathologic findings in skeletal radiology*. 4th English ed. Stuttgart, New York: Thieme, 1993.)

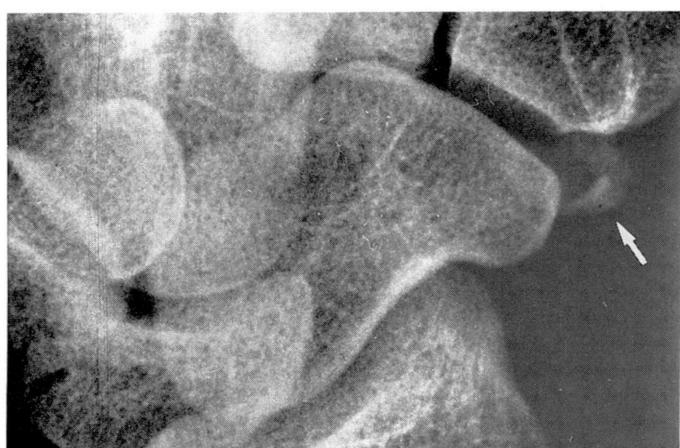

FIGURE 10–58. Calcifying tendinitis (arrow). (Note the amorphous structure.)

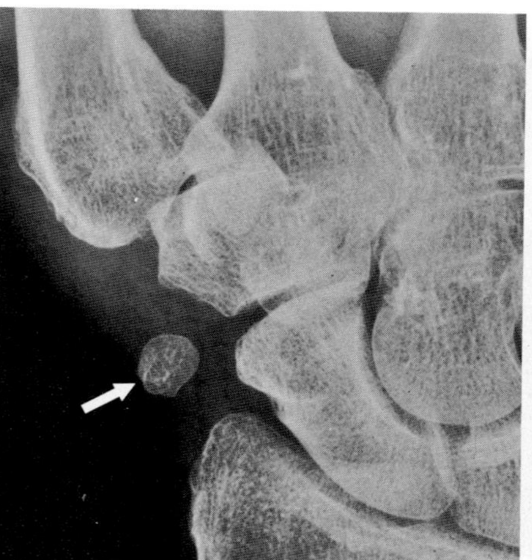

A

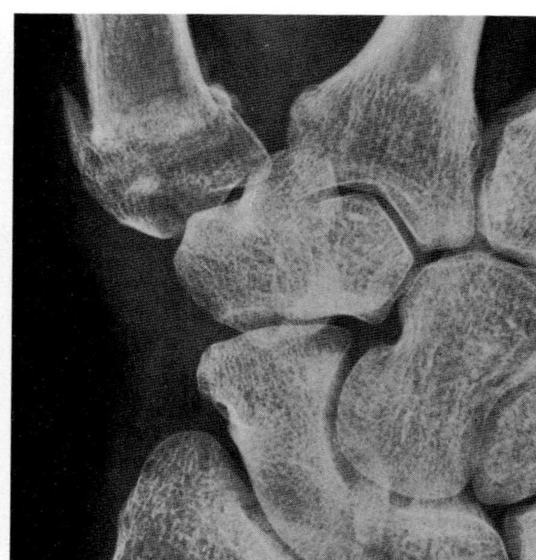

B

FIGURE 10–57. A: Well-defined bony element on the radial side of the distal pole of the scaphoid (arrow). It may be an old fragment, os radiale externum, or os epitrapezium. **B:** Seventeen years earlier. No bony element is visible but the first metacarpal is fractured. We assume the bony element in question is the result of a posttraumatic soft-tissue ossification. (Reprinted with permission from Schmidt H, Freyschmidt J, eds. *Borderlands of normal and early pathologic findings in skeletal radiology*. 4th English ed. Stuttgart, New York: Thieme, 1993.)

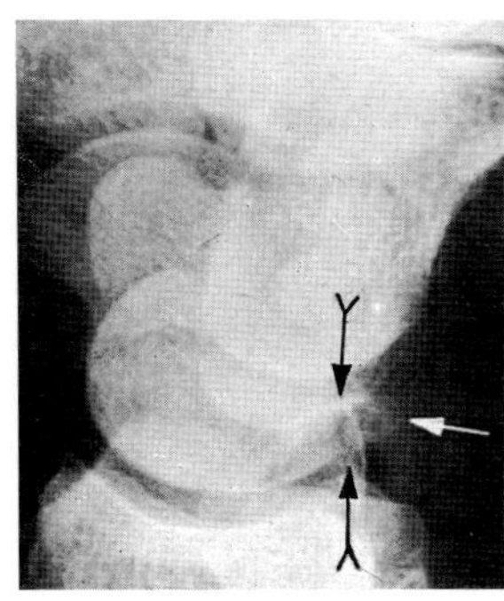
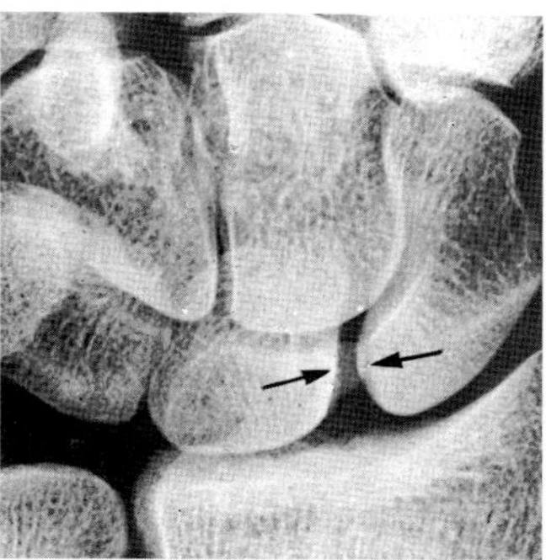

FIGURE 10–59. A and **B:** Epilunate (arrows). A cleft (between arrows with tails) separates this bone from the lunate. (Reprinted with permission from Schmidt H, Freyschmidt J, eds. *Borderlands of normal and early pathologic findings in skeletal radiology.* 4th English ed. Stuttgart, New York: Thieme, 1993.)

dioscaphoid space can be mistaken for chondrocalcinosis because of its amorphous appearance.

Lunate

At the dorsal pole of the lunate, the so-called epilunate (see Figs. 10–54/*6* and 10–59) may be mistaken for an avulsion from the triquetrum. This bony element is a small, round ossicle of low density. Therefore it is not visible on every projection, in contrast to almost any other ossicle. The hypolunate (Fig. 10–54/*17*), located on the distal radial and somewhat palmar side of the lunate, can occur symmetrically in both hands. Because of its possibly triangular form it should not be misinterpreted as a flake fragment of the lunate (Fig. 10–60) or, in an oblique position, of the scaphoid.

Triquetrum

Two bony elements have been described in the intercarpal space between the triquetrum and the adjacent distal row of the carpal bones. The os epitriquetrum (Fig. 10–54/*18*) on the dorsal side must be distinguished from avulsions of the triquetrum. The epipyramis (Figs. 10–54/*19* and 10–61) is located on the palmar side. Bony structures, unnamed partly because of their little clinical relevance, and undefined calcifications can occur in the ulnocarpal space. As visible in Fig. 10–62A, some ossicles are located close to the styloid process of the ulna. Others are located more distal in the region of the triquetrum (Fig. 10–62B). These findings are often caused by nonunited older fractures of the styloid (Fig. 10–63), although a corresponding defect is not found in every case. Complete reossification of periosteal lesions and hypertrophy of chip fragments is possible. Degenerative changes because of nonunited fractures of the ulnar styloid process are commonly observed. Large, well-defined ossicles in the ulnocarpal space may be classified as persistent ossification centers of the styloid process (Fig. 10–54/*2*).

Such ossicles have been reported as "posttraumatic ossa triangularia" (Fig. 10–54/*2*).[34] Location, shape, and structure are not specific and therefore they cannot be differentiated from nonunited fractures of the styloid process. The os triangulare, like the os centrale carpi, is a congenital skeletal element, which normally disappears at birth. It can be visible in congenital malformation syndromes overlying the distal ulna.[7]

Pisiform

If there are multiple ossification centers (Fig. 10–54/*10*) of the pisiform, difficulties in interpretation can arise in the adolescent. These must be distinguished from avulsion fractures, especially if a shell-like configuration is found (Fig. 10–64). The clinician should also take care not to misinterpret these physiologic findings as osteochondrotic changes.

Hamate

A congenital absence of the hamulus may occur.[25] In these cases, the typical dense ring of the base of the hamulus in the dorsopalmar projection is absent (Fig. 10–54/*20*). If nonfusion of the hamulus occurs, the hook-shaped isolated "accessory bone" is called os hamuli proprium. It is visible and accessible in the lateral view or in a tangential projection of the carpal tunnel.

Another accessory bone occurring between the hamate and the fifth metacarpal is the os vesalianum (Fig. 10–54/*8*). It could be mistaken for either a chip fragment from the base of the fifth metacarpal or an avulsion from the ulnar part of the hamulus (Fig. 10–65). Köhler and Zimmer[6] described the os ulnare externum, which may be differentiated from the os vesalianum, although this is of little clinical importance.

Capitate

A capitatum secundarium (Fig. 10–54/*13*), best seen on oblique views (Fig. 10–66), can occur in the CMC space between the bases of the third and fourth metacarpals and the distal part of the capitate and hamate. This ossicle is easily identifiable by its mostly rounded shape and its typical location. Differential diagnosis should include the ossiculum Gruberi (Fig. 10–54/*13*), which is only a tiny calcified structure and occurs in the same region.

The os styloideum (Figs. 10–54/*5*, 10–67, 10–68A, and 10–68B) occurs as a normal variant and arises from an accessory ossification center at the base of the second or third metacarpal. It is found between these bases and the capitotrapezoid space. The best radiographic projection is in profile with 30-degree supination and ulnar deviation of the wrist. Clinically a fixed dorsal prominence on the second and third metacarpal bases is palpable. This clinical finding, however, can have explanations other than an os styloideum. Often exostosis-like changes at the CMC joints, sometimes with degenerative changes, are found (Figs. 10–68A and 10–68B). The os styloideum as well as the exostosis-like changes can cause the carpe bossu or "carpal boss" condition. Patients

Text continued on page 288

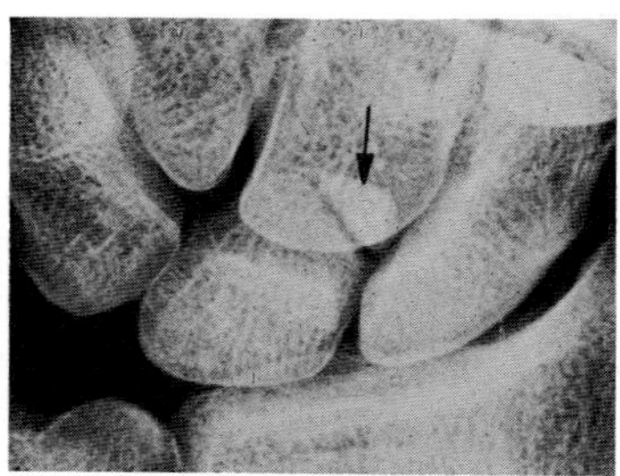

FIGURE 10–60. Hypolunate (arrow). (Reprinted with permission from Schmidt H, Freyschmidt J, eds. *Borderlands of normal and early pathologic findings in skeletal radiology.* 4th English ed. Stuttgart, New York: Thieme, 1993.)

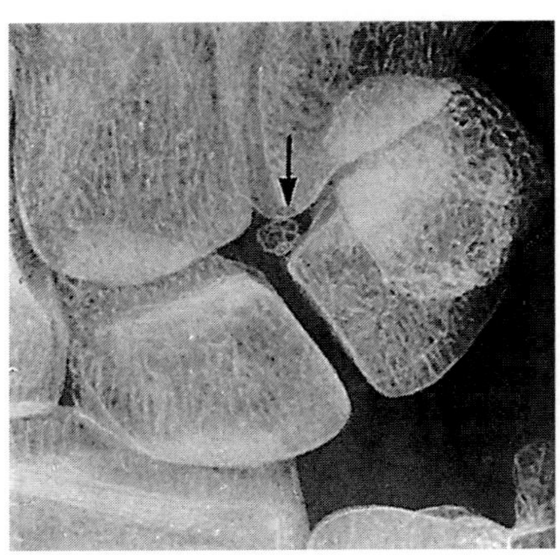

FIGURE 10–61. Epipyramis (arrow). (Reprinted with permission from Schmidt H, Freyschmidt J, eds. *Borderlands of normal and early pathologic findings in skeletal radiology.* 4th English ed. Stuttgart, New York: Thieme, 1993.)

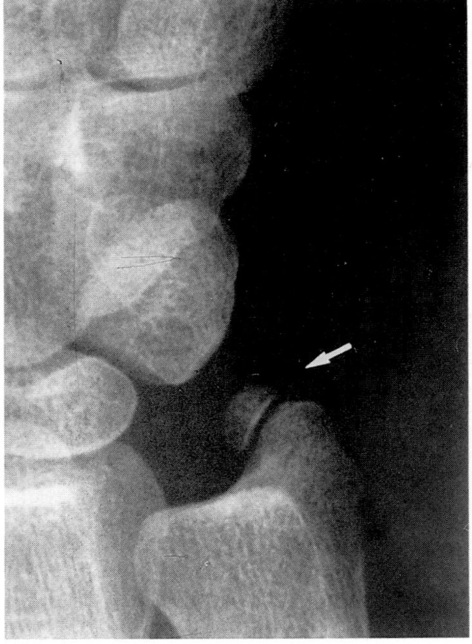

A

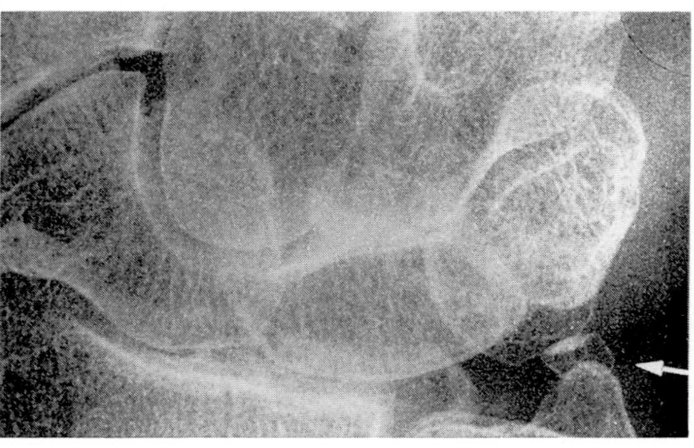

B

FIGURE 10–62. A: This may depict a persistent ossification center (arrow) or old avulsion. **B:** Possibly an os ulnare externum (arrow), old avulsion, or persistent ossification center.

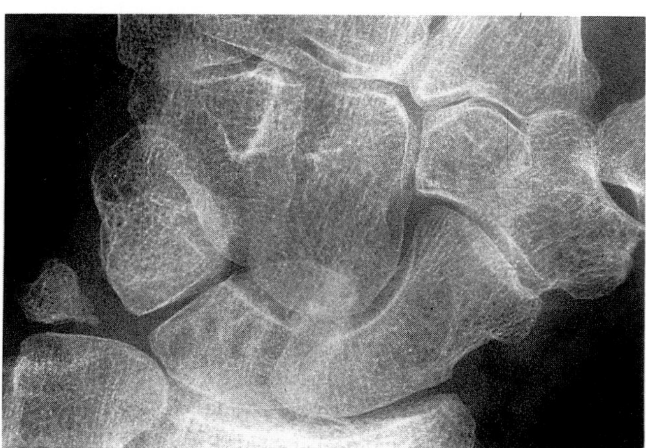

FIGURE 10–63. Nonfusion of a fractured ulnar styloid process.

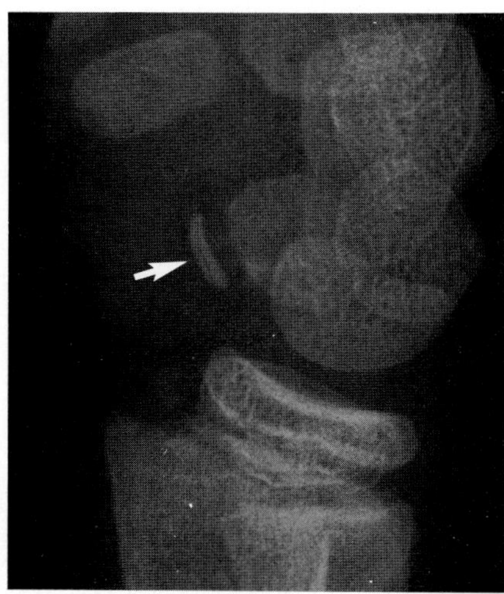

FIGURE 10–64. Epiphysiolysis of the distal radius. Shell-like ossification center (arrow) of the pisiform. (Reprinted with permission from Schmidt H, Freyschmidt J, eds. *Borderlands of normal and early pathologic findings in skeletal radiology.* 4th English ed. Stuttgart, New York: Thieme, 1993.)

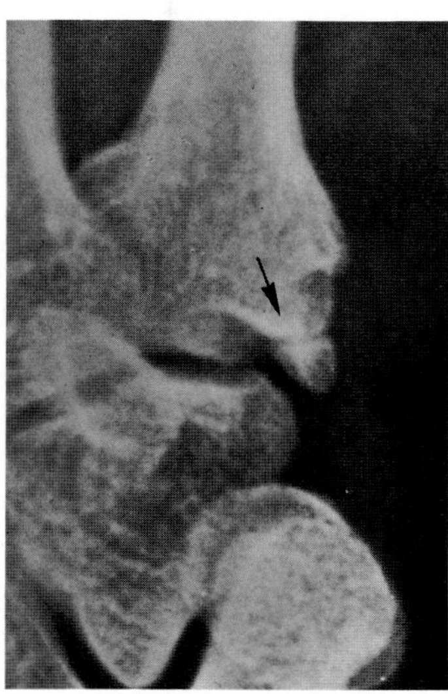

FIGURE 10–65. Os vesalianum (arrow). (Reprinted with permission from Schmidt H, Freyschmidt J, eds. *Borderlands of normal and early pathologic findings in skeletal radiology.* 4th English ed. Stuttgart, New York: Thieme, 1993.)

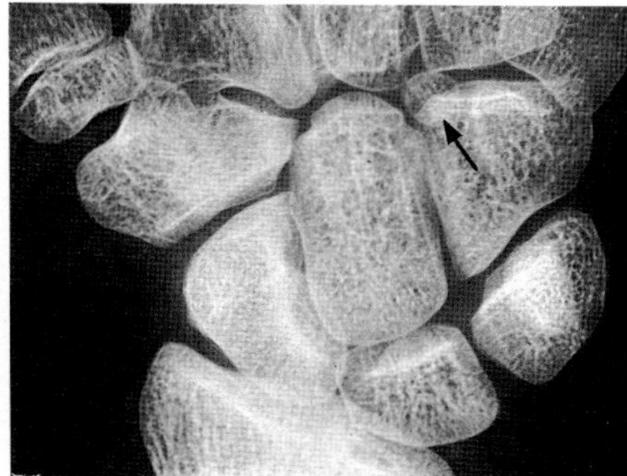

FIGURE 10–66. Capitatum secundarium (arrow). (Reprinted with permission from Schmidt H, Freyschmidt J, eds. *Borderlands of normal and early pathologic findings in skeletal radiology.* 4th English ed. Stuttgart, New York: Thieme, 1993.)

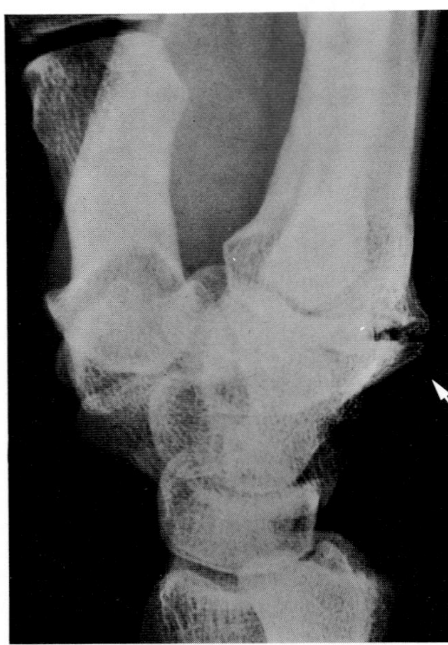

FIGURE 10–67. Osseous ridges (arrow) at the bases of the second and third metacarpal bones. A separate os styloideum is not identifiable. (Reprinted with permission from Schmidt H, Freyschmidt J, eds. *Borderlands of normal and early pathologic findings in skeletal radiology.* 4th English ed. Stuttgart, New York: Thieme, 1993.)

with this condition suffer from painful reduction of the mobility of the hand caused by an overlying ganglion or a bursitis with pressure on the external tendinous sheaths, moving over those osseous prominences. An os styloideum was found in 33% of patients suffering from carpe bossu disease, compared with an occurrence of about 3% in asymptomatic wrists.[35]

In his anatomic studies, Pfitzner described an os metastyloideum and an os parastyloideum in the same region as the os styloideum.[31] A differentiation between these ossicles and an os styloideum is not conceivable on plain film radiography of the hand.

Trapezium

The epitrapezium has been mentioned previously. Four different accessory ossicles close to the trapezium, which are rather impossible to distinguish radiologically, were described on Pfitzner's anatomic studies.[31] An os paratrapezium (Figs. 10–54/*3* and 10–69) and the os praetrapezium on the radial side of the trapezium should be recognized and not be considered as flake fractures from the trapezium or avulsions from the first metacarpal base. The same is true for the trapezium secundarium (Fig. 10–54/*4*) and the trapezoides secundarium, located in the space between the bases of the first and second metacarpals and the trapezium and trapezoid.

Variants in Carpal Angle

The normal carpal angles, palmar slope, and distal radial inclination,[36] which are discussed in Chapter 9, show relatively small variances. Alterations are usually posttraumatic. When standard projections are not available because of distressed patients in the emergency room, a subluxation should not be diagnosed. To determine carpal instabilities plain films should be repeated promptly under standard conditions.

Acquired diseases such as rheumatoid arthritis may cause an obvious change in carpal angles, especially

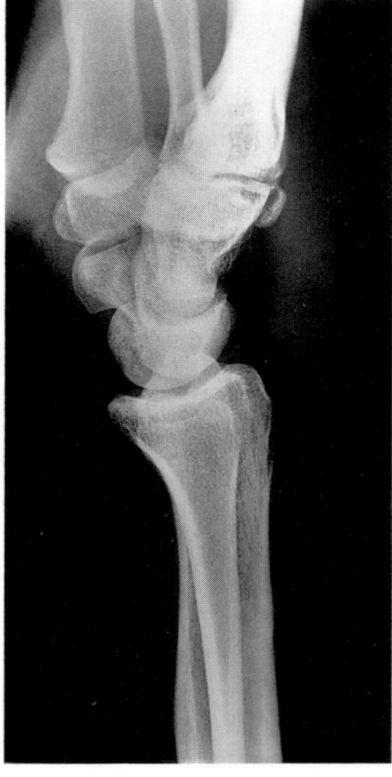

A

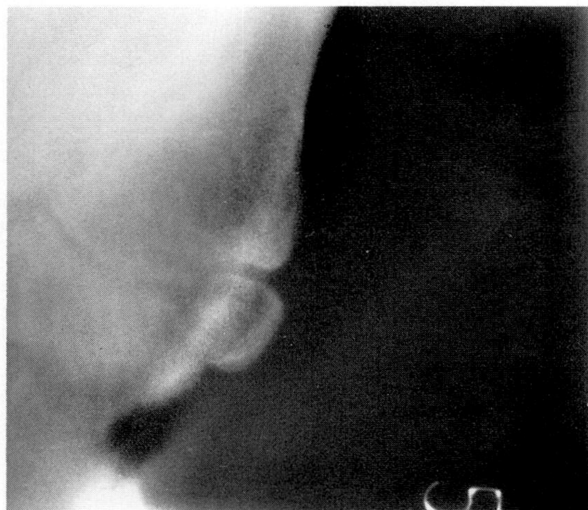

B

FIGURE 10–68. A and **B:** Possibly an os styloideum. No trauma in patient's history. Painful reduction in mobility.

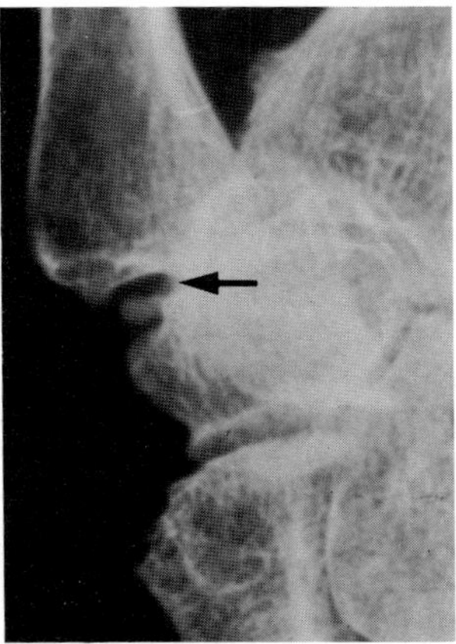

FIGURE 10–69. It is not possible to distinguish if this is a paratrapezium or praetrapezium bone. (Reprinted with permission from Schmidt H, Freyschmidt J, eds. *Borderlands of normal and early pathologic findings in skeletal radiology.* 4th English ed. Stuttgart, New York: Thieme, 1993.)

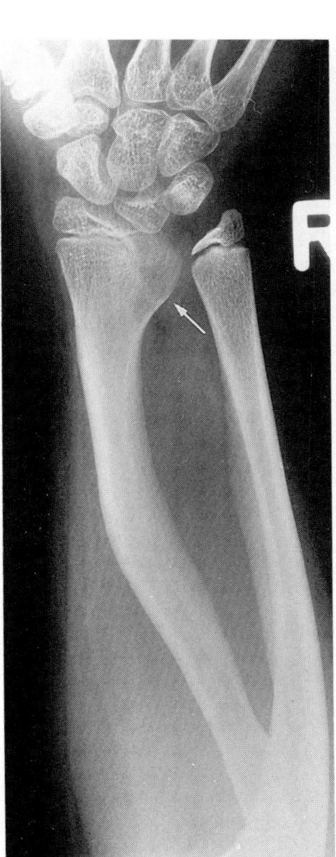

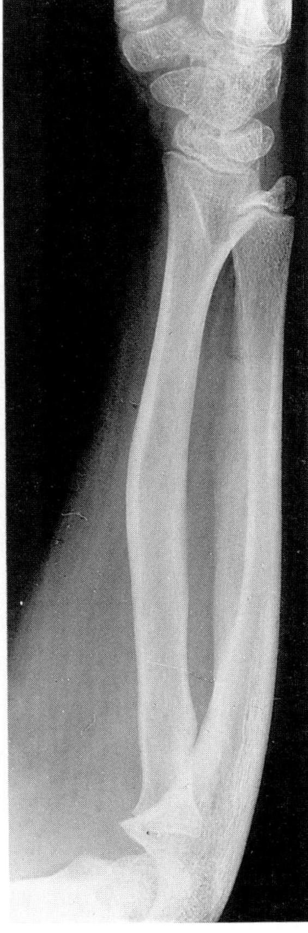

A B

FIGURE 10–70. PA (**A**) and lateral (**B**) views. Typical findings in Madelung deformity (bayonet position of the wrist, dorsal prominence of the distal ulna, increased angle or steeper slope of the distal radius on the PA view accompanied with decreased carpal angle, and decreased bony density (arrow) on the distal ulnar border of the radius).

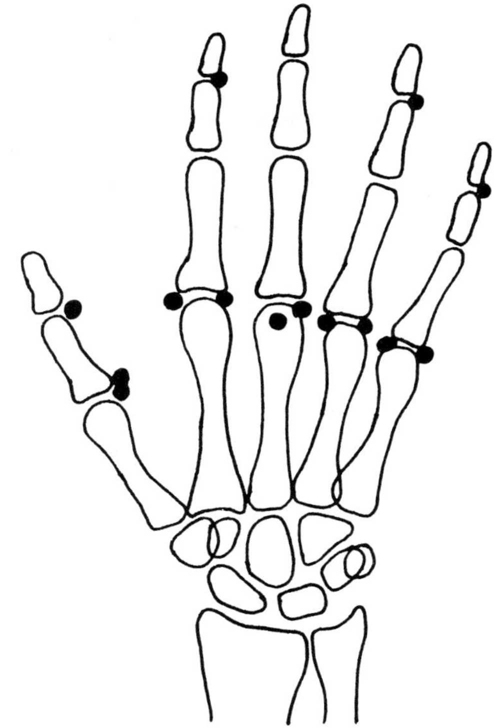

FIGURE 10–71. Sesamoids in the healthy adult. Usually two sesamoids are present at the metacarpophalangeal joint of the thumb. In about 80% of people sesamoids near the distal joint of the thumb and the metacarpophalangeal joint of the fifth digit are observed. Occurrence of sesamoids at other joints is more or less rare.

in later stages. Other causes are congenital anomalies, such as the Madelung deformity, in which a shortening of the radius causes a decrease of the carpal angle and a palmar and proximal displacement of the carpus. Erroneous interpretation of the lucency at the distal radius in this deformity as a bone tumor has been described (Figs. 10–70A and 10–70B).[34]

SESAMOID BONES

Normal Findings and Minor Variants

Singular or multiple sesamoid bones occur at various metacarpophalangeal and interphalangeal joints (Fig. 10–71). Two sesamoids are always visible at the metacarpophalangeal joint of the thumb. Frequently one sesamoid occurs at the interphalangeal joint of the thumb and at the fifth metacarpophalangeal joint, while sometimes additional sesamoids can appear in those regions. More or less often sesamoids are found at the metacarpophalangeal joints. Rarely sesamoids may be seen at the distal interphalangeal joints of the index finger, the ring finger, or the small finger.

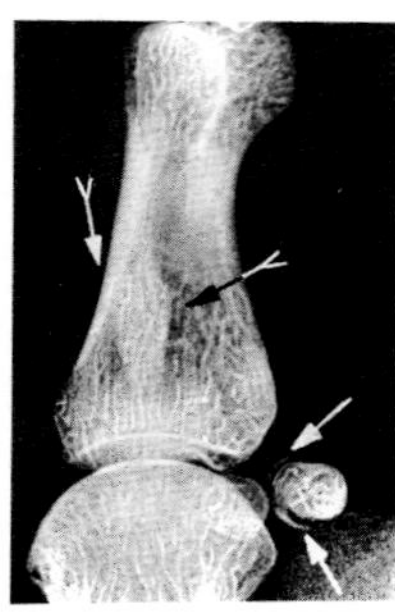

FIGURE 10–72. Shell fracture of a sesamoid (arrows). A benign sclerotic foci (arrows with tail) is in the shaft. (Reprinted with permission from Schmidt H, Freyschmidt J, eds. *Borderlands of normal and early pathologic findings in skeletal radiology.* 4th English ed. Stuttgart, New York: Thieme, 1993.)

Sesamoid bones must be differentiated from heterotopic ossifications or fractures of the adjacent bones, especially in unusual locations. This is easily possible when a well-organized spongious bone surrounded by a compact shell is detected in larger sesamoids, especially in typical locations such as the base of the proximal phalanx of the thumb. Fractures of the thumb sesamoids are seen after abduction trauma, such as a fall on the outstretched hand. These fractures are rare and might be detected because of a cortical avulsion (Fig. 10–72). These intrasesamoidal fractures should be differentiated from bipartite sesamoids (Fig. 10–73). Small sesamoids with a homogeneous calcified density can be misinterpreted as a bone island when projected over the adjacent bone, which is only of academic interest. Traumatic trapping of a sesamoid into the metacarpophalangeal joint at the thumb is not infrequently observed. Rarely this occurs at the metacarpophalangeal joint of the fifth digit.[19]

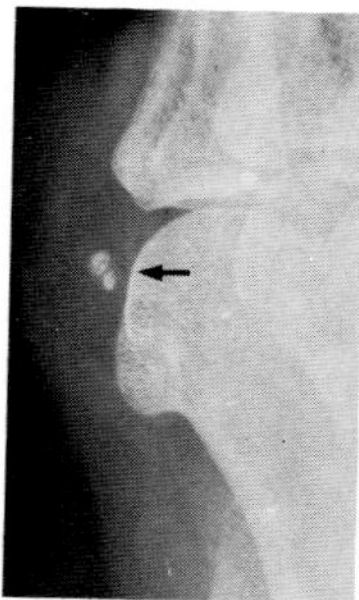

FIGURE 10–73. Bipartite sesamoid (arrow). (Reprinted with permission from Schmidt H, Freyschmidt J, eds. *Borderlands of normal and early pathologic findings in skeletal radiology.* 4th English ed. Stuttgart, New York: Thieme, 1993.)

REFERENCES

1. Van der Laan JG, Thijn CJP. Ivory and dense epiphyses of the hand: Thiemann's disease in three sisters. *Skeletal Radiol* 1986;15:117–122.
2. Kuhns LR, Poznanski AK, Harper HAS, Garn SM. Ivory epiphyses of the hands. *Radiology* 1973;109:643–648.
3. Pitt MJ. Rachitic and osteomalacic syndromes. *Radiol Clin North Am* 1981;19:581–599.
4. Giedion A. Zapfenepiphysen. Naturgeschichte und diagnostische Bedeutung einer Störung des enchondralen Wachstums. In: Glauner R, Rüttimann A, Thurn P, Vogler E, eds. *Ergebnisse der medizinischen Radiologie.* Bd.I. Stuttgart: Thieme. 1968:59–124.
5. Riggs W Jr, Wilroy RS Jr, Etteldorf JN. Neonatal hyperthyroidism with accelerated skeletal maturation, craniosynostosis, and brachydactyly. *Radiology* 1972;105:621–625.
6. Köhler A, Zimmer EA. *Borderlands of normal and early pathologic findings in skeletal radiography.* 4th English ed. Schmidt H, Freyschmidt J, eds. Stuttgart, New York: Thieme, 1993.
7. Poznanski AK. *The hand in radiologic diagnosis.* 2nd ed. Philadelphia: WB Saunders, 1984.
8. Metz VM, Schimmerl SM, Gilula LA, et al. Wide scapholunate joint space in lunotriquetral coalition: A normal variant? *Radiology* 1993;188:557–559.
9. Taylor GA, Jordan CE, Dorst SK, et al. Polycarpaly and other abnormalities of the wrist in chondroectodermal dysplasia: The Ellis-van Creveld syndrome. *Radiology* 1984;151:393–396.
10. Kosowicz J. The roentgen appearance of the hand and wrist in gonadal dysgenesis. *Am J Roentgenol* 1965;93:354–361.
11. Archibald RM, Finby N, De Vito F. Endocrine significance of short metacarpals. *J Clin Endocrinol* 1959;19:1312–1322.
12. Bloom RA. The metacarpal sign. *Brit J Radiol* 1970;43:133–135.
13. Freyschmidt J, Ostertag H. *Knochentumoren: Klinik, Radiologie, Pathologie.* Berlin: Springer, 1988.
14. Freyschmidt J. *Skeletterkrankungen: Klinisch-radiologische Diagnose und Differentialdiagnose.* Berlin: Springer-Verlag, 1993.
15. Resnick D, Niwayama G. *Diagnosis of bone and joint disorders,* Vol. 4. 2nd ed. Philadelphia: WB Saunders, 1988.
16. Fischer E. Früh-und Minimalformen des Hyperparathyreoidismus am Rande der Tuberositas phalangis distalis der Finger. *Fortschr Röntgenstr* 1990;153:289–295.
17. Yune HY, Vix VA, Klatte EC. Early fingertip changes in scleroderma. *JAMA* 1971;215:1113–1116.
18. Wilson RH, McCormick WE, Tatum CF, et al. Occupational acroosteolysis. *JAMA* 1967;201;577–581.
19. Inada Y, Tamai S, Kawanishi K, et al. Fifth digit sesamoid fracture with tendosynovitis. *J Hand Surg* 1992;17A:915–917.
20. Fischer E. Weichteilverkalkungen am Rand der Tuberositas phalangis distalis der Finger. *Fortschr Röntgenstr* 1983;139:150–157.
21. Norgaard F. Earliest roentgenological changes in polyarthritis of the rheumatoid type: Rheumatoid arthritis. *Radiology* 1965;85:325–329.
22. Stelling CB, Keats MM, Keats TE. Irregularities at the base of the proximal phalanges: False indicator of early rheumatoid arthritis. *AJR* 1982;138:695–698.
23. Eiken O, Jonsson K. Carpal bone cysts. *Scand J Plast Reconstr Hand Surg* 1980;14:285–290.
24. Ravelli A. Anatomisch-röntgenologische Handgelenksstudien. *Z Orthop* 1955;86:70–89.
25. Wiss DA, Reid BS. Painless osteoid osteoma of the fingers: Report of three cases. *J Hand Surg* 1983A;8:914–917.
26. Tiel-van Buul MMC, van Beek EJ, Broekhuisen AH, et al. Diagnosing scaphoid fractures: Radiographs cannot be used as a gold standard! *Injury* 1992;23:77–79.
27. Staniforth P. Scaphoid fractures and wrist pain: Time for new thinking. *Injury (Br)* 1991;22:435–436.
28. Norman A, Nelson J, Green S. Fractures of the hook of hamate: Radiographic signs. *Radiology* 1985;154:49–53.
29. Seeger LL, Bassett LW, Gold RH. Case report 464: Bilateral congenital absence of the hook of the hamate. *Skeletal Radiol* 1988;17:85–86.

30. Uchiyama S, Terayama K. Radiographic changes in wrists with ulnar plus variance observed over a ten-year period. *J Hand Surg* 1991;16A:45–48.
31. Pfitzner W. Beiträge zur Kenntnis des menschlichen Extremitätenskeletts. Dritte Abteilung. Die Varietäten VI. Die Variationen im Aufbau des Handskeletts. *Morph. Arb Hrsg. von G. Schwalbe IV,* 1895:347–570.
32. Georgy HU, Hillger H. Beobachtung eines ungewöhnlich großen os radiale externum. *Fortschr Röntgenstr* 1969;111:715–716.
33. Freyschmidt J. *Knochenerkrankungen im Erwachsenenalter.* Berlin: Springer, 1980.
34. Thomas RD, Fairhurst JJ, Clarke NMP. Madelung's deformity masquerading as a bone tumour. *Skeletal Radiol* 1993;22:329–331.
35. Cuono CB, Watson HK. The carpal boss: Surgical treatment and etiological considerations. *Plas Reconstr Surg* 1979;63:88–93.
36. Mann FA, Wilson AJ, Gilula LA. Radiographic evaluation of the wrist: What does the hand surgeon want to know? *Radiology* 1992;184:15–24.

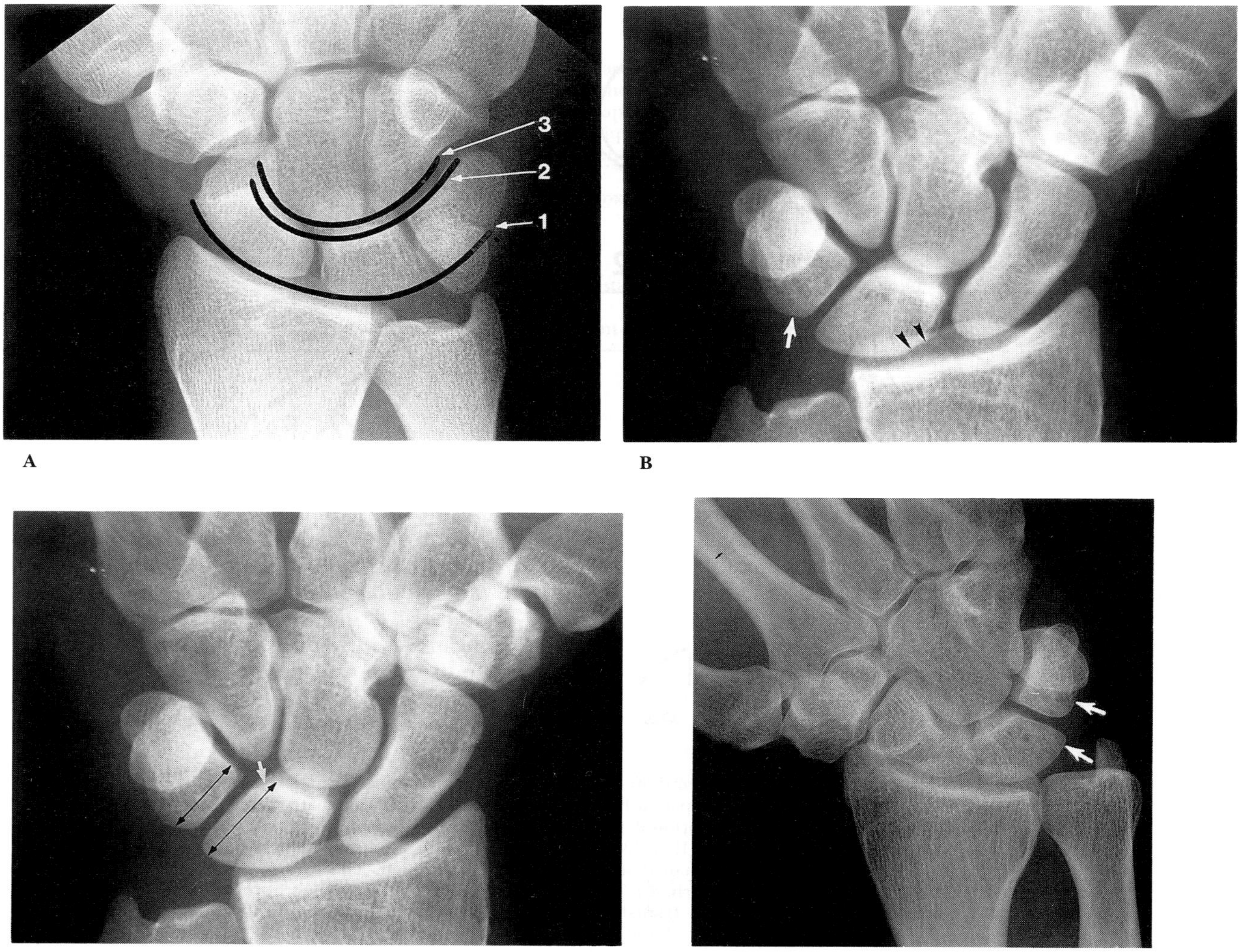

A

B

C

D

FIGURE 11–3. Three normal arcs on the PA view of a wrist. **A:** Standard PA view of the right wrist demonstrates three arcs (Arcs I, II, III). Arc I joins the outer curvatures of the proximal articular surfaces of the scaphoid, lunate, and triquetrum (the proximal carpal articular surfaces of the proximal carpal row). Arc II connects the distal smooth curves of these same three bones (the distal carpal articular surfaces of the proximal carpal row). No hamate facet of the lunate is evident (see Fig. 11–3C). Arc III identifies the proximal surfaces of the capitate and hamate. (Modified with permission from Gilula LA. Carpal injuries: Analytic approach and case exercises. *AJR* 1979;133:503–517.) **B:** PA view of the left wrist demonstrates a normal round corner at the lunate (black arrowheads) and triquetrum (white arrow). **C:** PA view of the left wrist demonstrates an offset between the lunate and triquetrum distally breaking Arc II caused by the shorter distance between the proximal and distal surfaces of the triquetrum than that of the lunate (double-headed arrows). A small facet of the lunate (hamate facet) that articulates with the proximal pole of the hamate is present (arrow). This is called a Type II lunate by Viegas et al.[12] **D:** PA view of the right wrist in radial deviation demonstrates that Arcs I and II are interrupted at the LT joint (arrows). However Arc I is not applicable at this joint because the proximal–distal lengths of the adjacent portions of the lunate and triquetrum are congenitally different. **E:** PA view of the left wrist in ulnar deviation demonstrates about 1 mm offset at the SL joint, seen more easily along Arc II (arrowheads).

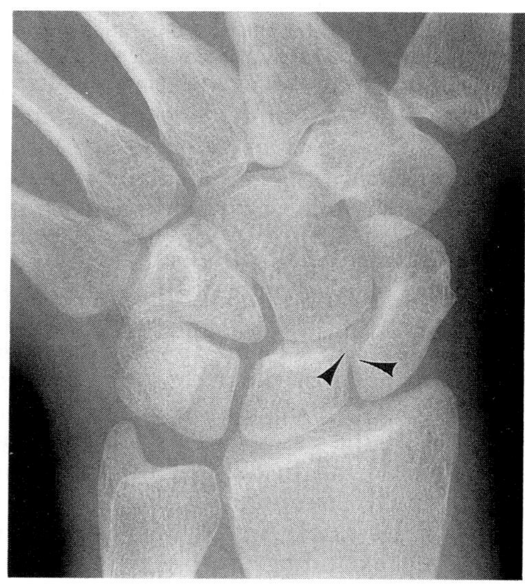

E

is not located within either carpal row, abnormalites of the pisiform alone do not interrupt the continuity of the carpal arcs. Disruption of Arc III with or without intact Arcs I and II implies an abnormality located between the capitate and hamate (Fig. 11–5). When all three arcs are "broken," both proximal and distal rows are abnormal.

Parallelism is another feature of normal alignment.[1,4,15] In general all the carpal bones can be observed in two ways. The first is to examine all the bones separately and try to remember the shapes of all the bones in every conceivable position of the wrist (Figs. 11–6A and 11–6B). In the opinion of these authors, that approach is very difficult. The second method to look at the carpal bones and articulating metacarpals, radius, and ulna is to recognize the concept of "parallelism." When joints are tangentially profiled, the apposing subchondral articulating cortices should be parallel. Parallelism can be easily understood by thinking of a jigsaw puzzle. If one piece of the puzzle is sitting on top of other pieces, it can be recognized easily as out of place or "dislocated." Similarly if articulating bones are examined by looking at their normally parallel articulating cortices, abnormally positioned bones can be recognized easily (Figs. 11–6A and 11–6C). This principle of parallelism can be used for nearly any joint in the body. The only difficult part of using parallelism is learning to recognize what are "profiled" cortices, because if a cortex is profiled, that adjacent joint should be visible. In that situation the cortex on the opposite side of the joint should also be visible and parallel, even though portions of these bones may be overlapping each other (Fig. 11–6). Therefore, in the normal wrist, parallelism should be seen at any profiled joints: between the radius, scaphoid, and lunate; between the bones of the proximal and distal carpal rows; at the intercarpal joints; and at the CMC joints (see Fig. 11–1).

On a neutral PA view of the normal wrist, routinely the pisotriquetral and scaphotrapeziotrapezoidal joints are not profiled. Usually some overlap of the proximal portions of the scaphoid and lunate by the dorsal lip of the radius will be evident, as well as that between the dorsal lip of the lunate and the head of the capitate. In these circumstances, there remains a clear profile of the "joint spaces." However, when overlap exists between both the palmar and dorsal parts of apposing bones, a subluxation or dislocation is probable (Fig. 11–7).

All RC, intercarpal, and CMC joint spaces should be similar in width and are about 1 to 2 mm wide. Occasionally, normal joint spaces may be slightly wider and symmetric, but their widths do not exceed 4 mm. Arkless suggested that if a joint space is more than 1 mm greater or less in width than that of the other joints, further evaluation is indicated.[16] However, in a normal wrist it is common for the RC joint to be slightly wider than the intercarpal and CMC joints. Symmetric narrowing of joint spaces usually represents loss of articular cartilage. This may be a normal variant, such as LT coalition (Fig. 11–8), or

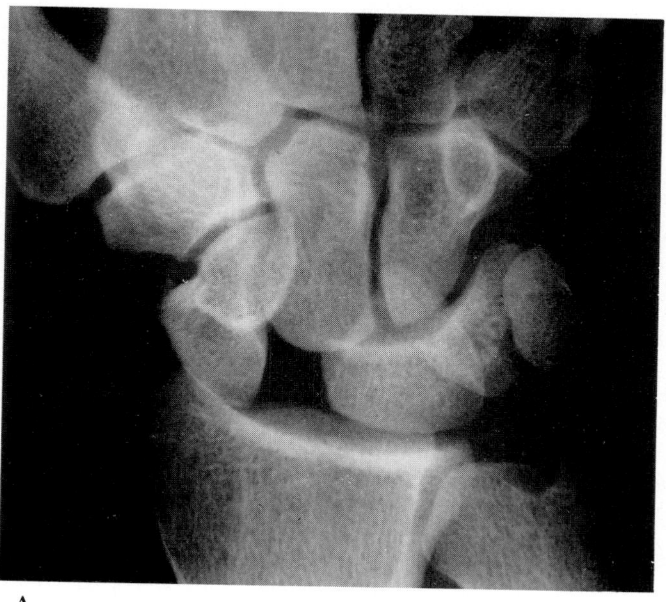

A

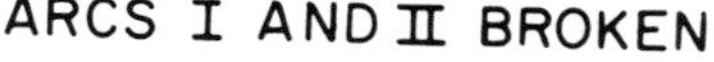

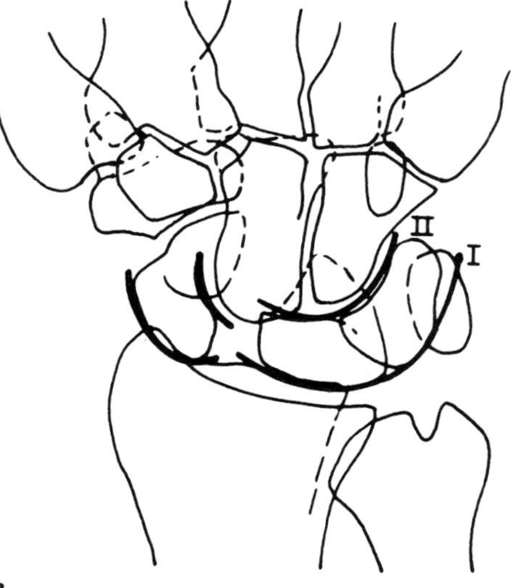

B

FIGURE 11–4. "Broken" Arcs I and II. **A:** PA view of the right wrist demonstrates that both Arcs I and II are broken at the SL joint. SL joint widening is present. The lunate is triangular in shape and tilts palmarly. **B:** A diagram of this wrist demonstrates the broken Arcs I and II. (Reprinted with permission from Gilula LA. Carpal injuries: Analytic approach and case exercises. *AJR* 1979;133: 503–517.)

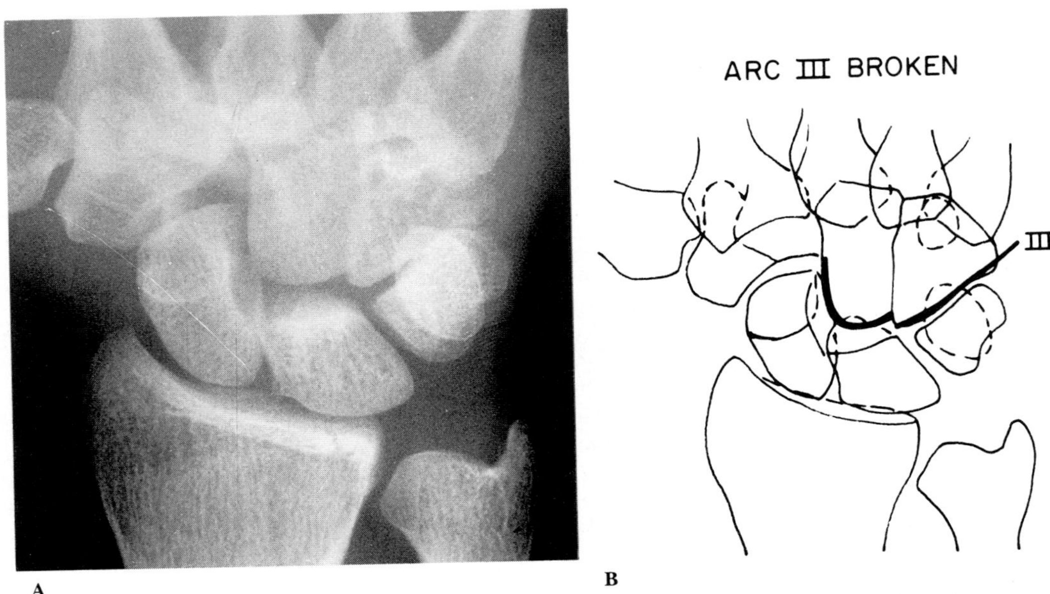

FIGURE 11–5. PA view of the right wrist shows broken Arc III. **A:** PA view of the right wrist demonstrates that Arc III is disrupted, especially at the capitohamate articulation, indicating abnormality at this joint. The joint space between the capitate and the lunate is widened. **B:** A line diagram illustrates the broken Arc III. (Reprinted with permission from Gilula LA. Carpal injuries: Analytic approach and case exercises. *AJR* 1979;133:503–517.)

result from various synovial disorders, for example, arthritis destroying articular cartilage (Fig. 11–9). Caution is recommended, since a joint may appear narrowed or even fused when not in profile (Fig. 11–10). Subluxation or dislocation should be considered when "joint space" narrowing is not symmetric, and normally apposing cortices do not articulate with each other (Fig. 11–11). Similarly, abnormally wide "joint spaces," even if adjacent cortices are parallel, suggest that a dissociation is present (Fig. 11–12). In the carpus, however, it has been recognized that with LT coalition, normally there can be slight widening of the SL joint (Fig. 11–13).[17]

On a standard PA wrist radiograph, the CMC joint spaces consist of segmentally parallel cortical surfaces which form an M-shaped set of parallel lines from the second to the fifth CMC joint (Fig. 11–14). Fisher, Rogers, and Hendrix suggested a systematic approach to the diagnosis of CMC joint dislocation on standard radiographic views.[18] The normal CMC joint shows symmetric parallel cortical lines at the opposing bone margins on a neutrally positioned standard PA view with the palm flat on the x-ray film cassette or table. If there is any wrist extension during the x-ray exposure (how some technologists are taught to obtain wrist radiographs or as occurs with clenched-fist views), the parallel cortical margins of the CMC joints may not be visible. Any break of the parallel cortical lines, changes in joint width, overlap of two normally parallel joint margins, blurring, or loss of definition of one of the normally opposing surfaces indicates subluxation, dislocation,[18,19] or other pathology. Lateral or off-lateral views will help profile a CMC subluxation or dislocation and better display the sagittal-plane relationships of any associated abnormalities (Fig. 11–15). If the sagittal plane information is still not clear, sagittal plane computed tomography (CT) of the CMC joint(s) in question may provide the desired anatomic information (see Chapter 16).

If less than half of the proximal articular surface of the lunate is in contact with the distal articular surface of the radius in the neutral PA position (the third metacarpal shaft central axis is coaxial with the central axis of the radius), a subluxation, dislocation, or ulnar translocation should be considered. In ulnar translocation (translation), the carpus migrates to the ulnar side of the forearm. The radiographic diagnosis of ulnar translocation is based on the routine PA radiograph.[6,11,20–22] Normally more than half of the lunate is in contact with the radius on a neutral PA projection (see Figs. 11–1 and 11–3B). The pathognomonic finding of ulnar translocation is abnormal translation of the lunate in an ulnar direction (Fig. 11–16).[23] The key visual measure of ulnar translocation is provided by the position of the lunate in relation to the lunate facet of the radius on a PA view of the wrist. In addition, the radioscaphoid joint width radially at the level of the radial styloid may become wider than the ulnar side of the radioscaphoid joint and radiolunate joint (ulnar translocation Type I). However, since the lunate normally moves in an ulnar direction with radial deviation (Fig. 11–17), before making a diagnosis of ulnar translocation, the

Text continued on page 302

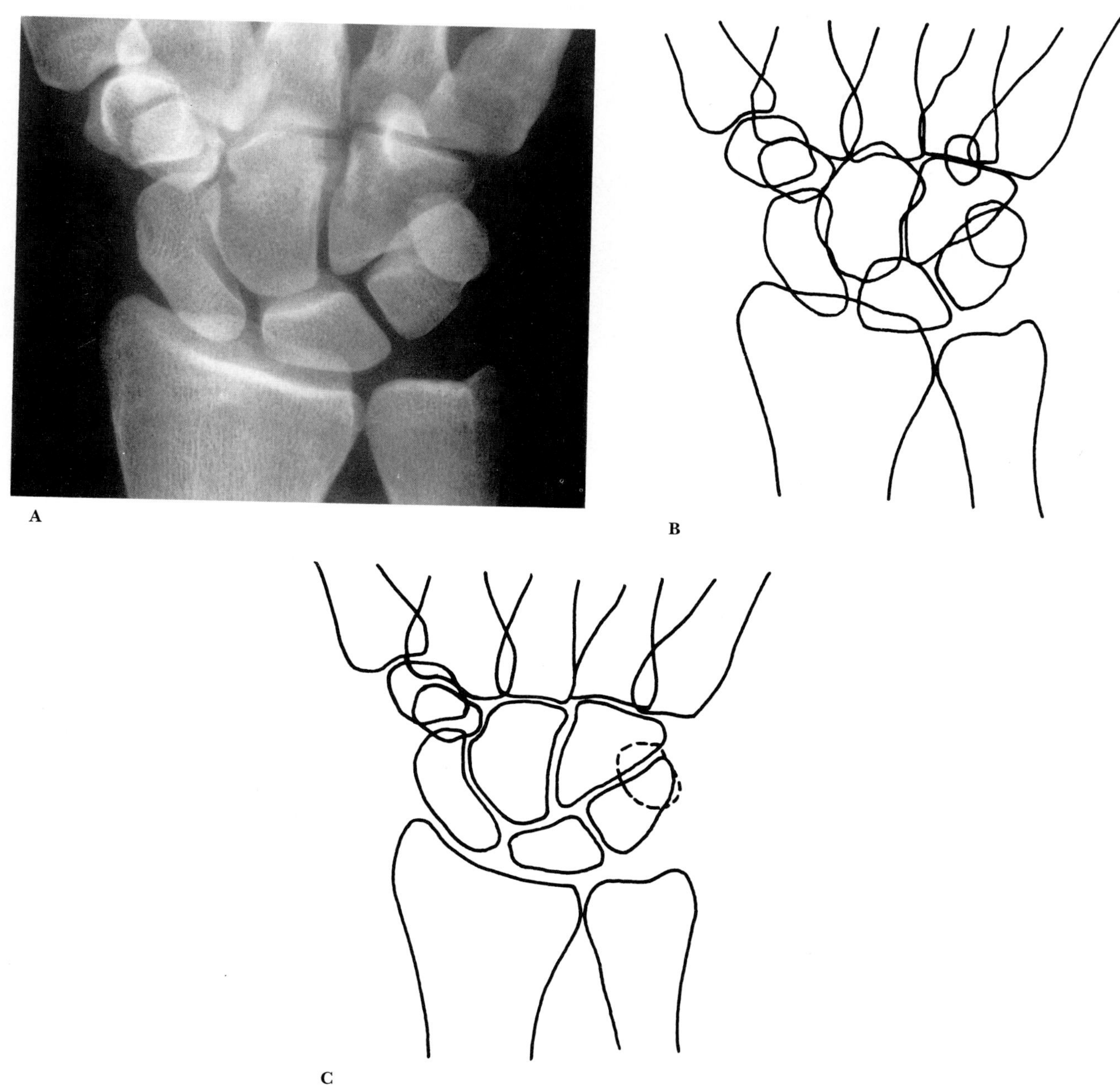

FIGURE 11–6. Two ways to observe the same carpus. **A:** PA radiographic view of a left carpus. **B:** Tracing the outer curvatures of the carpus shows the shapes of the carpal bones as well as the metacarpals and the adjacent radius and ulna. **C:** "Parallelism" concept of jigsaw puzzles. Tracing parallel articulating cortical surfaces of the same bones in panels A and B provides immediate determination if the bones in the carpus are fitting together, similar to pieces of a jigsaw puzzle. (Reprinted with permission from Gilula LA, Totty WG. Wrist trauma: Roentgenographic analysis. In: Gilula LA, ed. *The traumatized hand and wrist: Radiographic and anatomic correlation*. Philadelphia: WB Saunders, 1992:223.)

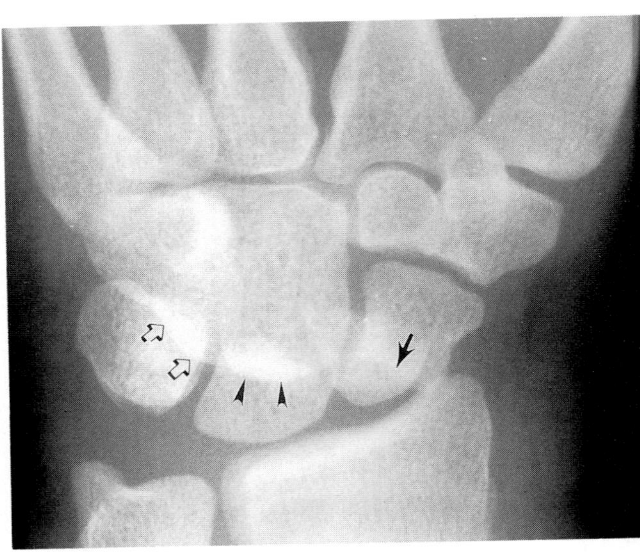

A

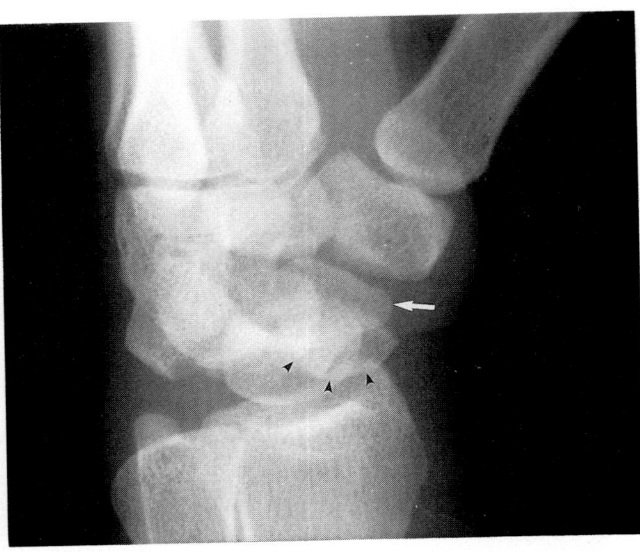

B

FIGURE 11–7. Transscaphoid dorsal perilunate dislocation. **A:** PA view of the left wrist demonstrates overlapping articular cortices and obliteration of lunocapitate joint (arrowheads) and triquetrohamate joint (open arrows) spaces. A scaphoid fracture (arrow) is present. **B:** Obliqued lateral view of the wrist demonstrates that the capitate has displaced dorsally from the lunate. The lunate remains in line with the distal radius. The proximal scaphoid fracture fragment (arrowheads) remains attached to the lunate; the distal scaphoid fracture fragment (arrow) has migrated dorsally with the other carpal bones.

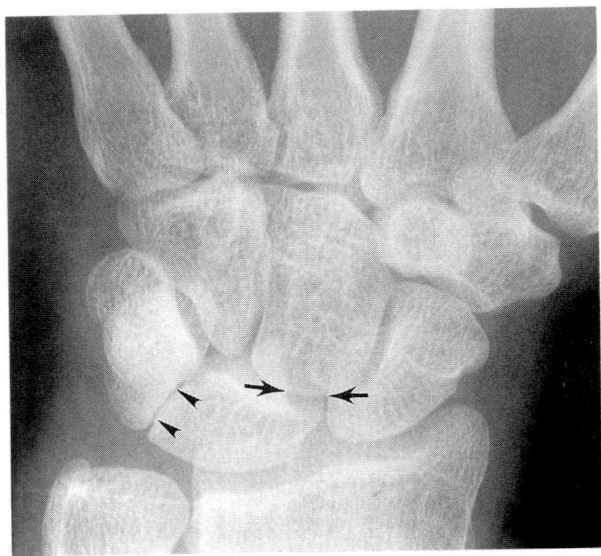

FIGURE 11–8. LT coalition. PA view of the left wrist demonstrates irregular joint space narrowing at the lunotriquetral joint (arrowheads). No osteophytes or subcortical sclerosis suggestive of osteoarthritis are present at the LT joint. The SL joint space may be widened (arrows) but this joint is not profiled well enough to be certain that these cortical structures represent parallel articular surfaces of the lunate and scaphoid (see Fig. 11–13).

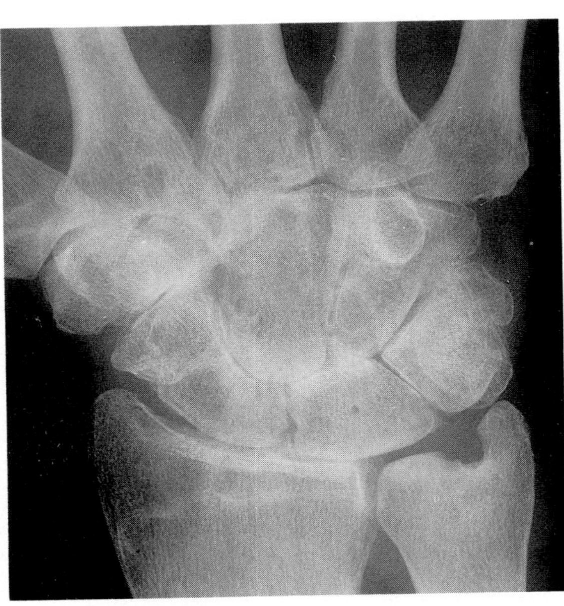

FIGURE 11–9. Rheumatoid arthritis of the wrist. PA view of the right wrist demonstrates generalized joint space narrowing with parallelism preserved among the carpal bones and at the radiocarpal joint, except for slight ulnar translocation type I, recognized by noting that the radioscaphoid joint space is radially wider than the other intercarpal joints, and/or that more than half of the width of the lunate lies ulnar to the ulnar edge of the radius (see Chapter 8).

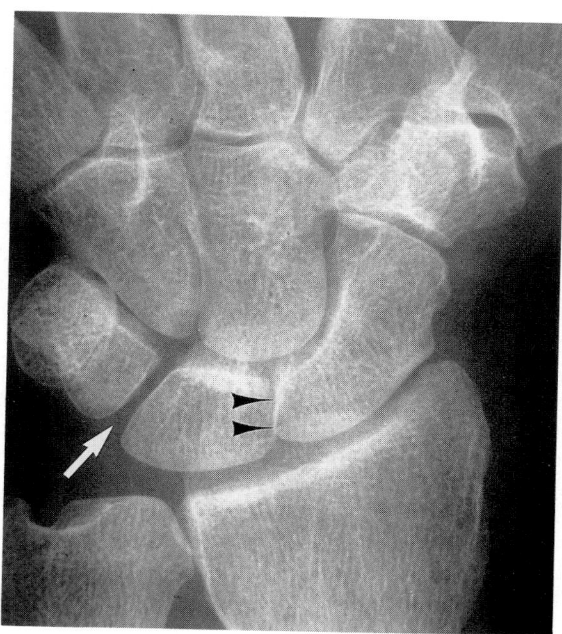

FIGURE 11–10. PA view of a normal left wrist. The SL joint is not profiled (arrowheads) on the PA view of a left wrist taken with central beam slightly angled toward the radial side; however, the LT joint is perfectly profiled (arrow). Similarly, the capitotrapezoidal joint is not profiled and simulates fusion, but this cannot be accurately ascertained without specific profile of that joint.

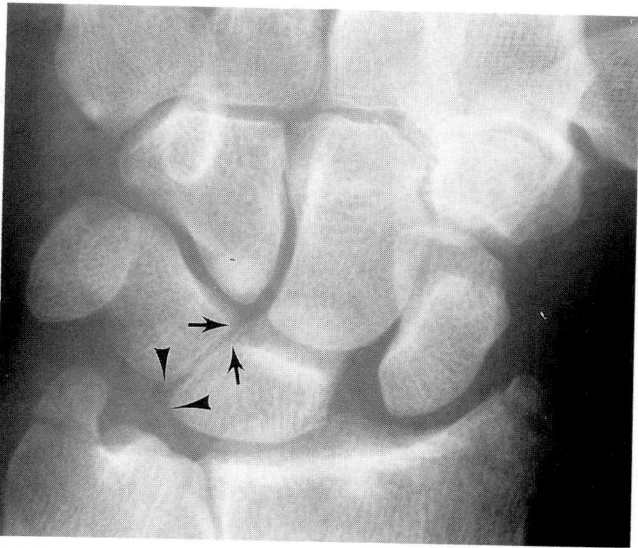

FIGURE 11–12. SL dissociation with dissociation also at the LT joint. PA view of the left wrist demonstrates SL joint space widening. Arcs I (between arrowheads) and II (between arrows) are questionably broken with apparent narrowing at the LT joint. It is uncertain if the offset in Arc II is due to a small hamate facet of the lunate and if the offset at Arc I is due to a slightly narrower proximal distal length of the triquetrum compared to the lunate. Both the radial and ulnar styloids are fractured.

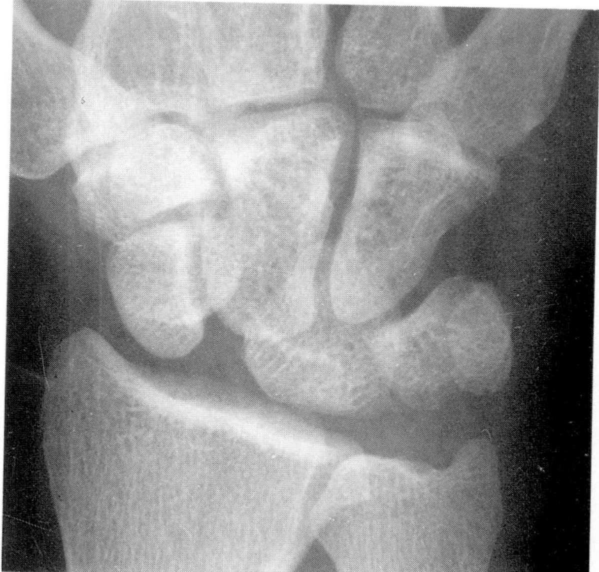

FIGURE 11–11. Dislocation between the lunate and other carpal bones with prominent tilting of the lunate. On a PA right wrist view, the lunocapitate joint space is absent and normally parallel cortices of the articulating cortices of the lunate and capitate are overlapping. The lunate is triangular in shape, indicating tilting of this bone. Arc II is broken at both the SL and LT joints. The scaphoid is foreshortened, SL joint diastasis is present, and normally adjacent cortices of the scaphoid and lunate are not parallel. (Reprinted with permission from Gilula LA. Carpal injuries: Analytic approach and case exercises. *AJR* 1979;133:503–517.)

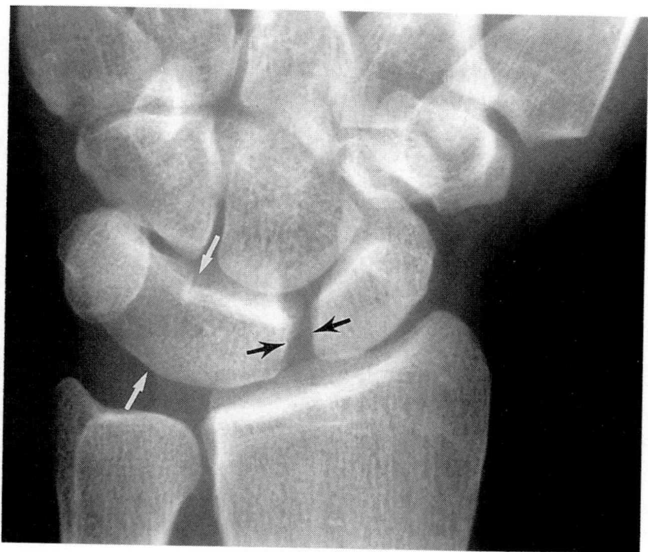

FIGURE 11–13. LT coalition with normal widening of the SL joint. PA roentgenogram of a 28-year-old man who has bony LT coalition (between white arrows) and widening of the SL joint space (between black arrows). The opposite side was identical and arthrography was normal (see also Fig. 11–8). (Reprinted with permission from the Radiological Society of North America from Metz VM, Schimmerl SM, Gilula LA, Viegas SF, Saffar P. Wide scapholunate joint space in lunotriquetral coalition: A normal variant? *Radiology* 1993;188:557–559.)

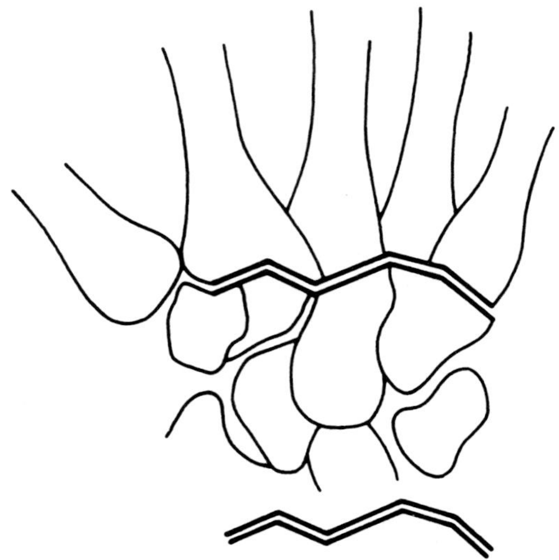

FIGURE 11–14. A diagram shows that parallel "M" lines are formed by CMC joints two through five. The width of the CMC joint spaces is uniform. The distal ends of the trapezoid, capitate, and hamate form the proximal parallel "M" line, and the bases of the second through fifth metacarpals form the distal parallel "M" line. (Reprinted with permission from Fisher MR, Rogers LF, Hendrix RW. Carpometacarpal joint dislocation. *Crit Rev Diag Imaging* 1984;22:95–126. Copyright CRC Press, Boca Raton, Florida.)

examiner should ascertain the position of the third metacarpal with respect to the radius.

At least three methods have been reported for measuring ulnocarpal translation.[6,11,20,24,25] Depending on the position of the scaphoid, two types of ulnar translocation may occur. In Type I, the entire carpus including the scaphoid migrates ulnarly. The distance between the radial styloid and the scaphoid is widened (see Fig. 11–16). In Type II, the relationship and the distance between the scaphoid and the radial styloid process remains normal but the SL space is widened. The distal carpal row translates ulnarly with the lunate. Only the scaphoid remains in normal position; the rest of the carpus migrates ulnarly.[22] However, since the scaphoid also retains its trapeziotrapezoidal attachments, the scaphoid must be in some stage of rotation to maintain these attachments while the remainder of the carpus is ulnar in position. In our anecdotal experience, this situation is most commonly encountered in the scapholunate advanced collapse (SLAC) pattern of wrist malalignment (Chapter 20). The differential between the two types of ulnar translocation is important, because the appearance of a wide SL gap may lead to a misdiagnosis of an isolated SL dissociation. If treated as SL dissociation, efforts to stabilize the scaphoid and lunate may fail to correct either the underlying ulnocarpal translocation or the apparent SL diastasis. Similarly, if a

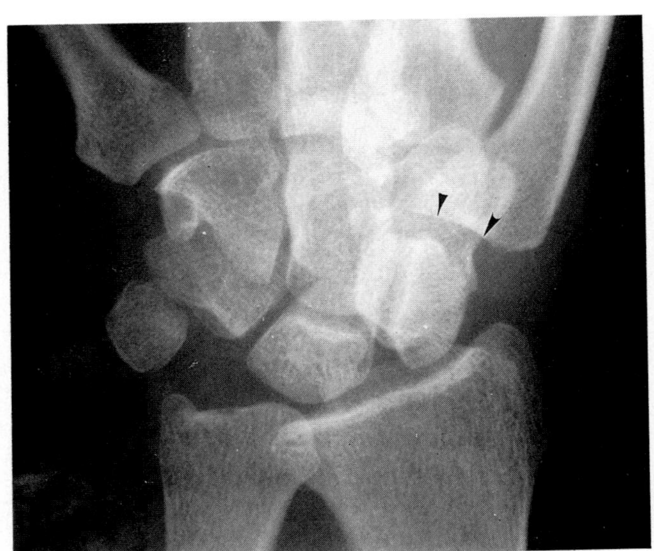

A

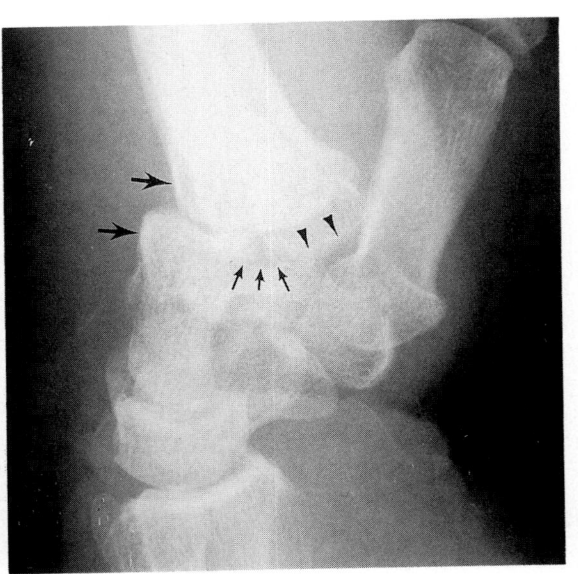

B

FIGURE 11–15. Palmar dislocation of the first, second, and third CMC joints. **A:** PA view of the left wrist demonstrates disruption of normally parallel cortices at the first, second, and third CMC joints and questionable pathology at the fourth and fifth CMC joints. The base of the first metacarpal (arrowheads) overlaps the trapezium and is migrated proximally. The second CMC joint is not well seen. At the third CMC joint, the metacarpal base cortex is sharply profiled; however, the adjacent articular surface of the capitate is not seen. Asymmetry of the fourth and fifth CMC joints is present with the fifth CMC joint wider than the fourth; the cortical base of the fourth metacarpal is much sharper in profile than the opposing articular surface of the hamate. **B:** A lateral view demonstrates palmar displacement of metacarpal bases at the dorsal aspect of the wrist (arrows). The base of metacarpal II (arrowheads) is palmar to the trapezoid (small arrows).

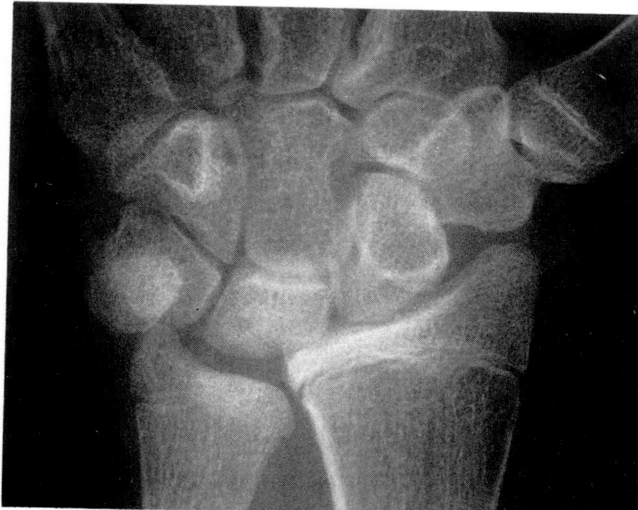

FIGURE 11–16. Ulnar translation (Type I). PA view of the left wrist demonstrates the ulnar position of the whole carpus as well as the lunate. Two-thirds of the lunate is ulnar to the lunate facet of the distal radius. The distance between the radial styloid and scaphoid is wider than the rest of the radiocarpal joint and intercarpal joints. Radiolunate joint narrowing indicates cartilage loss.

SLAC wrist with unrecognized ulnar translocation Type II with osteoarthritis of the radioscaphoid joint is treated for the osteoarthritis, as is commonly done by removing the scaphoid combined with another procedure such as intercarpal arthrodeses, an unsatisfactory result can be obtained because of persistant ulnar translocation.

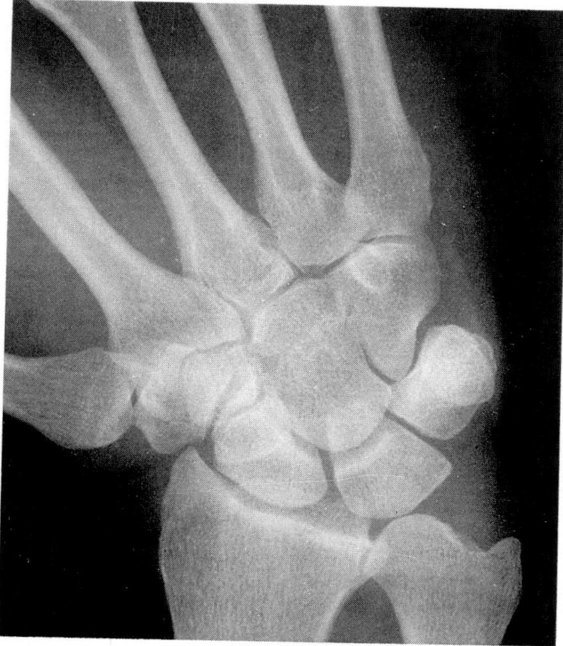

FIGURE 11–17. PA view of a normal wrist in radial deviation demonstrates that more than half of the proximal surface of the lunate has moved to the ulnar side of the distal radius. (Reprinted with permission from Gilula LA. Carpal injuries: Analytic approach and case exercises. *AJR* 1979;133:503–517.)

LATERAL PROJECTION

The lateral view should be obtained with the dorsum of the metacarpals in a straight line with the dorsum of the radius and ulna (Fig. 11–18). Such standardization of wrist positioning makes it easier to recognize alignment abnormalities. A true lateral projection is present when the palmar cortex of the pisiform overlies the mid portion of the scaphoid, which projects palmar to the palmar surface of the head of the capitate. In other words, a neutral lateral view projects the ventral cortex of the pisiform approximally halfway between the ventral tip of the distal scaphoid tubercle and the ventral margin of the capitate head. The long axes of the capitate and lunate are collinear with the long axis of the radius. This method uses the overlap of an ulnar-sided structure on a radial-sided structure to verify a true lateral projection. Merely using the ulna with respect to the radius can be misleading, since some normal wrists have a prominent ulna dorsally. The lateral view should be obtained at right angles to the PA view to provide a true orthogonal view of the ulna. This can be performed by adducting the arm to the patient's side with the patient standing erect, flexing the elbow 90 degrees, and placing the ulnar surface of the hand and wrist on the cassette. Alternatively, two right-angled views can be obtained with the forearm fixed in a holder, with the patient's forearm flexed 90 degrees at the elbow and the arm kept next to the patient's side.[26] One view is taken with a horizontal beam to get the PA view. A second view is obtained by redirecting the x-ray tube by 90 degrees so that the beam is directed from the ceiling toward the floor to get the lateral view.

Normal Lateral View of the Wrist

On the standard neutral lateral radiograph, a normal wrist is characterized by near collinear longitudinal axes of the radius, lunate, capitate, and third metacarpal. In previously published work, it was shown that the situation in which all three of these axes are exactly collinear is present in only about 10% of patients and therefore is not too common.[4,27] In the lateral view depending on the wrist, most of or all the carpal and metacarpal bones project palmar to a line extended from the dorsum of the third metacarpal to the dorsum of the radius.[1] This line is fairly parallel to a line drawn through the center of the third metacarpal, and this line should intersect the longitudinal axis of the scaphoid at an angle between 30 to 60 degrees (Fig. 11–18C).[4,6,11,27–29] Alterations in these normal relationships may indicate antecedent trauma and/or wrist instability (see Chapter 8).

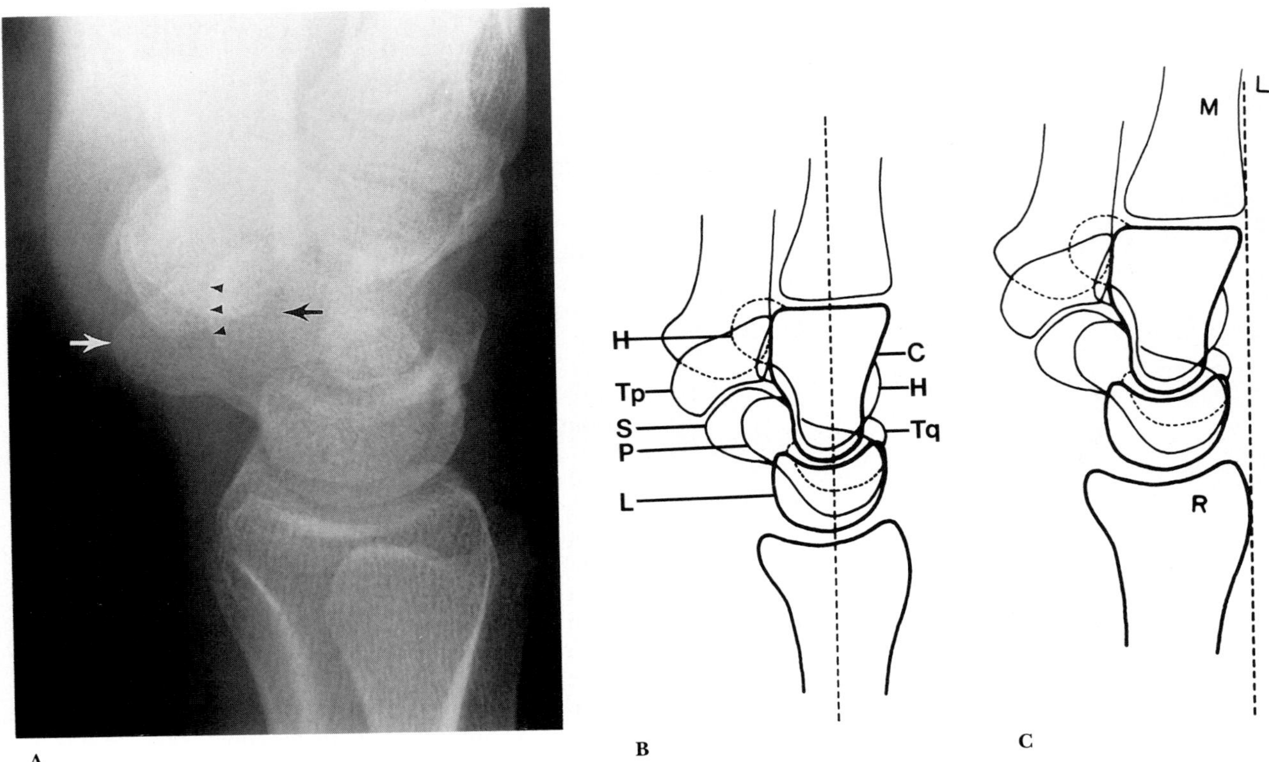

FIGURE 11–18. Standard lateral view of the wrist. **A:** The dorsum of the third metacarpal is in line with the dorsum of the radius. The ventral surface of the pisiform (arrowheads) lies midway between the ventral surface of the capitate head (black arrow) and the ventral distal pole of the scaphoid (white arrow). **B:** A diagram of the lateral wrist view shows the major cortical surfaces seen in all adequately exposed and positioned radiographs (C, capitate; H, hamate; L, lunate; P, pisiform; S, scaphoid; Tp, trapezium; Tq, triquetrum). (Modified with permission from Gilula LA. Carpal injuries: Analytic approach and case exercises. *AJR* 1979;133:503–517.) **C:** A diagram of the lateral wrist view shows all the carpal and metacarpal bones project palmar to a line (L) extended from the dorsum of the third metacarpal (M) to the dorsum of the radius (R).[1] This line is fairly parallel to a line drawn through the center of the third metacarpal and should intersect the longitudinal axis of the scaphoid at an angle between 30 and 60 degrees.

While the carpal bones partly or completely overlap each other, the articulations between the capitate and lunate, between the lunate and radius, and between the capitate and third metacarpal are usually profiled. In the lateral view, the axis of the capitate is mostly parallel or continuous with the longitudinal axis of the third metacarpal to which the capitate is firmly attached. The joint space between the scaphoid and trapezium is occasionally profiled in this projection.

If there is any offset at the CMC joints, especially dorsally, a subluxation or dislocation should be considered (see Fig. 11–15B). The mid axis of the lunate may be centered at the middle of the distal articular surface of the distal radius and be parallel with the central axes of the radius and capitate. However, this situation is true in only about 10% of wrists.[27] It is common for small degrees of angulation to exist between these three axes. The proximal surface of the lunate should be congruent with the distal radius surface. Any migration and/or prominent angulation of the lunate represents a potential abnormality. If the lunate tilts dorsally or palmarly sufficiently to create an abnormal SL and/or capitolunate angle (Fig. 11–19 and Chapter 8), a pattern of dorsiflexion ligament instability (DISI) or palmar-flexion instability (VISI) exists. Dorsal or palmar translation with or without abnormal intercarpal angulation potentially indicates a dorsal or palmar carpal instability. Abnormal intercarpal angulation with translation and loss of capitolunate congruence occurs in lunate or perilunate dislocations. Because the position of the lunate is a key to recognizing many common static carpal instabilities, Fig. 11–19 is included to show its appearance on lateral views in major different conditions (Figs. 11–19B through 11–19G).

FRACTURES, DISLOCATIONS, AND INSTABILITIES

Wrist trauma can result in an array of different combinations,[30,31] which on occasion can be very subtle and result in significant wrist derangement and func-

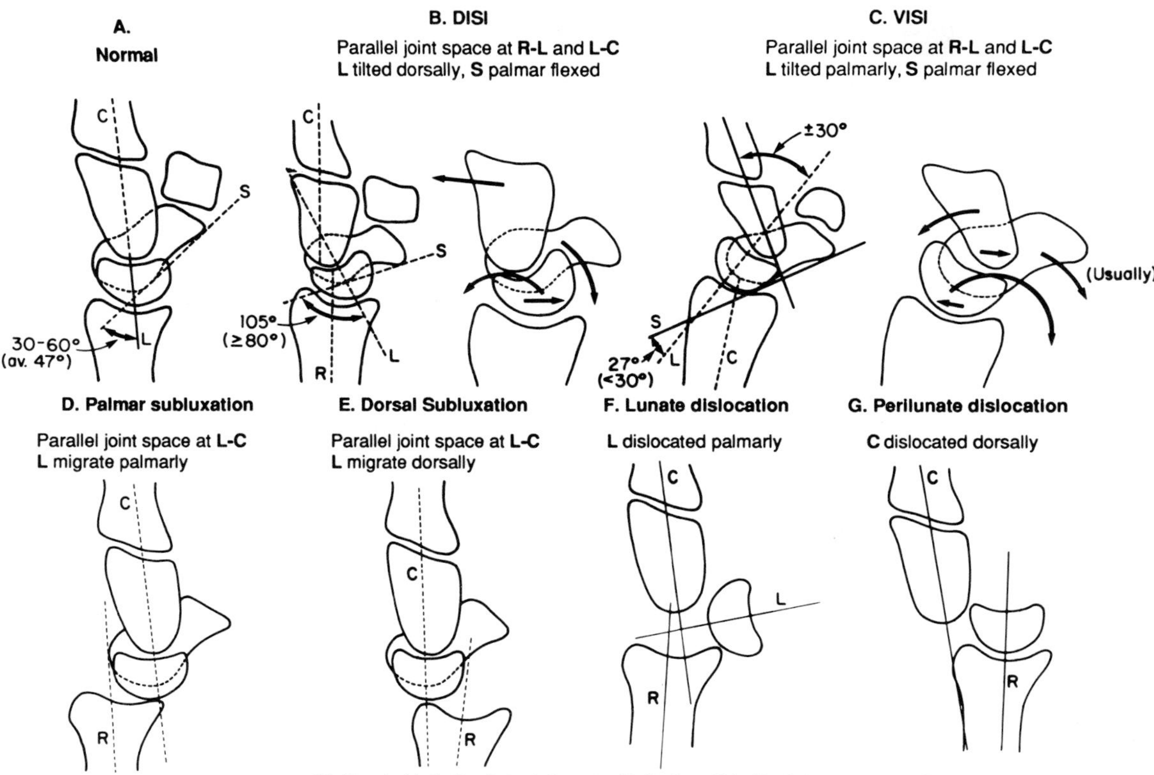

FIGURE 11–19. Diagrams show various lunate appearances in major different static instability patterns. (Modified with permission from the Radiological Society of North America from Gilula LA, Weeks PM. Post-traumatic ligamentous instabilities of the wrist. *Radiology* 1978;129:641–651.)

tional impairment.[31,32] Most carpal fractures and dislocations occur within the "vulnerable zone," an area that involves the scaphoid, capitate, hamate, triquetrum, and joints around the lunate. The vulnerable zone is bounded by two arcs, the lesser arc (consisting of the joints around the lunate) and the greater arc (a distally convex arc that crosses the middle or proximal portions of the scaphoid, capitate, hamate, and triquetrum).[31] A pure lesser-arc injury would be a perilunate or lunate dislocation. A pure greater-arc injury would be a transscaphoid, transcapitate, transhamate, transtriquetral fracture-dislocation. When a lunate dislocation occurs, the injury involves not only the lesser arc, but also the structures of radiolunate joint. Any combination of these two patterns can occur and are the most common of the fractures and dislocations of the carpus (Fig. 11–20).[31,33]

The terminology of fracture-dislocations may sometimes seem complicated. However, a few general principles can make understanding it easier. When there is a dislocation, the dislocation commonly occurs around the lunate as described above, resulting in a lunate or perilunate dislocation. Any bone that is fractured is named first, followed by the dislocation type (lunate or perilunate). Another type of dislocation described elsewhere in more detail is the axial fracture-dislocation, which refers to a longitudinal disruption of the carpus, such as between the capitate and hamate.[34,35] Finally, to complete the terminology it is most advisable to clarify if the abnormality is acute, subacute, or chronic and specify if there is an underlying cause, such as rheumatoid arthritis.[36,37]

Therefore, if a fracture exists without dislocation, the name of the abnormality is the bone fractured. When the injury involves the capitolunate joint, which is a fairly common injury in the wrist, either lunate or perilunate dislocation is suspected. Distinction between these two entities is made by determining which bone is centered over the distal radial articular surface. When the lunate is more centered on the distal radial articular surface than the capitate, which is dislocated with the rest of the carpus from the lunate, a perilunate dislocation is diagnosed (Fig. 11–21A). When the capitate is more centered on the distal radius and the lunate is dislocated from both the capitate and the distal radius, a lunate dislocation is diagnosed (Fig. 11–21B). Although both the lunate and perilunate dislocations are actually "midcarpal dislocations," if neither the lunate nor the capitate is centered over the radius, the terminology of a midcarpal dislocation can be used (Fig. 11–21C).

When a dislocation is associated with a fracture, the descriptive nomenclature includes the fractured

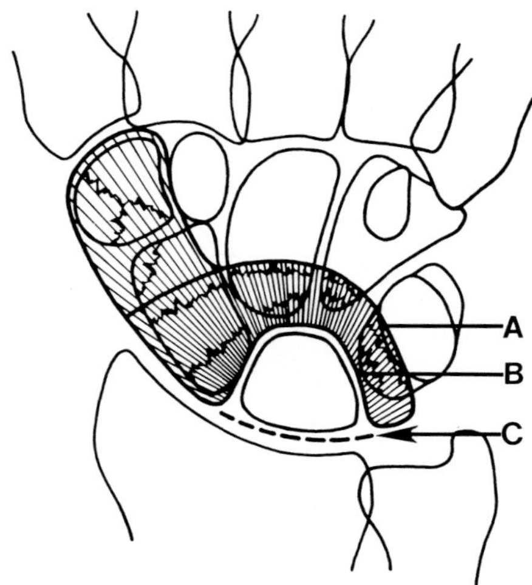

FIGURE 11–20. A diagram shows the greater (A) and lesser arcs (B). When a lunate dislocation occurs, the injury not only involves the lesser arc, but also the radiolunate joint through the dotted line (C). The shaded area represents the vulnerable zone of the carpus. Most carpal injuries seen clinically involve the structures within the shaded area. A pure greater-arc injury would be a transscaphoid, transcapitate, transtriquetral fracture-dislocation. A pure lesser-arc injury would be a perilunate or lunate dislocation. However, in lunate dislocation, the injury involves not only the lesser arc, but also the radiolunate joint (dashed line). (Modified with permission from Johnson RP. The acutely injured wrist and its residuals. *Clin Orthop* 1980;149:33–44.)

bone(s).[4,38–46] Therefore, a dorsal perilunate dislocation with a scaphoid fracture is called a transscaphoid dorsal perilunate fracture dislocation. Similarly, if fractures of multiple carpal bones (such as the scaphoid, capitate, and hamate) are associated with a dorsal perilunate dislocation, this combination is called a transscaphoid, transcapitate, transhamate dorsal perilunate fracture-dislocation. When a dorsal perilunate dislocation is accompanied by a radial and/or ulnar styloid fracture, the term is transradial (and/or transulnar) styloid, dorsal perilunate fracture-dislocation. The words *dorsal* and *palmar* are added before perilunate to indicate the direction of the dislocation. Many other types of carpal instabilities are recognized and the related terminology is addressed in Chapter 8.

Some authors believe that palmar dislocation of the lunate is the end stage of a progressive perilunate dislocation.[47–54] This stepwise spectrum has been named progressive perilunate instability (PLI). The four stages of PLI describe the progressive disruption of ligaments and anatomic relationship of the lunate. The radiologic patterns showing findings of the four stages of perilunar instability are given below (Fig. 11–22).[55]

Stage I. Scapholunate (SL) Instability—Rotary Scaphoid Subluxation

PA View of the Wrist: Foreshortening of the scaphoid producing the "ring" sign, SL gap widening, and disruption of Arcs I and/or II at the SL joint.

Lateral View of the Wrist: Dorsal subluxation of the scaphoid with narrowing of the radioscaphoid angle.

Stage II. Capitate Dislocation

PA View of the Wrist: The same as Stage I; abnormal capitolunate joint overlap may be present.

Lateral View of the Wrist: The capitate is dislocated dorsally at the capitolunate articulation.

Stage III. Triquetral Dislocation

PA View of the Wrist: In addition to the changes seen in Stage II, triquetrolunate dissociation is present with disruption of Arcs I and/or II at the SL and/or LT joints.

Lateral View of the Wrist: The capitate and triquetrum are dislocated dorsally with carpal bones other than the lunate.

Stage IV. Lunate Dislocation

PA View of the Wrist: The lunate projects a triangular shape and overlaps the SL, LT, and capitolunate articular surfaces.

Lateral View of the Wrist: The lunate is dislocated palmarly and usually is rotated such that its distal articular surface faces the palmar aspect of the distal radius.

CASE ILLUSTRATIONS OF PLI

The following cases are included to illustrate principles of analyzing complex carpal problems. Soft-tissue abnormalities accompanying these bone fractures and malalignments are detailed elsewhere.[55,56] In addition, these cases are used to illustrate the importance of recognizing as many abnormalities as possible on the PA view, because recognition of all the abnormalities on this view will more likely lead to a correct interpretation of the malalignments. The major value of the lateral view thus becomes recognition of the direction of bone displacements and confirmation and further understanding of abnormalities seen on the PA view.

Case 1: Acute Posttraumatic, Transradial Styloid, Dorsal Perilunate Fracture-Dislocation (Fig. 11–23)

Perilunate dislocation with or without fracture is a common injury of the wrist. In this example, an overlap of the capitate and lunate is present on the PA view of the wrist. Arc 1 is broken at the LT joint. Abnormal diastasis exists between the scaphoid and lunate. These features can appear in both perilunate and lunate dislocation. In perilunate dislocation, however, the lunate retains its articulation with the more anatomic at the radiolunate than at the radioscaphoid joint. Perilunate dislocations are commonly associated with carpal fractures as well as radial and ulnar styloid fractures.[30,32,57] Finally, on the lateral view of the wrist, the capitate is dorsally dislocated from the articular surface of the lunate, and its long axis is dorsal to the radius. The lunate usually tilts palmarly (see Fig. 11–21B). The magnitude of sub-

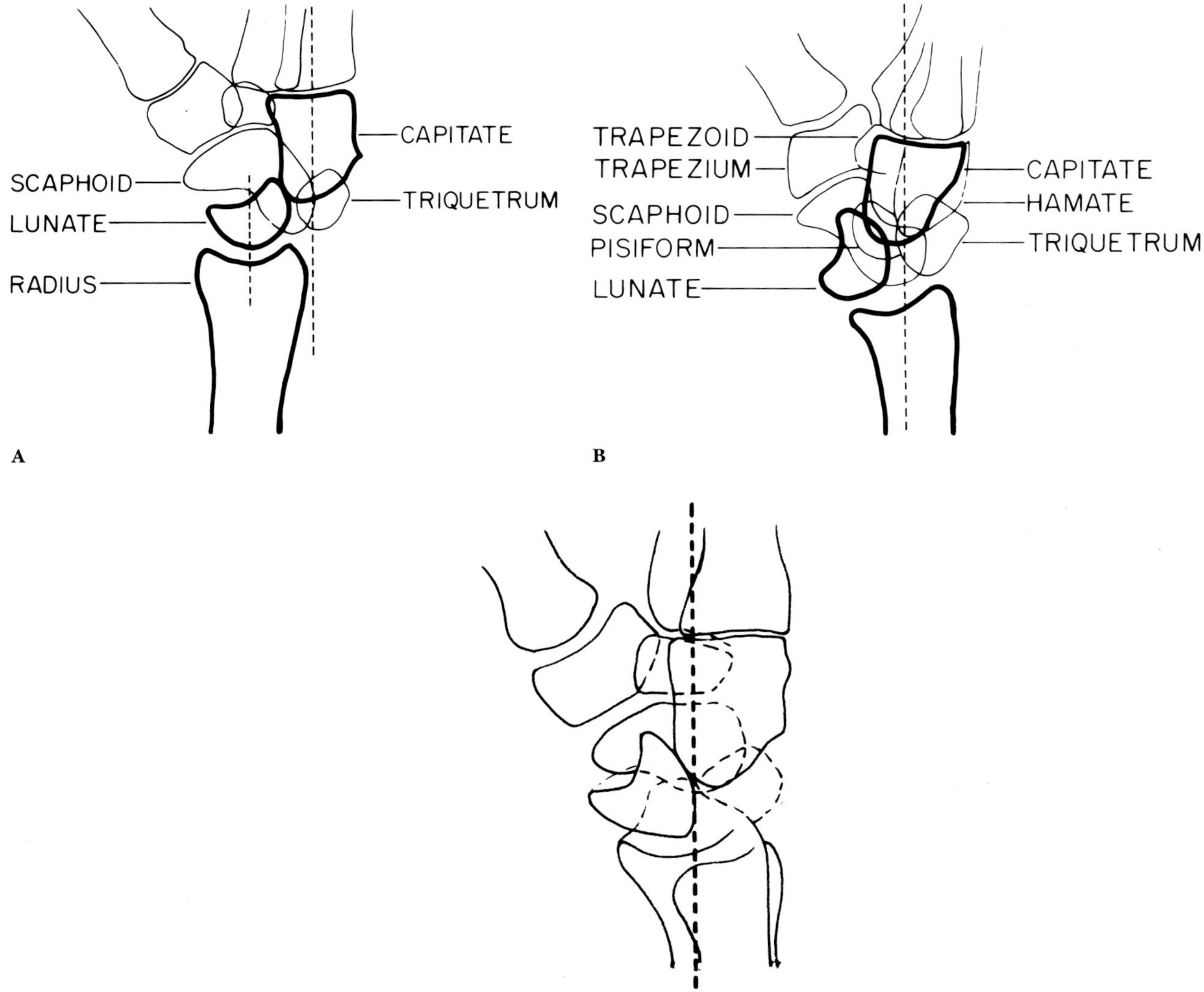

FIGURE 11–21. Diagrams show the relationship among the distal radius, lunate, and capitate with dislocations. **A:** Dorsal perilunate dislocation. A diagram shows that the capitate and the other carpal bones are dislocated dorsally. **B:** Ventral lunate dislocation. A diagram shows ventral tilting and displacement of the lunate with the capitate and other carpal bones in relatively anatomic position with respect to the radius. **C:** Midcarpal dislocation. A diagram shows dislocation between the lunate and other carpal bones, but neither the lunate nor capitate is centered over the radius. (Reprinted with permission from Gilula LA. Carpal injuries: Analytic approach and case exercises. *AJR* 1979;133:503–517.)

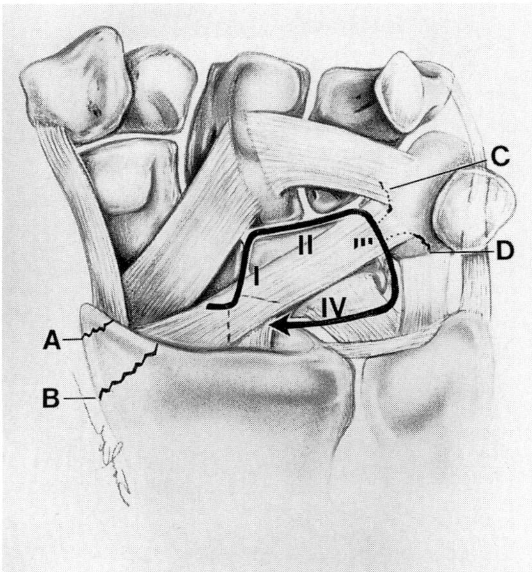

FIGURE 11–22. A diagram of four stages (I to IV) of perilunar instability (Palmar wrist view: **A:** radial styloid tip fracture; **B:** radial styloid body fracture; **C:** palmar radiolunotriquetral ligament chip fracture; **D:** avulsion fracture of palmar ulnotriquetral ligament; Stages I to IV of perilunate instability). (Reprinted with permission from Mayfield JK, Gilula LA, Totty WG. Carpal fracture-dislocations. In: Gilula LA, ed. *The traumatized hand and wrist: Radiographic and anatomic correlation.* Philadelphia: WB Saunders, 1992:288.)

luxation of scaphoid at the radius is greater than that of the lunate, even if the lunate has changed its position (Fig. 11–23B).

Case 2: Acute, Posttraumatic, Transscaphoid, Transradial Styloid, Transulnar Styloid Dorsal Perilunate Fracture-Dislocation (Fig. 11–24)

On a PA view of the wrist, Arcs I and II are broken at both the SL and LT joints. Arc III is normal. These signs indicate an abnormality involving the proximal carpal row. Overlap of articular surfaces involves the capitolunate, hamatolunate and triquetrolunate joints. The slight triangular shape of the lunate indicates tilting of the lunate, but parallelism is still present at the radiolunate joint. The capitate is dislocated from the lunate fossa. The distal surface of the proximal scaphoid fracture fragment is corticated, which means this fracture fragment is rotated, probably 180 degrees. Radial and ulnar styloid fractures are present (Fig. 11–24A). On the lateral view, the lunate remains centered on the distal radius, and the capitate and the other carpal bones are displaced dorsally (Fig. 11–24B).

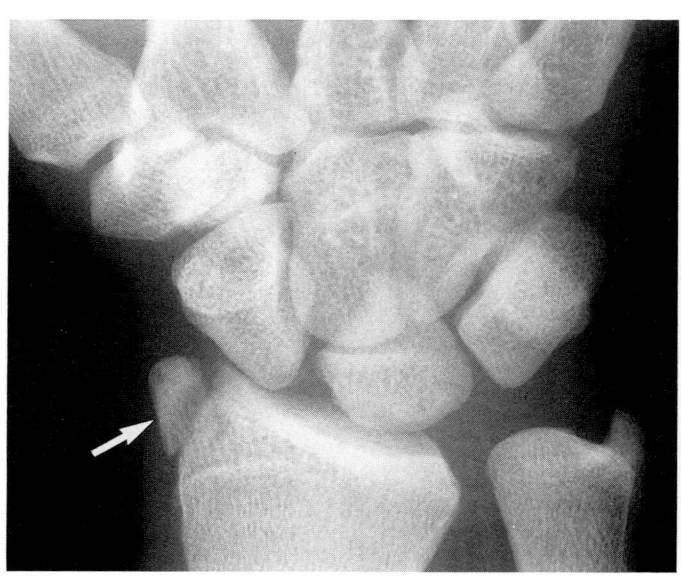

A

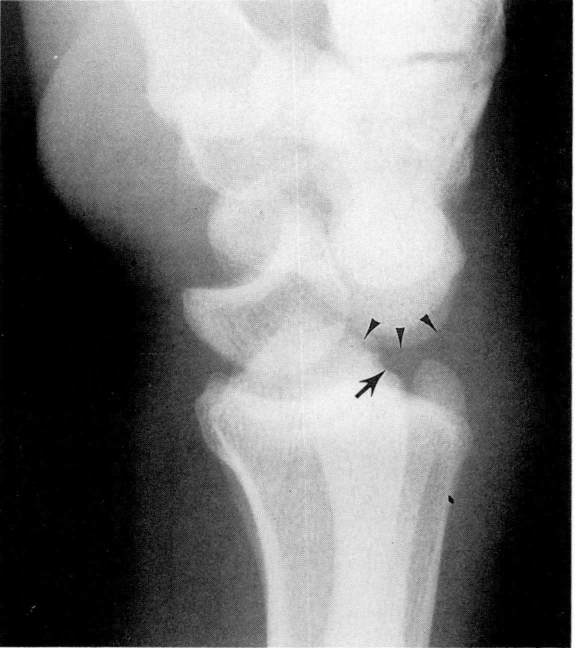

B

FIGURE 11–23. Transradial styloid dorsal perilunate fracture-dislocation. **A:** PA view of the right wrist demonstrates that Arc I is broken at the LT joint. The lunocapitate joint space is narrowed and the lunate has a triangular shape. The SL joint space is widened with lack of parallelism between cortices at this joint, and small chip fractures overlie this joint. The radioscaphoid joint is narrowed, with an associated radial styloid fracture (arrow). **B:** On the lateral view of the wrist the capitate along with other carpal bones except the lunate, have migrated dorsally. The lunate remains articulating with the radius and faces palmarly. Arrowheads outline the proximal cortex of the triquetrum, which is proximal to the proximal scaphoid pole, both of which are dislocated dorsal to the dorsal rim of the radius (arrow).

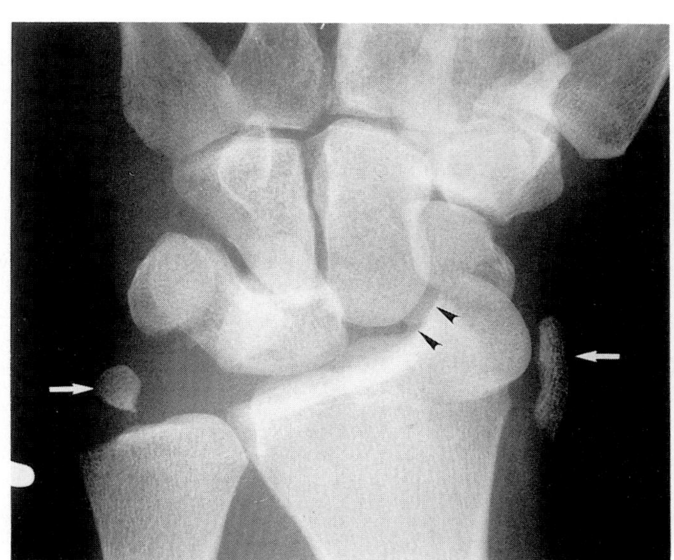

A

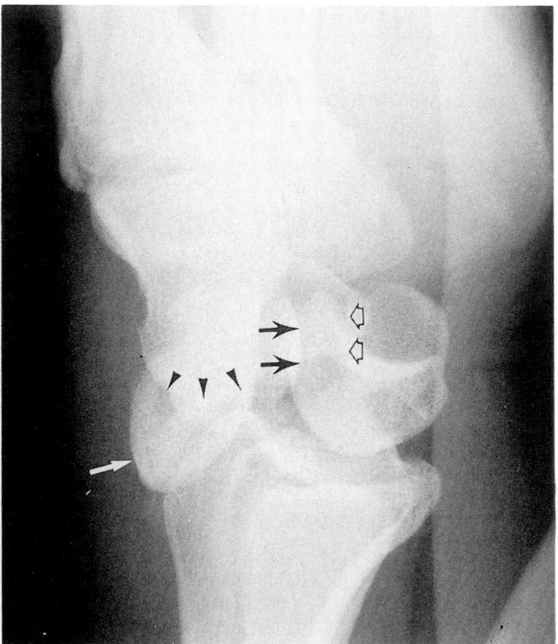

B

FIGURE 11–24. Transscaphoid, transradial styloid, transulnar styloid dorsal perilunate fracture-dislocation. **A:** PA view of the left wrist demonstrates a scaphoid waist fracture. The proximal fracture fragment overlaps the distal radius and therefore is displaced out of the distal radial fossa. Concavity with cortication (arrowheads) involves the distal surface of this proximal fracture fragment, which indicates that this corticated surface is probably the proximal pole of the scaphoid flipped 180 degrees. The capitate has migrated proximally and radially. Overlap of capitolunate, hamatolunate, and triquetrolunate joints is present. Both radial and ulnar styloids are fractured (arrows). The lunate still articulates with the radius and has a triangular shape. **B:** The capitate head (arrowheads) is displaced dorsally out of the lunate fossa with the other carpal bones and metacarpals. A dorsal ossicle (white arrow) is the proximal scaphoid fragment. The lunate remains articulating with the distal radius and faces palmarly. Widening between the dorsal cortex of the pisiform (open arrows) and ventral surface of the triquetrum (black arrows) results from the pisiform remaining in the flexor carpi ulnaris tendon as the triquetrum moves dorsally with the other carpal bones.

Case 3: Acute, Posttraumatic, Palmar Lunate Dislocation with Ulnar Translocation

(Fig. 11–25)

On the PA view, Arcs I and II are broken while Arc III is intact. Thus, the abnormality is within the proximal row of the carpus. The lunate is triangular in shape with nearly half of its distal portion overlapping the capitate, hamate, and triquetrum. Parallelism is lost at the SL joint, and overlapping of articulating surfaces is present at the capitolunate, hamatolunate, and triquetrolunate joints. The radiolunate joint is wider with less normal parallelism than the radioscaphoid joint. The distal articular surface of the lunate is not seen. All of those findings together indicate malpositioning of the lunate. Except for the lunate, intercarpal relationships are normal. No fracture is present. Asymmetry at the radioscaphoid joint supports the finding of ulnar carpal translocation. According to the PA-view analytic approach to the wrist, a probable diagnosis of lunate dislocation should be considered. Determination of whether the lunate is dislocated palmarly or dorsally requires a lateral view. On the lateral view, the lunate is palmarly displaced and rotated anteriorly 90 degrees (Fig. 11–25B). This confirms the diagnosis of palmar lunate dislocation.

Case 4: Acute, Posttraumatic, Transradial Styloid Palmar Lunate Fracture-Dislocation with Chip Fractures of the Lunate

(Fig. 11–26)

On the PA view, Arcs I and II are broken while Arc III is intact. This places the abnormality in the proximal carpal row. The lunate has a triangular shape overlapping the profiled articular surfaces of the capitate, hamate, and triquetrum with loss of parallellism between the lunate and these three bones, as well as the scaphoid. Although there is some gross parallelism between the lunate and the radius, the radiolunate joint is much wider than the radioscaphoid joint, which has a normal appearance of parallelism. The proximal articular surface of the lunate is flat and small chip fractures are present radially and ulnarly, compatible with lunate fractures. Except for

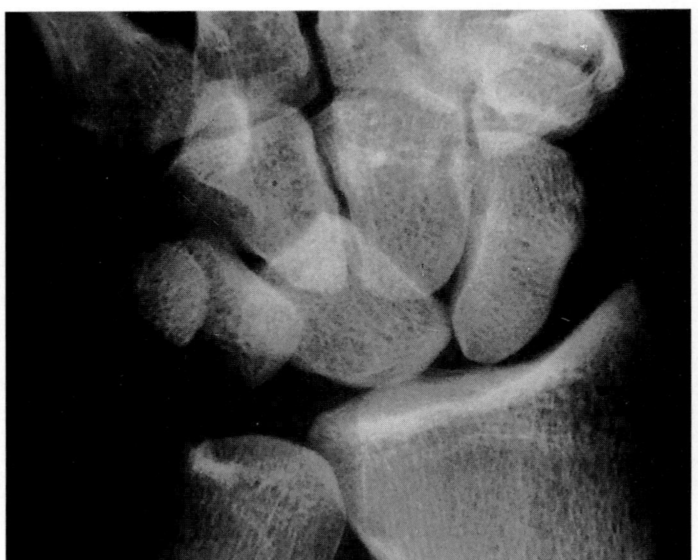

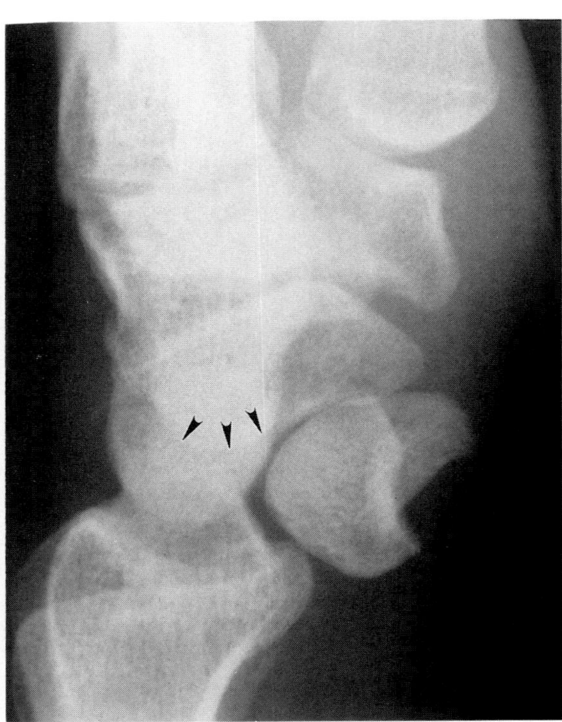

A B

FIGURE 11–25. Palmar lunate dislocation with ulnar carpal translocation. **A:** PA view of the left wrist demonstrates a triangularly shaped lunate and loss of the normally parallel articular relationship with the adjacent capitate, hamate, triquetrum, and scaphoid. Arcs I and II are broken at both the SL and LT joints. The distal articular surface of the lunate is not visible. The radioscaphoid joint width at the level of the radial styloid is much wider than the radioscaphoid joint width at the proximal scaphoid pole, indicating ulnar carpal translocation. **B:** A lateral view of the wrist demonstrates that the lunate is displaced out of the lunate fossa of the distal radius anteriorly and rotated more than 90 degrees palmarly. The head of the capitate (arrowheads) is centered to the concavity of the distal radius.

articulations involving the lunate, other intercarpal relationships are radiographically normal. A fracture of the radial styloid is present. Given the PA view, a diagnosis of transradial styloid lunate fracture-dislocation is most likely. On the lateral view, the lunate is displaced palmarly and rotated anteriorly nearly 90 degrees (Fig. 11–26B). The head of the capitate remains centered to the concave distal surface of the radius. This confirms the diagnosis of transradial styloid palmar lunate fracture-dislocation with chip fractures of the lunate.

Case 5: Acute, Posttraumatic Transscaphoid Lunate Palmar Fracture-Dislocation

(Fig. 11–27)

On the PA wrist view, Arcs I and II are disrupted (Figs. 11–27A and 11–27B). Both the scaphoid and lunate fossae of the distal radius are empty. The scaphoid is fractured through its waist and the distal scaphoid fragment articulates normally with the trapezium and trapezoid. Two bones overlap the triquetrum and hamate. One of these two bones is larger, and since a lunate is larger than half of a scaphoid, the larger bone must be the lunate and the smaller one the proximal half of the scaphoid. The fact that the capitate concavity of the scaphoid faces proximally supports the fact that the proximal scaphoid fragment and probably the lunate are flipped at least 90 degrees. The capitate, hamate, triquetrum, distal scaphoid fragment, trapezium, and trapezoid have maintained their normal interrelationships and position. On a lateral view (Figs. 11–27C and 11–27D) the lunate fossa is empty and the capitate is centered on the radius. The lunate and proximal pole of the scaphoid are in the palmar soft tissues of the wrist. Their concave articular surfaces face proximally, implying rotary malpositioning of approximately 180 degrees from their original orientation.

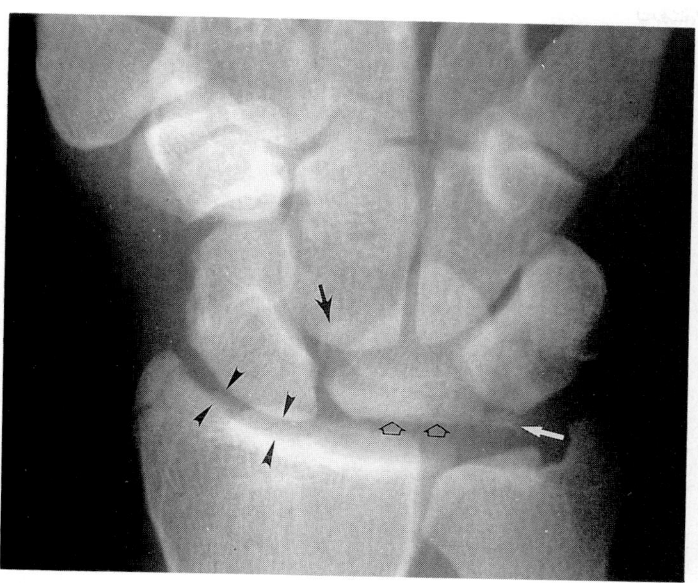

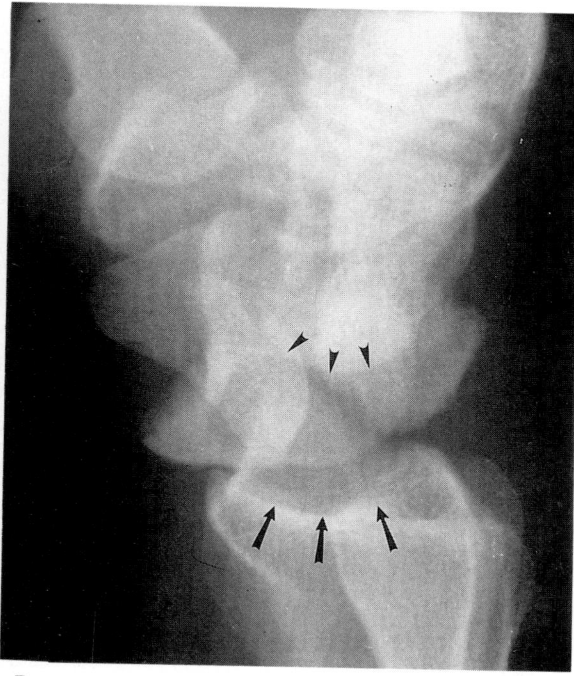

A B

FIGURE 11–26. Transradial styloid palmar lunate fracture-dislocation with lunate chip fractures. **A:** PA view of the right wrist demonstrates that the lunate is triangular in shape with loss of its parallel articular relationship with the adjacent scaphoid, capitate, hamate, and triquetrum. The proximal articular surface of the lunate is flat (open arrows) and its distal articular surface is not visible. Arcs I and II are broken at both the SL and LT joints. Small chip fracture fragments (arrows) project at the proximal ulnar and distal radial edges of the lunate, and a radial styloid fracture is evident. The radiolunate is wider than the radioscaphoid joint. Normal parallelism is present at the radioscaphoid joint (between arrowheads). **B:** A lateral wrist view demonstrates that the lunate is displaced out of the lunate fossa of the distal radius anteriorly and rotated approximately 90 degrees palmarly. The head of the capitate (arrowheads) is centered to the distal articular concavity of the radius (arrows).

Case 6: Acute, Posttraumatic Transscaphoid, Transcapitate, Dorsal Perilunate Fracture-Dislocation (Fig. 11–28)

This condition is also known as the naviculocapitate syndrome.[58–62] On the PA wrist view, both the scaphoid and capitate are fractured. The proximal fragments of both the scaphoid and capitate have rotated about 180 degrees with their proximal articular surfaces facing distally. Both Arcs I and II are broken at the SL and LT joints. Arc III is also broken. Chip fractures project over the SL and capitolunate joint spaces. The abnormalities involve both the proximal and distal carpal rows (Figs. 11–28A and 11–28B). On the lateral view, the lunate is centered over and parallel to the distal articular concavity of the distal radius, and the distal fragment of the capitate is displaced dorsally. The proximal fracture fragments of the capitate and scaphoid are rotated over 180 degrees (Figs. 11–28C and 11–28D). Failure to recognize all the radiographic features on the PA view can easily allow the triquetrum on the lateral view to be called the head of the capitate.

ILLUSTRATIONS OF "JUXTACARPAL" DISLOCATIONS

Case 1: Acute, Posttraumatic Transhamate, Transmetacarpal, Fourth and Fifth CMC Fracture-Dislocation (Fig. 11–29)

On the oblique PA view of the wrist, the three carpal arcs are intact. Overlap of and loss of parallellism at CMC joints four and five are present (Fig. 11–29A). Loss of smooth cortical margin of the fourth metacarpal is evident radially suggestive of acute fracture. Although the displacement direction of the metacarpals may not be well demonstrated on the PA view of the wrist, on the lateral view dorsal displacement of the metacarpals is seen at the CMC joints with a hamate chip fracture. Both views are absolutely nec-

Text continued on page 314

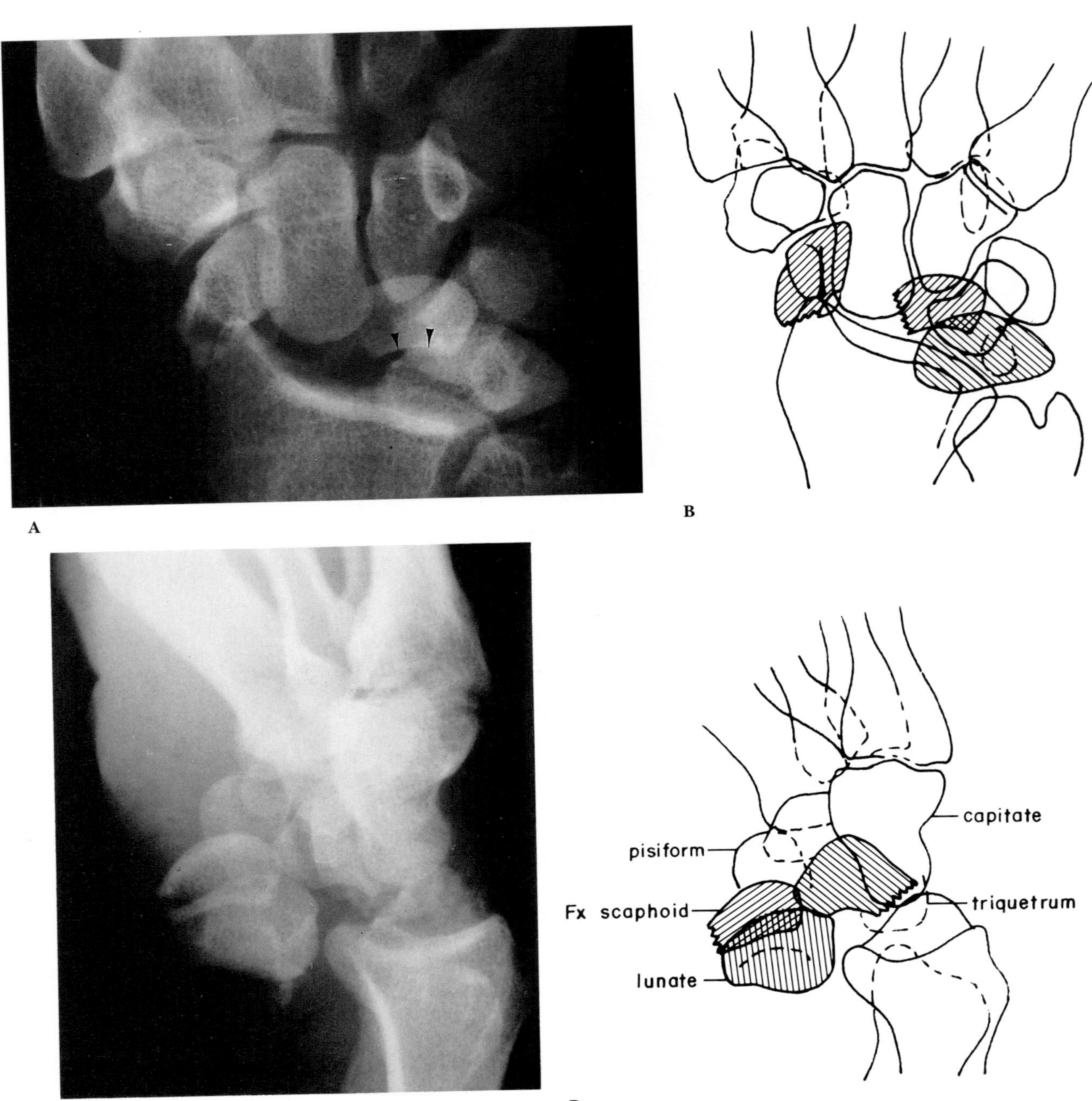

FIGURE 11–27. Transscaphoid lunate palmar fracture-dislocation. **A:** PA view of the right wrist. **B:** Diagram of A demonstrates disruption of the proximal carpal row. Both the scaphoid and lunate fossae of the distal radius are empty, which means that both the scaphoid and lunate are out of their normal position. Two bones overlap the triquetrum and hamate. The smaller, more distal bone has a concave articular surface (arrowheads), which is diagnostic for the concave surface of the scaphoid that articulates with the capitate. This concavity faces proximal. The more proximal bone is larger, and therefore should be the lunate. This larger bone overlaps the articular cortices of the radius as well as the triquetrum. The scaphotrapeziotrapezoidal joint has a normal appearance, which indicates that part of the distal scaphoid fragment has normal attachments with the trapezium and trapezoid. The capitate, hamate, triquetrum, trapezoid, and CMC joints two through five have normal parallelism to each other and are in near-normal position. **C:** The lateral view. **D:** Diagram of **C** demonstrates an empty lunate fossa with the capitate centered distal to the radius. Two semilunar-shaped bones are in palmar soft tissues of the wrist. Their concave articular surfaces face proximally, indicating that these bones flipped about 180 degrees from their original position. (Reprinted with permission from Gilula LA. Carpal injuries: Analytic approach and case exercises. *AJR* 1979;133:503–517.)

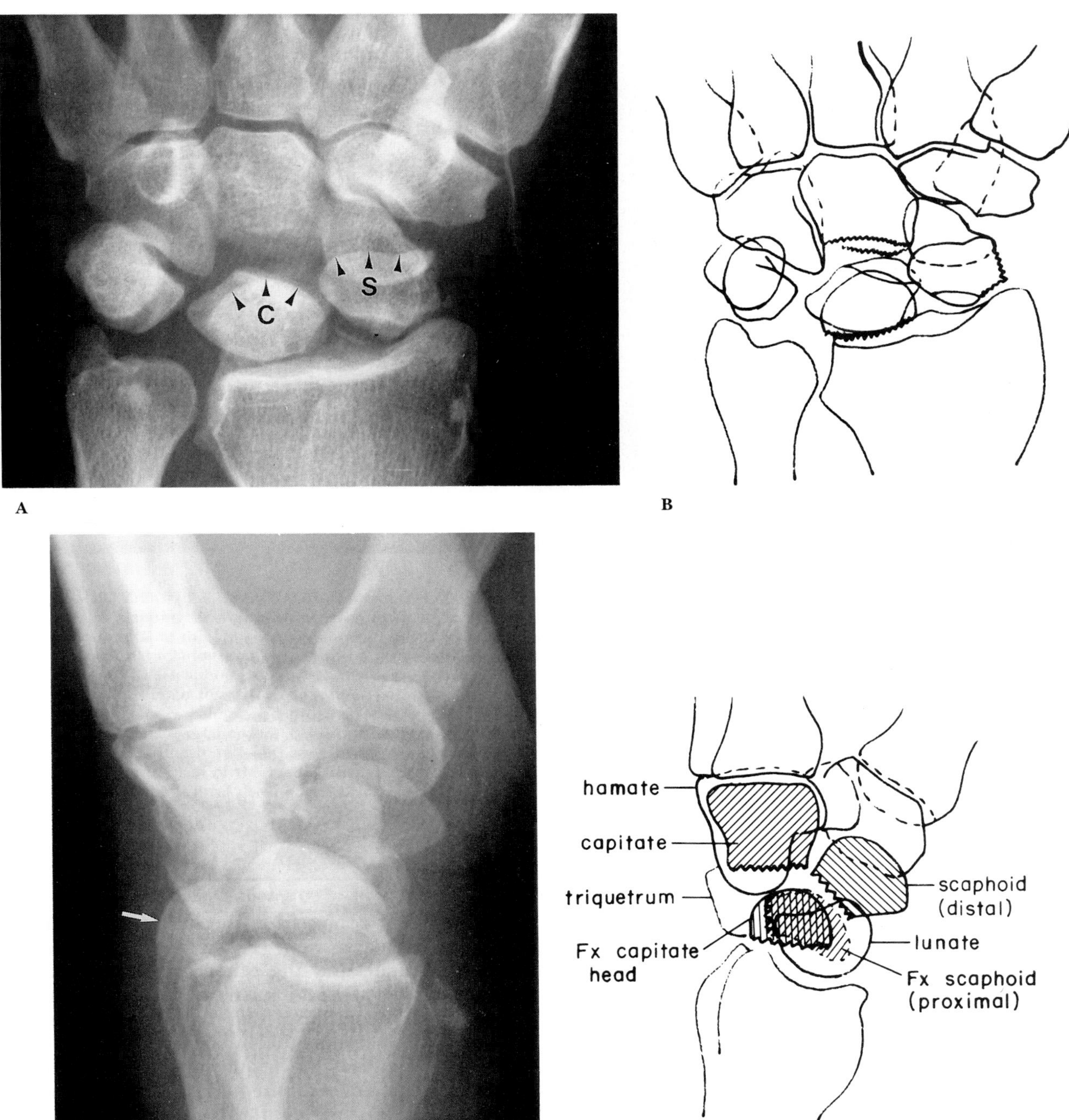

FIGURE 11–28. Transscaphoid, transcapitate, dorsal perilunate fracture-dislocation (scaphocapitate syndrome). **A:** PA view of the left wrist. **B:** Diagram of A demonstrates scaphoid and capitate fractures. Both proximal fragments of the scaphoid (S) and capitate (C) have flipped at least 180 degrees with their proximal articular surfaces (arrowheads) facing distally. Arcs I and II are broken at both the SL and LT joints. Arc III is also broken along the capitate head. Chip fracture fragments overlie the SL, capitolunate, and probably the radial styloid scaphoid joint spaces. **C:** Lateral view. **D:** Diagram of **C**. The lunate is centered over the concavity of the distal radius with slight dorsal tilting of the lunate. The capitate is displaced dorsally, and its proximal pole, which overlies the lunate, is flipped about 180 degrees. The proximal articular surface of the capitate faces distally. A fracture fragment of undefined origin (arrow) projects dorsally over the ulnar styloid. (Reprinted with permission from Gilula LA. Carpal injuries: Analytic approach and case exercises. *AJR* 1979;133:503–517.)

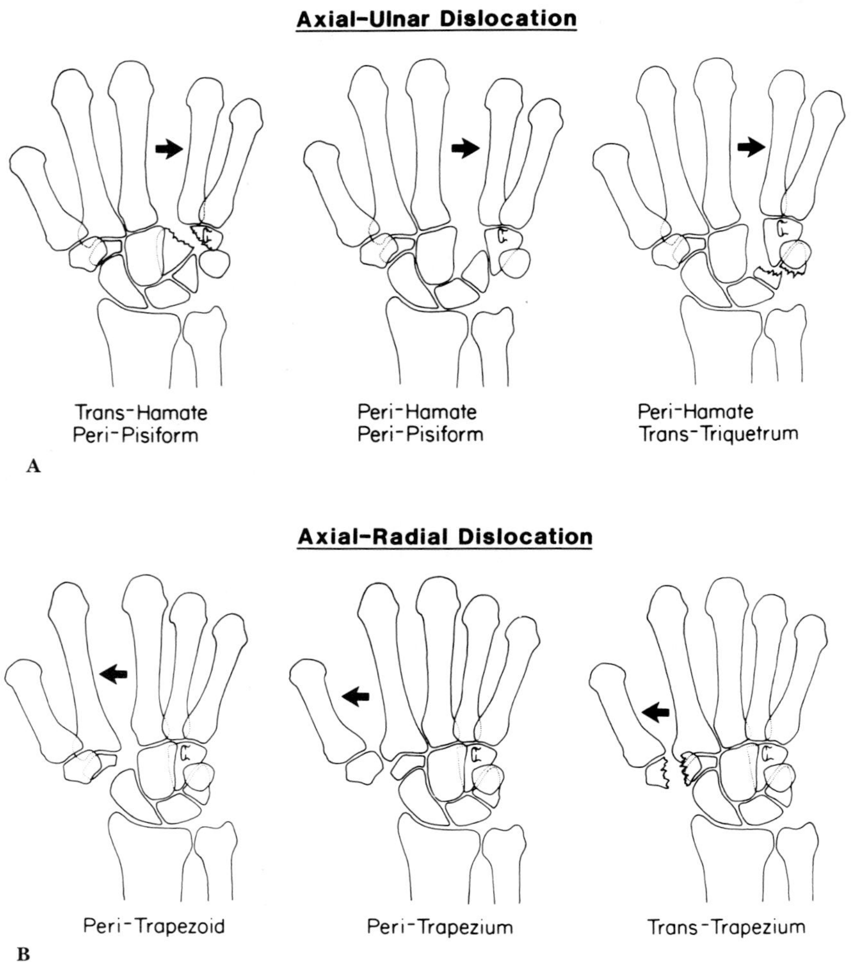

Axial-Ulnar Dislocation

Trans-Hamate Peri-Pisiform

Peri-Hamate Peri-Pisiform

Peri-Hamate Trans-Triquetrum

A

Axial-Radial Dislocation

Peri-Trapezoid

Peri-Trapezium

Trans-Trapezium

B

FIGURE 11–31. Drawing of the most common types of axial disruption of the carpus. **A:** Axial-ulnar dislocation. **B:** Axial-radial dislocation. (Modified from Garcia-Elias M et al. Traumatic axial dislocations of the carpus. *J Hand Surg* 1989;14A:446.)

fracture-dislocations uses the prefixes peri- or trans- depending on whether there is a dislocation around a bone ("peri-") or a fracture through a bone ("trans-") with dislocation of the carpus.

The three most common axial ulnar types (Fig. 11–31) are the transhamate fracture-dislocation (a distal fracture fragment of the hamate moving together with the fourth and fifth metacarpals, which are dislocated from the rest of the metacarpals and CMC joints), the perihamate, peripisiform dislocation (the hamate and pisiform with the fourth and fifth metacarpals are dislocated ulnarly), and the perihamate transtriquetral fracture-dislocation (a distal triquetral fracture fragment has moved ulnarly with the pisiform, hamate, and attached fourth and fifth metacarpals). In the axial radial group, the most common types (see Fig. 8–19) are the peritrapezial dislocation (the trapezium and the first metacarpal are dislocated from the carpal and metacarpal bones), the peritrapezoidal dislocation (the trapezium and the trapezoid are dislocated with the first and second metacarpals from the other carpal and metacarpal bones), and the transtrapezial fracture dislocation (dislocation of the first metacarpal with a fracture fragment of the trapezium)

Carpal instabilities are discussed in Chapter 8. A summary of the appearances of static carpal instability on radiography is presented in Table 11–2.

REFERENCES

1. Curtis DJ. Injuries of the wrist: An approach to diagnosis. *Radiol Clin North Am* 1981;19:625–644.
2. Schernberg F. Roentgenographic examination of the wrist: A systematic study of the normal, lax and injured wrist. Part 1: The standard and positional views. *J Hand Surg* 1990; 15B:210–219.
3. Schernberg F. Roentgenographic examination of the wrist: A systemic study of the normal, lax and injured wrist. Part 2: The stress views. *J Hand Surg* 1990;15B:220–228.

4. Gilula LA. Carpal injuries: Analytic approach and case exercises. *AJR* 1979;133:503–517.
5. Cantor RM, Braunstein EM. Diagnosis of dorsal and palmar rotation of the lunate on a frontal radiograph. *J Hand Surg* 1988;13A:187–193.
6. Gilula LA, Weeks PM. Post-traumatic ligamentous instabilities of the wrist. *Radiology* 1978;129:641–651.
7. Curtis DJ, Downey EF Jr, Brower AC, Cruess DF, Herrington WT, Ghaed N. Importance of soft-tissue evaluation in hand and wrist trauma: Statistical evaluation. *AJR* 1984;142:781–788.
8. Harris JH. The significance of soft tissue injury in the roentgen diagnosis of trauma. *Crit Rev Clin Radiol Nucl Med* 1975; 44:295–338.
9. Terry DW Jr, Ramin JE. The navicular fat stripe: A useful roentgen feature for evaluating wrist trauma. *AJR* 1975; 124:25–28.
10. MacEwan DW. Changes due to trauma in the fat plane overlying the pronator quadratus muscle: A radiologic sign. *Radiology* 1964;82:879–886.
11. Dobyns JH, Linscheid RL, Chao EYS, Weber ER, Swanson GE. Traumatic instability of the wrist. *AAOS Instructional Course Lectures.* St. Louis: CV Mosby, 1975:182–199.
12. Viegas SF, Wagner K, Patterson R, Peterson P. Medial (hamate) facet of the lunate. *J Hand Surg* 1990;15A:564–571.
13. Peh WCG, Gilula LA. Normal disruption of carpal arcs of the wrist. *J Hand Surg* 1995, in press.
14. Taleisnik J. Post-traumatic carpal instability. *Clin Orthop* 1980;149:73–82.
15. Linn MR, Mann FA, Gilula LA. Imaging the symptomatic wrist. *Orthop Clin North Am* 1990;21:515–543.
16. Arkless R. Cineradiography in normal and abnormal wrists. *AJR* 1966;96:837–844.
17. Metz VM, Schimmerl SM, Gilula LA, Viegas SF, Saffar P. Wide scapholunate joint space in lunotriquetral coalition: A normal variant? *Radiology* 1993;188:557–559.
18. Fisher MR, Rogers LF, Hendrix RW. Systematic approach to identifying fourth and fifth carpometacarpal joint dislocations. *AJR* 1983;140:319–324.
19. Fisher MR, Rogers LF, Hendrix RW, Gilula LA. Carpometacarpal joint dislocations. *Crit Rev Diagn Imaging* 1984;22:95–126.
20. DiBenedetto MR, Lubbers LM, Coleman CR. A standardized measurement of ulnar carpal translocation. *J Hand Surg* 1990;15A:1009–1010.
21. Taleisnik J. Classification of carpal instability. *Bull Hosp Joint Dis* 1984;44:511–531.
22. Taleisnik J. Carpal instability. *J Bone Joint Surg* 1988;70A:1262–1268.
23. Rayhack JM, Linscheid RL, Dobyns JH, Smith JH. Posttraumatic ulnar translation of the carpus. *J Hand Surg* 1987; 12(A):180–189.
24. McMurtry RY, Youm Y, Flatt AE, Gillespie TE. Kinematics of the wrist: II. Clinical applications. *J Bone Joint Surg* 1978;60A:955–961.
25. Green DP. Carpal dislocation and instabilities. In: Green DP, ed. *Operative hand surgery.* Vol. 1. 3rd ed. New York: Livingstone, 1993:861–928.
26. Larsen CF, Stigsby B, Mathiesen FK, Lindequist S. Radiography of the wrist: A new device for standardized radiographs. *Acta Radiol* 1990;31:459–462.
27. Sarrafian SK, Melamed JL, Goshgarin GM. Study of wrist motion in flexion and extension. *Clin Orthop* 1977;126: 153–159.
28. Armstrong GWD. Rotational subluxation of the scaphoid. *Can J Surg* 1968;11:306–314.
29. Crittenden JJ, Jones DM, Santarelli AG. Bilateral rotational dislocation of the carpal navicular. Case report. *Radiology* 1970;94:629–630.
30. Russell TB. Inter-carpal dislocations and fracture-dislocations: A review of fifty-nine cases. *J Bone Joint Surg* 1949;31B: 524–531.
31. Johnson RP. The acutely injured wrist and its residuals. *Clin Orthop* 1980;149:33–44
32. Worland RL, Dick HM. Transnavicular perilunate dislocations. *J Trauma* 1975;15:407–412.
33. Yeager BA, Dalinka MK. Radiology of trauma to the wrist: Dislocations, fracture dislocations, and instability patterns. *Skeletal Radiol* 1985;13:120–130.
34. Garcia-Elias M, Abanco J, Salvador E, Sanchez R. Crush injury of the carpus. *J Bone Joint Surg* 1985;67B:286–289.
35. Garcia-Elias M, Dobyns JH, Cooney WP, Linscheid RL. Traumatic axial dislocations of the carpus. *J Hand Surg* 1989; 14A:446–457.
36. Hodge JC, Larsen CF, Gilula LA, Amadio P. Analysis of carpal instability: Part II. Clinical application. *J Hand Surg* 1995A; in press.
37. Larsen CF, Gilula LA, Amadio P, Hodge JC. Analysis of carpal instability: Part I. Description. *J Hand Surg* 1995; in press.
38. Aitken AP, Nalebuff EA. Volar transnavicular perilunate dislocation of the carpus. *J Bone Joint Surg* 1960;42A:1051–1057.
39. DePalma FA. Fractures and dislocations of the carpal bones. In: DePalma FA, ed. *The management of fractures and dislocations, an atlas.* 2nd ed. Philadelphia: WB Saunders, 1970:952–1022.
40. Weiss C, Laskin RS, Spinner M. Irreducible trans-scaphoid perilunate dislocation. *J Bone Joint Surg* 1970;52A:565–568.
41. Cave EF. Retrolunar dislocation of the capitate with fracture or subluxation of the navicular bone. *J Bone Joint Surg* 1941;23:830–840.
42. Hill NA. Fractures and dislocations of the carpus. *Orthop Clin North Am* 1970;1:275–284.
43. Key JA, Conwell HE. Injuries of wrist and hand. In: Key JA, Conwell HE, eds. *Management of fractures, dislocations and sprains.* 5th ed. St. Louis: CV Mosby, 1951:716–737.
44. Dunn WA. Fractures and dislocations of the carpus. *Surg Clin North Am* 1972;52:1513–1538.
45. Botte MJ, Gelberman RH. Fractures of the carpus, excluding the scaphoid. *Hand Clinics* 1987;3:149–161.
46. Weissenborn W, Sabri W. Complex fracture dislocation of the wrist: Transscaphoid-transulnar-transstyloid fracture dislocation (in German). *Handchir Mikrochir Plast Chir* 1988;20:107–110.
47. Mayfield JK. Patterns of injury to carpal ligaments: A spectrum. *Clin Orthop* 1984;187:36–42.
48. Mayfield JK. Mechanism of carpal injuries. *Clin Orthop* 1980;149:45–54.
49. Mayfield JK, Johnson RP, Kilcoyne RK. Carpal dislocations: Pathomechanics and progressive perilunate instability. *J Hand Surg* 1980;5A:226–241.
50. Mayfield JK. Wrist ligamentous anatomy and pathogenesis of carpal instability. *Orthop Clin North Am* 1984;15:209–216.
51. Peltier LF. The Classic: Destot É. Injuries of the wrist: A radiological study. *Clin Orthop* 1986;202:3–11.
52. Wagner CJ. Perilunar dislocations. *J Bone Joint Surg* 1956;38A:1198–1207.
53. Wagner CJ. Fracture-dislocations of the wrist. *Clin Orthop* 1959;15:181–196.
54. Tanz SS. Rotation effect in lunar and perilunar dislocations. *Clin Orthop* 1968;57:147–152.
55. Mayfield JK, Gilula LA, Totty WG. Carpal fracture-dislocations. In: Gilula LA, ed. *The traumatized hand and wrist: Radiographic and anatomic correlation.* Philadelphia: WB Saunders, 1992:297–314.
56. Curtis DJ, Downey EF. Soft tissue evaluation in trauma. In: Gilula LA, ed. *The traumatized hand and wrist: Radiographic and anatomic correlation.* Philadelphia: WB Saunders, 1992:45–63.
57. Green DP, O'Brien ET. Open reduction of carpal dislocations: Indications and operative techniques. *J Hand Surg* 1978;3A:250–265.
58. Monahan PRW, Galasko CSB. The scapho-capitate fracture syndrome: A mechanism of injury. *J Bone Joint Surg* 1972;54B:122–124.
59. El-Khoury GY, Usta HY, Blair WF. Naviculocapitate fracture-dislocation. *AJR* 1982;139:385–386.
60. Fenton RL. The naviculo-capitate fracture syndrome. *J Bone Joint Surg* 1956;38A:681–684.
61. Resnik CS, Gelberman RH, Resnick D. Transscaphoid, trans-

capitate, perilunate fracture dislocation (scaphocapitate syndrome). *Skeletal Radiol* 1983;9:192–194.

62. Stein F, Siegel MW. Naviculocapitate fracture syndrome: A case report. New thoughts on the mechanism of injury. *J Bone Joint Surg* 1969;51A:391–395.
63. Linscheid RL, Dobyns JH, Beabout JW, Bryan RS. Traumatic instability of the wrist: Diagnosis, classification, and pathomechanics. *J Bone Joint Surg* 1972;54A:1612–1632.
64. Bellinghausen HW, Gilula LA, Young LV, Weeks PM. Post-traumatic palmar carpal subluxation: Report of two cases. *J Bone Joint Surg* 1983;65A:998–1006.
65. Gilula LA, Totty WG. Wrist trauma: Roentgenographic analysis. In: Gilula LA, ed. *The traumatized hand and wrist: Radiographic and anatomic correlation.* Philadelphia: WB Saunders, 1992:221–239.

CHAPTER 12

BONE SCINTIGRAPHY

Lawrence E. Holder

Three-phase radionuclide bone imaging (TPBI) has become a standard tool in the diagnostic armamentarium of the hand surgeon. The current techniques and applications of radionuclide bone imaging are dramatically different from those of the bone scans performed in the early 1970s chiefly to evaluate primary and metastatic bone tumors. Bone imaging in the routine practice of hand surgery has taken several directions: (1) the noninvasive evaluation and demonstration of vascular lesions and blood vessel patency, such as the diagnosis of arteriovenous malformations; (2) the recognition of expected bone changes prior to their radiographic appearance, such as bone pain secondary to occult fracture or inflammatory disease; (3) the detection and localization of pain of potentially osseous origin with direction of subsequent anatomic imaging; (4) the differential diagnosis, age, or metabolic activity of lesions seen on radiographs, such as evaluation of "lucent" or "cyst-like" lesions in the carpals and metacarpals; (5) the recognition of osseous disease entities that can occur without radiographic changes, such as reflex sympathetic dystrophy; and (6) the exclusion of osseous disease in the medicolegal and worker's compensation settings. In this chapter, the technique of TPBI as applied to the hand and wrist is introduced. The physiology underlying the images is described, and the ability of the study to provide anatomic localization of lesions, even if a specific diagnosis cannot always be made, is emphasized. Information about the historical development of radionuclide bone imaging (RNBI) can be found in texts,[1] monographs,[2] and review articles.[3,4]

Figures 12–1 to 12–16, 12–18, 12–20, 12–22, 12–24, 12–25, 12–27 to 12–30, 12–32, and 12–34 are reprinted with permission from Holder LE. Radionuclide bone imaging in surgical problems of the hand. In: Gilula LA. ed. The traumatized hand and wrist: Radiographic and anatomic correlation. *Philadelphia: WB Saunders, 1992.*

TECHNICAL ASPECTS OF RADIONUCLIDE BONE IMAGING

Nuclear Medicine Instrumentation

Textbooks provide detailed discussions of modern instrumentation, radiopharmaceuticals, radiation dosimetry, and the physiology of bone imaging.[5–7] Nuclear medicine imaging devices use a sodium iodide scintillation crystal to detect gamma photons, which are emitted by the radionuclides that have been administered to the patient. The system's electronics convert the photon energy sequentially into a light scintillation, an electron, and finally an electric signal, which is then processed to create an anatomic image. Introduced in the early 1970s, the Anger gamma scintillation camera is the imaging device used almost exclusively in clinical nuclear medicine practice. Gamma cameras simultaneously view areas of the body 25 to 50 cm in diameter, with camera electronics providing resolution of approximately 1.7 mm at the surface, with a clinically useful resolution of 5 to 6 mm. Collimators are interposed between the organ being imaged and the detector. The collimator is a device that restricts the field of view and, depending on its design, creates high-resolution images, magnified images, and in certain circumstances, images in which rapid data collection takes precedence over spatial resolution. Positron emission tomography (PET) requiring special scanners has been used to image bone with fluorine-18 as the tracer.[8] Single photon emission tomographic imaging (SPECT) devices equipped with high-energy collimators have also recently been investigated for use with fluorine-18. Routine SPECT imaging with technetium-labeled tracers has not proved diagnostically helpful in the hand and wrist and is rarely performed in the hand and wrist.

Radiopharmaceuticals

In 1971, Subramanian and McAfee attached the radioisotope technetium-99m to a phosphorus moiety, initiating modern bone imaging.[9] Technetium is a Group VIIA element that does not exist in nature in a nonradioactive form. Technetium-99m, which is the radioactive daughter of radioactive molybdenum-99m, was introduced into clinical practice in 1964. A short (six-hour) half-life, a favorable monoenergetic disintegration energy of 140 keV, and ready availability make this radioisotope nearly ideal. Its short half-life allows higher doses to be administered to the patient, which provides improved diagnostic images and, coupled with the pure gamma emission, results in very low absorbed doses.

A variety of phosphorus-based compounds have been tested over the past 15 years. The diphosphonate analogs with P-C-P bonding instead of the P-O-P sequence of pyrophosphates have become the most popular. The diphosphonate bonding is more stable chemically and is not subject to enzymatic hydrolysis in vivo. Methylene disphosphonate has been the most widely used of these new agents for many years because of its rapid blood disappearance and relatively low concentrations in the major viscera and other soft tissues.

The specific mechanisms of skeletal localization of the phosphate tracers are still poorly understood. The major factors probably responsible for the locally increased uptake in lesions are increased bone blood flow, including opening of more blood vessels per unit volume, and increased extraction efficiency. It is thought that these radiotracers localize by a chemisorption or an adsorption phenomenon that occurs in the hydration shell around the hydroxyapatite crystals and amorphous calcium phosphate. It has been suggested that in areas of rapid bone turnover or increased metabolism with high osteoblastic activity, newly deposited bone mineral contains a larger number of smaller crystals with greater surface area, and hence have a relatively greater probability of absorbing the radiotracer.[10] Following an intravenous injection of these tracers, the half-time for distribution from the vascular to the extravascular space is 2 to 4 minutes. By 3 hours after injection, in the normally hydrated patient, approximately 35% of the injected dose has been excreted by the kidneys, 30% to 40% is associated with bone, 10% to 15% is in other tissues, and 5% is in the blood.[3]

Although all of the above factors have combined to allow relatively precise gross anatomic localization of abnormal metabolic activity, there has been only minimal progress in the more histologic localization of tracer accumulation. Some studies have suggested that diphosphonates localize in the mineral phase of bone at active sites of bone formation or resorption, particularly at the osteoid–mineral interfaces. A macroautoradiographic study of samples obtained at surgery on osteoarthritic femoral heads demonstrated that tracer accumulation occurred in subchondral cyst walls and osteochondral junctions in osteophytes —areas of enchondral ossification.[11]

Radiation Dosimetry

The estimated absorbed radiation doses are measured for the whole body, including the bones, the bladder (which, as the organ receiving the highest relative dose, is called the critical organ), and the gonads (which, in patients of childbearing age, account for the genetically significant dose and, as such, allow for comparison with other techniques). The absorbed radiation doses to a 70-kg adult receiving an average 20 mCi administered dose of technetium-labeled phosphorus compound are 0.13 rads, total body; 2.6 to 6.2 rads, bladder wall (voiding after 2 to 4.8 hours); 0.24 to 0.34 rads, ovaries (voiding after 2 to 4.8 hours); and 0.16 to 0.22 rads, testes (voiding after 2 to 4.8 hours).[12] Most patients who are seen in the orthopedic setting can void normally; therefore, the lower dose estimates apply because the radiotracer is excreted rapidly. By comparison, a barium enema gives a 0.2-rad to a 0.5-rad dose to the ovaries and an anteroposterior (AP) and lateral lumbar spine radiographic examination gives a 0.225-rad dose to the ovaries.[12] Nuclear physicians and radiologists, in comparison, are allowed an occupational exposure of up to 5 rads per year. The doses given to patients are low and well within the accepted ranges for diagnostic examinations, so one should not hesitate to use RNBI when clinically indicated.

Imaging Technique

The three-phase examination follows the previously described passage of the tracer from the blood vessels (phase one) to the extravascular extracellular spaces (phase two) to the hydration shell of the bone crystal (phase three). These phases are termed, respectively, the radionuclide angiogram or intravascular phase (RNA); the blood pool, tissue phase, or extracellular space images (BP); and the delayed or metabolic images. A fourth phase consisting of 18- to 24-hour delayed images has been reported to increase the specificity from 73% to 87% as well as the overall accuracy in diagnosing osteomyelitis, especially in patients with diabetes mellitus and/or peripheral vascular disease.[13] In patients with osteomyelitis underlying superficial ulcers or soft-tissue infection, the relative increased tracer accumulation on the fourth-phase image continues to increase. Some authors have recently questioned the value of routine three-phase imaging in general orthopedic imaging in children, but in our experience, especially in the hand and wrist, the technique has been invaluable.[14,15] The RNA (phase one) demonstrates the perfusion to a lesion. The patient is seated in front of the gamma camera and the hands are placed palm down on the collimator face. Two-by-two gauze pledgets are used to separate the fingers and paper-type tape is placed over the hands and wrists to maintain close contact between the hand and the collimator face (Fig. 12–1). Sequential images are obtained,

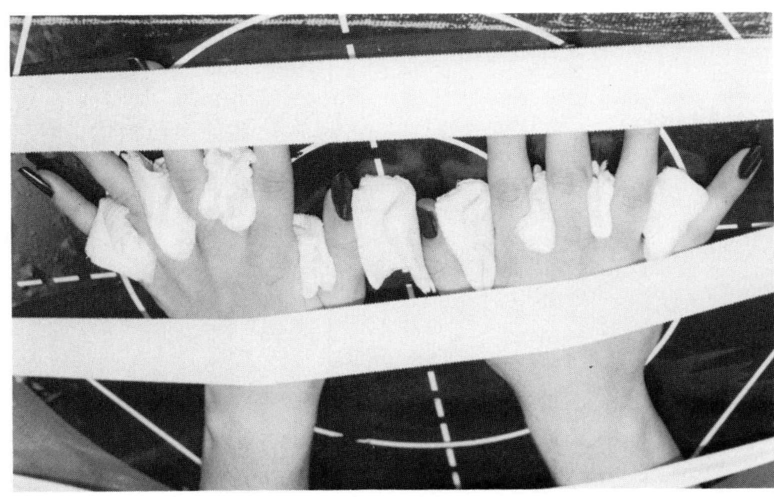

FIGURE 12–1. Position of patient's hands. To obtain images of anatomic detail, pledgets are used to separate fingers; to eliminate movement, tape is used to immobilize the hand.

each for a preset time following bolus injection of the tracer. In our institution, 5-second analog images have proved an adequate compromise between temporal and spatial resolution requirements. With digital acquisition of data, 60 1-second images can be obtained. Trial and error for each particular camera–computer configuration is then required to determine the optimum summing of images (3 to 10 seconds) to obtain adequate spatial resolution. Similar trials are also required to decide upon the most optimal acquisition matrix. Much controversy has existed about the technique of tracer injection in obtaining diagnostic RNAs.[16] In most patients, a routine tourniquet is placed proximal to the antecubital fossa of the asymptomatic extremity, a 20-gauge needle inserted, preferably into the medial antecubital vein, a high specific-activity (small volume) bolus injected, and the tourniquet released. Occasionally, a butterfly-type needle with a three-way stopcock at the end of the tubing is used, with a 5- to 10-ml saline flush used immediately after the injection of tracer. We have not felt the need to use a blood pressure cuff technique. We do use the external jugular vein, particularly if we want to compare elbows or forearms. We have not noticed diagnostically significant reactive hyperemia of the injected side, secondary to use of the tourniquet.

The BP images (phase two) demonstrate the relative vascularity of a lesion. These images are obtained immediately after the angiogram for a set number of counts rather than for a preset time. With standard large-field-of-view (LFOV) cameras, we obtain approximately 500,000 counts per image in the extremities, whereas jumbo cameras often require 1,000,000 or more counts per image for a satisfactory information density (ID). A minimum 128 × 128 acquisition matrix is used for digital data collection. Between the BP and delayed images, the patient is encouraged to drink at least six 8-ounce glasses of liquid. The delayed images (phase three) demonstrate the relative bone turnover in a particular anatomic area. These images are usually obtained 3 hours after injection of the tracer and use a high-resolution collimator instead of the high-sensitivity or general-purpose collimator used for accumulation of data in phases one and two. Between 800,000 and 1,500,000 counts are obtained, and, for digital data, a minimum matrix of 256 × 256 is used. Work continues to create camera and computer combinations that will allow even higher matrix resolutions to be used in an attempt to duplicate the quality of analog images obtained with older cameras using 0.25-inch crystals. Images obtained with the pinhole or converging collimator often supplement the high-resolution parallel hole collimator images. In patients with delayed clearance of tracer, which may be secondary to poor fluid intake, renal disease, cardiac disease, or technical factors, such as infiltration of the injected tracer, further 4- or 5-hour delayed images are obtained. In most cases, all three phases can be obtained without removing a plaster cast, although occasionally special views require cast removal.[17]

NORMAL THREE-PHASE BONE IMAGING[14]

Images produced using nuclear medicine techniques should be considered primarily physiologic images. Although improvements and advances in instrumentation and radiopharmaceutical design continue to increase resolution capabilities, the main purpose of these examinations is to define a locus of abnormal physiology, in many cases leaving the more precise anatomic description of these areas to detailed plain film radiography, polytomography, and in some instances computed tomography (CT) scanning, magnetic resonance imaging (MRI), or both.

Radionuclide Angiogram (Fig. 12–2)

Following the bolus injection of tracer, activity at the site of the radial and ulnar arteries appears as two

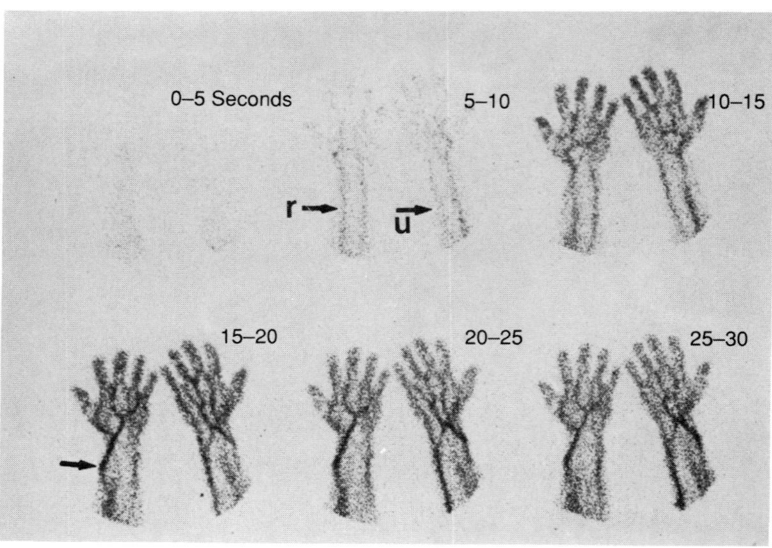

FIGURE 12–2. Normal radionuclide angiogram (RNA), dorsal view, 5-second sequential images recorded on x-ray film. Activity is represented by black dots on a white background. Radial (R) and ulnar (U) artery activity are seen on the 5- to 10-second image. Palmar arch blush and early digital perfusion are seen on the same frame but often are seen first on the next sequential image. Venous drainage (arrow) seen on the 15- to 20-second image is not always as prominent as in this patient.

distinct lines in the distal forearm and wrist, while flow through the palmar arches is seen as a blush in the palm that appears within one frame (5 seconds) after activity is noted in the wrist. Specific vessels in the palmar arches can be identified only occasionally.

Activity in the fingers normally appears either in the same frame as the palmar arch activity or in the next frame. When flow through the radial and ulnar arteries is equal, all fingers fill at the same time and with the same intensity. The digital arteries are usually not defined, although activity often appears early along the sides of the finger where the arteries are located. Most often, there is a homogeneous distribution of activity encompassing the soft tissues.

Approximately 25% of patients demonstrate either a "radial-dominant" (thumb plus index and long fingers, followed by ring and small fingers) or an "ulnar-dominant" (fifth plus ring and long fingers, followed by the index finger and thumb) perfusion pattern. These are normal variations, usually without clinical significance.[14]

Blood Pool or Tissue Phase Images (Figs. 12–3 and 12–4)

The 500,000-count images, obtained immediately after the last frame of the RNA, are usually acquired in 5 to 8 minutes. Occasionally, curvilinear structures, which correspond to intravascular activity in prominent veins and arteries, are seen. Usually tracer distribution is symmetrical in both hands with normally increased activity (no more than two or three times that of the other soft tissues) in the thenar and hypothenar areas and frequently in many fingertips. Occasionally, linear activity radiating outward from the palm to the web spaces between the fingers is seen and is thought to correspond to the smaller, intrinsic muscles of the hand.[14,15,18]

Delayed or Metabolic Images (Figs. 12–5 and 12–6)

These images, obtained three to four hours after injection of tracer, demonstrate the distal radius and ulna as well-defined linear structures. The wrist, including the radiocarpal joint, inferior radioulnar compartment, carpal bones, and the metacarpal bases, is seen as a homogeneous area of diffuse accumulation two to three times more intense than the distal third of either the radius or the ulna. In healthy subjects, the individual carpal bones cannot routinely be identified. The metacarpals and phalanges appear as linear structures. Juxtaarticular activity, which is two to three times that of the adjacent bone, defines the metacarpophalangeal and proximal interphalangeal joints, with the distal interphalangeal joints showing less activity. Patients who do not drink significant amounts of fluid or who have poor renal function, and occasionally some patients for unknown reasons, show low bone-to-soft-tissue ratios, with less optimal bone detail. In those cases, sometimes 5- to 7-hour delayed images are helpful.

In younger patients, tracer accumulation in the growth plate regions reflects the normal relative increase in bone metabolism in those areas (see Figs. 12–4 and 12–6). In our institution, we use a three-step grading system for the degree of abnormal flow, blood pool, or delayed tracer activity.[14,19,20] One plus (1 +) equals (=) minimally increased activity or flow, barely perceptible above the normal soft tissue or bone (1.5 to 2 times normal); 2 + = moderately increased activity, easily discernible above normal soft tissue or bone (still only 1.5 to 2.5 times normal); 3 + = intense activity, which in younger patients on delayed images is at least as intense as the growth plate regions (at least 3 times normal).

Text continued on page 325

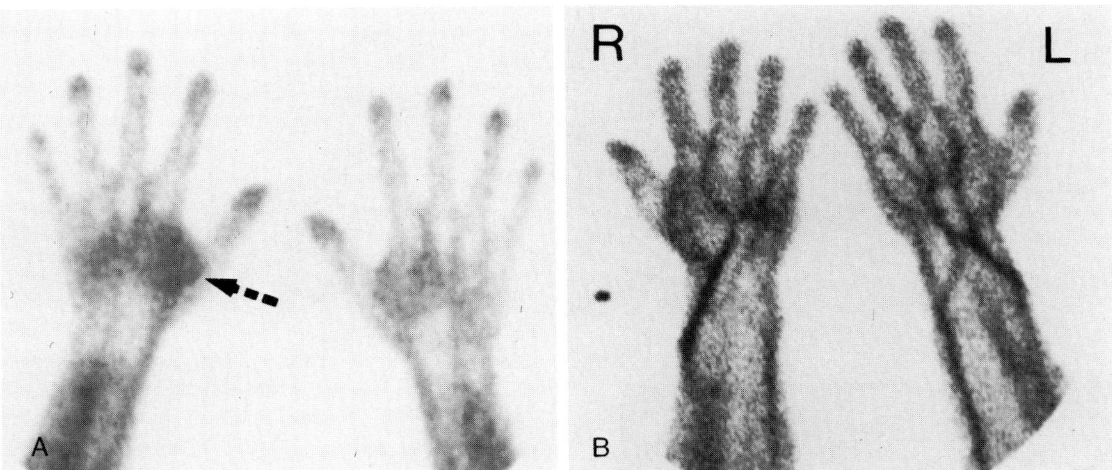

FIGURE 12–3. Normal blood pool (BP) images. Five hundred thousand counts were obtained immediately after RNA without moving the patient. The extracellular distribution of tracer reflects relative vascularity of the tissues. **A:** Palmar view. The thenar (arrow) and, to a lesser extent, the hypothenar muscles are also seen. **B:** Dorsal view, same patient as in Fig. 12–2. Veins are particularly prominent.

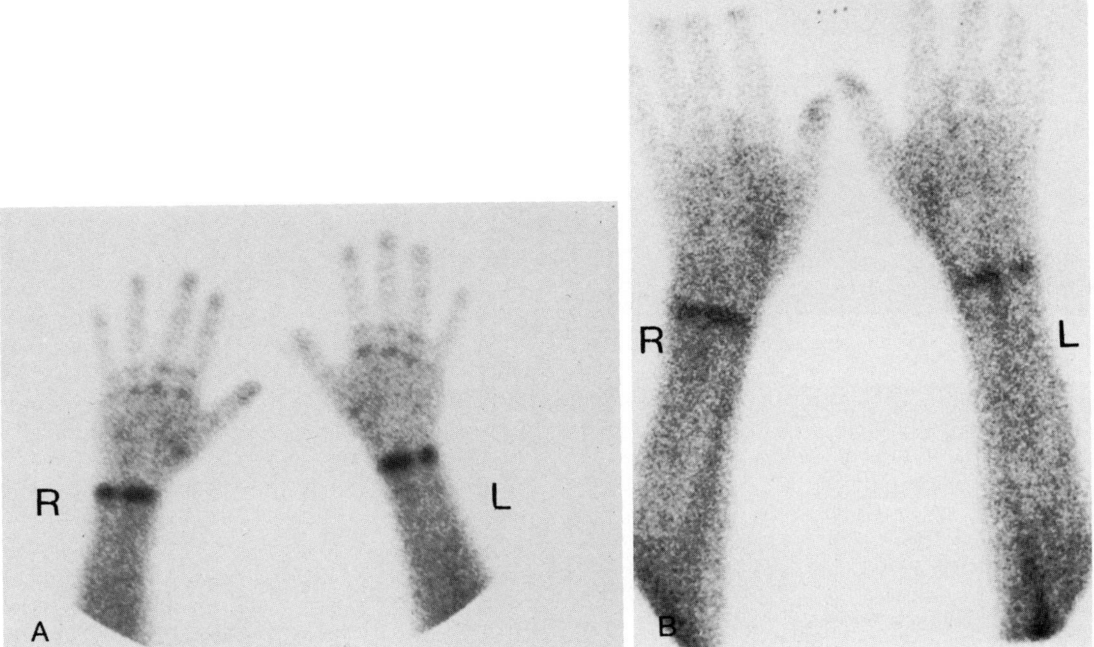

FIGURE 12–4. Normal BP images, young patients, palmar views. **A:** Seven-year-old. Increased relative vascularity in distal radial, ulnar, distal metacarpal, and proximal phalangeal growth plates. **B:** Sixteen-year-old. Vascularity is noted only in distal radial and ulnar growth plates.

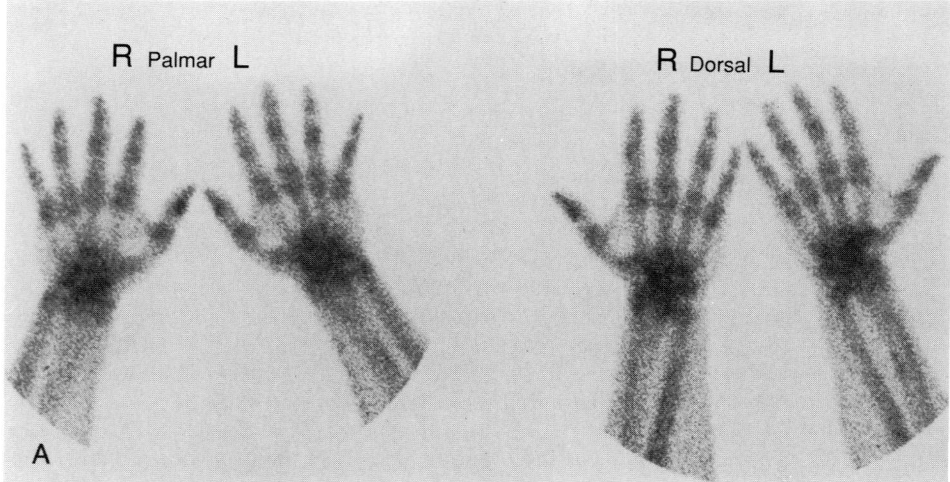

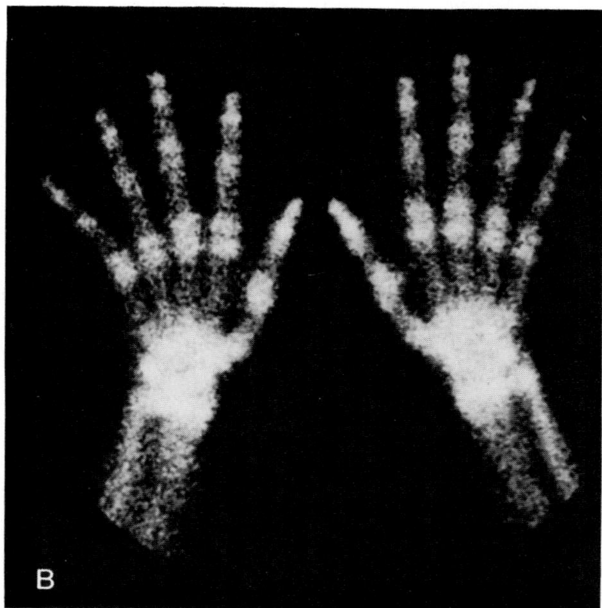

FIGURE 12–5. Normal delayed or metabolic images. Five hundred thousand counts were obtained 3–4 hours after injection of tracer. **A:** The radius and ulna are well visualized but normal carpals are not usually individually defined. Metacarpophalangeal and interphalangeal joints are defined by juxtaarticular activity 1.5–2.5 times more intense than that of individual phalanges. **B:** Image in another patient recorded on Polaroid film with activity represented as white dots on a black background. Juxtaarticular activity is more prominent than in **A**. The amount of activity progressively decreases from proximal to distal.

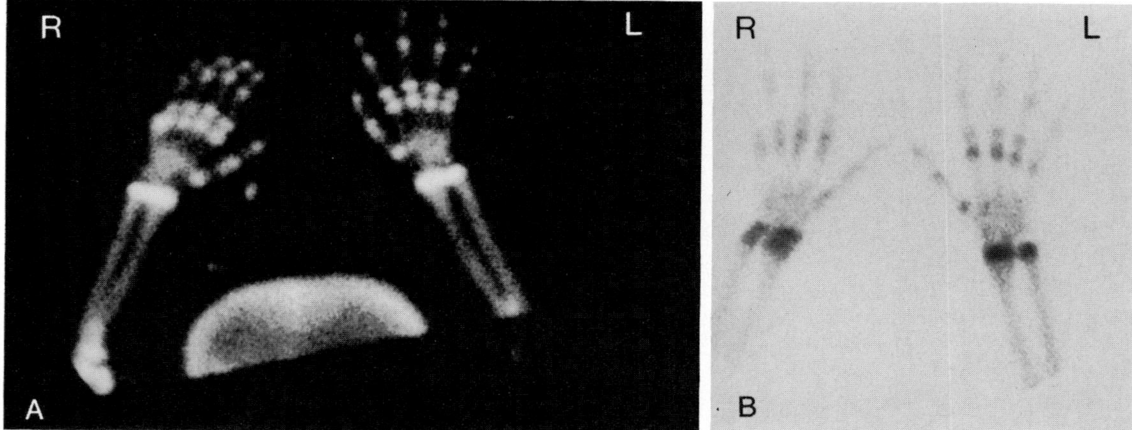

FIGURE 12–6. Normal delayed images, young patients, palmar views. **A:** Two-year-old. Intense tracer accumulation at growth plates associated with normally increased bone growth in these areas. **B:** Seven-year-old. Less prominent activity in distal areas reflects normal physiology.

VASCULAR LESIONS IN THE HAND

Although the anatomic detail of the RNA does not equal that of contrast angiograms, radionuclide evaluation of perfusion through blood vessels and the relationship of masses to the blood vessels and their vascularity, and its ability to rapidly and quickly image postoperative patients, many of whom are heavily bandaged (Fig. 12–7), continue to make RNA useful in the evaluation of vascular lesions.[14,21] In addition, vascular lesions can be unexpectedly encountered when patients are being imaged to diagnose pain of potentially osseous origin.

Vascular Occlusions

In most patients with occlusion of either the radial or ulnar artery, absent visualization of the vessel at the level of the occlusion is noted, increased flow is seen in the palmar arch of the affected hand, and there is delayed filling to the digits supplied primarily by that vessel (Fig. 12–8). Blood pool images can also show decreased relative vascularity in the digits supplied by the occluded vessel. In very severe lesions, delayed images can also show some decreased metabolic activity. Digital artery occlusions, often associated with Raynaud's phenomenon or other vasospastic conditions, appear as absent or decreased activity on the three phases, also proportionate to the severity of the lesion (Fig. 12–9). Once demonstrated, contrast arteriography, often with the intraarterial digital subtraction technique, is necessary to separate a focal occlusion from severe small vessel disease. In our institution, pulse volume recording is the primary diagnostic modality used to evaluate digital perfusion,[22] while color duplex ultrasound imaging[23] and more recently magnetic resonance angiography (MRA) have been introduced.[24]

Arteriovenous Malformation

Three-phase bone imaging can differentiate fast-flowing arteriovenous malformations (AVMs) from slow-flowing hemangiomas. In approximately 75% of patients with an AVM, a large dominant feeding artery can be seen, and in somewhat less than half, a prominent draining vein is visualized.[14] The AVM usually is seen as a focal area of increased perfusion on the earliest images, often before more proximal structures are visualized in the ipsilateral hand and well before perfusion to similar areas on the contralateral hand (Fig. 12–10). Activity becomes less intense on later angiographic images and even less intense on the BP images. Delayed images are usually normal unless the lesion is so large that a pressure-induced stress response is present. In those instances, the x-ray findings are usually abnormal. If large lesions are suspected, the angiographic data should be recorded digitally at a faster frame rate, and the analog images themselves should be obtained for less than 5 seconds each. Doppler ultrasound with newer color flow techniques,[23] and MRA are frequently used as the primary diagnostic tool when vascular lesions are suspected.[24]

Hemangiomas

Activity on the RNA in hemangiomas occurs in the capillary or venous phase rather than in the early arterial phase, as in AVMs (Fig. 12–11). Activity usually remains on the BP images, but the delayed images are again normal. By pure scintigraphic

Text continued on page 328

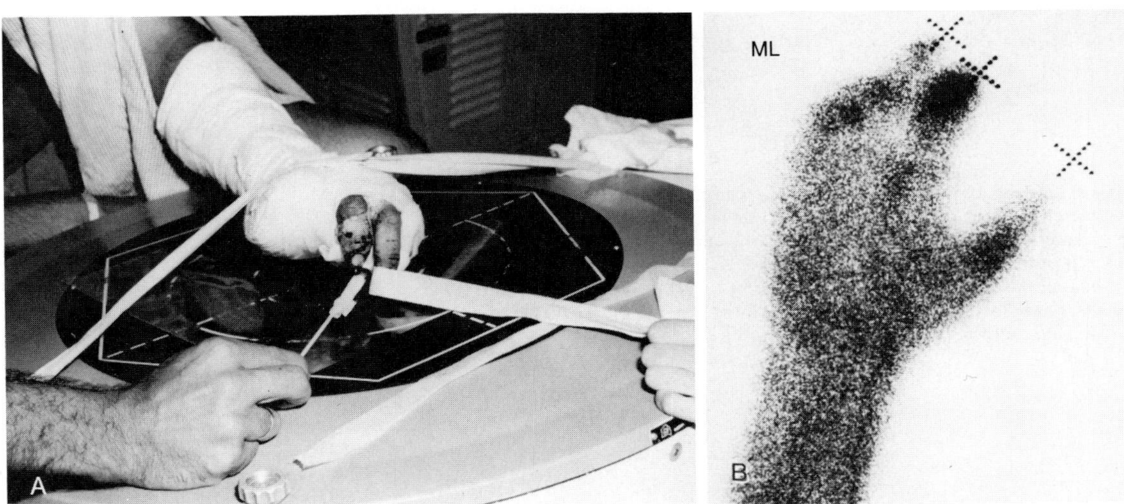

FIGURE 12–7. Imaging heavily bandaged patient after replantation. Often hands cannot be imaged simultaneously. **A:** Creative positioning is important to isolate the digit or area of interest. Marker (in this case a cobalt-57 point source) indicates the physical, anatomic extent of the digit. **B:** BP image shows vascularity extending to the fingertips with reactive hyperemia associated with the replantation site. X, marker points.

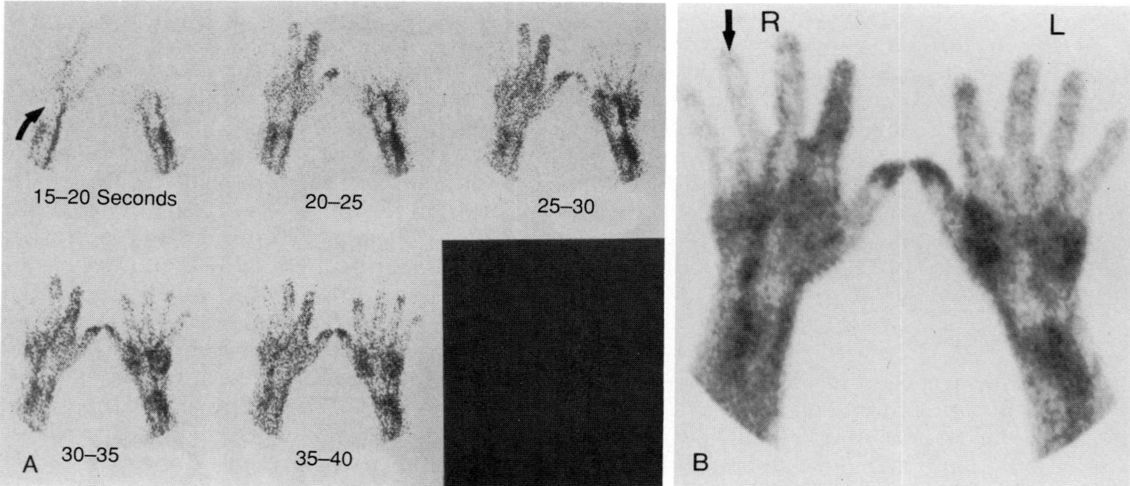

FIGURE 12–8. Ulnar artery occlusion. **A:** RNA. Right ulnar artery flow is absent (curved arrow), and there is persistent, decreased activity in the ulnar digits. Increased flow through the ipsilateral palmar arch is not prominent in this patient but is usually present, representing enhanced collateral supply from the radial artery. **B:** BP image, palmar view. Subtle decrease in the relative vascularity of the ulnar digits of the right hand (arrow).

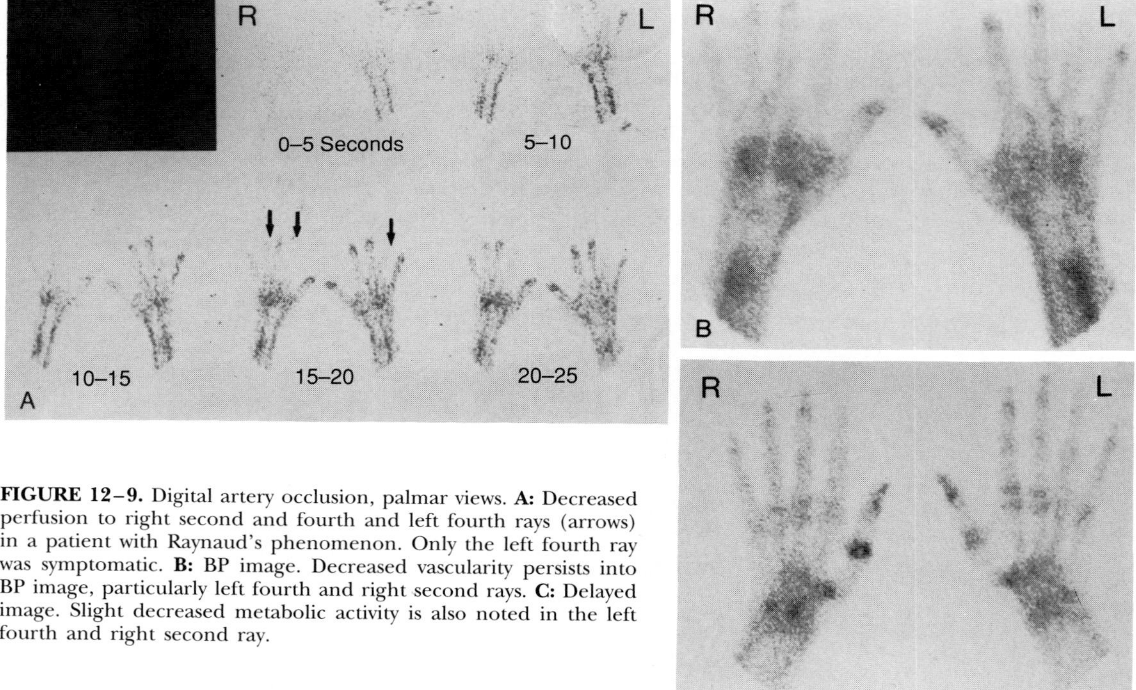

FIGURE 12–9. Digital artery occlusion, palmar views. **A:** Decreased perfusion to right second and fourth and left fourth rays (arrows) in a patient with Raynaud's phenomenon. Only the left fourth ray was symptomatic. **B:** BP image. Decreased vascularity persists into BP image, particularly left fourth and right second rays. **C:** Delayed image. Slight decreased metabolic activity is also noted in the left fourth and right second ray.

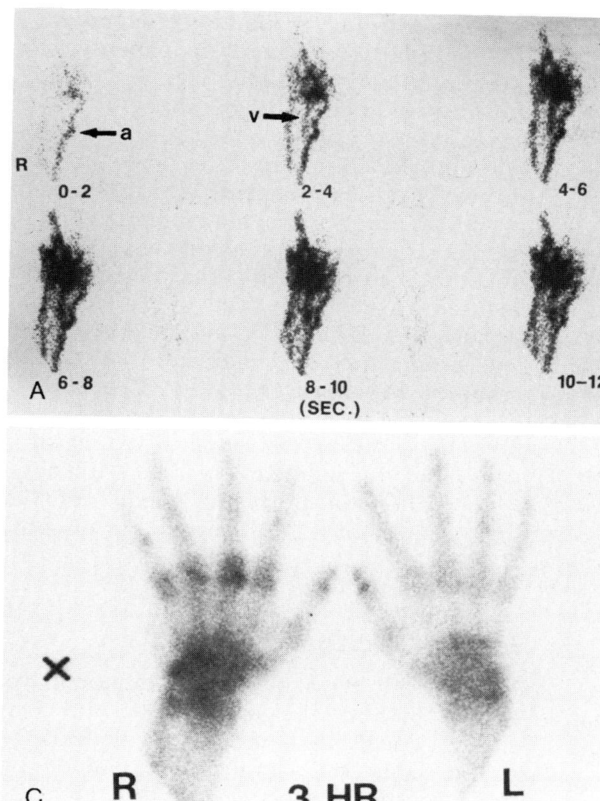

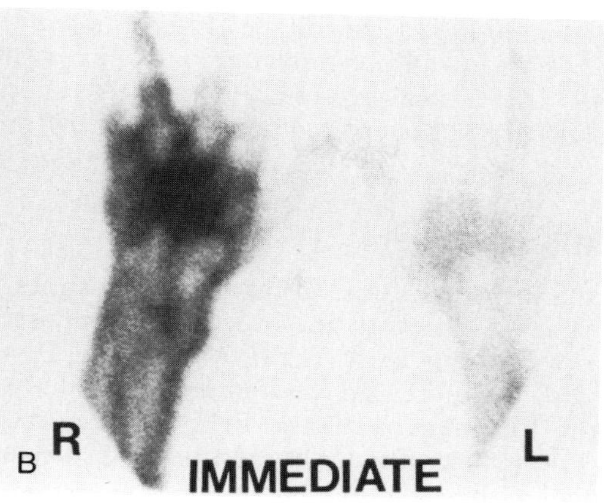

FIGURE 12–10. Arteriovenous malformation. **A:** RNA. Images were obtained at 2-second intervals because of a suspected vascular lesion with rapid flow. The tortuous feeding artery (a) and the early draining vein (V) are seen. At 12 seconds there is still no significant activity in the normal left hand. **B:** BP image. The lesion's extent is well defined. **C:** Delayed image. Asymmetric tracer uptake in bone is relatively minimal.

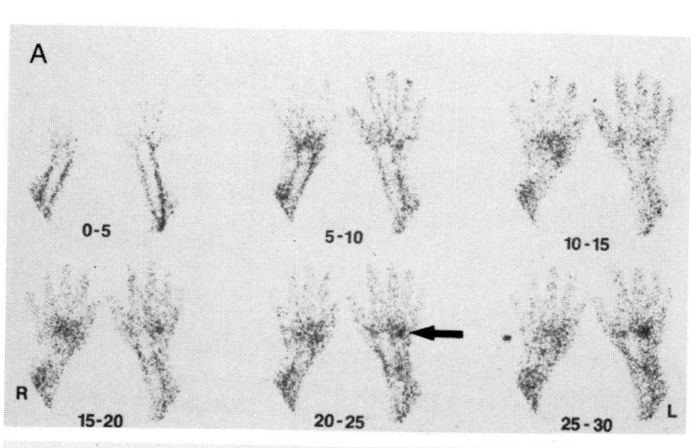

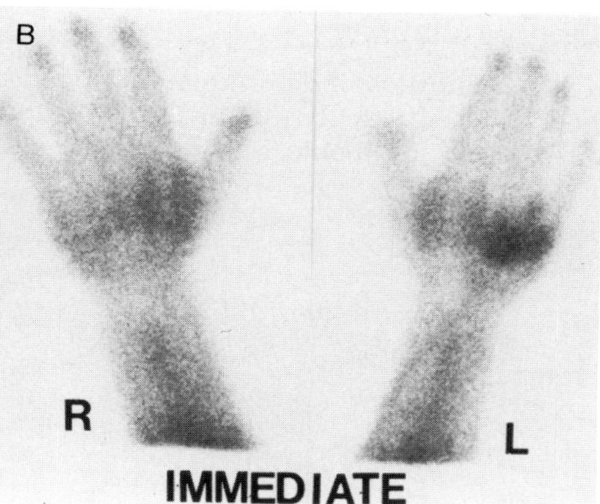

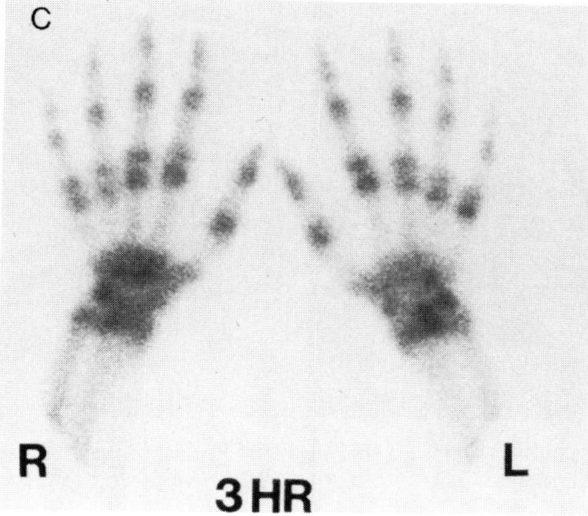

FIGURE 12–11. Cavernous hemangioma. **A:** RNA. Increased perfusion in the area of a left wrist palpable mass begins in the capillary phase and gradually becomes more defined (arrow). **B:** BP image. The extent of the left-sided vascular mass is defined. **C:** Delayed image. Minimal degenerative changes but no primary bone involvement is evident on plain radiographs.

criteria, hemangiomas cannot be differentiated from vascular soft-tissue lesions such as giant cell tumors, but usually the clinical presentation and the question being asked are sufficiently dissimilar to allow differentiation.

Traumatic Aneurysm

Posttraumatic aneurysms usually demonstrate increased focal perfusion in the arterial phase, although not quite as early as the AVMs (Fig. 12–12). A focal area of increased vascularity tends to persist during the BP image, with the delayed images being normal. Often the radionuclide estimate of the lesion size is smaller than is clinically or surgically apparent. This is secondary to the accumulation of tracer only in the flowing blood part of the aneurysmal compartment that communicates with the blood vessel. Surrounding clot within or adjacent to the aneurysmal compartment is not visualized.

True Aneurysms

In contrast to traumatic aneurysms, which usually result from penetrating trauma, blunt trauma has recently been reported to cause true aneurysms of the hand.[25] The radionuclide appearance of the true aneurysm is similar to that of the traumatic aneurysm, with a focal area of increased vascularity in the arterial phase, a BP blush, and a normal delayed image.[25]

Postoperative Viability

The rapid, noninvasive determination of patent versus compromised vascular supply to replants and transplants can be invaluable in the decision-making process regarding reoperation, aggressive drug therapy, or both.[14] Particularly in patients with bandages and postoperative wounds (see Fig. 12–7), Doppler and other flow techniques cannot be used. Although decreased perfusion and relative vascularity can be well defined in phases one and two, the delayed images have occasionally demonstrated minimal activity, which suggests some microcirculation to the osseous structures. The significance of this latter observation is currently uncertain. Demarcation of nonperfused areas is also used in patients with frostbite or burn-type injuries[26,27] and has been successful in determining sites of demarcation before their clinical or radiologic appearance (Fig. 12–13). To correlate the extent of perfusion (RNA) and relative vascularity (BP images) with the physical extent of the digits, the tips of the digits are marked with either a point source (often the tip of the needle and syringe used for injection) or a gel string source of cobalt-57 (Fig. 12–13B).

Vasospastic Diseases

Patients with Raynaud's phenomenon have been examined in both the symptomatic and asymptomatic states.[14] The RNA demonstrates decreased perfusion to the digits that cannot be explained by either a radial or ulnar artery lesion (see Fig. 12–9). Both symptomatic and asymptomatic digits can be detected, although no large study has been performed to define sensitivity and specificity. When decreased vascularity persists on the BP image and the delayed images are abnormal as well, consideration should be given to digital artery occlusion, which needs surgical attention.

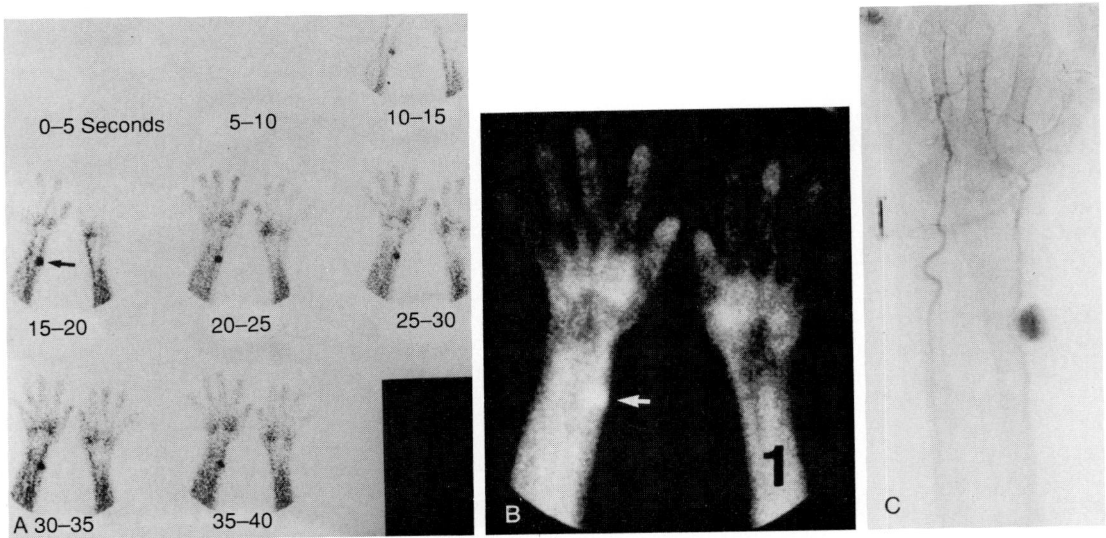

FIGURE 12–12. Traumatic aneurysm. **A:** RNA, palmar view. Focal increased perfusion associated with right radial artery (arrow) appears in arterial phase. **B:** BP image also defines vascular focus (arrow). **C:** Contrast angiogram confirms scintigraphic findings.

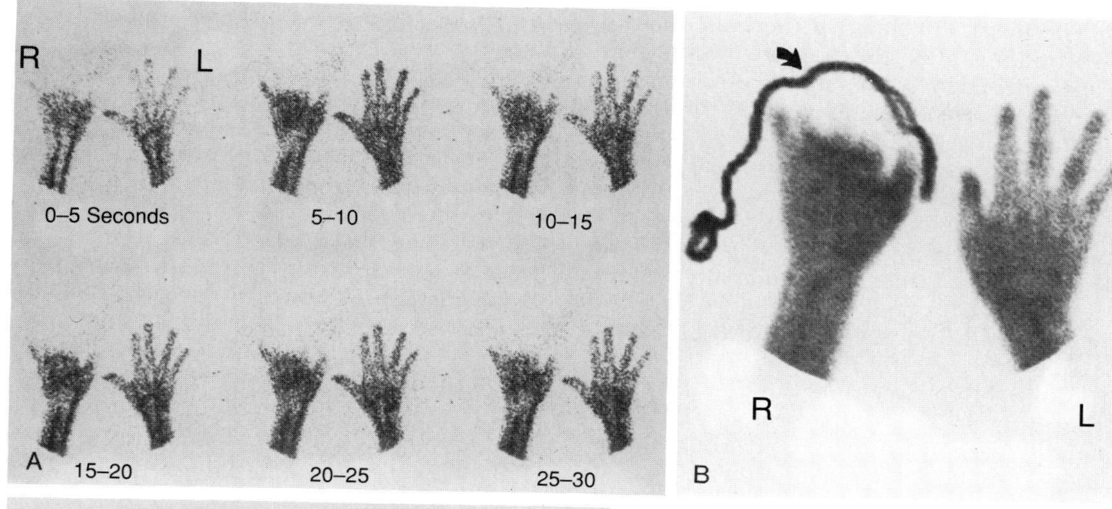

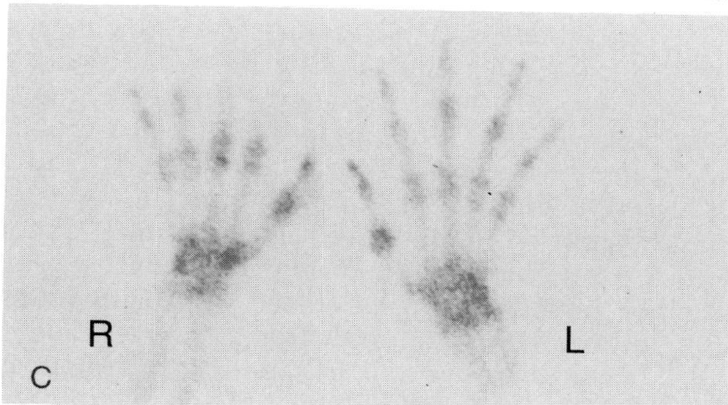

FIGURE 12–13. Frostbite injury, palmar views. **A:** RNA. Absent perfusion to distal aspects of all five rays on the right. **B:** BP image. Palmar view. Demarcation levels identified. Marker of cobalt-57 imbedded in gel (arrow) allows physical extent of digits to be related to extent of perfused tissue. **C:** Delayed image. Some residual metabolic activity exists, associated with preserved delayed microcirculation. The delayed image does not predict viability as accurately as does the blood pool image.

TRAUMATIC LESIONS

After known acute trauma, radiographs usually define the presence of a fracture, and often patients with significant clinical symptoms are treated even though standard radiographs fail to demonstrate a definite lesion. RNBI has been used in those situations in which objective evidence of fracture is desired before treatment and in those patients with pain in whom the presence of a fracture is suspected even though symptoms are not completely typical. In the subacute and even more chronic situations, when radiographs have been normal but symptoms remain, RNBI is used to localize a site of increased bone turnover. It is this ability to anatomically localize a physiologic process, which is not producing any demonstrable anatomic change, that gives the clinician information helpful in diagnosis and therapy.

Anatomic Localization

At our institution we have followed the dictum to define "where the lesion is before deciding what it is." In this regard, all of the comments described in the section on imaging techniques are applied here. Despite all the technical limitations of the procedure, in most instances the specific focus of abnormal tracer accumulation can be confidently identified. Especially with the advent of digital data acquisition and display, data manipulation is very often required to accurately define the site of abnormal uptake. Magnification views of various kinds, including electronic magnification during acquisition and the use of pinhole collimation, may prove useful. Background subtraction, contrast enhancement, inverse and other scaling variations, and the use of color display maps should be tried as needed. Hawkes et al reported a system for registration and combined display of the x-ray image and radionuclide bone scan; they concluded that in 12 to 16 of 18 cases (different observers) the registration technique improved localization.[28] All types of image fusion techniques are currently being investigated in an attempt to link the physiologic information provided by radionuclide imaging with the more detailed anatomic information provided by CT, MRI, and radiography. A variety of images have been chosen to illustrate localization in various anatomic areas (Figs. 12–14 through 12–22, 12–25, 12–30, 12–31, and 12–34).

Acute Fractures

RNBI can not only define an acute fracture when radiographs are nondiagnostic, but also, when the age of a fracture cannot be determined from a radiograph, it can distinguish a recent fracture from a healed fracture.[29,30] In general, fracture sites tend to show increased accumulation of tracer within hours after injury. The minimum time for the bone scan to show positive findings after the fracture occurs may be slightly age dependent with any effect secondary to underlying physiologic changes. In one study[30] involving only 20 patients, 95% of fractures in patients under 65 years of age were demonstrated by 24 hours, and 95% of fractures in all patients were demonstrated by 72 hours. In a combined prospective and retrospective study of hip fractures[31] no relationship was found between patient age, time after injury when scanning was performed, or type of fracture. In the 145 patients with normal or equivocal radiographs, the sensitivity was 0.978, the specificity was 0.950, the positive predictive value 0.896, and negative predictive value 0.990. In equivocal cases, particularly in patients over 70 years of age when therapeutic decisions are made based on the results, at our institution we repeat any study performed within the first 24 hours after injury at 48 to 72 hours. Matin also emphasized that 95% of simple fractures return to normal by 2 years after injury and outlined the general delayed scintigraphic image appearance of fractures at various times following trauma.[30] In another study, Rupani et al, working in our department, described the RNA and BP appearances.[20] A monograph by Deutsch and Gandsman also reviews aspects of scintigraphy as it relates to fracture healing.[32] In the acute phase, which lasts 3 to 4 weeks, all three phases of the study are positive (Fig. 12–14). On the delayed images, the fracture site shows very intense activity, which, in the carpal bone areas in particular, blurs the margins of individual bones. In the subacute phase, which lasts 10 to 12 weeks, the RNA becomes normal, the BP image activity stays positive 6 to 8 weeks, and the delayed images, although still very intense, become more focal, with greater correspondence to the fracture line or carpal bone (Fig. 12–15). The chronic phase corresponds to the end stages of healing and remodeling. RNA and BP activity is usually normal, with activity on the delayed images slowly decreasing over 3 to 8 months but often demonstrating minimal activity for several years, depending on the amount of focal stress present (see Figs. 12–14 and 12–15).

Fracture Nonunion and Posttraumatic Bone Pain

Many patients present with pain and have radiographs that demonstrate normal findings or nonspecific changes of uncertain clinical significance. RNBI is extremely valuable in detecting the presence of any abnormal metabolic activity in those patients with normal x-ray findings and in detecting the current state of metabolic activity associated with an anatomic lesion defined on a radiograph. However, RNBI has diagnostic limitations. For example, abnormal increased activity demonstrated on delayed images can be physiologically associated with many different conditions. In addition, bone tracer accumulation may be qualitatively similar and only quantitatively different through a wide physiologic continuum of the same condition, such as in the various stages of fracture healing.

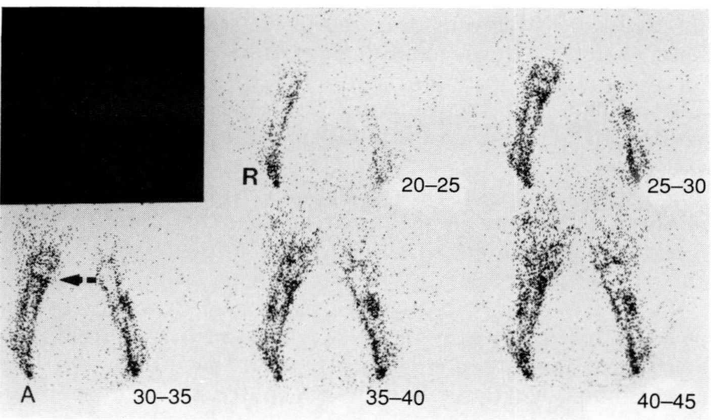

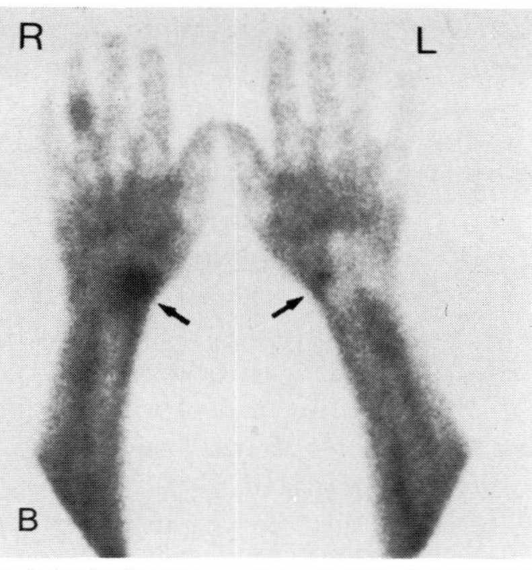

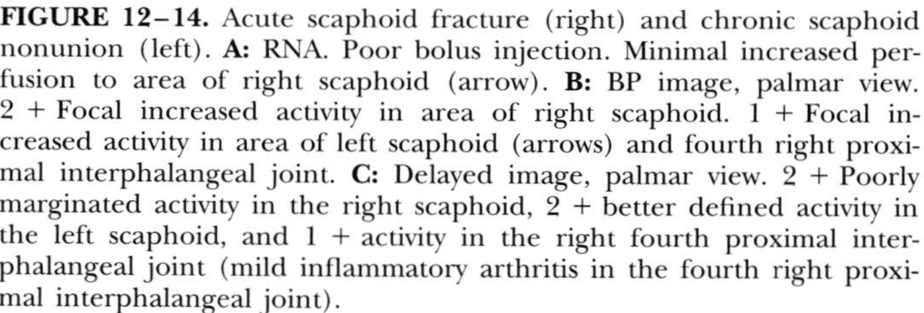

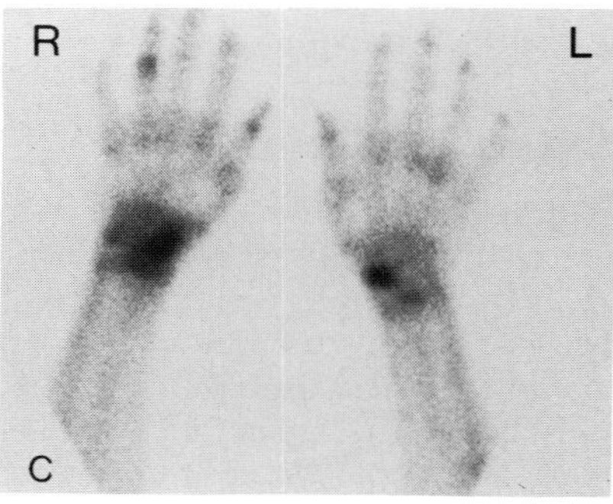

FIGURE 12–14. Acute scaphoid fracture (right) and chronic scaphoid nonunion (left). **A:** RNA. Poor bolus injection. Minimal increased perfusion to area of right scaphoid (arrow). **B:** BP image, palmar view. 2 + Focal increased activity in area of right scaphoid. 1 + Focal increased activity in area of left scaphoid (arrows) and fourth right proximal interphalangeal joint. **C:** Delayed image, palmar view. 2 + Poorly marginated activity in the right scaphoid, 2 + better defined activity in the left scaphoid, and 1 + activity in the right fourth proximal interphalangeal joint (mild inflammatory arthritis in the fourth right proximal interphalangeal joint).

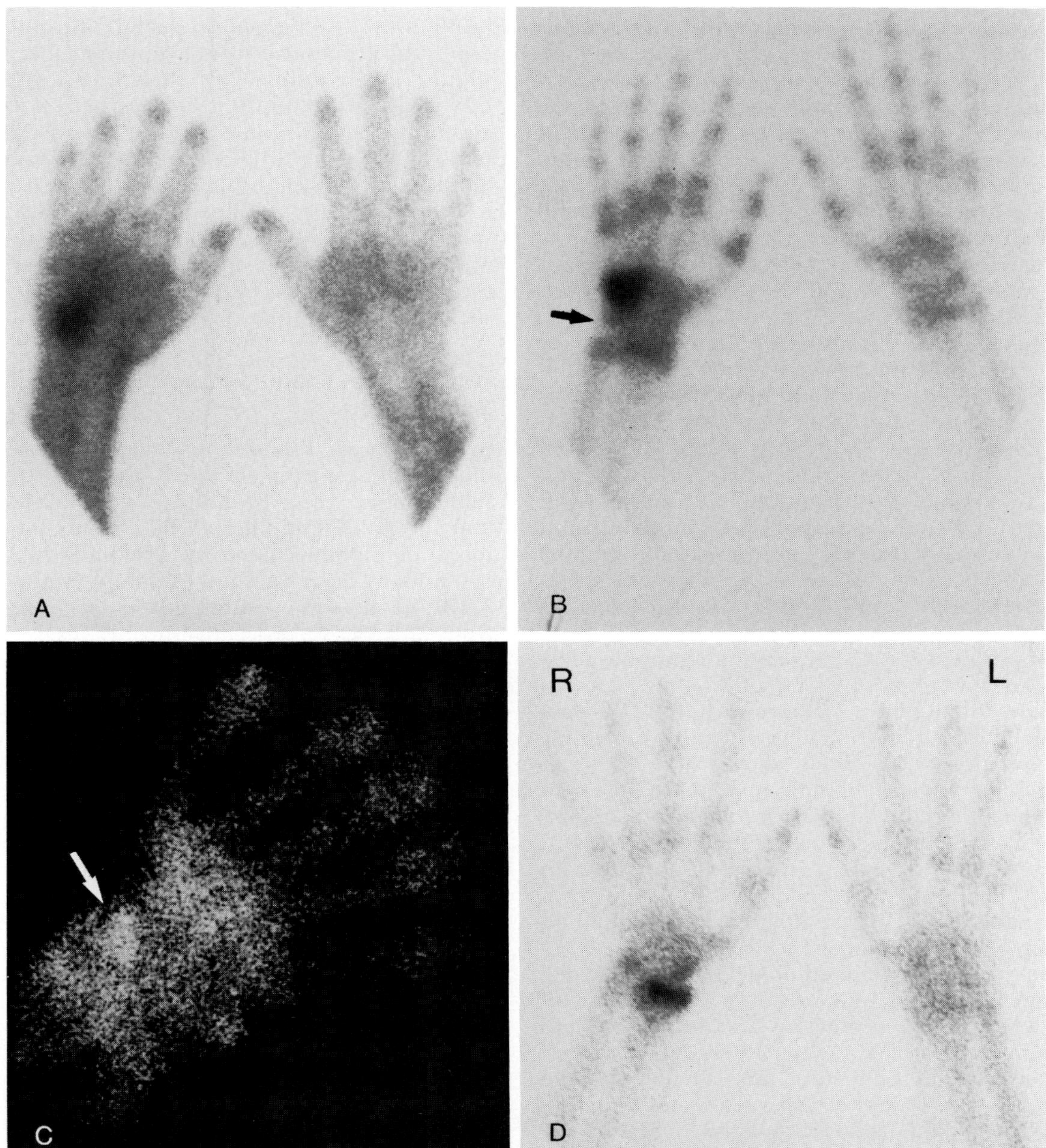

FIGURE 12–15. Subacute fractures. **A:** Seven-week-old hamate fracture, BP image. 2 + Increased activity. **B:** Delayed images, same patient as A. 3 + Increased activity is still so great that exact borders of carpal bones are obscured. Location relative to proximal carpal row (arrow) allows anatomic localization. **C:** Six-month-old scaphoid fracture. Magnified view, ulnar deviation. Minimal scaphoid activity remains (arrow). Magnified, converging, and pinhole collimator views can be used to aid in anatomic localization. Relative intensity of tracer accumulation is judged only on parallel hole collimator views. **D:** Four-month-old distal radial fracture, delayed, palmar view.

Trauma to bone results in a spectrum of bone injury from frank fracture and hematoma to minimal intraosseous bleeding or periosteal elevation. Such minimal bone injury may be termed a "bone bruise" for want of a better phrase to explain a complicated physiologic process to patients.[33] We conceptualize normal fracture healing as beginning with hematoma formation around the fracture site, which acts as a substrate upon which the healing process proceeds. This process includes the deposition of osteoid, fracture callus, consolidation, and remodeling. Healing that does not proceed normally may result in delayed union, fibrous union, or nonunion. For the purposes of our descriptions we define delayed union as a prolongation of the time ordinarily necessary for solid healing to occur. The potential for spontaneous healing must still be considered to be present to use this classification. Fibrous or cartilaginous union occurs when nonmineralized fibrous or cartilaginous tissue bridges a fracture, after which no further evidence of bony consolidation can be seen. Nonunion is defined as that point in time after which spontaneous healing can no longer be expected to occur and after which there is no fibrous or cartilaginous union. It is not surprising that the nuclear physician has been asked to use a physiologic study (RNBI) to help elucidate this physiologic spectrum of healing.

Patients in all of these categories seek treatment days to months after the injury. Early radiographs may be normal, so that the differential diagnosis includes occult fracture, nonspecific "bone bruise," or soft-tissue injury. In the subacute situation, also often with normal radiographs, noninflammatory arthritis (i.e., inflammatory but not necessarily infectious) must be considered.

Patients with a "bone bruise" usually have a normal RNA, variable activity on the BP images with minimal to moderate increased tracer accumulation relatively well defined to the bony area, and minimal to moderate increased tracer on the delayed images (Figs. 12–16 and 12–17). Often in this subacute group of patients, once the abnormal bone has been identified scintigraphically, special radiographic techniques such as slightly obliqued plain films, directed fluoroscopy, tomography, CT scanning, or MRI identify osteochondral abnormalities, fractures, or subtle marrow variations not initially demonstrated or suspected.[34] Since nonspecific fatty marrow replacement is often encountered during MRI, the physiologic significance may still be better documented by RNBI. It is still not clear whether it is efficacious to obtain MRI in all patients with subacute unexplained pain, normal radiographs, and a focus of abnormal increased uptake on bone scan.

Patients with reactive nonunion also have normal RNA images, a variable amount of activity on the BP images ranging from normal to 2 + increased, and delayed images with 1 + to 3 + focal increased tracer activity in the bone (Fig. 12–18). On a single examination, delayed union can usually not be confidently differentiated from reactive nonunion. If the BP images are normal, however, and the amount of activity associated with the delayed images is minimal, the lesion is more likely to be in the end stages of healing. In patients whose radiographs demonstrated a typical nonunion pattern of separation of the fragments with well-defined sclerotic borders, the RNBI examination can be used to demonstrate the degree of nonspecific stress change taking place (by the degree of activity on the delayed image) and the amount of synovial-type inflammation present (by the degree of activity on the BP images). A more detailed discussion of this concept has been published elsewhere.[33]

Biomechanical Stress Lesions

Although many traumatic lesions can be described in terms of biomechanical loading or stress, when the insult is of lower grade, and more chronic, the general term "repetitive stress syndrome" has come into vogue. The potential for such a lesion should be considered when there is a focus of abnormal tracer accumulation on a scan performed for pain of potentially osseous origin with normal radiographs. Similarly, the bone scan can be used to assess the metabolic activity and hence the potential for a nonspecific lesion seen on a radiograph to be associated with increased bone turnover and be the source of the patient's pain. The ulnar impaction syndrome is such a lesion (Fig. 12–19).[35]

Aseptic Necrosis (Avascular Necrosis)

Most adult patients with pain from aseptic necrosis present during the revascularization phase when radiographic appearances are abnormal. In some instances, there are only minimal, equivocal changes, so that the RNBI examination documents the abnormal focus of metabolic activity (Fig. 12–20). In other cases, when the x-ray study is definitely abnormal, the RNBI examination differentiates an active process from an inactive process with only residual changes. The degree of metabolic activity present is reflected in the RNBI examination. All three phases can be positive, the BP and delayed images can be positive, and near the end stages of healing, just the delayed images can be abnormal. These patterns are similar to those associated with acute fracture healing and they give indirect support to the hypothesis that suggests that repeated microtrauma with interruption of blood supply is the etiology for all osteonecrotic-type lesions.[36] MRI has been used to demonstrate diffuse marrow replacement in aseptic necrosis of the lunate (Kienböck's disease), occasionally separating patients with abnormal tracer secondary to a nonspecific bone response to stress or other anatomic abnormalities, such as an intraosseous ganglion, from those with underlying aseptic necrosis.[37] In a study by Sowa et al, all of the patients with pain who had replaced marrow compatible with avascular necrosis (AVN) on the MR examination also had abnormal increased tracer accumulation on delayed RNBI. We have recently seen a stick-sport patient believed to have AVN of the hook of the hamate (Fig. 12–21) in whom high-resolution CT scanning was used to provide further anatomic detail about the demonstrated physiologic abnormality.[38]

Synovitis and Arthritis

Although the etiology of synovitis can be varied and often remains uncertain, this entity is often found following trauma, and because the hand surgeon evaluates the posttraumatic hand, he or she must be aware of the entire gamut of inflammatory and noninflammatory arthropathies that may be present. One review[39] summarizes the status of radionuclide joint imaging. Again, the RNBI examination reflects the physiology present. In inflammatory but nonin-

Text continued on page 336

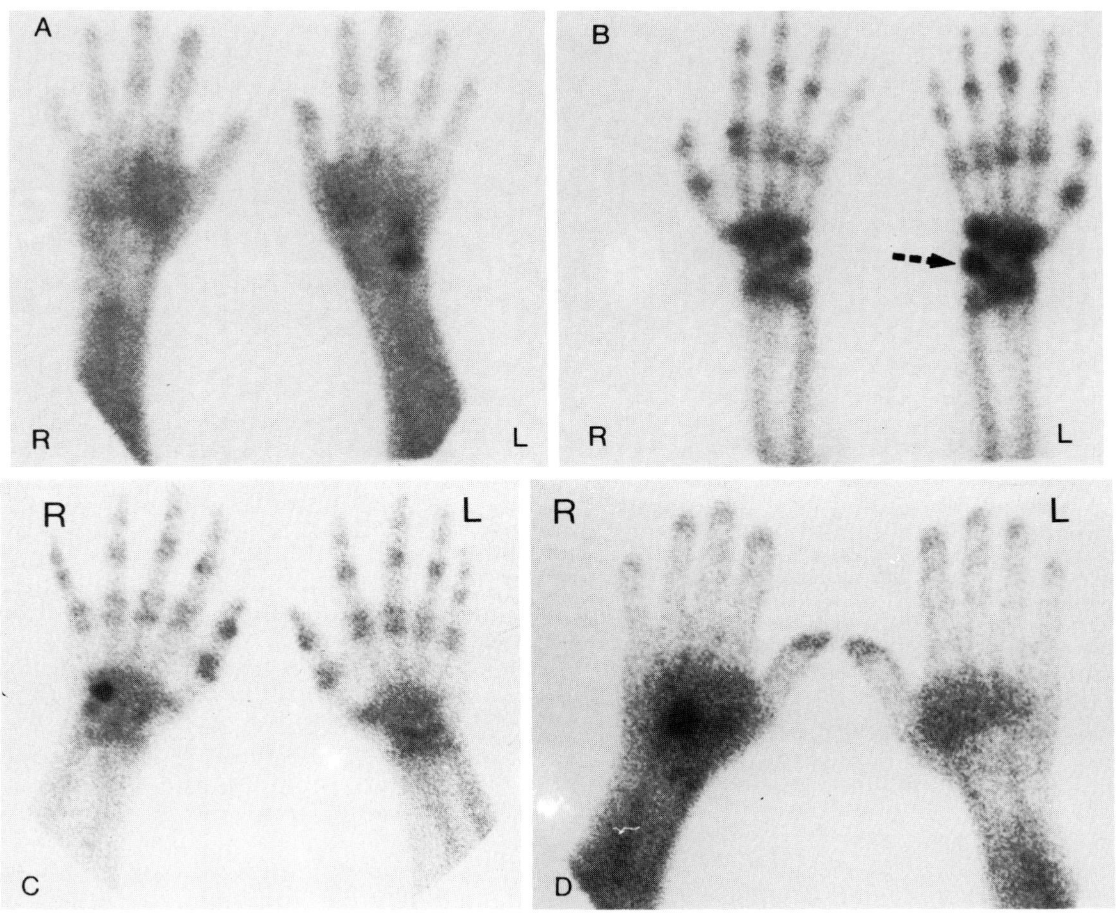

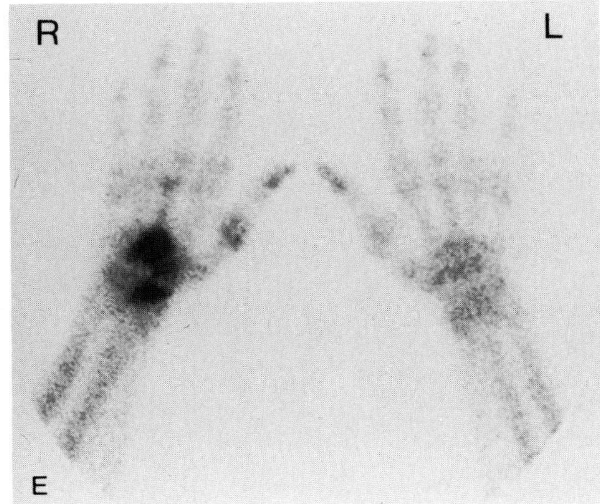

FIGURE 12–16. Bone bruise (abnormal scan, radiographically unexplained focal bone uptake). The radiographs of all patients were normal 4 or more months after trauma. **A:** BP image, palmar view. **B:** Delayed image, dorsal view, left pisiform bruise (arrow). 1 + blood pool and 2 + delayed activity. **C:** Hamate bruise, delayed image, palmar view. This 2 + activity near base of metacarpals can be compared with the more proximal pisiform activity in **B**. **D:** BP image, palmar view. **E:** Delayed image, palmar view, right capitate bruise. 2 + BP and 3 + delayed activity involves the capitate. Also, the distal right radius has 2 + activity.

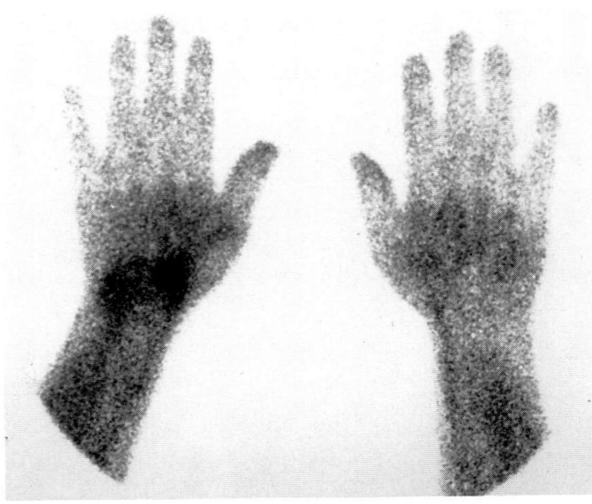

A

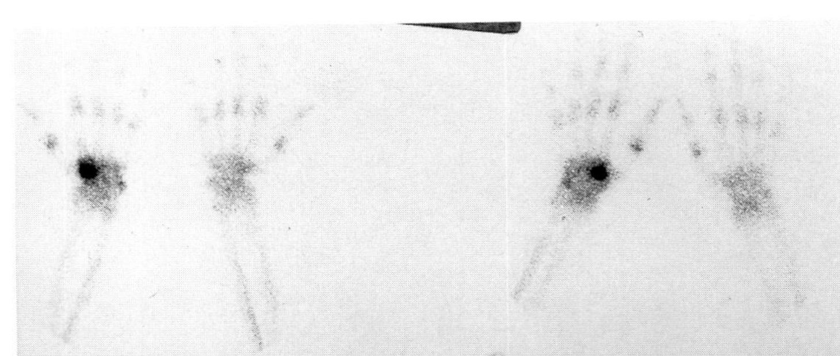

B

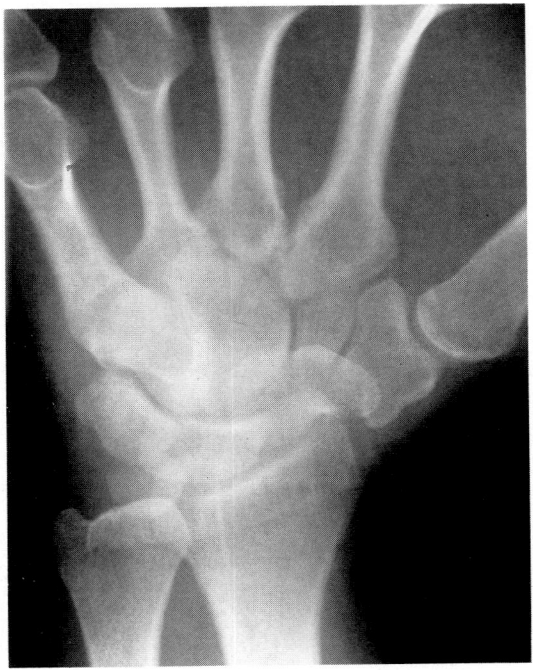

C

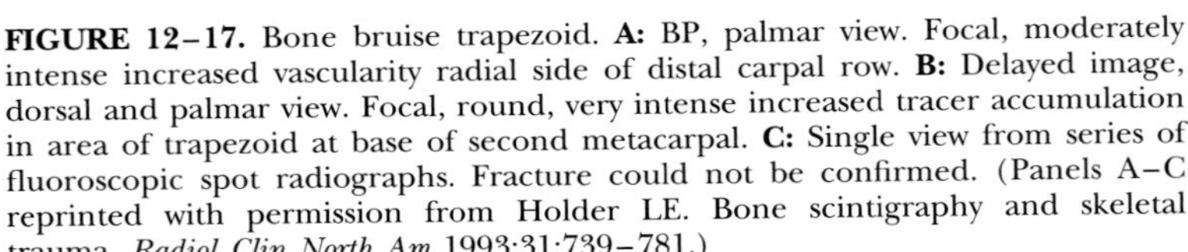

FIGURE 12–17. Bone bruise trapezoid. **A:** BP, palmar view. Focal, moderately intense increased vascularity radial side of distal carpal row. **B:** Delayed image, dorsal and palmar view. Focal, round, very intense increased tracer accumulation in area of trapezoid at base of second metacarpal. **C:** Single view from series of fluoroscopic spot radiographs. Fracture could not be confirmed. (Panels A–C reprinted with permission from Holder LE. Bone scintigraphy and skeletal trauma, *Radiol Clin North Am* 1993;31:739–781.)

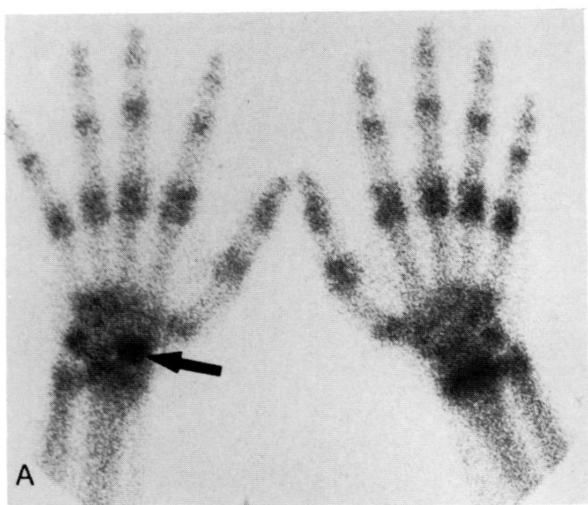

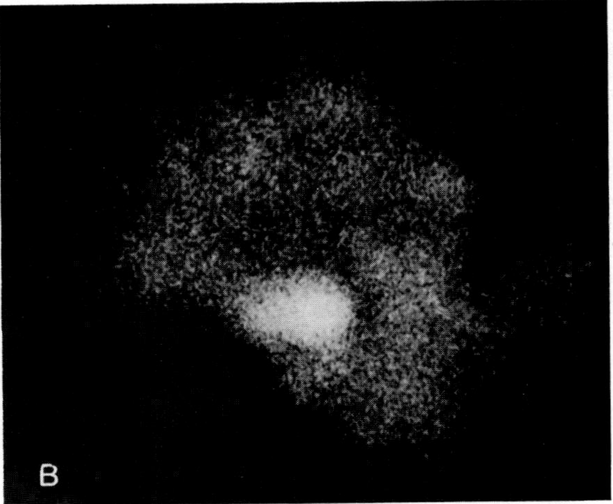

FIGURE 12–18. Reactive nonunion scaphoid. Normal RNA results (not shown) excluded the possibility of an acute fracture in this 17-year-old football player. **A:** Delayed image. 2 + Well-defined increased scaphoid activity (arrow). **B:** The magnified left dorsal view better localizes increased tracer to the scaphoid.

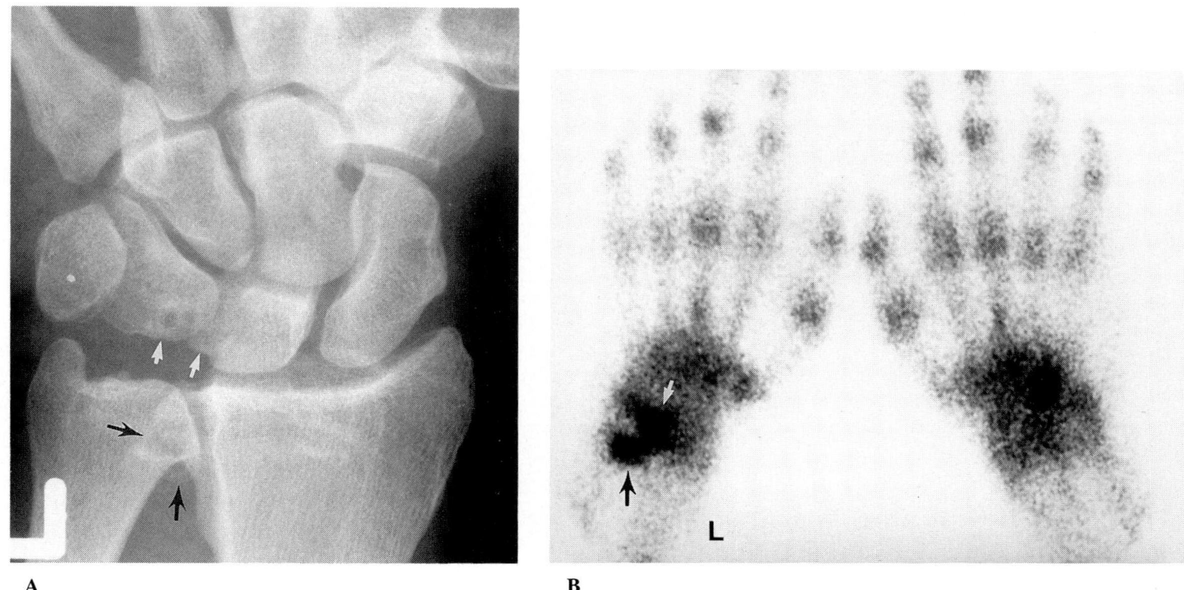

A B

FIGURE 12–19. Ulnar impaction syndrome. **A:** Radiograph. Radiolucent areas involve the radial aspect of the triquetrum and flattening or depression of the proximal surface of the triquetrum and lunate (white arrows). Degenerative joint disease also involves the distal ulna (black arrows). **B:** Delayed bone image, palmar view. Intense abnormal increased uptake at left lunotriquetral area (white arrow), and also distal ulna (black arrow). (Reprinted with permission from the Radiological Society of North America from Mann FA, Wilson AJ, Gilula LA. Radiographic evaluation of the wrist: What does the hand surgeon want to know? *Radiology* 1992;184:15–24.)

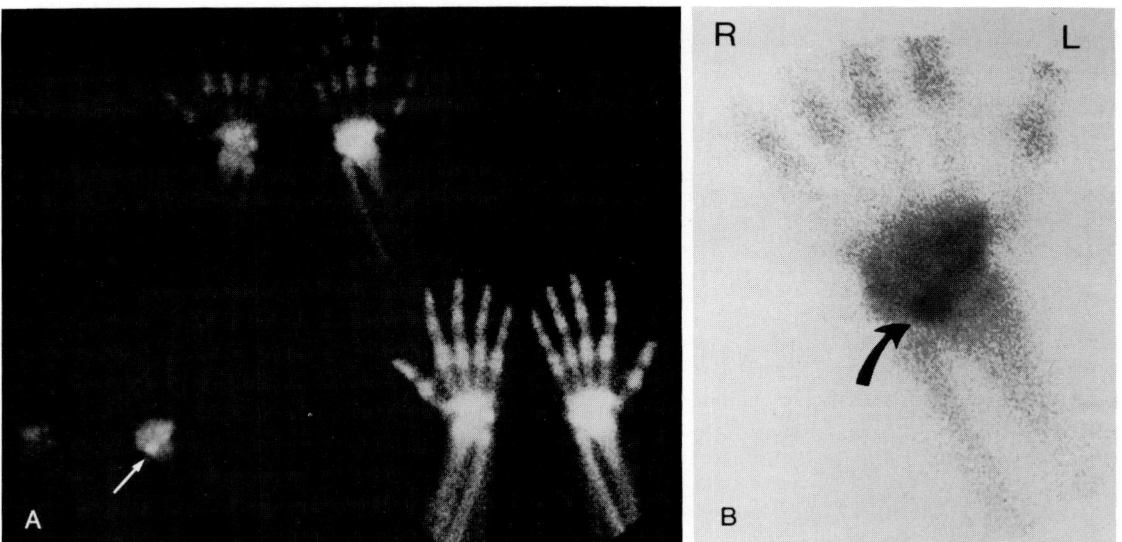

FIGURE 12–20. Revascularization phase of Kienböck's disease, left lunate, delayed images. **A:** Triple lens Polaroid display provides background subtraction and often allows more precise anatomic localization. Diffuse increased activity is seen in the left wrist, and more focal lunate activity (arrow) is seen best in the lower left image. **B:** Magnified left dorsal view. Lunate localization of increased activity is clear (arrow).

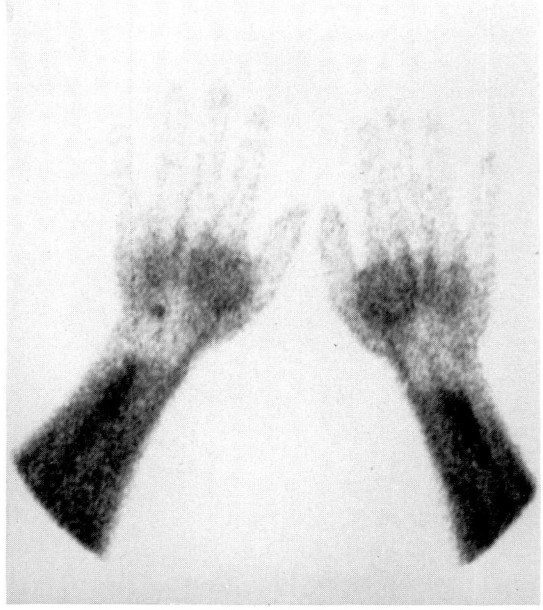

A

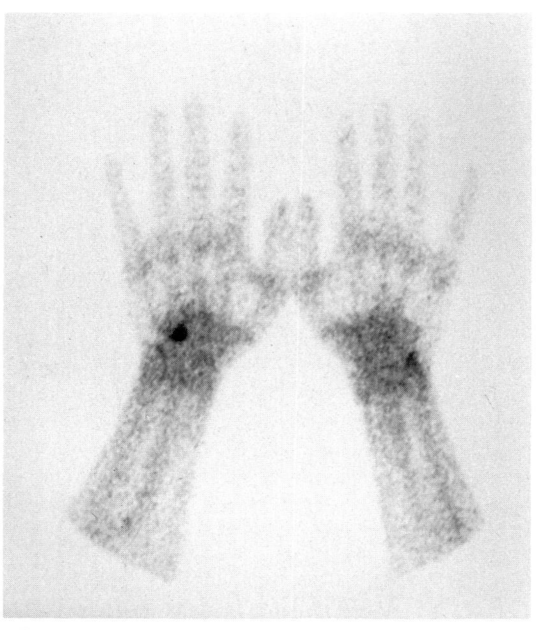

B

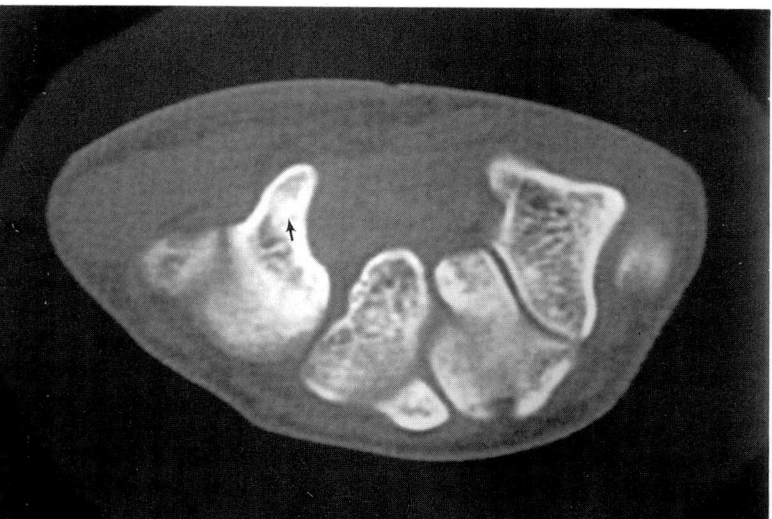

C

FIGURE 12–21. Hook of hamate. **A:** BP image, palmar view. Moderately intense, very focal increased tracer accumulation in the hamate area. **B:** Delayed image, palmar view. Intense focal increased tracer accumulation in the hamate area. **C:** CT scan, transaxial through hook of hamate. Sclerosis with marrow replacement (arrow).

fectious arthritis, the RNA, BP, and delayed images can all be abnormal with diffuse increased vascularity, hyperemia, and delayed metabolic activity present throughout the periarticular regions of the radial and ulnar carpal, intercarpal, and carpometacarpal articulations (Fig. 12–22). Schneider found delayed RNBI helpful in the management of patients with polyarthralgias by providing objective evidence of disease activity when there was no clinical synovitis, normal radiographs, and nondiagnostic laboratory evaluations.[40] Pin and his colleagues found that only 9 of 14 patients diagnosed with synovitis had abnormal bone scans, and the 5 with normal scans had only ''mild'' synovitis clinically. They believed this degree of sensitivity to be less valuable.[41] We have used a more generalized algorithm for the role of radionuclide imaging in the evaluation of pain of potentially osseous origin and find it very valuable (Fig. 12–23). We emphasize, however, that if a primary soft-tissue or vascular abnormality is strongly suspected, MRI, often with MRA, can be the initial diagnostic examination.[24]

ter Meulen and Majd reported the value of RNBI in 358 children with obscure skeletal pain.[42] Although bone scans were positive in 36% of patients with the final diagnosis suggested by the findings (including 14 with juvenile rheumatoid arthritis [JRA]), and of the 227 patients with normal scans 187 had symptoms resolve spontaneously and 17 were treated successfully as synovitis, 23 were later diagnosed with JRA. They concluded therefore that bone scintigraphy was not the test of choice in establishing the

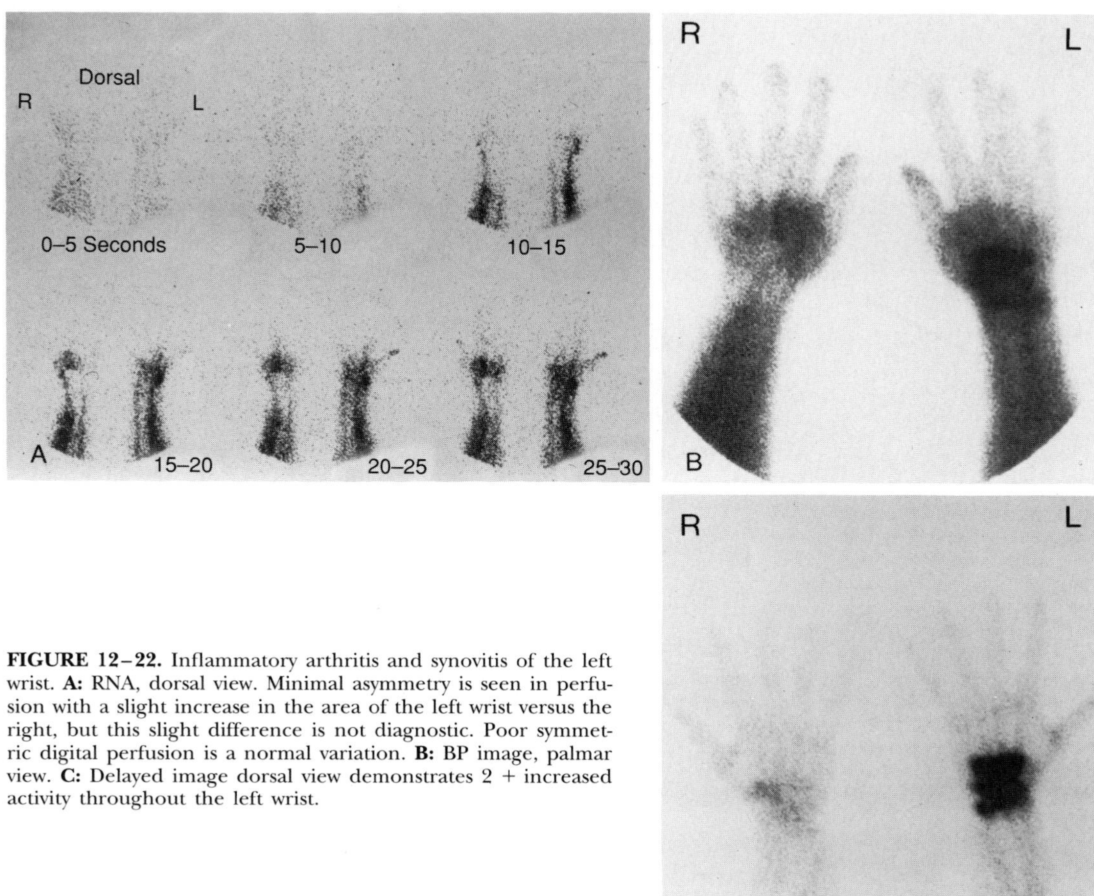

FIGURE 12–22. Inflammatory arthritis and synovitis of the left wrist. **A:** RNA, dorsal view. Minimal asymmetry is seen in perfusion with a slight increase in the area of the left wrist versus the right, but this slight difference is not diagnostic. Poor symmetric digital perfusion is a normal variation. **B:** BP image, palmar view. **C:** Delayed image dorsal view demonstrates 2 + increased activity throughout the left wrist.

diagnosis of JRA; rather its role was in excluding malignancy or other lesions that may mimic JRA. Some authors have found that technetium-99m-labeled lysosomes accumulate only in clinically active inflammatory disease, and were thus more specific than technetium-MDP RNBI, which continued to show increased activity during healing and remodeling after the active inflammation had resolved.[43] Labeled lysosomes are not routinely available in most nuclear medicine departments, nor are they offered by central radiopharmacies.

Negative delayed images accurately predict the absence of synovial disease, because even mild synovial inflammation causes increased periarticular bone blood flow and deposition of radiotracer. In patients with noninflammatory arthritis, the RNA is usually normal and the BP or tissue phase images, if positive, are only minimally abnormal, whereas the delayed images may show the same degree of intense abnormal activity as inflammatory arthritis (Fig. 12–24). In a prospective study reported by Buckland-Wright et al involving 32 patients examined every 6 months for 18 months, technetium-99m-MDP uptake correlated only with osteophyte size among the various parameters evaluated. The physiologic nature of this imaging technique is emphasized by the fact that the size of growing or remodeling osteophytes did increase significantly at joints with increased isotope uptake.[44] Hutton et al described acute arthritis in a patient with mixed connective tissue disease (MCTD) associated with intraarticular deposition of carbonated hydroxyapatite crystals. Synovial fluid analysis demonstrated uptake of the radiotracer directly onto the crystals.[45]

Often, the RNBI is performed to assess the degree of activity of a lesion seen on a radiograph. Most lucent carpal defects are normal; however, some defects are not and on occasion may need to be evaluated further with MRI, CT, or even surgery to deal with the painful lucent defect (Fig. 12–25). In one study,[46] no correlation with intensity of symptoms and tracer uptake could be made. Some patients with grossly abnormal radionuclide studies had totally normal radiographs. We believe this reflects increased bone turnover, but not enough imbalance in either osteoblastic or osteoclastic activity to be manifest on radiographs. The etiology of focal abnormal accumulation in these patients often remains uncertain because treatment is conservative and usually no biopsy or surgical material is available for analysis. If biopsy

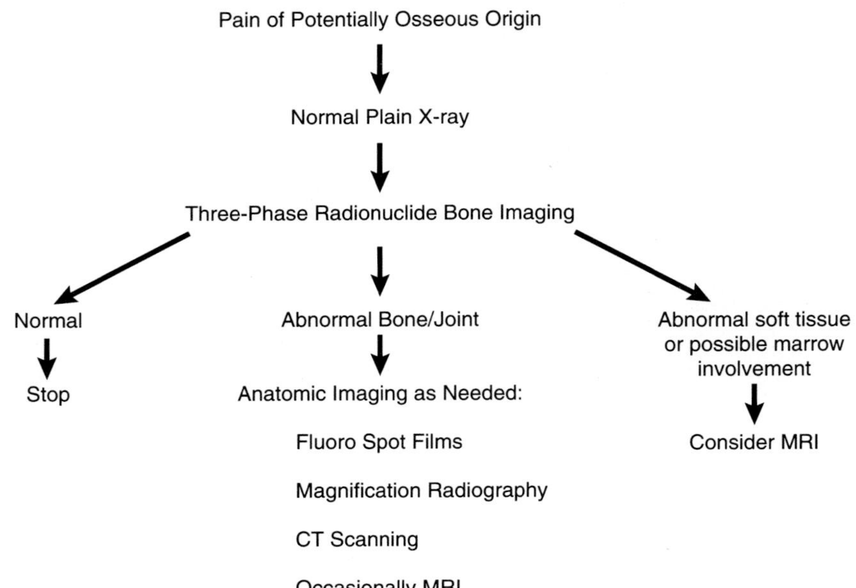

FIGURE 12–23. Pain of potentially osseous origin. Decision tree after normal plain radiograph. (Reprinted with permission from Holder LE. Bone scintigraphy and skeletal trauma. *Radiol Clin North Am* 1993;31:739–781.)

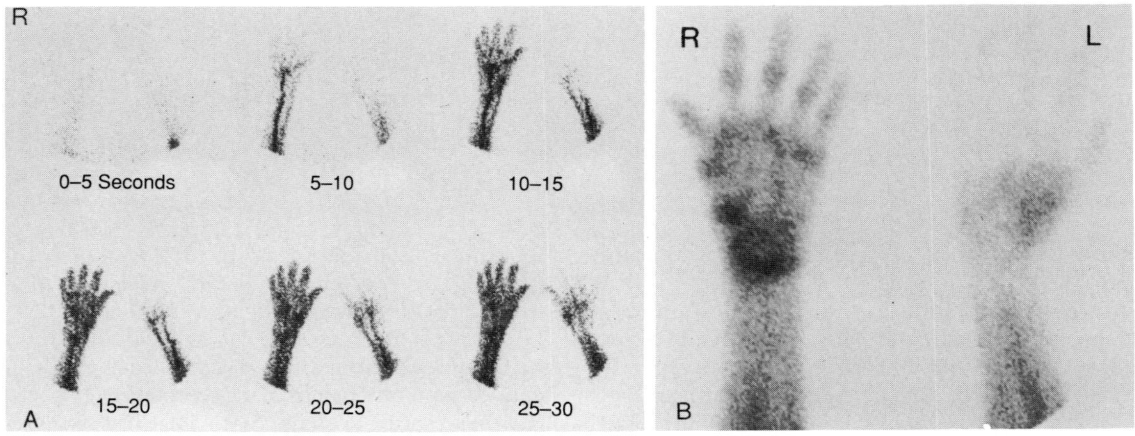

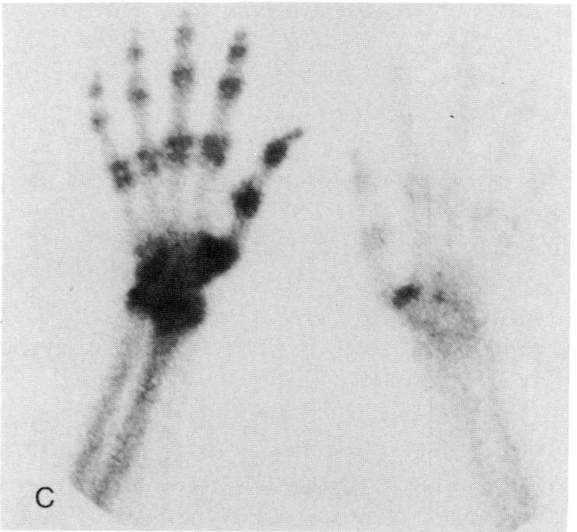

FIGURE 12–24. Inflammatory arthritis of the right basal (trapezial metacarpal) joint, noninflammatory arthritis of the left basal joint, and reflex sympathetic dystrophy of the right hand. **A:** RNA. Diffuse increased perfusion of the right forearm, wrist, and hand. **B:** BP image, dorsal view. Diffuse increased activity in the right side, with more focal increased right radial carpal and basal joint area. **C:** Delayed image, palmar view. On the right, diffuse increased activity occurs throughout the hand and wrist, with superimposed 2 + focal activity in the basal joint and distal radius. On the left, 1 + increased activity in the basal joint (see text).

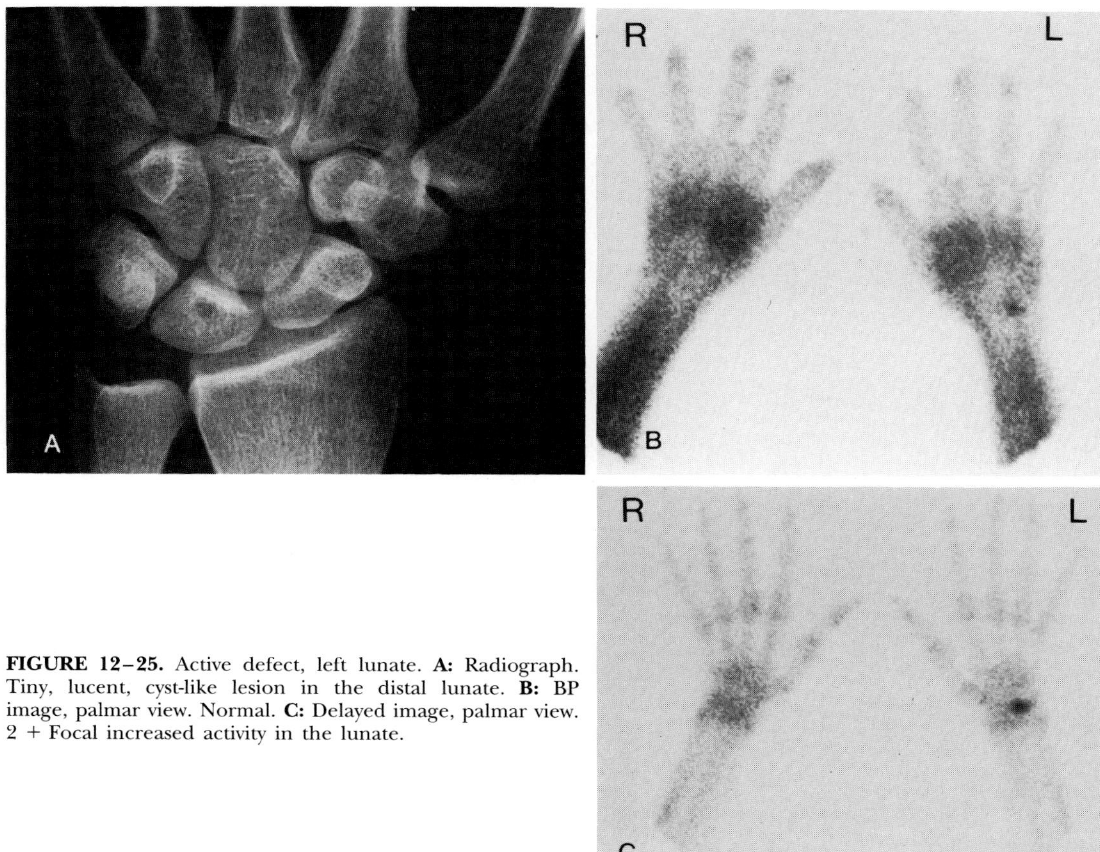

FIGURE 12–25. Active defect, left lunate. **A:** Radiograph. Tiny, lucent, cyst-like lesion in the distal lunate. **B:** BP image, palmar view. Normal. **C:** Delayed image, palmar view. 2 + Focal increased activity in the lunate.

or curettage is performed because of persistent intolerable pain, cyst fluid, fibrous tissue, or intraosseous ganglia material may be found.[47] The abnormal tracer uptake in these cases does suggest to the clinician an anatomic site responsible for the patient's pain, especially if this site correlates with clinical symptoms. However, as described above, in the appropriate clinical setting, a prominent focal abnormality should probably be investigated further with CT, MRI, or both before a bone can be called radiographically normal.

Tendinitis and Tenosynovitis

Most often patients with chronic tendinitis, tenosynovitis, or both have normal RNBI examinations.[14] Occasionally, when a patient is examined in the acute phase, the RNA and BP images are abnormal, demonstrating increased perfusion and vascularity corresponding to the particular tendon area involved. Stein, Miale, and Stein have also reported this pattern, but they did not describe the exact temporal relationship of the bone scan to the time of injury in their group of patients.[48]

Heterotopic Bone Formation (Myositis Ossificans)

Heterotopic bone formation (HBF) or myositis ossificans is a disorder characterized by an initial inflammatory lesion of muscles and other soft tissues followed by heterotopic ossification. Although it has been reported in the upper arm, it is relatively uncommon in the hands and wrists. Maurer, Paczolt, and Myers reported on a patient thought to have a traumatic myositis only of the intrinsic muscles of the hand with more prominent tracer accumulation on BP than on delayed images (Fig. 12–26).[18] Orzel and Rudd also reported that in many cases the flow and BP study become abnormal prior to the delayed images.[49] In our practice, in which patients are imaged more often in the subacute or chronic phases, ossification and inflamed or traumatized muscle is associated with more intense tracer uptake on delayed images. Ogilvie-Harris, Hons, and Fornassier reviewed a group of patients with pseudomalignant myositis ossificans who had a localized deposit of heterotopic bone developing without antecedent trauma.[50] One of those patients was an 18-year-old man with a circumscribed bone lesion adjacent to the first metacarpal. These lesions consist of rapidly

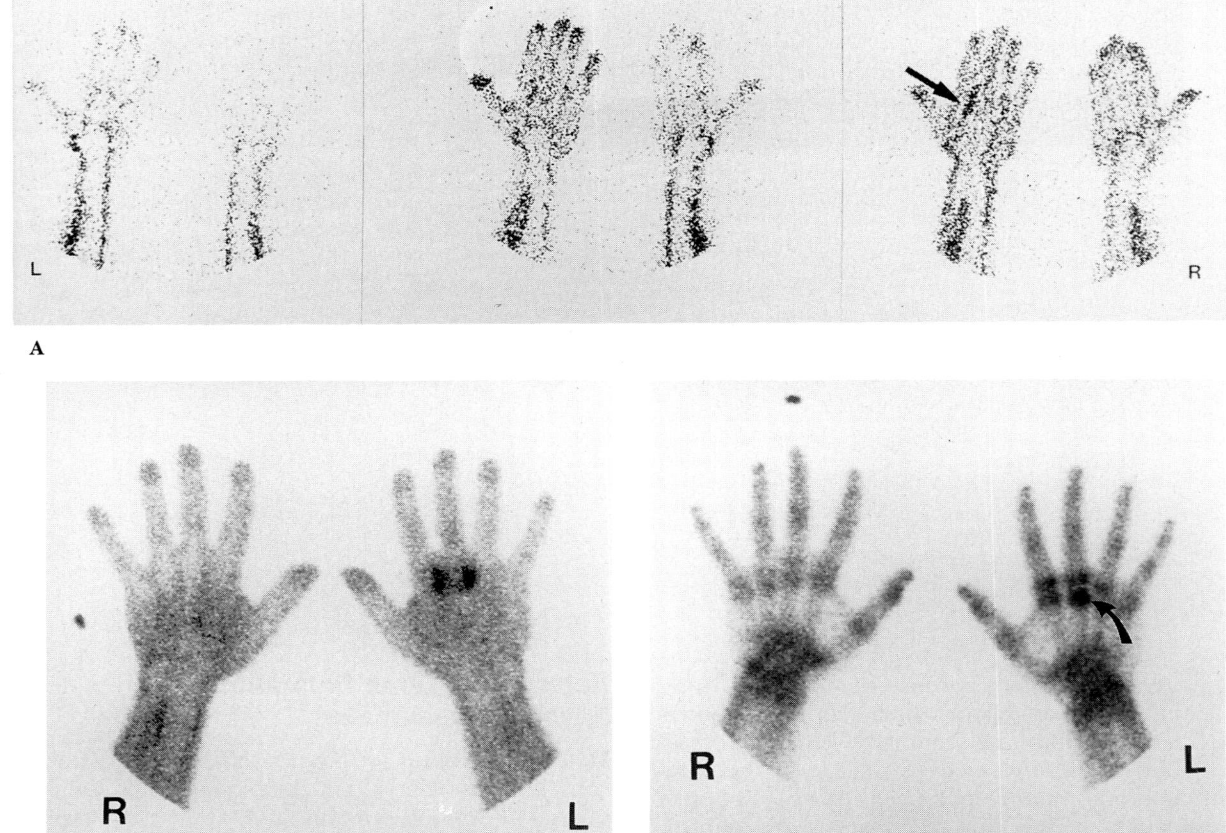

A

B

C

FIGURE 12–26. Traumatic myositis ossificans intrinsic muscles. **A:** RNA, dorsal view. Linear area of mild to moderately increased perfusion on the lateral aspect of the third metacarpal corresponds to the position of lumbrical and/or interossei muscles (arrow). **B:** BP, palmar view. Localized hyperemia on both medial and lateral sides of left third metacarpal. **C:** Delayed image palmar view. Probable "augmented" uptake associated with head of third metacarpal rather than primary soft-tissue/muscle uptake. (Panels A–C reprinted with permission from Maurer AH, Paczolt EA, Myers AR. Diagnosis of traumatic myositis of the intrinsic muscles of the hand by the use of three-phase skeletal scintigraphy. *Clin Nucl Med* 1990;15:535–538.)

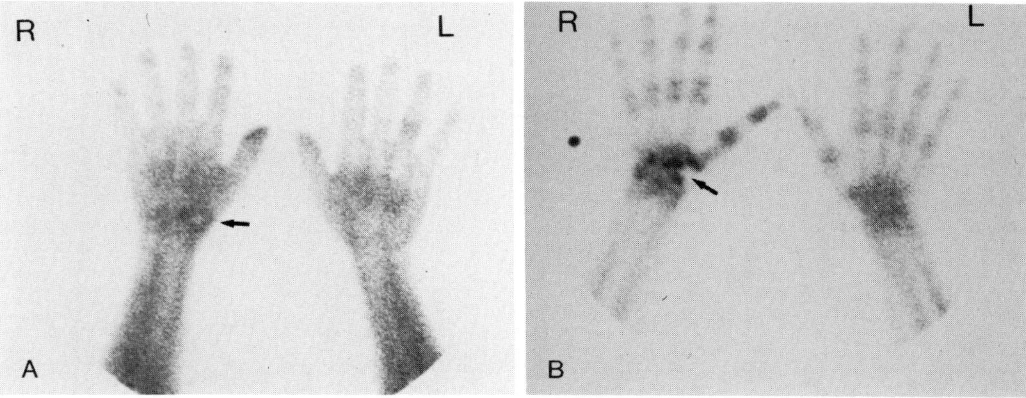

FIGURE 12–27. Normal trapezium prosthesis, mild nonspecific stress change in adjacent carpal bones, and reflex sympathetic dystrophy. **A:** BP image, palmar view. Less than 1 + increased activity surrounds area of trapezium prosthesis (arrow). **B:** Delayed image, palmar view. Prosthesis is photon deficient (arrow). Adjacent carpals show 1 + increased activity in all metacarpophalangeal and interphalangeal joints on the right when compared with the normal left.

proliferating mesenchyme that differentiates to form bone. Awareness of this lesion, which has maximum radiographic opacity at the periphery with the central zone being relatively radiolucent, is important so that radical procedures are not undertaken.[50]

Prosthesis Evaluation

RNBI evaluation most often has been performed to evaluate prostheses in the hip and knee for loosening, infection, or heterotopic bone formation.[3,4] Although there has been less experience with the procedure for evaluation of the hand, the same principles should apply, i.e., abnormal stress and movement cause increased metabolic activity on the delayed images, whereas infections, which will be discussed subsequently, cause increased activity on all three phases of the examination. More recent reports suggest that abnormal activity on the bone scan may represent normal repair for up to one year postoperatively.[51,52] A normal prosthesis appears as a photon-deficient area of activity (Fig. 12–27).

INFECTIONS

The appearance on the RNBI of cellulitis, osteomyelitis, and septic arthritis, as well as the differentiation between cellulitis and the latter two entities, has been well described.[53] Maurer reported a 92% sensitivity for the detection of osteomyelitis, with the three-phase examination decreasing the false-positive rate to 0.06. In patients with osteomyelitis or septic arthritis, the RNA is focally abnormal, the BP images show diffuse increased vascularity, and the delayed images demonstrate more intense and more focal accumulation of radiotracer in the abnormal osseous or articular region. Osteomyelitis cannot normally be differentiated from septic arthritis except for location. In patients with cellulitis (although the RNA and BP images can also be abnormal) the delayed image shows less rather than more tracer accumulation (Fig. 12–28). In patients with underlying abnormalities, such as healing fractures, which in themselves could lead to increased bone turnover, the diagnosis of osteomyelitis must be made with caution. In these instances, additional imaging with another radiotracer, such as gallium-67 citrate, or indium-111 or technetium-99m-HMPAO-labeled white blood cells would have to be considered.[54,55] Although both of these radiotracers are more sensitive and specific for infection, they provide less anatomic detail and often need to be supplemented by the phosphorus moiety bone scan, radiographs, or MRI.

BONE TUMORS

Benign bone tumors are most often encountered either when the nuclear radiologist is asked to determine the significance of a lesion detected on a radiograph or as an incidental finding on a whole-body bone scan performed to detect metastatic disease. Similarly malignant lesions are usually first detected clinically and confirmed with a radiograph. The three-phase RNBI examination is performed to evaluate metabolic activity, and a whole-body bone scan is performed to determine if the disease is monostotic or polyostotic. At the outset, it should be made clear that there are no absolute scintigraphic criteria to distinguish benign from malignant lesions. Even the addition of RNA and BP images, although helpful, is not absolute. A lesion demonstrated on a radiograph that has no increased perfusion on RNA, has normal BP images, and has normal or only minimally increased tracer accumulation on delayed images is almost certainly benign. Because many lesions of

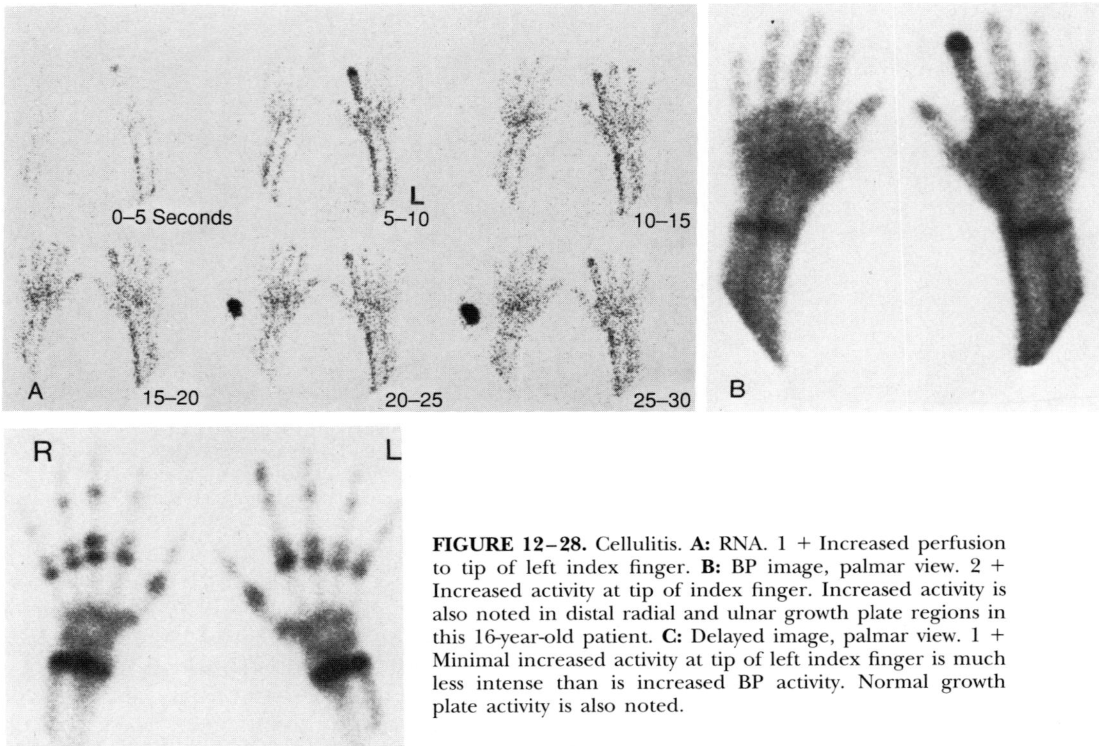

FIGURE 12–28. Cellulitis. **A:** RNA. 1 + Increased perfusion to tip of left index finger. **B:** BP image, palmar view. 2 + Increased activity at tip of index finger. Increased activity is also noted in distal radial and ulnar growth plate regions in this 16-year-old patient. **C:** Delayed image, palmar view. 1 + Minimal increased activity at tip of left index finger is much less intense than is increased BP activity. Normal growth plate activity is also noted.

multiple myeloma and very destructive metastases can be normal scintigraphically, when these entities are clinically or roentgenographically suspected additional evaluation should be considered. Otherwise, criteria such as the relative uptake of tracer, the number of lesions, the location of lesions, the radiographic appearance, and the clinical setting must always be considered together to help the referring physician plan any further diagnostic or therapeutic efforts.[56] Metastatic disease of the hands is relatively uncommon, but in the appropriate clinical setting a metastasis would have to be considered (Fig. 12–29).[3]

The diagnosis of osteoid osteoma, which is being increasingly reported in the hand both as a cause for general pain and even articular pain,[57–59] has been greatly facilitated by RNBI, which demonstrates an intense focal area of increased tracer accumulation on the delayed images (Fig. 12–30). Some specificity is possible, since BP images often demonstrate a rounded focal area of increased tracer accumulation, presumably representing the vascular nidus (Fig. 12–31).[57,60] The lack of intense increased perfusion on the radionuclide angiogram and the focal round activity on the other phases make infection less likely, but not totally excludable. Some additional benign lesions with significant abnormal tracer accumulation but recognizable radiographic findings to aid in differential diagnosis include osteoblastomas, chondroblastomas, aneurysmal bone cysts, and fibrous dysplasia.[61]

REFLEX SYMPATHETIC DYSTROPHY

RNBI plays a pivotal role in the diagnosis of reflex sympathetic dystrophy (RSD). In another publication,[19] we reported a specific scintigraphic pattern for RSD, established by using strict clinical criteria in a group of patients specifically referred to experienced hand surgeons. These patients had complaints of diffuse hand pain, diminished hand function, joint stiffness, and skin and soft-tissue trophic changes with or without vasomotor instability. Most sensitive (96%) and specific (97%) in the diagnosis of RSD is the delayed bone image, in which diffusely increased activity involves the radiocarpal, intercarpal, carpometacarpal, metacarpophalangeal, and interphalangeal joints (Fig. 12–32). Although in some patients RNA demonstrates diffusely increased perfusion to the hand and wrist, and the BP images demonstrate diffusely increased relative vascularity, neither of these phases is nearly as sensitive (45% and 52%, respectively) as the delayed images. This sensitivity has been confirmed by others,[62,63] some of whom have tried to relate activity to the particular phase of the syndrome.[63] Although some authors have questioned the sensitivity of this study, it has been generally accepted.[62] A discussion of possible etiologies for this syndrome and its scintigraphic findings has been published,[64] yet both remain uncertain and continue to provide research opportunities. Very occasionally, patients will have clinical signs and symptoms suggesting RSD, but involving only one, two, or three

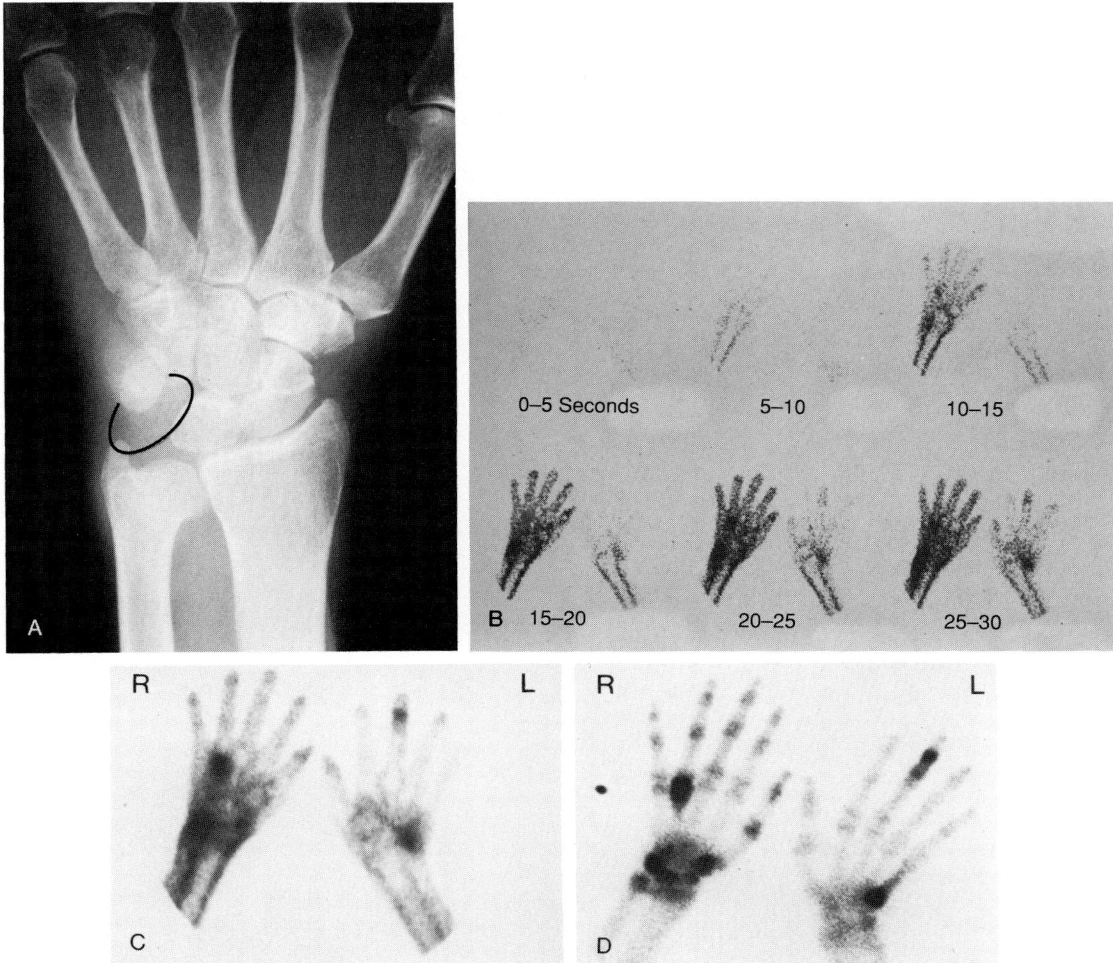

FIGURE 12–29. Metastatic transitional cell renal carcinoma. **A:** Radiograph. Soft-tissue fullness, lytic involvement of triquetrum (within circled area) and fourth metacarpal head. There are also questionable lytic changes of the lunate, radial-proximal aspect of the trapezium, and proximal radial aspect of the ulnar head. This radiograph is oriented to correlate with the palmar orientation of the scan. **B:** RNA. Diffuse increased perfusion of the right hand and wrist, with slightly more focal increased activity involving right medial proximal carpal row, fourth metacarpal head, and left fifth metacarpal base. **C:** BP image. **D:** Delayed image, palmar view. Focal 3 + increased activity in multiple areas.

rays. When the radionuclide bone scan demonstrates diffuse increased activity involving all of the metacarpal and metacarpophalangeal joints, phalanges, and interphalangeal joints of a ray regardless of the site, proximal or distal of the underlying inciting injury, a diagnosis of segmental RSD should be considered (Fig. 12–33).[65] ter Meulen and Majd reported decreased tracer on delayed images in children with potential RSD.[42] Since the RSD syndrome as it is usually recognized by hand surgeons is not seen in children, other neurovascular or neuroregulatory causes or perhaps other variants of sympathetically maintained pain syndromes should be considered.[66] Patients with disuse secondary to hemiplegia have decreased flow and decreased blood pool images with normal delayed images, whereas when RSD is superimposed, the delayed images are abnormal.[67]

PAIN OF UNCERTAIN ETIOLOGY

Although this chapter for organization and discussion purposes groups encountered lesions etiologically, in routine clinical practice most referrals for RNBI evaluation of the hand occur in patients with pain of unknown etiology. A normal TPBI examination excludes an osteochondral abnormality as the cause of the patient's symptoms and for the most part excludes any of the recognizable lesions reported and discussed in this chapter that have specific abnormal scintigraphic patterns.[14,46]

In addition, when TPBI examination is abnormal,

Text continued on page 348

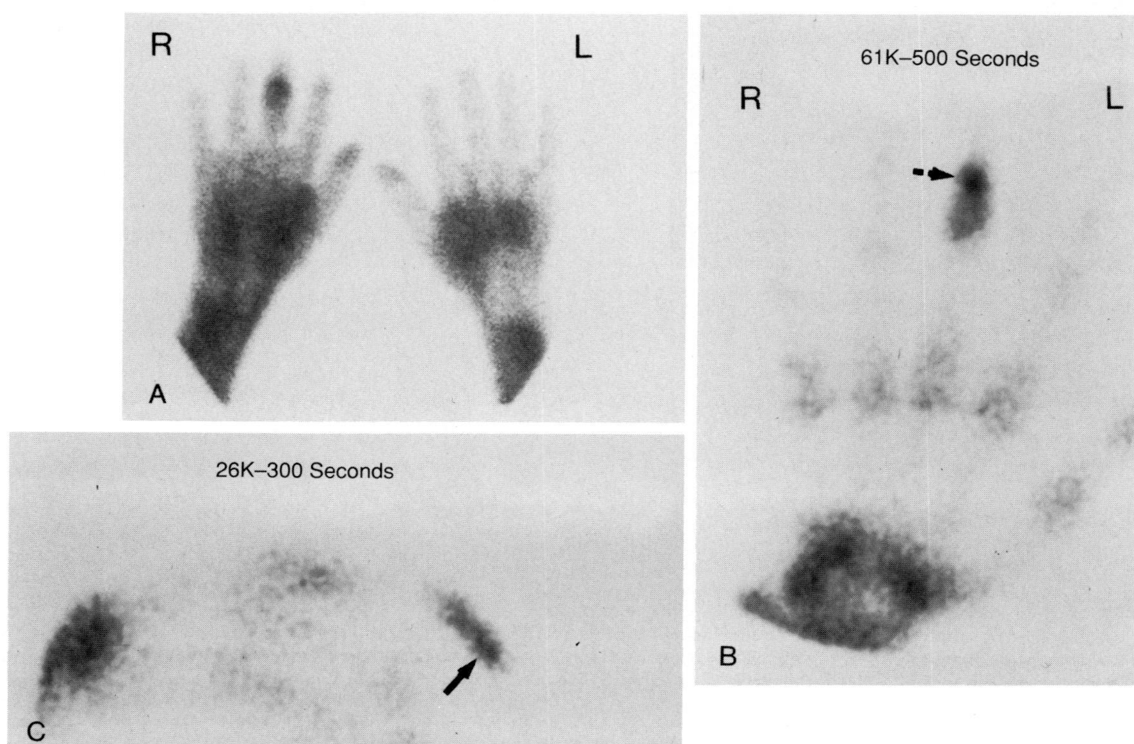

FIGURE 12–30. Osteoid osteoma, right long finger. **A:** BP image, palmar view. Focal increased activity of the long finger, middle phalanx. **B:** Delayed converging right palmar view. **C:** Right lateral view localizes activity to correspond to the osteoid osteoma nidus (arrow). The extended adjacent uptake is associated with a chronic reactive process; however, this activity is not fully explained. Magnified, converging, and pinhole collimator views, taken to obtain better anatomic detail, often have fewer counts, since acquisition time is limited by the patient's ability to remain immobilized.

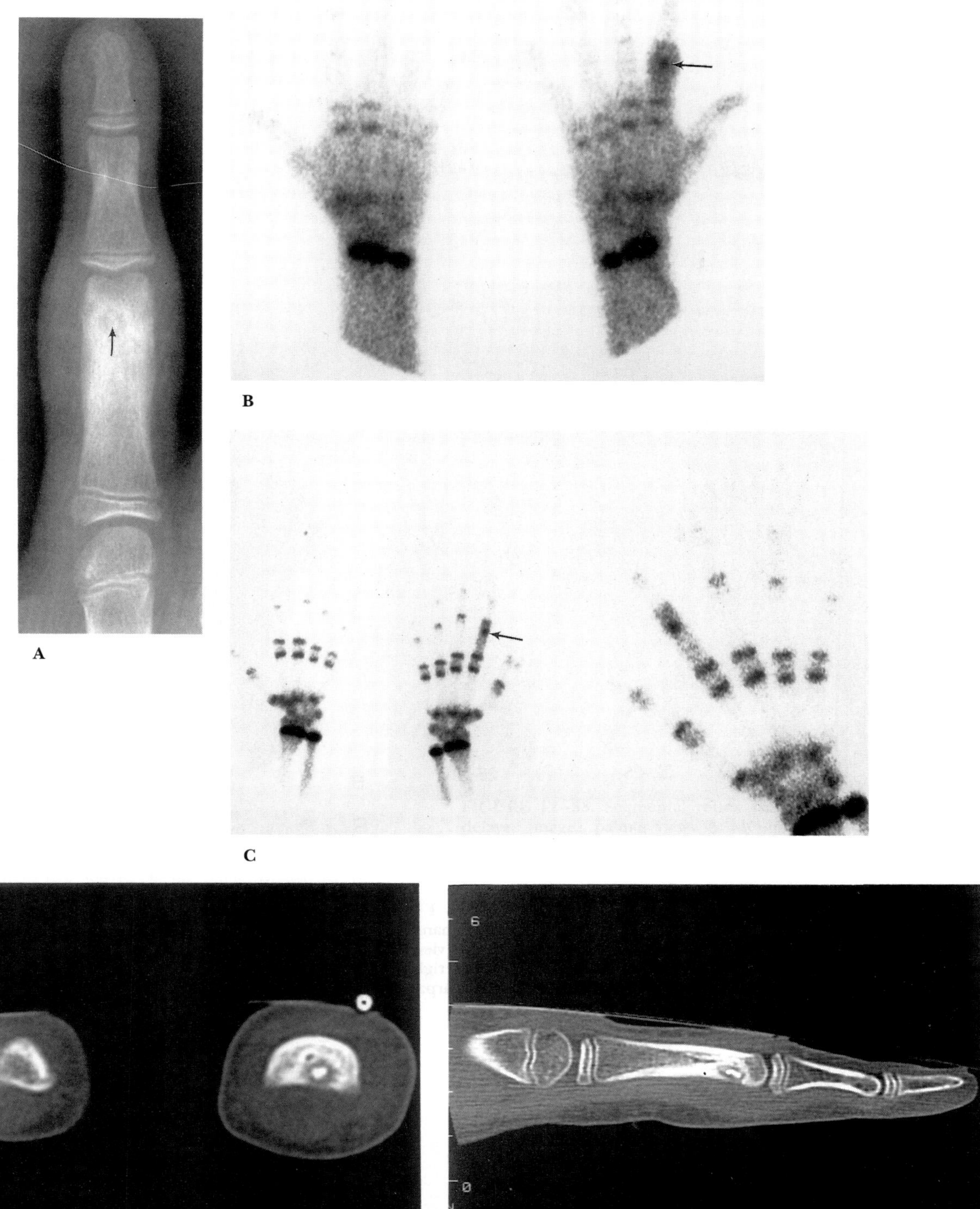

FIGURE 12–31. Osteoid osteoma, second proximal phalanx. **A:** Plain radiograph. Area of lucency with possible sclerotic center (arrow). The entire phalanx is enlarged with chronic cortical thickening. **B:** BP image. Tiny focus of more intense rounded activity distally (arrow) corresponding to area of lucency on the radiograph. Note the general increased vascularity associated with the diffuse soft-tissue swelling that is often seen in osteoid osteoma in fingers of children. **C:** Delayed image. Intense rounded area of increased tracer accumulation (arrow). Transaxial **(D)** and direct sagittal **(E)** CT delineates extent of reactive sclerosis, the lucent lesion, and the calcified central nidus. (Panels A–E reprinted with permission from Holder LE, Bright RW. Osteoid osteoma in a phalanx. *Maryland Med J* 1992;41:157–158.)

images, while sections in the lateral projection provide sagittal images.

To perform the tomogram, seat the patient in a chair next to the tomographic table, or alternatively, place the patient in a prone position on the tomographic table (Fig. 13–1). The technologist can then position the wrist or hand for both PA and lateral tomography. Performing tomography with the patient standing or leaning over the table is not advisable because this position quickly becomes uncomfortable, increasing the risk of patient motion during the examination.

For evaluation of the scaphoid, a special oblique view of the wrist is often required; this view brings the long axis of the scaphoid parallel to the cassette. The oblique view is obtained by slightly supinating and ulnarly deviating the wrist from the straight PA position (Fig. 13–2). Although tomography can be performed through a cast, optimal positioning may be difficult, necessitating removal of the cast before the examination.

Since the exposure time is often long and multiple exposures may be required, immobilization is therefore crucial. Adequate immobilization can usually be obtained with the placement of sandbags on either side of the wrist. Taping the wrist and hand to the table can be helpful, but this is not always necessary.

Our tomographic technique for the wrist and hand typically consists of 360-degree circular motion at 10 mA, 54 kVp, and 2- to 3-mm intervals. We prefer the 360-degree circular motion over the hypocycloidal or trispiral motion because it achieves similar resolution and better tissue contrast with shorter exposure times and therefore less radiation to the patient.

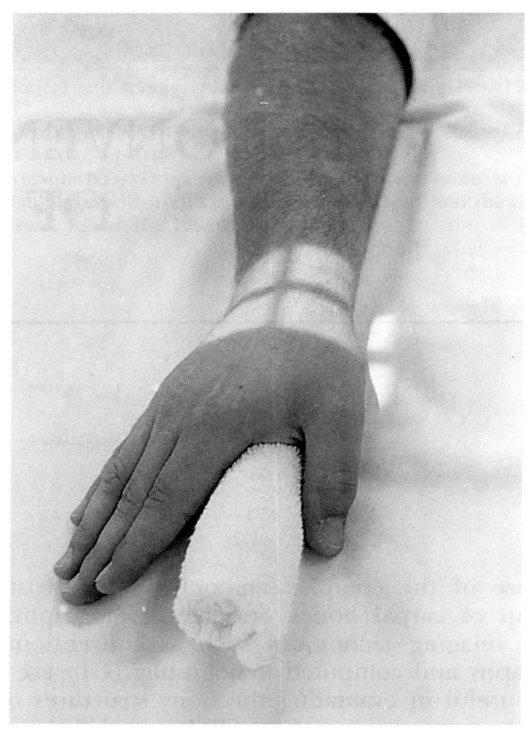

FIGURE 13–2. Oblique view. This position is obtained by placing a rolled-up washcloth or angled sponge on the table under the patient's hand between the thumb and index finger and positioning the cloth or sponge coaxial to the long axis of the forearm.

APPLICATIONS

Conventional tomography has largely been supplanted by CT and magnetic resonance (MR) imaging; however, conventional tomography is well suited for the evaluation of tissues with inherent tissue con-

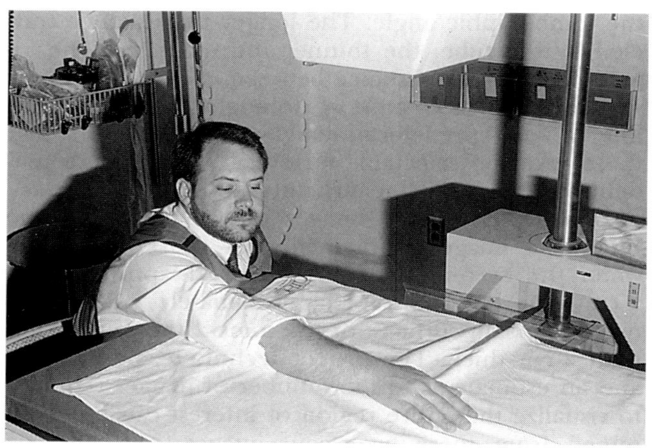

A

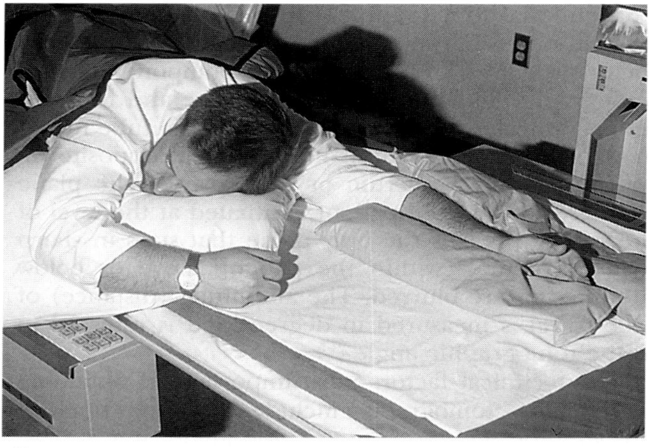

B

FIGURE 13–1. Positioning for tomography. **A**: Sitting: patient sits at the end of the table, arm resting on the table and elbow extended. For PA tomography, the hand and wrist should be placed flat on the table with no deviation of the wrist. **B**: Prone: patient lies prone with the arm above the head, and the elbow extended. For lateral tomography, the ulnar aspect of the hand and wrist should be placed on the table, thumb up. Sandbags placed adjacent to the forearm and wrist are usually adequate immobilization for wrist tomography.

trast, such as bone.[3] Coronal and sagittal sections of the wrist obtained directly by conventional circular tomography are routinely of very high quality, easier to interpret than axial CT sections, and aesthetically more pleasing than reformatted sagittal and coronal CT images.

Conventional tomography is especially useful in the detection, staging, and follow-up of bony injuries of the wrist, because adequate visualization of the distal radius, carpal bones, and proximal portions of the metacarpal bones on plain radiographs can be difficult.[3–11] Conventional tomography is generally not used in the evaluation of soft-tissue disorders of the wrist and hand; however, some authors have used wrist arthrotomography to study the interosseous ligaments of the wrist.[12,13] In addition to trauma, conventional tomography is often used to evaluate other bony disorders such as avascular necrosis of the lunate (Kienböck's disease), neoplasms, the bony sequella of arthropathies, premature physeal fusion, and congenital anomalies.

Traumatic Injuries

Because there is marked overlap of the carpal bones on plain radiographs, conventional tomography is an ideal modality to use in the diagnosis of questionable or occult fractures of the carpus (Figs. 13–3 and 13–4).[8,9] Another area that is difficult to assess on plain radiographs is the carpometacarpal (CMC) joints. Conventional tomography, particularly lateral tomography, is beneficial in cases of suspected CMC fracture, subluxation, or dislocation (Fig. 13–5).

While PA and lateral tomograms are usually obtained, the examination can be tailored to the clinical history. The wrist and hand can be imaged in any degree of pronation, supination, flexion, extension, and radial or ulnar deviation (see Figs. 13–2 and 13–3C).

Treatment of intraarticular fractures of the distal radius and ulna is often dependent on the degree of impaction and displacement of the fracture fragments.[14] Although CT or conventional tomography can easily assess the articular surface of the distal radius and ulna, it is often easier to position patients, particularly those with multiple injuries, on the tomographic table rather than in the CT gantry (Fig. 13–6).

Fracture Follow-Up and Postsurgical Assessment

Displaced or angulated scaphoid fractures with carpal instability frequently proceed to nonunion or malunion.[15] These malunited fractures are predisposed to premature arthrosis.[16] Assessing the extent of healing, angulation, or displacement of scaphoid fractures on plain radiographs is often difficult. CT has been used to evaluate these fractures; however, it may be uncomfortable or impossible for patients with associated ipsilateral arm or shoulder injuries to assume the positions required to visualize scaphoid fractures on CT. In addition, sagittal and coronal reconstructions may be of limited value because of motion artifact.[16] Conventional tomography readily demonstrates the extent of displacement, malunion, or healing of scaphoid fractures and can invariably be comfortably performed in multitrauma patients (Figs. 13–7 and 13–8).

Visual inspection is often all that is required in the evaluation of fracture healing or malunion; however, techniques to quantify scaphoid fracture malunion and nonunion have been described. Smith et al devised a method to assess displaced or malunited scaphoid fractures on tomography using measurements of an intrascaphoid angle on sagittal and coronal images.[16] Tehranzadeh, Davenport, and Pais recommended measuring the intrascaphoid angle on sagittal tomograms performed in flexion and extension to document suspected fracture motion and therefore nonunion.[17] They propose drawing a line through the midportion of the scaphoid, parallel to the ventral cortex of the proximal pole, and a second line parallel to the dorsal surface of the distal pole. The angle between the two fragments of the scaphoid is measured in flexion and extension. A difference between the two angles of greater than 10 degrees indicates nonunion (Fig. 13–9).[17]

Conventional tomography is also valuable in the postoperative assessment of surgical fusion of the wrist joint. Tomography readily demonstrates areas of bony bridging or nonunion that might otherwise go undetected on plain radiography (Fig. 13–10).

Kienböck's Disease

Although Kienböck's disease is readily diagnosed with plain radiography, the integrity of the remaining bone stock of the lunate can be underestimated. Conventional tomography provides detailed information regarding the amount of fragmentation and collapse of the lunate (Fig. 13–11).

Neoplasm

A plain radiograph of the hand and wrist is often sufficient to formulate a differential diagnosis for bone tumors. Osteoid osteomas of the carpal bones, however, are notoriously difficult to visualize on plain films. Because it can conclusively demonstrate the nidus, conventional tomography is extremely helpful in cases where osteoid osteoma is suspected (Fig. 13–12).[18]

Recent literature suggests that focal radiolucent intraosseous defects that communicate with the joint are more likely to be symptomatic than those lesions that do not.[19] Conventional tomography can readily distinguish between these two types of intraosseous defects (Fig. 13–13).

Text continued on page 365

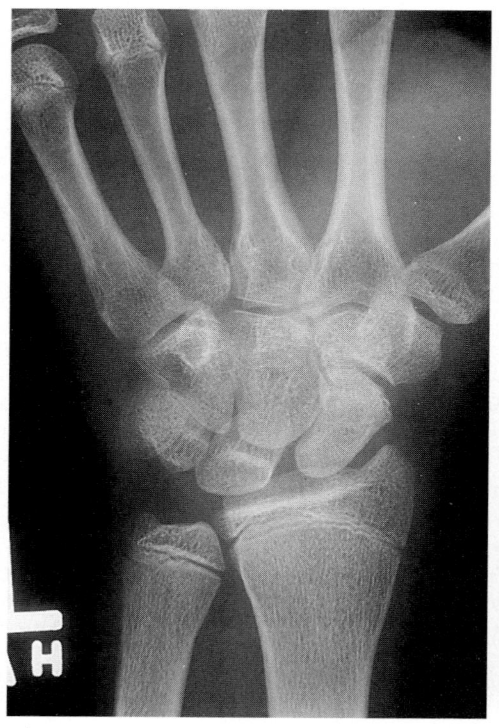

A

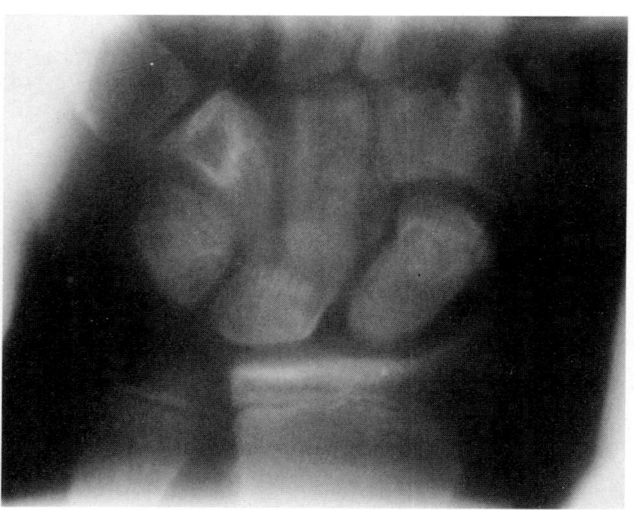

B

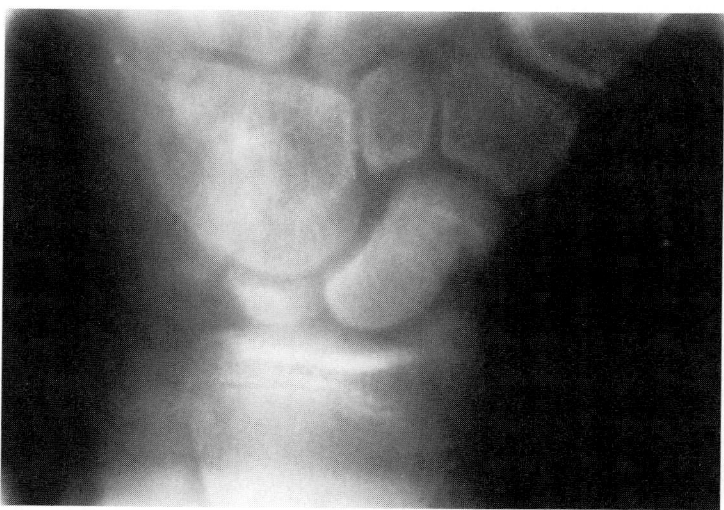

C

FIGURE 13–3. Twenty-seven-year-old man with wrist pain after a fall. **A**: PA and lateral (not shown) radiographs of the wrist several weeks after the injury show no definite evidence of scaphoid fracture. **B**: PA tomograms clearly demonstrate a subacute scaphoid fracture. **C**: Oblique tomogram of the scaphoid shows to better advantage the scaphoid fracture.

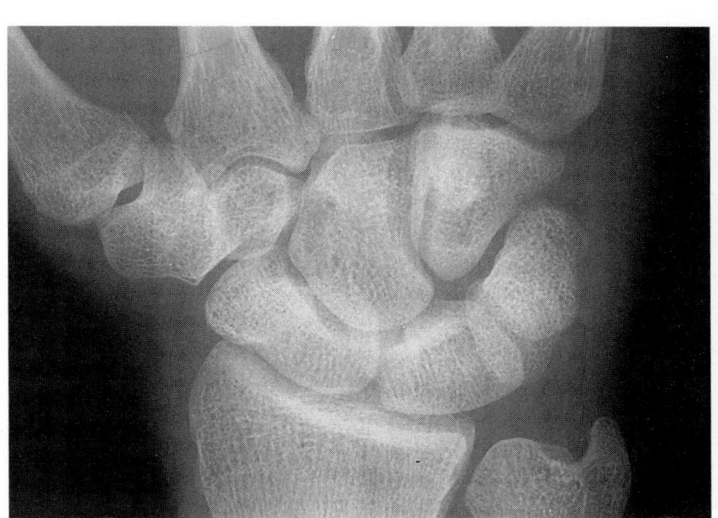

A

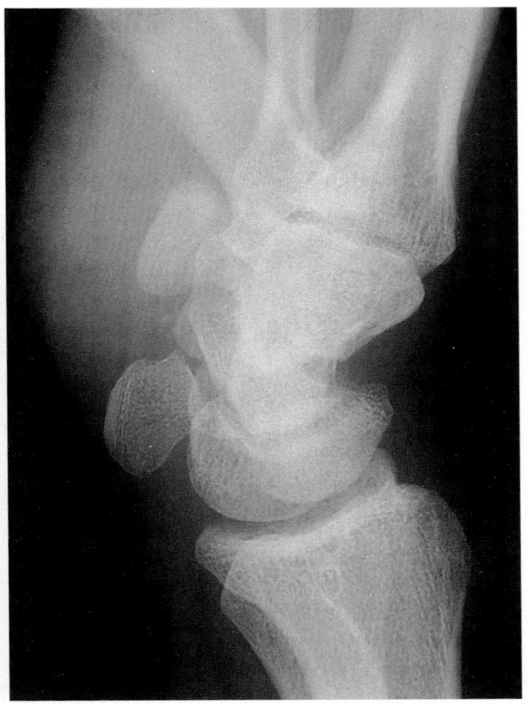

B

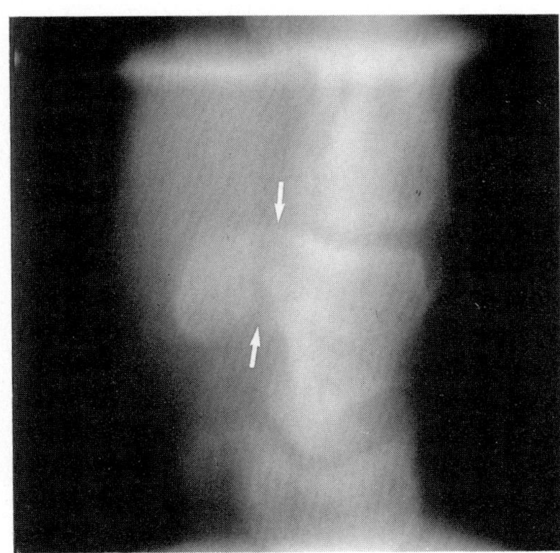

C

FIGURE 13–4. Occult hamate fracture. PA (**A**) and lateral (**B**) radiographs fail to clearly demonstrate a fracture. **C**: Lateral tomogram shows a hook of the hamate fracture (between arrows).

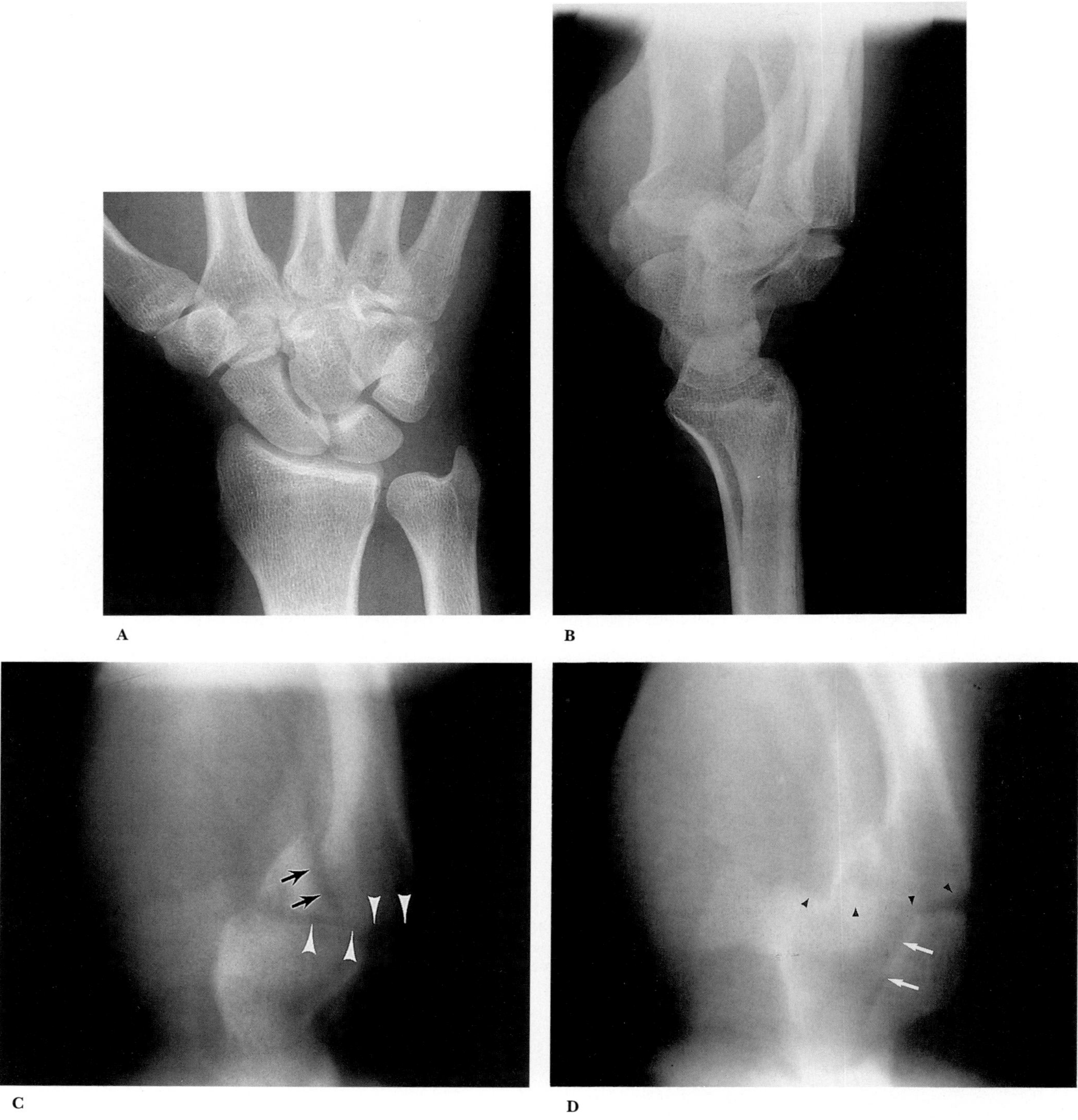

FIGURE 13–5. CMC fracture-dislocation. PA **(A)** and lateral **(B)** radiographs of the wrist show abnormal alignment in the region of the hamate, third, fourth, and fifth CMC joints; however, the nature of the fractures and degree of subluxation or dislocation at the CMC joints is difficult to determine. **C**: Lateral tomograms show an unsuspected fracture of the third metacarpal (arrows) with subluxation at the third CMC joint (between arrowheads) and **(D)** a vertical fracture through the hamate (arrows) with subluxation of the fourth CMC joint (between arrowheads).

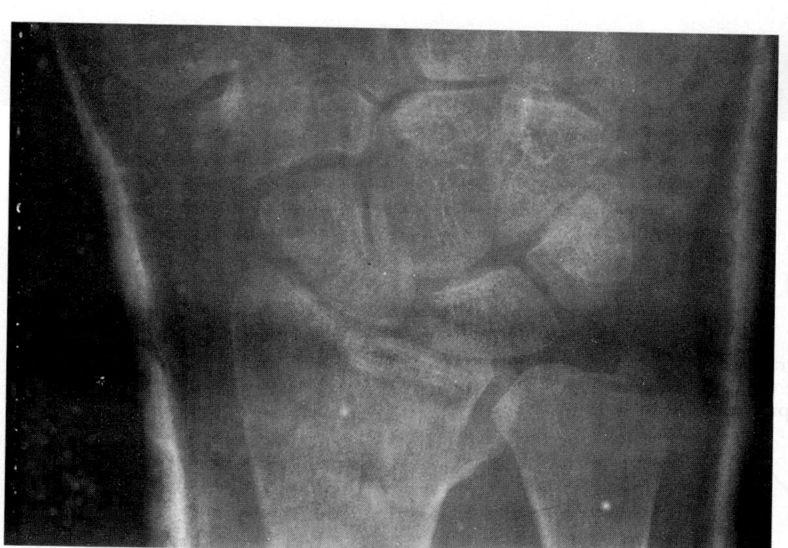

A

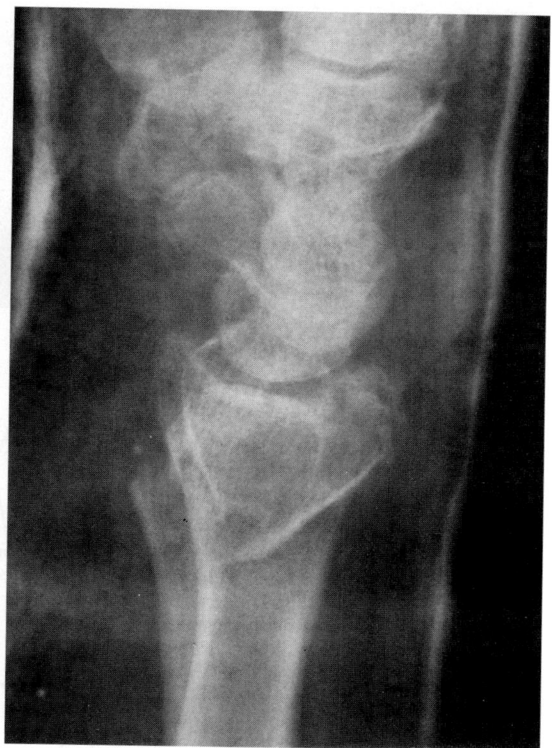

B

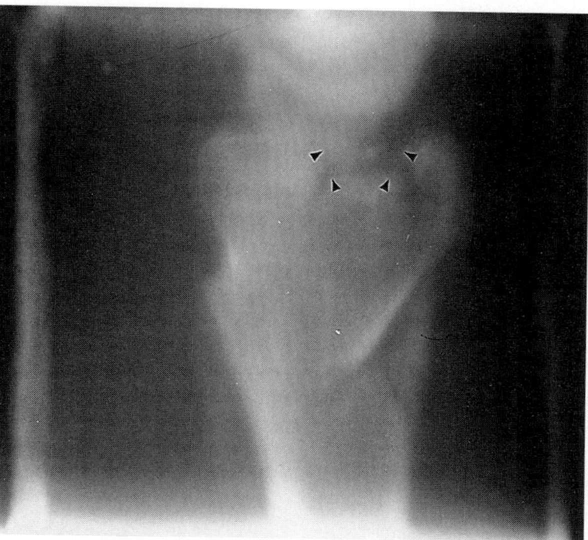

C

FIGURE 13–6. Distal radial fracture in multitrauma patient. PA (**A**) and lateral (**B**) radiographs of a distal radial fracture show no convincing evidence of depression at the radial articular surface. **C**: Lateral tomogram, obtained through a cast, clearly shows central articular surface depression (between arrowheads).

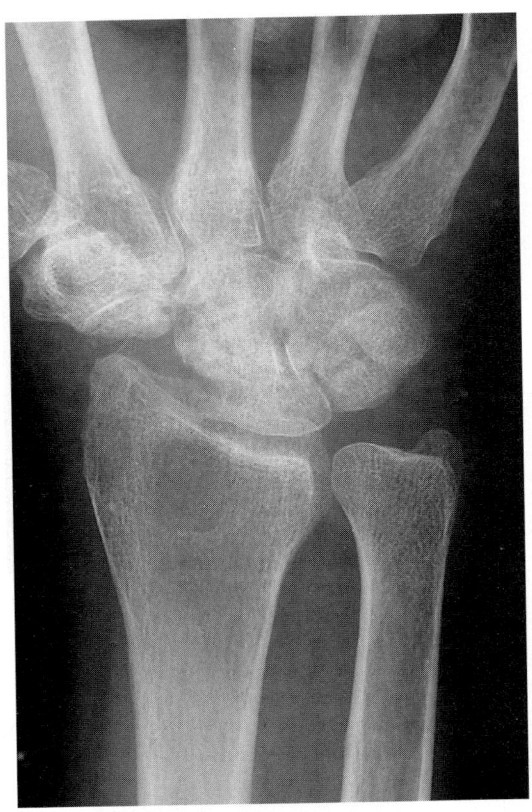

A

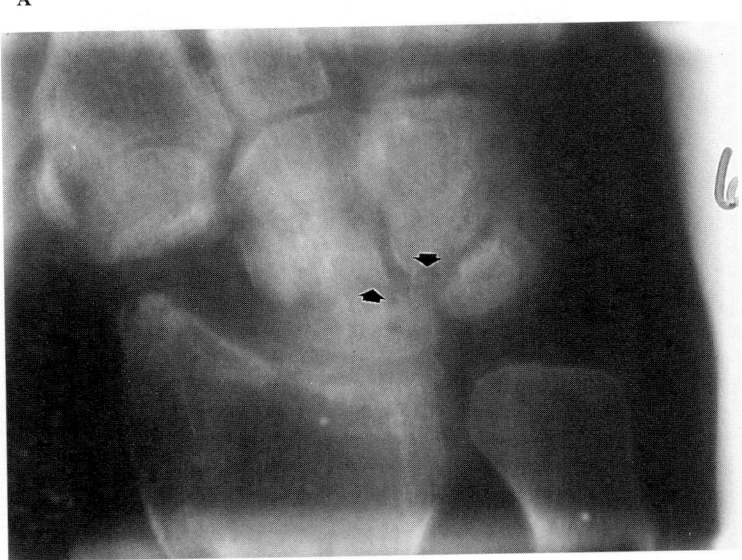

B

FIGURE 13–10. Nonunion after wrist fusion. **A**: PA radiograph of the wrist after scaphoid resection and carpal fusion shows no evidence of nonunion. **B**: PA tomogram obtained on the same day shows areas of nonunion between the capitate, hamate, triquetrum, and lunate (arrows).

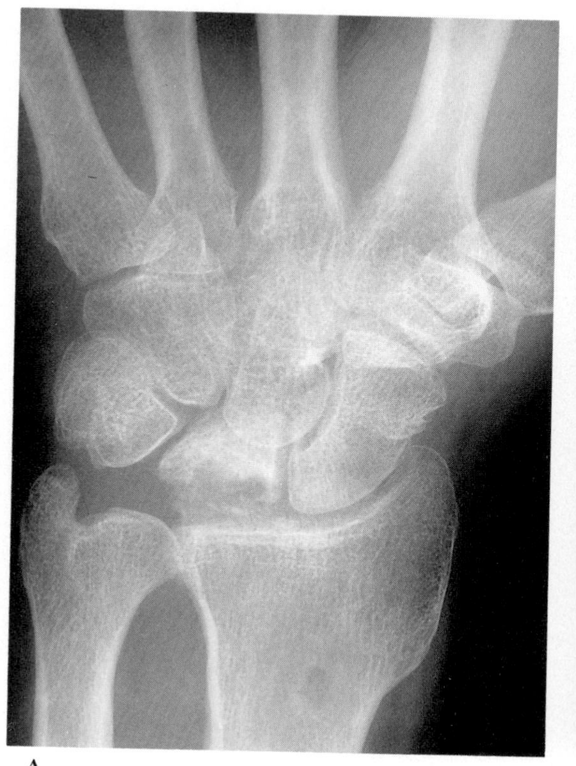

A

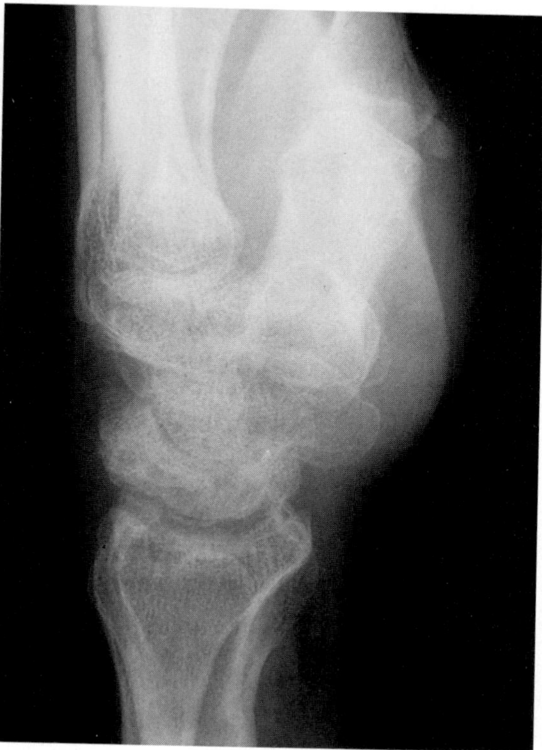

B

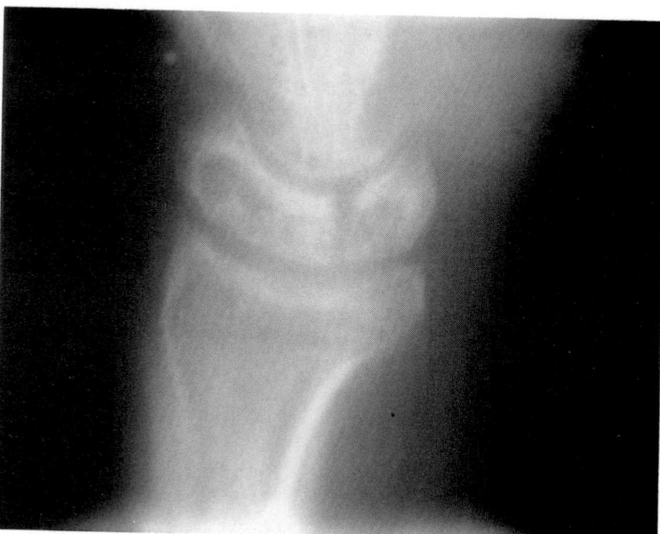

C

FIGURE 13–11. Kienböck's disease. PA (**A**) and lateral (**B**) radiographs show Kienböck's disease; however, the amount of fragmentation and cystic degeneration is better appreciated with lateral tomography (**C**).

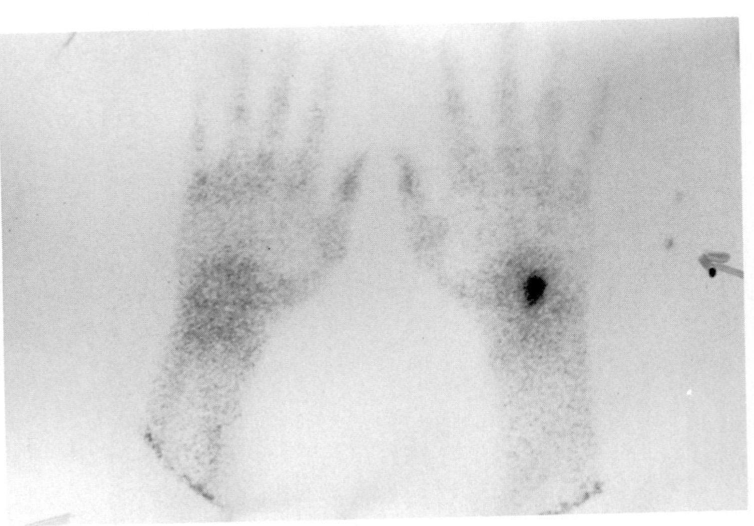

A

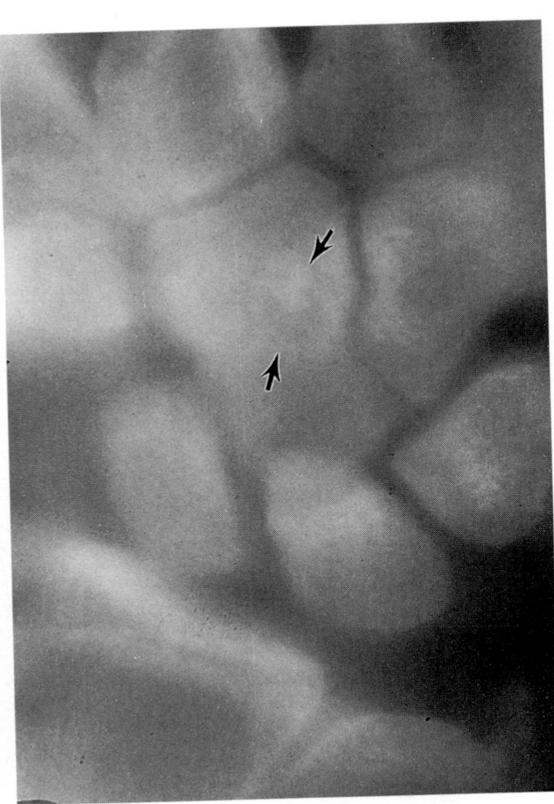

B

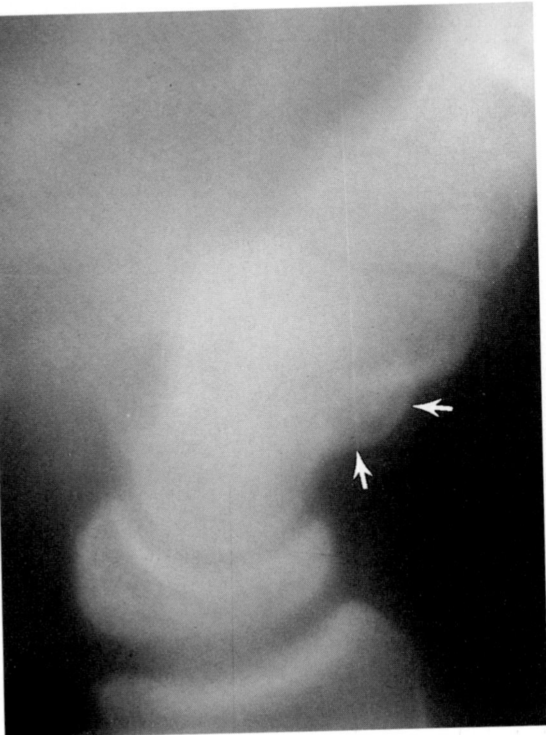

C

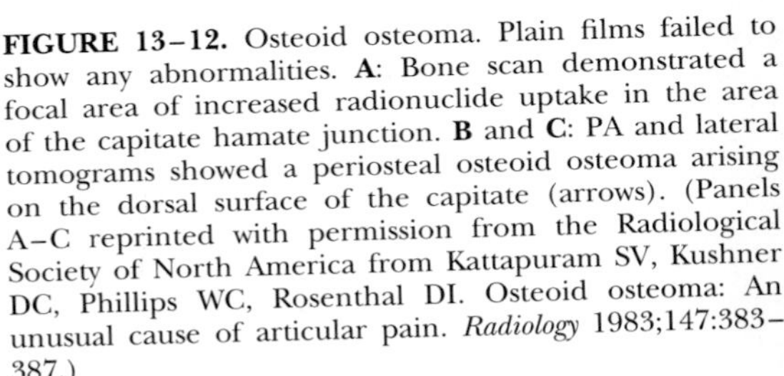

FIGURE 13–12. Osteoid osteoma. Plain films failed to show any abnormalities. **A**: Bone scan demonstrated a focal area of increased radionuclide uptake in the area of the capitate hamate junction. **B** and **C**: PA and lateral tomograms showed a periosteal osteoid osteoma arising on the dorsal surface of the capitate (arrows). (Panels A–C reprinted with permission from the Radiological Society of North America from Kattapuram SV, Kushner DC, Phillips WC, Rosenthal DI. Osteoid osteoma: An unusual cause of articular pain. *Radiology* 1983;147:383–387.)

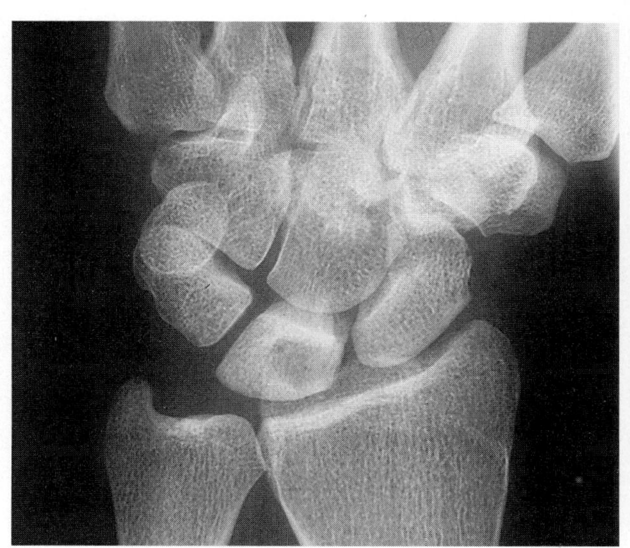

A

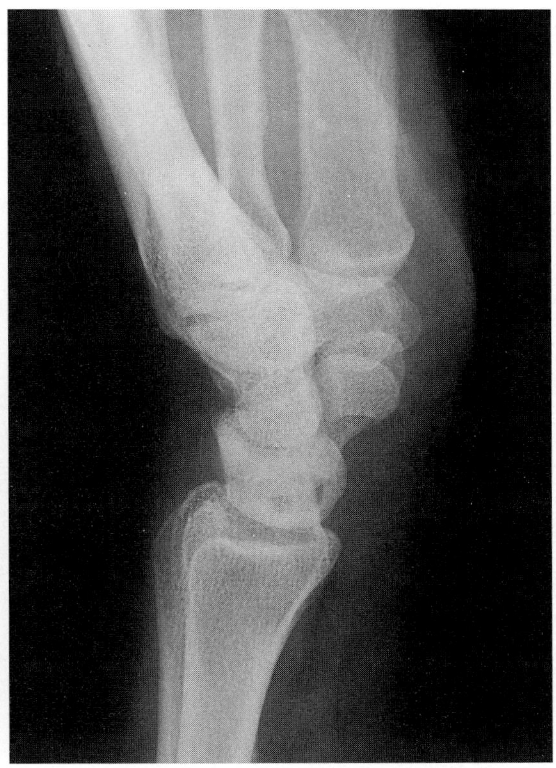

B

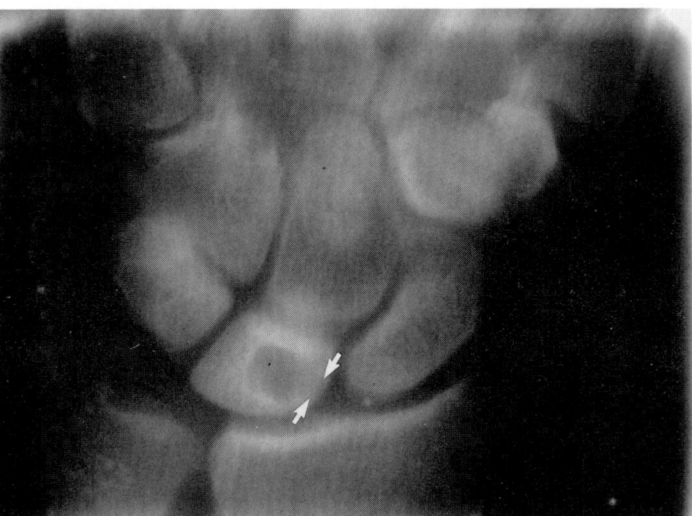

C

FIGURE 13–13. Intraosseous defects. PA (**A**) and lateral (**B**) radiography show an intraosseous defect within the lunate. **C**: PA tomogram confirms that the lesion communicates with the scapholunate joint (between arrows).

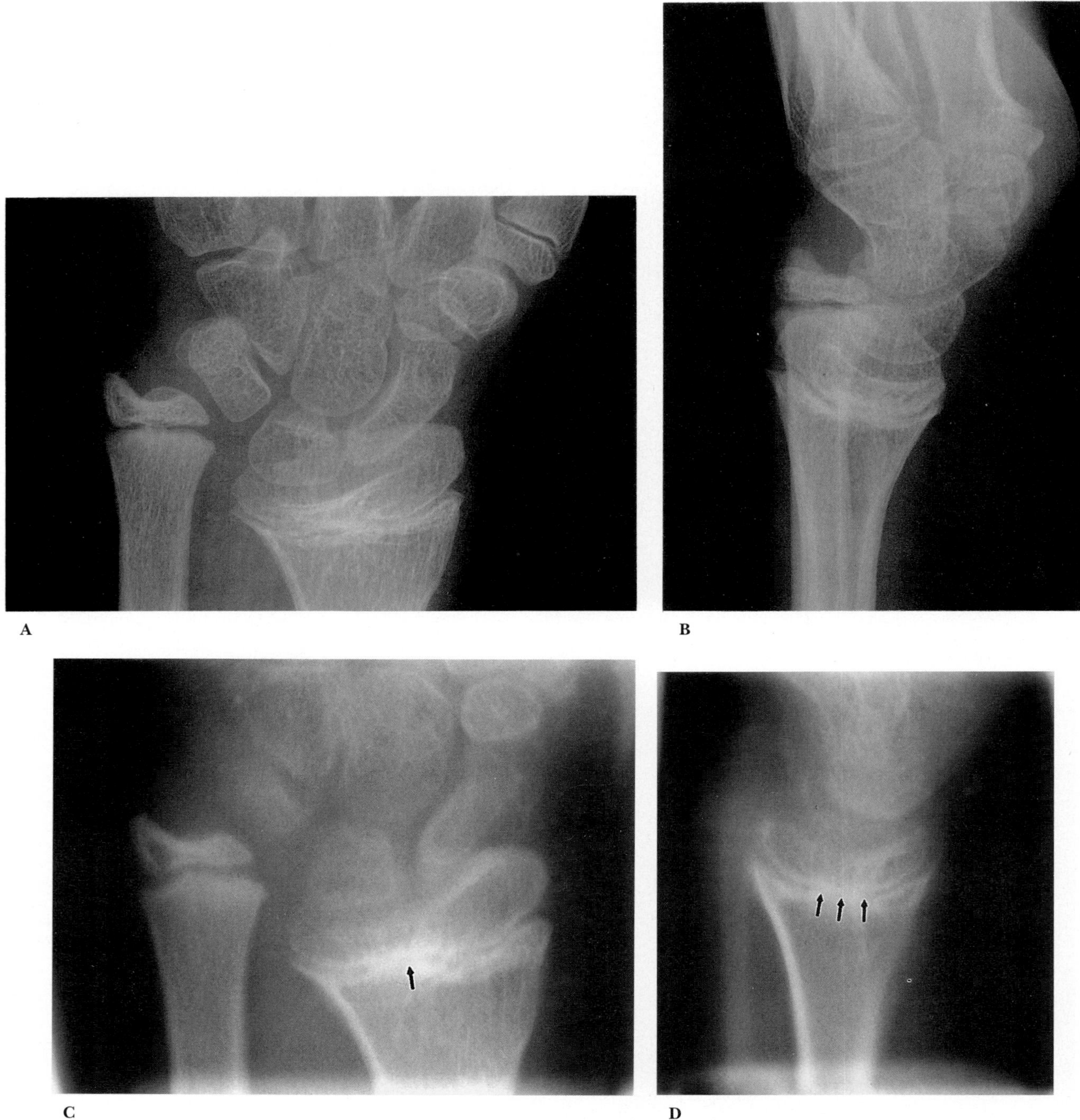

FIGURE 13–14. Premature physeal fusion. PA (**A**) and lateral (**B**) radiographs of the distal radius show partial physeal fusion with subsequent growth arrest. The radius is shortened relative to the ulna. PA (**C**) and lateral (**D**) tomograms are required to precisely demonstrate the areas of physeal fusion (arrows).

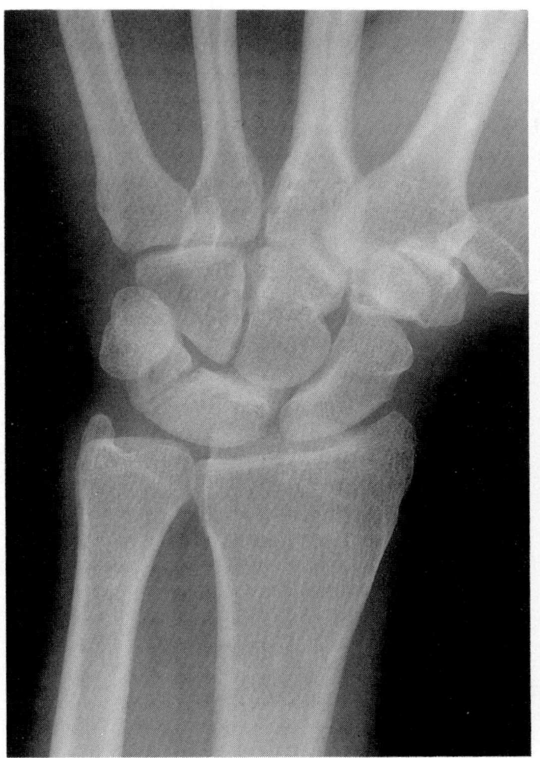

A

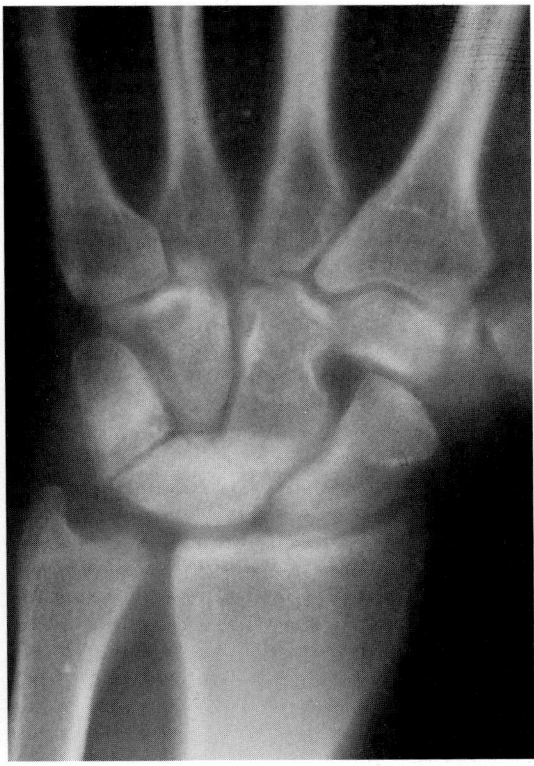

B

FIGURE 13–15. Carpal coalition. **A**: PA radiograph suggests coalition between the lunate and triquetrum. **B**: PA tomogram confirms fibrous or cartilaginous coalition since no bony coalition is demonstrated. This verifies joint space narrowing without subcortical sclerosis or marginal osteophytes, which would be seen with degenerative joint disease.

Arthropathies

Although visualization of the wrist ligaments and cartilage has been described using arthrotomography, MR imaging and arthrography are currently the imaging modalities of choice in the evaluation of the soft tissues of the wrist and hand.[12,13,20–23] Conventional tomography can be used to assess bony manifestations of arthropathies, such as posttraumatic degenerative disease that is not well appreciated on plain radiographs.

Premature Epiphyseal Growth Plate Fusion

The epiphyseal growth plate (physis) of the distal radius is the most frequently injured physis in children. Fortunately, it is estimated that the incidence of premature fusion of the physis following trauma is less than 10%. Most premature fusions of the physis occur in children who sustain injury to the physis with less than 2 years of physeal remodeling potential remaining, or in children who have undergone repetitive, forceful fracture reduction attempts. Surgical correction of deformities related to partial fusion of the physis requires knowledge of the exact area of fusion of the physis or physeal bar.[24–28] Thin-section tomography (2-mm intervals), in two orthogonal planes, accurately delineates areas of premature physeal fusion (Fig. 13–14).

Congenital Anomalies

Carpal coalition is a relatively rare entity, with the lunotriquetral joint involved most frequently.[29,30] Complete osseous coalition between carpal bones can be easily identified on plain radiographs. Fibrous or cartilaginous coalition, however, may be difficult to assess without sectional imaging; conventional tomography is ideally suited for this purpose (Fig. 13–15).

CONCLUSION

Although it has been supplanted by CT and MR imaging in the evaluation of most disorders of the musculoskeletal system, conventional tomography remains a cost-effective method of imaging the wrist and hand. In some centers conventional tomography is frequently used in the evaluation of bony disorders of the wrist and hand where the overlap of bony structures on plain radiographs makes interpretation difficult. Currently, conventional tomography of the wrist and hand is most often used in the evaluation and follow-up of traumatic carpal bone injuries, but it can also be used during the assessment of surgical fusion, Kienböck's disease, neoplasm, bony manifestations of arthropathy, premature physeal fusion, and congenital anomalies.

REFERENCES

1. Littleton JT. Conventional tomography in perspective. *RadioGraphics* 1986;6:336–339.
2. Curry TS III, Dowdey JE, Murry RC Jr. Body section radiography. In: Curry TS III, Dowdey JE, Murry RC Jr, eds. *Christensen's introduction to the physics of diagnostic radiology,* 3rd ed. Philadelphia: Lea & Febiger, 1984;243–261.
3. Ho C, Sartoris DJ, Resnick D. Conventional tomography in musculoskeletal trauma. *Radiol Clin North Am* 1989;27:929–932.
4. Norman A. The value of tomography in the diagnosis of skeletal disorders. *Radiol Clin North Am* 1970;8:251–258.
5. Norman A. The use of tomography in the diagnosis of skeletal disorders. *Clin Orthop* 1975;107:139–145.
6. Posner MA, Greenspan A. Trispiral tomography for the evaluation of wrist problems. *J Hand Surg* 1988;13A:175–181.
7. Bell MS. Linear tomography and the injured wrist. *Injury* 1977;8:303–306.
8. Apple JS, Martinez S, Khoury MB, Nunley JA. Occult carpal pathology: Tomographic evaluation. *Skeletal Radiol* 1986;15: 228–232.
9. Greenspan A, Posner MA, Tucker M. The value of carpal tunnel trispiral tomography in the diagnosis of fracture of the hook of the hamate. *Bull Hosp Jt Dis Orthop Inst* 1985;45:74–79.
10. Linscheid RL, Dobyns JH, Younge DK. Trispiral tomography in the evaluation of wrist injury. *Bull Hosp Jt Dis Orthop Inst* 1984;44:297–308.
11. Kerr R. Diagnostic imaging of upper extremity trauma. *Radiol Clin North Am* 1989;27:891–908.
12. Berger RA, Blair WF, El-Khoury GY. Arthrotomography of the wrist. *Clin Orthop* 1983;172:257–264.
13. Berger RA, Blair WF, El-Khoury GY. Arthrotomography of the wrist: The palmar radiocarpal ligaments. *Clin Orthop* 1984;186:224–229.
14. Knirk JL, Jupiter JB. Intra-articular fractures of the distal end of the radius in young adults. *J Bone Joint Surg* 1986;68A:647–659.
15. Amadio PC, Berquist TH, Smith DK, et al. Scaphoid malunion. *J Hand Surg* 1989;14A:679–687.
16. Smith DK, Linscheid RL, Amadio PC, et al. Scaphoid anatomy: Evaluation with complex motion tomography. *Radiology* 1989;173:177–180.
17. Tehranzadeh J, Davenport J, Pais MJ. Scaphoid fracture: Evaluation with flexion-extension tomography. *Radiology* 1990;176:167–170.
18. Kattapuram SV, Kushner DC, Phillips WC, Rosenthal DI. Osteoid osteoma: An unusual cause of articular pain. *Radiology* 1983;147:383–387.
19. Stewart NR, Gilula LA. CT of the wrist: A tailored approach. *Radiology* 1992;183:13–20.
20. Binkovitz LA, Berquist TH, McLeod RA. Masses of the hand and wrist: Detection and characterization with MR imaging. *AJR* 1990;154:323–326.
21. Cerofolini E, Luchetti R, Pederzini L, et al. MR evaluation of triangular fibrocartilage complex tears in the wrist: Comparison with arthrography and arthroscopy. *J Comput Assist Tomogr* 1990;14:963–967.
22. Gundry CR, Kursunoglu-Brahme S, Schwaighofer B, et al. Is MR better than arthrography for evaluating the ligaments of the wrist? *AJR* 1990;154:337–341.
23. Kang HS, Kindynis P, Brahme SK, et al. Triangular fibrocartilage and intercarpal ligaments of the wrist: MR imaging. *Radiology* 1991;181:401–404.
24. Carlson WO, Wenger DR. A mapping method to prepare for surgical excision of a partial physeal arrest. *J Pediatr Orthop* 1984;4:232–238.
25. Lee BS, Esterhal JL Jr, Das M. Fracture of the distal radial epiphysis. *Clin Orthop* 1984;185:90–96.
26. Peterson CA, Peterson HA. Analysis of the incidence of injuries to the epiphyseal growth plate. *J Trauma* 1972;12:275–281.
27. Peterson HA. Partial growth plate arrest and its treatment. *J Pediatr Orthop* 1984;4:246–258.
28. Salter RB, Harris WR. Injuries involving the epiphyseal plate. *J Bone Joint Surg* 1963;45A:587–622.
29. Graham CE, Mehta MC. Bilateral congenital carpal fusion in a champion golfer. *Clin Orthop* 1972;83:70–72.
30. O'Rahilly R. A survey of carpal and tarsal anomalies. *J Bone Joint Surg* 1953;35A:626–642.

CHAPTER 14

ARTHROGRAPHY AND CT–ARTHROGRAPHY OF THE WRIST AND HAND

I. ARTHROGRAPHY OF THE WRIST AND HAND

V. M. Metz

WRIST ARTHROGRAPHY

Because of the heightened interest in clinical evaluation of the painful wrist, wrist arthrography has become an important preoperative imaging modality. The most common indication for wrist arthrography is evaluation of persistent wrist pain and posttraumatic abnormalities in wrist motion. Arthrography may be helpful in identifying interosseous ligament defects and perforations of the triangular fibrocartilage (TFC), capsular defects and inflammatory synovial diseases, cartilage thinning, and ganglions. A positive finding on wrist arthrography must be carefully correlated with patients' symptoms and physical findings, however, since intercompartmental communicating defects increase in number with advancing age and, even when located at the site of symptoms, may not be the source of patients' pain.

Normal Arthrogram—Anatomy of Wrist Joints

The wrist consists of several synovial lined major and minor compartments that usually do not communicate (Fig. 14–1).[1–3] The major compartments are the radiocarpal joint (RCJ) or compartment, the distal radioulnar joint (DRUJ) or compartment, and the midcarpal joint (MCJ) or compartment. Minor compartments are the first carpometacarpal compartment of the thumb, the pisotriquetral compartment, and the common carpometacarpal and intermetacarpal compartments.

The radiocarpal compartment is bordered proximally by the distal radial articular cartilage and the triangular fibrocartilage complex (TFCC). The TFCC consists of the TFC (also known as the articular disc), the meniscus homologue, the ulnar collateral ligament, and the tendon sheath of the extensor carpi ulnaris muscle. Distally the radiocarpal compartment is bordered by the cartilaginous surfaces of the bones of the proximal carpal row (scaphoid, lunate, and triquetrum) and the interosseous ligaments between these bones (scapholunate and lunotriquetral ligaments). The radiocarpal compartment has a C shape between the radius and the proximal carpal row and, when a meniscus is present, has a Y-shaped configuration at its ulnar aspect (Fig. 14–2). Under normal conditions the synovial surfaces are smooth and three recesses[4–7] are commonly filled (Fig. 14–2): (1) the prestyloid recess, which is anterior to the ulnar styloid, (2) the prescaphoid (or ventral radial) recess, ventral to the scaphoid waist and distal radius, and (3) finally the dorsoscaphoid (dorsal radial) recess. As mentioned above, normally there should be no communication between the RCJ and other compartments of the wrist except to the pisotriquetral compartment. A communication between these two joints is a common finding, occurring in up to 75% of normal subjects.[8,9]

The DRUJ (Fig. 14–3) outlines the proximal surface of the TFCC, which extends a variable distance from its radial attachment on the distal radius to the base of the ulnar styloid, outlining the articulation between them. Contrast outlines the articular cartilage of the ulnar head. The entire synovial contour is smooth, without recesses.

The midcarpal compartment (Fig. 14–4) extends

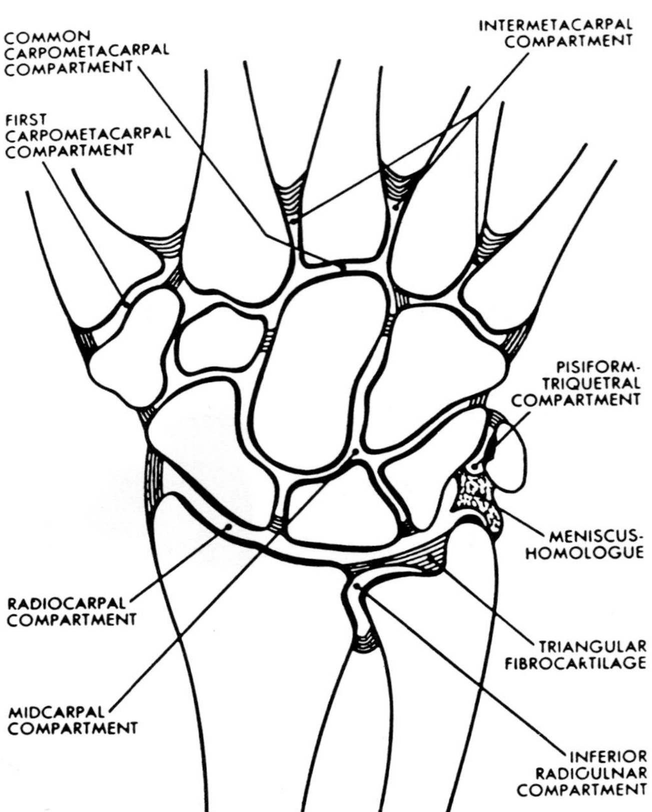

FIGURE 14–1. Illustration of different major and minor compartments of the wrist. (Reprinted with permission from Gold RH. Arthrography of the wrist. In: Arndt RD, Horns JW, Gold RH, Blaschke DD, eds. *Clinical arthrography.* 2nd ed. Baltimore: Williams & Wilkins, 1985:222.)

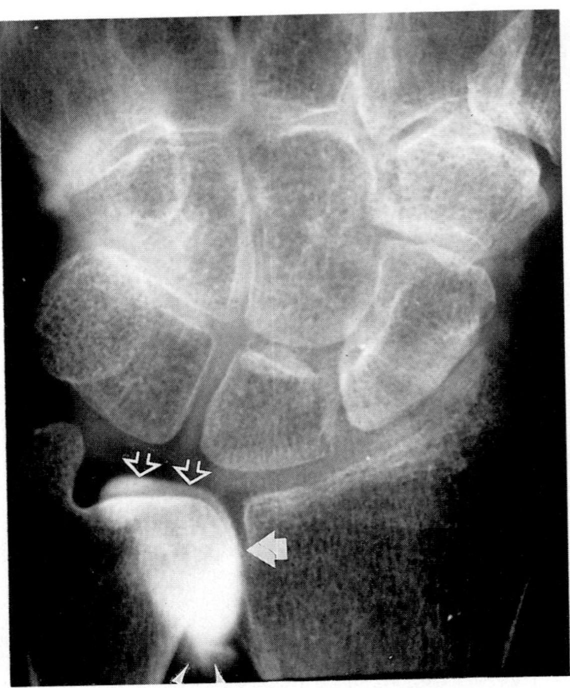

FIGURE 14–3. Normal PA view of a DRUJ arthrogram. The proximal ulnar border is formed by the ulnar head, the radial border by the ulnar notch of the radius (white arrow), and the distal border by the proximal surface of the TFC (open arrows). Minimal extravasation (white arrowheads) involves the proximal DRUJ capsule. This is a common site of extravasation with the fully distended DRUJ. Contrast in the MC and RC joints is from an earlier injection. No connection existed between the DRUJ and the RCJ.

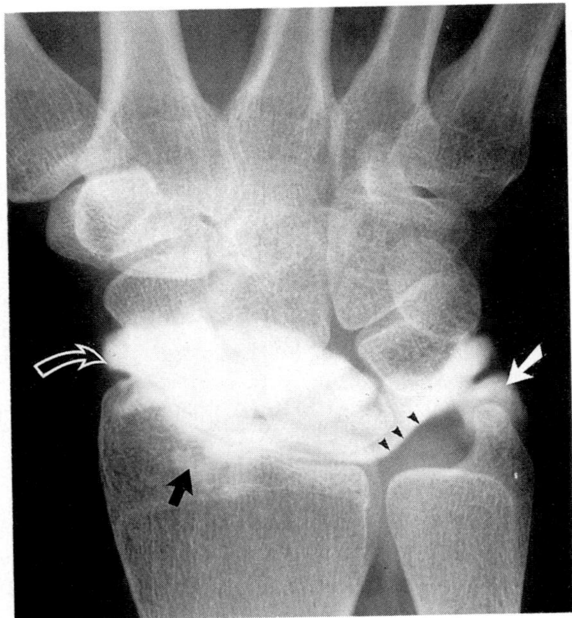

FIGURE 14–2. Normal radiocarpal joint (RCJ) arthrogram (PA view). White arrow, prestyloid recess; black arrowheads, distal surface of the TFC; black arrow, ventral radial recess; open arrow, dorsoscaphoid recess. Residual contrast from an earlier injection is in the DRUJ; no communication was present between the DRUJ and the RCJ.

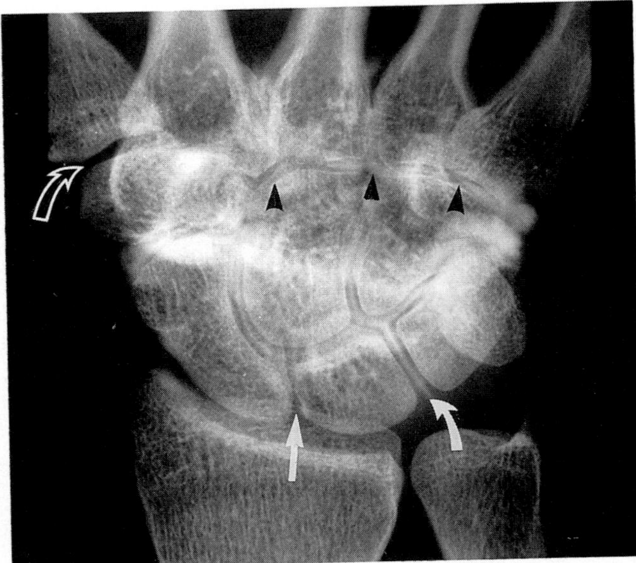

FIGURE 14–4. Normal MCJ arthrogram (PA). Contrast fills the space between the carpal bones and extends into the scapholunate (straight white arrow) and lunotriquetral joint spaces (curved white arrow) to outline the distal surface of the scapholunate and lunotriquetral ligaments, respectively. There is communication into carpometacarpal joints II to V (black arrowheads) but not into carpometacarpal joint I (open arrow).

between the proximal and distal carpal rows. Although normally there is no communication between the MCJ and the RCJ, there is commonly a communication between the MCJ and the common carpometacarpal and the second to fifth intermetacarpal joints.[1–3] The carpometacarpal joint of the thumb is completely enclosed by a capsule and does not communicate with the MCJ or the common carpometacarpal joint in most cases, as discussed later in this chapter.

Opacification of tendon sheaths and lymphatics, other than in the needle track site, is generally not observed in normal wrist arthrograms, although it is stated in the literature that filling of tendon sheaths may be apparent in 6% of normal individuals.[10,11]

General Comments

Ligamentous, cartilaginous, or capsular communicating defects may be complete (through and through) and seen on both adjacent compartments injected (bidirectional communication). A communicating defect may also occur in a "one-way valve" behavior (unidirectional communication) and can therefore be overlooked when only one compartment is injected (Fig. 14–5).[12–14] Some controversy exists in the literature as to whether one-way valve behavior of interosseous ligaments and TFC defects may be artifacts dependent on the degree of distention of the joint capsule and the sequence of injection[15,16] or represent real pathologic features.[12–14,17] A ligamentous or cartilaginous defect may also occur as an incomplete defect (not through and through or not communicating between two adjacent compartments) and can therefore be detected only by injecting both adjacent wrist compartments. For example, an incomplete perforation of the TFC or a proximal avulsion of the TFC from the base of the ulnar styloid can only be seen with distal radioulnar arthrography and not with radiocarpal arthrography (Fig. 14–6). In addition, patients may have more than one abnormality in different compartments; this would be missed on single-compartment arthrography alone. Therefore, as supported by some literature,[12–14] in our opinion an arthrographic study of the wrist should include injection of all three major compartments: the RCJ, the MCJ, and the DRUJ, if all abnormal findings (significant or not) are to be shown.

The use of the word "tear" should not be used when describing defects, since it implies acute trauma to some people, and arthrography cannot differentiate types or causes of communicating or noncommunicating defects.[18]

Technique

Our technique generally uses fluoroscopic control[19,20] with the patient prone on the fluoroscopy table, the arm raised above the head, the elbow extended, and the wrist prone. The skin of the dorsum of the wrist is cleansed sterilely and draped. Local anesthesia is placed superficially in the site to be injected. A 2:1 mixture of dilute water-soluble contrast (Conray-43 Iothalamate meglumine, Mallinckrodt, Inc., St. Louis, Mo.) to 1% lidocaine is used. The use of a diluted, less dense contrast medium allows easier observation of underlying bone, ligament, and cartilage details and decreases the possibility of contrast-induced

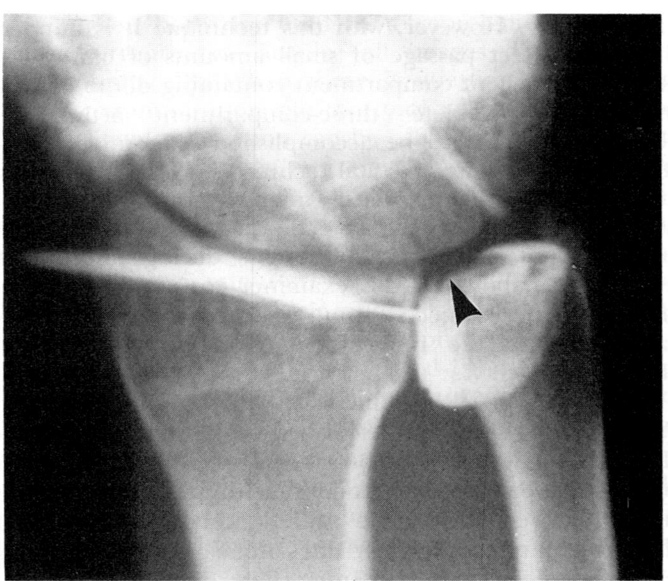

A

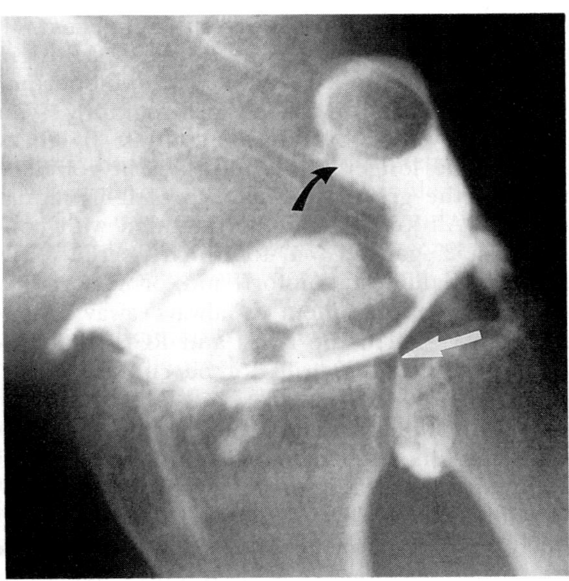

B

FIGURE 14–5. On DRUJ arthrography **(A)** performed immediately after MCJ injection, irregular demarcation of the proximal surface of the TFC (arrow) is visible (or this can also represent incomplete distention of the DRUJ), but there is no communication to the RCJ. After RCJ injection **(B)** contrast passes through a small radial-sided defect of the TFC (white arrow) into the DRUJ. There is also filling of the pisotriquetral joint (black arrow) as a common, normal variant of RCJ injection.

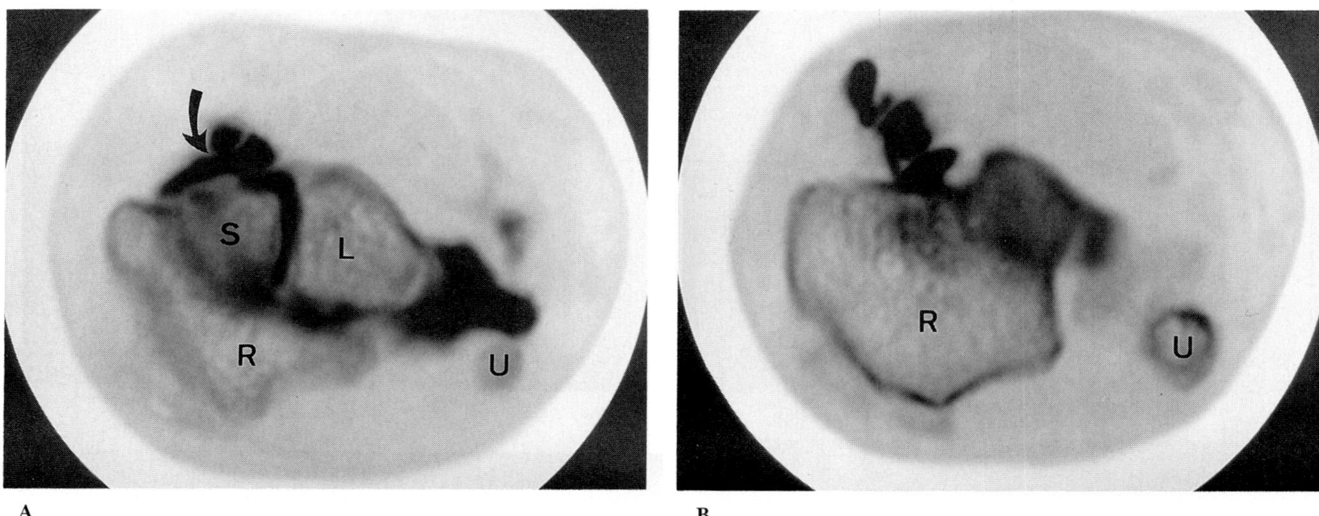

A B

FIGURE 14–41. Acute perforation of the scapholunate ligament associated with palmar intracapsular ligament perforations. **A** and **B:** Axial slices performed after arthrography shows the location of the capsular leak (arrow). R, radius; U, ulna; S, scaphoid; L, lunate.

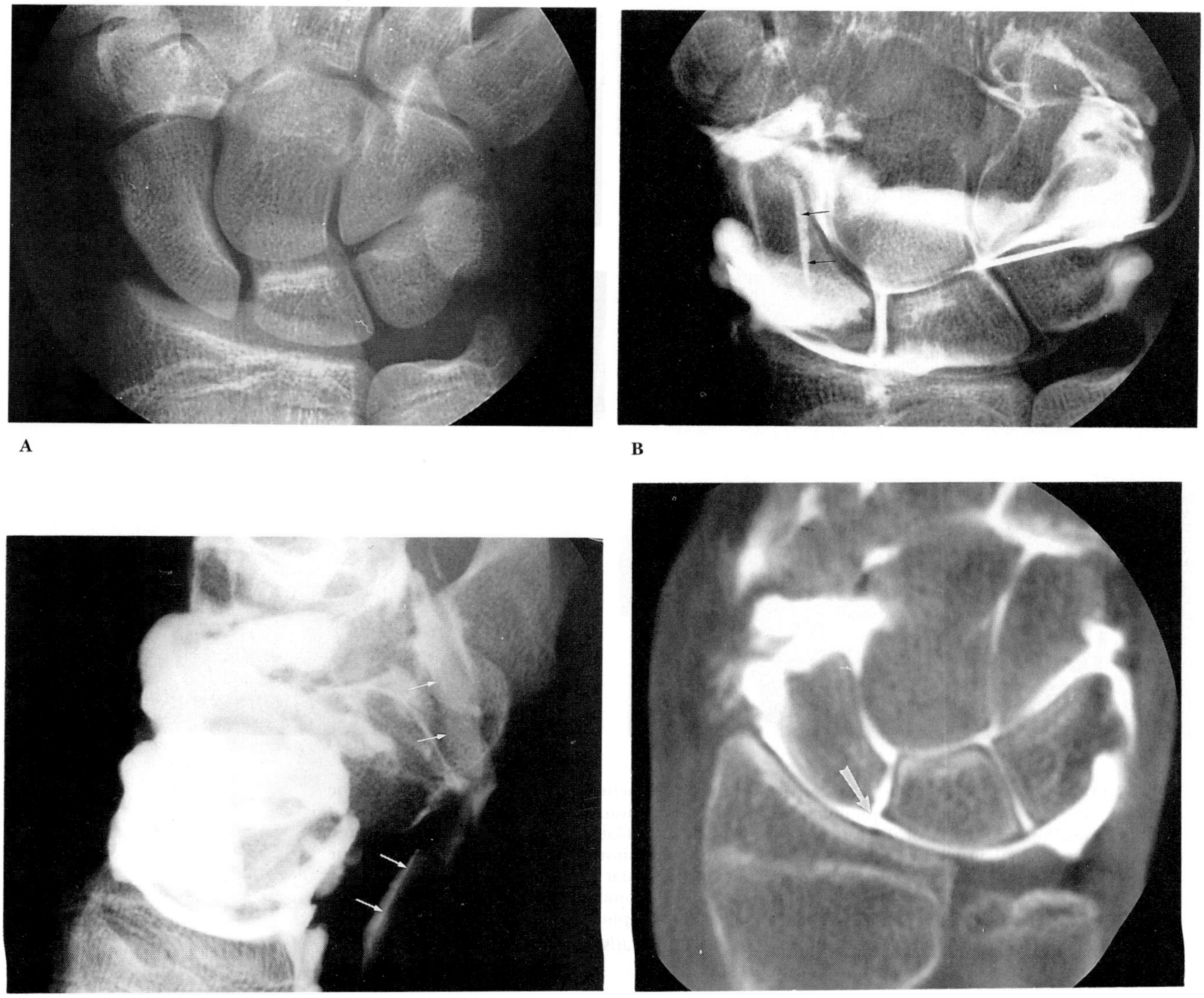

A B

C D

FIGURE 14–42. (A–D) *See legend on opposite page*

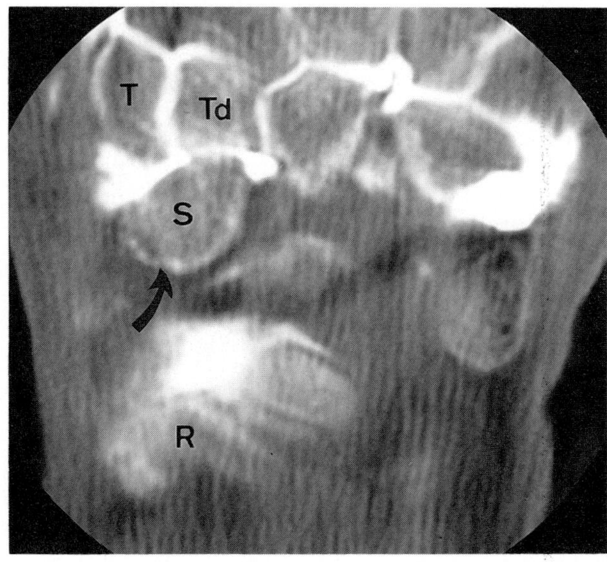

E

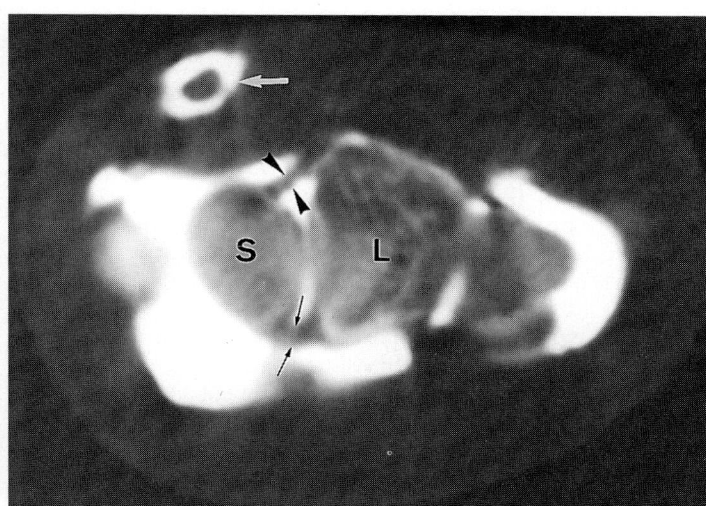

F

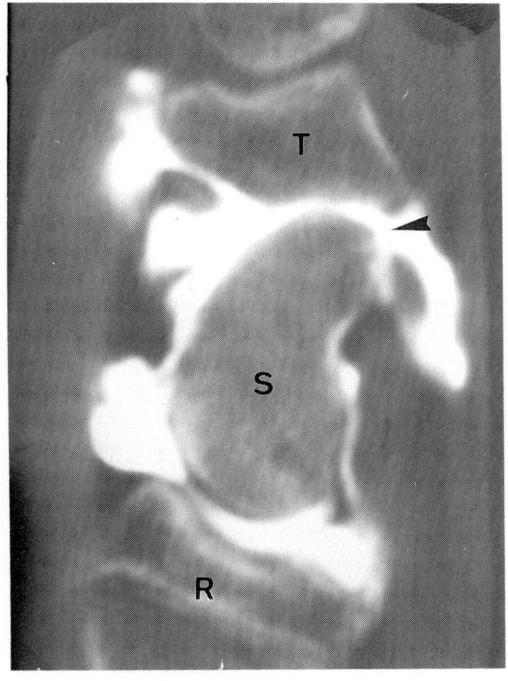

G

FIGURE 14–42. *Continued* Scaphoid fracture with perforations of the scapholunate ligament and ventroradial capsule. **A:** PA radiograph interpreted as normal. **B** and **C:** MCJ arthrogram shows a scapholunate ligament perforation and a communication with the sheath of the flexor carpi radialis (arrows). **D:** Coronal slice shows a scapholunate ligament perforation (arrow). **E:** Coronal slice illustrates a small fracture of the distal scaphoid (curved arrow). **F:** Axial slice shows the integrity of the palmar (between arrowheads) and dorsal (between small arrows) portions of the scapholunate ligament. Some contrast material is in the sheath of the flexor carpi radialis (white arrow). **G:** Slice performed along the long axis of the scaphoid demonstrates the location of the capsule perforation and the exact site of communication with the tendon sheath (arrowhead). In this case, CT–arthrography detected an occult fracture of the scaphoid and helped to precisely locate the site of a ligament perforation and a capsule leak not clearly detected with arthrography. R, radius; L, lunate; S, scaphoid; T, trapezium; Td, trapezoid.

Triangular Fibrocartilage

The TFC is well identified on coronal slices. The location and size of the TFC perforations are well appreciated. However, the fine anatomic detail obtained does not significantly modify the appreciation of lesions of the TFC made with arthrography, and therefore does not influence the clinical management of the patient.[30]

Ulnocarpal Impingement Syndrome

Ulnocarpal impingement has been noted in many disorders that decrease the height of the carpus and bring the ulnar carpal bones to a position in which they may abut the ulna. Ulnocarpal impingement has also been noted in disorders that decrease the relative length of the radius, such as idiopathic positive ulnar variance, fractures of the distal radius, and rheumatoid arthritis.[83,84]

The diagnosis of idiopathic ulnocarpal impingement is made on plain films when a positive ulnar variance and geodes (lucent defects) of the ulnar side of the lunate are present. Arthrography is performed to detect TFC or lunotriquetral ligament perforations and thinning or erosions of the cartilage of the lunate.[38] CT–arthrography demonstrates the bone lesions well but does not modify the diagnosis or the treatment (Fig. 14–43).

When ulnocarpal impingement is induced by a deformity due to a fracture of the distal radius, arthrography demonstrates the ligament perforations and CT is indicated to search for incongruity, degenerative changes or subluxation of the DRUJ.[66,85]

Scaphoid Nonunion

Wrist arthrography can be used to demonstrate if contrast passes through the fracture site of the scaphoid, showing communication between the MCJ and the RCJ as evidence of nonunion. On the contrary, the absence of contrast passing through the fracture line indicates a fibrous or a cartilaginous union.[86] In addition, arthrography demonstrates associated interosseous ligament perforations and the early signs of osteoarthritis such as thinning or erosions of cartilage.

Coronal and long parasagittal axes of the scaphoid are usually demonstrated with CT using the Pennes or the Sanders positions, respectively.[66,76,77] The former position shows radial or ulnar displacement of the distal fracture fragment. The latter also provides information about the position of fracture fragments and especially about any dorsal angulation of the proximal fragment or palmar or dorsal translation of the distal fragment. It can show development of a ''humpback'' deformity (dorsal exostosis) at the healed or healing scaphoid fracture site,[77] the status of graft incorporation to aid fracture union, and the status of healing or nonunion. Abutment of dorsal exostoses against the dorsal rim of the radius can also be evaluated.[66] Coupling arthrography and CT allows evaluation of all these features and is especially useful for determining the development of nonunion at fracture or arthrodeses sites (Figs. 14–44 and 14–45).

Ligament Perforations and Occult Fractures

The chronically or subacutely symptomatic wrist is a common challenge for the clinician since most of the

Text continued on page 399

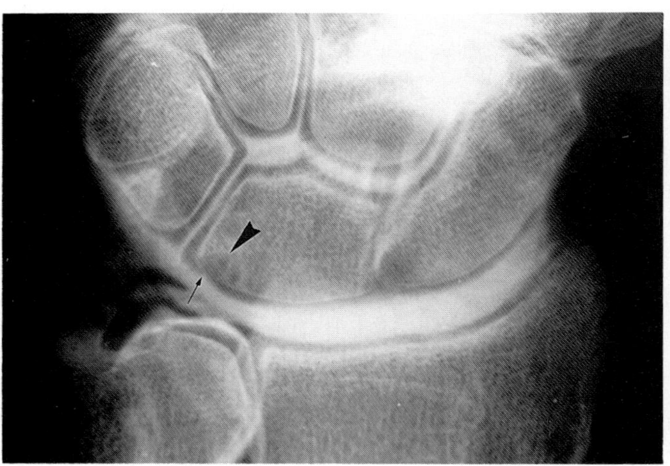

A

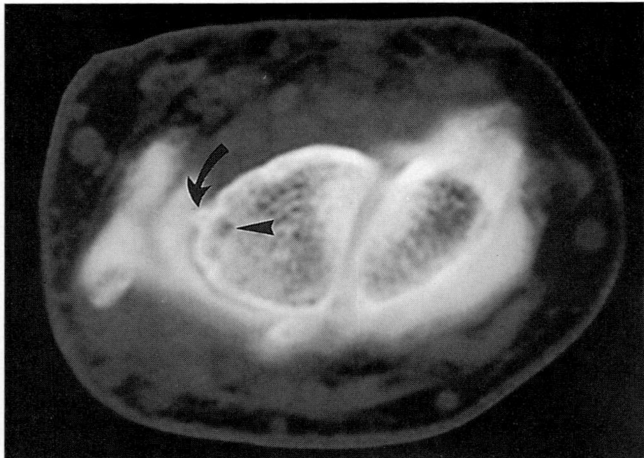

B

FIGURE 14–43. Ulnocarpal impingement syndrome. **A:** Arthrogram (view obtained with traction applied to the wrist) shows a lunotriquetral perforation, a central TFC perforation, lucent defects (geodes?) of the lunate (arrowhead), and an erosion of the cartilage of the lunate (arrow). **B:** Axial slice shows lucent defects (geodes?) of the lunate (arrowhead) and a small spur on its ulnar side (curved arrow).

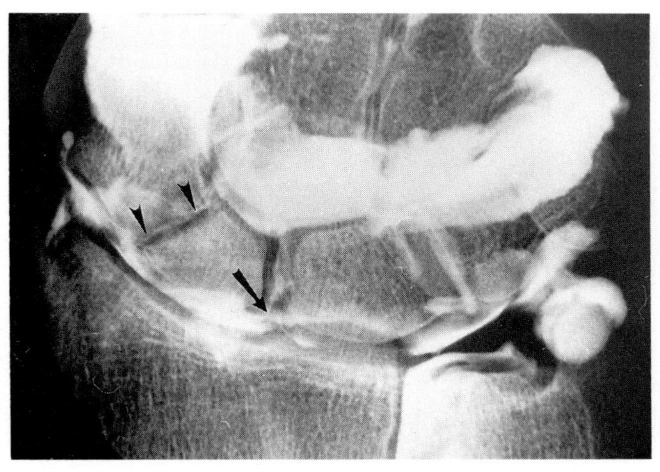

A

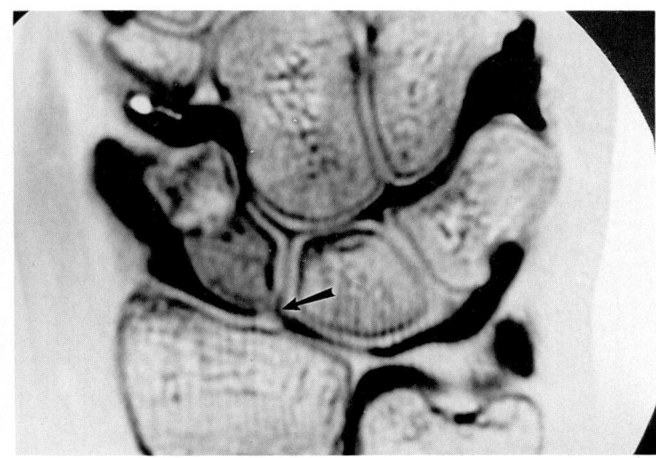

B

C

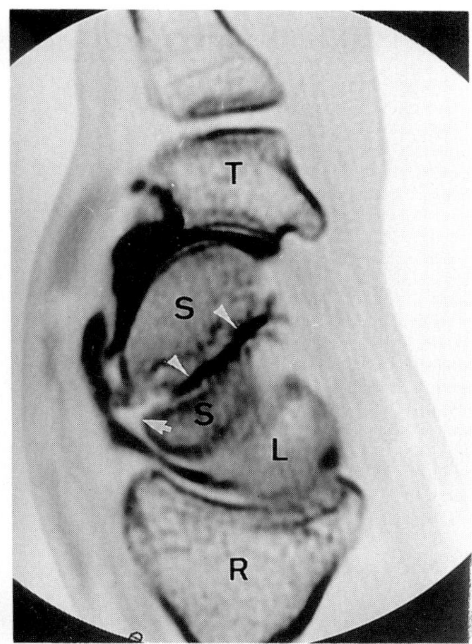

D

FIGURE 14–44. Nonunion of the scaphoid and perforation of the scapholunate ligament. **A:** Arthrogram demonstrates communication between the MCJ and the RCJ through the fracture line (arrowheads) and through a perforation of the scapholunate ligament (arrow). **B:** Coronal slice shows a perforation of the scapholunate ligament (arrow) and some fibrous or cartilaginous tissue within the fracture line. **C** and **D:** Slices performed along the long axis of the scaphoid show the presence of fibrous or cartilaginous tissue (white arrows), contrast material along the ventral portion of the fracture site (white arrowheads), a dorsal exostosis of the distal fragment of the scaphoid (arrow), palmar angulation of the distal fragment, and thinning of the cartilage of the proximal pole of the scaphoid. R, radius; L, lunate; S, scaphoid; T, trapezium.

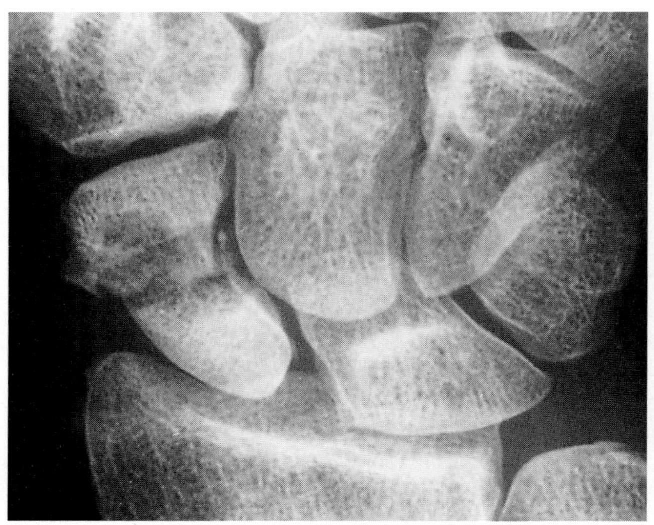
A

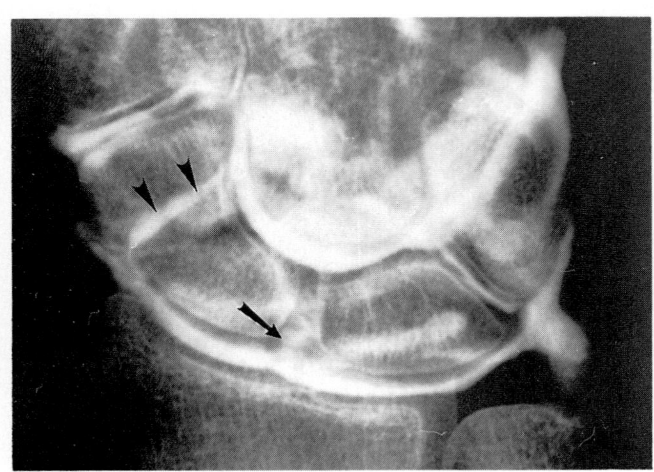
B

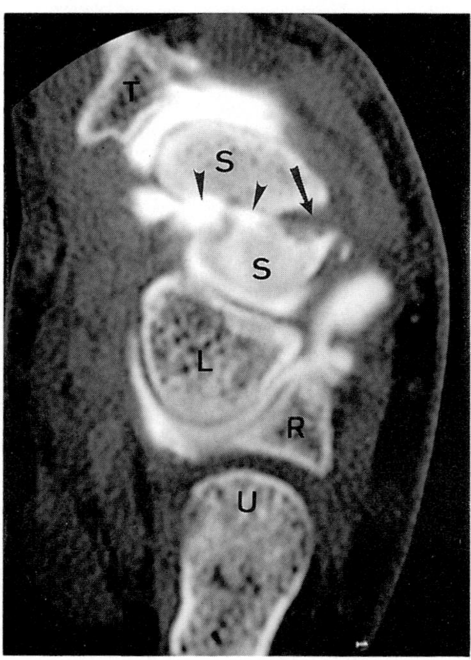

C

FIGURE 14–45. Scaphoid nonunion and perforation of the scapholunate ligament. **A:** PA radiograph shows a scapholunate gap, nonunion of the scaphoid, increased density of its proximal fragment, and radial displacement of the distal scaphoid fracture fragment. **B:** Arthrogram (view obtained with traction applied to the wrist) demonstrates a scapholunate ligament perforation (arrow) and the scaphoid nonunion as evidenced by contrast in the scaphoid fracture site (arrowheads). **C:** Slice performed along the long axis of the scaphoid shows fibrous or cartilaginous tissue at the dorsal portion of the fracture line (arrow) and contrast media at its palmar portion (arrowheads). Palmar tilt of the distal fragment is well demonstrated. R, radius; L, lunate; S, scaphoid; U, ulna.

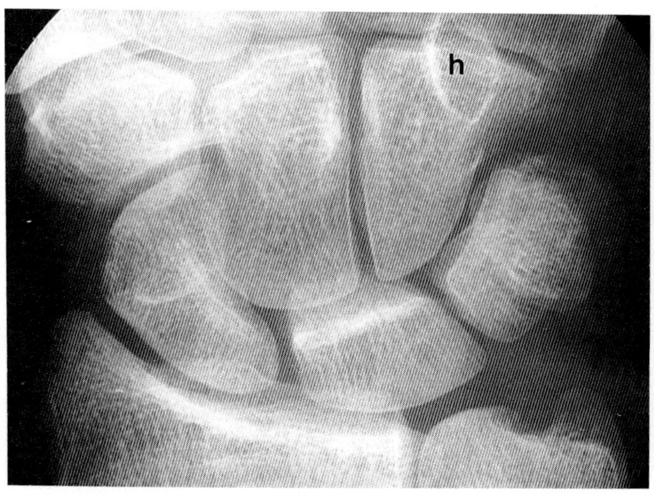

A

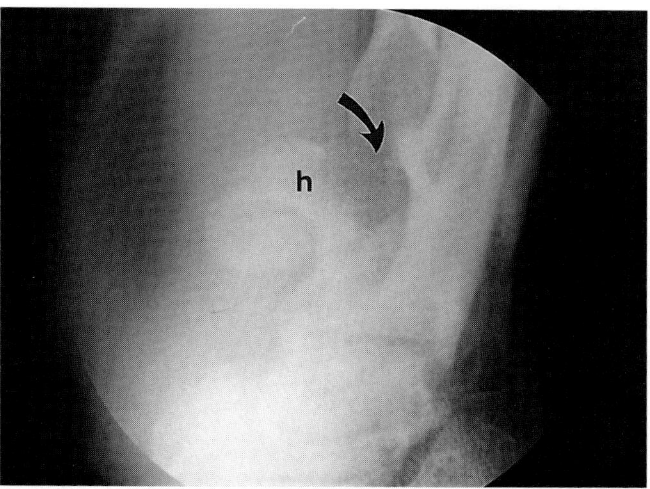

B

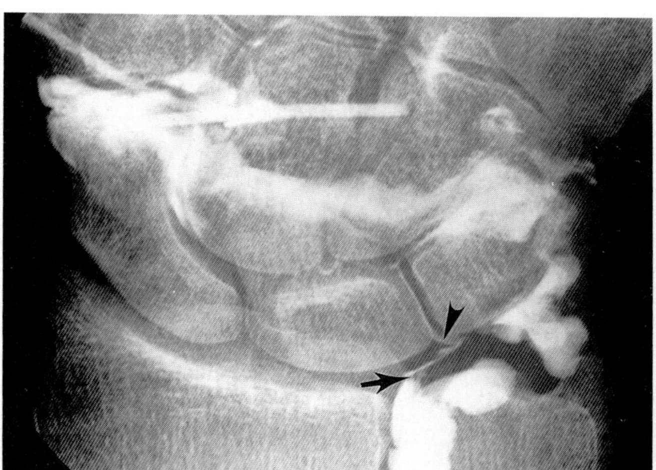

C

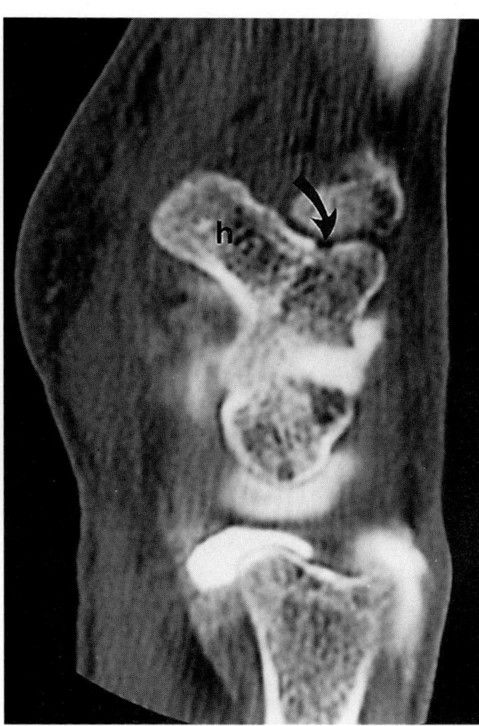

D

FIGURE 14–46. Fracture of the hamate associated with perforations of the lunotriquetral ligament and the TFC. **A:** PA view of the wrist does not show any abnormality. The hook of the hamate (h) is well defined. **B:** A small fracture at the base of the hook of the hamate (arrow) is suspected with the view described by Papilion et al.[89] **C:** TFC (arrow) and lunotriquetral (arrowhead) perforations are demonstrated with an MCJ injection. **D:** The fracture of the hook of the hamate base (arrow) is demonstrated with sagittal slices. h, hook of the hamate. (Panels A–D reprinted with permission from Papilion JD, DuPuy TE, Aulicino PL, Bergfield TG, Gwathmey FW. Radiographic evaluation of the hook of the hamate: A new technique. *J Hand Surg* 1988;13A:437–439.)

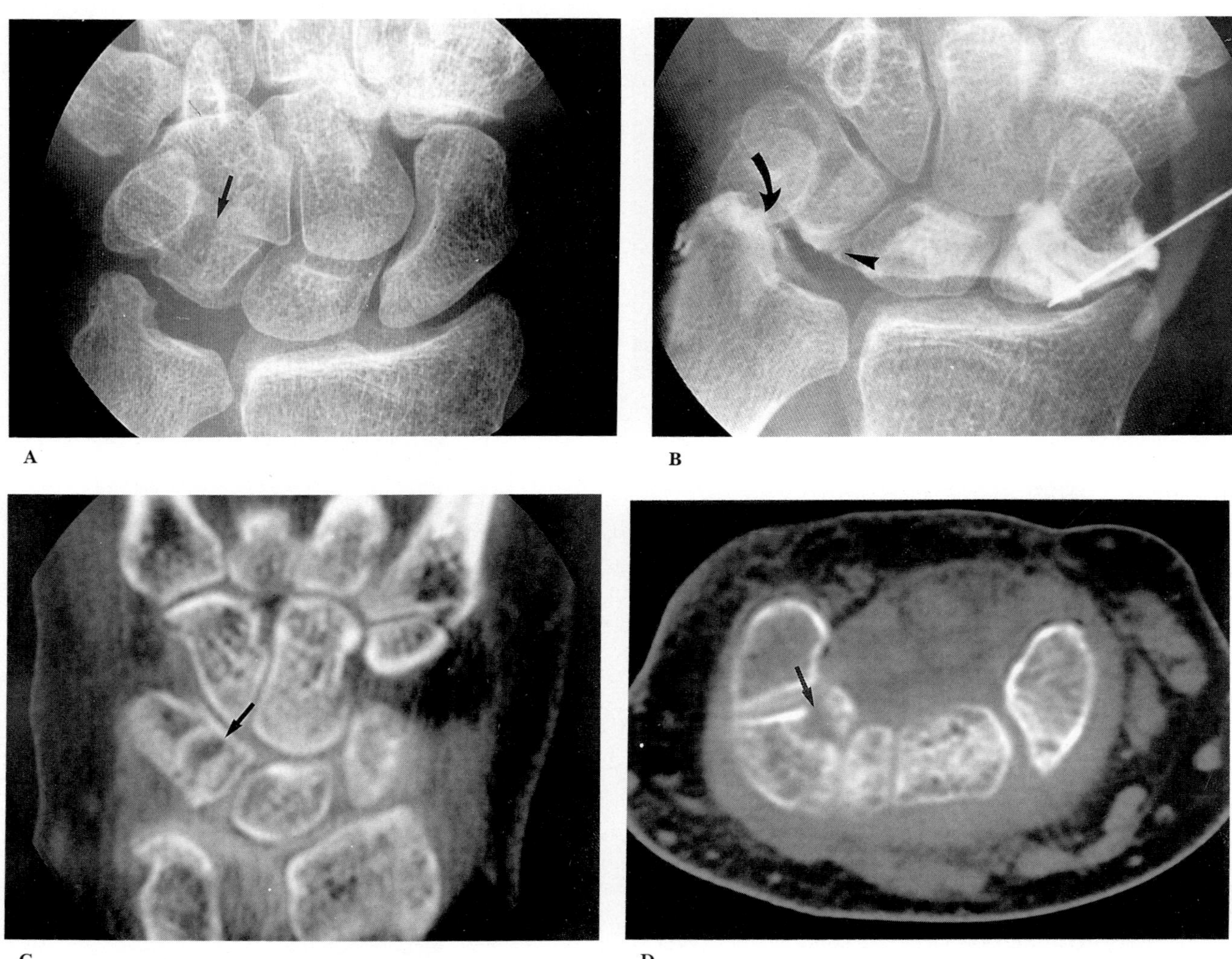

FIGURE 14–47. Triquetral fracture associated with a perforation of the lunotriquetral ligament and an avulsion of the TFC. **A:** Suspicion of a triquetral fracture (arrow) on the PA radiograph of the wrist. **B:** RCJ arthrography shows an ulnar avulsion of the TFC (curved arrow) and a lunotriquetral perforation (arrowhead). **C** and **D:** Coronal and axial slices. The rapid resorption of contrast media in this patient makes analysis of the ligaments difficult; however, the fracture of the triquetrum (arrow) is well demonstrated.

patients display nonspecific clinical findings with normal plain films and stress views. In such cases, some authors propose performing arthrography first, whereas others advocate the use of a bone scan. When prominent focal increased uptake is noted, a CT or an MRI examination is then performed.[87,88]

In our experience, in these particular patients an arthrographic and CT–arthrographic examination has proved efficient to detect both ligament tears and occult fractures of the wrist. With this procedure, a quick and accurate as well as less costly diagnosis is obtained, avoiding the use of additional examinations to reach the same diagnosis. Therefore, using this approach could thus simplify the decision algorithm.

In our experience, fractures of the hamate and triquetrum can be difficult to diagnose with plain films. Since these fractures are often associated with perforations of the TFC and the lunotriquetral ligament, we believe CT–arthrography is the examination of choice to demonstrate all these findings (Figs. 14–46 and 14–47).

CONCLUSION

Arthrography and CT are two common and reliable techniques for examination of the wrist. In our practice, use of both together proves to be more efficient than each of these techniques used separately. CT–arthrography is indicated in the chronically symptomatic wrist, in the overall evaluation of the scapholunate ligament tears, and in scaphoid nonunion. Until improved MRI techniques provide as good or better contrast-to-noise ratio and spatial resolution as CT–arthrography, the latter will continue to be a valuable diagnostic tool in the detection of bone and ligament lesions.

REFERENCES

1. Gold RH. Arthrography of the wrist. In: Arndt RD, Horns JW, Gold RH, Blaschke DD, eds. *Clinical arthrography.* 2nd ed. Baltimore: Williams & Wilkins, 1985:221–245.
2. Gilula LA, Hardy DC, Totty WG. Wrist arthrography: An updated review. *J Med Imag* 1988;2:252–266.
3. Resnick D. Arthrography and tenography of the hand and wrist. In: Dalinka MK, ed. *Arthrography.* New York: Springer Verlag, 1980:165–175.
4. Blair WF, Berger RA, El-Khoury GY. Arthrotomography of the wrist: An experimental and preliminary clinical study. *J Hand Surg* 1985;10A:350–359.
5. Kessler I, Silberman Z. An experimental study of the radiocarpal joint by arthrography. *Surg Gynecol Obstet* 1961;112:33–40.
6. Lewis OJ, Hamshere RJ, Bucknill TM. The anatomy of the wrist joint. *J Anat* 1970;106:539–552.
7. Mikic Z. Arthrography of the wrist joint: An experimental study. *J Bone Joint Surg* 1984;66A:371–378.
8. Palmer AK, Levinsohn EM, Kuzma GR. Arthrography of the wrist. *J Hand Surg* 1983;8:15–23.
9. Levinsohn EM, Palmer AK. Arthrography of the traumatized wrist: Correlation with radiography and carpal instability series. *Radiology* 1983;146:647–651.
10. Harrison MO, Freiberger RH, Ranawat CS. Arthrography of the rheumatoid wrist joint. *AJR* 1971;112:480–486.
11. Trentham DE, Hamm RL, Masi AT. Wrist arthrography: Review and comparison of normals, rheumatoid arthritis and gout patients. *Semin Arthritis Rheum* 1975;5:105–120.
12. Zinberg EM, Palmer AK, Coren AB, Levinsohn EM. The triple injection wrist arthrogram. *J Hand Surg* 1988;13A:803–809.
13. Tirman RM, Weber ER, Snyder LL, Koonce TW. Midcarpal wrist arthrography for detection of tears of the scapholunate and lunatotriquetral ligaments. *AJR* 1985;144:107–108.
14. Levinsohn EM, Rosen ID, Palmer AK. Wrist arthrography: Value of the three-compartment injection method. *Radiology* 1991;179:231–239.
15. Wilson AJ, Gilula LA, Mann FA. Unidirectional joint communications in wrist arthrography: An evaluation of 250 cases. *AJR* 1991;157:105–109.
16. Manaster BJ. The clinical efficacy of triple-injection wrist arthrography. *Radiology* 1991;178:267–270.
17. Viegas SF, Ballantyne G. Attritional lesions of the wrist joint. *J Hand Surg* 1987;12A:1025–1029.
18. Gilula LA, Palmer AK. Is it possible to call a "tear" on arthrography or MRI? Letter to the editor. *Radiology* 1993; 187:582.
19. Braunstein EM, Louis DS, Greene TL, Hankin FM. Fluoroscopic and arthrographic evaluation of carpal instability. *AJR* 1985;144:1259–1262.
20. Gilula LA, Totty WG, Weeks PM. Wrist arthrography: The value of fluoroscopic spot viewing. *Radiology* 1983;146:555–556.
21. Gunther SF. The medial four carpometacarpal joints. In: Lichtman DM, ed. *The wrist and its disorders.* Philadelphia: WB Saunders, 1988:199–210.
22. Hall FM, Goldberg RP, Wyshak G, Kilcoyne RF. Shoulder arthrography: Comparison of morbidity after use of various contrast media. *Radiology* 1985;154:339–341.
23. Resnick D, Andre M, Kerr R, Pineda C, Guerra J Jr, Atkinson D. Digital arthrography of the wrist: A radiographic-pathologic investigation. *AJR* 1984;142:1187–1190.
24. Quinn SF, Pittman CC, Belsole R, Greene T, Rayhack J. Digital subtraction wrist arthrography: Evaluation of the multiple-compartment technique. *AJR* 1988;151:1173–1174.
25. Manaster BJ. Digital wrist arthrography: Precision in determining the site of radiocarpal-midcarpal communication. *AJR* 1986;147:563–566.
26. Yin YM, Wilson AJ, Gilula LA. *The value of digital subtraction images in three compartment wrist arthrography.* Presented at the ASSH National Meeting, Cincinnati, OH, 1994.
27. Conway WF, Hayes CW. Three-compartment wrist arthrography: Use of low-iodine-concentration contrast agent to decrease study time. *Radiology* 1989;173:569–570.
28. Berger RA, Blair WF, El-Khoury GY. Arthrotomography of the wrist. *Clin Orthop* 1984;186:224–229.
29. Blum AG. *New indicator of scapholunate ligament tear: Fibrosis within the scapholunate joint.* Abstract. Presented at RSNA, Chicago, IL, December 1992.
30. Quinn SF, Belsole RS, Greene TL, Rayhack JM. Work in progress: Postarthrography computed tomography of the wrist: Evaluation of the triangular fibrocartilage complex. *Skeletal Radiol* 1989;17:565–569.
31. Dalinka MK, Turner ML, Osterman AL, Batra P. Wrist arthrography. *Radiol Clin North Am* 1981;19:217–226.
32. Gilula LA, Hardy DC, Totty WG, Reinus WR. Fluoroscopic identification of torn intercarpal ligaments after injection of contrast material. *AJR* 1987;149:761–764.
33. Metz VM, Gilula LA. Is this scapholunate joint and ligament abnormal? *J Hand Surg* 1993;18A:746–755.
34. Mikic Z. Age related changes in the triangular fibrocartilage of the wrist. *J Anat* 1978;126:367–384.
35. Ganel A, Engel J, Ditzian R, Militeanu J. Arthrography as a method of diagnosing soft-tissue injuries of the wrist. *J Trauma* 1979;19:367–380.
36. Manaster BJ. Digital wrist arthrography: Precision in determining the site of radiocarpal-midcarpal communication. *AJR* 1986;147:563–566.
37. Reinus WR, Hardy DC, Totty WG, Gilula LA. Arthrographic evaluation of the carpal triangular fibrocartilage complex. *J Hand Surg* 1987;12A:495–503.

38. Palmer AK. Triangular fibrocartilage lesions: A classification. *J Hand Surg* 1989;14A:594–606.
39. Hardy DC, Totty WG, Carnes KM, et al. Arthrographic surface anatomy of the carpal triangular fibrocartilage. *J Hand Surg* 1988;13A:823–829.
40. Resnick D. Arthrography in the evaluation of arthritic disorders of the wrist. *Radiology* 1974;113:331–340.
41. Andren L, Eiken O. Arthrographic studies of wrist ganglions. *J Bone Joint Surg* 1971;53A:299–301.
42. Maloney MD, Sauser DD, Hanson EC, Wood VE, Thiel AE. Adhesive capsulitis of the wrist: Arthrographic diagnosis. *Radiology* 1988;167:187–190.
43. Bottke CA, Louis DS, Braunstein EM. Diagnosis and treatment of obscure ulnar-sided wrist pain. *Orthopedics* 1989;12:1075–1079.
44. Manaster BJ, Mann RJ, Rubenstein S. Wrist pain: Correlation of clinical and plain film findings with arthrographic results. *J Hand Surg* 1989;14A:466–473.
45. Metz VM, Mann FA, Gilula LA. Three compartment wrist arthrography: Correlation of pain site with location of uni- or bidirectional communications. *AJR* 1993;160:819–822.
46. Metz VM, Mann FA, Gilula LA. Lack of correlation of wrist pain with noncommunicating defects of the interosseous ligaments, triangular fibrocartilage, and joint capsules demonstrated by three-compartment wrist arthrography. *AJR* 1993;160:1239–1243.
47. Herbert TJ, Faithfull RG, McCann DJ, Ireland J. Bilateral arthrography of the wrist. *J Hand Surg* 1990;15B:233–235.
48. Cantor RM, Stern PJ, Wyrick JD. *Selective bilateral wrist arthrography.* Abstract. Presented at the ASSH National Meeting, Phoenix, AZ, November 1992.
49. Yin Y, Evanoff B, Gilula LA, Littenberg G, Pilgram T. *The role of bilateral three compartment wrist arthrography in surgeon's decision making with chronic wrist pain patients: A prospective study.* Submitted to AUR (American University Radiologist) Annual Meeting, 1995.
50. Schweitzer ME, Brahme SK, Hodler J, et al. Chronic wrist pain: Spin-echo and short tau inversion recovery MR imaging and conventional and MR-arthrography. *Radiology* 1992;182:205–211.
51. Kang HS, Kindynis P, Brahme SK, et al. Triangular fibrocartilage and intercarpal ligaments of the wrist: MR-imaging. *Radiology* 1991;181:401–404.
52. Zlatkin MB, Chao PC, Osterman AL, Schnall MD, Dalinka MK, Kressel HY. Chronic wrist pain: Evaluation with high resolution MR-imaging. *Radiology* 1989;173:723–729.
53. Metz VM, Schratter M, Dock WI, et al. Age-associated changes of the triangular fibrocartilage of the wrist: Evaluation of the diagnostic performance of MR-imaging. *Radiology* 1992;184:217–220.
54. Rosenthal DI, Murray WT, Smith RJ. Finger arthrography. *Radiology* 1980;137:647–651.
55. Gerber NJ, Dixon A. Synovial cysts and juxtaarticular bone cysts (geodes). *Semin Arthritis Rheum* 1974;3:323–348.
56. Resnick D, Danzig LA. Arthrographic evaluation of injuries of the first metacarpophalangeal joint: Gamekeeper's thumb. *AJR* 1976;126:1046–1052.
57. Weston WJ. The normal arthrogram of the metacarpophalangeal, metatarsophalangeal and interphalangeal joints. *Australas Radiol* 1969;13:211–234.
58. Linscheid RL. Arthrography of the metacarpophalangeal joint. *Clin Orthop* 1974;103:91–96.
59. Bowers WH, Hurst LC. Gamekeeper's thumb: Evaluation by arthrography and stress roentgenography. *J Bone Joint Surg* 1977;59A:519–524.
60. Stener B. Displacement of the ruptured ulnar collateral ligament of the metacarpophalangeal joint of the thumb. *J Bone Joint Surg* 1962;44B:869–879.
61. Kraemer BA, Gilula LA. Metacarpal fractures and dislocations. In: Gilula LA, ed. *The traumatized hand and wrist: Radiographic and anatomic correlation.* Philadelphia: WB Saunders, 1992:171–219.
62. Weston WJ, Palmer DG. *Soft tissues of the extremities: A radiologic study of rheumatoid disease.* New York: Springer-Verlag, 1977.
63. Ono H, Gilula LA, Marzke MW, Obermann WR. Bicompartmentalization of the radiocarpal joint. *J Hand Surg,* submitted.
64. Gundry CR, Brahme SK, Schwaighofer B, Kang HS, Sartoris DJ, Resnick D. Is MR better than arthrography for evaluating the ligaments of the wrist? In vitro study. *AJR* 1990;154:337–341.
65. Berger RA, Blair WF, El-Khoury GY. Arthrotomography of the wrist: The triangular fibrocartilage complex. *Clin Orthop* 1983;172:257–264.
66. Stewart NR, Gilula LA. CT of the wrist: A tailored approach. *Radiology* 1992;183:13–20.
67. Biondetti PR, Vannier MW, Gilula LA, Knapp R. Wrist: Coronal and transaxial CT scanning. *Radiology* 1987;163:149–151.
68. Bush CH, Gillespy T, Dell PC. High-resolution CT of the wrist: Initial experience with scaphoid disorders and surgical fusions. *AJR* 1987;149:757–760.
69. Cone RO, Szabo R, Resnick D, Gelberman R, Taleisnik J, Gilula LA. Computed tomography of the normal soft tissues of the wrist. *Invest Radiol* 1983;18:546–551.
70. Egawa M, Asai T. Fracture of the hook of the hamate: Report of six cases and the suitability of computerized tomography. *J Hand Surg* 1983;8:393–398.
71. Friedman L, Yong-Hing K, Johnston GH. Forty degree angled coronal CT scanning of scaphoid fractures through plaster and fiberglass casts. *J Comput Assist Tomogr* 1989;3:1101–1104.
72. Hindman BW, Kulik WJ, Lee G, Avolio RE. Occult fractures of the carpals and metacarpals: Demonstration by CT. *AJR* 1989;153:529–532.
73. Merhar GL, Clark RA, Schneider HJ, Stern PJ. High-resolution computed tomography of the wrist in patients with carpal tunnel syndrome. *Skeletal Radiol* 1986;15:549–552.
74. Muren C, Nygren E, Svartegren G. Computed tomography of the scaphoid in the longitudinal axis of the bone. *Acta Radiol* 1990;31:110–111.
75. Brody AS, Ball WS, Towbin RB. Computed arthrotomography as an adjunct to pediatric arthrography. *Radiology* 1989;170:99–102.
76. Pennes DR, Jonsson K, Buckwalter KA. Direct coronal CT of the scaphoid bone. *Radiology* 1989;171:870–871.
77. Sanders WE. Evaluation of the humpback scaphoid by computed tomography in the longitudinal axial plane of the scaphoid. *J Hand Surg* 1988;13A:182–187.
78. Linscheid RL, Dobyns JH, Beabout JW, Bryan RS. Traumatic instability of the wrist: Diagnosis, classification and pathomechanics. *J Bone Joint Surg* 1972;54A:1612–1632.
79. Mayfield JK, Johnson RP, Kilcoyne RK. The ligaments of the human wrist and their functional significance. *Anat Rec* 1976;186:417–428.
80. Taleisnik J. The ligaments of the wrist. *J Hand Surg* 1976;1:110–118.
81. Cooney III WP, Linscheid RL, Dobyns JH. Fractures and dislocations of the wrist. In: Rockwood CA, Green DP, Bucholz RW, eds. *Fractures in adults,* Vol. 1. 3rd ed. Philadelphia: JB Lippincott Company, 1991:563.
82. Blum AG, Claudon M, Regent D, Boyer B, Grignon B, Bazin C. New indicator of scapholunate ligament tear: Fibrosis within the scapholunate joint. *Radiology* 1992;185:115.
83. Bell MJ, Hill RJ, McMurtry RY. Ulnar impingement syndrome. *J Bone Joint Surg* 1985;67B:126–129.
84. Bowers WH. The distal radio-ulnar joint. In: Green DP, ed. *Operative hand surgery,* Vol. 2. New York: Churchill Livingstone, 1988:939.
85. Mino DE, Palmer AK, Levinsohn EM. Radiography and computerized tomography in the diagnosis of incongruity of the distal radioulnar joint: A prospective study. *J Bone Joint Surg* 1985;67A:247–252.
86. Roy C, Godin C, Dussault RG. Complementary role of wrist arthrography in non-union of scaphoid fractures. *J Can Assoc Radiol* 1985;36:870–871.
87. Pin PG, Semenkovich JW, Young VL, et al. Role of radionuclide imaging in the evaluation of wrist pain. *J Hand Surg* 1988;13A:810–814.
88. Wilson AJ, Mann FA, Gilula LA. Imaging the hand and the wrist. *J Hand Surg* 1990;15B:153–167.
89. Papilion JD, DuPuy TE, Aulicino PL, Bergfield TG, Gwathmey FW. Radiographic evaluation of the hook of the hamate: A new technique. *J Hand Surg* 1988;13A:437–439.

CHAPTER 15

LIGAMENTOGRAPHY A Method of Imaging Intracapsular Wrist Ligaments*

Richard A. Berger and Willem R. Obermann

INTRODUCTION

To fully understand normal and pathologic wrist joint mechanics, the contribution of the intracapsular ligaments must be accounted for. This requires accurate imaging of the ligaments in a way that ideally will not disturb the normal mechanics of the wrist. The first attempts to study the association of the intracapsular wrist ligaments with joint function were dependent on direct visualization.[1–4] This method, however, has an indeterminate effect on the mechanics of the wrist by virtue of disturbing the in situ anatomy. Arthrography and arthrotomography have been employed in the wrist and other joints to counter the detrimental effects of gross dissection by outlining various intraarticular soft-tissue structures, such as menisci and intraarticular ligaments.[5–9] A major drawback to these techniques, however, is that only the joint surface of the structure being studied is outlined by the contrast material in the joint space. Therefore, no information regarding the substance of the structure can be obtained from the radiographs unless a communication between the abnormality and the surface of the structure exists. Magnetic resonance imaging (MRI) has introduced the potential for viewing intraarticular soft tissues in a noninvasive manner.[10–15] In the laboratory, several methods of radiographically imaging intracapsular ligaments have been employed, including coating the outer surface of the ligament with titanium paint,[16] implanting wires within the substance of the ligament,[17,18] implanting metal pellets within the substance of the ligament,[19] and marking the bony origins of the ligament with metal pellets. Each method has technical drawbacks, including an inability to show the three-dimensional substance of the ligament, and ethical constraints in studying the behavior of the structures in vivo. It has been demonstrated that the capsular wrist ligaments are "ensheathed" by fibrous laminae on their superficial surfaces and by synovial cells lining their joint surfaces.[20] Using this information, we developed the hypothesis that capsular ligaments can be directly injected with radiographic contrast material, a process we have defined as *ligamentography,* which potentially allows radiographic imaging of the entire course and depth of an injected ligament. This chapter defines the histologic features of capsular ligaments that allow ligamentograms to be obtained, describes the methods of producing ligamentograms, and presents representative images of the major carpal ligaments, which have been targeted in a recent research study.

** Figures 15–1 to 15–5, 15–7, and 15–11 to 15–15 reprinted with permission of the Mayo Foundation, Rochester, MN.*

LIGAMENT ARCHITECTURE

Histologic Organization of Ligaments

There are three basic categories of ligaments in the human wrist: capsular, intraarticular, and mesocapsular.[20–22] Capsular ligaments are arranged histologically in a manner analogous to all other laminated connective tissues in the human body, such as nerve, muscle, and tendon. Variably sized collagen bundles, or fascicles, are oriented in a relatively parallel fashion throughout the length of the ligament. Often these fascicles course in parallel bundles or fascicles slightly offset to each other. These fascicles are surrounded by perifascicular "spaces" composed of loosely organized (areolar) connective tissue (Fig. 15–1). Through these spaces course blood vessels and nerves. The usual pattern found consists of three or four major collagen fascicles surrounding a neurovascular bundle in the perifascicular space. Near the

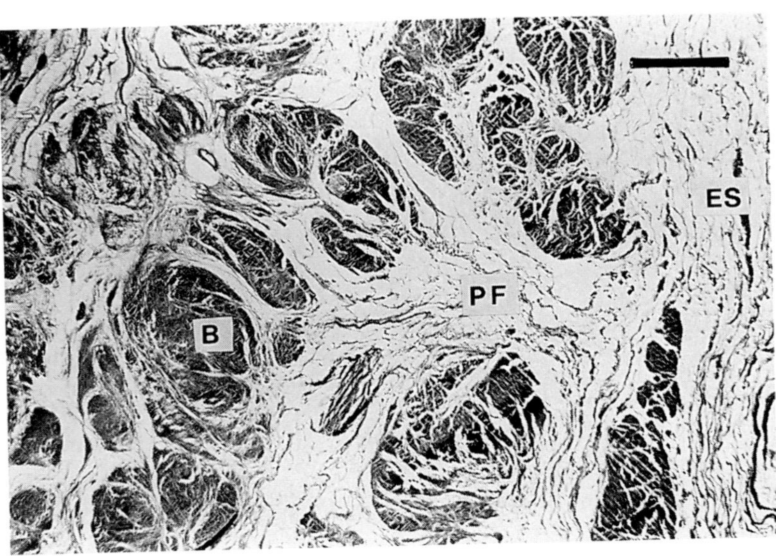

FIGURE 15–1. Histologic cross-section of the superficial (nonjoint) epiligamentous zone of the radioscaphocapitate ligament, a capsular ligament. Dense collagen fascicles (B) and parallel collagen fibers are surrounded by a loosely organized perifascicular zone (PF) of connective tissue. This perifascicular zone transmits longitudinally oriented nerves and blood vessels and superficially coalesces to form the epiligamentous zone (ES). The epiligament zone is composed of loose connective tissue with nerves and blood vessels. Hematoxylin and eosin, 100×.

surface of the capsular ligament, the perifascicular spaces coalesce to form the epiligamentum, which is also composed of loose areolar connective tissue with numerous large nerves and blood vessels. On the superficial surface of the ligament, the epiligamentum is lined by dense connective tissue representing the fibrous lamina of the joint capsule (Fig. 15–1). On the deep, or joint, surface of the ligament, synoviocytes line the epiligamentum as cuboidal cells, generally two to three cells thick, as a continuous lamina of cells (Fig. 15–2). In those areas where two or more capsular ligaments merge, the perifascicular space diminishes dramatically and the collagen fascicles delaminate as they interweave (Fig. 15–3). This same pattern occurs at a bony insertion of a capsular ligament, where the perifascicular space diminishes, the bundled appearance of the collagen fascicles is lost, and a transition from collagen to fibrocartilage to mineralized (calcified) fibrocartilage to bone is found.[6]

Intraarticular ligaments are different from capsular ligaments in several ways. First, intraarticular ligaments are generally lined on exposed surfaces of perifascicular tissue by synoviocytes, with no dense connective tissue layer consistent with the fibrous lamina of the joint capsule. Additionally, the intraarticular ligaments of the wrist are generally shorter than their capsular counterparts. Finally, intraarticular ligaments are prone to mixed composition, incorporating fibrocartilage into their structure, particularly if they extend into the actual intraarticular space.

Gross Organization of Carpal Ligaments

The carpal ligaments can be divided into several groupings, defined by their location within the carpus and within the organization of the joint capsule. The capsular ligaments are defined as crossing the radiocarpal joint, the midcarpal joint, or both. Additionally, designations are made regarding the dorsal or palmar location of the ligament. The short ligaments between the bones of either the proximal

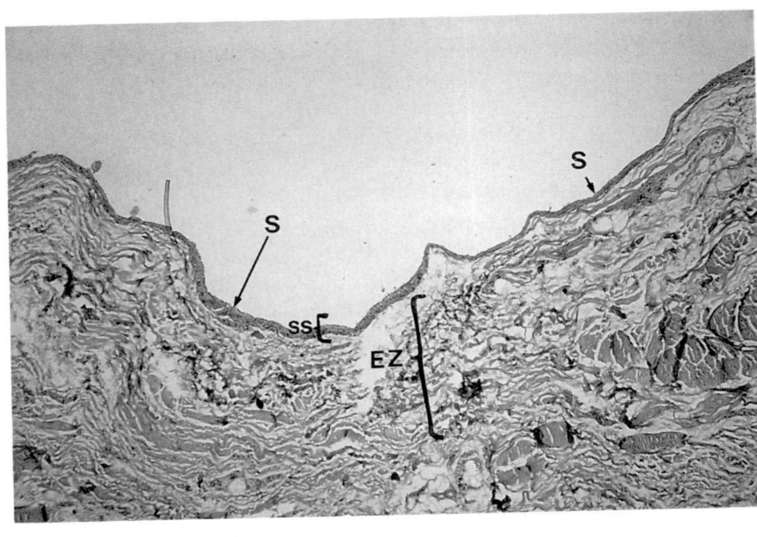

FIGURE 15–2. The deep (joint) epiligamentous zone of a capsular ligament such as the radioscaphocapitate ligament shown here is encapsulated by synoviocytes (S), characterized by one or more continuous layers of cuboidal cells with prominent central round nucleoli. This layer of synoviocytes forms the synovial stratum (SS) of the joint capsule. The epiligamentous zone (EZ) persists between the synovial stratum and the collagen fascicles (CF) of the true ligament. Hematoxylin and eosin, 100×.

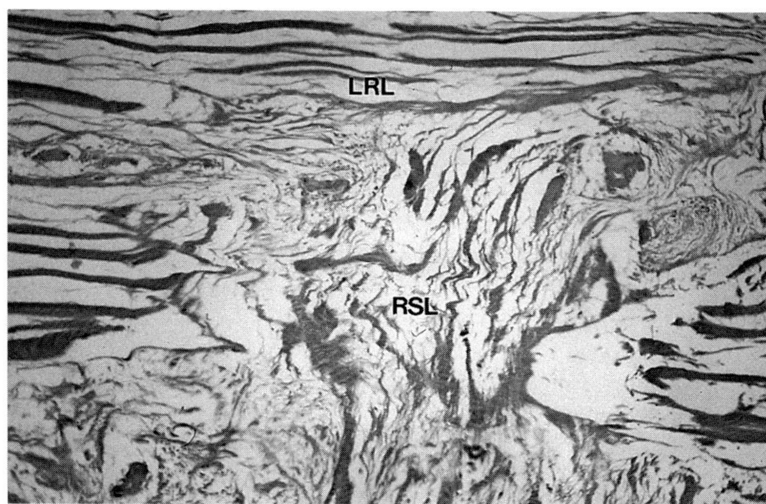

FIGURE 15–3. Merger zone between the long radiolunate (LRL) ligament and the radioscapholunate (RSL) ligament. There is loss of continuity of the fascicular architecture and subsequent loss of the perifascicular space. Hematoxylin and eosin, 100×.

or distal carpal rows are called interosseous or intrinsic ligaments. The principal name of each ligament stems from the major bones to which it attaches. Although not entirely analogous to muscular descriptions, the terms *origin* and *insertion* may be used to designate the proximal and distal attachments, respectively, of a ligament. If more than one ligament connects two bones, a modifying term, (e.g., *short, long, dorsal, palmar, deep*) is added to the name.

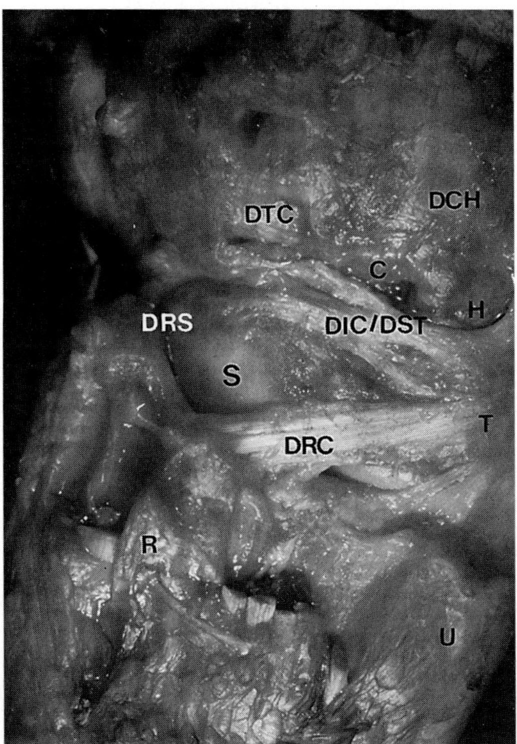

FIGURE 15–4. Photograph of a fresh cadaver wrist showing the dorsal carpal ligament complex. R, radius; U, ulna; S, scaphoid; T, triquetrum; H, hamate; C, capitate; DRC, dorsal radiocarpal ligament; DIC, dorsal intercarpal ligament; DST, dorsal scaphotriquetral ligament; DRS, dorsal radioscaphoid ligament; DTC, dorsal trapezoid-capitate interosseous ligament; DCH, dorsal capitohamate interosseous ligament.

The dorsal capsular wrist ligaments are readily appreciated as distinct structures from an extraarticular perspective after elevating the extensor retinaculum (Fig. 15–4). In contrast, the palmar carpal ligaments are not visible until a thin, vascular adventitial lining of the carpal tunnel is removed (Fig. 15–5). Even with this tissue removed, the individual ligaments are difficult to discern and appear to merge and blend in flattened sheets of collagen. However, when viewed from within the radiocarpal and midcarpal joint spaces, peering palmarward from a dorsal perspective, several ligaments are seen protruding into the joint space as distinct structures (Fig. 15–6). Additionally, these ligaments have specific features that serve as convenient landmarks when arthroscopically evaluating the radiocarpal and midcarpal joint spaces. The specific ligaments that have been successfully targeted for ligamentography are illustrated in Fig. 15–7 and listed in Table 15–1. It should be acknowledged, however, that any capsular ligament with an epiligamentous sheath is amenable to ligamentography.

UNDERLYING CONCEPT OF LIGAMENTOGRAPHY

The underlying concept of ligamentography was developed from observations made during routine arthrography, where numerous joint capsule indentations and irregularities are identified in a number of normal joints. In the radiocarpal joint, two such irregularities are consistently seen in the palmar capsule, corresponding to the radioscaphocapitate and long radiolunate ligaments. When viewed in the sagittal plane, the two ligaments project into the radiocarpal joint space as hemicylindrical structures separated by the interligamentous sulcus (Fig. 15–8). Contrast

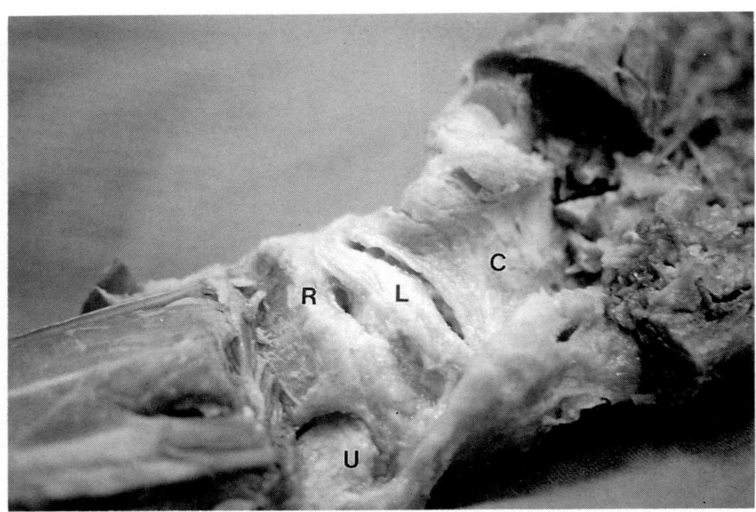

FIGURE 15–5. Photograph of a fresh cadaver wrist after excision of the adventitia covering the palmar carpal ligaments. The ligaments are grossly indistinct from the superficial perspective. However, general directional trends of the ligaments can be appreciated coursing obliquely distally and toward the midline of the carpus. R, radius; U, ulna; L, lunate; C, capitate.

material introduced into the radiocarpal joint through a dorsal approach fills the joint space, outlining the deep (joint) surface of the two ligaments, and fills the interligamentous sulcus (Fig. 15–9). This essentially provides a "negative" image of the two ligaments as they project into the radiocarpal joint space. If a defect in the synovial lamina of the epiligamentous sheath exists, contrast material introduced into the radiocarpal joint may enter the substance of the ligament through this defect and disperse through the ligament (Fig. 15–10). This dispersion presumably takes place though the perifascicular tissue planes. Additionally, if a disruption exists in the fibrous lamina of a ligament highlighted with intrasubstance contrast material, contrast material may extravasate out of the joint capsule into the pericapsular tissues and spaces.

With these observations in mind, the concept of ligamentography was developed (Fig. 15–11). Its principle is based on the intentional bypass of the laminae of the epiligamentous sheath of capsular ligaments with a small needle, allowing the controlled introduction of contrast material into the substance of the ligament. With minimal injection pressure, the contrast material is forced to diffuse throughout the

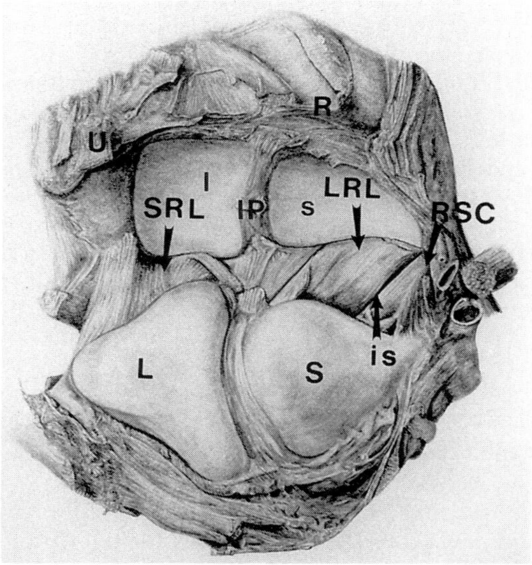

FIGURE 15–6. Drawing of the radiocarpal joint from a dorsal and distal perspective with the dorsal radiocarpal joint capsule completely divided and the proximal carpal row maximally palmarflexed. R, radius; U, ulna; S, scaphoid; L, lunate; s, scaphoid fossa; l, lunate fossa; IP, interfacet prominence; RSC, radioscaphocapitate ligament; LRL, long radiolunate ligament; SRL, short radiolunate ligament; is, interligamentous sulcus. (Reprinted with permission from Berger RA, Landsmeer JMF. The palmar radiocarpal ligaments: A study of adult and fetal human wrist joints. *J Hand Surg* 1990;15A:847–854.)

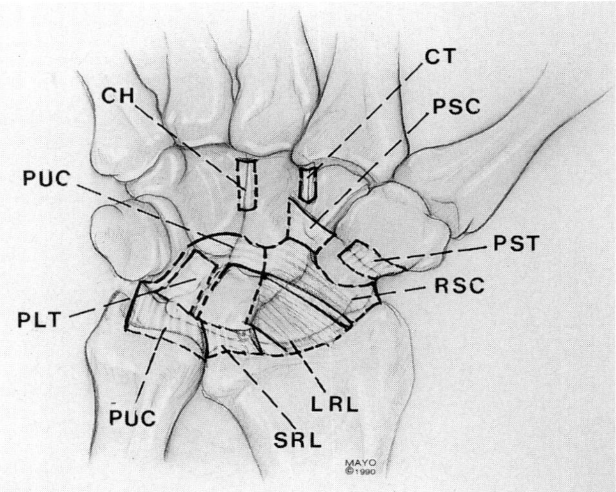

FIGURE 15–7. Drawing of some of the major wrist ligaments successfully highlighted by ligamentography. The palmar (anterior) perspective of the wrist is illustrated. RSC, radioscaphocapitate; LRL, long radiolunate; SRL, short radiolunate; PST, palmar scaphotrapezial; CT, palmar capitotrapezoidal; CH, capitohamate; PLT, palmar lunotriquetral; PUC, palmar ulnocarpal; PSC, palmar scaphocapitate.

TABLE 15–1. *Carpal Ligaments Successfully Targeted for Ligamentograms*

Joint/Surface	Ligament	Abbreviation
Radiocarpal: palmar	Radioscaphocapitate*	RSC
	Long radiolunate†	LRL
	Short radiolunate	SRL
Ulnocarpal: palmar	Ulnotriquetral	UT
Midcarpal: palmar	Scaphotrapeziotrapezoid‡	STT
	Scaphocapitate	SC
	Triquetrocapitate	TC
	Triquetrohamate	TH
Interosseous: deep	Capitohamate§	DCH

* *See Fig. 1–12.*
† *See Fig. 15–13.*
‡ *See Fig. 15–14.*
§ *See Fig. 15–15.*

length of the ligament, limited only by the extent of the perifascicular spaces.

The technique of ligamentography, including the use of a dorsal approach, evolved from several empirical experiences. In standard arthrography, it is well known that the contrast material often "leaks" around the needle track during the injection process. If the needle is introduced from a palmar approach, this may obscure small pathologic extravasations from the joint capsule. Additionally, the dorsal approach avoids passing the needle through the contents of the carpal tunnel. Finally, the dorsal approach allows the delivery of a test bolus of contrast material as the needle is advanced palmarly into the joint capsule. This has few detrimental effects on the quality of the ligamentogram by virtue of the diffusion of the contrast material into the joint fluid.

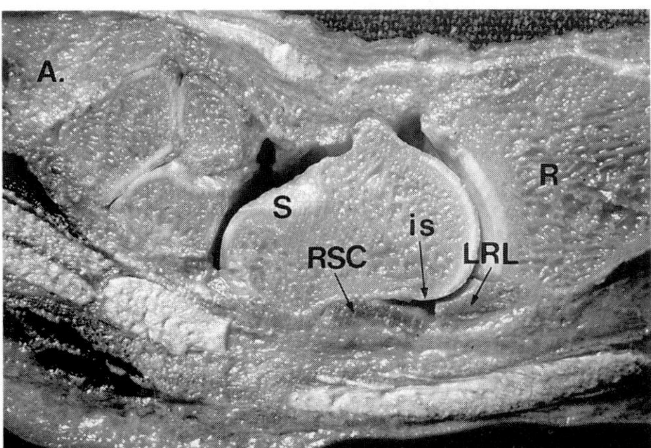

FIGURE 15–8. Parasagittal section through a cadaver wrist at the level of the scaphoid (S) and radius (R). Two of the palmar radiocarpal ligaments are shown in cross-section, the radioscaphocapitate (RSC) and the long radiolunate (LRL) ligaments, separated by the interligamentous sulcus (is). The ligaments appear to protrude into the radiocarpal joint space. (Reprinted with permission from Berger RA, Blair WF. Arthrotomography of the wrist: The palmar radiocarpal ligaments. *Clin Orthop* 1984;186:224–229.)

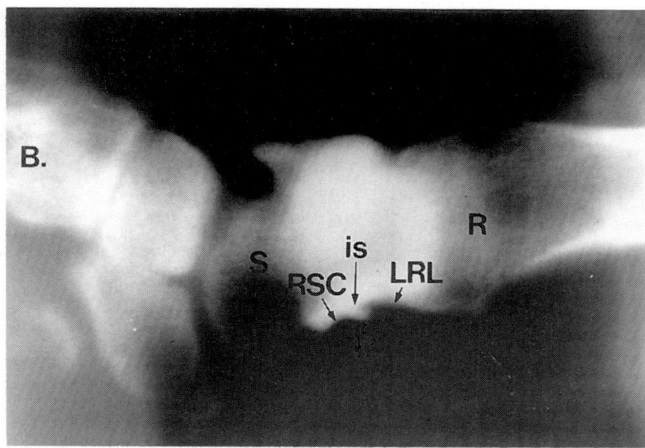

FIGURE 15–9. Lateral arthrotomogram of the radiocarpal joint. Protrusion of the palmar radiocarpal ligaments into the radiocarpal joint space appears as two serial hemispheres. S, scaphoid; R, radius; RSC, radioscaphocapitate ligament; LRL, long radiolunate ligament; is, interligamentous sulcus. (Reprinted with permission from Berger RA, Blair WF. Arthrotomography of the wrist: The palmar radiocarpal ligaments. *Clin Orthop* 1984;186:224–229.)

The 25-gauge spinal needle was chosen because of its small diameter, which reduces the potential for creating a tear in the epiligamentous sheath, which may in turn promote extravasation of the contrast material into the joint space. Additionally, the stylette is in place during needle advancement, minimizing the potential of soft tissue becoming entrapped in the cannula of the needle tip.

METHOD OF LIGAMENTOGRAPHY

Basic Equipment

Ligamentograms are performed under fluoroscopic monitoring. This is necessary for needle placement as well as for monitoring of the dispersion of contrast material through the substance of the ligament. The use of videotape adds substantially to image analysis potential, since the contrast material tends to resorb quite quickly and dispersion patterns may require review after the ligamentographic series is complete.

Water-soluble contrast material is used and may be diluted up to 1:4 with a local anesthetic or saline solution. A 25-gauge spinal needle, preferably with the tip slightly blunted, is used to penetrate the ligament, and we have found delivery of the contrast material to the needle facilitated by the use of extension tubing. Generally, a 5-mL syringe is sufficient as a reservoir for the contrast material.

Basic Technique

For most carpal ligamentograms, the hand is positioned prone on the fluoroscopy table and prepared for the injection as for an arthrographic injection. Based on thorough understanding of the normal lig-

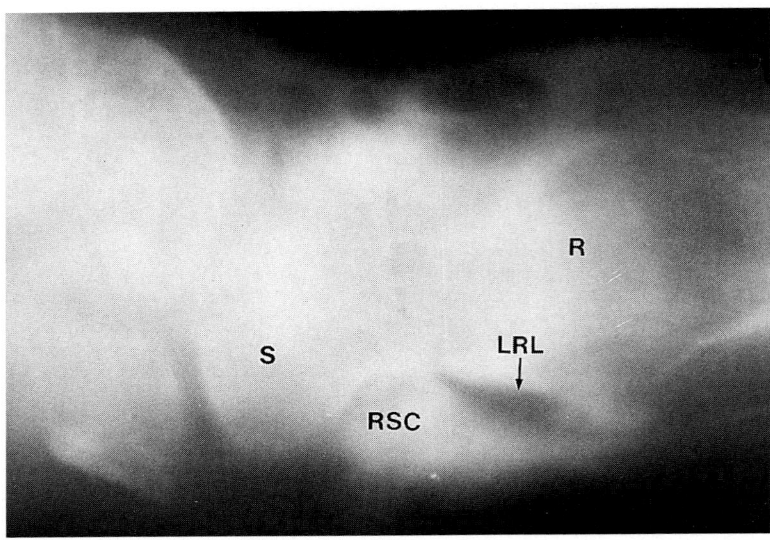

FIGURE 15–10. Because of a disruption of the synovial lamina of the radioscaphocapitate (RSC) ligament, the ligament is highlighted following a standard radiocarpal joint arthrographic injection. The long radiolunate (LRL) ligament is left free from contrast penetration due to an intact epiligamentous sheath. (Reprinted with permission from Berger RA, Blair WF. Arthrotomography of the wrist: The palmar radiocarpal ligaments. *Clin Orthop* 1984;186:224–229.)

amentous anatomy of the joint, the entrance point of the needle is established directly dorsal to the most accessible portion of the target level using fluoroscopic guidance. The needle is advanced through the dorsal skin and joint capsule to rest within the appropriate joint space.

The forearm is repositioned for lateral fluoroscopy, and the needle is slowly advanced palmarward. All ligamentograms are produced by passing the needle through the joint space before entering the substance of the target ligament to facilitate the concept of test bolus delivery. As the needle is advanced toward the target ligament, periodic removal of the stylette and delivery of one or two drops of contrast material allows the examiner to determine if the needle is in the joint space or within the substance of the target ligament. If the tip of the needle is in the joint space, the contrast material will diffuse into the surrounding joint fluid. Conversely, if the tip of the needle is in the substance of the target ligament or other soft tissue, a small bolus of contrast material will stay in the neighborhood of the needle tip, indicating that the needle is embedded in soft tissue.

Once the examiner is convinced that the needle

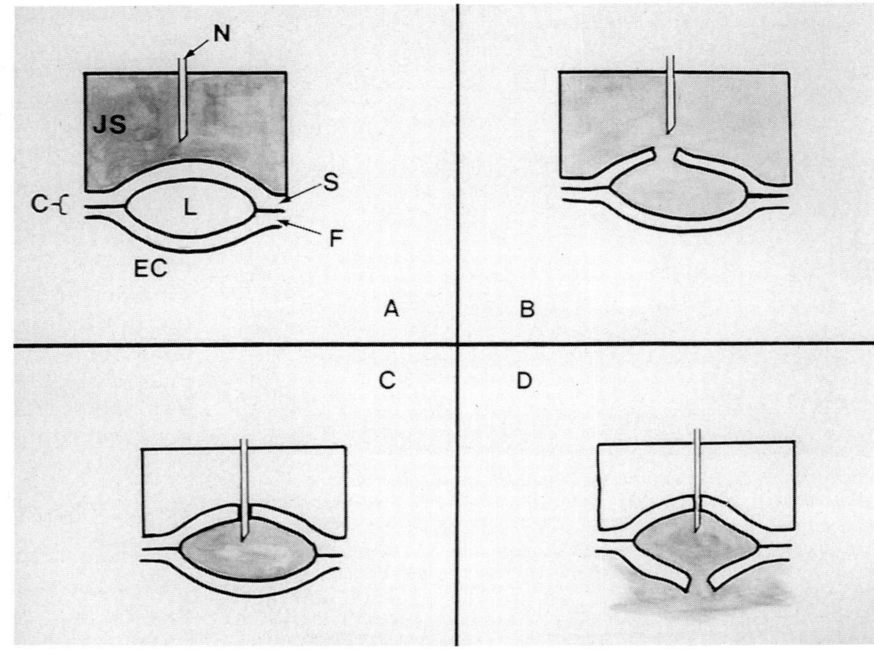

FIGURE 15–11. Schematic concept of ligamentography. **A:** The epiligamentous sheath (S) of the ligament (L) forms a semipermeable membrane surrounding the ligament as part of the joint capsule (C). In a simple arthrogram, the synovial stratum (S) of the joint capsule prevents the contrast material injected into the joint space (JS) through the needle (N) from passing into the substance of the ligament. The fibrous stratum (F) normally prevents the contrast material from extravasating into the extracapsular space (EC). **B:** If a defect exists in the synovial stratum of the epiligamentous sheath, contrast material injected into the joint space may enter into the substance of the ligament, creating a "passive" ligamentogram. **C:** A needle can be passed through an intact synovial stratum until the tip is within the substance of the ligament. Contrast material can then be injected into the ligament, creating an "active" ligamentogram as the contrast material spreads within the space defined by the epiligamentous sheath. **D:** If a defect in the fibrous stratum of the epiligamentous sheath exists, contrast material injected into the substance of the ligament through passive or active ligamentography may extravasate through the defect into the pericapsular area.

tip has penetrated the epiligamentous sheath of the target ligament, the stylette is removed and the forearm is repositioned prone on the fluoroscopy table. Under continuous fluoroscopic imaging, contrast material is slowly infused using steady but not excessive pressure. Fluoroscopy should confirm that the contrast material is flowing along the fibers of the ligament throughout its length. It is expected that the contrast material may not fill out the ligament to its bony insertion, since the fascicular pattern of collagen organization is lost as the insertion zone is approached. Additionally, a merger between ligaments may prevent the continuation of contrast material flow due to the same phenomenon of loss of fascicular organization.

Generally, approximately 0.5 mL of contrast material solution will be required to highlight a short ligament, such as an interosseous or midcarpal capsular ligament. Up to 1.5 mL may be necessary to highlight a longer capsular ligament, such as the radioscaphocapitate ligament. No extravasation of contrast material should normally take place. If an extravasation is seen, it indicates one of three possibilities: (1) the placement of the needle tip is faulty, either such that it is outside the confines of the epiligamentous sheath or a rent in the sheath has occurred as a result of needle placement; (2) a disruption in the substance of the ligament other than that produced during needle placement has occurred, presumably due to a traumatic disruption of the ligament; or (3) a nontraumatic condition of the ligament exists that results in loss of integrity of the epiligamentous sheath, most frequently seen in the wrists of the elderly.

Once the fluoroscopic placement of contrast material within the substance of the target ligament is complete, standard radiographs are obtained. We find that multiple views are beneficial, especially with the wrist placed in the "cardinal" positions of radial deviation, ulnar deviation, palmar-flexion, and dorsiflexion. Clearance of the contrast material is quite rapid, allowing serial ligamentograms to be performed if desired.

RESULTS AND EXAMPLES

The list of successful target ligaments by the authors is shown in Table 15–1. Generally, the larger ligaments, such as those found in the palmar radiocarpal joint capsule, are easier to target and highlight. For example, the radioscaphocapitate (Fig. 15–12) and long radiolunate (Fig. 15–13) ligaments are easily accessible through the radiocarpal joint space and have sufficient depth to allow placement of the tip of the spinal needle fully within the substance of the ligament, thereby minimizing the risk of extravasation about the needle. Conversely, thin capsular ligaments, such as the palmar scaphotrapeziotrapezoidal (STT) ligament (Fig. 15–14), although readily accessible through the STT joint space, are difficult to

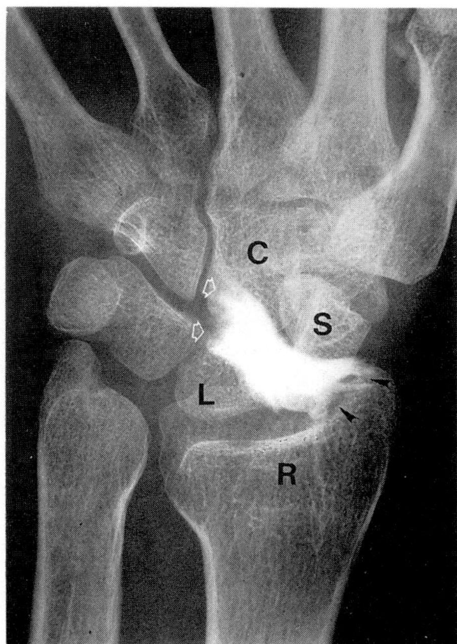

FIGURE 15–12. Posteroanterior ligamentogram of the radioscaphocapitate ligament. The ligament is well defined from origin to insertion. The contrast material does not penetrate the insertion of the ligament into the radius (black arrows), nor does it course beyond the region where the ligament merges with another ligament (white arrows). R, radius; S, scaphoid; L, lunate; C, capitate.

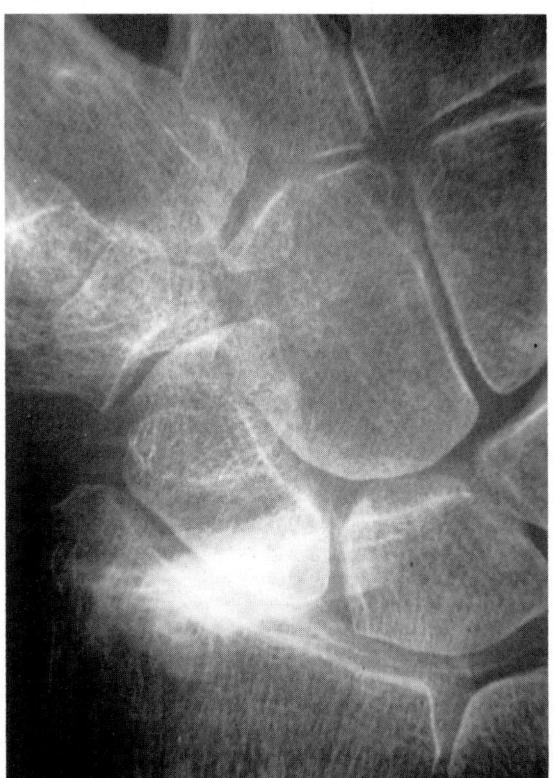

FIGURE 15–13. Posteroanterior ligamentogram of the long radiolunate ligament. The contrast material does not penetrate beyond the insertion of the ligament into the radius or the lunate and does not cross over into surrounding ligaments, such as the radioscaphocapitate and radioscapholunate ligaments.

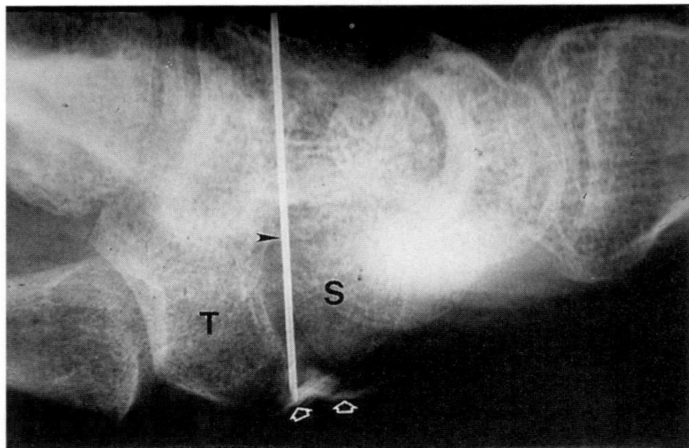

FIGURE 15–14. Lateral ligamentogram of the palmar scaphotrapezial ligament, with the needle (black arrowhead) in the substance of the ligament (white arrowheads), introduced from a dorsal approach. Precise placement of the needle tip is mandatory for thin ligaments such as this. S, scaphoid; T, trapezium.

image because the height of the needle bevel may exceed the thickness of the ligament. This makes extravasation of contrast material much more likely. Finally, thick ligaments, such as the deep capitohamate ligament (Fig. 15–15) may be relatively well suited for completely embedding the tip of the needle within the substance of the ligament but may be difficult to access due to a narrow or obliquely oriented joint surface.

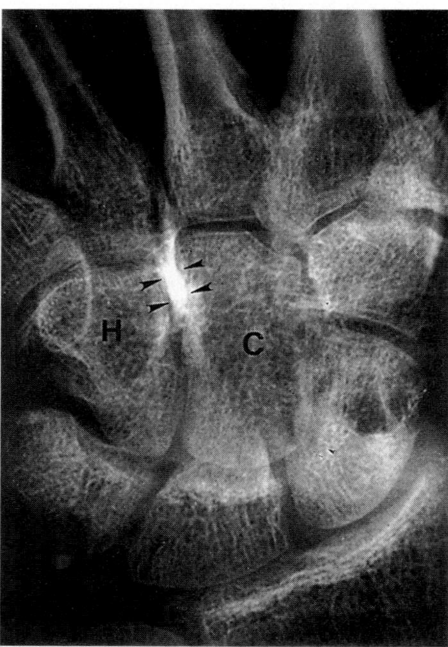

FIGURE 15–15. Posteroanterior ligamentogram of the capitohamate interosseous ligament (black arrowheads). Unlike the capsular wrist ligaments, the capitohamate ligament is ensheathed in a synovial stratum with no fibrous stratum and is therefore an intraarticular ligament. The principles of ligamentography, however, apply as they do with capsular ligaments. Note the lack of contrast material in the midcarpal and carpometacarpal joint spaces. C, capitate; H, hamate.

Generally, the thin or narrow ligaments will accept 0.5 ml of injected contrast material, while the larger capsular ligaments may take up to 1.5 to 2.0 mL of contrast solution to highlight their entire length. Active observation of the filling process fluoroscopically is mandatory; the examiner must be ready to cease injecting when the ligament is maximally highlighted or extravasation begins. Extravasation is more likely with increasing age of the wrist, presumably due to loss of competency of the synovial laminae lining the joint space. Additionally, recordings of the ligamentograms should be made expeditiously, since the contrast material is rapidly and actively resorbed from the ligament, rendering the ligamentogram less useful.

The technique of ligamentography is straightforward, but the ligamentographer requires practice to become comfortable with its application. A thorough understanding of the normal relationships of the target ligaments is necessary to readily identify radiographic landmarks. Finally, it is suggested that practice trials of ligamentography be carried out on fresh adult cadaver wrists before in vivo applications are considered.

SUMMARY OF TECHNIQUE

1. Approach target ligament over the most accessible portion from a dorsal approach.
2. A 25-gauge spinal needle, with stylette, is advanced through the dorsal joint capsule toward the target ligament, with the wrist positioned for lateral fluoroscopic monitoring.
3. As the region of the target ligament is approached, a series of small test boluses are delivered as the needle is advanced until dispersion of the contrast material ceases.
4. The wrist is repositioned for posteroanterior fluoroscopic viewing and between 0.5 and 1.5 mL of diluted water-soluble contrast material is slowly advanced until the entire predicted length of the target ligament is highlighted.

REFERENCES

1. Horwitz T. An anatomic and roentgenographic study of the wrist joint. *Surgery* 1940;7:773–783.
2. Lewis OJ, Hamshere RJ, Bucknill TM. The anatomy of the wrist joint. *J Anat* 1970;106:539–552.
3. MacConaill MA. The mechanical anatomy of the carpus and its bearing on some surgical problems. *J Anat* 1941;75:166–175.
4. Mayfield JK, Johnson RP, Kilcoyne RF. The ligaments of the wrist and their functional significance. *Anat Rec* 1976;186:417–428.
5. Berger RA, Blair WF, El-Khoury GY. Arthrotomography of the wrist: The palmar radiocarpal ligaments. *Clin Orthop* 1984;186:224–229.

6. Blair WF, Berger RA, El-Khoury GY. Arthrotomography of the wrist: An experimental and preliminary clinical study. *J Hand Surg* 1985;10A:350–359.
7. El-Khoury GY, Albright JP, Abu Yousef MM, Montgomery WJ, Tuck SL. Arthrotomography of the glenoid labrum. *Radiology* 1979;131:333–337.
8. Eto RT, Anderson PW, Harley JD. Elbow arthrography with the application of tomography. *Radiology* 1975;115:283–288.
9. Pavlov H, Warren RF, Sherman MF, Cayea PD. The accuracy of double-contrast arthrographic evaluation of the anterior cruciate ligament. *J Bone Joint Surg* 1983;65A:175–183.
10. Gundry CR, Kursunoglu-Brahme S, Schwaighofer B, Kang HS, Sartoris J, Resnick D. Is MR better than arthrography for evaluating the ligaments of the wrist? An in-vitro study. *AJR* 1990;154:337–341.
11. Hodler J, Kursunoglu-Brahme S, Snyder S, et al. Rotator cuff disease: Assessment with MR imaging in 36 patients with arthroscopic confirmation. *Radiology* 1992;182:431–436.
12. Kaplan PA, Bryans KC, Davick JP, Otte M, Stinson WW, Dussault RG. MR imaging of the normal shoulder: Variants and pitfalls. *Radiology* 1992;184:519–524.
13. Lawson TL, Middleton WD. MRI and ultrasound evaluation of the shoulder. *Acta Orthop Belg* 1991;57(suppl.):62–69.
14. Mink JH, Levy T, Crues JV. Tears of the anterior cruciate ligament and menisci of the knee: MR imaging evaluation. *Radiology* 1988;167:769–774.
15. Victor J, Gielen J, Martens M, et al. Correlation between magnetic resonance imaging and arthroscopy in the diagnosis of anterior cruciate ligament and meniscus lesions. *Acta Orthop Belg* 1991;57(suppl.):56–61.
16. Kaye JJ, Bohne WHO. A radiographic study of the ligamentous anatomy of the ankle. *Radiology* 1977;125:659–667.
17. Trent PS, Walker PS, Wolf B. Ligament length patterns, strength, and rotational axes of the knee joint. *Clin Orthop* 1976;117:263–270.
18. Wang C, Walker PS, Wolf B. The effects of flexion and rotation on the length patterns of ligaments of the knee. *J Biomech* 1973;6:587–596.
19. de Lange A, Huiskes R, Kauer JMG. Wrist-joint ligament changes in flexion and deviation of the hand: An experimental study. *J Orthop Res* 1990;8:722–730.
20. Berger RA, Blair WF. The radioscapholunate ligament: A gross and histologic description. *Anat Rec* 1984;210:393–405.
21. Berger RA, Landsmeer JMF. The palmar radiocarpal ligaments: A study of adult and fetal human wrist joints. *J Hand Surg* 1990;15A:847–854.
22. Berger RA, Kauer JMG, Landsmeer JMF. The radioscapholunate ligament: A gross anatomic and histologic study of fetal and adult wrists. *J Hand Surg* 1991;16:350–355.
23. Cooper RR, Misol S. Tendon and ligament insertion: A light and electron microscopic study. *J Bone Joint Surg* 1970;52A:1–21.

CHAPTER 16

COMPUTED TOMOGRAPHY
Applications and Tailored Approach

Yuming Yin, Kevin W. McEnery, and Louis A. Gilula

INTRODUCTION

Because of its high resolution and fast scan capabilities, computed tomography (CT) has become increasingly popular for diagnosing wrist problems. Wrist CT can be performed in multiple planes including sagittal, axial, coronal, or other oblique planes.[1–4] Previous reports have shown that CT scanning is useful in evaluating complex carpal trauma;[4] diagnosing and localizing foreign bodies,[5–9] intra-articular loose bodies,[10] loss of articular cartilage, intraosseous lucent defects ("cysts"), bone defects, bone irregularities, and soft-tissue abnormalities;[11] visualizing bone graft material; and determining the degree of bone healing.[12] CT is helpful in determining bony union, especially in the presence of advanced osteoporosis[12] and is particularly advantageous in its ability to obtain diagnostic information in the presence of metal fixation or cast immobilization.[13] Axial CT scan can demonstrate overgrowth of Lister's tubercle and has been used to evaluate distal radioulnar joint (DRUJ) subluxation,[14] incongruity,[15–17] and carpal tunnel syndrome.[18–23] Three-dimensional CT of the wrist has demonstrated carpal volume, contour, and spatial position.[15,16] Three-dimensional surface reconstruction has demonstrated the vascular anatomy of the carpus.[24] Three-dimensional reconstruction of CT scan data has been used for surgical planning.[25] Spiral CT has the advantages of faster scans and multiple plane reconstructions with good resolution.[26–28]

General Technical Factors

Setting the correct imaging parameters will markedly improve the resultant examination. The field of view should be as small as possible to include the anatomy in question and adjacent bones. Zooming should be set before acquisition of images to ensure the highest possible detail. In general, zooming after acquisition of the CT images with a large field of view will cause loss of potential CT detail. The imaging algorithm for bone that gives highest practical detail should be used. This can be the one selected by the machine manufacturer for "bone," or it can be the one established for bone examination in the skull. The forearm and/or metacarpals should be positioned out of the same plane as the carpal bone(s) in question to diminish streak artifacts. Section thickness and interval should be selected according to the presenting clinical question. Since all information within a slice thickness is averaged to produce one image, sections thicker than 2 mm may produce images that are not truly representative of anatomy when looking for detail within a carpal bone or wrist structure that is only 10 to 15 mm wide. Slice interval should not allow space between sections to be skipped when maximal detail is desired within a wrist structure. If three-dimensional reconstruction is contemplated, some images are better when overlapping sections are obtained, e.g., 2-mm thick sections at 1-mm intervals. When more than one plane will be obtained, one plane can be very high detail and the other can be more of a survey. An example of this is an examination of the scaphoid where oblique sagittal sections are obtained at 2-mm thick sections at 1-mm intervals and coronal sections of the scaphoid and entire wrist structures are obtained at 2-mm slice thickness and 2-mm intervals. If the extent of a process, such as a lipoma or a angiovenous dysplasia, is questioned, thicker slices with space between slices could be obtained purely for mapping purposes.

In general we prefer to use higher kilovolts and to optimize lower MAS. Field of view should be limited to the immediate area of the wrist. A bone- or edge-enhancing filter should be employed to optimize visualization of subtle bone alterations. The patient should be as comfortable as possible and the wrist and/or hand immobilized. This is particularly important because small fields of view will accentuate any movement during scanning and therefore adversely affect image quality. Comfort can be enhanced by

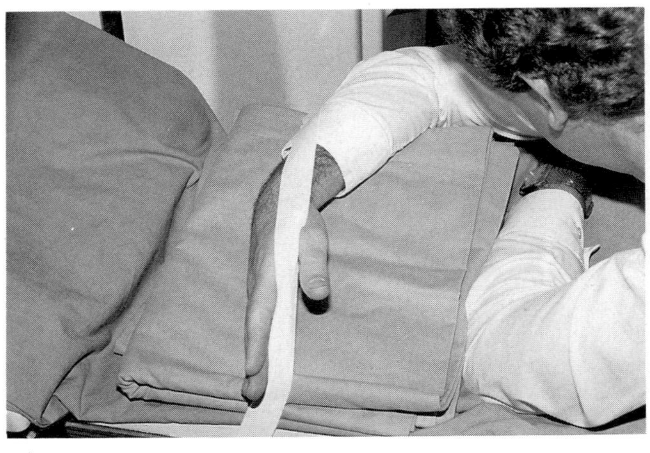

A

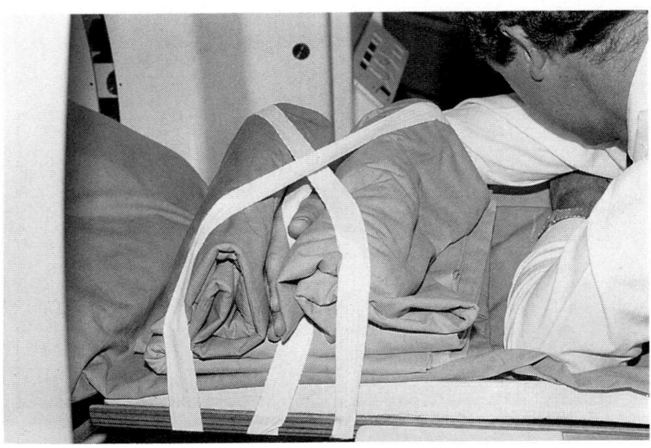

B

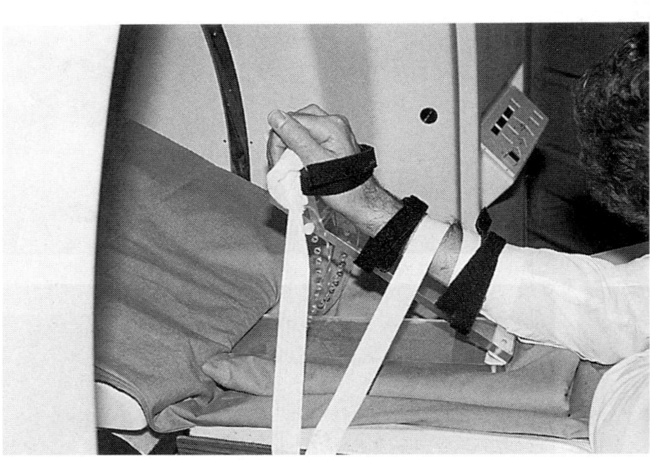

C

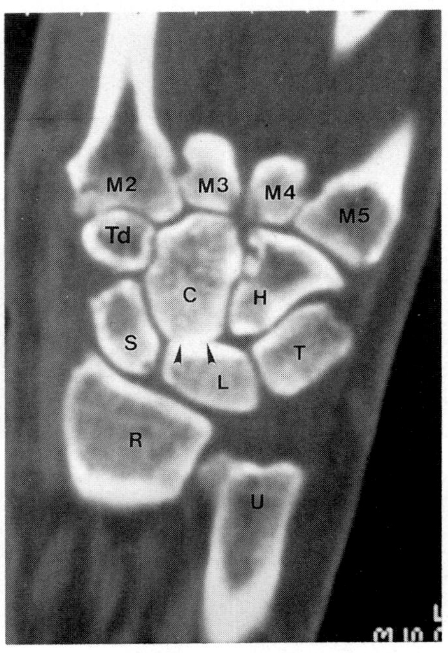

D

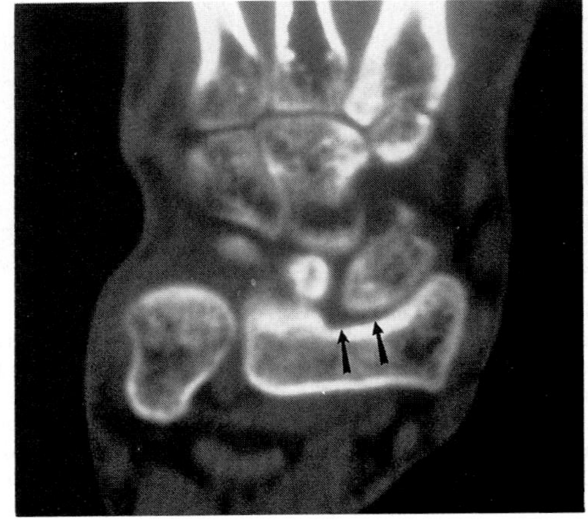

E

FIGURE 16–2. Coronal positioning. Pennes's positioning **(A)** before and **(B)** after securing forearm for coronal scan. Slight flexion (or extension) at the radiocarpal joint and positioning the proximal portion of the forearm and elbow out of the scan plane may reduce the beam hardening artifact. Bed sheets or other objects placed along both sides of the hand and wrist can help keep the wrist from rolling out of position during the procedure. **C:** A wrist is supported for coronal scanning using the Vannier wrist holder. The gantry has not yet been angled. **D:** Coronal CT image shows anatomy of the wrist including the radiocarpal, intercarpal, and CMC joints. Loss of cartilage between the lunate and capitate is shown (black arrowheads). **E:** Coronal image of the left wrist demonstrates a depression fracture deformity in the scaphoid fossa of the distal radius (arrows). (S, scaphoid; L, lunate; C, capitate; H, hamate; L, lunate; M2–5, second to fifth metacarpal bones; R, radius; S, scaphoid; T, triquetrum; Td, trapezoid; U, ulna. (Panels B and C reprinted with permission from the Radiological Society of North America. Stewart NR, Gilula LA. CT of the wrist: A tailored approach. *Radiology* 1992; 183:13–20.)

ing most scaphoid pathology. However, adding a coronal plane examination, especially in Vannier's position (uses fewer sections than Pennes's position for scaphoid) is necessary to recognize radial or ulnar displacement of fracture fragments.

Oblique STT Plane

This scan position, described by Stewart and Gilula,[1] was developed for the sole purpose of improving visualization of the scaphotrapeziotrapezoidal (STT) joints. The wrist is placed above the head with the patient prone as for the sagittal plane scan, then the wrist is overpronated 45 degrees (Fig. 16–5A) or, as another option, the wrist could be in 45-degree supination. A CT section in this position passes through the scaphoid, trapezium, trapezoid, and bases of the first and second metacarpal bones in the same section. It is excellent for demonstrating the interrelation of these joints, particularly for assessing STT joint fusion (Fig. 16–5B).[1] If there is question about whether a bone union could be bridging this joint area dorsally or palmarly, then a second CT plane, such as the sagittal, may be appropriate to use so that CT sections are performed at right angles to the dorsal or palmar surface of this joint complex.

In practice, usually two and sometimes three planes are obtained to formulate a three-dimensional picture (Figs. 16–6A and 16–6B).[13] Sagittal imaging best demonstrates longitudinal or intercompartmental relationships (radiocarpal, midcarpal, and carpometacarpal joints) and alignment along coronal or axial planes.[13] Axial scanning best defines side-to-side relationships of the DRUJ, carpal bones within a specific row (proximal and distal rows), and between the adjacent metacarpal bones. The oblique sagittal plane is specific for scaphoid detail, and the oblique STT plane is specific for demonstrating the STT joints as for fusion.

Spiral (Helical) CT

The availability of spiral (helical) CT gives the wrist imager more flexibility in CT evaluation of the wrist, especially in the evaluation of acute fractures of the distal radius and carpus. Given the ability to complete an examination during a 24- to 40-second continuous acquisition, spiral CT provides the capability of acquiring an examination optimized for multiplanar reconstructions.[27,28] Routinely, 2-mm collimation with 2 mm/second table increments is used. The length of spiral scan coverage is determined by the time available for imaging. A 32-second examination with a 2 mm/second table increment scan images approximately 6 cm of tissue volume. This is sufficient for imaging the carpus in either the coronal or axial plane. The sagittal plane may be problematic because some patients cannot be entirely imaged in a single scan. This situation is addressed by focusing scan coverage on the affected portion of the wrist. For instance, when imaging in the sagittal plane to assess a radius fracture, one should initiate the scan at the radial aspect of the wrist and scan in the direction of the ulna. This will ensure complete coverage of the radius.

Spiral CT is best used to assess the acutely traumatized wrist. These patients are typically protected by a cast and are not always able to assume an optimal imaging position. In these cases, multiplanar reconstructions can help determine fracture relationships (Fig. 16–7). Spiral CT provides thin collimation with maximal overlap, which provides an ideal image data

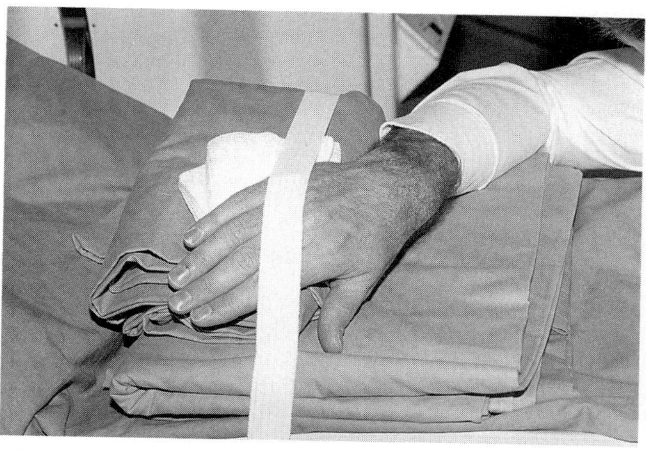
A

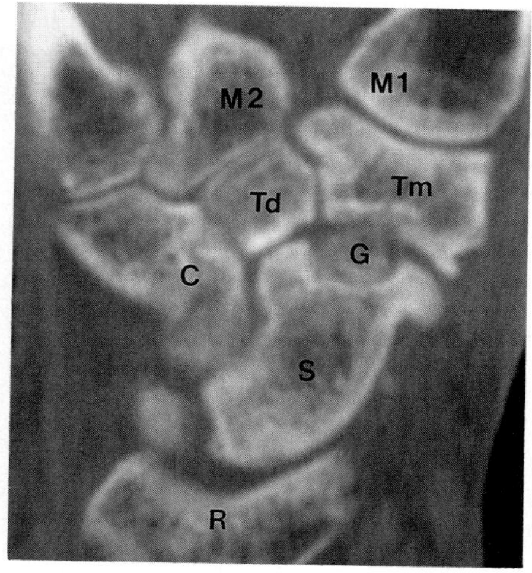

B

FIGURE 16–5. A: Slightly overpronated positioning of the wrist for the STT joint. **B:** STT joint CT image of left wrist shows a surgical defect with only questionable areas of bone graft (G) incorporation involving the distal scaphoid (S) and no definite bridging between graft and the trapezium (Tm). C, capitate; G, graft; M1, M2, first and second metacarpals; R, radius; S, scaphoid; Td, trapezoid; Tm, trapezium. (Reprinted with permission from the Radiological Society of North America. Stewart NR, Gilula LA. CT of the wrist: A tailored approach. *Radiology* 1992;183:13–20.)

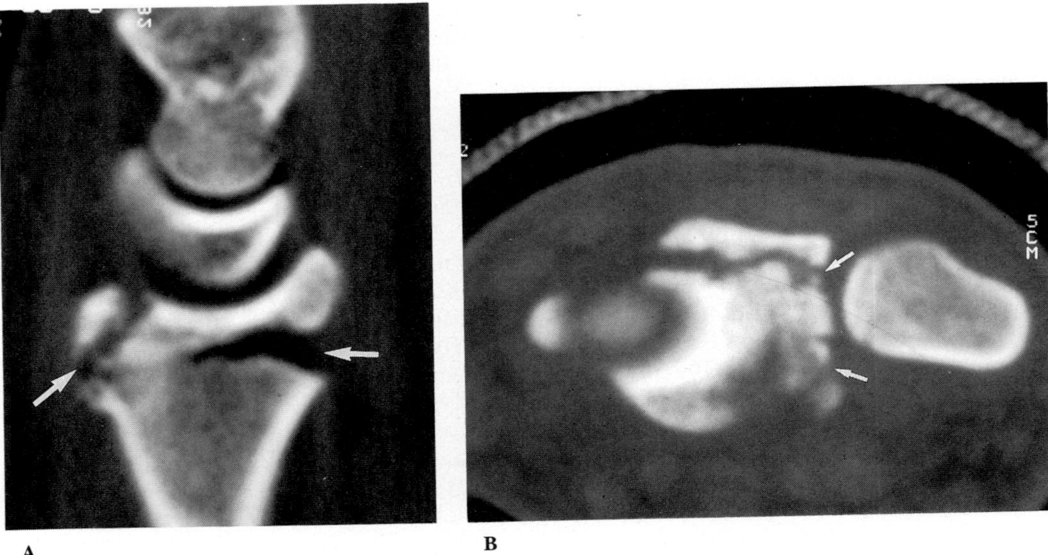

FIGURE 16–6. A: Sagittal CT image of left wrist shows comminuted intraarticular fracture of the distal radius (arrows) (dorsal is to the reader's left). **B:** Axial CT image shows the fracture involves the distal radioulnar joint (arrows) and demonstrates the fracture pattern of the distal articular surface of the radius.

set for multiplanar images. The efficiency in obtaining the image data set minimizes the potential of patient movement. Although the same diagnostic information could be obtained with conventional CT, and multiplanar reconstructions created from the conventional CT images, there is a great likelihood that subtle patient movement during an extended conventional CT examination would diminish the clinical usefulness of the reconstructions. In our clinical practice, we attempt to scan trauma patients in the axial plane (Fig. 16–8A). Then reconstruction images can be obtained in the coronal or sagittal planes or both if necessary (Figs. 16–8B through 16–8D). Axial imaging is not always practical for those patients with long arm casts, although it can be obtained,[1] and the sagittal plane usually serves as an alternative. Reconstructed images can substitute for direct planar images that would otherwise have not been acquired. Conventional CT direct planar imaging will likely remain the preferred imaging method for those instances in which a subtle bone abnormality is anticipated, especially in the context of evaluation of a traumatized patient with negative plain radiographs and a positive bone scan. An exception to this statement is the situation where bone marrow edema ("bone bruise") or an intraosseous, nondisplaced fracture is possible. In that situation, MRI would usually be preferable to CT.

FRACTURE

Although most fractures of the carpus usually do not require a CT scan, complete evaluation of complex wrist fractures, especially comminuted fractures of the radius or the scaphoid, may be difficult to interpret on plain films alone. The multiplanar capability, high contrast, and special resolution of CT allow assessment of complex anatomy and detection of subtle fractures. In addition, CT is useful in the detection of occult fractures suspected on the basis of physical examination findings and/or bone scintigrams when plain films are normal (Fig. 16–9).[1] CT may provide the necessary information for clinical management: whether the fracture affects the articular cartilage, how much articular cortex is involved, the number and size of fragments, amount of displacement, rotation and location of the fragments (whether a fragment is within the space of the joint). All of this information may help determine whether to perform closed or open reduction and fixation. Generally, the best plane to show a fracture is the anatomic plane perpendicular to the fracture plane. Usually, two scan planes are optimal to accurately assess complex fracture relationships.

Scaphoid Fracture

Scaphoid fracture is the most common carpal bone fracture.[34] Two-thirds of the scaphoid fractures are through the waist. In most cases, the fracture plane is nearly parallel or slightly oblique to the axial axis. It rarely occurs in the sagittal or coronal plane. The best scan plane for evaluating the scaphoid fracture is along the long axis of the scaphoid, i.e., either direct coronal plane[2] or oblique scaphoid long axial plane. The sagittal plane is also more valuable than the axial plane because it is generally more closely perpendicular to the predominant fracture plane pattern.[2]

The long sagittal axial scaphoid scan plane is ex-

Text continued on page 423

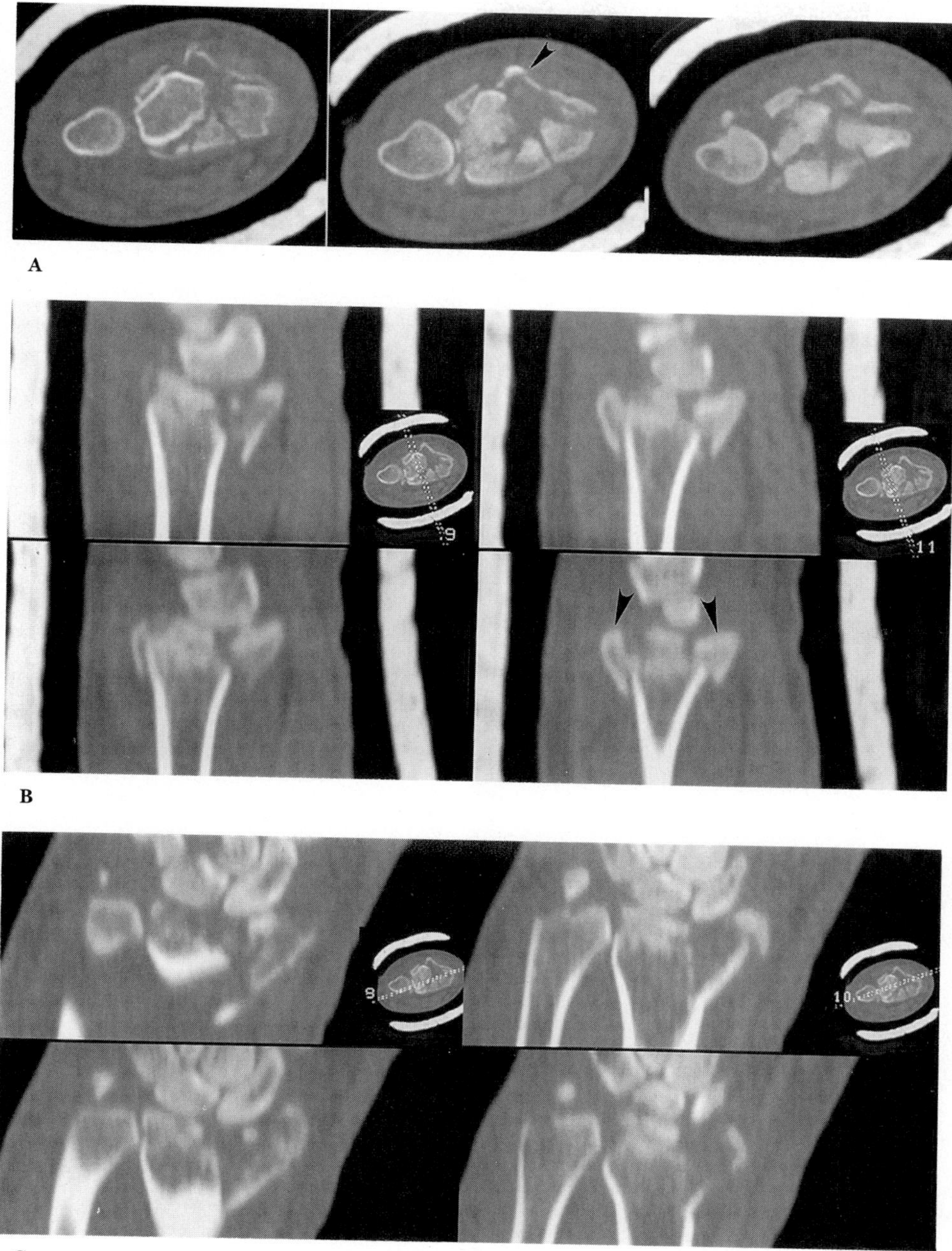

FIGURE 16–7. Axial images in a 70-year-old man following a fall. **A:** Axial images demonstrate a complex intraarticular fracture of the distal radius with extension into the DRUJ as well as Lister's tubercle (arrowhead). Sagittal reconstructions **(B)** demonstrate outward displacement of both dorsal and ventral fracture fragments (arrowheads). (Ventral is to the reader's right.) Coronal reconstructions **(C)** show impaction of central part of the radiocarpal joint (also seen on sagittal images) and displacement of fractures of both the radial and ulnar styloids.

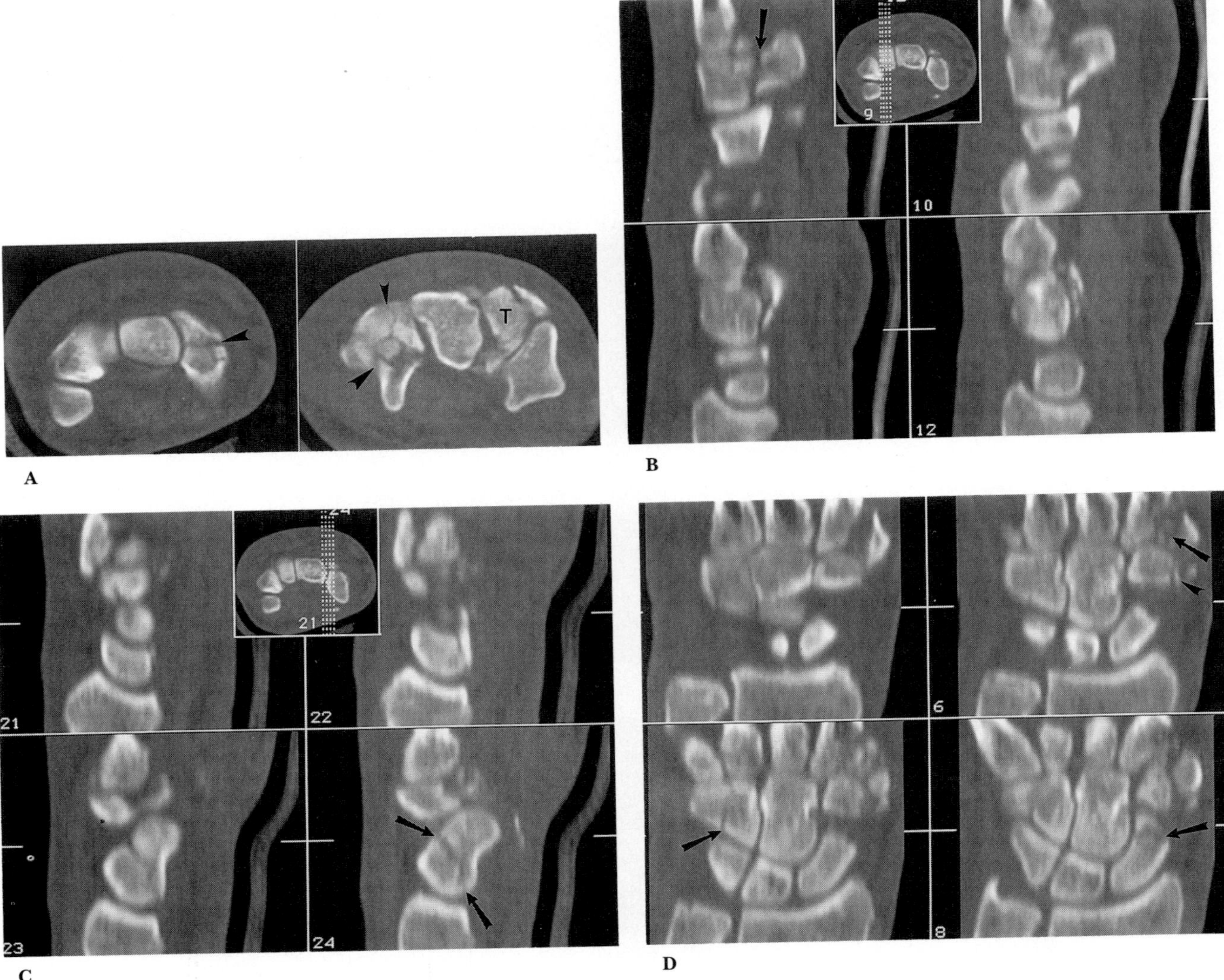

FIGURE 16–8. Axial spiral CT examination of wrist in patient following motorcycle accident. Axial images **(A)** from proximal (left image) and distal carpus (right image) demonstrate complex fractures of the scaphoid (arrowhead on left), hamate (arrowheads on right), and trapezoid (T). Sagittal reconstructions **(B)** at the ulnar side of the wrist demonstrate comminuted fracture through the hamate hook (arrow) and sagittal images from the radial side of the wrist **(C)** demonstrate a 1- to 2-mm displaced fracture (between arrows) through the scaphoid waist. Coronal reconstructions **(D)** show fractures extending through the midportion of the hamate (arrow in lower left image), fracture of the scaphoid (arrow in lower right image), shattering of the radial aspect of the base of the second metacarpal (arrow in upper right image), and fracture through the radial cortex of the trapezoid (arrowhead).

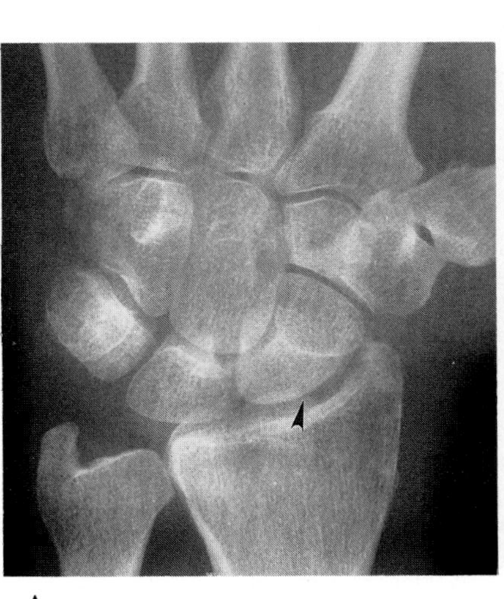

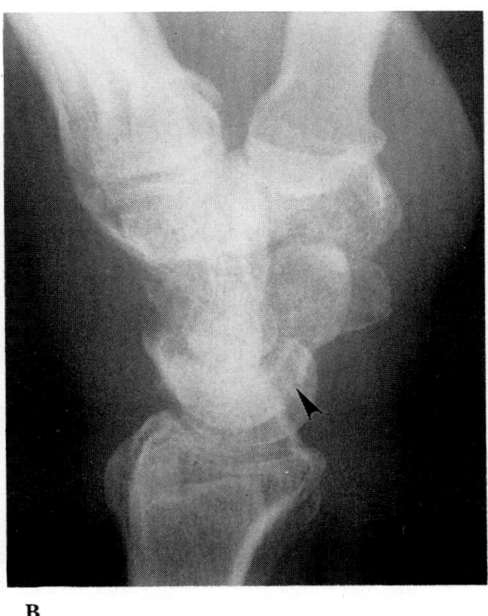

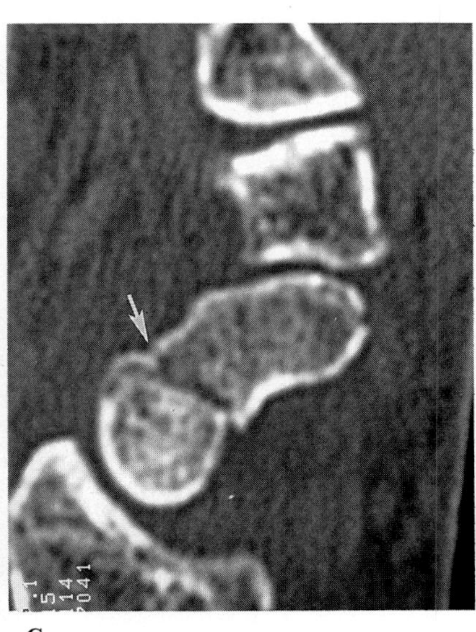

A B C

FIGURE 16–9. PA (**A**) and lateral (**B**) views of the left wrist show a questionable scaphoid fracture (arrowheads). **C:** Long axial scaphoid CT image shows a fracture line across the scaphoid waist with about 2 mm of palmar displacement of the distal fracture fragment (arrow).

cellent for evaluating scaphoid fractures (Figs. 16–10A and 16–10B).[1] Because the images in one scan plane may not clearly demonstrate an occult fracture, a second scan is usually necessary, either by reformation or by another set of scans, to adequately display needed information. The second scan plane images may also provide additional information, such as how much displacement of a scaphoid fracture is present in a direction additional to that shown on the first CT scan plane. The displacement of a scaphoid waist fracture in the radial and ulnar direction may show up best (or only) on coronal plane CT (Fig. 16–10C).[34] Dorsal and palmar fracture fragment displacement is best shown on long axial scaphoid CT images (Fig. 16–10D). A fracture displacement of 1 to 2 mm or more indicates a need for internal manipulation and fixation.

Direct coronal plane images can be obtained in most patients. It may be slightly more difficult to perform a direct coronal CT after trauma because of difficulty for the patient to move the injured part and diminished capability to maintain the part in a fixed position for the examination.[34] Using a Vannier's wrist holder, a direct coronal CT scan can be obtained by placing the injured wrist on a lucite holder (see Fig. 16–2C) in maximum tolerable extension. With the gantry paralleling the extended wrist, the rest of the forearm may be placed out of the scanning plane to minimize beam hardening artifacts. If coronal plane CT is performed in a Vannier's holder or in this position of wrist extension, a coronal plane will be obtained down the longest axis of the scaphoid. In the injured patient who has limited mobility or who has a long arm cast, a modification of the Pennes's position can usually be obtained to provide a coronal plane view. This can be accomplished by keeping the elbow flexed 90 degrees (as in a long arm cast) and putting the wrist above the head with thumb down (toward the floor) and the ulnar side of the wrist directed toward the ceiling with the patient supine. The gantry can be angled to parallel the coronal axis of the wrist and not to produce images that pass obliquely through the carpus. The cast can be secured to the table with tape. Similarly, coronal plane images can be obtained by placing the hand and wrist in a saluting position over the head; or in a small person or a person lying on the affected shoulder, the elbow and shoulder can be flexed 90 degrees and the fingers pointed to the ceiling. In this position, the dorsum of the arm (not the forearm) lies flat on the table.

A common complication of scaphoid fractures is development of the dorsal humpback deformity, commonly found with an exostosis-like prominence on the dorsal surface of the healed fracture line, which is caused by palmar angulation of the distal pole after fracture (Fig. 16–11A).[33] This configuration may lead to foreshortening of the healed scaphoid fracture, which may be predisposed eventually to degenerative radiocarpal arthritis and long-term functional impairment.[35] A routine lateral wrist radiograph may not clearly demonstrate this deformity because of overlap of the carpal bones.[36] CT can display the individual carpal bones.[35,37] Sagittal and long axis (as well as polytomography) scaphoid plane CT scans are the preferred ways to demonstrate this deformity (Figs. 16–11B and 16–11C).[34]

A common use of CT is to assess fracture healing, malunion, nonunion, or possible avascular necrosis.[34] A previous CT study may be useful to determine the optimal plane to be used. To evaluate a known or suspected scaphoid fracture, a long sagittal axial

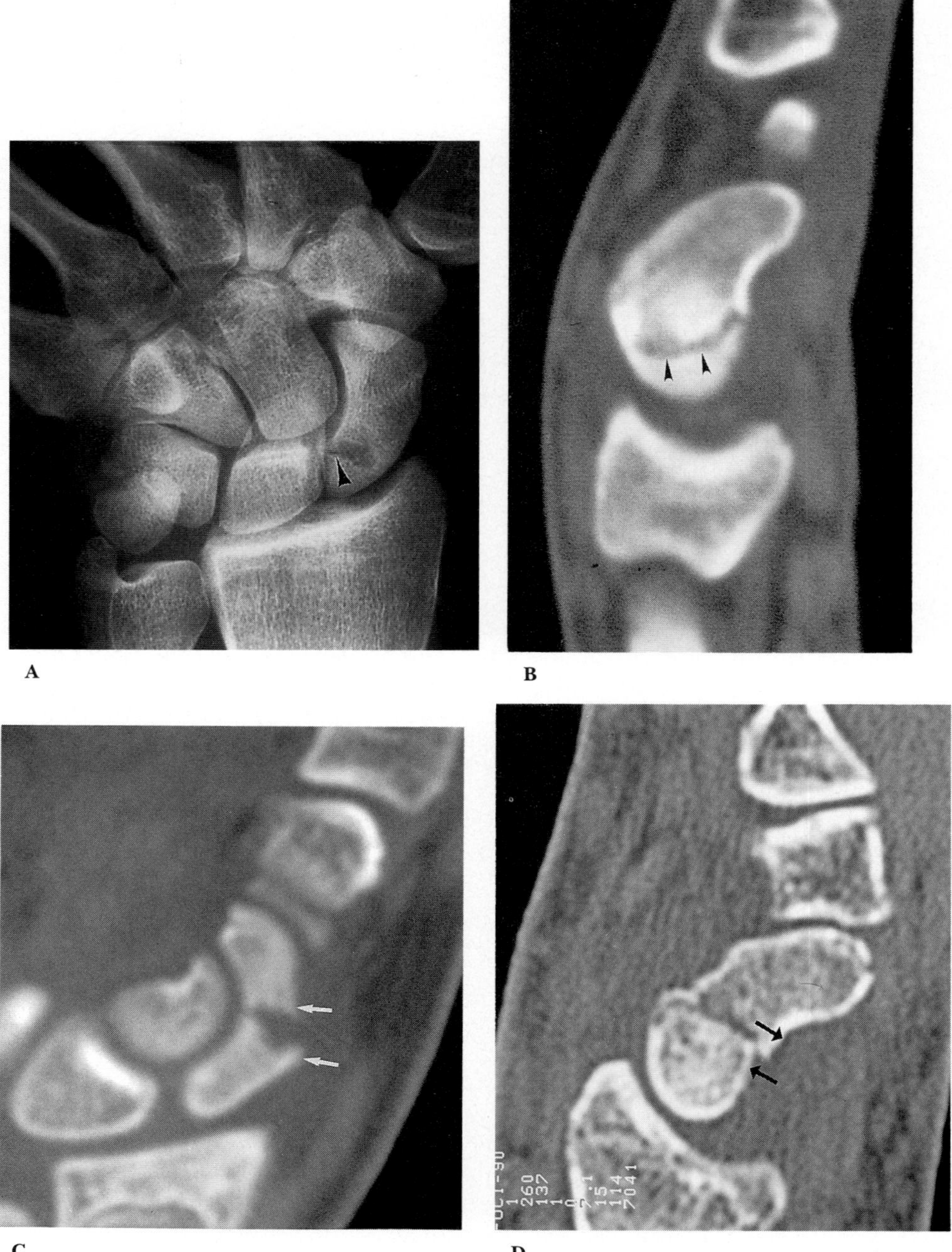

FIGURE 16–10. A: PA view of the left wrist in ulnar deviation demonstrates a radiolucent defect at the proximal pole of the scaphoid with a questionable fracture at this point (arrowhead). **B:** Long axial scaphoid CT image shows fracture (arrowheads) of the scaphoid with sclerosis on both sides of the fracture. **C:** In another patient a coronal image shows radial separation of scaphoid waist fracture fragments (between arrows). **D:** Long axial scaphoid CT image of the left scaphoid of the patient in **C** demonstrates palmar displacement of the distal fracture fragment evidenced by an offset between the two fracture fragments (arrows). (Reprinted with permission from the Radiological Society of North America. Stewart NR, Gilula LA. CT of the wrist: A tailored approach. *Radiology* 1992;183:13–20.)

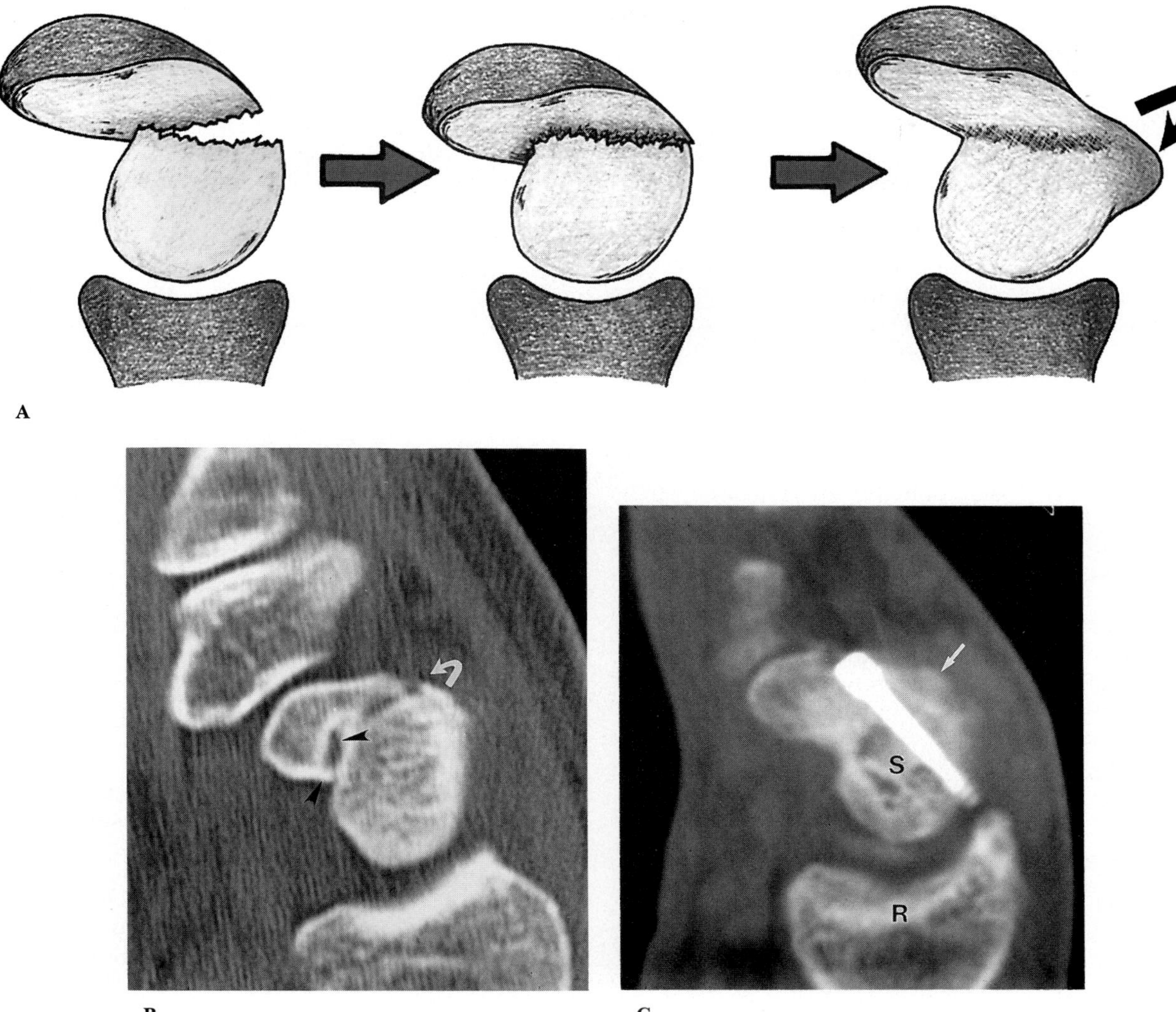

FIGURE 16–11. A: A diagram shows development of a dorsal humpback deformity (curved arrow) caused by ventral angulation of the distal pole after fracture. **B:** Long axis scaphoid CT image shows a developing dorsal humpback deformity (curved arrow), which is caused by ventral angulation of the distal scaphoid fracture fragment and late exostosis formation at the fracture site dorsally. A nonunion is evident with cortical margins (arrowheads) along the ventral half of the fracture line. **C:** Long axis scaphoid CT image demonstrates palmar angulation of the distal pole of the scaphoid after healed fracture with exostosis or dorsal humpback deformity (arrow). Passing the CT plane down the long axis of the fixating Herbert's screw results in very little metallic streak artifact. R, radius; S, scaphoid.

scaphoid plane is mandatory. It can demonstrate whether there is bony bridging of the fracture site, nonunion, humpback deformity, and/or DISI configuration (lunate tilted dorsally).[36] Displacement and dorsal tilting of a scaphoid fracture may be manifested as dorsal tilting of lunate, creating a DISI configuration. In other words, any dorsal tilting of the lunate may reflect dorsal tilting of the proximal scaphoid fragment with palmar tilting of the distal fragment[36] because of an intact scapholunate and adjacent extrinsic ligaments. This is called "bony DISI." The configuration can be better shown on the long sagittal axial scaphoid plane.[36] Images in the coronal plane are most helpful if further characterization of the scaphoid fracture is desired, as with radioulnar displacement of fracture fragments and bone healing along the radial and/or ulnar sides of the fracture site. In addition, congruency of the scaphocapitate joint can be best evaluated with coronal plane CT.

For those patients who have the carpus casted in a set position, the angulation of the gantry can be adjusted to obtain the true coronal plane,[34] or a 40-degree angled coronal CT is possible by adjusting both the gantry and the patient position.[38] This procedure has proven to be a reliable method of displaying scaphoid fractures and assessing healing without removing the cast.[38]

CT scans can clearly demonstrate the presence

(Fig. 16–12A) or absence (Fig. 16–12B) of bony healing of the scaphoid fracture.[30,39] In early union, partial bony bridging superimposes on residual fracture gap. CT may demonstrate bony bridging between fragments that cannot be confirmed on plain radiographs (Fig. 16–12C). Some partial bony healing of a scaphoid fracture may present as a radiolucent line on plain radiographs, which may be interpreted as nonunion, whereas CT scans can demonstrate partial or complete bony healing (Figs. 16–12C and 16–13). Some radiographs may demonstrate apparent total bony healing of the fracture, whereas CT demonstrates only partial bony healing or complete nonunion, because of the lack of profile and display of an entire fracture line on a plain radiograph. CT can show whether there is bony healing and, if so, its exact location (Fig. 16–13). Thin section tomography may be helpful in instances when CT is unavailable. But focal bone bridging may not be as easily detected with thin section tomography as with CT scans because of the tomographic blur. In the case of a Herbert screw or other metallic fixation, CT is also an excellent way to evaluate the presence or absence of bony union. Careful positioning of the wrist by aligning the Herbert screw parallel to the scan plane usually enables the images to avoid the metal artifact and obtain satisfactory information about healing (Figs. 16–11C, 16–12A, 16–12B, and 16–13D).

Capitate Fracture

Capitate fractures are uncommon. A review article by Adler and Shaftan[40] reported that 91 cases were found in the literature. These included 48 isolated capitate fractures, 11 cases of scaphocapitate syndrome, and 32 capitate fractures associated with other carpal injuries.[40] Because the proximal pole of the capitate is entirely intraarticular, capitate waist fractures often result in nonunion and avascular necrosis.[40–42] CT examination of the capitate usually requires two complementary planes to more fully evaluate the capitate. Coronal imaging may show waist fractures nicely (Fig. 16–14). Direct sagittal plane imaging may demonstrate a fracture in the coronal plane and show the longitudinal anatomy of the carpal and metacarpal bones as well as dorsal/ventral displacement of the fragments. A second plane is usually needed to demonstrate additional displacement and/or rotation, e.g., the coronal plane will show radial and/or ulnar displacement of the fragments.

Hamate Hook Fracture

Hamate hook fracture is the most common fracture of the hamate. These fractures frequently result from direct force. A plain-film diagnosis is usually difficult. An axial CT scan is particularly useful to assess hamate fractures as well as trapezial bone fractures (Fig. 16–15A).[30] Sagittal imaging may also show hamate body fractures (Fig. 16–15B). Bilateral axial scans of the wrist allow exclusion of congenital anomalies of the hamate hook or other abnormalities, especially when the plain film is normal while the bone scan is prominently abnormal (Figs. 16–16A through 16–16C).[29] In one case, an unusual erosive lesion of the hamate hook without soft-tissue mass was characterized by CT scan, confirming it as a benign lesion.[43]

Lunate Fracture

Lunate fracture is uncommon, accounting for 1.2–3% of carpal fractures.[44,45] When fractures occur, they are usually palmar (Fig. 16–17A) or dorsal (Fig. 16–17B) chip fractures caused by either axial compression or hyperextension.[45] Sagittal CT images best demonstrate this fracture.[45] When evaluating Kienböck's disease, coronal scanning is an excellent plane for quantifying the degree of sclerosis and compression of the lunate, the presence of the fracture, fragmentation, and cyst formation. This plane also shows the relationship between the carpal rows, carpal bone, radius, metacarpals, and the radioulnar joint.[46] Direct sagittal plane CT scan is valuable to show coronal plane fractures of the lunate.

Distal Radius Fracture

Distal radius fractures are very common, especially in elderly patients. Diagnosis of most of these fractures does not require a CT scan; however, in cases when the fracture is intraarticular or severely comminuted, or an intraarticular fragment is suspected, CT imaging may be helpful (Fig. 16–18). Coronal or sagittal plane CT scans are excellent for demonstrating depression fractures of the distal radius (Fig. 16–19A), whereas sagittal CT images may help demonstrate palmar or dorsal chip fractures of the distal radius (Fig. 16–19B) as well as depressions and diastases between fragments. In addition, sagittal plane CT images are valuable to show how much bone void exists along the dorsal (or ventral) portions of the distal radius for dorsal (or ventral) impacted fractures of the distal radius. CT may help detect a subtle fracture in the case of a "normal" appearance on plain films (Fig. 16–20A) especially when further examination is indicated by a "very hot" bone scan (Fig. 16–20B).

Fracture and/or Dislocation of a Metacarpal Base

Carpometacarpal (CMC) joint dislocations or subluxations associated with metacarpal base fracture are uncommon but not rare. Subtle radiographic findings may result in failure to recognize these dislocations or subluxations. Such joint subluxations are reported to be the most frequently overlooked wrist joint dislocations.[47–49] Dorsal dislocations are more common than ventral dislocations, and these are frequently associated with fractures, either from the

Text continued on page 429

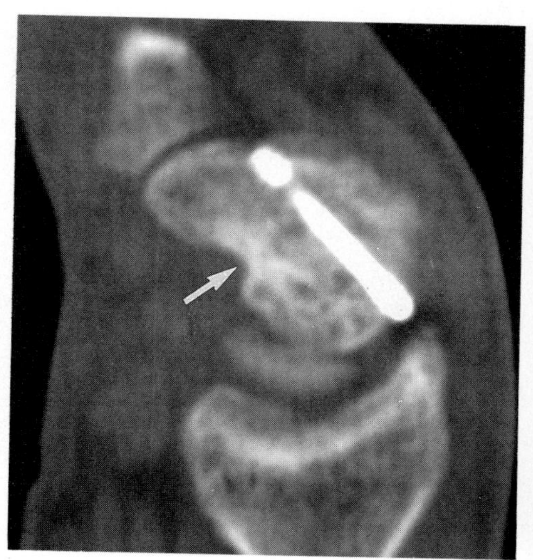

A

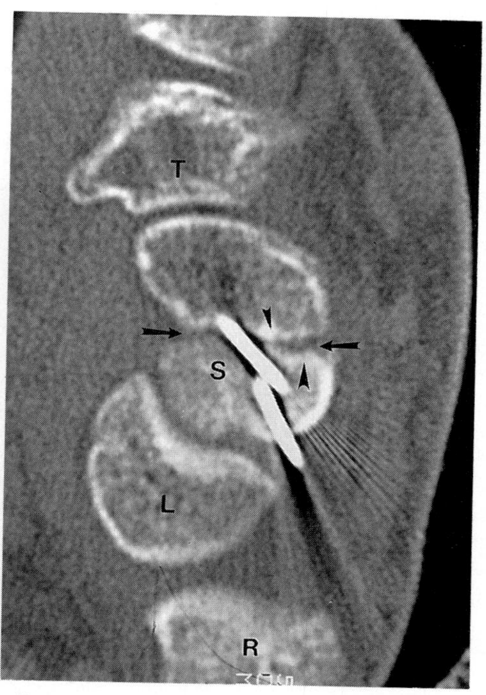

B

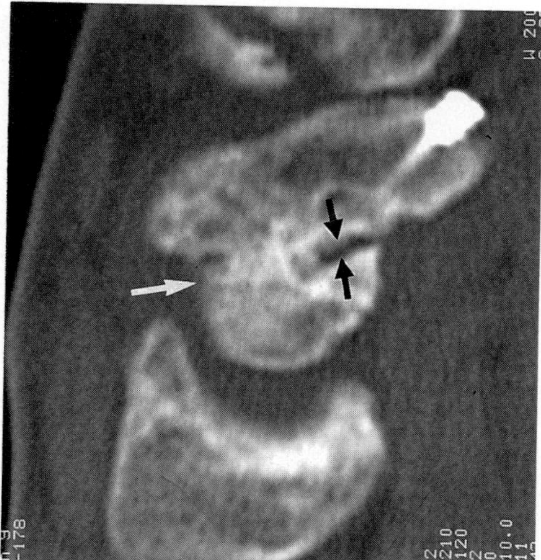

C

FIGURE 16–12. A: Long sagittal axial CT image of a right fractured scaphoid demonstrates solid bony healing (arrow) of the scaphoid fracture even with a Herbert screw present. **B:** Long sagittal axial CT image of a right scaphoid fracture in another patient demonstrates nonunion of the scaphoid fracture (arrows) after 4 months of internal pin fixation. A gap and sclerosis involves both fracture ends (between arrowheads). Minimal streak artifacts project proximally from the pins, but diagnostic detail is not lost. The lunate is tilting dorsally; however, sectioning the lunate obliquely may create a pseudo dorsal tilting of the lunate, and such "dorsal tilting" should be confirmed with a standard neutral lateral plain film view before definite dorsal tilting is diagnosed. L, lunate; R, radius; S, scaphoid; T, trapezium. **C:** Long sagittal CT image of a scaphoid fracture demonstrates solid bony healing of the dorsal part of the scaphoid fracture (white arrow). The distal end of a Herbert screw is present without streak artifacts. A nonunion fracture gap involves the palmar half of the scaphoid (between black arrows). (Reprinted with permission from the Radiological Society of North America. Stewart NR, Gilula LA. CT of the wrist: A tailored approach. *Radiology* 1992;183:13–20.)

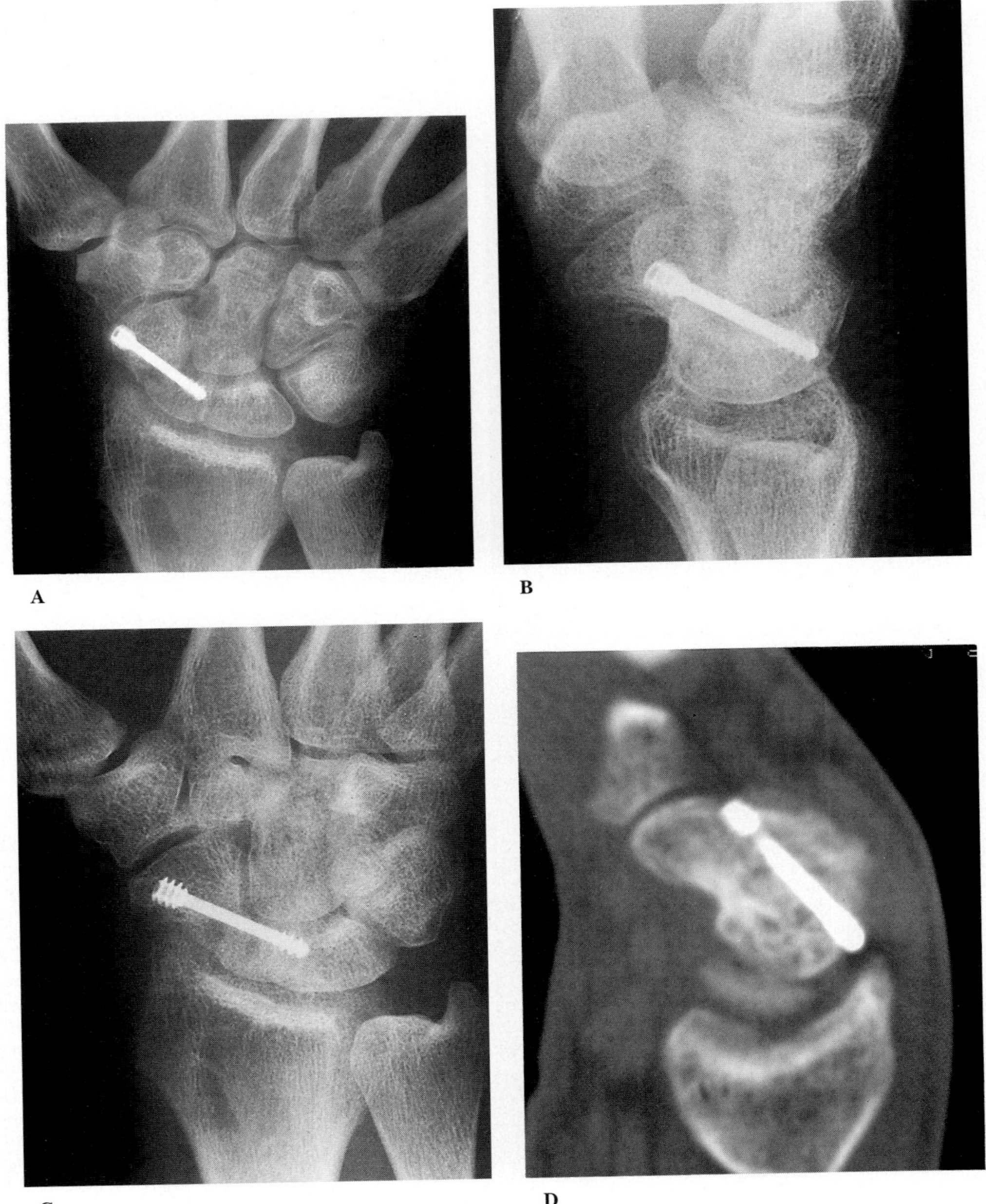

FIGURE 16–13. PA **(A)**, lateral **(B)**, and oblique **(C)** views of the right wrist after Herbert's screw internal fixation demonstrates a radiolucent line visible at the scaphoid waist. **D:** Long sagittal axial CT image of the scaphoid demonstrates solid healing with humpback deformity of the scaphoid. The Herbert's screw creates no appreciable streak artifact.

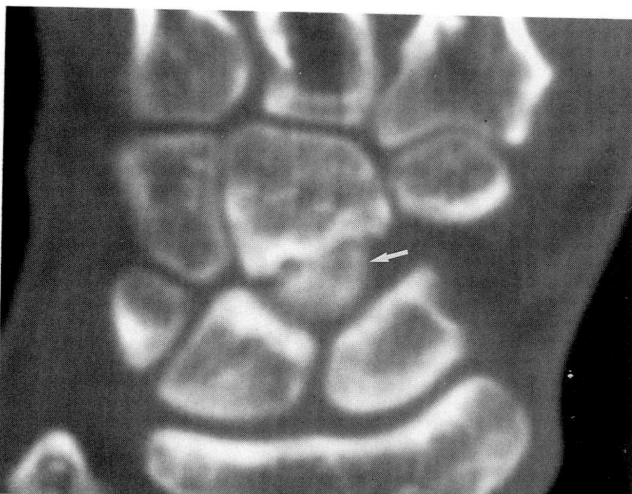

FIGURE 16–14. Coronal image of the left wrist demonstrates fracture of the capitate. The proximal fragment is much smaller (arrow) than the distal fragment, which means there is either dorsal or palmar displacement or rotation of the proximal fragment, or less commonly, the proximal fracture fragment has lost volume, such as from avascular necrosis.

metacarpal bases or small avulsions from the carpal bones.[48,50,51] Fracture of an adjacent metacarpal shaft is a common associated dislocation or subluxation. These entities are usually best demonstrated on the coronal and/or sagittal plane (Fig. 16–21).[30]

DRUJ

CT is ideal for evaluation of either subluxation or dislocation of the distal radioulnar joint (DRUJ) and the rotational mobility of the radioulnar articulation, which may prove valuable in identifying postoperative and posttraumatic changes.[52] Anatomically, the distal ulna is considered the relatively fixed structure at the DRUJ around which the radius and carpus rotate. However, clinically and radiographically, instabilities and translations are usually described by the distal ulnar position.[53–56] Motion at the DRUJ is comprised of about 150 degrees of radius rotation around the ulnar head with sliding or translation of the ulnar head in the sigmoid notch of the distal radius. The ulnar head will slide in the radial sigmoid notch from a dorsal distal position to a palmar proximal position as the forearm rotates from full pronation into full supination.

Injury of the DRUJ is usually associated with many other disorders, including ulnar styloid fracture, radial diaphyseal fracture, Colles's fracture, and so on. Occasionally it may be subjected to isolated traumatic subluxation or dislocation. Dislocation can often be diagnosed on plain films; however, it may be difficult to obtain a true lateral view, because pain or immobility may be a limiting factor.[17] The diagnosis of DRUJ subluxation usually is difficult on plain films.[57]

Axial CT through the head of the ulna provides an excellent method to observe normal and abnormal

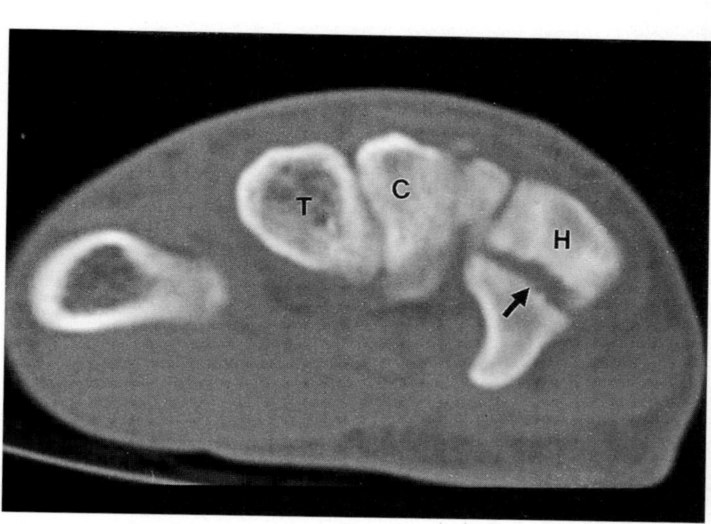

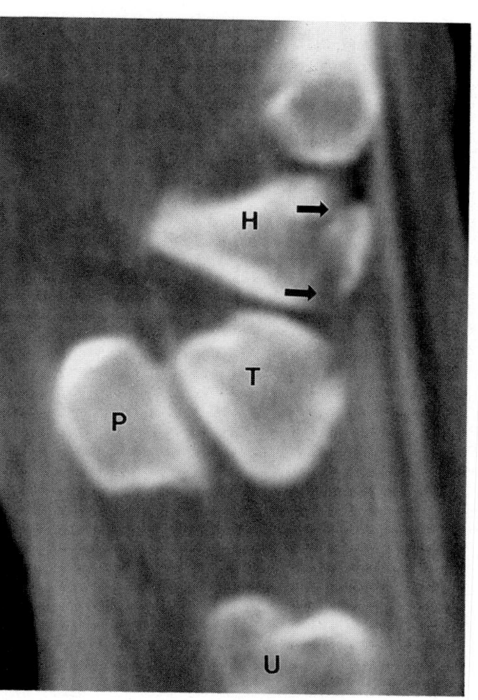

FIGURE 16–15. A: An axial CT image of a right wrist shows a transverse fracture of the base of the hamate hook (arrow). T, trapezoid; C, capitate; H, hamate. **B**: Sagittal image of a right wrist demonstrates a fracture of the hamate along the coronal plane (arrows). The fragment has migrated dorsally and proximally. H, hamate; T, triquetrum; P, pisiform; U, ulna.

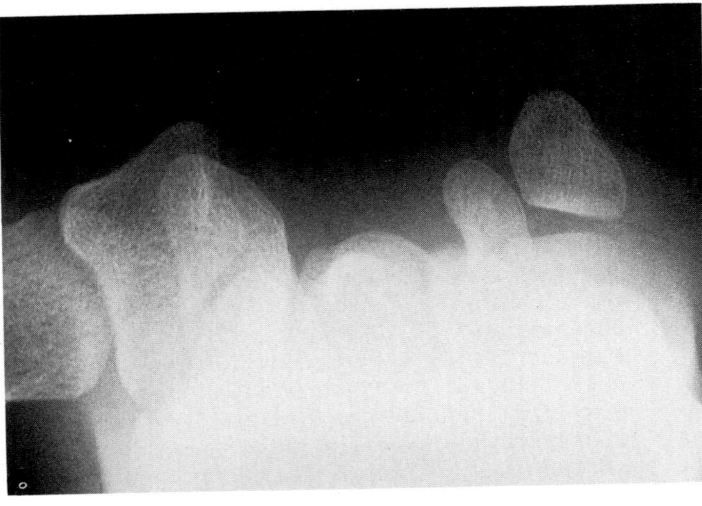

A

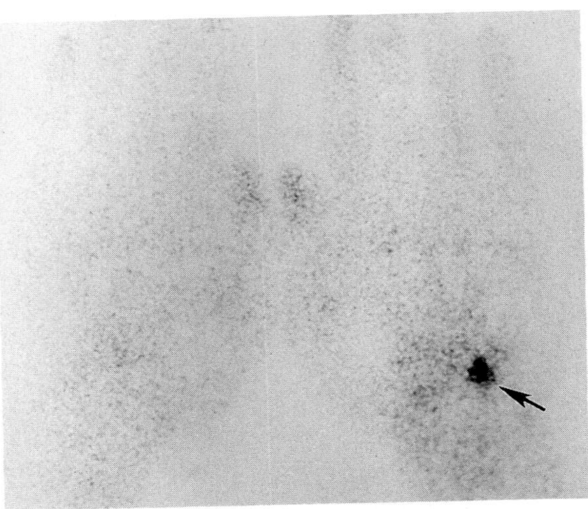

B

FIGURE 16–16. A: A carpal tunnel view of the right wrist is normal. **B:** On the palmar bone scan of both wrists increased uptake of Tc^{99m} is in the right hamate (arrow). **C:** An axial CT scan image of bilateral wrists shows a small high-density calcification near the hook of the hamate (arrowhead) most consistent with calcific tendonitis. H, hamate; C, capitate; Td, trapezoid.

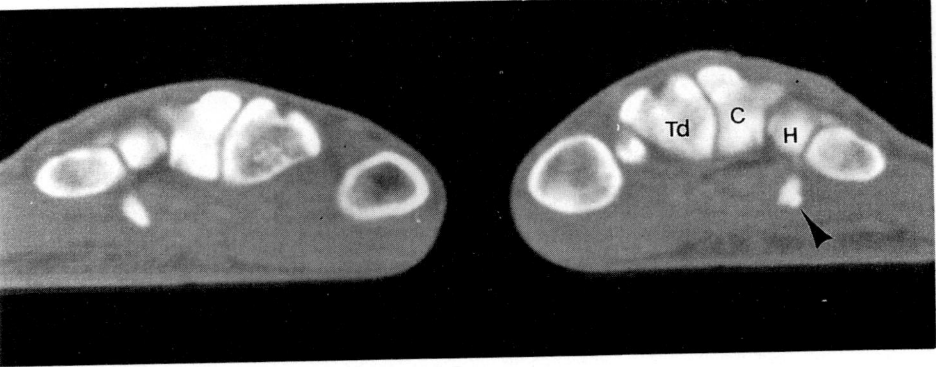

C

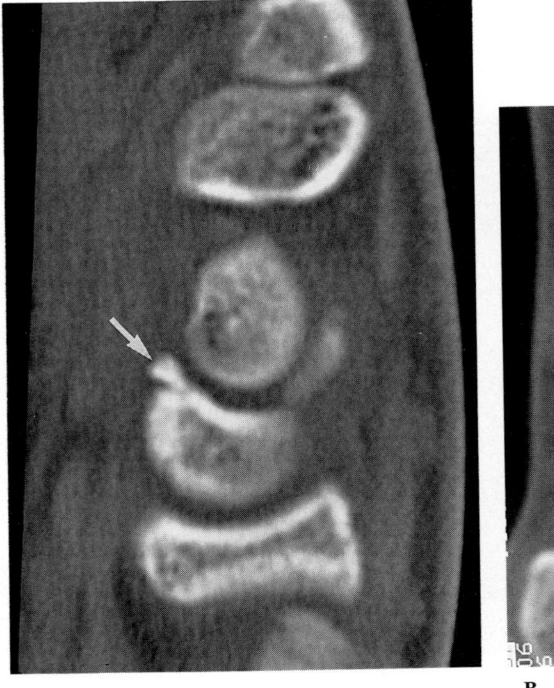

A

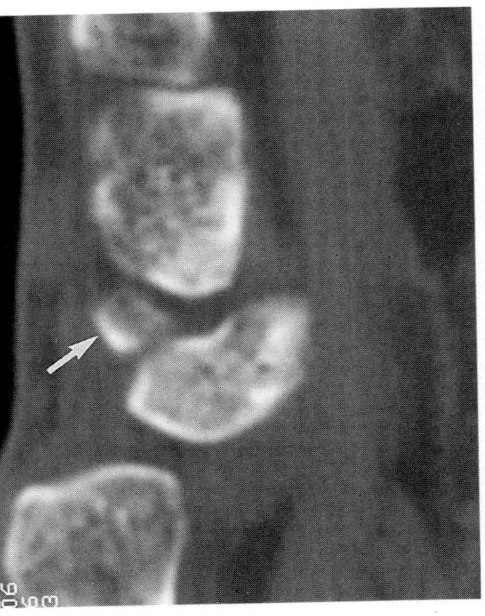

B

FIGURE 16–17. A: Sagittal CT image of the right wrist demonstrates a small chip fracture fragment off the anterior distal edge of the lunate (arrow). **B:** Sagittal CT image of the left wrist demonstrates a chip fracture fragment off the posterior distal edge of the lunate (arrow).

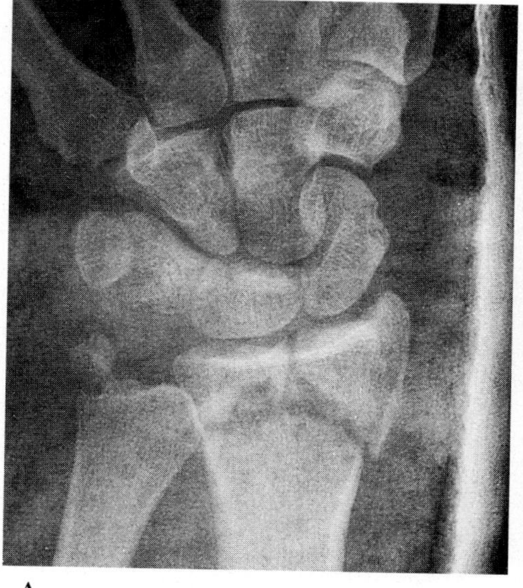

A

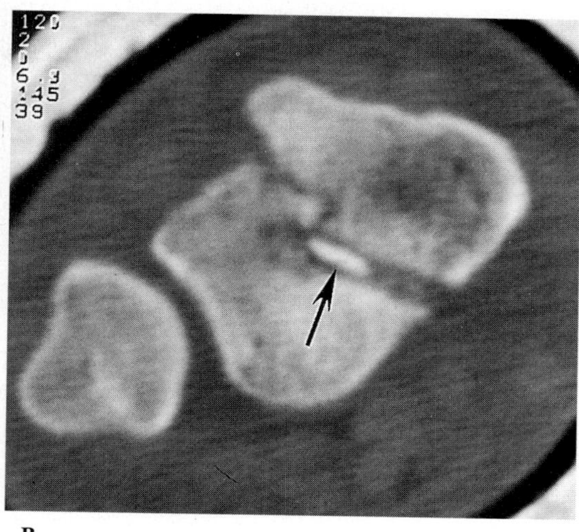

B

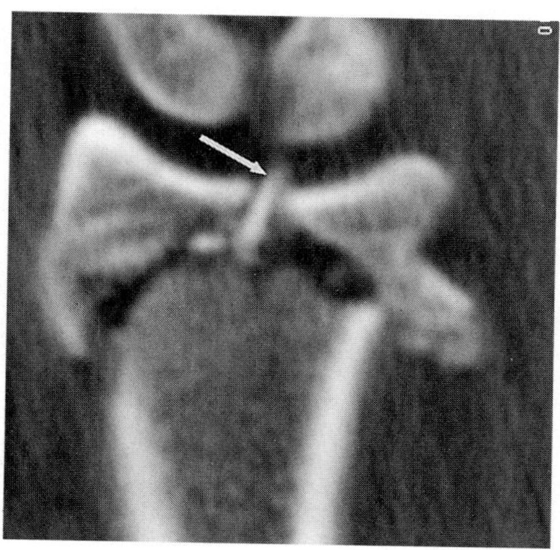

C

FIGURE 16–18. Distal radius fracture. **A:** An obliqued posteroanterior view of the left wrist (in a cast) demonstrates a comminuted distal radius and ulnar styloid fractures. **B:** Axial image of the wrist shows a distal radius fracture. A cortical fragment (black arrow) is located in the fracture gap. **C:** An obliqued sagittal image demonstrates a fragment (arrow) located between the two distal radius fragments projecting into the radiocarpal joint space.

rotational relationships of the DRUJ and to measure the distal radioulnar angle through a range of motion. Axial CT can be performed on both wrists simultaneously, allowing comparison with the contralateral wrist. The comparison of bilateral DRUJs provides a good method to detect subtle abnormalities (Fig. 16–22).[1,34] Some authors recommend that in evaluating subluxation of the DRUJ, axial plane images should be obtained in three positions: full supination, neutral, and full pronation. We recommend at least two scans in different positions. The hands are initially positioned prone and the thumbs side by side with the DRUJs of both wrists at the same level for symmetry. The hands and forearms are taped securely to the CT table. Because DRUJ abnormalities are often dynamic and may appear reduced at some point in the arc from full pronation to full supination, images in a second position are recommended with the hands placed symmetrically in the position that reproduces the patient's symptoms, typically pain or limited range of movement. Once the painful position is identified, e.g., oversupination or overpronation, both hands and wrists are taped together to maintain this "symptomatic" position. Then the hands and wrists are taped securely to the table.[1] Familiarity of the radiologist with the normal rotation and translation that occurs between the distal radius and ulna is important.[52,58]

Rotation of the radius around the ulna is accompanied by ulnar translation, so that in supination the ulna is somewhat palmar, whereas in pronation the ulna is more dorsal relative to the radius.[58] The plain film examination usually requires careful positioning to identify instability; subluxations may still be difficult to recognize on plain films. A CT scan can be performed with the hand in any position.[59] The result of the CT scan does not depend as much on position as the plain film examination.[59] Some authors recog-

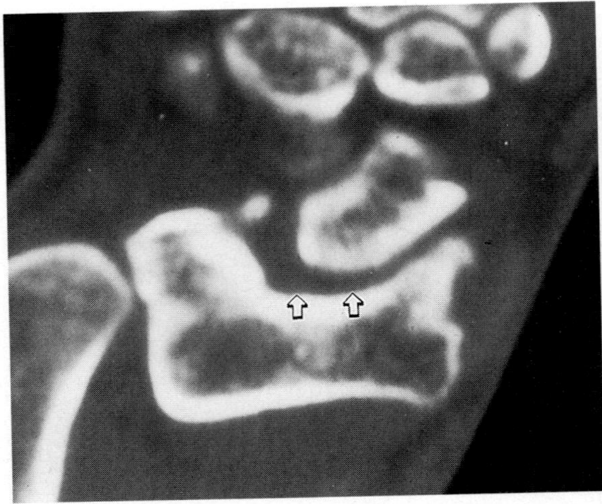

A

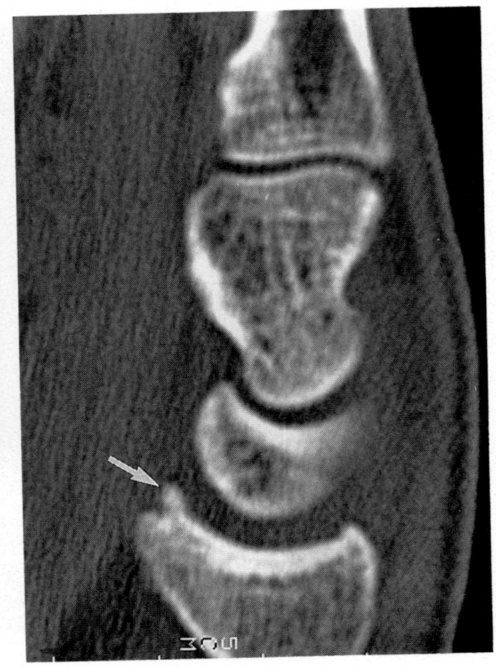

B

FIGURE 16–19. A: A coronal plane CT image shows depression fracture of the scaphoid fossa (arrows). (Reprinted with permission from the Radiological Society of North America. Stewart NR, Gilula LA. CT of the wrist: A tailored approach. *Radiology* 1992;183:13–20.) **B:** In another patient a sagittal plane CT image demonstrates a chip fracture from the palmar rim of the distal radius (arrow).

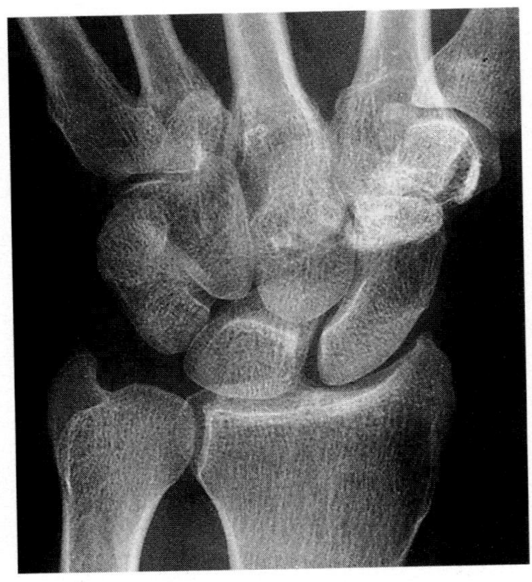

A

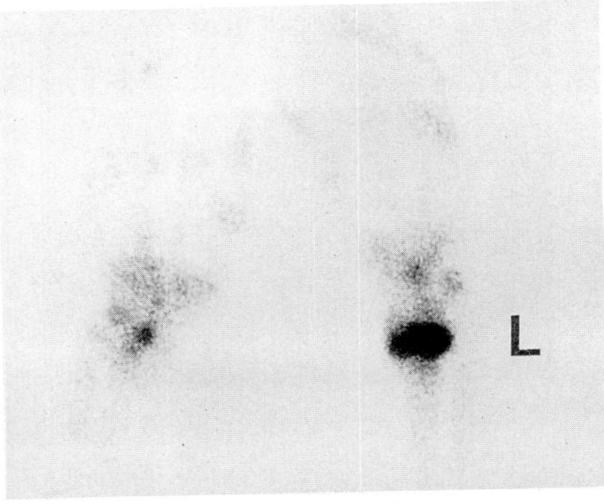

B

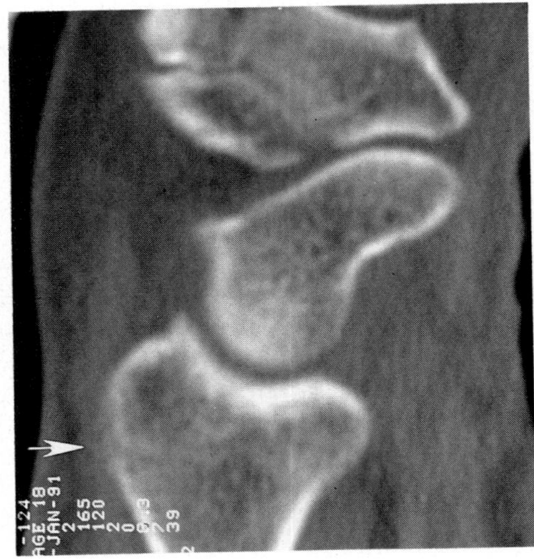

C

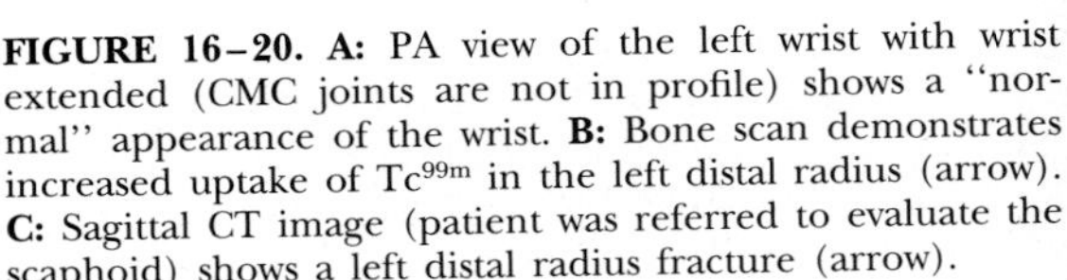

FIGURE 16–20. A: PA view of the left wrist with wrist extended (CMC joints are not in profile) shows a "normal" appearance of the wrist. **B:** Bone scan demonstrates increased uptake of Tc^{99m} in the left distal radius (arrow). **C:** Sagittal CT image (patient was referred to evaluate the scaphoid) shows a left distal radius fracture (arrow).

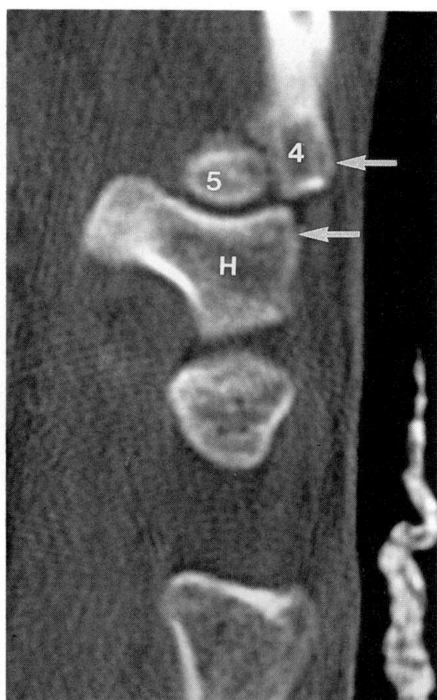

FIGURE 16–21. Sagittal CT image of a right wrist shows dorsal subluxation of the fourth metacarpal base (arrows). 4, fourth metacarpal bone; 5, fifth metacarpal bone; H, hamate.

nize that supination and pronation may change the relationship between distal radius and ulna at the DRUJ, but it is not necessary to put the hand in a certain position for the examination, as is necessary for the lateral plain film.[59] However, it is valuable to keep both DRUJs in identical positions for ease of interpreting CT results. Occasionally a CT scan performed under stress on the DRUJ may be helpful in finding the dynamic instabilities.[60]

CARPAL TUNNEL SYNDROME

The carpal tunnel is formed by the carpal bones and a ligament through which the flexor tendons of the fingers and median nerve pass. The ventral surface of the carpus has a concave shape. The transverse carpal ligament is a thick fibrous band that passes superficial to the concave surface of the carpal bones, the flexor tendons, and the median nerve, attaching radially to the distal scaphoid tuberosity and a portion of the trapezium and ulnarly to the pisiform and hook of the hamate. Usually the normal carpal tunnel is smaller in women than in men.[18]

The best scan plane in which to see the above relationships in the carpal tunnel is axial through the hamate hook (Fig. 16–23).[19] Using a soft-tissue window, the window and level setting should be adjusted for adequate visualization of the median nerve. The median nerve in normal wrists is a well-defined round structure surrounded by fat lying in the palmar superficial aspect of the carpal tunnel underneath the retinaculum.[19,20] It appears as a lower-density structure than the flexor tendons surrounding it. In flexion the median nerve usually moves dorsally, away from the flexor retinaculum.[19] Any process that increases the volume within the carpal tunnel may lead to compression of the median nerve and result in carpal tunnel syndrome. Axial CT may demonstrate carpal tunnel stenosis caused by thickening of the flexor retinaculum, synovial hyperplasia, edema, inflammation of the flexor tendons, neoplasm, and congenital abnormalities.[20,21,61] CT can demonstrate clearly enlargement of the carpal tunnel after operation.[22,61]

FOREIGN BODIES

CT is valuable for distinguishing subtle differences in densities, such as wood fragments, thorns, and

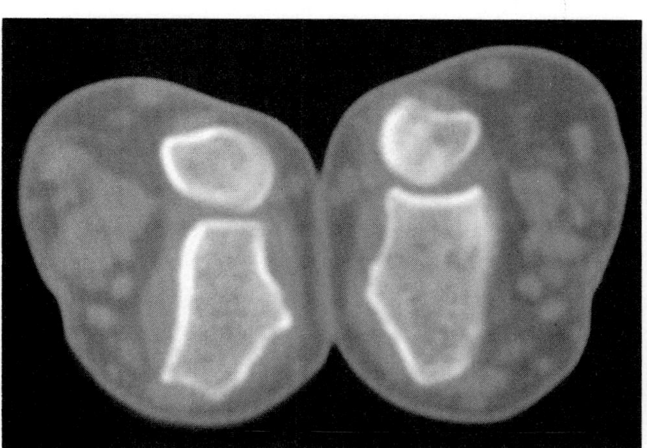

A

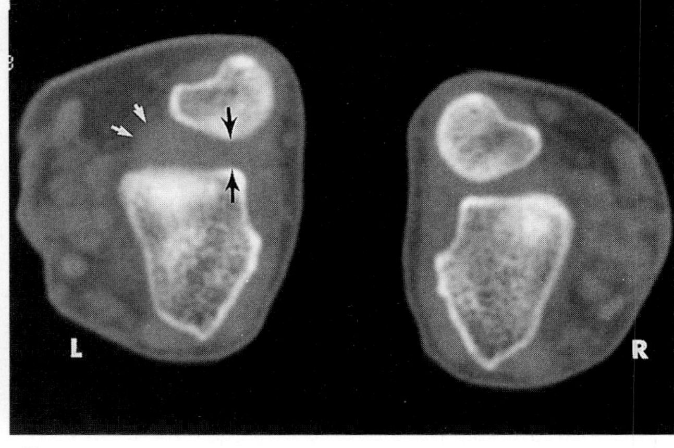

B

FIGURE 16–22. A: Axial images of both overpronated wrists demonstrates normal DRUJs. **B:** In another patient axial images of both overpronated wrists show left DRUJ widening (between black arrows) and soft-tissue swelling (white arrows). R, right; L, left.

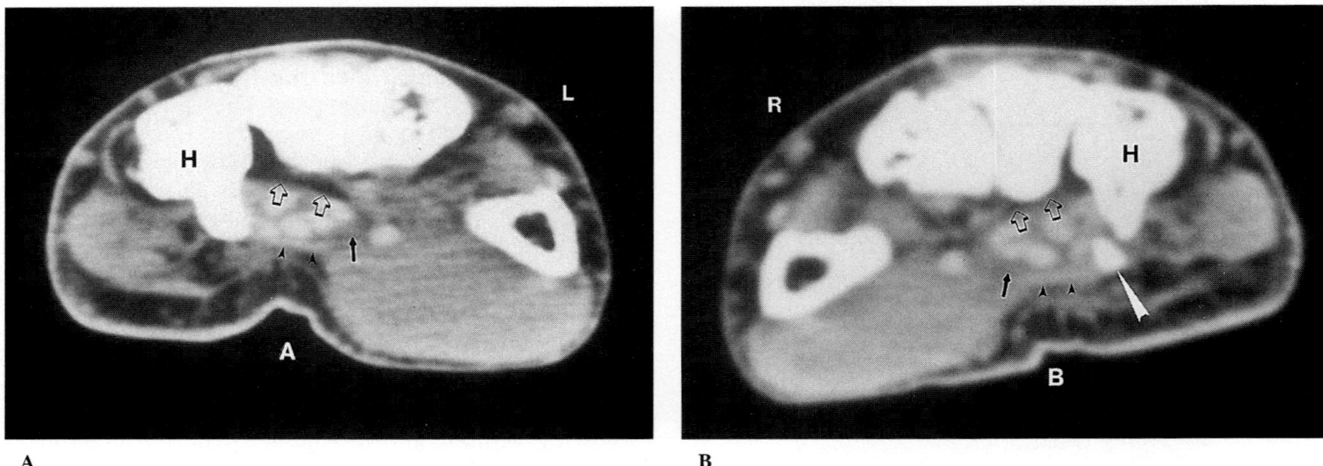

A B

FIGURE 16–23. Axial images of left (**A**) and right (**B**) wrists demonstrate a right hamate hook fracture (white arrowhead) and carpal tunnel swelling of the right wrist evidenced by loss of fat tissue on the right (compare open black arrows). H, hamate; black arrowheads, transverse ligament; small black arrows, median nerve.

A B

C

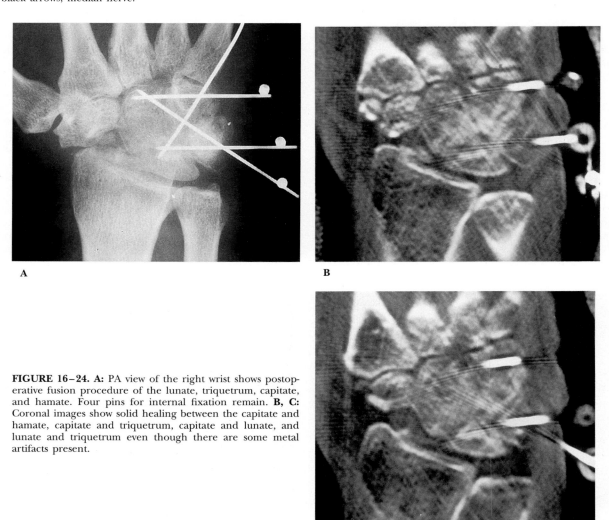

FIGURE 16–24. A: PA view of the right wrist shows postoperative fusion procedure of the lunate, triquetrum, capitate, and hamate. Four pins for internal fixation remain. **B, C:** Coronal images show solid healing between the capitate and hamate, capitate and triquetrum, capitate and lunate, and lunate and triquetrum even though there are some metal artifacts present.

splinters as well as glass, plastic, and metallic fragments. These can be detected readily by CT imaging.[5,7] A retained wood fragment usually contains air after injury and may appear as low attenuation in CT scanning, while the fragment may acquire high attenuation after remaining in the soft tissues for an extended period of time.[6,13] CT scans may show the exact location of the foreign material and its relationship to joints, tendons, the neurovascular bundle, and the carpal tunnel. This information helps define the surgical approach to the foreign body and preoperatively may help determine the extent of the debridement required.[5] CT may show a foreign-body granuloma when a thorn is too small or is radiotransparent. CT can exclude the presence of the foreign body within soft tissue.[22] Ultrasound can also be used to identify foreign bodies; when an experienced ultrasonographer is available, ultrasonography may be preferable since it is usually less expensive than CT (see Chapter 18). With either CT or ultrasound, a localizing mark or needle can be placed next to the foreign body for ease of body removal.

ARTHRODESIS AND POSTSURGICAL CHANGES

CT is better than plain radiography and conventional tomography for evaluating the amount of bone healing after osteotomy and/or arthrodesis. This is because thin section CT (1- to 2-mm thick sections at 1- to 2-mm intervals) can avoid the overlapping bone surfaces and other structures seen on plain radiography and allow direct imaging of the postsurgical appearance.[1,62]

The best plane for evaluation of joint fusion is perpendicular to the fusion plane. Axial or coronal planes work well when evaluating the scapholunate joint or lunate, capitate, and hamate fusion.[11,13,62] Coronal images can usually provide enough information about the status of an intercarpal arthrodesis even with the presence of K-wire pins (Fig. 16–24) to make clinical decisions. STT fusion is shown better on the oblique STT plane than on the coronal or axial planes (Fig. 16–5B).[1,62] Coronal CT image may also be used to evaluate joint fusion (Fig. 16–25); however, as mentioned, only an oblique semipronated or semisupinated position will show all three bones simultaneously well (Fig. 16–5).

CT can demonstrate clearly the amount of bone bridging or graft incorporation.[62] The best plane for showing the status of graft incorporation or fusion is perpendicular to the arthrodesis or graft–bone interface.[1] CT can show the exact position of the fixation screws and K-wires relative to joints and soft-tissue structures. Metal artifacts can be reduced if the scan plane is positioned carefully parallel to the metal (Fig. 16–26B).[1] Even when metal fixation devices are present, the CT scans usually provide more useful information than plain radiography or conventional tomography (Figs. 16–24 and 16–26A). Because conventional tomography procedures blur and conventional radiographs have too many overlapping osseous structures, four bone fusion (lunate, triquetrum, capitate, hamate) can be evaluated well by coronal images (Figs. 16–24 and 16–26A). Some sites of four bone fusions or STT fusion can be evaluated by sagittal and axial images (Figs. 16–26C and 16–26D). CT images may demonstrate whether there is a large or small area of osseous union between the bones postoperatively (Figs. 16–26E and 16–26F).

Evaluating Potentially Clinically Significant Lucent Defects Seen at Plain Radiology

Focal radiolucent intraosseous defects that communicate with the joint are thought to be more likely symptomatic than purely intraosseous lesions, especially when the defect has focal tenderness and focal increased uptake on the bone scintigram.[2] CT is useful for identifying whether a lucent defect communicates with an articular surface or if it is entirely intraosseous (Fig. 16–27). This can be assessed by obtaining scans perpendicular to the joint surfaces adjacent to the defect. Two-millimeter thick sections at 1-mm intervals are preferred for maximal resolution. The coronal plane is our preferred plane and is often sufficient to characterize the anatomic appearance of these defects. If the defect is large enough, some assessment of whether it contains fat, fluid, or fibrous tissue may be made by determining region of interest attenuation. Magnetic resonance imaging (MRI), or rarely arthrography,[63] can also be useful to characterize the nature of the defect.[1]

TUMOR

In general, CT cannot make a specific diagnosis of tumor; that is usually accomplished better with plain radiography. However, since CT has the ability to quantify the density of tissue, it may identify fatty tissue, fluid, and calcification.[64–67] CT scans of patients with neoplasms in the wrist and hand are most useful in defining the osseous extent of the lesion, its relationship with surrounding tissue, the exact location, and the integrity of the surrounding cortical bone if the lesion is within the bone.[68,69] It can also demonstrate the presence of bony erosion in an extraskeletal soft-tissue mass, which is not seen in the plain films.[70] Some authors have reported that CT scans can demonstrate the nidus better than plain films in osteoid osteoma.[71] In general, however, if MRI is available, it should be used to evaluate neoplasia because MRI can show marrow space involvement and soft-tissue details better than CT.

SOFT-TISSUE MASS

CT provides the ability to analyze soft-tissue abnormalities; with CT it is possible to differentiate fat, muscles, tendons, larger ligaments, and blood vessels.

Text continued on page 438

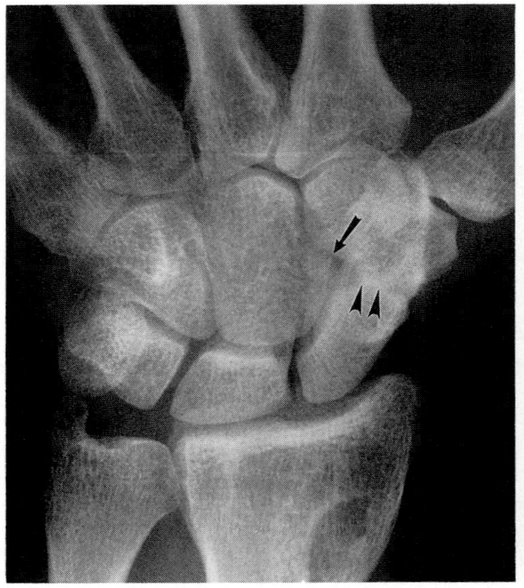

A

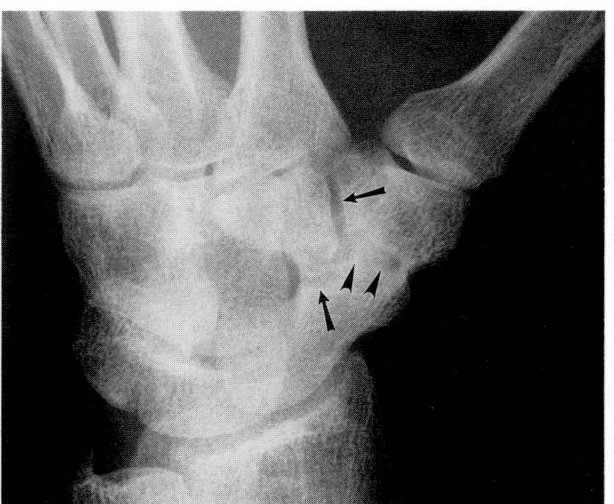

B

FIGURE 16–25. PA **(A)** and oblique **(B)** views of the left wrist after STT joint fusion demonstrate bony bridging across the scaphotrapezial joint (arrowheads). A radiolucent space is visible at the scaphotrapezoidal and trapeziotrapezoidal joints (arrows); however, there is still questionable fusion at the scaphotrapezoidal joint. **C:** Coronal CT image demonstrates no bony union between the trapezoid and scaphoid. Solid scaphotrapezial fusion was verified on more ventral sections. Defect in the radius is a bone graft donor site. T, trapezoid; S, scaphoid; L, lunate; C, capitate; arrowhead, bone graft attaching to scaphoid and not to trapezoid.

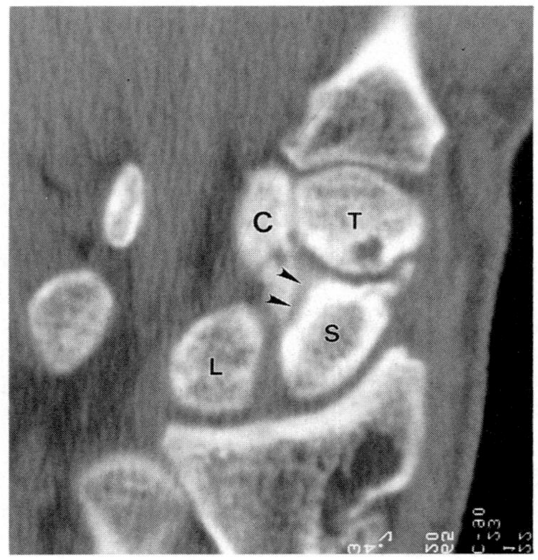

C

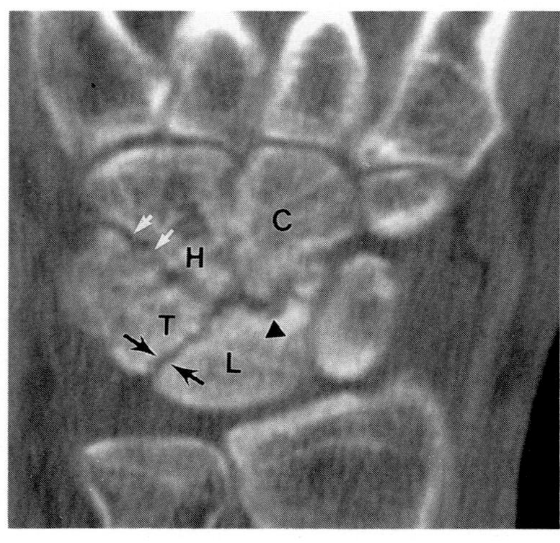

A

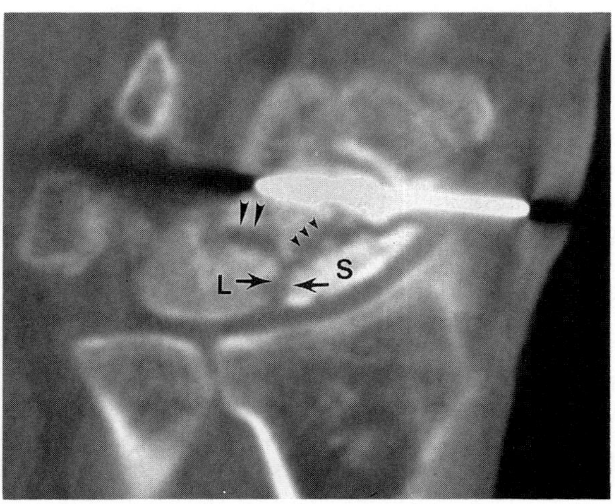

B

FIGURE 16–26. *See legend on opposite page*

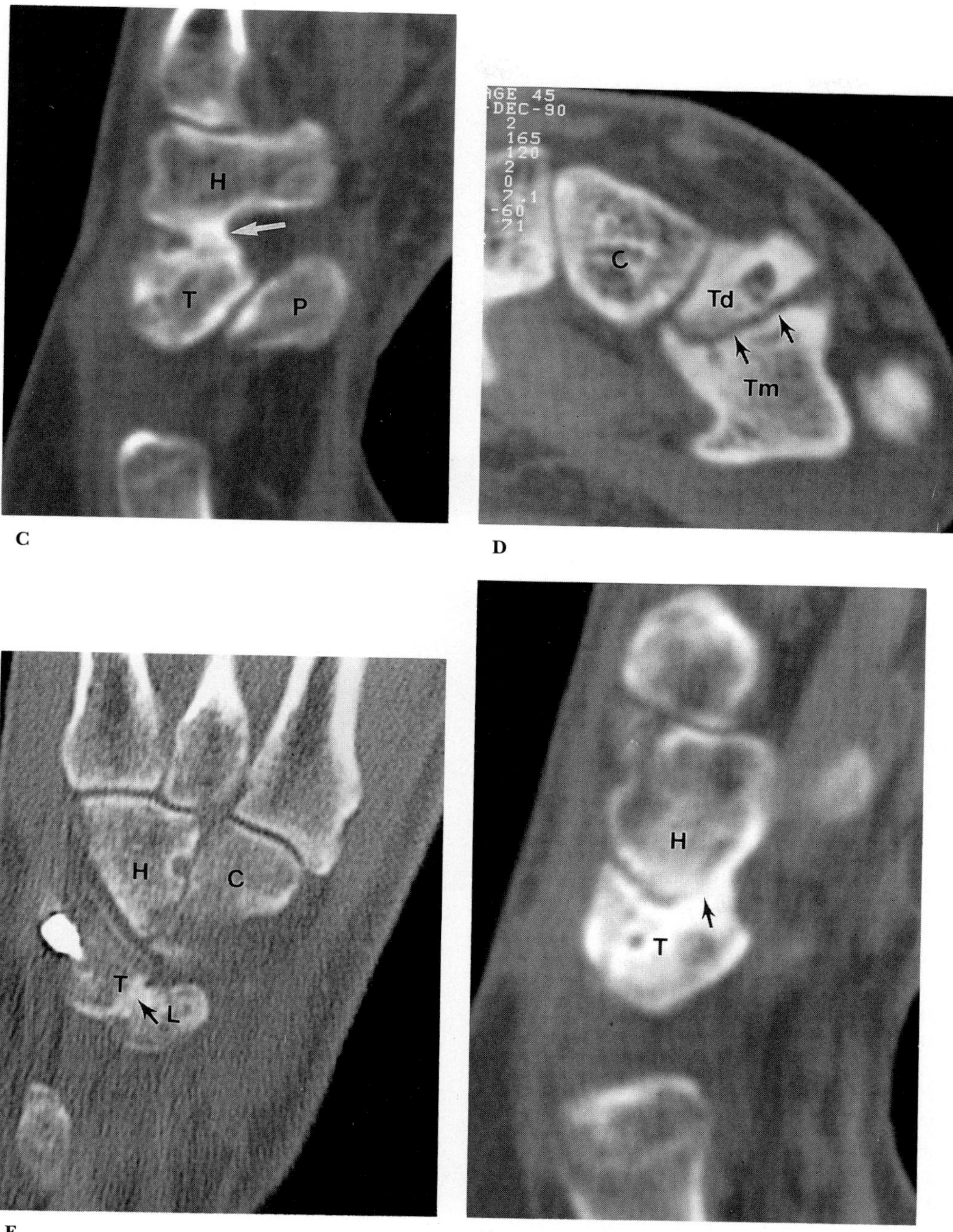

FIGURE 16–26. A: Four bone fusion. Coronal image of wrist shows no solid bone healing at the lunotriquetral (black arrows), capitolunate (black triangle), capitohamate, and triquetrohamate (white arrows) joints after a four joint (four bone) fusion. C, capitate; H, hamate; T, triquetrum; L, lunate. **B:** Scaphocapitolunate fusion procedure performed for scaphoid waist fracture. Coronal CT image demonstrates no healing between the scaphoid and lunate (black arrows), scaphoid and capitate (small arrowheads), and lunate and capitate (large arrowheads) even though a large metal pin is present. The scaphoid fracture site is evident proximal to the pin radially. Probably some fusion is present at the distal scaphoid fragment capitate articulation (around the pin site). S, scaphoid; L, lunate. **C:** Sagittal CT image of a left wrist after a triquetrohamate joint fusion procedure demonstrates solid bony union between the hamate and triquetrum (arrow). H, hamate; T, triquetrum; P, pisiform. **D:** Axial CT image of a left wrist after STT joint fusion demonstrates nonunion between the trapezium and trapezoid (arrows). C, capitate, Td, trapezoid; Tm, trapezium. **E:** Coronal image after lunotriquetral joint fusion demonstrates solid fusion between the lunate and triquetrum (arrow). C, capitate; H, hamate; L, lunate; T, triquetrum. **F:** Sagittal CT image of a left wrist after surgical fusion demonstrates fusion of the anterior portion of the triquetrohamate joint (arrow). H, hamate; T, triquetrum.

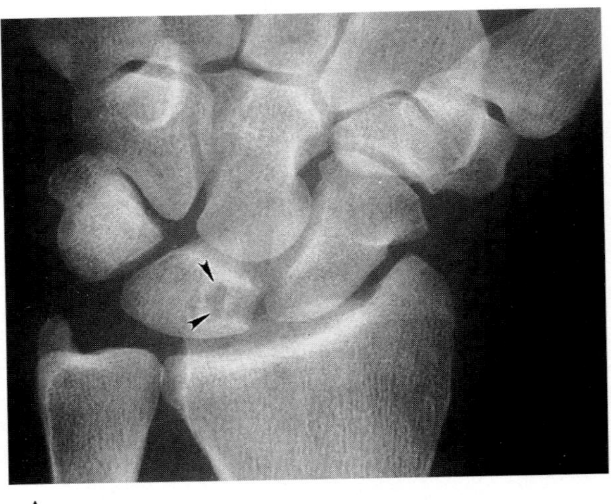

A

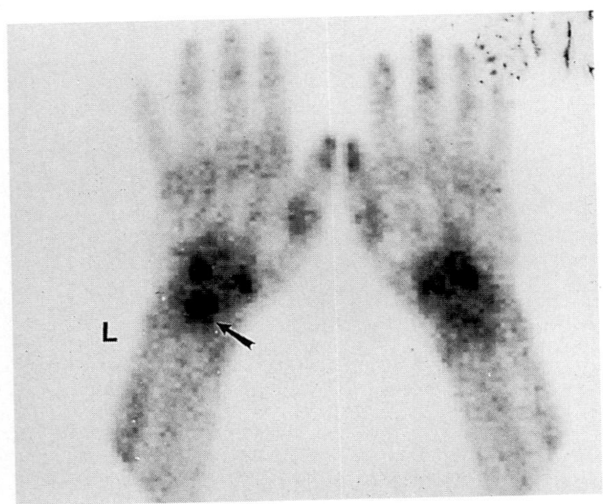

B

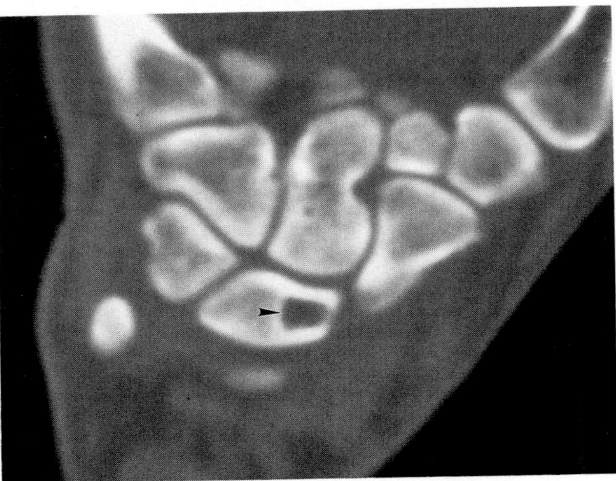

C

FIGURE 16–27. A 32-year-old man with chronic wrist pain. **A:** Posteroanterior view of the left wrist shows a radiolucency at the radial side of the lunate (arrowheads) that communicates to the scapholunate joint. **B:** Bone scan of both wrists demonstrates the most prominent increased uptake of Tc^{99m} at the lunate area of the left wrist (arrow). **C:** Coronal CT image demonstrates a well-defined defect in the radial side of the lunate (arrowhead) with the remaining lunate being normal in appearance.

In selected cases injected intravenous contrast medium is especially helpful to differentiate the blood vessels from tendons and ligaments.[70] MRI is superior to CT for detecting soft-tissue pathology.[3,11,72] However, CT may not only display soft tissue, but also provide more bone detail than MRI. CT offers direct demonstration of the soft-tissue mass and allows accurate evaluation of the relationships between the mass and the adjacent structures and possible compression or infiltration of the muscular bundles, vascular trunks, and subcutaneous fatty tissue. This is of considerable value when planning surgery.[73] CT is able to demonstrate certain pathologic features such as lipoma, fibrolipoma, and cyst.[68,73–75] The margin, delineation, presence of invasion, and pattern of contrast enhancement may suggest whether the mass is benign or malignant.[22] CT can confirm tendon rupture by demonstrating absence of tendon in one or more slices and demonstrating the location of the rupture.[22] The main value of CT in evaluation of soft-tissue masses of the hand is in determining the location, local extension, and relationship of the mass to adjacent structures rather than defining its nature (except that of lipoma and cyst). Despite the value of CT for soft-tissue processes in the hand and wrist, MRI is preferable, when available, because of its superiority in demonstrating soft-tissue and marrow detail.

CONGENITAL ANOMALIES

The carpal boss, an immobile bony protuberance, is located on the dorsum of the wrist at the base of the second and third metacarpals adjacent to the capitate and trapezoid bones. This bony prominence may represent degenerative osteophyte formation and/or the presence of an os styloideum, an accessory ossification center that occurs during embryonic development.[76] When this condition is symptomatic, patients complain of pain and limitation of motion of the affected hand. The symptoms of carpal boss may result from an overlying ganglion or bursitis, an exterior tendon slipping over this bony prominence, or from osteoarthritic changes at this site.[76] Radiographically, the view that best profiles the separate os styloideum is a lateral view using 30 degrees of supination and ulnar deviation of the wrist.[76] Once a diagnosis has been made, treatment can range from the use of nonsteroidal anti-inflammatory medication and limited use of the wrist to surgical excision of the anatomic abnormality.[77,78] CT scan may better demonstrate the presence and location of a carpal boss. The relationship of the capitate, trapezoid, second and third metacarpals, and os styloideum is best demonstrated with sagittal imaging,[11] sometimes complemented with axial images. Due to the close apposition of carpal bones, CT in various planes could also be of value in understanding complex bone relationships in other wrist anomalies.

POSTARTHROGRAPHY CT

Coronal and axial CT scans postarthrography can show better the configuration of the triangular fibrocartilage (TFC) and its attachments as well as interosseous ligaments (see Chapter 14). It may also show perforations of the TFC.[11] Postarthrography CT can also help in evaluation of the ulnar capsular disruptions.[13] Postarthrography CT may help demonstrate loose bodies within the joint and differentiate air bubbles from loose bodies.[10]

REFERENCES

1. Stewart NR, Gilula LA. CT of the wrist: A tailored approach. *Radiology* 1992;183:13–20.
2. Biondetti PR, Vannier MW, Gilula LA, Knapp R. Wrist: Coronal and transaxial CT scanning. *Radiology* 1987;163:149–151.
3. Aaron JO. A practical guide to diagnostic imaging of the upper extremity. *Hand Clin* 1993;9:347–358.
4. Patel RB. Evaluation of complex carpal trauma: Thin-section direct longitudinal computed tomography scanning through a plaster cast. *J Comput Assist Tomogr* 1985;9:107–109.
5. Bodne D, Quinn SF, Cochran CF. Imaging foreign glass and wooden bodies of the extremities with CT and MRI. *J Comput Assist Tomogr* 1988;12:608–611.
6. Donaldson JS. Radiographic imaging of foreign bodies in the hand. *Hand Clin* 1991;7:125–134.
7. Kuhns LR, Borlaza GS, Seigel RS, Paramagul C, Berger PE. An in vitro comparison of computed tomography, xeroradiography, and radiography in the detection of soft-tissue foreign bodies. *Radiology* 1979;132:218–219.
8. Nyska M, Pomeranz S, Porat S. The advantage of computed tomography in locating a foreign body in the foot. *J Trauma* 1986;26:93–95.
9. Rhoades CE, Soye I, Levine E, Reckling FW. Detection of a wooden foreign body in the hand using computed tomography: Case report. *J Hand Surg* 1982;7:306–307.
10. Tehranzadeh J, Gabriele OF. Intra-articular calcified bodies: Detection by computed arthrotomography. *South Med J* 1984;77:703–710.
11. Quinn SF, Belsole RJ, Greene TL, Rayhack JM. Advanced imaging of the wrist. *RadioGraphics* 1989;9:229–246.
12. Quinn SF, Murray W. Watkins T, Kloss J. CT for determining the results of treatment of fractures of the wrist. *AJR* 1987;149:109–111.
13. Quinn SF, Belsole RJ, Greene TL, Rayhack JM. CT of the wrist for the evaluation of the traumatic injuries. *Crit Rev Diag Imag* 1989;29:357–380.
14. Scheffler R, Armstrong D, Hutton L. Computed tomographic diagnosis of distal radio-ulnar joint disruption. *J Canad Assoc Radiol* 1984;35:212–213.
15. McNiesh LM. Unique musculoskeletal trauma. *Radiol Clin North Am* 1987;25:1107–1132.
16. Sclafani SJA. Dislocation of the distal radioulnar joint. *J Comput Assist Tomogr* 1981;5:450.
17. Mino DE, Palmer AK, Levinsohn EM. Radiography and computerized tomography in the diagnosis of incongruity of the distal radio-ulnar joint: A prospective study. *J Bone Joint Surg* 1985;67A:247–252.
18. Dekel S, Papaioannou T, Rushworth G, Coates R. Idiopathic carpal tunnel syndrome caused by carpal stenosis. *Brit Med J* 1980;31:1297–1299.
19. Jessurun W, Hillen B, Zonneveld F, Huffstadt AJC, Beks JWF, Overbeek W. Anatomical relations in the carpal tunnel: A computed tomographic study. *J Hand Surg* 1987;12B:64–67.
20. Jetzer T, Erickson D, Webb A, Heithoff K. Computed tomography of the carpal tunnel with clinical and surgical correlation. *CT Clin Symposium* 1984;7:2–7.
21. Hindman BW, Avolio RE. High resolution scanning of the hand and wrist. *CT Clin Symposium* 1985;8:2–11.
22. Hauser H, Rheiner P. Computed tomography of the hand. Part II: Pathological conditions. *Medicamundi* 1983;28:129–135.
23. Merhar GL, Clark RA, Schneider HJ, Stern PJ. High-resolution computed tomography of the wrist in patients with carpal tunnel syndrome. *Skeletal Radiol* 1986;15:549–552.
24. Oberlin C, Salon A, Pigeau I, Sarcy JJ, Guidici P, Treil N. Three-dimensional reconstruction of the carpus and its vasculature: An anatomic study. *J Hand Surg* 1992;17A:767–772.
25. Weeks PM, Vannier MW, Stevens WG, Gilula LA. Three dimensional imaging of the wrist. *J Hand Surg* 1985;10:32–39.
26. Zeman RK, Fox SH, Silverman PM, et al. Helical (spiral) CT of the abdomen. *AJR* 1993;160:719–725.
27. Fishman EK, Wyatt SH, Bluemke DA, Urban BA. Spiral CT of musculoskeletal pathology: Preliminary observations. *Skeletal Radiol* 1993;22:253–256.
28. McEnery KW, Wilson AW, Murphy WA. *Spiral CT evaluation of wrist trauma.* Exhibit presented at ARRS meeting. San Francisco, April 1993.
29. Egawa M, Asai T. Fracture of the hook of the hamate: Report of six cases and the suitability of computerized tomography. *J Hand Surg* 1983;8:393–398.
30. Hindman BW, Kulik WJ, Lee G, Avolio RE. Occult fractures of the carpals and metacarpals: Demonstration by CT. *AJR* 1989;153:529–532.
31. Pennes DR, Jonsson K, Buckwalter KA. Direct coronal CT of the scaphoid bone. *Radiology* 1989;171:870–871.
32. Hauser H, Rheiner P, Gajisin S. Computed tomography of the hand. Part I: Normal anatomy. *Medicamundi* 1983;28:90–94.
33. Sanders WE. Evaluation of the humpback scaphoid by computed tomography in the longitudinal axial plane of the scaphoid. *J Hand Surg* 1988;13A:182–187.
34. Magid D, Thompson JS, Fishman EK. Computed tomography of the hand and wrist. *Hand Clin* 1991;7:219–233.
35. Amadio PC, Berquist TH, Smith DK, Ilstrup DM, Cooney WP, Linscheid RL. Scaphoid malunion. *J Hand Surg* 1989;14A:679–687.
36. Smith DK, Gilula LA, Amadio PC. Dorsal lunate tilt (DISI configuration): Sign of scaphoid fracture displacement. *Radiology* 1990;176:497–499.
37. Cooney WP, Linscheid RL, Dobyns JH. Scaphoid fractures: Problems associated with nonunion and avascular necrosis. *Orthop Clin North Am* 1984;15:381–391.
38. Friedman L, Yong-Hing K, Johnston GH. Forty degree angled coronal CT scanning of scaphoid fractures through plaster and fiberglass casts. *J Comput Assist Tomogr* 1989;13:1101–1104.
39. Bresina SJ, Vannier MW, Logan SE, Weeks PM. Three-dimensional wrist imaging: Evaluation of functional and pathologic anatomy by computer. *Clin Plastic Surg* 1986;13:389–405.
40. Adler JB, Shaftan GW. Fractures of the capitate. *J Bone Joint Surg* 1962;44A:1537–1547.
41. Kimmel RB, O'Brien ET. Surgical treatment of avascular ne-

crosis of proximal pole of the capitate: Case report. *J Hand Surg* 1982;7A:284–286.
42. Rand JA, Linscheid R, Dobyns JH. Capitate fractures: A long-term follow-up. *Clin Orthop* 1982;165:209–216.
43. Foster EJ, Palmer AK, Levinsohn EM. Hamate erosion: An unusual result of ulnar artery constriction. *J Hand Surg* 1979;4:536–539.
44. Leslie IJ, Dickson RA. The fractured carpal scaphoid: Natural history and factors influencing outcome. *J Bone Joint Surg* 1981;63B:225–230.
45. Meyer S. Radiographic evaluation of wrist trauma. *Semin Roentgenol* 1991;26:300–317.
46. Friedman L, Yong-Hing K, Johnston GH. The use of coronal computed tomography in the evaluation of Kienbock's disease. *Clin Radiol* 1991;44:56–59.
47. Fisher MR, Rogers LF, Hendrix RW, Gilula LA. Carpometacarpal dislocations. *Crit Rev Diagn Imag* 1984;22:95–126.
48. Fisher MR, Rogers LF, Hendrix RW. Systematic approach to identifying fourth and fifth carpometacarpal joint dislocations. *AJR* 1983;140:319–324.
49. Hsu JD, Curtis RM. Carpometacarpal dislocations on the ulnar side of the hand. *J Bone Joint Surg* 1970;52A:927–930.
50. Helal B, Kavanagh TG. Unstable dorsal fracture dislocation of the fifth carpometacarpal joint. *Injury* 1977;9:138–142.
51. Kraemer BA. Metacarpal fractures and dislocations. In: Gilula LA, ed. *The traumatized hand and wrist: Radiographic and anatomic correlation.* Philadelphia: WB Saunders, 1992:178–216.
52. Cone RO, Szabo R, Resnick D, Gelberman R, Taleisnik J, Gilula LA. Computed tomography of the normal radioulnar joints. *Invest Radiol* 1983;18:541–545.
53. Palmer AK, Werner FW. The triangular fibrocartilage complex of the wrist: Anatomy and function. *J Hand Surg* 1981;6A:153–162.
54. Palmer AK. The distal radioulnar joint. *Orthop Clin North Am* 1984;15:321–335.
55. Bowers W. Distal radioulnar joint. In: Green DP, ed. *Operative hand surgery.* New York: Churchill Livingstone, 1975:734–769.
56. Bowers WH. Distal radioulnar joint arthroplasty: Current concepts review. *Clin Orthop* 1992;275:104–109.
57. Space TC, Louis DS, Francis I, Braunstein EM. CT findings in distal radioulnar dislocation. *J Comput Assist Tomogr* 1986;10:689–690.
58. King GJ, McMurtry RY, Rubenstein JD, Ogston NG. Computerized tomography of the distal radioulnar joint: Correlation with ligamentous pathology in a cadaveric model. *J Hand Surg* 1986;11A:711–717.
59. Levinsohn EM. Imaging of the wrist. *Radiol Clin North Am* 1990;28:905–921.
60. Pirela-Cruz MA, Goll SR, Klug M, Windler D. Stress computed tomography analysis of the distal radioulnar joint: A diagnostic tool for determining translational motion. *J Hand Surg* 1991;16A:75–82.
61. Merhar GL, Clark RA, Schneider HJ, Stern PJ. High-resolution computed tomography of the wrist in patients with carpal tunnel syndrome. *Skeletal Radiol* 1986;15:549–552.
62. Bush CH, Gillepsy III T, Dell PC. High-resolution CT of the wrist: Initial experience with scaphoid disorders and surgical fusions. *AJR* 1987;149:757–760.
63. Luke DL, Pruitt DL, Gilula LA. Intraosseous ganglion of the lunate. *J Canad Radiol* 1993;44:304–306.
64. Azouz EM, Kozlowski K, Masel J. Soft-tissue tumors of the hand and wrist of children. *Can Assoc Radiol J* 1989;40:251–255.
65. Patel MR, Zinberg EM. Pigmented villonodular synovitis of the wrist invading bone: Report of a case. *J Hand Surg* 1984;9A:854–858.
66. Halldorsdottir A, Ekelund L, Rydholm A. CT-diagnosis of lipomatous tumors of the soft tissues. *Arch Orthop Traumat Surg* 1982;100:211–216.
67. Hogeboom WR, Hoekstra HJ, Mooyaart EL, et al. MRI or CT in the preoperative diagnosis of bone tumours. *Eur J Surg Oncol* 1992;18:67–72.
68. Wilson JS, Korobkin M, Genant HK, Bovill EG. Computed tomography of musculoskeletal disorders. *AJR* 1978;131:55–61.
69. Preisser P, Buck GD. Computerized tomography of the hand with high resolution technique. *Handchir Mikrochir Plast Chir* 1992;24:136–144.
70. Stackhouse TG, Weiland AJ. Extraosseous chondrosarcoma of the wrist: A case report. *J Hand Surg* 1984;9A:338–342.
71. McConnell III B, Dell PC. Localization of an osteoid osteoma nidus in a finger by use of computed tomography: A case report. *J Hand Surg* 1984;9A:139–141.
72. Baker LL, Hajek PC, Bjorkengren A, et al. High-resolution magnetic resonance imaging of the wrist: Normal anatomy. *Skeletal Radiol* 1987;16:128–132.
73. Adani R, Calò M, Torricelli P, Squarzina PB, Caroli A. The value of computed tomography in the diagnosis of soft-tissue swellings of the hand. *J Hand Surg* 1990;15B:229–232.
74. Heiken JP, Lee JKT, Smathers RL, Totty WG, Murphy WA. CT of benign soft-tissue masses of the extremities. *AJR* 1984;142:575–580.
75. Egund N, Ekelund L, Sako M, Persson B. CT of soft tissue tumors. *AJR* 1981;137:725–729.
76. Conway WF, Destouet JM, Gilula LA, Bellinghausen HW, Weeks PM. The carpal boss: An overview of radiographic evaluation. *Radiology* 1985;156:29–31.
77. Kaulesar Sukul DM, Steinberg PJ, Lichtveld PL. The carpal boss. *Neth J Surg* 1986;38:90–92.
78. Cuono CB, Watson HK. The carpal boss: Surgical treatment and etiological considerations. *Plast Reconstr Surg* 1979;63:88–93.

CHAPTER 17

MRI OF THE WRIST AND HAND

Saara M. S. Totterman and Richard J. Miller

Magnetic resonance imaging (MRI) of the musculoskeletal system in general, and of the wrist and hand in particular, is a rapidly evolving technology. As such, there are numerous exciting possibilities to pursue, as well as many challenging problems to resolve, before the full capabilities and limitations of this imaging modality are thoroughly understood. The rate at which new hardware and software are being developed is such that today's high-quality images will necessarily give way to even higher-tech images tomorrow. As technologic advances permit improved contrast and increasingly detailed resolution of small anatomic structures, the clinician finds that he or she must strive to develop a new and more refined knowledge of the infrastructure of the anatomic parts being imaged. Nowhere in the musculoskeletal system is this challenge to the imaging and understanding of fine anatomic detail more applicable than in the wrist and hand. Here, clinically important structures such as the intrinsic and extrinsic ligaments and triangular fibrocartilage (TFC) are typically only 1 to 2 mm thick. Therefore, present-day magnetic resonance (MR) techniques that generate 3- to 5-mm thick slices will likely be of limited value in imaging those structures. As the resolving capabilities of MR steadily improve, the indications for MRI in the assessment of hand and wrist pathology will continue to evolve. For now, the indications for this imaging modality must necessarily be closely linked to both the available scanning technology and the interest and knowledge of the people requesting and interpreting the studies.

Of particular note at this time is the conflict of interest between the need for high resolution in the imaging of small structures such as the hand and wrist and the demand for containment of ever-increasing medical costs. High-resolution MRI is expensive, and ultimately outcome-oriented research will be required to determine the cost effectiveness of this as well as other new medical technologies. Nevertheless, it is the feeling of the authors that while the cost effectiveness of high-resolution imaging of the wrist and hand may be open to question, the worthlessness of low-resolution studies of these structures is not. We maintain that high resolution in imaging the hand and wrist is a definite necessity rather than a luxury.

The first section of this chapter is devoted to a brief overview of those aspects of the imaging parameters and protocols that we have found to be most important to the enhancement of image quality and resolution. Although imaging procedures will change with the acquisition of new hardware and software, the MR anatomy of the wrist and hand will not. In the second section of the chapter we review our current understanding of the normal MR anatomy of this region. In the third section, illustrations of applications and the authors' current assessment of indications for MRI of the wrist and hand are discussed. Most MR applications in the distal upper extremity have been at the level of the wrist, and both our experience and that recorded in the literature with respect to the hand and digits are limited. Thus, the focus of this chapter will be on the wrist.

WRIST

Technical Considerations

Imaging Sequences

Our experience indicates that the minimum in-plane resolution required to adequately visualize the extrinsic and intrinsic ligaments of the wrist is 0.3 × 0.3 mm, combined with 1.0- to 1.5-mm slice thickness.[1,2] Support for this resolution requires excellent signal-to-noise performance of the hardware; this, in turn, implies a high field magnet and a dedicated receiver or transmitter–receiver coil.[1–3] The images shown in this chapter were obtained using a 1.5 tesla clinical imager (GE Signa) and custom-built receiver coils.[2] Universally applied imaging parameters for the wrist included field of view 8 cm, matrix 256 × 256 or 256 × 192, and NEX 1. Sequence specific parameters for three-dimensional (3D) gradient recall echo (GRE) imaging were TR 69 ms, TE 17 ms, and flip angle 20 degrees with 1-mm slice thickness. Parameters for spin echo (SE) sequences were TR/TE of 2000 ms/27, 70 ms with 1.5-mm slice thickness, and for fat-suppressed sequences were TR/TE of 2000 ms/20, 80 ms with 3-mm slice thickness. The resolution achieved with this technique results in excellent visualization of the normal structures such that aspects of the infrastructural detail of many tissues including ligaments, tendons, and nerves can often be appreciated. With developing technology, even-higher-resolution imaging will be available in the future, which should further enhance the visualization of ligament–cartilage interfaces and degenerative changes in cartilaginous joint surfaces.[3,4]

Several different pulse sequence protocols in MR applications in the hand and wrist have been found useful. These include 3D GRE, standard SE, and fat-suppressed spin echo. Each sequence protocol has certain advantages and disadvantages.

Although conceptually SE imaging using proton density (PD) and T2-weighted (T2W) images is probably the most useful protocol for visualizing both the normal and pathologic anatomy of the wrist and hand, the hardware (surface coils) and software (1.5-mm slice thickness sequence) required for the degree of high resolution needed in these applications may not be available. In that event, we have found that 3D GRE imaging offers the best means for acquiring data with appropriate resolution.[2,5] Of particular note with respect to the resolving properties of 3D GRE acquisitions is the capability of this technique to generate slices that are both thin (0.7–1.0 mm) and contiguous. These features of the whole-volume acquisition technique result in small structures and small lesions being visualized on more than one slice, thereby significantly enhancing the diagnostic potential of the imaging process. Although 3D GRE sequences provide excellent signal-to-noise ratio (and thereby support high resolution), the use of these sequences results in inherently less contrast (compared with SE imaging) between various anatomic structures of interest. Thus, when using a 3D GRE sequence, one must carefully tailor the specific imaging parameters to the clinical problem for which the study is being done. An advantage of 3D GRE acquisition using very thin slices is that the data acquired from a single plane in this manner can be reformatted in any other plane.[5] Although this offers the potential of avoiding the need to image in more than one plane,[5,6] the resolution in reconstructed planes is significantly less than that in the plane of acquisition.

In the evaluation of soft-tissue masses and tumors, very high resolution may not be as critical as it is in the assessment of soft and hard tissue mechanical integrity. In this situation, excellent contrast information can usually be obtained using standard SE sequences with 3-mm thick slices.

If available, fat-suppressed SE imaging can be particularly useful in the evaluation of soft-tissue tumors, soft-tissue inflammations, and certain types of bony lesions and bone tumors.[7] With suppression of the high signal associated with fat, further enhancement of contrast between certain types of tissues can often be achieved.[7] The resolution, however, is lower than with standard SE sequences.

In summary, at this time, the highest-resolution images are being obtained with 3D imaging, but optimal contrast information requires SE data. Further experience in light of constantly improving technical capabilities will be required to determine which sequence will provide the best demonstration of specific pathologic changes in various clinical settings. For the present, we believe that the information inherent in the two studies is often complementary, and for many applications we continue to obtain both 3D and SE sequences.

Positioning of Hand and Wrist

Careful positioning of the hand for evaluation of the wrist is critical. With the hand in a gently fisted position, the hand, wrist, and forearm are supported on their ventral aspect by the surface coil platform such that the long finger metacarpal rests in 15 degrees of extension relative to the forearm. For evaluation of the hand and fingers, the fingers are allowed to rest in near full extension with just a few degrees of flexion at the interphalangeal (IP) and metacarpophalangeal (MCP) joints. Taping the hand and wrist to the supporting platform may provide additional stabilization and minimize motion artifact.

The configuration of the surface coil that we have been using for imaging the wrist and hand is such that the long axis of the forearm and wrist must be perpendicular to the axis of the main magnetic field.[2] This requirement dictates that the hand and wrist be overhead with the patient supine. Somewhat surprisingly, this position has been tolerated quite well even by patients with significant arthritis in the proximal joints of their upper extremity. Problems due to shoulder stiffness have been circumvented by using a chest support beneath the supine patient such that the wrist position can be achieved without full forward flexion of the shoulder. Obviously, imaging with the hand and wrist at the patient's side would be preferred, but we do not know of any surface coils presently available that allow imaging in this position while delivering comparable resolution. Future developments in coil designs may resolve this problem.[4]

Normal MR Anatomy

As has already been emphasized, the anatomic structures of the hand and wrist are small enough to challenge the resolving capabilities of even the best of MR imagers. Because the important extrinsic and intrinsic carpal ligaments are typically no more than 2–3 mm thick, neither the normal anatomy nor pathologic alterations in these ligaments can be fully appreciated without carefully evaluating all of the thinly sliced and closely spaced images obtained through the structure of interest. Constraints on space in this chapter, however, require that the number of images used for the purpose of illustrating both the normal and pathoanatomy be limited.

Discussion of the normal anatomy of the wrist will be organized according to the imaging plane. The coronal plane has proven to be the most useful in assessing the integrity and pathoanatomy of the ligaments and triangular fibrocartilage complex (TFCC), and most of our comments regarding these important soft tissues will be made with respect to this plane. The axial plane images are obviously most relevant in evaluating longitudinal structures including the tendons, nerves, and vessels. This plane is also of particular value in assessing the mechanical status and stability of the distal radioulnar joint (DRUJ). Sagittal images permit a different (and more difficult to interpret) perspective on the extrinsic ligaments and TFCC. The sagittal plane is also useful for measuring intercarpal alignment angles in the assessment of carpal stability. All three planes are useful in assessing bone lesions (including fractures) and soft-tissue neoplasms.

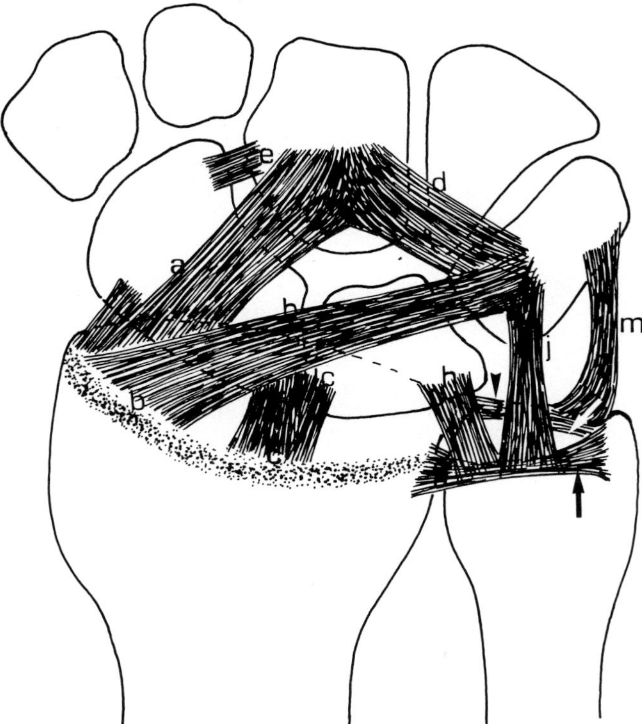

FIGURE 17–1. Schematic drawing showing the ventral capsular and intrinsic wrist ligaments: radioscaphocapitate (a), radiolunotriquetral (b), radioscapholunate (c), capitotriquetral (d), and capitoscaphoid (e) arms of the deltoid ligament. The disc of the TFCC (white arrow) ulnolunate (h) and ulnotriquetral (j) ligaments, meniscus homologue (m), and ventral (black arrow) and dorsal (arrowhead) radioulnar ligaments are demonstrated.

Correlations of MR images with normal anatomy are provided with diagrammatic illustrations of normal ligaments (Fig. 17–1), selected gross dissections (Fig. 17–2), histologic cryosection (Fig. 17–3), and selected cross-sectional specimens (Fig. 17–4).

As previously mentioned, the imaging protocols should be tailored to the clinical questions that dictated the study. Beyond this, we have found that for the coronal plane, both 3D GRE and SE images are required to extract the maximum anatomic information from the series. Axial images are generally obtained with SE sequences both with and without fat suppression. Sagittal images are obtained using 3D GRE.

Wrist Coronal Plane Anatomy

Although 3D GRE series in the coronal plane has been our "workhorse" series for most diagnostic problems in the wrist, SE images have provided important additional information. We anticipate a time in the near future when SE images will be available with very thin and essentially contiguous slices, and at that time the 3D GRE series may become less essential. Figure 17–5 shows selected images of a coronal plane series obtained using a 3D GRE technique (TR 69 ms, TE 17 ms, flip angle 20 degrees) with 1-mm thick contiguous slices, 256 × 256 matrix, and 8 cm field of view. Although the 3D protocol in the coronal plane provides superior contrast between cartilage, ligament, and bone, the SE sequence provides better contrast information with respect to soft tissues and fluid.

Ventral (Volar) Ligaments

The terminology regarding the ventral ligaments is confusing partly because various authors have used different terms to describe the same structures, and partly because our understanding of the details of the anatomy in this difficult to access area is still evolving. In 1976, Taleisnik[8] and Mayfield and associates[9] independently published studies describing the ligamentous anatomy of the ventral surface of the wrist. These studies have provided the major foundation for the hand surgeons' understanding of the carpal ligamentous anatomy over the past decade. Unfortunately, their terminology was not identical even though most of their observations were consistent. A concise current discussion of these terminology issues as well as a review of the ligamentous anatomy as currently accepted by most hand surgeons has been provided by Green.[10] Berger and associates[11–13] have recently reported additional gross and histologic observations with respect to some of the finer details of the extrinsic ventral ligaments. The interested reader is referred to their work, but should be forewarned that both their terminology and interpretation of the anatomy is at some variance with that of Taleisnik and Mayfield et al. At the time of this writing, most hand surgeons continue to accept Taleisnik's termi-

A

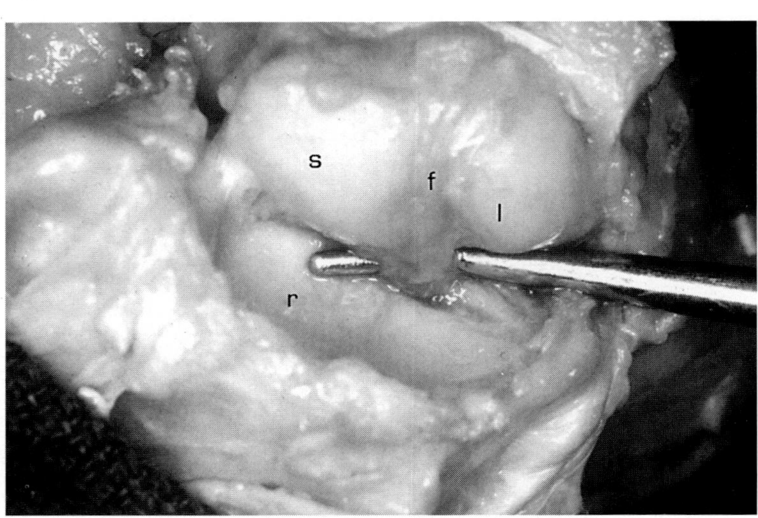

B

FIGURE 17–2. Dorsal radiocarpal arthrotomy demonstrating the ventral extrinsic ligaments. **A:** Radioscaphocapitate ligament (a), radiolunate portion of radiolunotriquetral (b) ligament, and radial attachment of radioscapholunate ligament (c) are visualized. The scapholunate ligament (f) and ventral portion of the TFCC disc (white arrow) are evident, as are the radius (r), scaphoid (s), lunate (l). **B:** Radioscapholunate ligament outlined by probe. Notice the width of radioscapholunate ligament and its attachment to the lunate and scaphoid. The scapholunate ligament (f) extends between the scaphoid and lunate.

nology, and we have adopted it (with minor variations) for our purposes here.

The line drawing in Fig. 17–1 reviews the major ventral carpal ligaments according to Taleisnik with minor modifications.[8] Although these ligaments cannot be appreciated on gross anatomic dissection from the ventral aspect of the wrist, they are well visualized using dorsal arthrotomy (Fig. 17–2) and arthroscopy. Of particular note are the well-defined fascicles of the larger radiocarpal ligaments. MR images showed an excellent correlation on cryosection (Fig. 17–3) with the major extrinsic ligaments appearing on MRI as striated structures with alternating bands of low- and intermediate-signal intensity. With 3D GRE imaging (contiguous 1-mm slices), the major ventral capsular ligaments (radioscaphocapitate, radiolunotriquetral, and deltoid ligaments) are consistently visualized on at least three contiguous slices (Fig. 17–5).[2]

Ventral (Volar) Extrinsic Ligaments

The *radioscaphocapitate (RSC) ligament* is the most radial of the major ventral ligaments. It originates from the ventral aspect of the styloid process of the radius, continues across the waist of the scaphoid, and attaches to the head of the capitate (Figs. 17–2, 17–3, and 17–5). Because of its relatively large size and obliquity, its configuration and course can usually be followed through four or five contiguous 1-mm slices.[2] The most dorsal portion of this ligament crosses the waist of the scaphoid bone. Slightly more dorsal slices show those portions of the ligament that originate from the radial styloid and

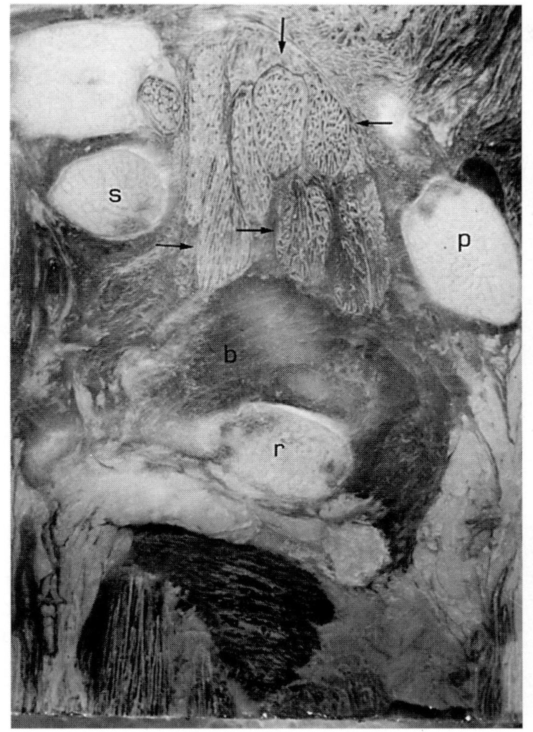

A

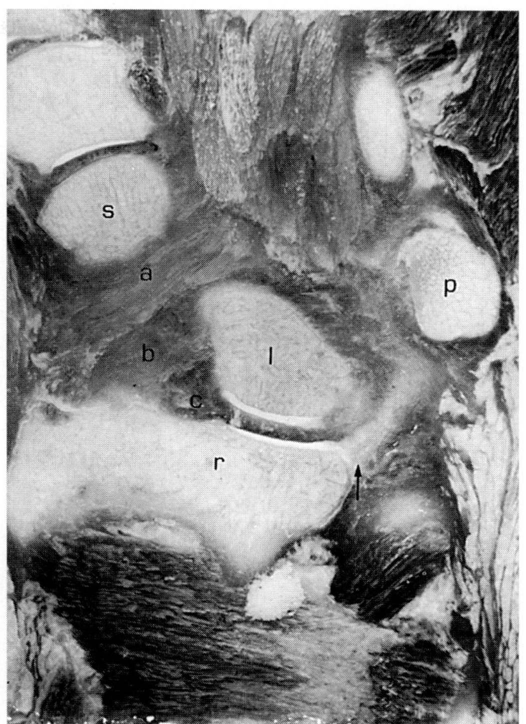

B

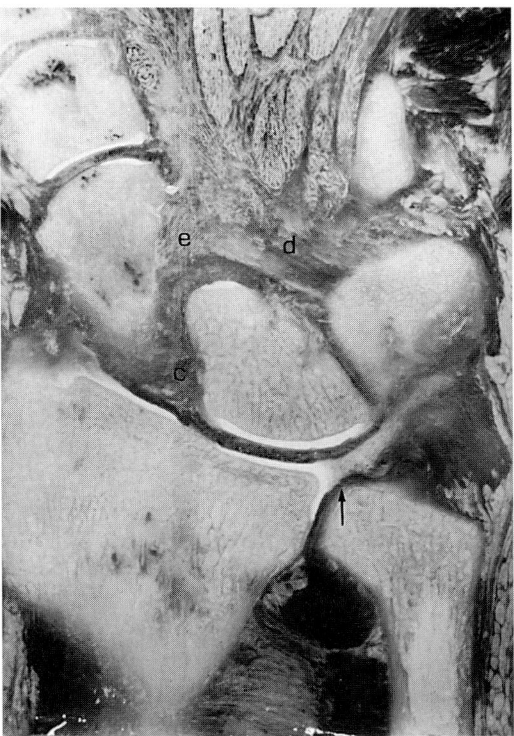

C

FIGURE 17–3. Cryosections from ventral to dorsal through the palmar carpal ligaments. **A:** The most ventral fascicles of the radiolunotriquetral ligament (b) are visualized. Flexor tendons cut tangentially (arrows) appear as speckled structures. r, radius; s, scaphoid; p, pisiform. **B:** Ventral fascicles of the radioscaphocapitate ligament (a) are shown. The more dorsal fascicles of the radiolunate portion of the radiolunotriquetral ligament (b) are visualized. The radioscapholunate ligament (c) is behind the radiolunate portion of the radiolunotriquetral ligament. The ventral attachment of the TFCC (black arrow) to the radius is demonstrated. **C:** Only the most ventral fascicles of the capitoscaphoid (e) and capitotriquetral (d) arms of the deltoid ligament are shown. More dorsal portions of the radioscapholunate ligament (c) attaching to the scaphoid and lunate are visualized. The TFC disc attachments (black arrow) to the hyaline cartilage of the radius are evident.

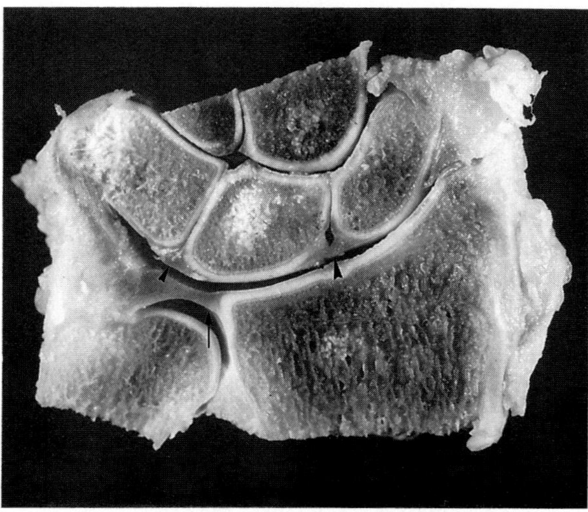

FIGURE 17–4. Cross-section through the midline of the wrist demonstrating the intrinsic ligaments and TFC. The scapholunate ligament (large arrowhead) attaches directly to the cartilage of the scaphoid and lunate at this level. The cartilage has a different appearance from the ligament. The lunotriquetral ligament (small arrowhead) attaches directly to the corresponding hyaline cartilage of the lunate and triquetrum. The TFC disc (arrow) attaches radially to the radius cartilage and at this level ulnarly sends fibers to the base and the tip of the ulnar styloid.

those that insert on the capitate head (Figs. 17–3 and 17–5).

The *radiolunotriquetral (RLT) ligament* originates on the radius just ulnar to the RSC ligament (Figs. 17–2, 17–3, and 17–5). The most superficial fascicles of this ligament can be followed from the radius over the lunate to the triquetrum (Figs. 17–3 and 17–5). The deeper fibers of the RLT ligament attach to the ventral surface of the lunate, securing the radius to the lunate and the lunate to the triquetrum (Figs. 17–3 and 17–5).[2] These radiolunate and lunotriquetral portions of the ligament are visualized in two or three additional (1-mm thick contiguous) more dorsal slices.[2]

The *radioscapholunate (RSL) ligament* is a less substantial structure than the other ventral extrinsic ligaments. It originates on the radius more dorsally and ulnarly than the RLT ligament (Figs. 17–2, 17–3, and 17–5).[12,13] Although the anatomic detail of this ligament has been the subject of considerable study in recent years, its function and role in the mechanics of the wrist remain controversial.[8,9,11–15] Its origin on the ventral indentation of the cortical surface of the radius can often be appreciated on high-resolution MR images (Fig. 17–5). On MR, this structure has areas of mixed high- and intermediate-signal intensity, a finding believed to be consistent with its histology.[11,12] The striations prominent in the other ventral ligaments are not present.[2] The ventral fibers of the RSL ligament attach to the ventral cortex of the scaphoid and lunate, whereas the more dorsal fibers merge with the fibers of the intrinsic scapholunate ligament (Figs. 17–2, 17–5, and 17–6).

Ulnar to the RSL ligament a thick capsule connects the ventral lip of the lunate fossa to the ventral proximal aspect of the lunate bone. Berger and Landsmeer called this tissue the *short radiolunate ligament,*[12] distinguishing it from the radiolunate portion of the RLT ligament radially (described above) and the ulnolunate ligament ulnarly (to be described in reference to the TFCC below). For reasons that are unclear, we have not been able to identify this ligament either in dissections or on MR images.

The reader may be interested to note that Berger and Landsmeer[12] refer to the radiolunate portion of Taleisnik's[8] RLT ligament as the long radiolunate ligament, whereas Mayfield and coworkers[9] referred to this portion of the RLT ligament as simply the radiolunate ligament.

The *deltoid ligament* consists of a fan-shaped array of fascicles extending from the capitate to the triquetrum, scaphoid, and lunate (Figs. 17–1, 17–3, and 17–5). The lunate fascicle is frequently absent[8] and is neither illustrated in Fig. 17–1, nor demonstrated in Fig. 17–3 or Fig. 17–5. With the hand in the fisted imaging position, the most ventral portion of the capitate bone is located dorsal to the most ventral aspect of the lunate bone. Consequently, the capitotriquetral arm of the deltoid ligament is usually visualized at the same anteroposterior (AP) level as the deeper fibers of the RLT and RSC ligaments (Fig. 17–5).[2] The scaphocapitate arm of the deltoid ligament is shorter than the capitotriquetral component (Figs. 17–3 and 17–5).[8] It is located dorsal to the RSC ligament and this feature, together with its steeper obliquity in both the coronal and sagittal planes, distinguishes it from the RSC ligament.

Of note is the fact that the most proximal fibers of the RSC ligament and capitotriquetral ligament do not attach to the capitate, but rather pass ventral to the head of the capitate, attaching to each other. These ligamentous elements are joined by fibers reflected distally from the TFC[12] to effect a sling-like ventral support for the head of the capitate and hamate. These features of the ventral ligaments account for the appearance on axial images obtained at this level of a thick band of low-signal ligamentous tissue extending from the triquetrum to the scaphoid (Fig. 17–7).

Intrinsic Ligaments

The *intrinsic scapholunate (SL) ligament* is horseshoe shaped in the sagittal plane and connects the ventral, proximal, and dorsal borders of the scaphoid to the lunate (Figs. 17–4 and 17–5).[16] The most ventral and dorsal portions are stout structures, but the midcoronal part may be thin and membranous. The proximal–distal dimension of the midcoronal portion of the ligament varies from 2 mm in some wrists to as much as one-third the height of the lunate bone in others. On 3D GRE MR images, the SL ligament is visualized as a structure with low- to intermediate-signal intensity (Fig. 17–5). The most ventral and dorsal portions of the ligament attach directly to the scaphoid and lunate bones.[2] The midportion of the SL ligament has variable attachment to bone and articular cartilage with corresponding variable MR signal intensities in this middle attachment region (Figs. 17–4 and 17–5). A familiarity with the normal blend of signal in this area on high-resolution 3D GRE and PD and T2W SE images is necessary to correctly distinguish normal SL ligaments from those with degenerative changes or partial or full thickness perforations.[2] Histologic correlation with MR images of the midcoronal insertion of the intrinsic SL ligament has been helpful in developing an understanding of the MR appearance of the normal anatomy.

The *intrinsic lunotriquetral (LT) ligament* is also horseshoe shaped in the sagittal plane and, like the SL ligament, it connects the ventral, proximal, and dorsal margins of the two bones (Fig. 17–5). The proximal–distal dimension of the LT ligament in the midcoronal plane is usually much less than that of the SL ligament and is often membranous, making this portion of the ligament difficult to consistently visualize. Like the SL ligament, the ventral and dorsal portions of the LT ligament attach directly to the cortical surfaces of the lunate and triquetrum with the corresponding low MR signal intensity of the ligament blending directly with the low-signal intensity of the bone (Fig. 17–5).[2] The middle portion of this ligament, however, virtually always attaches to the lunate and triquetral bones through hyaline cartilage (Figs. 17–4 and 17–5). Because of this, on 3D GRE images the homogeneous low-signal intensity of this midportion of the ligament always blends into the higher-signal intensity of the articular cartilage at the margin of the two carpal bones. As commented on in reference to the SL ligament above, familiarity with the appearance of the LT intrinsic ligament at its midcoronal attachment to the adjacent proximal row bones is necessary to avoid the error of interpreting the normal high signal of the hyaline cartilage as a perforation (communicating defect) of the ligament at its point of attachment to either the lunate or triquetrum. Again, as mentioned above with respect to the SL ligament, because the hyaline cartilage has low- or intermediate-signal intensity on T2W imaging, any high signal on T2W images that extends completely through the lunotriquetral interval must represent a full-thickness perforation (Fig. 17–8) of the ligament.[2]

Dorsal Carpal Ligaments

The gross anatomy of the dorsal carpal ligaments and extensor retinaculum has been detailed in literature.[17,18] Smith has shown a good correlation between the gross anatomic description of these dorsal structures and high-resolution whole-volume MRI.[5] Our experience with thin-section (1-mm slice thickness) 3D GRE imaging provides confirmation that these structures can be readily visualized (Figs. 17–5 and 17–29). We have not, however, had experience documenting injury or disease within these tissues (other than dorsal ganglia).

TFCC

The TFCC consists of ventral and dorsal radioulnar ligaments, a central fibrocartilaginous disc (the TFC), the extensor carpi ulnaris (ECU) tendon sheath, the so-called meniscus homologue, and the ulnolunate and ulnotriquetral ligaments (Fig. 17–5).[19] It is important to appreciate the fact that this complex is not made up of discrete anatomic structures, but rather is found histologically to consist of a blending confluence of structures connecting the ulnar aspect of the sigmoid notch of the distal radius to the ulnar head and styloid, and the ulnar styloid to the ulnar aspect of the carpus. The details of the gross and histologic anatomy of this complex of collagenous and fibrocartilaginous structures has been described in the literature[19–21] and is further elaborated in Chapter 4. We have found that the normal MR appearance of the various components of the TFCC is dependent on the imaging resolution.

Ventral (Volar) and Dorsal Radioulnar Ligaments

The ventral and dorsal radioulnar ligaments are thick, collagenous structures that extend from the ventral and dorsal margins of the sigmoid notch of the radius to the ulnar head and styloid process. On high-resolution images, these ligaments are visualized as striated low to intermediate signal bands (Fig. 17–5).[22] The appearance correlates well with the collagenous bundles that histologically constitute these structures.[20,21] These bands blend directly with the low signal of the cortical bone at their ventral and dorsal attachments to the sigmoid notch of the radius (Fig. 17–5).[22] The ulnar attachments of the ligaments to the styloid process is variable, but generally fibers from these ligaments find insertions at both the tip and base of the process (Fig. 17–5). The tip of the styloid process may have a thin cap of hyaline cartilage, and in this case the insertion of the TFCC fibers in this location will be through cartilage.[19] The MR appearance on high-resolution spin density and 3D GRE coronal images in this event will show a thin intermediate to intermediate high-signal line just radial to the tip of the styloid; this should not be confused with a perforation of the TFCC insertion at this location. With lower resolution, the ventral and dorsal radioulnar ligaments appear as

Text continued on page 451

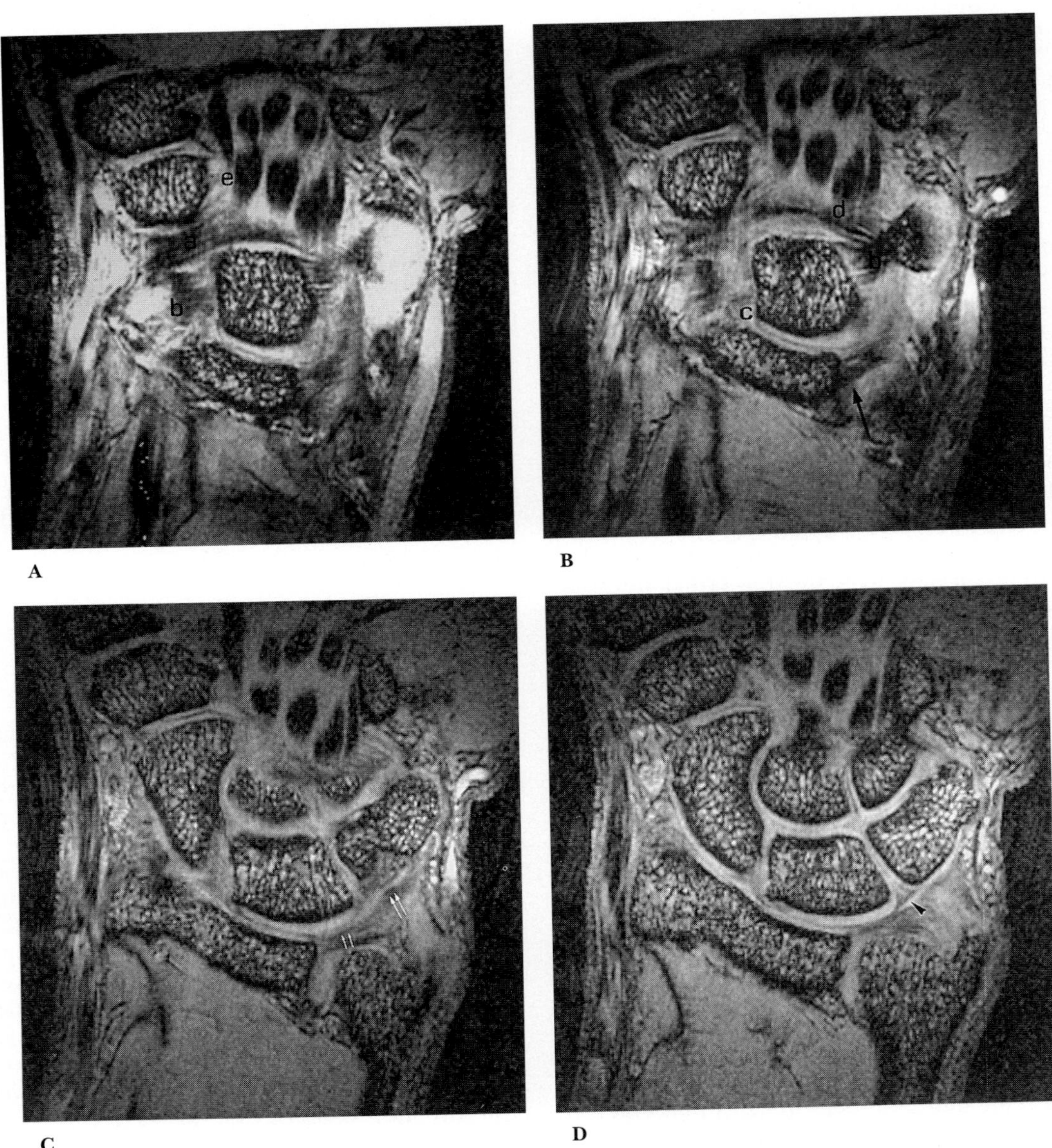

FIGURE 17–5 (panels **A–D**) *See legend on opposite page*

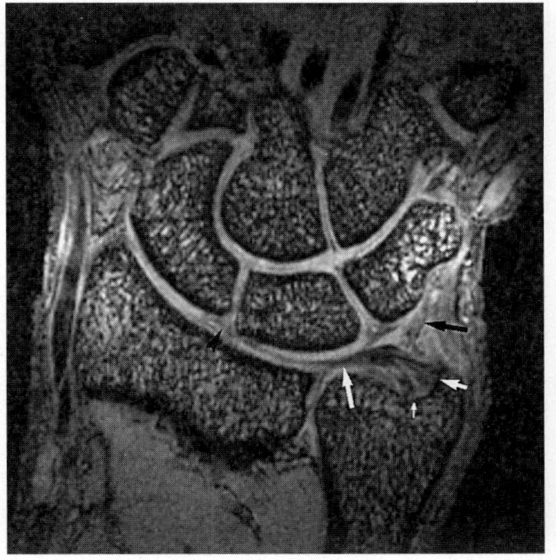

E

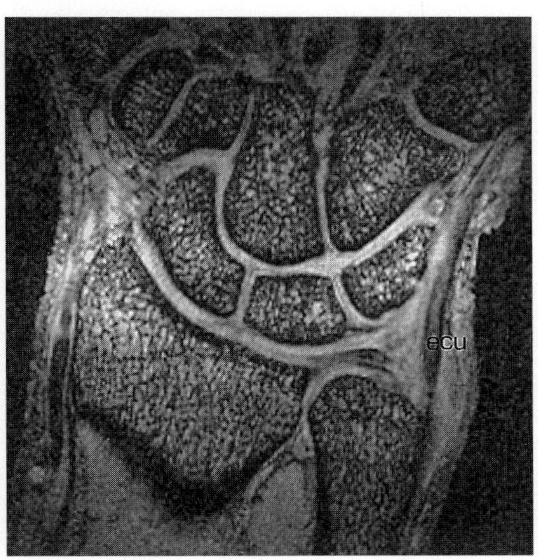

F

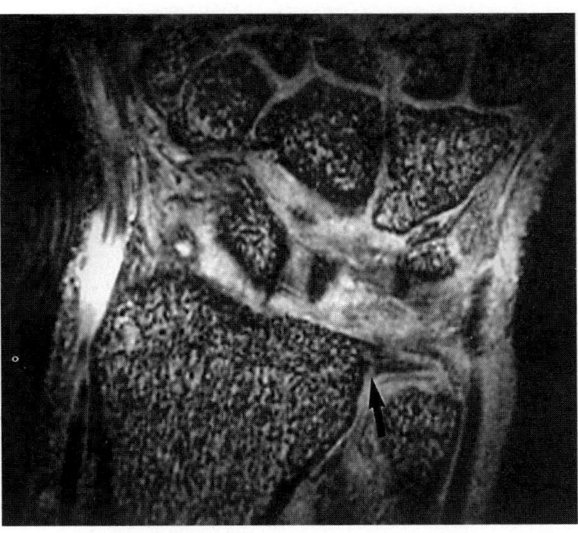

G

FIGURE 17–5. Selected coronal 3D GRE images from palmar to dorsal through the wrist demonstrating the extrinsic and intrinsic ligaments as well as the TFCC and its components (**A** to **G**). The flexor tendons are seen as speckled, low-signal intensity structures. The radioscaphocapitate ligament (a), the radiolunate and lunotriquetral components of the radiolunotriquetral ligament (b), the capitoscaphoid (e) and capitotriquetral (d) arms of the deltoid ligament, and the radioscapholunate ligament (c) are visualized. The signal behavior of the scapholunate ligament (large arrowhead) differs from that of the lunotriquetral ligament (small arrowhead). The ventral (long black arrow in **B**) and dorsal (large black arrow in **G**) radioulnar ligaments, ulnolunate (small white arrows in **C**) and ulnotriquetral ligament (larger white arrows in **C**), meniscus homologue (black arrow in **E**), TFC disc (large white arrow in **E**), and its attachment to the tip of the styloid (short large white arrow in **E**) and to the base of the styloid (small white arrow in **E**) are visualized. The extensor carpi ulnaris tendon (ecu in **F**) and radiocarpal and carpocarpal cartilage surface interfaces are demonstrated.

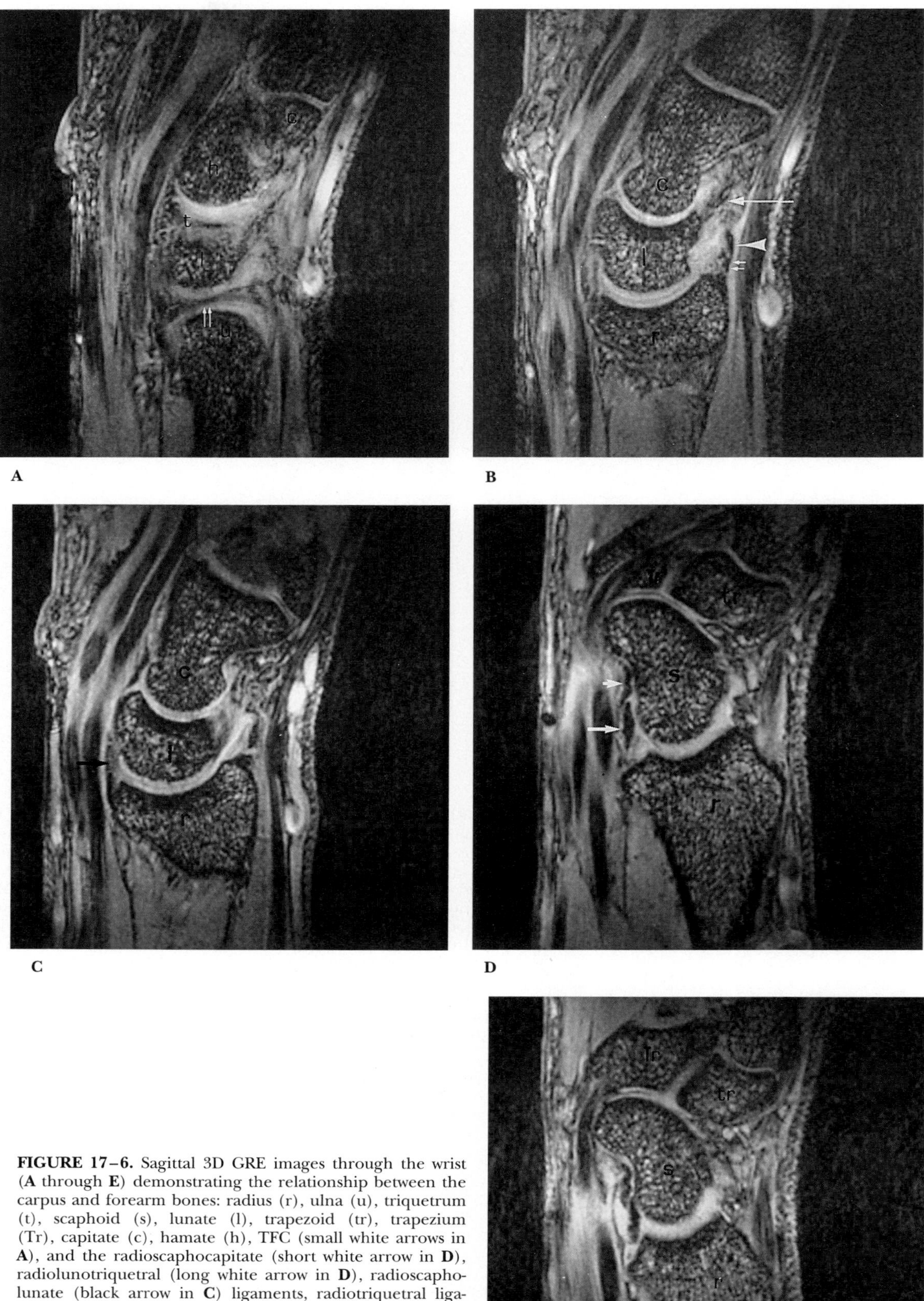

FIGURE 17–6. Sagittal 3D GRE images through the wrist (**A** through **E**) demonstrating the relationship between the carpus and forearm bones: radius (r), ulna (u), triquetrum (t), scaphoid (s), lunate (l), trapezoid (tr), trapezium (Tr), capitate (c), hamate (h), TFC (small white arrows in **A**), and the radioscaphocapitate (short white arrow in **D**), radiolunotriquetral (long white arrow in **D**), radioscapholunate (black arrow in **C**) ligaments, radiotriquetral ligament (white arrowhead in **B**), triquetroscaphoid ligament (double small white arrows in **B**), and triquetrotrapezial ligament (long white arrow in **B**).

thick, homogeneous, low-signal bands extending from the ventral and dorsal aspects of the sigmoid notch to the ulnar styloid.[23–28] With this technique, the finer details at the ulnar styloid attachment are rarely appreciated.[22]

Central TFCC Disc (Triangular Fibrocartilage, TFC)

The central disc is a fibrocartilaginous structure that spans the interval between the ventral and dorsal radioulnar ligaments and fills the void between the ulnar head proximally and the triquetrum and lunate distally (Figs. 17–4 and 17–5).[19–21]

Thus the thickness of the disc varies directly with the degree of negative ulnar variance.[29] If the ulnar variance is neutral or positive, then the disc is necessarily thin, and both traumatic and degenerative perforations of the disc are more likely to occur. Central disc perforations and virtually all traumatic tears of the central disc are readily visualized on high-resolution MRI.[23–26,28,30]

The radial attachment of the central disc to the sigmoid notch of the radius is through hyaline cartilage that wraps around the margin of the radius at this location from the lunate fossa to the distal radioulnar joint (DRUJ).[20,21] The MR appearance on 3D GRE and SE coronal images at this site always shows a thin intermediate to high-signal line that should not be mistaken for a marginal tear of the disc (Fig. 17–5).[2,28]

The appearance of the central disc on lower-resolution images is similar to that described above.[28] In those images, smaller perforations may be missed.

Meniscus Homologue and ECU Sheath

The meniscus homologue is an ill-defined band-like thickening of the TFCC that extends from the dorsal margin of the sigmoid notch distally, ulnarly, and ventrally to blend with the ventral surface of the thick ECU sheath, the triquetrum, and base of the fifth metacarpal.[19] It has intermediate signal on MRI and is usually difficult to appreciate as a discrete structure both on MRI and at gross dissection.

The thickened ventral aspect of the ECU sheath and its relationship to the ulnar styloid can usually be appreciated on MR images.

Ulnolunate and Ulnotriquetral Ligaments

The ulnolunate and ulnotriquetral ligaments are thickenings of the capsular tissue that extends from the ventral radioulnar ligament and ventral surface of the ulnar styloid base to the ventral aspect of the lunate and triquetrum.[8] This tissue does not show the prominent discrete fascicular bundles that characterize the radiocarpal ligaments. The MR appearance reflects a less-defined capsular structure of low to intermediate signal (Fig. 17–5).

Bone and Cartilage

The yellow marrow of the carpal bones has high signal on T1W, PD, and T2W images. Visualization of details of the trabecular bone and hyaline cartilage requires very-high-resolution imaging. Although trabecular detail can be visualized with 0.3-mm in-plane resolution and 1.5- to 1.0-mm slice thickness, our experience to date suggests that degenerative cartilaginous disease and other hyaline cartilage lesions cannot be reliably detected unless in-plane resolution is at least 0.15×0.15 mm and slice thickness is 1.0 mm or thinner.[31]

With 3D imaging all cartilages in the radiocarpal joint, midcarpal joint, and DRUJ appear as high-signal intensity areas with fine low-signal intensity outer borders (Fig. 17–5).[2] The articular ridge between the scaphoid and lunate fossae on the articular surface of the radius is covered by a thin layer (1 to 2 mm thick) of soft tissue.[2] This tissue has low-signal intensity on MR images (Fig. 17–5). Low-signal intensity synovial tissue is commonly seen in the more dorsal sections of the midcarpal joints at the level of the triquetrohamate articulation (Fig. 17–5).

Wrist Axial Plane Anatomy

Satisfactory imaging of the wrist in the axial plane does not require the very thin slice thickness that we have found critical for successful imaging in the coronal plane. The obvious reason for this is that the cross-sectional anatomy does not change as rapidly within scans through the volume of wrist in the axial plane compared with the coronal plane. We have found that SE and fat-suppression imaging (TR/TE 2000 ms /20,80 ms) with 3-mm slice thickness and 0.5- to 1.0-mm interslice gap provides for efficient imaging in this plane with satisfactory contrast and resolution in most clinical applications.[32] 3D imaging is used in special situations.

The cross-sectional gross anatomy of the wrist is outlined in Chapter 4. For the most part, high-resolution MR cross-sectional anatomy of the normal wrist is readily apparent and there is little need for elaborate comment to supplement the representative illustrative images provided (Fig. 17–7). Only selected salient features of the MR cross-sectional anatomy are mentioned here. In our opinion, while the extrinsic and intrinsic ligaments can be visualized on axial images, we have not found these images to be particularly helpful in assessing ligamentous problems, and do not routinely obtain them for this application.

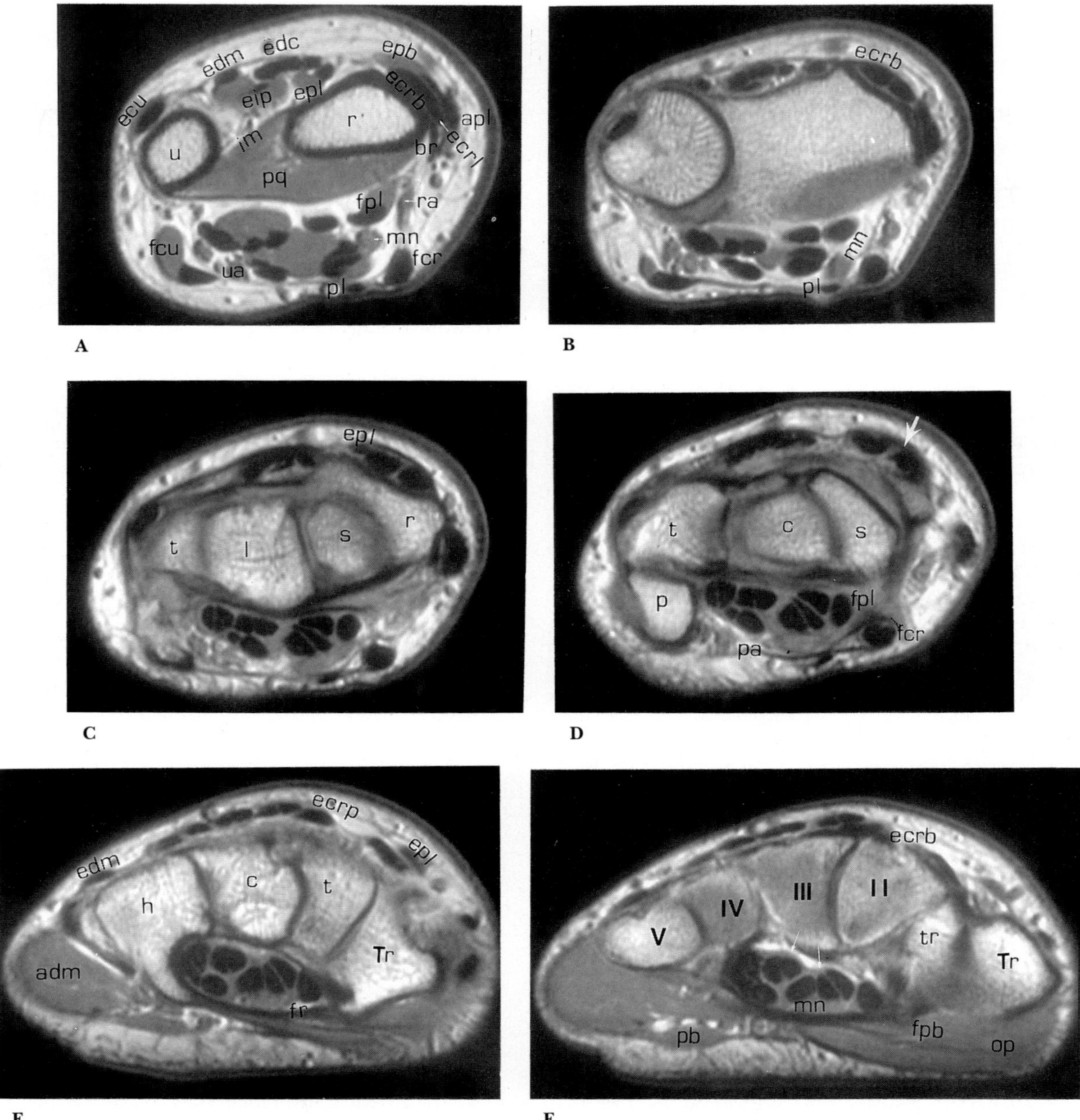

FIGURE 17–7. Axial PD images from proximal to distal, through the normal wrist and hand demonstrating their soft-tissue components (**A** through **K**). Ventral wrist structures outside the carpal tunnel include the flexor carpi radialis (fcr), flexor carpi ulnaris (fcu), and palmaris longus (pl) tendons. The flexor pollicis longus (fpl) is the most radial tendon in the carpal tunnel. Deep and superficial finger flexor tendons and their courses through the carpal tunnel are easily followed. In the distal forearm the pronator quadratus (pq) lies deep to the flexor tendon muscle. The posterior interosseous artery, veins, and nerve are dorsal to the interosseous membrane (im).

The speckled appearance of the tendons reflects the tendon fascicles. The relationship between the superficial and the deep flexor digitorum communis muscles and tendons changes from the distal forearm through the carpal tunnel. The radial artery (ra) accompanied by the radial nerve and veins can be followed radially to the flexor carpi radialis. The ulnar artery (ua), accompanied by veins and nerve, is located deep to the flexor carpi ulnaris muscle. Their course in Guyon's canal is easily appreciated deep to the palmar aponeurosis (pa). The median nerve (mn) is identified deep to the flexor retinaculum (fr).

Dorsal compartment tendons: extensor carpi ulnaris (ecu), extensor digiti minimi (edm), extensor digitorum communis (edc), extensor indicis proprius (eip), extensor pollicis longus (epl), extensor carpi radialis brevis (ecrb) and longus (ecrl), extensor pollicis brevis (epb), abductor pollicis longus (apl), and brachioradialis (br) muscle and tendons are identified. The signal intensity changes in the extensor pollicis longus are due to the magic angle effect (white arrow in **D**).

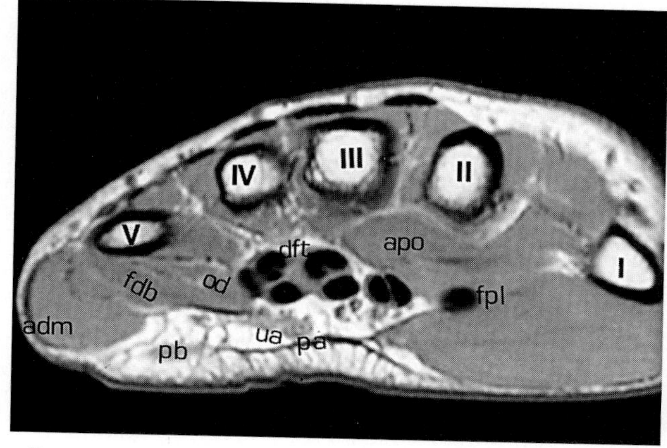

G

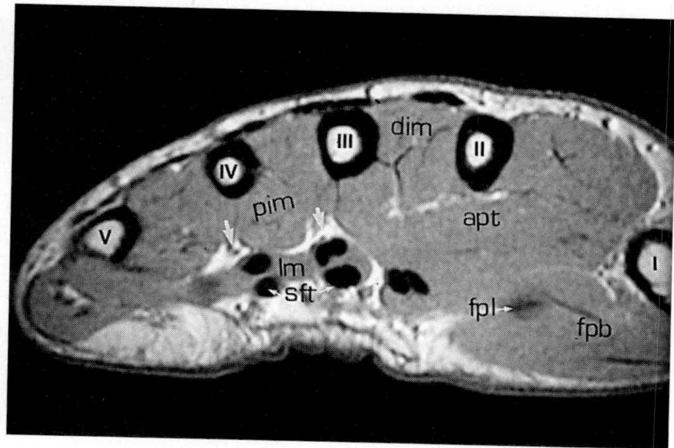

H

I

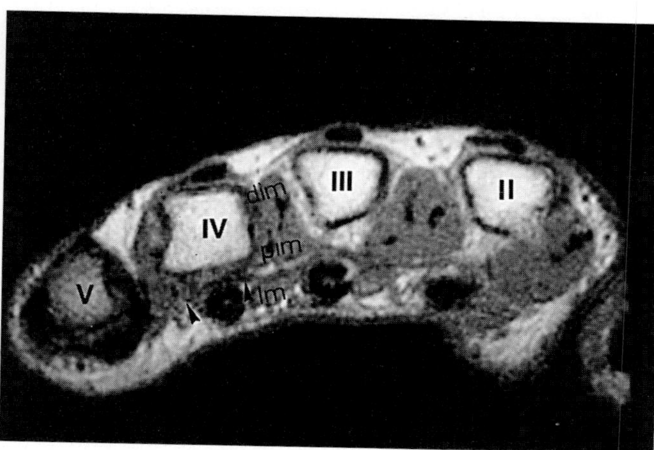

J

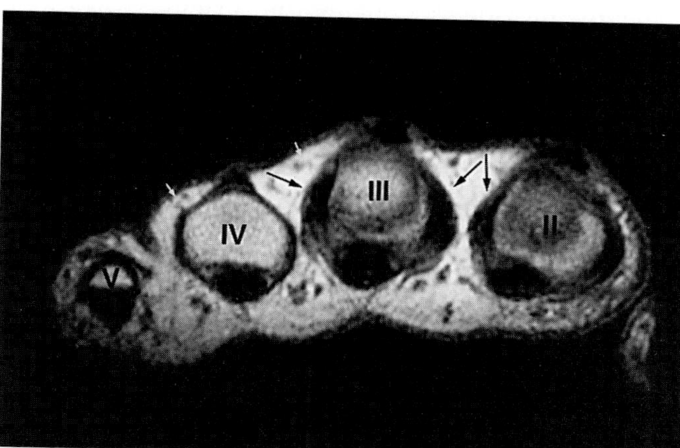

K

FIGURE 17–7 *Continued* Bones of the forearm, carpus, and hand: radius (r), ulna (u), scaphoid (s), lunate (l), triquetrum (t), trapezium (Tr), trapezoid (tr), capitate (c), lunate (l), pisiform (p), hamate (h), hamulus of hamate (hh), first (I), second (II), third (III), fourth (IV), and fifth (V) metacarpal bones.

The ventral soft-tissue structures of the hand on the radial side: abductor pollicis brevis (apb), opponens pollicis (op), flexor pollicis brevis (fpb), adductor pollicis with transverse (apt) and oblique (apo) heads, radial artery (ra), palmar interosseous muscles (pim), dorsal interosseous muscles (dim), lumbrical muscles (lm).

Ventral soft-tissue structures of the hand on the hypothenar side: lateral bands of extensor expansion (arrows), abductor digiti minimi (adm), flexor digiti minimi brevis (fdb), opponens digiti minimi (od), ulnar artery and veins (ua), superficial flexor tendons (sft), deep flexor tendons (dft), deep transverse metacarpal ligament (black arrowheads in **J**), palmaris brevis (pb), palmar aponeurosis (pa), tenosynovium of flexor tendons (white arrows in **F**), flexor pollicis longus tendon (fpl). The dorsal digital arteries (small white arrows) are illustrated (**K**). The black arrows indicate the extensor expansions.

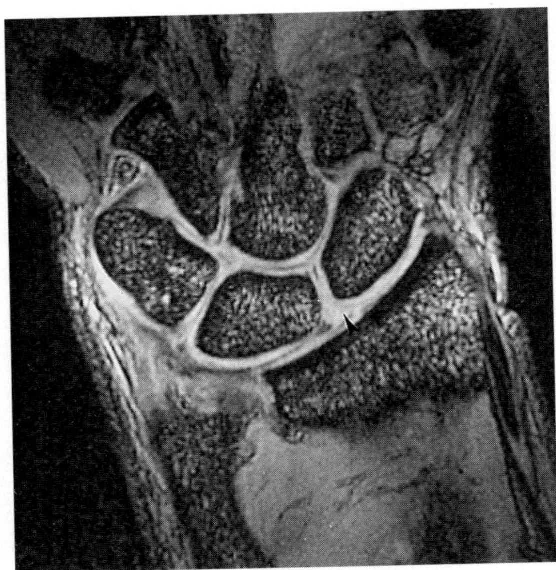

FIGURE 17–8. Scapholunate ligament disruption. A coronal 3D GRE image through the wrist demonstrates a full-thickness perforation (arrowhead) in the SL ligament showing as a high-signal intensity area. The ligament is detached from its origin on the scaphoid cartilage.

Carpal Tunnel and Ulnar Tunnel

Details of the MR anatomy of the carpal tunnel have been reviewed in the literature.[28,32–35] The deep fascia of the forearm thickens and divides at the level of the wrist to form the transverse and ventral carpal ligaments (Fig. 17–7). The carpal tunnel is bounded by the carpal bones on three sides and the firm transverse carpal ligament on the fourth. The ulnar tunnel (canal of Guyon) is bounded by the transverse ligament below, the ventral carpal ligament above, and the pisiform bone and hypothenar musculature ulnarly (Fig. 17–7). Although entrapment or compression of the median nerve in the carpal tunnel and ulnar nerve in the canal of Guyon are common clinical problems that usually can be diagnosed and treated without MRI, such imaging may be quite helpful in atypical cases and cases where mass lesions are suspected within the tunnels.[36] Familiarity with the normal appearance of the contents of these tunnels is obviously an important prerequisite to understanding pathologic states.

Nerves and Vessels

The median nerve lies beneath the flexor digitorum superficialis muscle mass in the distal forearm. At the level of the wrist, the nerve passes to a more superficial position adjacent to the superficial finger flexors and comes to lie just deep and ulnar to the palmaris longus.[32–34] In its normal state, the median nerve is visualized on MR cross-sectional imaging as a speckled intermediate-intensity ovoid structure on T1W and spin density images (Fig. 17–7). Although the normal signal intensity of the nerve on T2W images varies significantly from one patient to the next, the appearance of the nerve on these images is often distinctive with the intermediate to high signal of the nerve contrasting sharply against the low signal of the adjacent tendons and transverse carpal ligament.

Ventral (Volar) Tendons and Muscles

The MR axial plane appearance of the flexor tendons on spin density, T2W, and 3D images is that of discrete ovoid structures of low-signal intensity. With high resolution, a speckled infrastructural pattern is observed. All of the flexor tendons are enclosed in tenosynovial tissue as they pass through the carpal tunnel. The normal MR signal of tenosynovium on spin density images is intermediate and on T2W images is high. In inflammatory states such as infection or rheumatoid arthritis, the tenosynovial tissue becomes swollen and boggy, a change that is readily identified on MR images.[37]

Dorsal Extensor Compartments

The six extensor compartments on the dorsal aspect of the wrist are formed by fibrous septi extending from the dorsal retinaculum to the radius and ulna.[17,38] The first extensor compartment contains the abductor pollicis longus and extensor pollicis brevis; the second contains the extensor carpi radialis longus and brevis; the third contains the extensor pollicis longus; the fourth contains the extensor digitorum communis and extensor indicis proprius; the fifth contains the extensor digiti minimi; and the sixth contains the extensor carpi ulnaris tendon. All the extensor tendons found within these compartments are enclosed in tenosynovium (see Fig. 17–7). The normal MR appearance of these tissues on the dorsum is the same as that indicated above for the corresponding tissues on the ventral side of the wrist.[37] Of interest is the observation that the MR signal of the normal extensor pollicis longus tendon changes from low to intermediate or high as the tendon assumes an oblique course after passing Lister's tubercle (Fig. 17–7). This probably is related to the "magic angle" phenomena.[39] Like the situation on the ventral side, when the tendons become injured or otherwise "synovitic," the MR appearance is altered to reflect both the increased water content and the morphologic distortion of the inflamed tissues. This finding can be quite helpful in diagnosing and staging inflammatory conditions such as rheumatoid disease.[37]

WRIST PATHOLOGY

Ligament Tears

Injuries and degenerative conditions that involve the extrinsic and intrinsic ligaments of the wrist are common and can result in significant clinical symptomatology.[8,9] Evaluation of the anatomic and functional integrity of these ligaments can be difficult since clinical symptoms and signs are often nonspecific,[2] plain radiographs are frequently normal, and arthrograms can be difficult to correlate with clinical findings.[15,40] Because of these difficulties with conventional imaging modalities, high-resolution MRI is evolving as a useful tool for assessing the anatomic and functional integrity of these ligaments. It is important to emphasize, however, that at the time of this writing, the sensitivity and specificity of MRI with respect to wrist ligament injuries has not been determined, and the indications for the use of MRI in diagnosing these injuries has not been defined.

Extrinsic and intrinsic ligament tears (perforations) and degenerative lesions, like normal ligamentous anatomy, are best visualized on coronal-plane MR images. As mentioned previously, in our experience both 3D GRE and SE sequences are useful when analyzing the wrist in the coronal plane.[2]

SL Ligament Lesions

On MR images, a perforation (communicating defect or tear) of the SL ligament appears as a discontinuity in the normal signal intensity of the intact ligament. Perforations may involve either the middle substance of the ligament or its attachment to the lunate or scaphoid bone. In some cases in which the ligament has become detached the remnant retracts, making that portion of the ligament appear thicker.[2]

In our experience with cadaveric wrist and 3D GRE coronal-plane imaging, small perforations of the dorsal one-third of the membranous portion of the ligament were sometimes missed. In our clinical experience using SE in conjunction with 3D GRE, few false-negative or false-positive readings of full-thickness SL tears have been encountered.[2] Clinical experience, however, is still limited, and a determination of "true" sensitivity and specificity remains difficult during this time of constantly improving technology and resolution.[24,25,28,41]

One avoidable cause for a false-positive reading of a perforation of the SL ligament is misinterpretation of the normal low-signal intensity associated with the soft tissue that covers the ridge between the scaphoid and lunate fossae of the radius. If the low signal associated with this tissue is interpreted as being part of the SL ligament, the normal high-signal joint fluid visualized between this tissue and the adjacent SL ligament may be interpreted as a tear of the SL ligament. Again, a good appreciation of the somewhat complex normal MR anatomy of this region is essential for proper interpretation of images of abnormal wrists.

Partial-thickness perforations (noncommunicating defects) of the SL ligament occur with Grade II ligamentous sprains and with degeneration of the tissue in the absence of direct injury. These incomplete ligament lesions can produce troublesome clinical symptoms and can be particularly difficult to diagnose and document. The clinical examination is typically normal except for tenderness over the SL interval and pain when stressing the ligament. Ancillary studies are generally unrevealing, including plain films, bone scan, and arthrography, although midcarpal arthrography can show various appearances of the SL ligament including noncommunicating defects.[42] The role of MRI in this setting is unclear. We believe that certain degenerative changes in the SL ligament can be seen with MRI, and that with further refinements in technique and further clinical experience we will be able to detect at least some of these partial-thickness lesions (noncommunicating defects). For now, however, partial-thickness lesions of the SL ligament are often not detected by MRI.

Complete perforations of the SL ligament do not always result in physical dissociation of the two bones (Fig. 17–8). When scapholunate dissociation is apparent on plain radiographs, subtle cases may be surprisingly difficult to appreciate without the help of fluoroscopy.[42] However, MRI in the coronal plane always reveals the SL diastasis if it is present at the time of the MR scan, because any separation of the cartilage interface between the two bones is easily visualized (Fig. 17–9). If dorsal or ventral intercalated segmental instability (DISI/VISI) has developed, additional sagittal-plane MR views of the carpus will permit accurate evaluation of the abnormal intercarpal relationship and thereby further document this disorder (Figs. 17–10 and 17–17). In this situation the acquired images used for evaluation have to be true sagittal images acquired with the hand in neutral position. We know of no one who has compared measurements of intercarpal angles determined on plain films to those determined on MRI (or computed tomography [CT]) in cases of DISI and VISI. Since the wrist is positioned with some extension in MRI (Fig. 17–10C) the measurements that have been standardized on lateral views of the wrist where no extension or flexion has been allowed may not be directly applicable. If advanced SL collapse[43] has occurred (SLAC wrist disease), coronal and sagittal high-resolution MRI may show degenerative changes in the articular cartilage of either the scaphoid fossa of the radius and/or proximal pole of the scaphoid (Figs. 17–15 and 17–17).

LT Ligament Lesions

MR findings with respect to perforated (communicating) defects of the LT ligaments are similar to those noted for the SL ligament.[2] Perforations of the LT ligament appear as discontinuities in the normal homogeneous low-signal intensity of the intact structure (Fig. 17–11). Most perforations of the LT ligament

Text continued on page 458

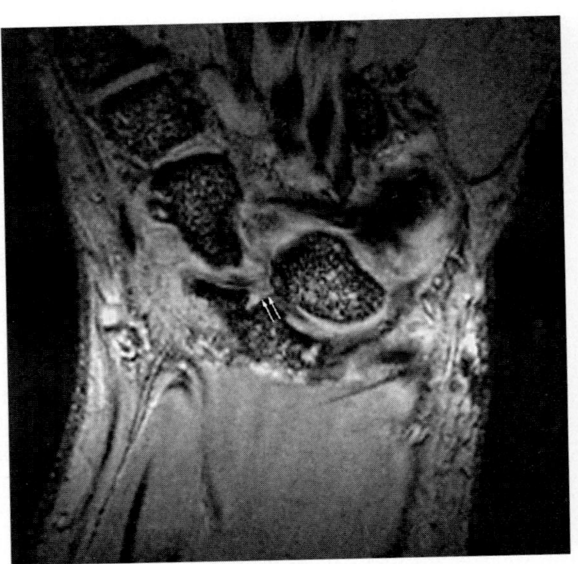

A

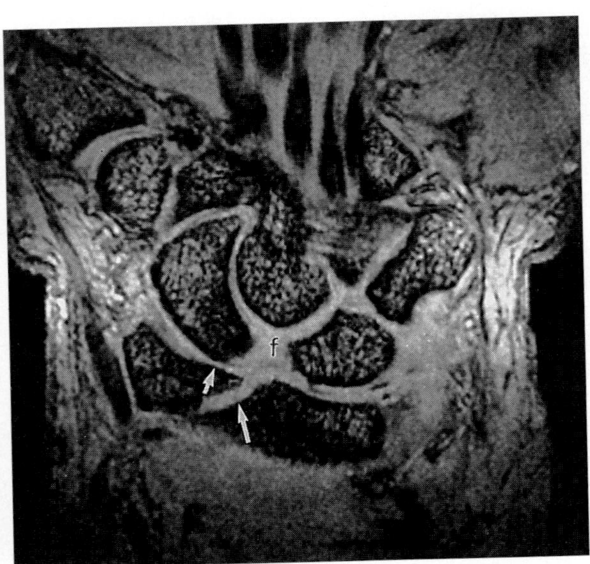

B

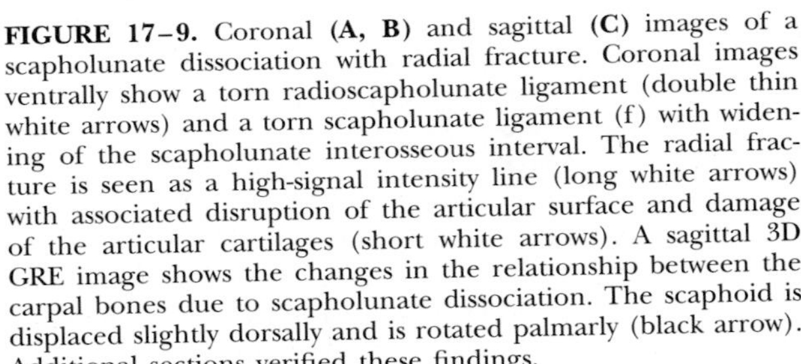

FIGURE 17–9. Coronal (**A, B**) and sagittal (**C**) images of a scapholunate dissociation with radial fracture. Coronal images ventrally show a torn radioscapholunate ligament (double thin white arrows) and a torn scapholunate ligament (f) with widening of the scapholunate interosseous interval. The radial fracture is seen as a high-signal intensity line (long white arrows) with associated disruption of the articular surface and damage of the articular cartilages (short white arrows). A sagittal 3D GRE image shows the changes in the relationship between the carpal bones due to scapholunate dissociation. The scaphoid is displaced slightly dorsally and is rotated palmarly (black arrow). Additional sections verified these findings.

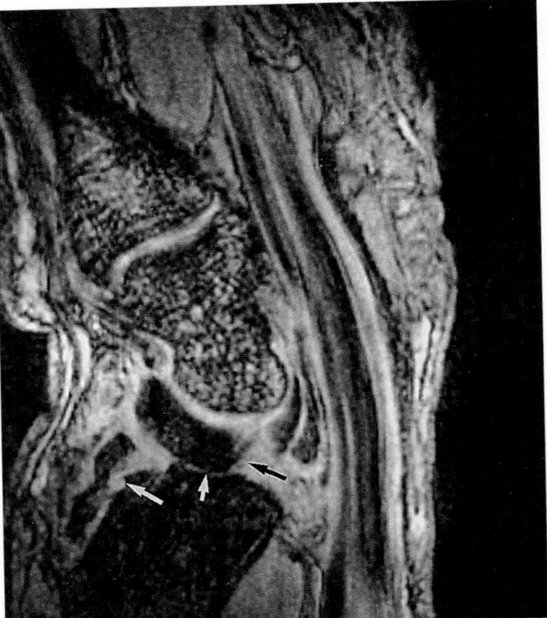

C

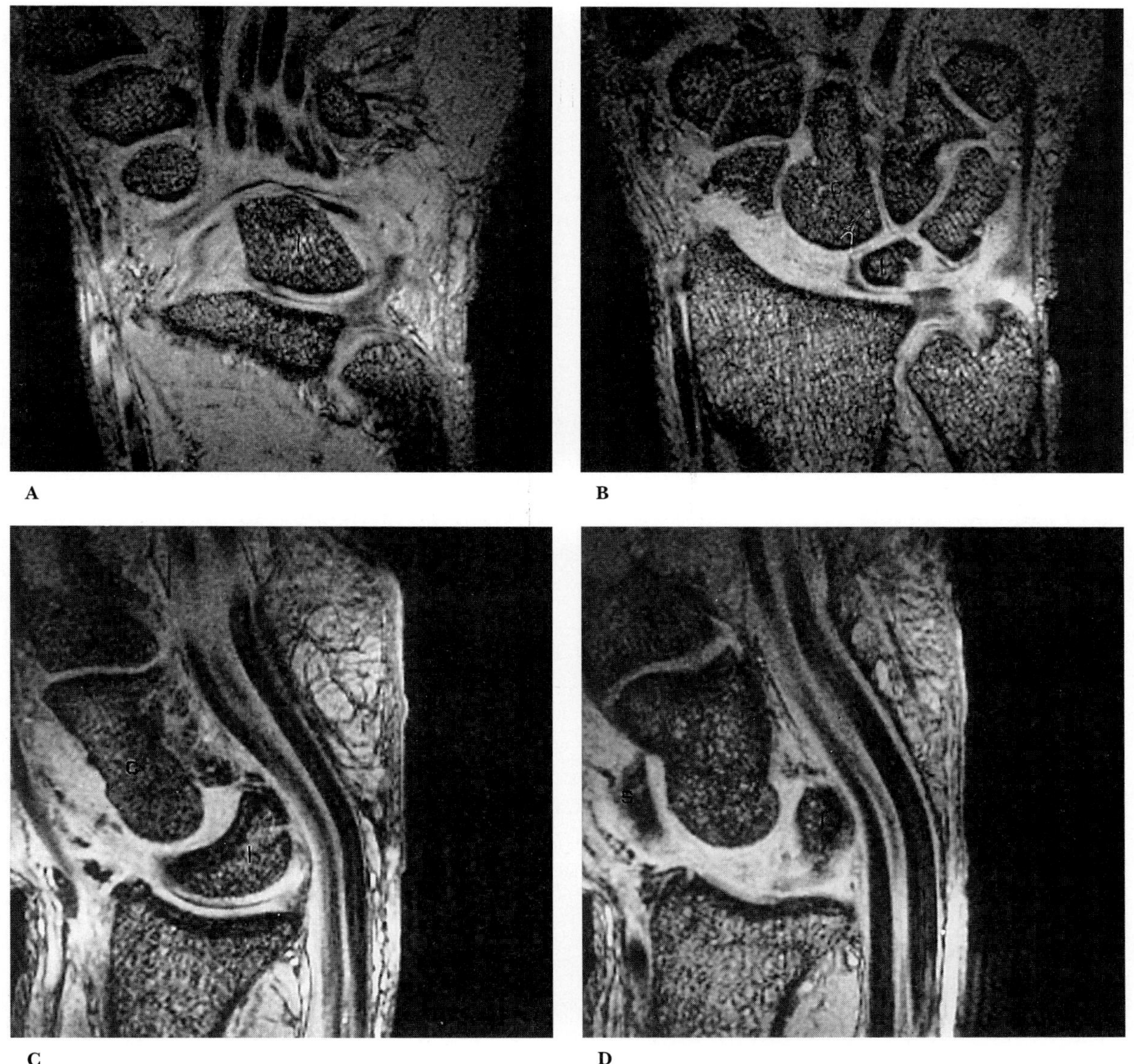

FIGURE 17–10. Old nonunion of displaced scaphoid fracture associated with scapholunate dissociation and DISI. In the ventral coronal image **(A)** the lunate appears much bigger than expected. This is the typical appearance of a dorsally tilted lunate. The dorsal coronal image **(B)** shows the proximally migrated capitate (c) and scapholunate dissociation. Sagittal images **(C, D)** show the DISI findings with dorsally tilted lunate (l) and dorsally dislocated proximal scaphoid fragment(s).

have been found in the midcoronal third of the ligament. Both middle-substance and ligament–cartilaginous junctional defects have been observed.[2] As previously mentioned, the part of the ligament that inserts into the bone through hyaline cartilage (midcoronal portion) may be visualized on 3D GRE images as high signal and should not be interpreted as a tear. This same area appears as low to intermediate signal on SE images; therefore, if thin-section high-resolution SE images are available, this potential problem will be minimized.

When 3D GRE imaging was used alone in a cadaveric study, we found some false-positive and false-negative readings for small LT tears.[2] In clinical practice (with surgical confirmation), however, we encountered only a few false-positive or false-negative readings when SE and 3D GRE sequences were used together and the studies were of good technical quality. Our comments regarding partial injury of the SL ligament apply equally to the LT ligament. In general, we have found the LT ligament to be somewhat more difficult to reliably image than the SL complex, and partial lesions to this ligament are difficult to detect with confidence. Problems visualizing the LT ligament have also been noted by other authors.[24,25,28,41]

Extrinsic Ligament Lesions

Although we have encountered few indications for imaging patients with extrinsic ligament disruption, we have found that this injury can definitely be visualized. Such disruptions often are combined with SL dissociation, midcarpal instability, and displaced scaphoid fractures. Because extrinsic ligaments are larger, better defined, and have less intricate infrastructure than the intrinsic ligaments, one would expect high-resolution MRI to discern any mechanical disruption or significant degenerative lesion within these tissues, which has been our experience (Figs. 17–9 and 17–12).

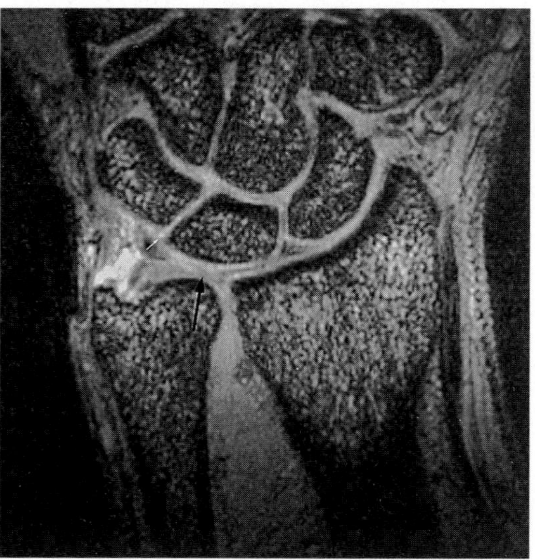

FIGURE 17–11. Lunotriquetral perforation (white arrow) in a patient with extensive TFCC perforation (black arrow).

One of the potential benefits of using MRI (as opposed to arthrography) to evaluate the ligamentous integrity of the carpus is the possibility of staging or quantifying ligamentous defects. Degenerative changes leading to small perforations of the intrinsic ligaments are common.[44–46] Inasmuch as many of the small central perforations are asymptomatic, MRI's potential for providing specific knowledge of the exact location and extent of a ligamentous lesion as well as associated bone or soft-tissue injuries may prove to be quite useful clinically.

TFCC Lesions

Tears or perforations of the TFC and TFCC are common.[44,46,47] Although many of these defects may be associated with significant clinical symptomatology, it is important to remember that there is a strong correlation between TFCC perforation and age.[44,47,48] Thus, the finding of a TFC or TFCC defect on MRI (or any other study) must always be correlated with clinical findings before judging the clinical significance of the lesion. There have been numerous reports in the literature as to the efficacy of MRI in the evaluation of the TFCC.[23–28,30,41,47] In our experience, MRI with the technical capabilities and resolution that we have detailed here yields studies that approach 100% sensitivity and specificity for full-thickness perforations.

TFCC lesions may be either traumatic or degenerative and involve one or more of a number of specific sites within the complex including the ventral or dorsal radioulnar ligaments; the ulnar attachment sites, especially about the ulnar styloid and fovea at the ulnar styloid base; the distal ulnolunate/ulnotriquetral ligament insertions; the central disc; or various combinations of these.[49,50] Palmer and others have reported a clinical classification for TFCC injuries based on both the etiology and location of the perforation as determined at arthroscopy or arthrotomy.[49] We believe that one of the evolving advantages of MRI over arthrography is its potential to localize a defect within the TFCC sufficiently to permit noninvasive staging and classification of the lesion.[22]

TFCC perforations or disruptions generally appear on the MR images as high-signal intensity areas interrupting the continuity of the low signal of an intact fibrocartilaginous central disc or the striated pattern of an intact ventral or dorsal radioulnar ligament. Complete perforations of the ventral or dorsal radioulnar ligament or ulnar attachments are easily appreciated (Figs. 17–13, 17–14, and 17–17). When assessing subtle lesions of the disc (TFC), it is important to recall that the origin of the central disc at the sigmoid notch is through high-signal hyaline cartilage, the thickness of the intact TFC varies di-

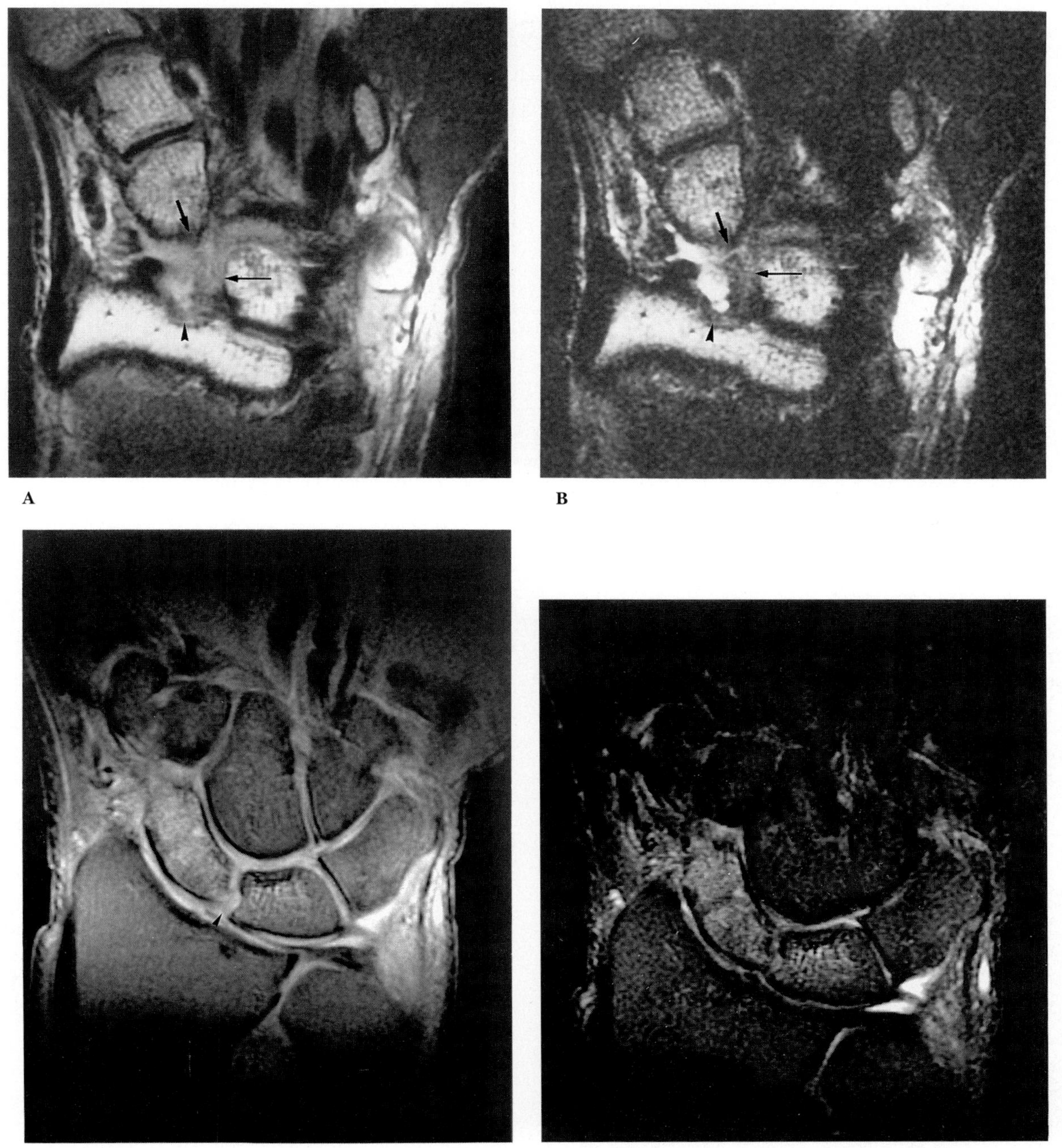

FIGURE 17–12. Extrinsic ligament disruptions in a patient with an old healed scaphoid fracture. PD **(A)** and T2W SE **(B)** images show absence of the intact linear fascicles of ligaments indicating torn deep fascicles of the radioscaphocapitate ligament (short thick arrows), radiolunate portion (long thin arrows) of the radiolunotriquetral ligament, and the torn radioscapholunate ligament (arrowheads in **A** and **B**). The scapholunate ligament (small arrowhead in **C**) has high-signal intensity on a fat-suppressed PD image **(C)** consistent with an old injury. The high-signal intensity of the lunate and scaphoid bone on PD and T2W fat-suppressed **(D)** images is consistent with old bone bruise without avascular necrosis (AVN).

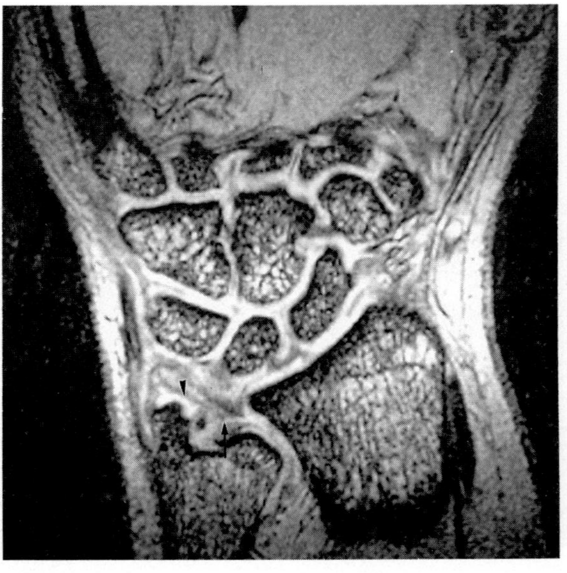

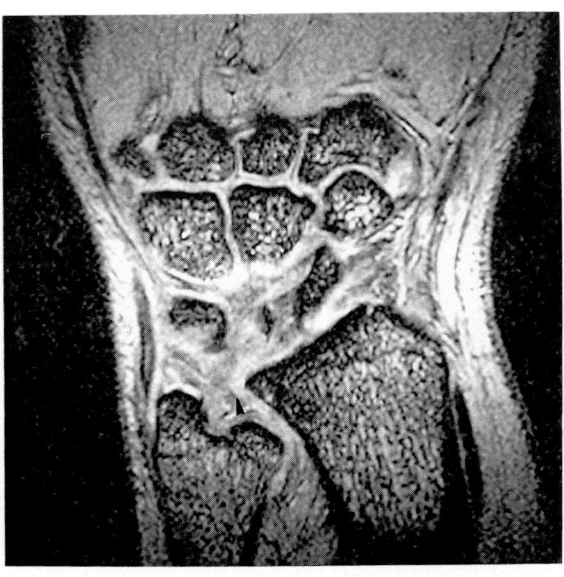

A B

FIGURE 17–13. Coronal images showing TFCC disruption **(A, B).** A patient with ulnar minus variance has extensive disruption of the central disc (arrow), the attachment of the TFC to the ulnar styloid (small arrowhead), and the dorsal radioulnar ligament (large arrowhead).

rectly with ulnar negative variance,[29] and in the normal state, the thin low-signal line of the superficial tangential layer on the surface of the lunate fossa cartilage joins seamlessly with the distal surface of the disc. With these MR anatomic points in mind, even short slit-like perforations of the disc adjacent to the sigmoid notch can be readily distinguished. As previously mentioned, the TFC may insert through hyaline cartilage at the level of the ulnar styloid tip returning high signal on 3D images and intermediate signal on T2W images. Care should be taken to avoid interpreting this normal variant as an insertional tear. An additional potential source of difficulty at the ulnar insertion site is fluid in the prestyloid recess. This recess, located anterior to the ulnar styloid, shows high-signal intensity on T2W images that could be considered a normal finding.

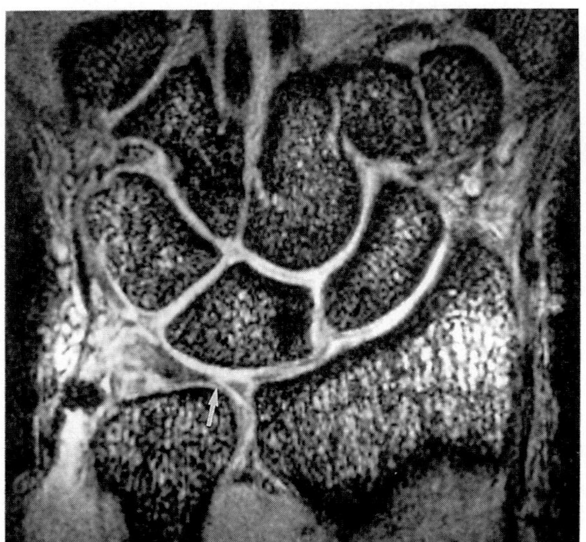

FIGURE 17–14. TFC perforation. A coronal image demonstrates a central disc (TFC) perforation (white arrow). The scapholunate and lunotriquetral ligaments are normal.

Partial-thickness perforations (noncommunicating defects) are recognized as irregular areas of higher signal intensity along the otherwise smooth proximal or distal surface of the TFC. Although some reports have claimed that MRI can distinguish degenerative lesions from partial thickness traumatic tears,[24] we have not been able to make this differentiation other than by inferring the cause based on the location of the defect.[50]

Fractures

Although fractures of the wrist and distal forearm can usually be satisfactorily evaluated with plain x-rays, there are some particularly complex fracture problems in the wrist that may warrant the effort and expense of an MR study. In these situations, MRI allows excellent multiplanar assessment of articular fracture alignment, while simultaneously providing useful information about associated soft-tissue injury, fragment vascularity, and (in the case of subacute injury) bone and soft-tissue healing (Figs. 17–9, 17–10, 17–12, 17–15 to 17–18, and 17–20). In such cases the information provided by MRI may be particularly useful, for example, to help make treatment decisions

Text continued on page 464

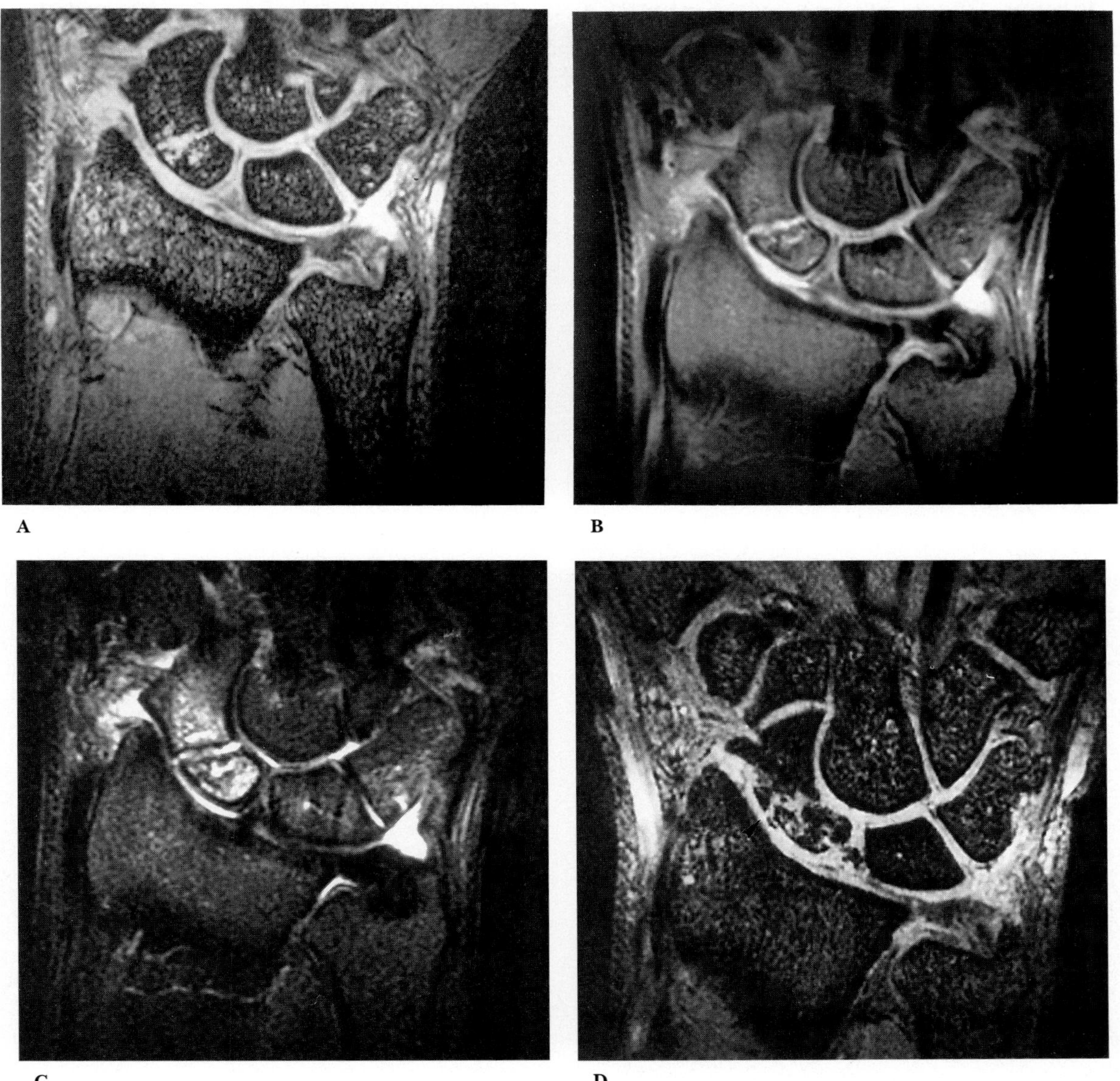

FIGURE 17–15. Nonunion of scaphoid fracture in an early phase: 3D GRE (**A**), PD (**B**), and T2W (**C**) fat-suppression images. The diffuse high-signal intensity in fat-suppression images both in the proximal and distal fragment of the scaphoid is consistent with a bone bruise induced by an injury. Cystic changes (**A**) involve the scaphoid at this stage. The same patient 1 year later after unsuccessful bone graft (**D**): both the proximal and distal fragments are cystic and fragmented. The cartilage in the radius and scaphoid is worn (arrowhead) with associated narrowing of the radioscaphoid joint space.

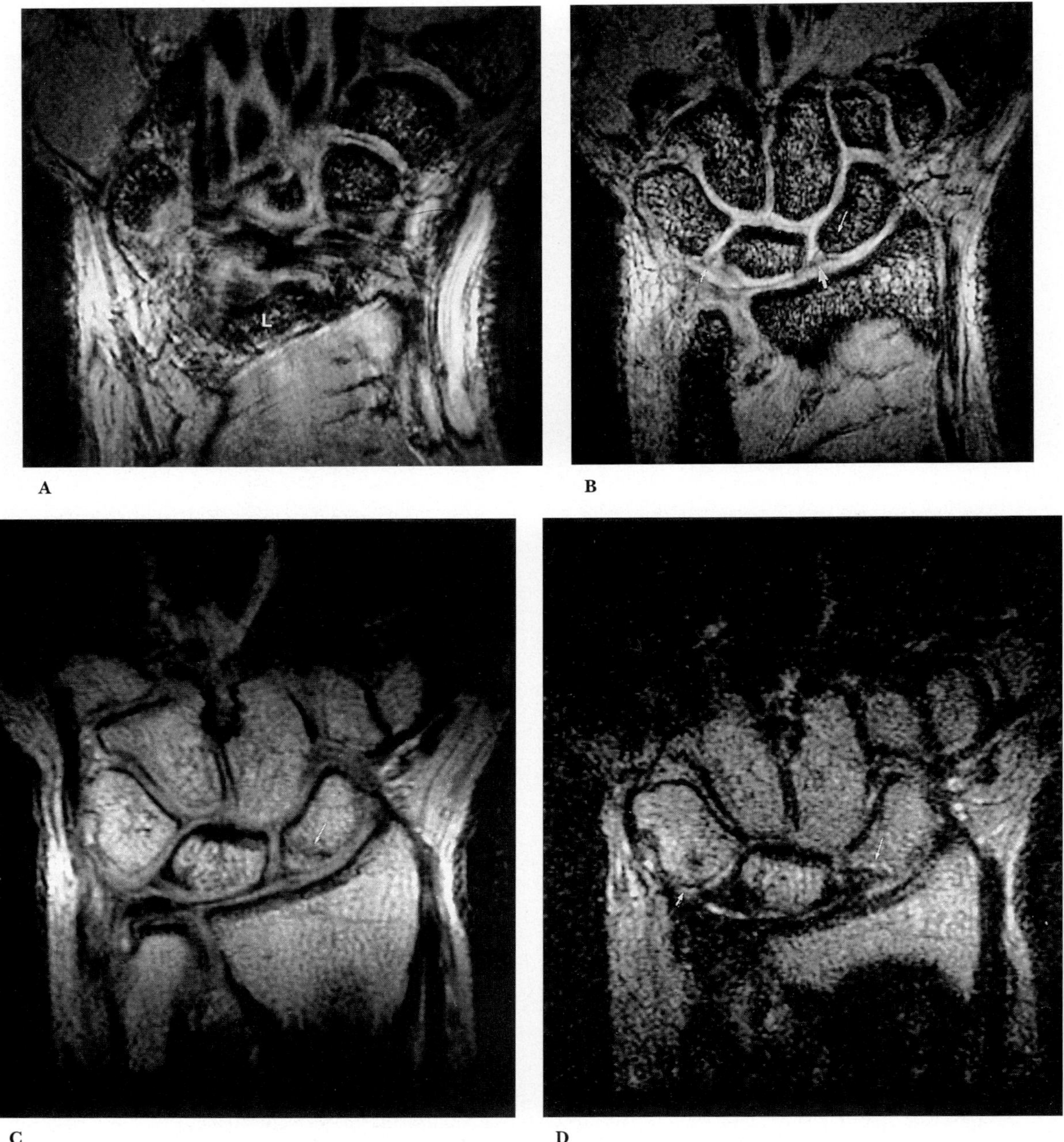

FIGURE 17–16. VISI associated with an old scaphoid fracture and lunotriquetral ligament perforation. This shows the typical appearance of a ventrally tilted lunate (L), which appears unusually prominent in ventral coronal images. The old fracture line in the scaphoid (thin white arrows) is not seen well on 3D GRE images **(A, B)** but is well seen on spin echo images **(C, D)**. The scapholunate ligament is intact (large white arrow) but the lunotriquetral ligament (small white arrow) is disrupted.

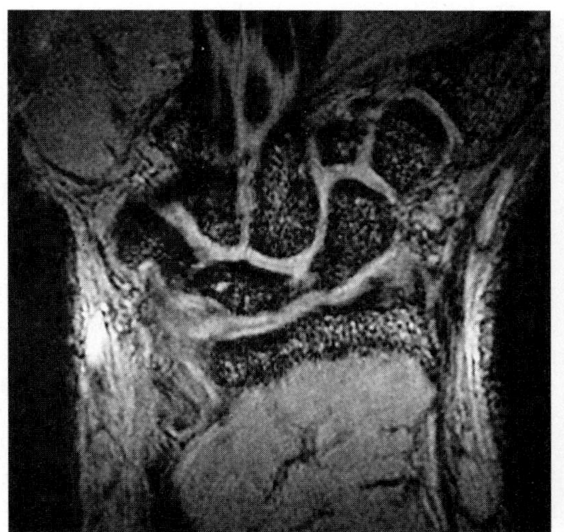

A

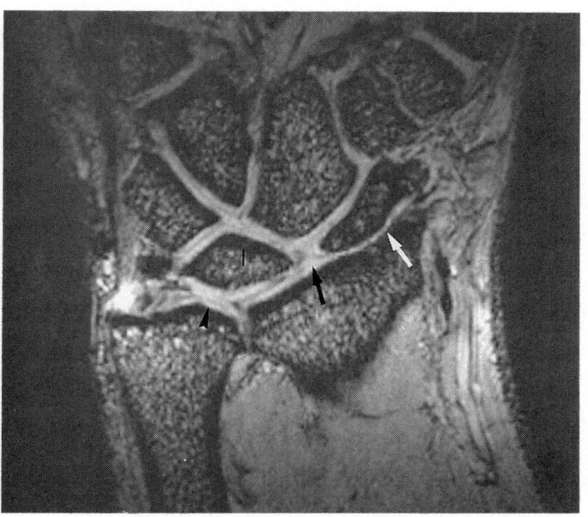

B

FIGURE 17–17. Coronal images of VISI found as a sequela of old scaphoid fracture and scapholunate dissociation **(A, B)** showing a ventrally tilted lunate (l) and scapholunate dissociation (black arrow). The scaphoid is deformed and rotated with resultant degeneration of the radioscaphoid cartilages (white arrow). Cartilage degeneration is evident by loss of the thin low-signal intensity interface of cartilages of the radius and scaphoid and thinning of the corresponding high-signal intensity cartilages. A more normal appearance of the cartilage can be seen at the radiolunate joint. A communicating defect involves the TFC (arrowhead) in a patient with positive ulnar variance.

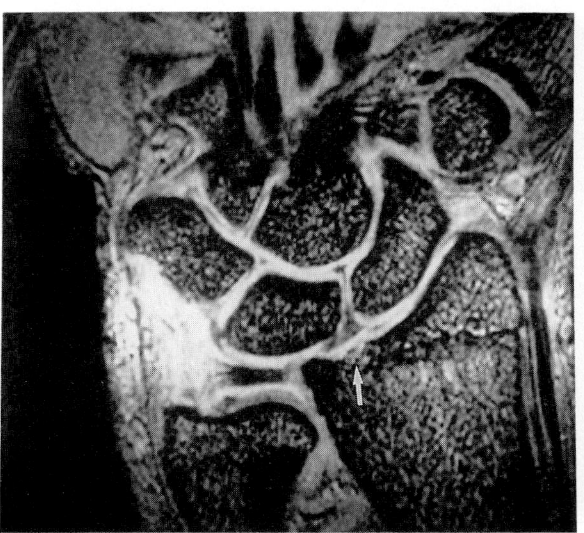

A

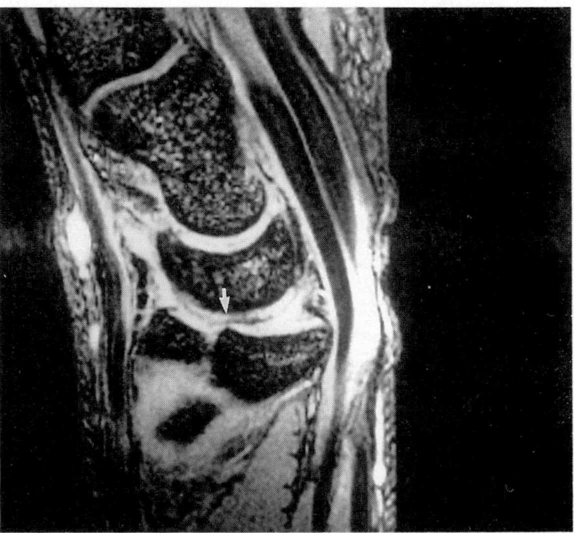

B

FIGURE 17–18. Intraarticular radial fracture with "stepoff" in subchondral bone and articular cartilage. A coronal image **(A)** shows extension of the fracture (white arrow) into the radiocarpal joint space. A sagittal image **(B)** shows a stepoff at the radial fracture site with associated damage (thinning) of the lunate fossa cartilage (short white arrow). The scapholunate and lunotriquetral ligaments are intact.

in cases of long-standing complex nonunions of scaphoid fractures with carpal collapse and associated lesions such as SL ligament tear, proximal pole avascularity, and radioscaphoid articular cartilage injury. Figure 17–15 shows a case in which MRI documented all of these complicating factors, resulting in an informed preoperative decision to proceed directly with proximal row carpectomy.

The complex intraarticular distal radius fracture is another injury that may sometimes warrant an MR study. Multiplanar fracture fragment displacement and angulation can be determined without resorting to image reconstructions or multiple positionings of the wrist as needed with CT (see Chapter 16). In addition, associated soft-tissue injuries to the carpal ligaments, cartilage surfaces, TFCC, and DRUJ can be assessed (Fig. 17–18). In the future, all of these structures should be assessable with increasing accuracy on MRI.

In all of these types of fracture cases use of 3D GRE imaging has been most appropriate because it provides high resolution with excellent contrast between the various structures of interest.

Avascular Necrosis

The sensitivity and specificity of MRI in the evaluation of avascular necrosis (AVN) of the lunate and other carpal bones is excellent, and many authors believe that this is now the imaging modality of choice for this problem.[51–57] In the evaluation of AVN, it is useful to use several sequences including T1W, PD, T2W SE and fat suppression, and thin-slice 3D images.

Kienböck's disease (AVN of the lunate) can be a debilitating wrist problem. Early identification and staging of this condition is important in that appropriate early institution of treatment may significantly affect the long-term prognosis. MRI is ideally suited for evaluation of Kienböck's disease because of its sensitivity in detecting the early stages of the condition, and its ability to demonstrate the 3D morphology of the lesion. Debate over the cause of the disorder persists, but it seems probable that in at least some of the cases, onset of the condition is associated with fracture of the lunate.[58] If there is no fracture, MR findings in the early stages of lunate AVN potentially can be limited to bone edema manifested by decreased signal intensity on 3D GRE images and T1W and PD SE images, and by increased signal intensity on both T2W SE images[56,57] and T2W fat-suppression images (Figs. 17–19A and 17–19B). Radiologists and other clinicians should know that some of these MR changes can also be seen with transient bone ischemia, a condition that is self-limiting and spontaneously resolves.[59]

Later, when Kienböck's disease is clearly evident, decreased signal intensity is seen not only on T1W, PD, and 3D GRE images, but also on T2W SE images[51,57] and T2W fat-suppression images (Figs. 17–19C and 17–19D). Lunate fractures associated with the AVN are best identified with thin-slice 3D images. AVN typically involves the lunate in a diffuse pattern, although focal high-signal intensity areas reflecting more fluid material could be present within a diffusely abnormal lunate.

Focal, well-defined lunate cysts of variable size appear as homogeneous high signal intensity on 3D GRE imaging and are easily distinguished from areas of AVN (Fig. 17–19F). Although these focal lesions with high-signal intensity areas may be cysts, they can also represent intraosseous ganglia. When the focal, well-defined lesion is of lower or intermediate signal on T2W or 3D GRE imaging, it represents a defect filled with fibrous tissue. A focal, ill-defined, low-signal intensity area on the proximal ulnar side of the lunate reflects the presence of sclerosis or another type of reactive bone alteration in ulnar impaction syndrome or senescent changes. Focal lesions of the proximal ulnar corner of the lunate may have high-, intermediate-, or low-signal intensity on T2W or 3D GRE, reflecting the presence of fluid, fibrous, or bony material. It is important to recognize that any of these focal lesions in the lunate will generally not progress to Kienböck's disease.

Scaphoid fractures are common and are sometimes complicated by AVN of the proximal fragment (Fig. 17–20). Early AVN of the scaphoid bone can be difficult to identify even with MRI. The MR changes associated with the bone marrow edema that accompanies early scaphoid fracture with AVN (low-signal intensity on T1W and PD and high-signal intensity on T2W SE images) are identical to those induced by any bone injury (Fig. 17–15). If these changes are observed in both the proximal and distal fragments and are restricted to an area adjacent to the fracture site, then they are probably due to the fracture and do not indicate AVN. On the other hand, if only the proximal pole shows areas of low-signal intensity on T1W and high-signal intensity on T2W images, AVN is likely present. If in suspected cases the signal changes mentioned above either persist or increase over time, the probability of AVN is markedly increased.

As a final note, although 3D GRE imaging of carpal AVN is quite sensitive and the morphologic information is usually clinically helpful, this imaging sequence is not particularly specific for avascularity. The low signal associated with AVN on this sequence can easily be confused with the low signal observed with non-AVN conditions such as bone edema, increased osseous blood flow, and simple increased ossification or calcification.

Carpal Tunnel Syndrome

The clinical entity known as carpal tunnel syndrome (CTS) is caused by compression of the median nerve beneath the transverse carpal ligament. It is undoubtedly the most common of all entrapment neuropa-

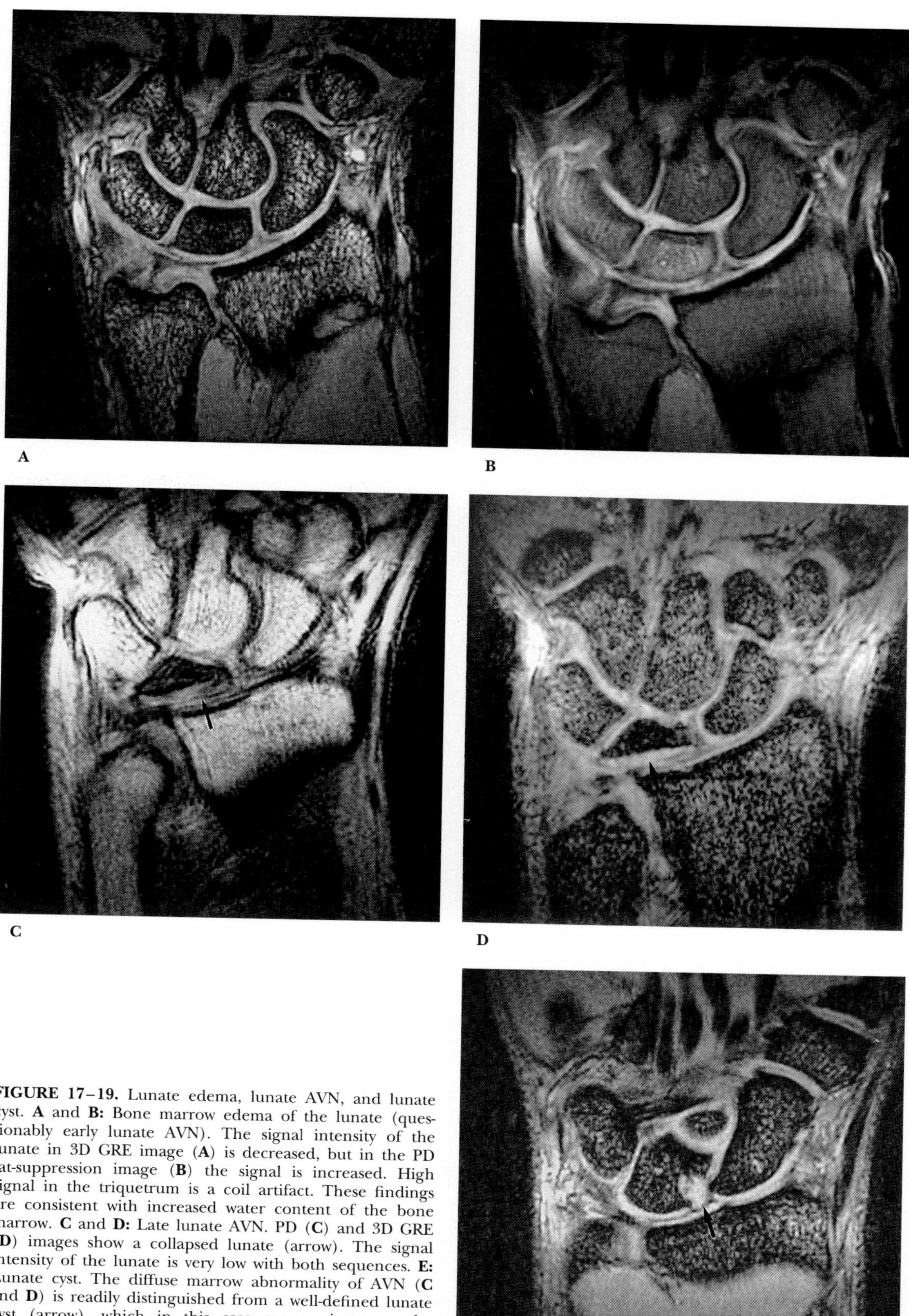

FIGURE 17–19. Lunate edema, lunate AVN, and lunate cyst. **A** and **B:** Bone marrow edema of the lunate (questionably early lunate AVN). The signal intensity of the lunate in 3D GRE image (**A**) is decreased, but in the PD fat-suppression image (**B**) the signal is increased. High signal in the triquetrum is a coil artifact. These findings are consistent with increased water content of the bone marrow. **C** and **D:** Late lunate AVN. PD (**C**) and 3D GRE (**D**) images show a collapsed lunate (arrow). The signal intensity of the lunate is very low with both sequences. **E:** Lunate cyst. The diffuse marrow abnormality of AVN (**C** and **D**) is readily distinguished from a well-defined lunate cyst (arrow), which in this case communicates to the scapholunate joint (see text).

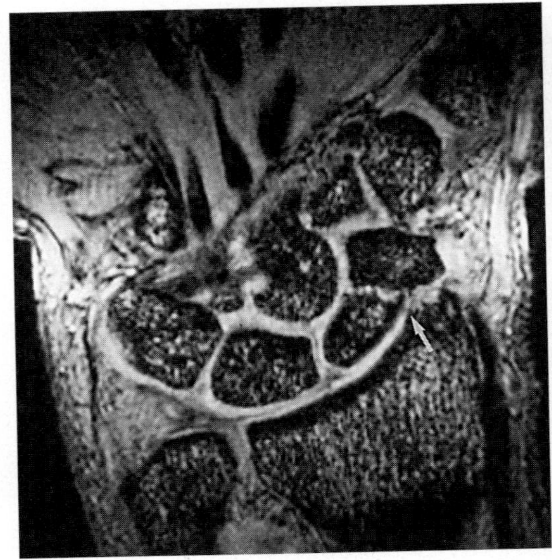

A

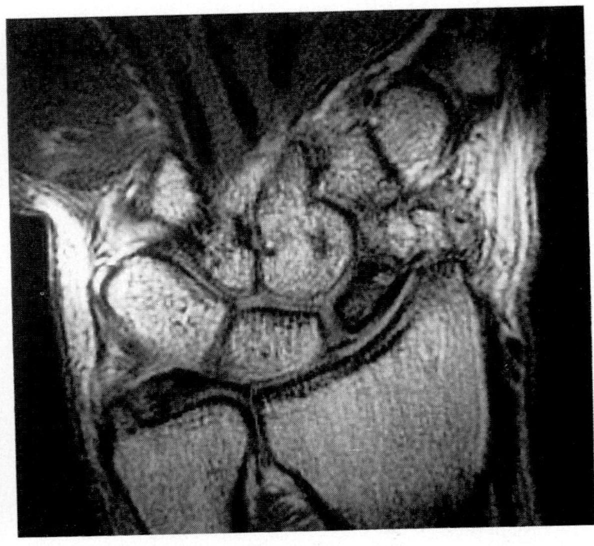

B

FIGURE 17–20. Old scaphoid fracture with AVN of proximal fragment. Low-signal intensity is present in a proximal scaphoid fragment on 3D GRE **(A)** and proton density SE **(B)** images. Thinning and loss (see comments in Fig. 17–17B) in the radial and scaphoid cartilages (white arrow) are best seen on the 3D GRE image.

thies, and for reasons that are not clear the incidence of this condition has been steadily increasing in recent years.[60] Occupational duties that require constant repetitive motion are believed to contribute significantly to the increasing incidence of this problem, but the mechanism by which this so-called overuse etiology exerts its damage on the neural function has not been fully elucidated. Aside from the overuse phenomena and direct trauma, there are a number of medical problems that predispose patients to CTS. These include diabetes mellitus, inflammatory arthritides (such as rheumatoid arthritis), certain metabolic disorders (such as thyroid disease), and amyloid deposition diseases.[61]

The clinical role of MRI in evaluating patients with suspected CTS is evolving. Although CTS can almost always be diagnosed accurately on the basis of clinical assessment and electrodiagnostic studies alone, there are some situations in which the diagnosis and/or cause may be obscure.[61] In that event, MRI may be useful as an adjunctive measure to confirm the suspected diagnosis. In addition, because CTS is often due to a space-occupying lesion with the carpal tunnel (such as hypertrophic tenosynovium), MRI may demonstrate a definitive cause for the condition.

MRI evaluation of CTS is best performed using axial images with either PD and T2W SE or fat-suppression sequences. Diffuse swelling of the median nerve, flattening of the median nerve at the level of hamate, palmar bowing of the flexor retinaculum, and increased signal in the median nerve on T2W images have been described as changes pathognomonic for CTS (Figs. 17–21 to 17–23).[28,36,62–64]

The synovial tissue that surrounds the nine tendons and the median nerve within the carpal tunnel is normally very thin and shows as an intermediate intensity tissue separate from the low-signal intensity bundles of tendon tissue. In rheumatoid disease or any other synovial process, the synovium appears as high-signal intensity on T2W images (Fig. 17–22).[37] In addition to this change in signal characteristic, the tenosynovial tissue is also hypertrophic in these synovitic disorders and with MRI this increase in bulk of synovial tissue within the carpal canal can be appreciated as the cause of the compressive neuropathy (Fig. 17–22).[36,62]

Aside from synovitis as a cause, any tumor or other space-occupying mass lesion within the carpal tunnel can precipitate CTS; these types of lesions can easily be demonstrated with MRI (Fig. 17–23). For example, a decrease in the potential space available for the median nerve can result from hypertrophic bone spurs or carpal malalignment associated with osteoarthritis. Malalignment of carpal bones sufficient to compress the median nerve can also result from ligamentous injury (such as SL ligament disruption), or as a consequence of erosive destruction from rheumatoid disease. In all these situations, MRI can provide both confirming diagnostic and definitive etiologic information.

Currently, although MRI is generally not required in the evaluation of CTS, it may be indicated when there is rapid onset of symptoms, if there are any symptoms suggesting that the cause may be due to a space-occupying lesion or some other abnormality that might require more extensive treatment than simple release of the retinaculum alone,[28] or if there is still uncertainty about the diagnosis of CTS, in which case MRI can potentially be of clinical value.

The surgical treatment of CTS is incisional release

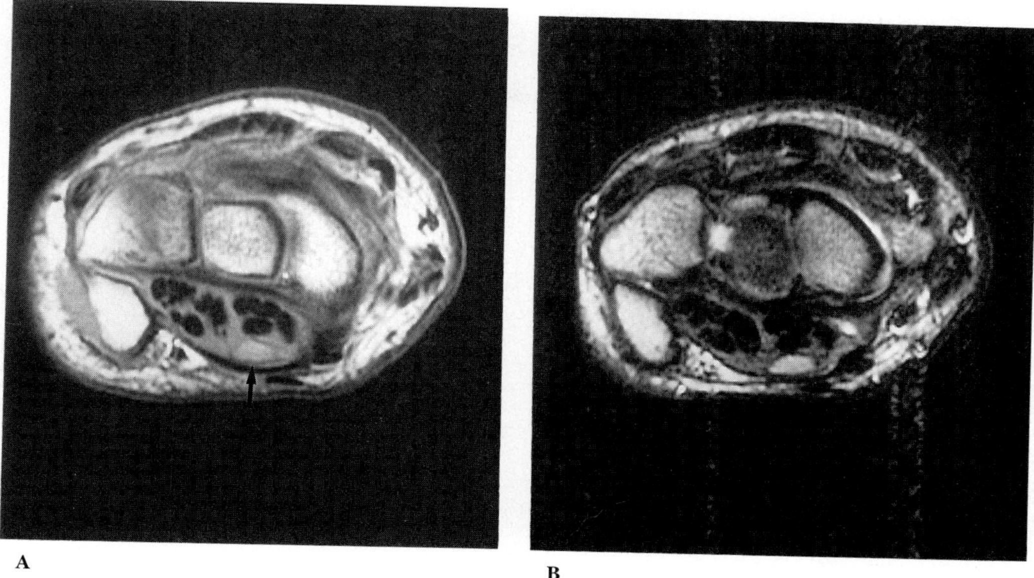

FIGURE 17–21. Carpal tunnel syndrome due to dorsal subluxation of the ulna. The signal intensity of the median nerve (arrow) is high intermediate on the first echo image (**A**) and high on the second echo image (**B**).

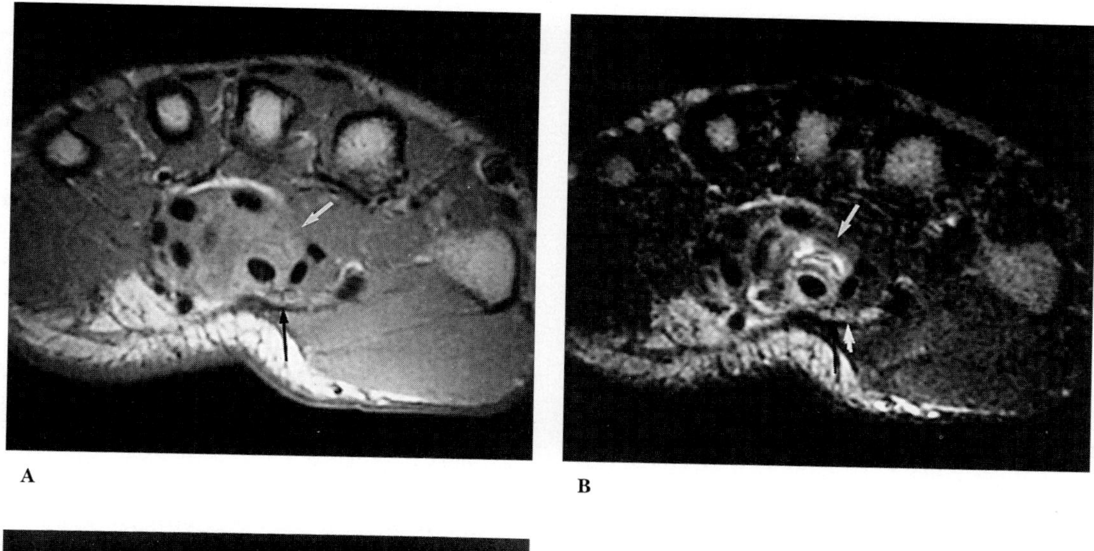

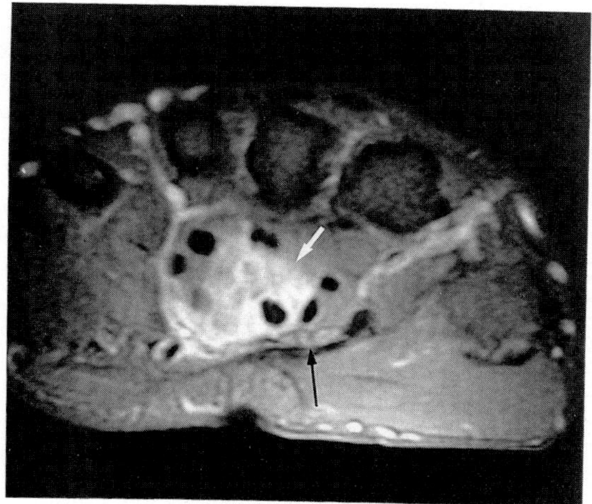

FIGURE 17–22. Carpal tunnel syndrome in a patient with inflammatory changes in the synovial tissue due to rheumatoid arthritis (**A** to **C**). The thick synovium (white arrow) acts as a space-occupying lesion leading to median nerve compression (black arrow). The signal intensity of the branches of the median nerve is increased, showing as high intermediate on PD (**A**), high on T2W SE (**B**), and intermediate on PD fat-suppression (**C**) image. Signal intensity is higher in the synovium than in the median nerve in the PD fat-suppression image (**C**).

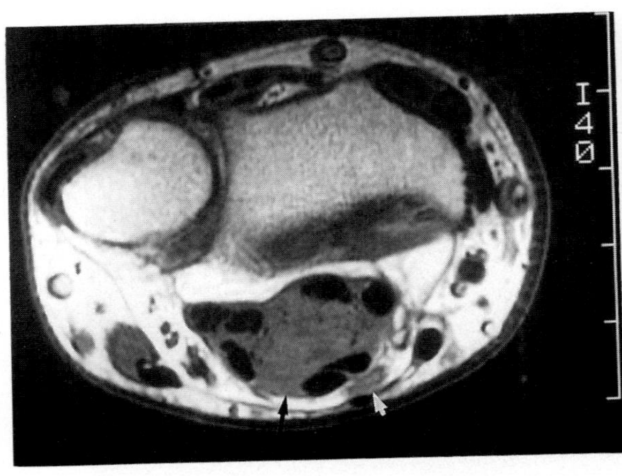

A

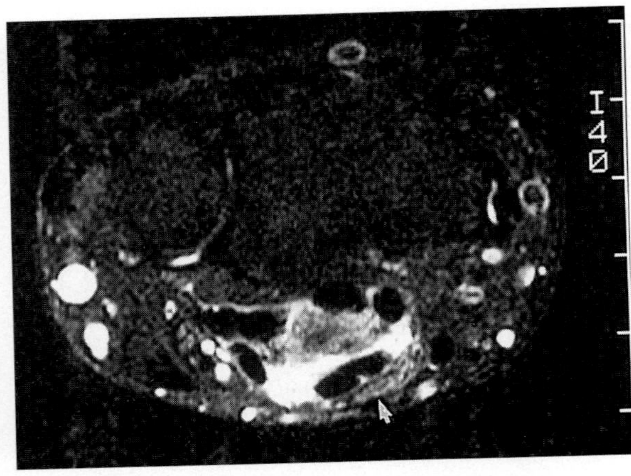

B

FIGURE 17–23. Carpal tunnel syndrome due to a space-occupying malignant fibrous histiocytoma. The axial T1W image **(A)** shows the tumor mass (black arrow). The patient had a 3-week history of carpal tunnel symptoms. The signal within the median nerve (white arrow) has not changed on a T2W fat-suppressed image **(B)**.

of the transverse retinaculum.[61] After the operation, the carpal tunnel contents migrate slightly palmarly into a larger volume, and thereby become decompressed.[65] Because incomplete division of the retinaculum, scar formation around the median nerve, and unrecognized anatomic anomalies are common causes of persistent symptoms after carpal tunnel surgery, MRI may be particularly helpful in evaluating patients who have persistent symptoms after surgical release.[66] If a postoperative MR study is required, it is important to realize that high-signal intensity within the median nerve on T2W images after release may persist, and that this finding alone is not a reliable indication of an unsuccessful operation.[28]

HAND

Normal Anatomy

As with the wrist, the intricate fine structures of the hand are best visualized with very-high-resolution MRI. Support for such imaging requires surface coils specifically built to conform to the shape and size of the part to be studied. We have used custom constructed receiver coils to generate the images shown here to illustrate the normal axial plane anatomy of the palm and fingers. The SE imaging parameters that we found most effective for use with these coils included TR 2000 ms, TE 20, 80 ms, field of view 8 cm, slice thickness 3 mm, interslice spacing 0.5 mm, and one excitation. 3D GRE imaging in the hand has also been useful with TR 60 ms, TE 17 ms, flip angle 20 degrees, slice thickness 1.0 mm, and one excitation. If the demands of the study do not require very high resolution (such as when imaging large mass lesions), then commercially available wrist coils are generally satisfactory.

Much of the descriptive MR anatomic detail outlined with respect to bone, joint, and ligaments in the section on the normal anatomy of the wrist carries over distally to the hand and fingers. The normal gross and cross-sectional anatomy of the hand is presented in Chapter 4. For the most part, this anatomy can be directly appreciated in the high-resolution illustrative MR images shown in Fig. 17–7. Certain features, however, are unique to the hand and warrant comment.[67–69] The intrinsic thenar muscles of the hand include the abductor pollicis brevis, the flexor pollicis brevis, and the opponens pollicis. The thenar fascia overlying these muscles has low-signal intensity in all pulse sequences. The hypothenar group is comprised of the flexor digiti minimi, the abductor digiti minimi, and the opponens digiti minimi. These muscles are covered by a substantial fascial layer and can be identified by their oblique course in all MR images (Fig. 17–7). The adductor pollicis has its origin on the palmar aspect of the third metacarpal. Like many of the intrinsic muscles, the tendon of this muscle has a complex insertion, in this case at the ulnar palmar aspect of the base of the proximal phalanx of the thumb, via direct attachment to the phalanx through the ulnar sesamoid and insertion into the extensor tendon (Fig. 17–7).

The four lumbrical muscles originate from the flexor digitorum profundus tendons and insert into the radial aspect of the extensor expansion. The palmar (volar) and dorsal interosseous muscles arise from the lateral aspects of the metacarpal bones and insert at the bases of the proximal phalanges and into the lateral bands of the extensor expansions (Fig. 17–7). Distally, at the level of the MCP joints, the interosseous tendons pass dorsal to the deep transverse metacarpal ligament, whereas the lumbricals pass palmar to this structure in a space referred to as the lumbrical canal.

The deep transverse metacarpal ligament is often referred to as the intermetacarpal plate ligament, because it connects the palmar (volar) plates at the MCP joint level (Fig. 17–7). The gross anatomy of the fine structure of the palmar (volar) plates and associated collateral and accessory collateral ligaments at the MCP and IP joint level have been detailed by Eaton.[70–72] With high-resolution MRI, the distal anatomic detail of both the intrinsic and extrinsic flexor and extensor tendon systems can be discerned. At the level of the proximal phalanx, for example, the bone is completely surrounded by tendon and related structures.

Although clinical indications for MRI of the hand have not been well defined at the time of this writing, this imaging modality is clearly the study of choice for evaluating soft-tissue and bone tumors with soft-tissue extension. The use of MRI for other soft-tissue abnormalities of the hand and fingers is developing.

TUMORS OF THE WRIST AND HAND

This section will discuss the role of MRI in the evaluation, staging, and characterization of soft-tissue and bone tumors in the wrist and hand. Although both soft-tissue and bone tumors in the wrist and hand are unusual, when they occur, MRI is generally critical to their clinical evaluation.

Soft-Tissue Tumors

Clinical symptoms and signs of soft-tissue tumors are determined by their location, size, and biologic nature. Most of them include either a palpable mass or pain. In the evaluation of a palpable mass, MRI is generally the imaging modality of choice. Although plain films in the evaluation of soft-tissue masses are mandatory, they usually provide very little clinical information, except to show if there is bone involvement and if areas of calcifications are present. CT is also of limited value in the evaluation of soft-tissue masses that do not involve bone except to show subtle calcifications. When MRI is not available, CT may show the extent of abnormal soft tissue if abundant fat planes are present. In those situations where pain is the only symptom, MRI often is the last investigation in a lengthy series of imaging studies. In these cases MRI may be the only study capable of demonstrating the lesion (see Chapter 18).

MRI is the most useful imaging modality in staging soft-tissue tumors.[73] It can provide exact information about the location and extent of the tumor and its relationship to the surrounding tissue in general and neurovascular structures in particular. All of this information is critical for treatment planning.[74] High-resolution PD and T2W SE and fat-suppression images are most useful.[75] Since invasion of neuromuscular bundles can significantly change treatment planning, the images must be acquired in planes that will provide that information.

The characterization of a tumor is keyed to changes in tissue appearance on different pulse sequences. Although MRI cannot provide the tissue diagnosis of most soft-tissue tumors, certain MR properties of tumors can be used to limit the differential diagnosis.[74,76–79] The enhancement pattern with gadolinium provides particularly helpful information for tumor characterization.

Benign Soft-Tissue Tumors

One of the most common tumors found about the wrist is a *lipoma.* On MRI benign lipomas demonstrate well-defined high-signal intensity on all sequences. They do not enhance after gadolinium administration and their signal is diminished with fat suppression sequences.

Giant-cell tumors of tendon sheath usually originate from a synovial sheath. They do enhance after gadolinium administration, and because of their hemosiderin component these tumors will have low-intermediate-signal intensity areas on PD images and low-signal intensity areas on T2W images (Fig. 17–24). Because of their inhomogeneous signal intensity they are easily distinguished from homogeneous, well-defined, high-signal intensity ganglia on T2W images (see upcoming discussion about ganglia).

Neurofibroma and neurilemmoma originate from neural tissue, and appear as well-capsulated tumors following the course of the corresponding nerve. Neurofibromas appear in typical cases to have a target pattern of increased peripheral signal intensity and decreased central-signal intensity on T2W images (Fig. 17–25).[78,80] The differential diagnosis distinguishing between malignant and benign tumors of

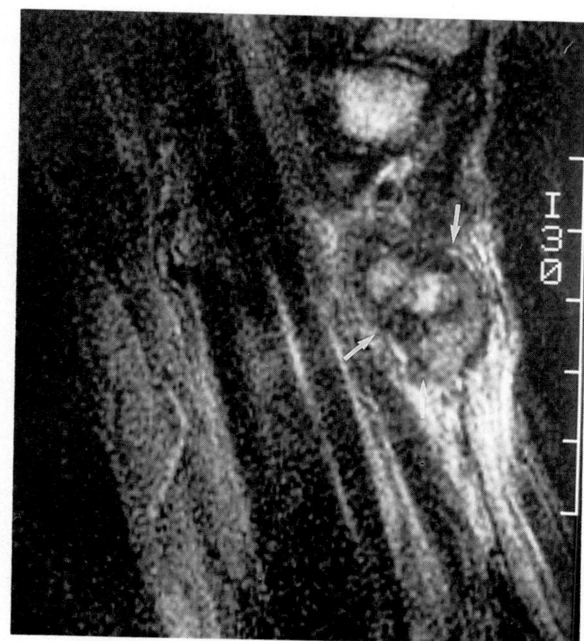

FIGURE 17–24. Giant-cell tumor of tendon sheath. T2W SE image showing signal intensity of recurrent giant-cell tumor (between arrows). The giant-cell tumor appears as an inhomogeneous signal intensity area having low-signal intensity on T2W images mixed with high-signal intensity areas. In this case the low-signal intensity was related to calcification of the tumor.

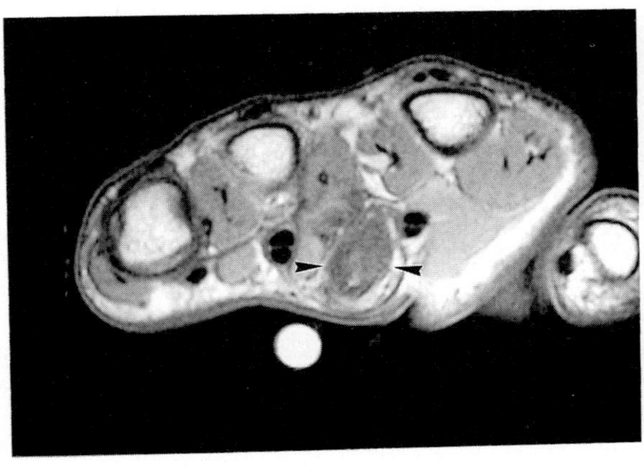

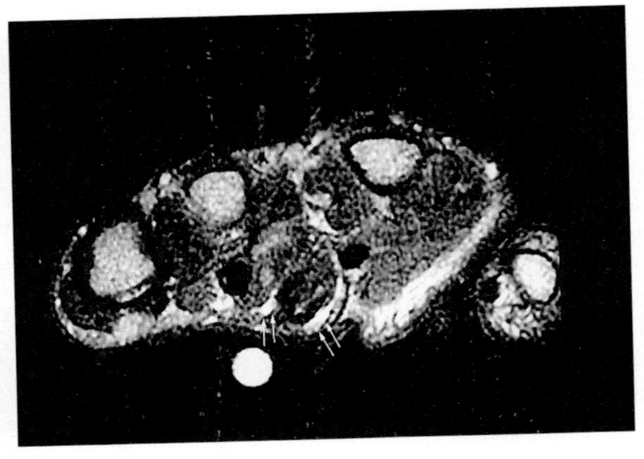

A B

FIGURE 17–25. Neurofibroma of a branch of the median nerve. This neurofibroma presented as a palpable mass affecting the function of the hand. PD **(A)** and T2W SE **(B)** images show low-signal intensity tissue combined with higher-signal intensity components, reflecting the fibrous constituents of this tumor (arrowheads). The tumor is displacing the common palmar digital arteries (white arrows) palmarly. The third metacarpal was previously resected due to severe trauma.

nerve cannot be made based on their MR appearance.[78]

Hemangioma, the most common vascular tumor in the hand, can occur either as a localized mass or as a process with extensive muscle invasion. It has a typical MR appearance, with homogeneous intermediate-signal intensity on T1W and PD images and very-high-signal intensity on T2W images (Fig. 17–26).[79] Hemangiomas are easily identified in fat-suppression images, where they appear as high-signal intensity lesions.

Arteriovenous malformations (AVM) are unusual. However, their serpentine appearance with a flow void in T1W and in T2W images makes their identification easy.

Malignant Soft-Tissue Tumors

Malignant fibrous histiocytoma is one of the most common malignant soft-tissue tumors. It has five subtypes: storiform pleomorphic, myxoid, giant cell, inflammatory, and angiomatoid.[81] Unfortunately, these different subtypes cannot be separated on the basis of their MR characteristics. As with any other soft-tissue tumor, they visualize with intermediate-signal intensity on T1W and PD images and with varying degrees

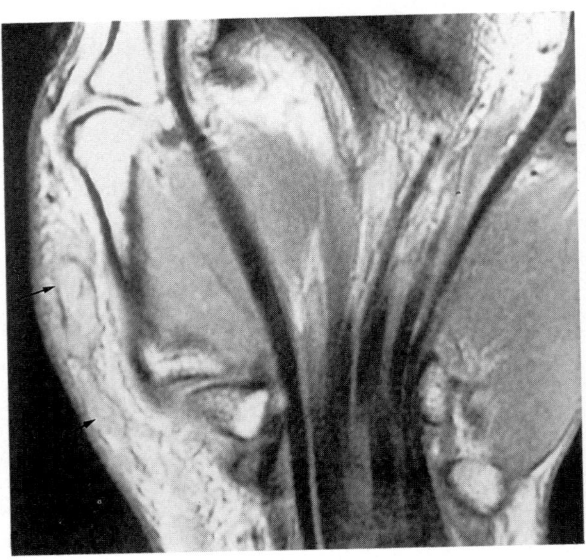

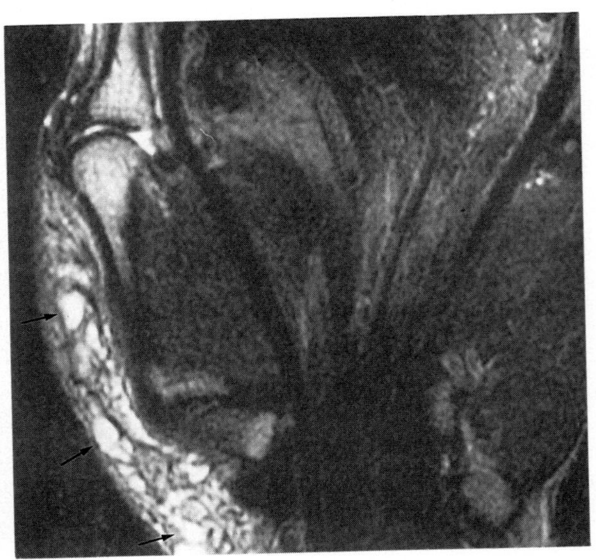

A B

FIGURE 17–26. Typical appearance of a hemangioma of the hand on PD **(A)** and T2W **(B)** images. On the PD image the hemangioma appears with intermediate-signal intensity (arrows). On the T2W image lacuna-like high-signal intensity areas are well defined (arrows).

of high-signal intensity on T2W images (Figs. 17–23 and 17–27). All of these tumor variants enhance after gadolinium administration.

Liposarcoma is another somewhat common tumor seen in the hand and wrist. The MR appearance of liposarcomas depends on the amount of fat in the tumor. While less aggressive fatty tumors have an appearance of septated fat, the myxoid type of liposarcoma appears as a high-signal intensity lesion on PD and T2W images, including fat-suppression sequences.[82]

Synovial sarcomas, angiosarcomas, malignant schwannomas, and *epithelioid sarcomas* are less common malignant soft-tissue tumors in the wrist and the hand; the authors of this chapter have no experience imaging these tumors distal to the elbow.

Bone Tumors

The role of MRI in bone tumor evaluation is different from that in soft-tissue tumor evaluation. Most bone lesions are detected by plain films, and usually the function of MRI is to help with their staging and characterization. Therefore all MR cases of bone tumors should be correlated with plain-film findings to diminish the chance of significant diagnostic errors. One exception to this generalization occurs when a bone tumor is restricted to the marrow and the patient complains of pain only. In this case, plain films may be ambiguous, and MRI may be very helpful to establish the diagnosis. In general, T1W, PD, and T2W SE imaging series are used in the evaluation of bone tumors. In the evaluation of marrow lesions, PD and T2W fat-suppression images are useful additions. With these fat-suppression images, the high-signal intensity marrow lesion is readily detected and its extent determined.

The evaluation of tumor extent in metaphyseal regions of long bones can be challenging. Architectural changes in the cancellous bone and erosions of both the periosteal and endosteal surfaces of the cortical bone need to be carefully assessed. These changes can be best evaluated with high-resolution thin-slice images, either on coronal or sagittal view. In the wrist and hand 1.5- to 2-mm slice thickness is appropriate. Gadolinium administration with high-resolution images will optimize visualization of these sometimes subtle changes.

Characterization of Bone Tumors

Although MRI can only occasionally make a definitive histologic diagnosis, certain MR features are useful to limit the differential. Although the appearance and signal characteristics of the infrastructure of the tumor are helpful in characterizing a lesion, of more importance is the observed behavior of the borders between the lesion and the surrounding trabecular bone or marrow. Usually the most important use of MRI is to precisely delineate the margins of a lesion.

The existence of calcium and the amount of calcium within the lesion further characterizes the tumor and may provide important diagnostic information. Thin-slice 3D GRE images, with their sensitivity to magnetic susceptibility effects are particularly useful in the evaluation of this aspect of infrastructural detail in bony lesions. Such thin slices can display a small amount of calcification in osteochondral and cartilaginous tumors. However, as mentioned above, all MRI examinations of neoplasia, as well as most other conditions that could potentially affect osseous structures, should be closely correlated with a current routine plain-film examination.

Benign Bone Tumors

Enchondroma is the most common benign bone tumor in the hand. It has a nearly diagnostic appearance on plain radiographs and MRI is generally not required in the clinical evaluation of these lesions. It does have a typical MR appearance. The cartilage matrix

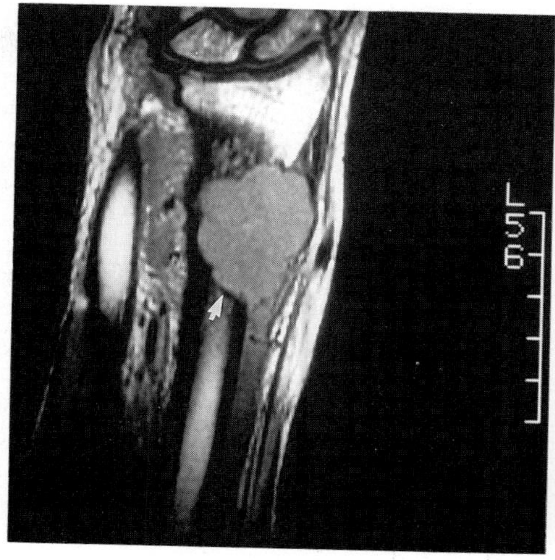

A

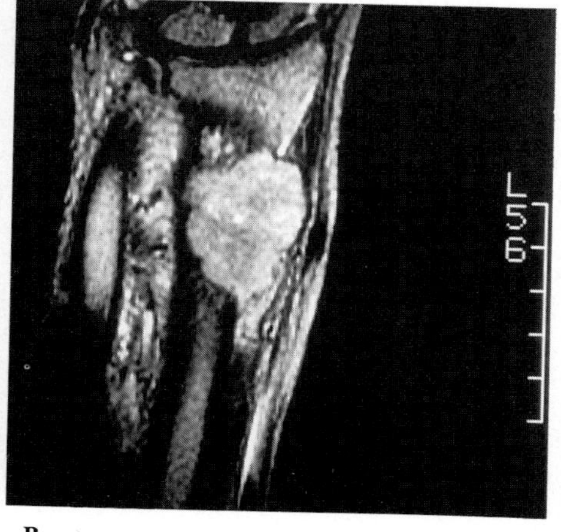

B

FIGURE 17–27. Malignant fibrous histiocytoma of the distal forearm. PD (**A**) and T2W (**B**) images in the coronal plane show an ill-defined, inhomogeneous, soft-tissue mass (arrow) invading and destroying the radius without bone reaction.

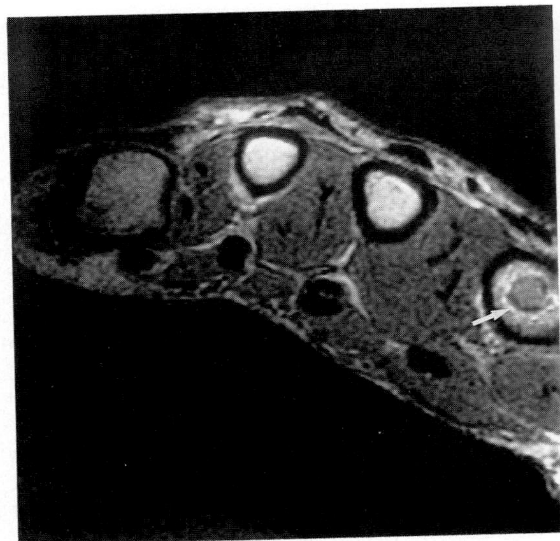
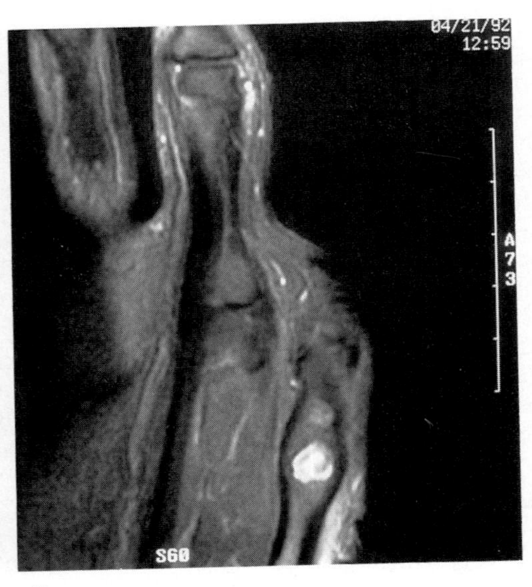

A B

FIGURE 17–28. Enchondroma, metacarpal. The lesion (white arrow) appears as an intermediate-signal intensity area on an axial PD SE image **(A)** and as a high-signal intensity area on a coronal fat-suppressed image **(B)** with a thickened, expanded adjacent cortex. The lesion is well defined with well-developed margins.

has intermediate-signal intensity on T1W and PD images and high-signal intensity on T2W images due to the intralesional cartilage (Fig. 17–28).[83,84] Low-signal intensity calcifications and high-signal intensity cartilage can give it a so-called strawberry appearance.

Bone islands are common. Their homogeneous very-low-signal intensity in both T1 and T2 makes identification easy.

In *osteoid osteomas,* low-signal intensity sclerotic bone surrounds the nidus, which has varying signal intensity on T1W and T2W images, depending on the constituents of the nidus.

The appearance of *osteochondromas* in MR images reflects the benign architecture of these lesions. The well-defined low-signal intensity cortex is interrupted by the cartilaginous cap, which has very-high-signal intensity on T2W images. The thickness of the cap and the relationship between the surrounding bone and osteochondroma itself are readily determined on MR images.

Malignant Bone Tumors

The most common malignant tumors in the wrist and hand are *metastases.* The MRI findings reflect the lytic or blastic nature of metastatic lesion.

Although osteoblastic lesions can have both bony and soft-tissue components, the osteolytic lesions have only soft-tissue components. In osteoblastic lesions the bone-forming components have low- to intermediate-signal intensity on T1W and PD images and lower-signal intensity on T2W images. The appearance of the soft-tissue components in both osteolytic and osteoblastic processes reflects the nature, whether it is fluid, blood, and so on, of that component.

Chondrosarcomas, although they are the most common malignant bone tumors in the hand, are still rare. This tumor tends to occur in patients between 40 and 70 years of age. The multilobulated appearance of chondrosarcomas can be seen best on T2W images.[83,84]

Ewing's sarcoma occurs primarily in a younger group of patients between the ages of 5 and 20 years. The MRI features of Ewing's sarcoma include ill-defined cortical destruction, periosteal reaction, and reactive new bone (not tumor bone) formation. These features reflect the aggressive nature of the tumor.[83,85]

MRI is useful in both the preoperative evaluation of these tumors and postoperative follow-up of the treatment site. The first baseline postoperative study done about 2 months after the operation typically shows extensive postoperative changes in both soft tissue and in bone. If there is no recurrence of the tumor, however, all of these reactive changes will decrease in size and intensity on subsequent follow-up studies.

MISCELLANEOUS LESIONS

Ganglion Cysts

Ganglion cysts are the most common soft-tissue lesions identified on MRI of the wrist. In many cases these cysts are incidental findings, and this fact simply underscores the need to correlate these findings (and all MR findings) with clinical information before drawing conclusions as to their significance. Ganglions appear as very-high-signal, single, multiple, or multiloculated fluid collections surrounded by a low-signal fibrous capsule (Fig. 17–29).[28,76,86,87] Although most ganglions are found dorsally and observed to communicate with the SL ligament, ganglions can occur in many locations both dorsally and

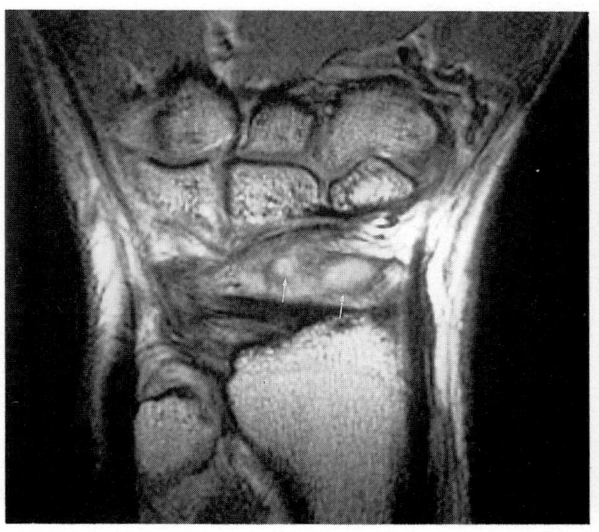

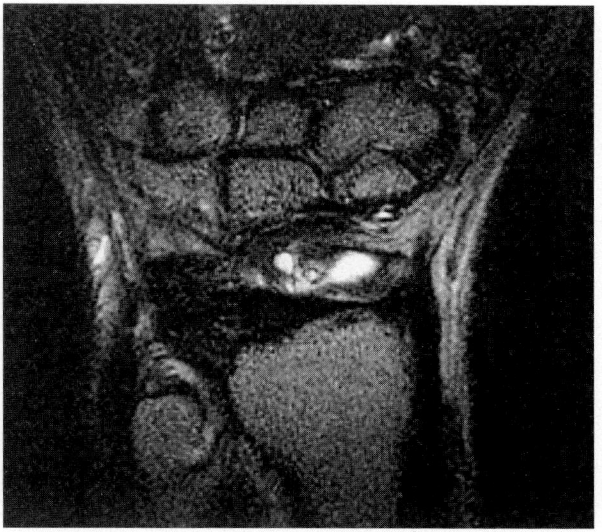

A B

FIGURE 17–29. Typical appearance of a multiloculated dorsal ganglion cyst protruding through and displacing the dorsal ligaments. On the PD image **(A)** the lesion appears as a multilocular, intermediate, high-signal intensity area (white arrows), whereas on the T2W image **(B)** it appears as a well-defined high-signal intensity area. The dorsal extrinsic ligaments are displaced distally.

ventrally and frequently arise in conjunction with tendon insertions and both intrinsic and capsular extrinsic ligaments. Smaller cysts such as those commonly seen adjacent to the abductor pollicis longus and flexor carpi radialis tendons may require high-resolution MRI to be visualized. Although many small ganglions are of questionable clinical significance, small intraligamentous or intracapsular cysts arising from the dorsal SL ligament may be associated with painful wrist symptoms.[88,89] These small intraligamentous lesions may be difficult to identify clinically; high-resolution MRI can be quite helpful in establishing this diagnosis.[90]

Although MRI is seldom required in the evaluation of ganglion cysts, it may be particularly useful in situations where symptoms persist after excision. Identification of a recurrent or residual ganglion is usually easy with T2W fat-suppression axial images where the high-signal intensity is readily detected against the very-low-signal intensity of suppressed fat.

Foreign Bodies

Localization of radiographically nonopaque foreign bodies is notoriously difficult. Here MRI can be exceptionally useful in planning surgical treatment. Most foreign bodies contain solid material that can be identified on 3D GRE images. Typically they appear as low-intensity structures that do not correspond to any normal anatomic structure in their location, shape, or course. Foreign bodies that have been present for a sufficient period of time will cause an inflammatory reaction in the surrounding soft tissues. These reactive changes are usually easy to identify on T2W fat-suppression images (Fig. 17–30), and thus this imaging sequence is often helpful for providing strong indirect evidence as to the location of a foreign body.

Rheumatoid Arthritis

Rheumatoid arthritis is a disease of the synovium and tenosynovium.[91,92] In the wrist, the progressive hypertrophy and inflammation of these tissues causes erosive destruction of cartilage, bone, intrinsic and extrinsic ligaments, TFCC, and tendons. Since all these structures are well visualized with MRI when they are free of rheumatoid disease, the role of MRI in the assessment of rheumatoid involvement of these tissues is currently under investigation.[37,93,94]

Both acutely and chronically inflamed synovium and tenosynovium are readily demonstrated with MRI using PD and T2W SE and fat-suppression sequences (Figs. 17–22 and 17–31). The signal intensity of these tissues on T2W images is lower than that of fluid[37] but higher than that of the adjacent normal structures (Figs. 17–22 and 17–31). Based on our experience with high-resolution images, ligamentous and TFCC erosive lesions are easily visualized. Bone erosions are visualized earlier with MRI than with plain films.[93–97] Tendons involved with rheumatoid disease appear with increased signal intensity on PD and T2W SE and fat-suppression images and can readily be distinguished from normal tendons.[37] Traditional teaching suggests that operative tenosynovectomy should be recommended to rheumatoid patients who have had no clinical response to medical treatment of tenosynovitis after several months.[91,98] When surgery is undertaken in accordance with these guidelines, many patients are found to have impending tendon ruptures. However, this is not always the case. An objective means to identify those patients

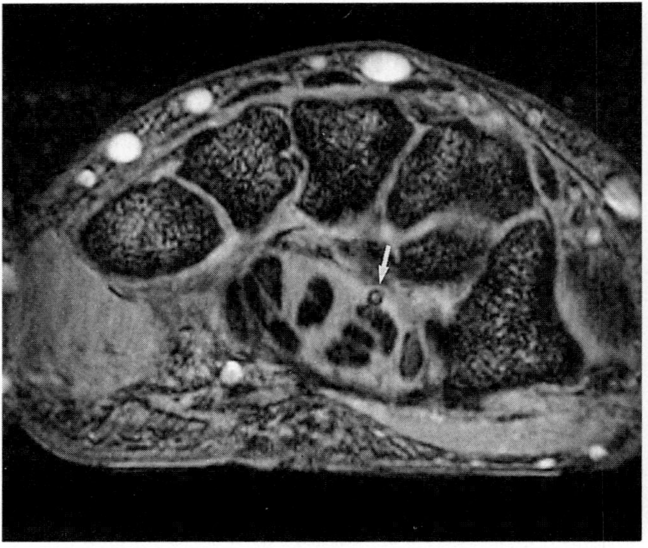

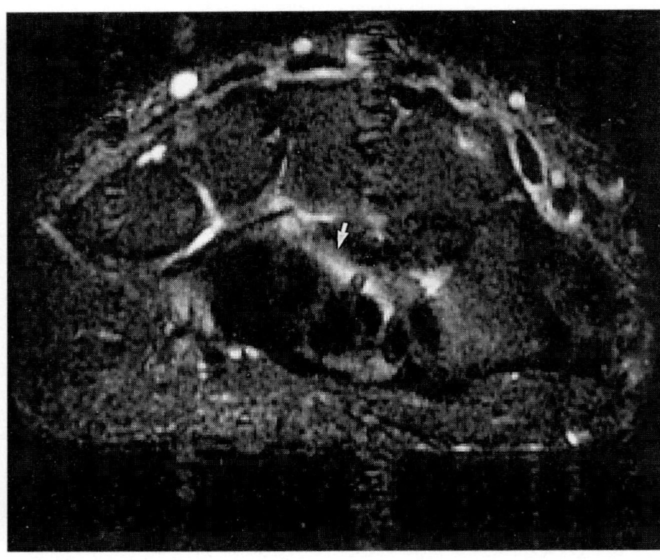

A B

FIGURE 17–30. Foreign body in the hand. 3D GRE (**A**) and T2W fat-suppression (**B**) images show a well-defined low-signal intensity foreign body (long white arrow) dorsal to the flexor tendons. The T2W image shows a thickened high-signal intensity synovium (short white arrow) reacting to the foreign body. This foreign body (a thorn) does not correspond to the location or course of any known anatomic structure.

who are at risk may be useful, because some operations could perhaps be avoided in deference to further medical management.[99] We have found MRI to be useful for identifying those patients who are indeed at increased risk for tendon rupture, and who therefore are candidates for urgent surgical intervention.[99]

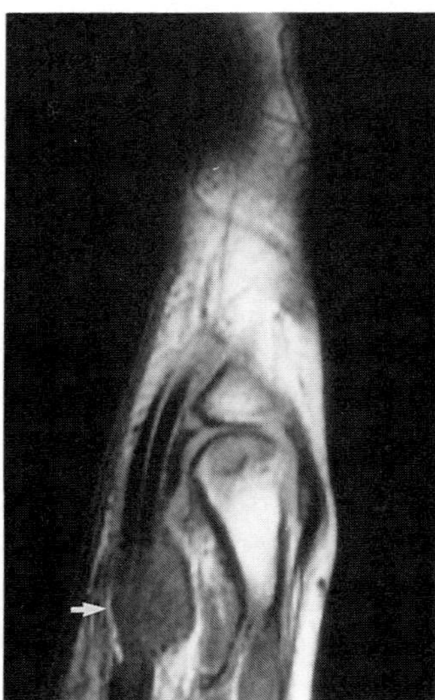

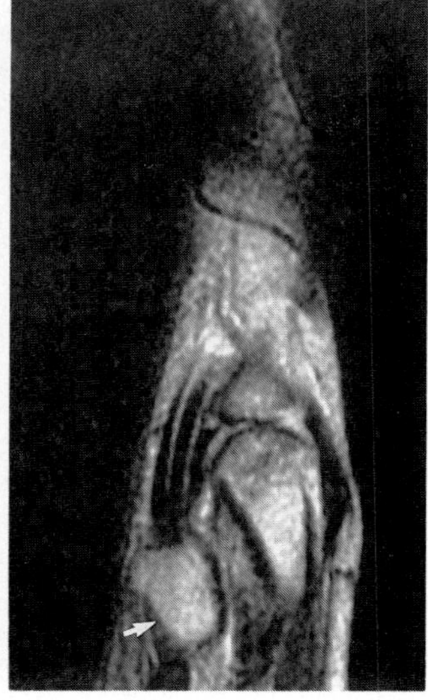

A B

FIGURE 17–31. Local pannus of the flexor tendon in a patient with rheumatoid arthritis. The signal intensity of the pannus (arrow) is low intermediate on the PD image (**A**) and intermediate on the T2W image (**B**).

Infections

The sensitivity of MRI to the existance of inflammatory changes both in soft tissue and bone marrow has made it very useful in evaluating musculoskeletal infections.[100–102] Based on our anecdotal experience, it reliably demonstrates the location of marrow changes in early phases and the extent of marrow and soft-tissue changes in late phases of osteomyelitis (Fig. 17–32). Although T1W SE images will demonstrate bone edema, T2W SE and fat-suppressed images are more sensitive to both bone-marrow and soft-tissue edema (Fig. 17–33). Axial images combined with either sagittal or coronal images will show the extent of infection.

Osteochondromatosis

Osteochondromatosis of the wrist is a rare entity. Osteocartilaginous bodies have a characteristic MR appearance with a high-signal intensity, cartilaginous outer layer surrounding an intermediate- to high-signal intensity bony center (Fig. 17–34). The lesions are located intracapsularly, either attached to the synovium or floating freely as loose bodies.

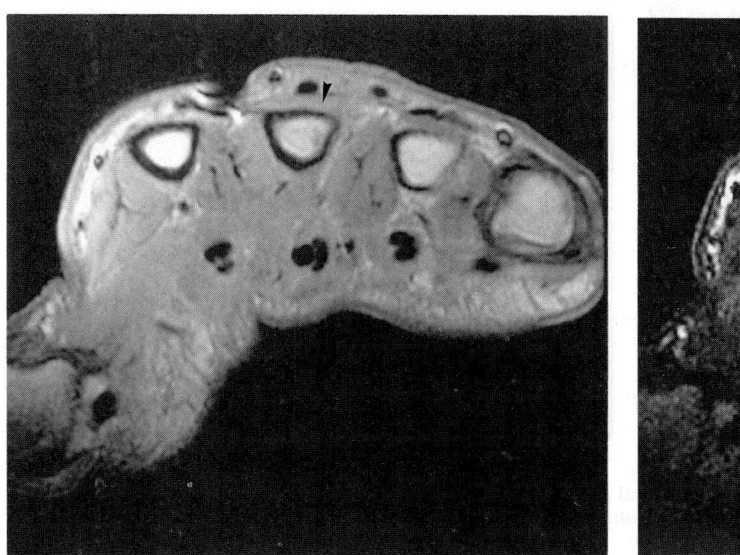
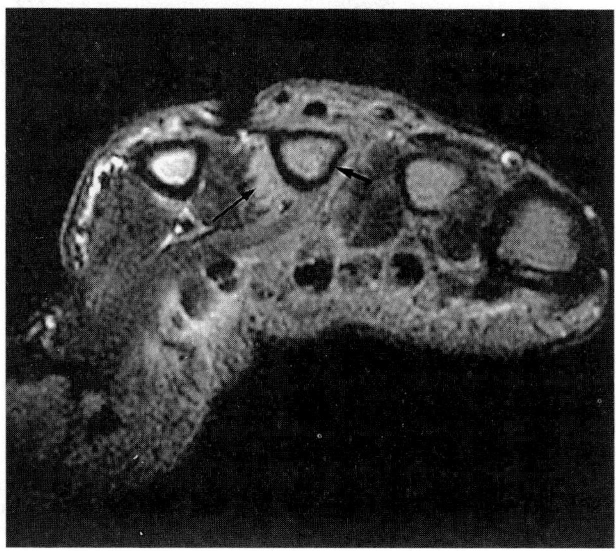

A B

FIGURE 17–32. Early osteomyelitis in a proximal phalanx. The patient had a phalangeal fracture with internal fixation. The bone marrow of the affected phalanx (arrowhead), compared with the IV phalanx, has an intermediate signal on PD **(A)** and higher signal (short arrow) on T2W images **(B)**. The signal intensity changes seen on the T2W image in the adjacent soft tissue (long arrow) are difficult to see using PD, even in retrospect. The decrease in marrow signal intensity from the index finger to little finger is coil dependent. After gadolinium administration (not shown), corresponding bone and soft tissue enhanced dramatically.

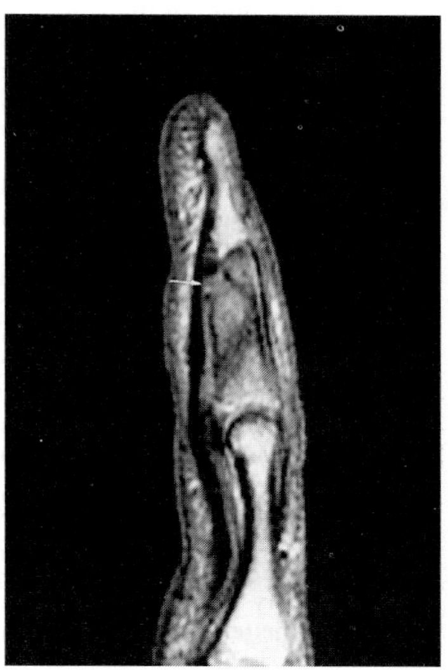
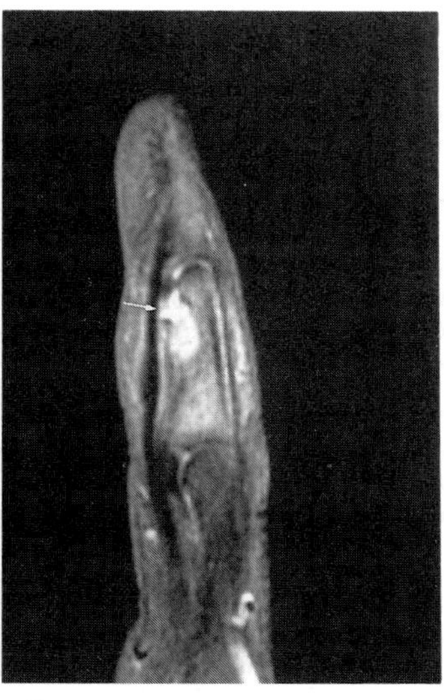

A B

FIGURE 17–33. Late osteomyelitis of a finger. PD SE **(A)** and gadolinium enhanced T1W fat-suppression images **(B)** show destruction of the cortex (white arrow) and trabecular bone in the middle phalanx in a patient with a history of several weeks of pain. After gadolinium administration the lesion enhances markedly, with enhancement of the adjacent bone marrow and most of the middle phalanx.

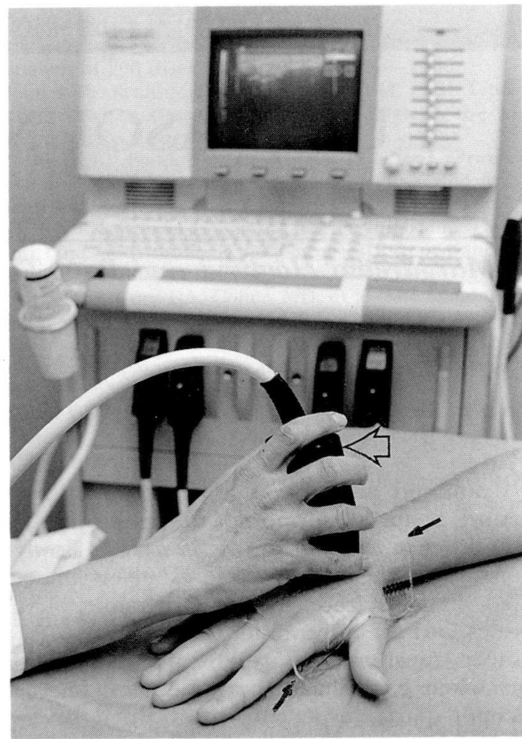

FIGURE 18–1. The patient is comfortably seated with the hand resting on a table. To smooth out the uneven skin surface and to make it easier to evaluate the most superficial parts, a thin stand-off pad (arrows) is used. The examiner holds the transducer (open arrow) in his or her hand.

described as hyperechoic, e.g., cortex of bones. As all energy is reflected back to the transducer or absorbed by the bone; there is no energy left and the area underneath the bone turns black. This phenomena is referred to as an acoustic shadow. The opposite situation is present when the ultrasound beam reaches a tissue that does not reflect the beam at all, e.g., a cyst, which appears black and is described as anechoic. As the beam passes through the cyst there is less energy loss than in the tissues adjacent to the cyst; therefore there will be acoustic enhancement, a whiter area, in the tissue underneath. When the ultrasound beam is partially reflected, it is referred to as hypoechoic, usually in relation to the surrounding tissues. Also noticed on the image is whether the echogenicity pattern is homogenous or inhomogenous.

THE NORMAL HAND

To evaluate pathological findings, the examiner must be well acquainted with the ultrasound image of the normal hand. A thorough knowledge of the normal anatomy is a prerequisite. With their typical forms and echogenic patterns, the different tissues in the hand, as in the rest of the body, are easy to recognize.

The *cutis,* or skin, is very thin, about 1 mm thick, and makes a white hyperechoic superficial border on ultrasound. The *subcutis,* or subcutaneous tissue, consists of a less-echoic zone composed of small longitudinal echoes (Fig. 18–2).

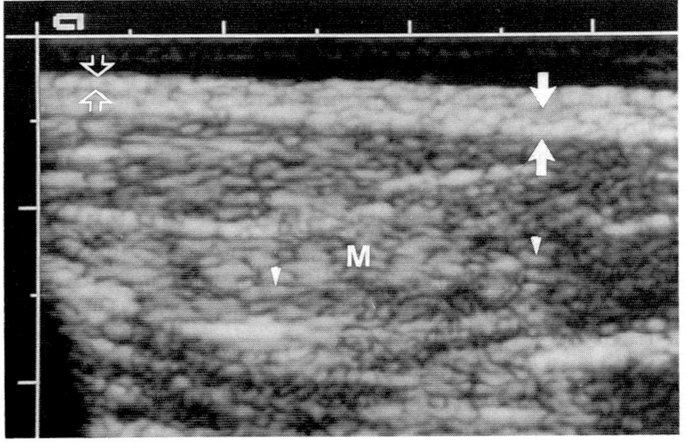

A

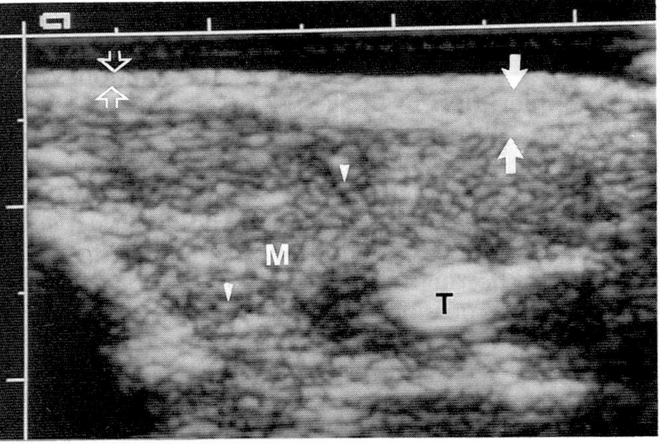

B

FIGURE 18–2. A: Normal hand with a longitudinal view of the thenar region. Cutis (between open arrows) gives a hyperechoic thin border. A thin layer of less-echoic subcutaneous tissue (between solid arrows) is seen as small longitudinal dots. The thenar muscle (M), musculus abductor pollicis brevis, and musculus flexor pollicis brevis contain fibroadipose septa (arrowheads) that are imaged as small scattered bands running in the same direction as the muscle. **B:** The transverse view where the cutis (between open arrows) and subcutis (between arrows) have the same image as on the longitudinal view. Here the fibroadipose septa (arrowheads) are square cut and seen as small dots, giving a speckled appearance to the muscle (M). The flexor pollicis longus tendon (T) as it passes through the thenar muscle has more of a square or even an oval cross-sectional shape.

Muscles are hypoechoic with scattered hyperechoic lines corresponding to the fibroadipose septa. On a longitudinal view these septa are seen as short scattered bands running in the same direction as the muscle. On a transverse view the muscle fibers are imaged in cross-section and the septa are seen as small dots, giving a speckled appearance (Fig. 18–2).[2,4]

When the ultrasound beam reaches the *tendons* at a right angle, they appear hyperechoic and their multiple longitudinal running internal fibers are seen. However, if the beam reaches them at an oblique angle, they turn hypoechoic (Fig. 18–3).[2,5] The extensor tendons over the fingers are very thin and just barely discernible. The flexor tendons are thicker and rounder and are therefore easier to visualize than the extensor tendons. Tendons lying close to each other, for example, the superficial and deep flexor tendons of the fingers, are well visualized but they usually are difficult to separate. At the level of the wrist, to determine which flexor tendon belongs to which finger, the patient is asked to gently bend the fingers one by one, making it possible to identify the individual tendons.

Vessels are easily seen on ultrasound examinations. The pulsations in the *arteries* are usually easily recognized and can be demonstrated beautifully with color as well as pulsed Doppler. The arteries can regularly be followed all the way to the fingertips. *Veins* are identified by their soft walls and are readily compressed by the transducer. When studying superficial parts of the hand, the examiner must be gentle, almost lifting the transducer from the surface to avoid compressing the veins (Fig. 18–4).

Nerves resemble tendons; their internal longitudinal fibers are seen but the echogenicity of the nerves is somewhat lower than that for tendons (Fig. 18–5).[5] The ulnar nerve's position adjacent to the ulnar artery helps identify the nerve, even in the narrow Guyon's canal. Since the nerves distal to the wrist are very thin, they are not visible with present equipment.

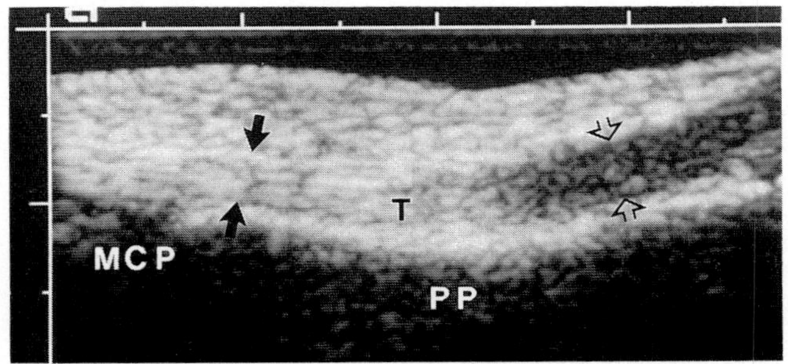

FIGURE 18–3. Normal hand with a palmar longitudinal view of a proximal phalanx (PP) with the flexor tendons (T). At the metacarpophalangeal joint (MCP), the ultrasound beam reaches the tendons at a perpendicular angle, resulting in a hyperechoic appearance (between arrows) that shows the multiple parallel internal fibers. More distally, the ultrasound beam reaches the tendons at an oblique angle, which results in a hypoechoic appearance (between open arrows).

Cortical bones reflect ultrasound a great deal, giving a hyperechoic border with a distinct acoustic shadow behind. The different bones are identified by their location and typical contours and serve as anatomic landmarks (Fig. 18–6).

Joints, the carpometacarpal, the metacarpophalangeal and the interphalangeal, are easily visualized from both palmar and dorsal views. The intercarpal joints are identified by the adjoining bones and can be easily seen from the dorsal aspect with a 7-MHz transducer. From the palmar side a 5-MHz transducer is sometimes preferable because of the thicker soft tissues palmarly. *Cartilage* is recognized as a thin anechoic zone, covering the cortical bones at the joints. The *joint capsules* are distinctly quite hyperechoic and are identified as thin structures surrounding the joints (Fig. 18–7). *Ligaments* are striped and hyperechoic. As with tendons, the appearance of ligaments depends on the direction of the ultrasound beam. In the normal hand, however, they are difficult to separate from the capsule.

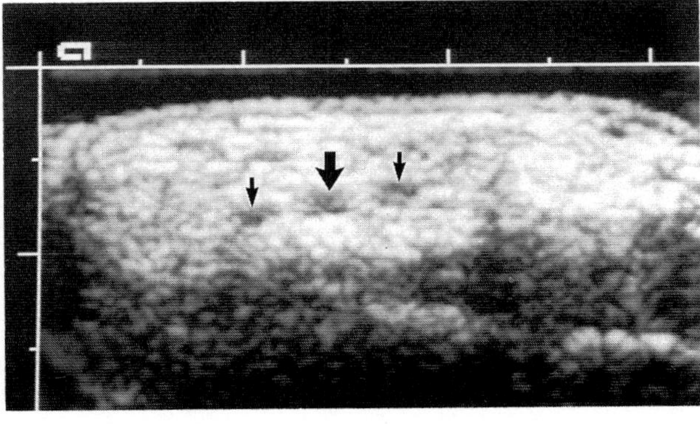

A

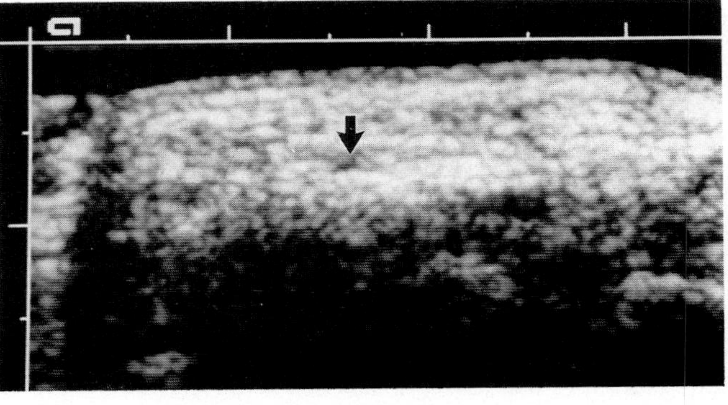

B

FIGURE 18–4. A: Normal hand with a palmar transverse view of the wrist. The radial artery (large arrow) is accompanied by two veins (small arrows). **B:** On this identical view moderate compression is performed with the transducer. The veins are easily compressed and are no longer visible, but the artery (large arrow) is unchanged.

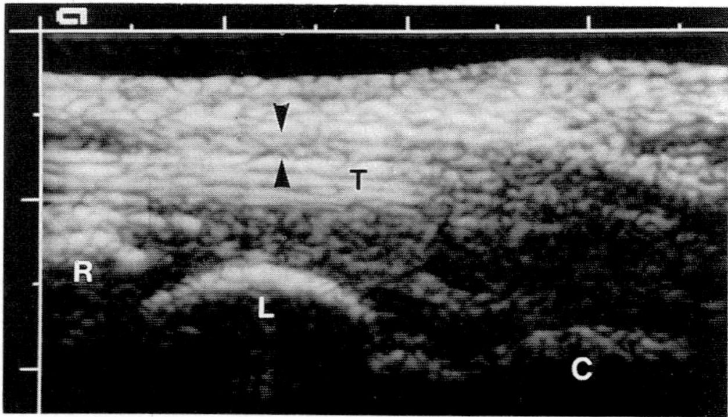

FIGURE 18–5. Normal hand with a longitudinal view of the carpal tunnel. The median nerve (between arrowheads) is superficial to the flexor tendons (T). The echogenicity of the nerve as well as the tendons changes with the angle of the ultrasound beam. Deep to these structures, the palmar surfaces of the radius (R), lunate (L), and capitate (C) bones are also discernible.

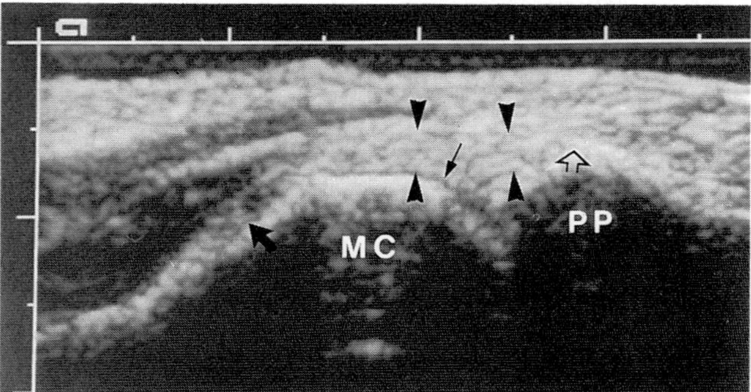

FIGURE 18–7. Normal hand with a dorsal longitudinal view of a metacarpophalangeal joint. The metacarpal bone (MC), the proximal phalanx (PP), and the hyperechoic capsule (between arrowheads) surrounding the joint are seen. The attachment sites of the capsule are on the metacarpal (thick arrow) and the phalanx (open arrow). A thin layer of anechoic cartilage (thin arrow) is also visualized surrounding the head of the metacarpal bone.

Documentation

It is difficult for the referring physician to demonstrate with static pictures conditions that were observed with a dynamic method. This circumstance makes it difficult for a radiologist to read films from someone else's examination. This is a well-known drawback to ultrasound. Therefore, it is even more important that the findings be well documented to ensure that other physicians, with the aid of a comprehensive report, can understand and demonstrate findings on the films. A standard method of documentation when recording pathology and other findings is therefore mandatory.

During our development of ultrasound examinations of the hand, we have found it advisable to use the following rules for documentation. As in all ultrasound examinations, the tissues next to the transducer are always at the top of the picture. In the *longitudinal image,* independent of which hand is examined, proximal is always kept to the left and distal to the right (Fig. 18–8).

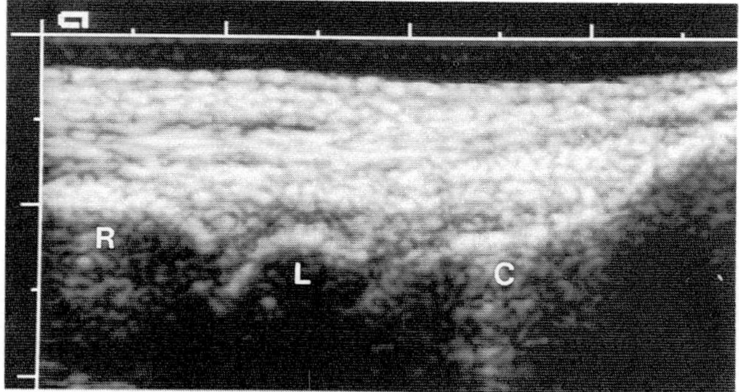

FIGURE 18–6. Normal hand with a dorsal longitudinal view of the carpal region. The cortex of the distal radius (R), lunate (L), and capitate (C) bones with their hyperechoic borders and distinct acoustic shadows behind are recognized by their typical contours.

In the *transverse image,* the hand is viewed as if the observer is looking in a direction from the fingertips toward the arm. This is the same procedure as in CT where the body is viewed from the feet. In a *palmar* transverse image of the right hand, radial is to the left and ulnar to the right. In a *dorsal* transverse image of the same hand, radial is to the right and ulnar to the left. When displaying the other hand, the reverse situations are present (Fig. 18–9).

PATHOLOGIC FINDINGS

Screening the entire hand is not helpful.[4] An accurate result depends on an accurate definition of the problem in question by the referring physician. Close cooperation between the radiologist and the clinician leads to a much more successful ultrasound examination.

Foreign Bodies

When foreign bodies are suspected but not identifiable by conventional radiography, ultrasound can verify and localize them, facilitating surgical extraction.[4,6] Usually there is distinct hyperechoic scar formation in the skin or slightly hypoechoic edema subcutaneously, indicating where to search for the object. A slow screening over the suspected area in all directions is necessary to detect a small foreign body. The first noticeable indication for the site of a foreign body is often an echo shadow. As the search is continued the hyperechoic foreign body can be identified superficial to the shadow. By turning the transducer back and forth over the object, the length and width of the object is determined. It should also be noted how deep under the skin the foreign body is located and how far down it extends (Fig. 18–10). Its relation to tendons, nerves, arteries, and other structures should be considered so that as much in-

Text continued on page 485

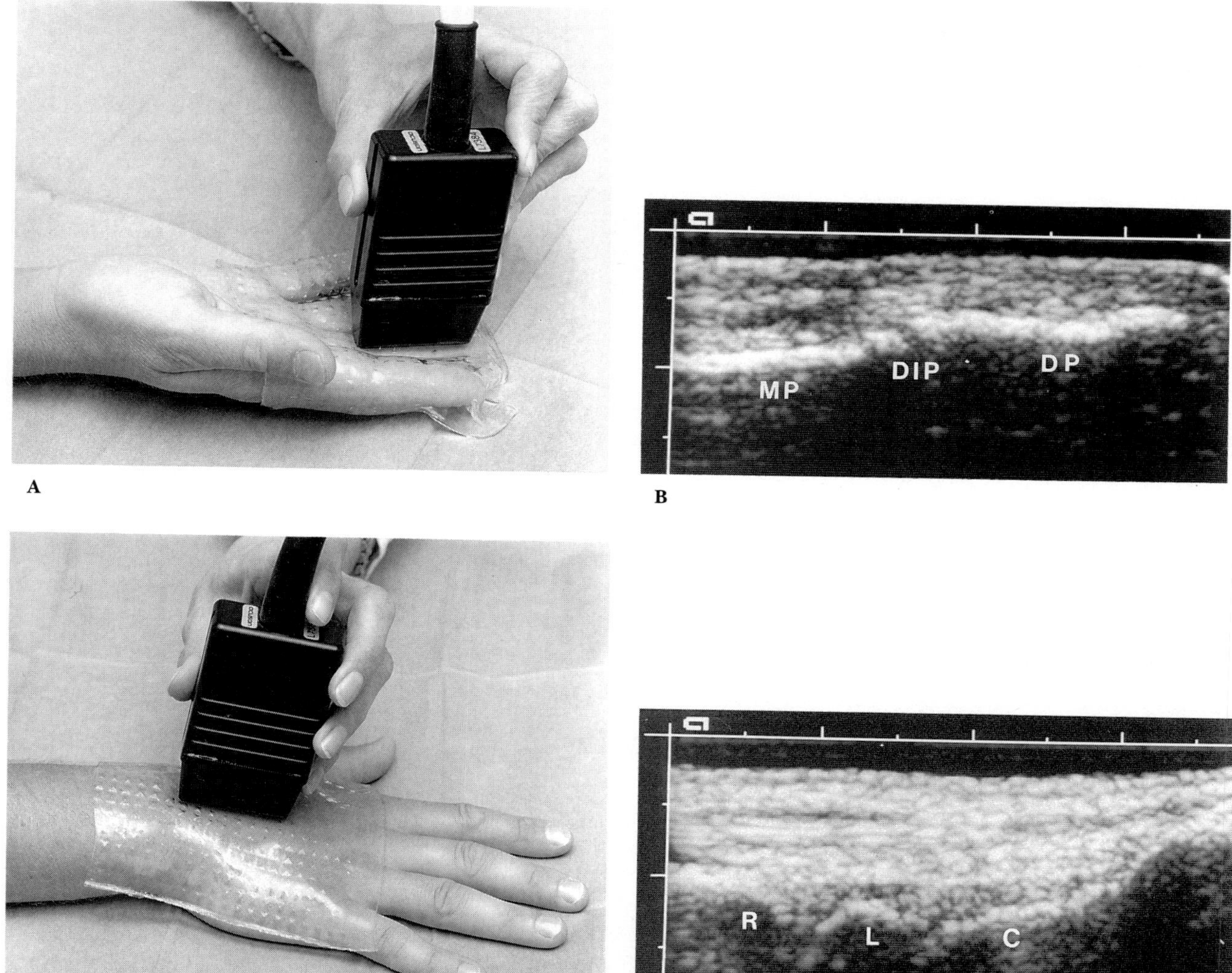

FIGURE 18–8. A: Position of hand and transducer for a longitudinal palmar view of the right long finger. **B:** Corresponding ultrasound picture. Palmar, which is next to the transducer, is uppermost. The middle (MP) and distal (DP) phalanges and the distal interphalangeal joint (DIP) are imaged. Proximal is to the left and distal to the right, even though the right hand is examined. **C:** Position of the hand and transducer for a dorsal longitudinal view of the right carpal region. **D:** Corresponding ultrasound picture. The dorsal aspect of the hand is uppermost, and below the dorsal cortices of the radius (R), lunate (L), and capitate (C) bones are seen. By convention, proximal is always to the left and distal to the right, irrespective of which hand or side is examined.

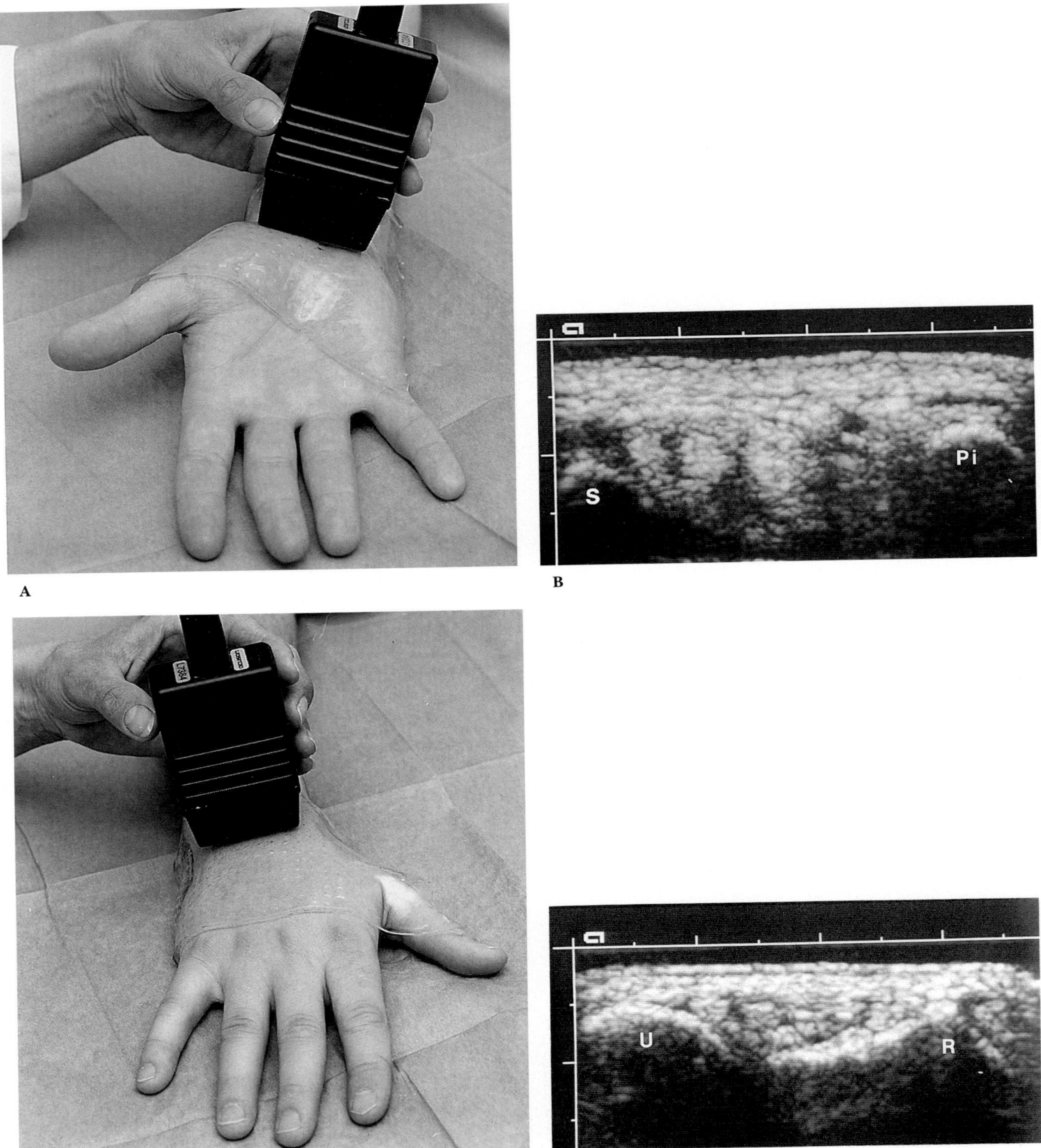

FIGURE 18–9. A: Position of hand and transducer for a palmar transverse view of the right carpal tunnel. **B:** Corresponding ultrasound picture. Palmar is uppermost and, because the hand is seen from the fingertips, the radial side and the scaphoid bone (S) are imaged to the left and the ulnar side and the pisiform bone (Pi) are to the right. **C:** Position of hand and transducer for a dorsal transverse view of the right wrist. **D:** Corresponding ultrasound picture. Dorsal is uppermost and, because the hand always is seen from the fingertips, the radius (R) is to the right and the ulna (U) is to the left. On the transverse view when picturing the left hand, the opposite situation will be present.

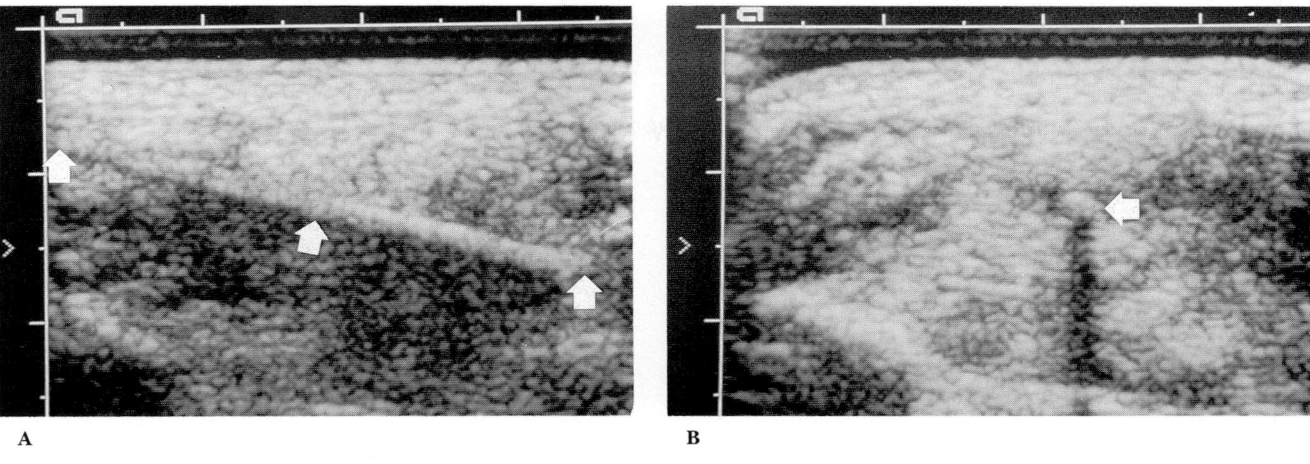

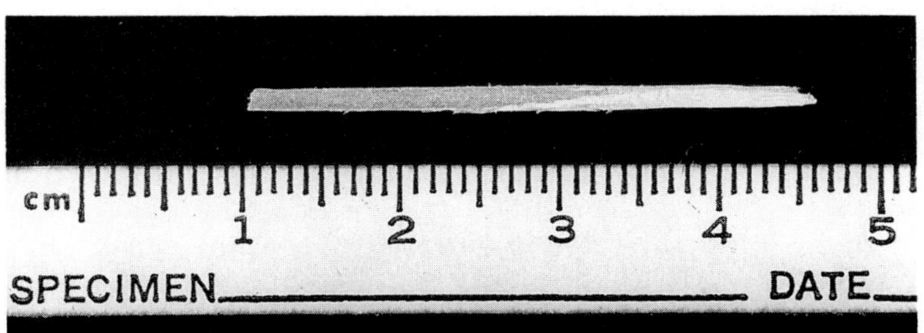

FIGURE 18–10. Longitudinal **(A)** and transverse **(B)** views of the thenar region. An almost–4-cm long and 3-mm thick hyperechoic foreign body (arrows) with a distinct anechoic area deep or behind the foreign body is imaged. The most superficial part is located 8 mm and the deepest part almost 18 mm under the skin. The foreign body extended proximal as well as distal to the small cutaneous wound. The location was marked on the skin preoperatively with a waterproof pen to guide the surgeon. The distance between each mark on the side and top of the ultrasound image is equal to 5 mm. **(C)** This was the foreign body that corresponded exactly to the ultrasound image.

formation as possible is available for the surgeon preoperatively. For ease of subsequent removal of the foreign body, we have found it valuable to use a waterproof pen to mark the skin site under which the foreign body is located and in which direction it extends.

Tumors

Many different tumors can be present in the hand, 95% of which are benign.[7,8] With ultrasound it is usually not possible to determine whether a tumor is benign or malignant. By defining the various characteristics of a tumor, however, it is possible to give a considered opinion of its origin and nature. One important factor is the absence or presence of a distinct capsule. Further observations include definition of the tumor extent, its relation to the surrounding soft tissues, and whether or not it displaces or invades other structures. It is also important to observe if the tumor destroys or impinges on the bone. With help of color and pulsed Doppler and by compression, it can be determined if the tumor contains arteries as well as veins.

Although we cannot list all the tumors that may occur in the hand, a description of the more common tumors follows. Their characteristics on ultrasound and specific features are given. Also included are some examples of rare malignant tumors with interesting ultrasonic features.

Benign Tumors

Ganglion Cysts

Ganglions represent about 60% of all soft-tissue tumors in the hand.[7,9] On ultrasound the cysts have a typical appearance of a well-circumscribed, hard-to-compress, and almost anechoic mass with acoustic enhancement deep to the lesion (Fig. 18–11).[1,5,10] Sometimes it is difficult to estimate the enhancement when the cyst is located adjacent to a cortical bone. If the ganglion is collapsed or has been operated on before, there may be a few hyperechoic irregular structures within it.

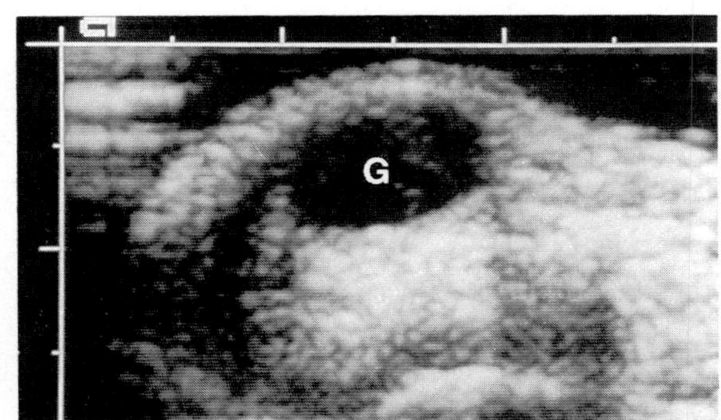

FIGURE 18–11. A ganglion cyst (G) with a typical appearance on ultrasound. It is well circumscribed, difficult to compress with the transducer, and is almost anechoic with echo enhancement behind the lesion.

Ganglions may be multilobulated. When they arise from a joint, they may have a long stalk and appear far from their origin. When the ultrasound examination is performed, to further help the surgeon, attempts should be made to follow this stalk and determine from which joint it originates. The risk of a recurrence after surgery is less if the stalk is properly extirpated,[11] which may require resection of part of the ligament at the involved joint.

Depending on their origin, ganglions can be divided into four different groups.[9] Ninety percent of hand and wrist ganglions belong to one of these four groups, but ganglions may appear at any site.

1. *Dorsal wrist ganglions* are the most common, usually emanating from the scapholunate joint and appearing at the dorsal aspect of the hand between the extensor tendons. Typical dorsal wrist ganglions are easy to identify clinically. Nevertheless, an ultrasound examination may supply valuable information, since even experienced surgeons are helped preoperatively by knowledge of the subcutaneous extension of the ganglions and their point of origin.[12] Tenosynovitis and supplementary muscles can also be clinically misinterpreted as dorsal ganglions, whereas their true nature is easily recognized with ultrasound.

   There are situations where the clinical diagnosis is more obscure, however. For example, when a patient has symptoms consistent with a dorsal ganglion, but none is found on the clinical examination, ultrasound may help by verifying or excluding a small ganglion (Fig. 18–12). In other cases a patient may still have a tender palpable mass after an earlier operation. It is then hard to decide clinically if the mass consists of scar formation or a recurrence. On ultrasound it is possible to differentiate between these diagnoses since, contrary to scar formations, even very small recurrences are anechoic.
2. *Volar (ventral, or palmar) wrist ganglions* are the second most common group and usually emanate from one of the joints at the base of the thumb. They are commonly secondary to osteoarthritis, for example, in the scaphotrapezial joint (Fig. 18–13).[13] The stalk of a palmar ganglion is often long and tortuous, therefore the ganglion usually appears proximal to its origin. Frequently the ganglion surrounds the flexor carpi radialis tendon and/or the radial artery (Fig. 18–14).[14] On ultrasound a small palmar wrist ganglion close to the artery may resemble an aneurysm. However, when one is conscious of this possibility, the diagnosis is not difficult because there is no circulation in the ganglion.
3. *Flexor tendon sheath or volar (ventral, palmar) retinacular ganglions,* as the name indicates, arise from the flexor tendon sheath and are most often seen at the base of the finger or along the proximal phalanx. These ganglions are often firm, round, and up to 1 cm in diameter. They are located close to but separate from the flexor tendons, and therefore do not follow the movements of the tendons (Fig. 18–15).[3]
4. *Mucous cysts* are also included in this classification of ganglions. Most often they appear dorsally at the distal interphalangeal joint, but

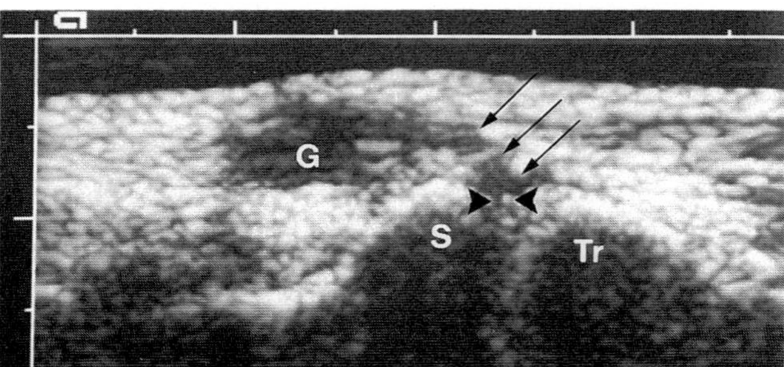

FIGURE 18–13. Palmar longitudinal view of the joint (between arrowheads) between the scaphoid (S) and the trapezium (Tr) bones. A small palmar ganglion (G) with a thin stalk (black arrows) is emerging from the joint.

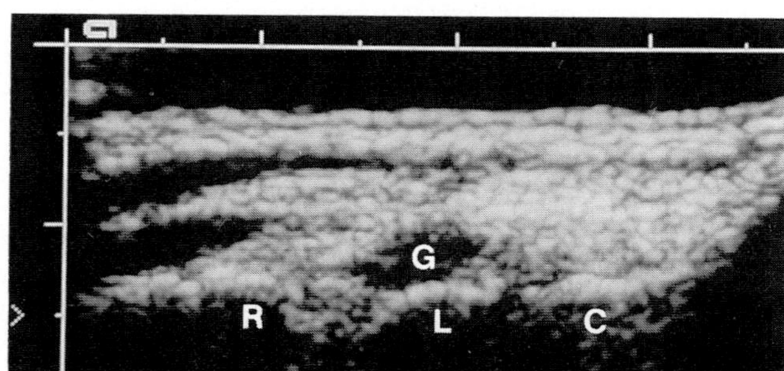

FIGURE 18–12. Dorsal longitudinal view of the carpal region with a 4 × 5–mm nonpalpable dorsal wrist ganglion (G) adjacent to the lunate bone (L). The radius (R) and capitate (C) bones are also evident.

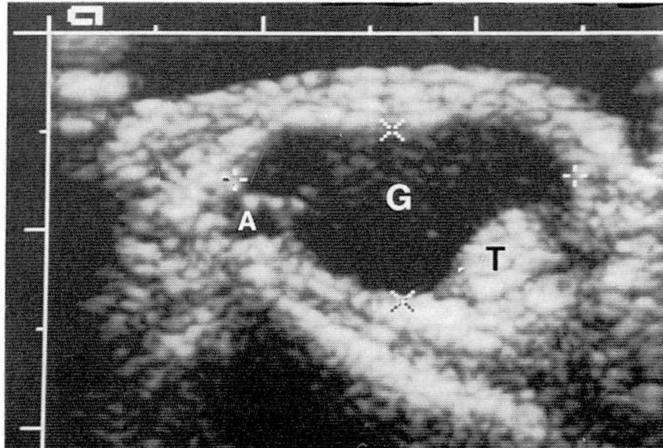

FIGURE 18–14. Palmar transverse view of a wrist ganglion (G) emanating from one of the joints at the base of the thumb. The ganglion is in close contact with the flexor carpi radialis tendon (T) and the radial artery (A).

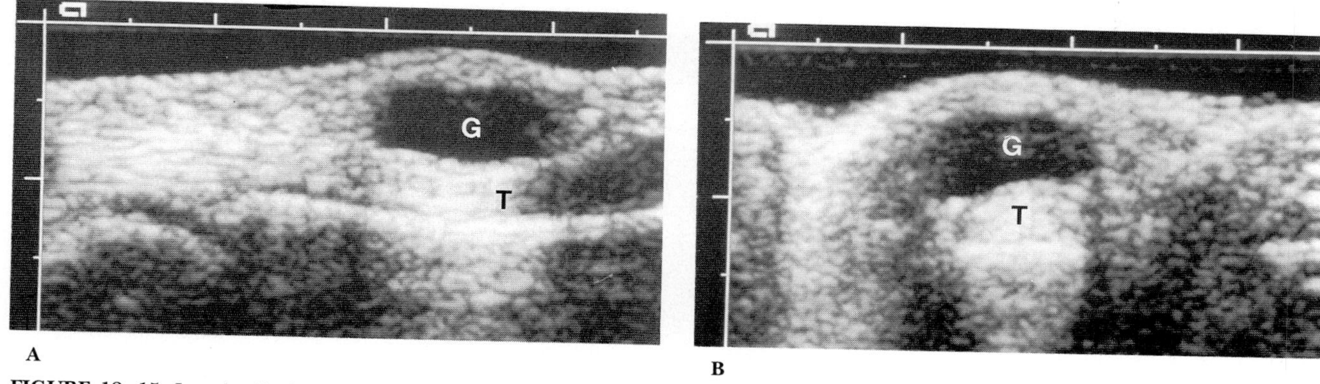

FIGURE 18–15. Longitudinal **(A)** and transverse **(B)** views of a flexor tendon sheath ganglion (G) located close to the flexor tendon (T). When the patient bends his or her finger, the tendon moves but not the ganglion, indicating that the mass is separate from the tendon.

when they appear on the palmar side the clinical diagnosis is more obscure. Not uncommonly they dissect away from the joint in the subcutaneous tissue and skin (Fig. 18–16). Osteoarthritis is often the underlying cause.[14]

Lipomas

Lipomas in the hand are usually well circumscribed by a thin capsule.[5,15] When they are deep seated, they may be rather large before the patient notices them. Their echogenicity varies from rather high, such as in subcutaneous fat, to quite low, but they are never anechoic. There is usually no echo enhancement behind the tumor (Fig. 18–17).

Vascular Tumors

Hemangiomas are clinically difficult to diagnose in the absence of typical skin alterations. They grow diffusely in the soft tissues, sometimes only subcutaneously and sometimes infiltrating the muscles.[16] They belong to a category of tumors that may be difficult to depict on ultrasound. The first impression on examination is that there is an excess of soft tissue, commonly with lower echogenicity than expected. When the tumor is huge the diagnosis is easy, because of the presence of large feeding arteries and dilated veins. Typically it is difficult to define its borders. A small lesion is easier to delineate, but the characteristic vessels are more difficult to identify. When compressed, the tissue diminishes and small anechoic parts, corresponding to locally dilated veins, disappear. With Doppler it is difficult to see any flow in the veins, but in the neighboring tissues diffusely scattered, small, pulsatile arteries can be observed (Fig. 18–18). Even if it is difficult to diagnose all hemangiomas with ultrasound, by excluding other more characteristic soft-tissue abnormalities on ultrasound, hemangioma may emerge as the most likely diagnostic alternative.

Glomus tumors arise from glomus bodies, which occur in great numbers in the digital artery walls. Typically they are painful and especially sensitive to low temperature.[17] They are usually located either subungually or on the palmar surface of the fingertip. Glomus tumors may be as small as a few millimeters and difficult to palpate. Ultrasound can be helpful since such a lesion is usually well demonstrated, even under the nail. A glomus tumor is hypoechoic with slight acoustic enhancement deep to

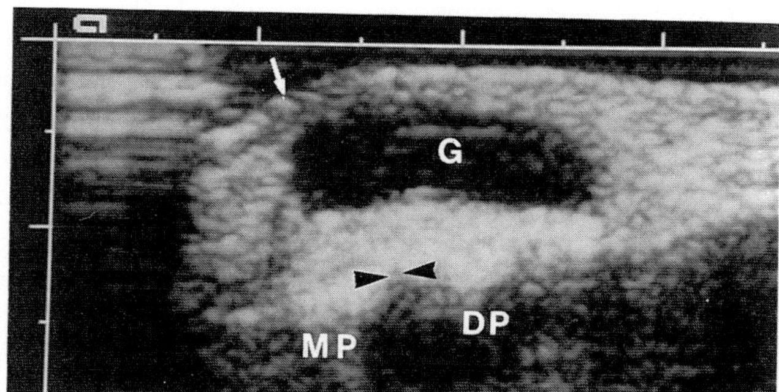

FIGURE 18–16. Longitudinal view of a mucous cyst (G) in close contact with the skin surface (white arrow) at the palmar aspect of the distal interphalangeal joint. The joint space (arrowheads) between the middle (MP) and distal (DP) phalanges is narrow, indicating an osteoarthritis as the underlying cause.

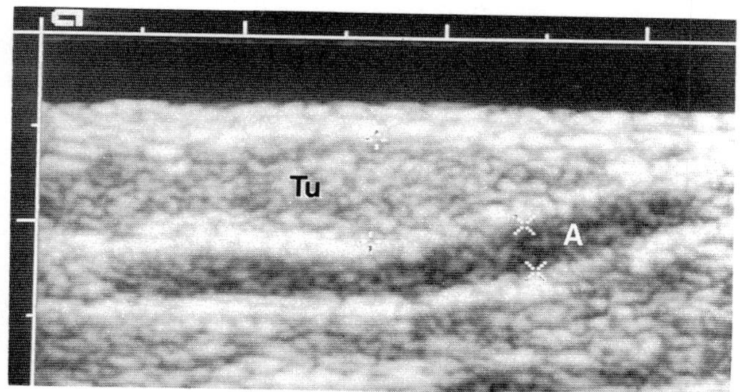

FIGURE 18–17. Longitudinal view of the radial part of the wrist. A subcutaneous, hyperechoic, rather well-defined tumor (Tu) without any obvious capsule is located adjacent to the radial artery (A). This is a subcutaneous lipoma.

FIGURE 18–18. **A:** Transverse view of the palmar aspect of the hand with a hypoechoic, poorly demarcated tumor (Tu) surrounding the superficial tendons (ST) and deep flexor tendons (DT). **B:** The identical view with compression by the transducer showing that the tumor (Tu) is easily compressed and diminishes in size. There were also many small arteries visible with Doppler in the surrounding tissues, suggesting the diagnosis of a hemangioma.

A

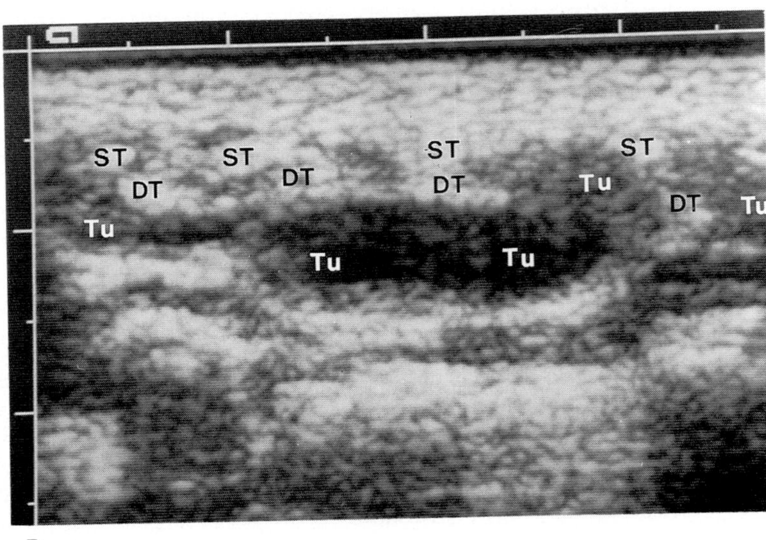

B

the lesion. It is well defined but without any visible capsule (Fig. 18–19).[5]

Villonodular Synovitis

The origin of these common but often misinterpreted benign giant cell tumors in the hand is the synovial membrane. Consequently, they may appear near any joint or tendon.[11,18] Commonly the size and extent of these lesions on ultrasound is greater than the clinically palpated mass. The tumor is often irregularly shaped, with a medium-low echogenicity. It is well separated from the adjacent tissues, but with a capsule difficult to discern (Fig. 18–20).[5]

Epidermoid Cysts

If they are not typically small and situated distally on the fingers that have a history of earlier trauma, epidermoid cysts can be difficult to differentiate from other soft-tissue masses. Such masses include early Dupuytren's contracture, lipomas, villonodular synovitis, or tendon sheath ganglions. On ultrasound epidermoid cysts are well recognized; they have a rather high and homogenous echogenicity, are well circumscribed, surrounded by a capsule, and quite firm on palpation (Fig. 18–21).

Nerve Tumors

There are three different benign nerve tumors. They rarely coexist, and their natural histories are different.[19–21]

Neuromas are also called traumatic or amputation neuromas. As the name indicates, most of these tumors appear when a nerve has been severed or crushed, either after a major trauma or repetitive minor traumas. The proximal end of a nerve fasciculus fails to meet with the distal end and a mass results. On ultrasound this tumor is quite hypoechoic with slight acoustic enhancement and without any visible capsule (Fig. 18–22).

Neurilemomas originate from the Schwann cells that

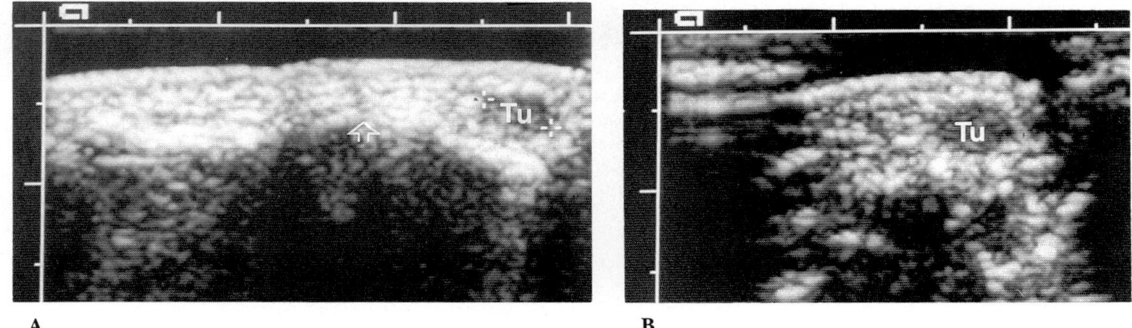

A B

FIGURE 18–19. Longitudinal **(A)** and transverse **(B)** views of the palmar aspect of a finger at the distal interphalangeal joint (open arrow). Subcutaneously there is a hypoechoic tumor (Tu) 4 mm in diameter with slight echo-enhancement deep to the lesion. The tumor is well circumscribed but there is no visible capsule. This is the typical appearance for a glomus tumor, which correlated to the site of the patient's complaint and symptom of pain aggravated by cold weather.

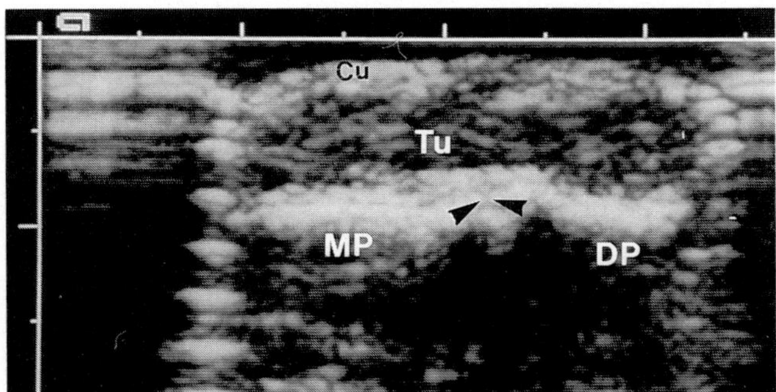

FIGURE 18–20. Dorsal longitudinal view of the distal interphalangeal joint (between arrowheads) of a finger. Adjacent to the joint an irregular, well-circumscribed tumor (Tu) is between the cutis (Cu) and the cortical bone of the middle (MP) and distal (DP) phalanges. It has a medium-low echogenicity, and is adjacent to the bone. This is a villonodular synovitis emanating from the synovial membrane.

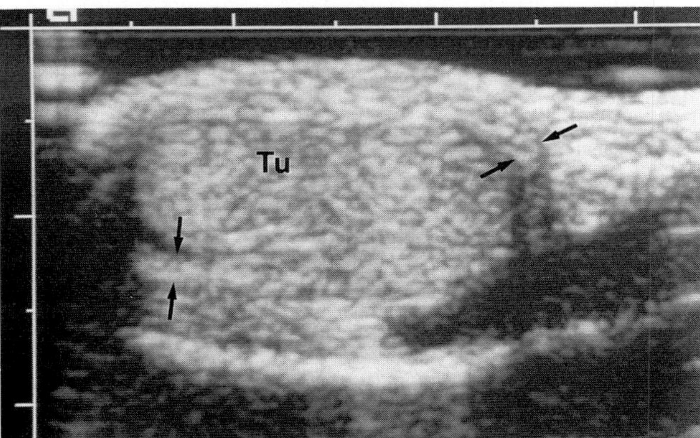

FIGURE 18–21. Longitudinal view of the palmar aspect of the hand. Situated in the subcutis is a homogenous hyperechoic tumor (Tu) with a well-marked capsule (between arrows) representing an epidermoid cyst.

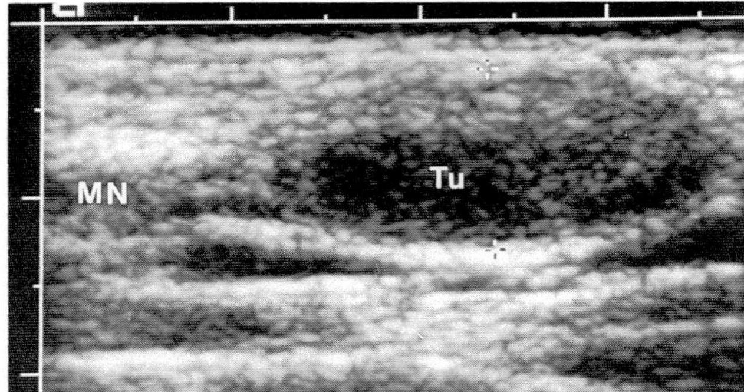

FIGURE 18–22. Longitudinal palmar view of the distal forearm with an inhomogenous, hypoechoic tumor (Tu) with slight echo-enhancement and without any clear capsule. The median nerve (MN) passes into the tumor. Earlier, the patient had had trauma to the median nerve. At the time of the examination, he had pain on palpation at the site of the earlier wound. This mass was found to be a neuroma at surgery.

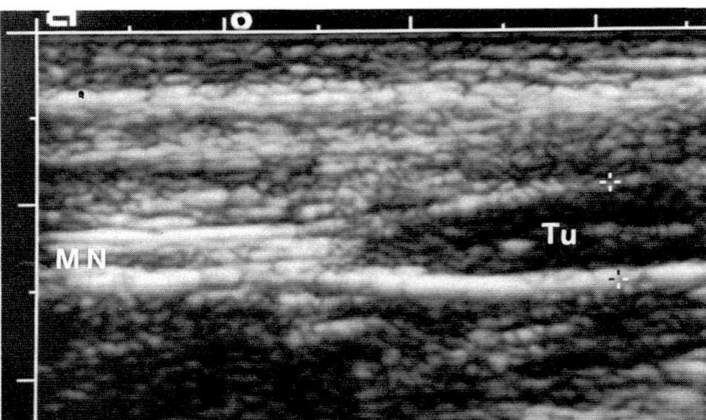

FIGURE 18–24. Longitudinal view of the palmar aspect of the wrist. The median nerve (MN) is continuous with the proximal aspect of a tumor (Tu) that totally replaces the nerve structure. This is one of multiple neurofibromas in a girl with von Recklinghausen's disease.

ensheath the peripheral nerves.[22] They are truly encapsulated tumors and appear on the flexor surface of the extremities. They are usually solitary and rarely become malignant. If the nerve of origin is not too small, on ultrasound one can identify the nerve proximal to the tumor and also follow the nerve when it passes by the edge of the tumor. There is an easily identifiable capsule and the echogenicity is medium-low and homogenous (Fig. 18–23).

Neurofibromas, such as in von Recklinghausen's disease, can be solitary or multiple. They consist of a mixture of all elements in the peripheral nerve.[20,21] Usually they are soft on palpation and not encapsulated. Deep tumors may grow large and result in plexiform neurofibromas. On ultrasound the tumor is rather hypoechoic with only slight acoustic enhancement. It is well defined and mostly without any visible capsule. If large enough, the nerve of origin may be visible proximal and distal to the tumor, but it is not possible to follow the nerve passing through the tumor (Fig. 18–24).

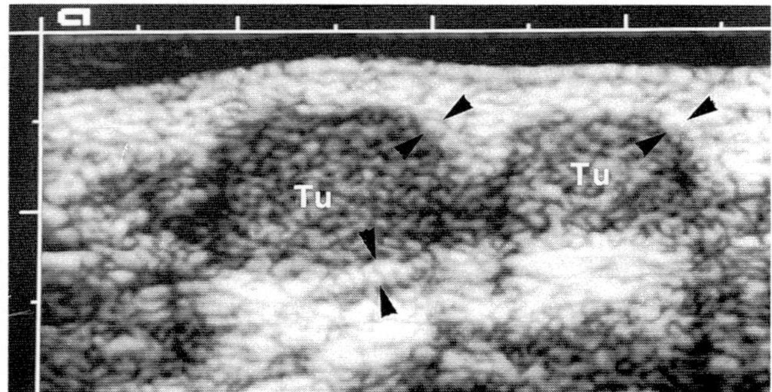

FIGURE 18–23. Longitudinal view of the ulnar part of the wrist. A multilobulated, homogenous, hypoechoic tumor (Tu) has a well-marked capsule (between arrowheads) and slight echo-enhancement behind. This is a neurilemoma growing off the ulnar nerve.

Malignant Tumors

Malignant soft-tissue tumors are rare in the hand, as are metastases, thus limiting experience with ultrasound.[23] In addition to detection and demonstration of the tumor, probably the most important observation that ultrasound can supply is to define the tumor margins.

Diffuse spread into soft tissues, without any possibility of defining a tumor border, can be demonstrated. Finding a poorly marginated lesion should lead to suspicion of malignancy as well as inflammation or synovitis (Fig. 18–25).

Cortical destruction of adjacent bones with ill-defined borders is also an ominous sign that can and should be observed on ultrasound (Fig. 18–26). Correlative routine radiographs can usually verify a cortical destructive area.

Recurrence of malignant tumors can be difficult to palpate, because frequently there is extensive scarring and postoperative deformation in the former tumor bed. Scar formations may be superficially situated and prevent the examiner from palpating deeper-located masses. Early scarring with persistent edema has a rather low echogenicity, whereas older fibrotic scars have high echogenicity. Ultrasound can penetrate the scar formations and evaluate the tissues underneath. Depending on the origin and echogenicity of the primary tumor, a recurrence can often be recognized and separated from the surrounding scarring. The fact that extension of a recurrence has a different appearance from scar formation is also helpful in evaluating the mass. On ultrasound it is thus possible to visualize a recurrence much earlier than when the mass becomes palpable (Fig. 18–27).

Tendons

Tenosynovitis

Inflammatory tenosynovitis is caused by inflammation of a tendon sheath and is sometimes difficult to delin-

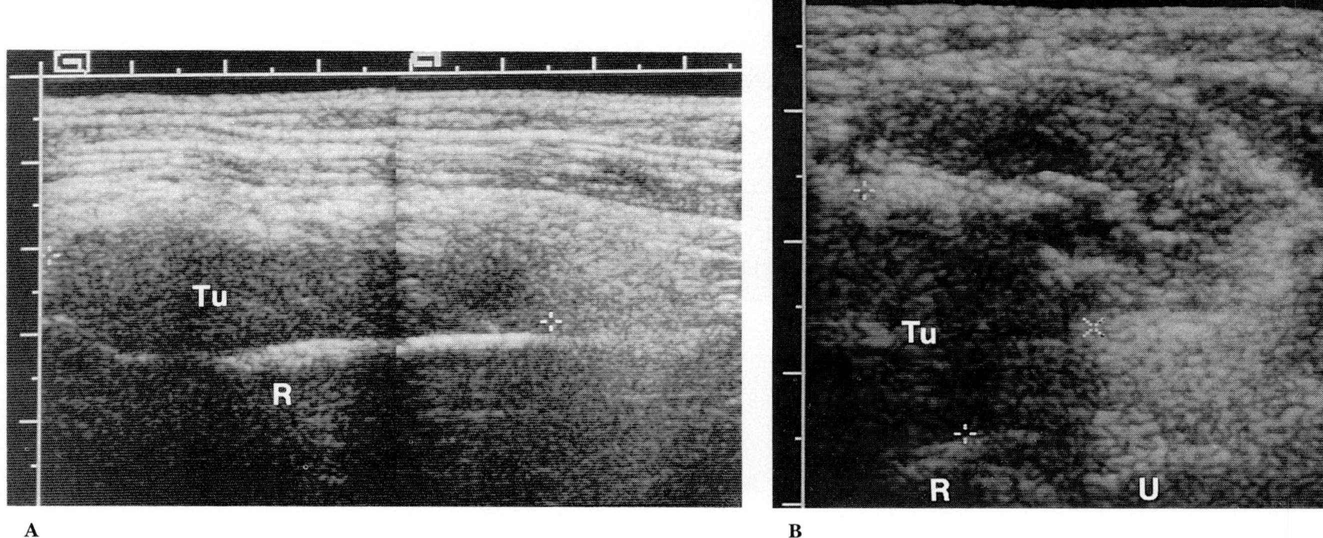

FIGURE 18–25. A: Longitudinal view of the palmar aspect of the proximal forearm with a hypoechoic tumor (Tu) in the soft tissue next to the proximal part of the radius bone (R). **B:** A magnified transverse view of the same tumor (Tu) with the radius (R) and ulnar (U) bones just discernible at the bottom of the print. The tumor is difficult to demarcate from the surrounding tissues, which leads to a suspicion of malignancy. This proved to be a fibrosarcoma.

eate on palpation.[4] On ultrasound there is an anechoic, often irregular zone encircling the tendon, representing fluid caused by the synovitis (Fig. 18–28). Even closely apposed tendons that normally are not separable on ultrasound can be discerned when they are separated by synovitis (Fig. 18–29). In more advanced cases the synovitis may invade the tendon and eventually cause a tendon rupture. With ultrasound the picture of an invading anechoic synovitis with a thin remaining part of the tendon, indicating an impending rupture, may be visualized (Fig. 18–30).

In *rheumatoid arthritis* the tenosynovitis is often extensive. It is usually not rewarding to screen the entire hand, but when there is a localized problem, ultrasound may be of value, e.g., to diagnose an impending rupture.

Pyogenic tenosynovitis may cause serious functional disabilities of the hand if left untreated.[24] It is often clinically difficult to differentiate a pyogenic tenosynovitis from arthritis or a more superficial infection. With ultrasound it is possible to distinguish subcutaneous hypoechoic edema from anechoic effusion

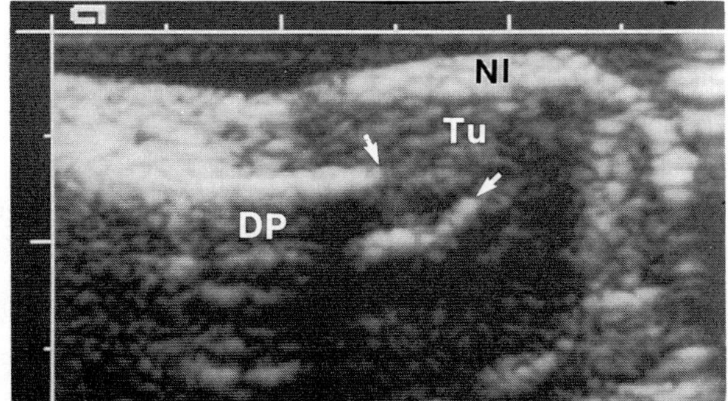

FIGURE 18–26. Dorsal longitudinal view of the distal phalanx (DP) of the thumb. The ultrasound is performed through the nail (Nl), which does not interfere with the examination. Subungually there is a homogenous hypoechoic tumor (Tu) without any capsule. The tumor is clearly destroying the bone (arrows), indicating a possible malignancy or an infection. This cortical destruction was verified on subsequent routine radiographs. Histologic examination demonstrated a squamous cell carcinoma.

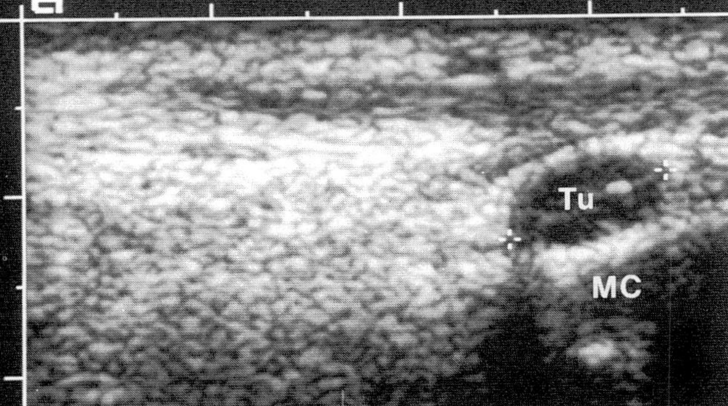

FIGURE 18–27. Palmar longitudinal view at the base of a metacarpal bone (MC). In the past 8 years this patient had been operated on several times for recurrences of an extraskeletal myxoid chondrosarcoma. Because of postoperative deformity and scar formation, it was difficult to palpate early recurrences, and therefore ultrasound examinations were performed regularly. This small low-echoic recurrence of the tumor (Tu) was found. To guide the surgeon at operation, its location was preoperatively marked on the skin with a waterproof pen.

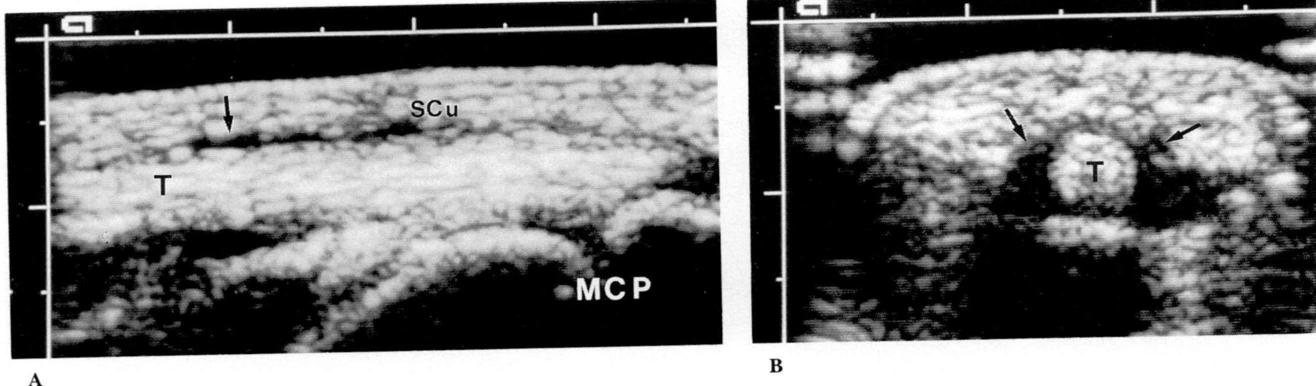

FIGURE 18–28. A: Palmar longitudinal view with the flexor tendons (T) passing the metacarpophalangeal joint (MCP). Superficial to the tendons and separating them from the subcutis (SCu) is an anechoic border of fluid (arrow), representing tenosynovitis. **B:** Transverse view with the anechoic fluid (arrows) surrounding the flexor tendons (T).

around a swollen tendon. When there is a suppurative tenosynovitis in the proximal part of the hand possibly passing from the thumb to the small finger, a so-called "horseshoe abscess," the involved area can be delineated with ultrasound. The different tissues are difficult to separate from each other because the tendons are thick, poorly delineated, and surrounded by a diffuse hypoechoic effusion. However, the abnormal can be differentiated from the normal tissues.

Localized Tendinitis

Before it leads to triggering or other typical clinical signs, localized tendinitis in *adults,* may be difficult to diagnose. This tendinitis is often subacute and can involve any tendon.[25–27] On ultrasound the tendon is locally thickened, fusiform, and exhibits lower echogenicity than normal parts of the tendon (Fig. 18–31).[4,5]

In *children* localized tendinitis most commonly affects the flexor pollicis longus tendon.[27] Although symptoms are commonly focused around an interphalangeal joint, the tendon thickening is regularly localized at the metacarpophalangeal joint level.[28] Unlike the adult form, on ultrasound this tendinitis is usually well delineated with a clearly defined, rather hypoechoic nodule formation of the tendon (Fig. 18–32).

Tendon Ruptures

Traumatic tendon ruptures are often clinically obvious, but if the patient cannot cooperate, or if a partial rupture is suspected, ultrasound can be helpful.[29] In a case of a subcutaneous rupture this examination can localize the site and possibly verify an additional rupture.[4] In the acute rupture there is an anechoic effusion at the site of the tear. In a *total* rupture the proximal portion of the tendon can be visualized in a retracted position and the diastasis demonstrated and measured (Fig. 18–33). In a *partial* rupture the remaining thin portion of the tendon can be visualized as continuous through the area of the injury, with an anechoic area in the tendon indicating the site of the partial rupture (Fig.

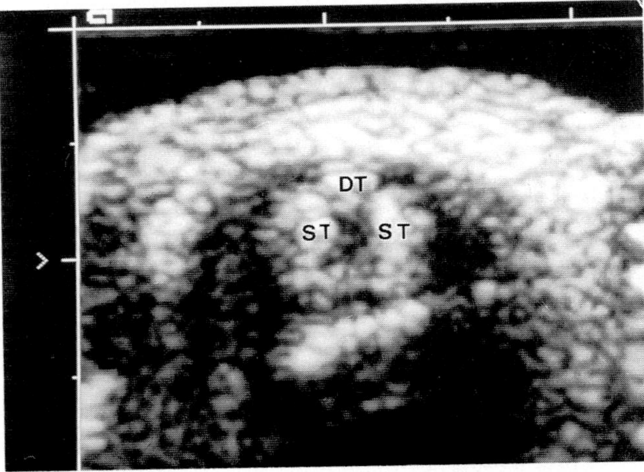

FIGURE 18–29. Palmar transverse view of the distal part of a proximal phalanx. Anechoic fluid due to synovitis separates the deep tendons (DT) and superficial tendons (ST) making them visible.

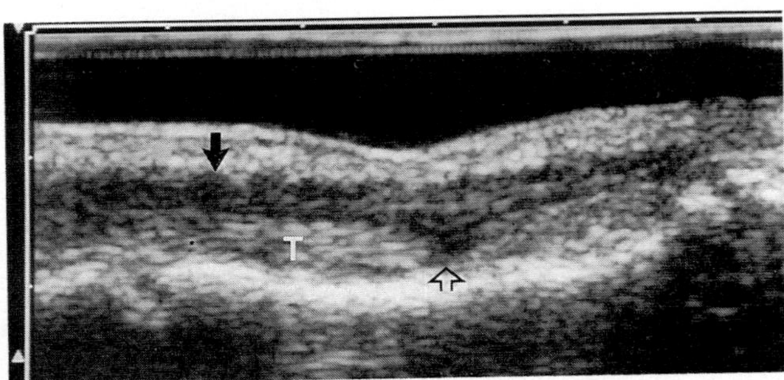

FIGURE 18–30. Palmar longitudinal view of a proximal phalanx. A hypoechoic synovitis (black arrow) covers the flexor tendons (T), and at one site the synovitis infiltrates the tendon (open arrow), indicating an impending rupture.

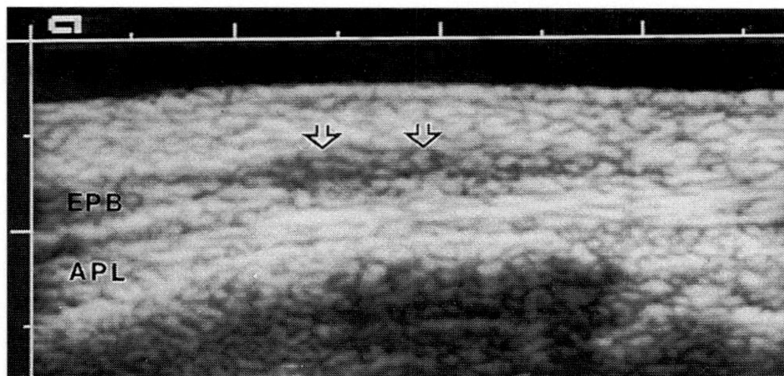

FIGURE 18–31. Dorsal longitudinal view of the extensor pollicis brevis tendon (EPB) at the wrist. The tendon is thickened and has a lower echogenicity (open arrows) compared with the underlying abductor pollicis longus (APL) tendon. This thickening represents de Quervain's disease, a localized tendinitis.

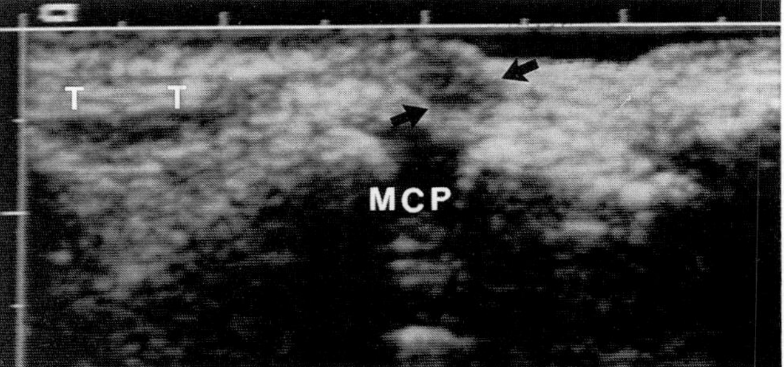

FIGURE 18–32. Palmar longitudinal view of the thumb in a toddler. Superficial to the metacarpophalangeal joint (MCP) is an easily-seen hypoechoic nodule formation (between arrows) of the flexor tendon (T). This is a localized tendinitis causing a "trigger finger."

18–34). When the patient is asked to gently bend his or her finger, ultrasound can show if tendon movement is impaired.

In *rheumatoid arthritis* and similar inflammatory diseases, the extensor tendons may dislocate ulnarly at the metacarpophalangeal joints. This may be difficult to differentiate clinically from tendon ruptures in the presence of a general inflammation. With ultrasound it is possible to see if a tendon is continuous and/or if it is dislocated (Fig. 18–35).

After *tendon suture,* function of the tendon is often impaired. When postoperative mobilization is prolonged, it can be difficult to clinically determine whether there is a rerupture or scar formation with adhesions. On ultrasound a rerupture with retraction of the tendon and diastasis between the two tendon parts can be visualized, as in the acute rupture. In the case of adhesion the tendon can be followed into an area where the tendon structure disappears and is replaced by a mass with inhomogenous echogenicity, representing a scar formation with the tendon caught onto it. If the patient is asked to initiate active flexion of the finger, it is often possible to determine if the tendon is continuous and/or fixed in this scar formation (Fig. 18–36).

Mapping of Tendons

In tendon transplantation, it is important when planning the operation to know if there is any suitable tendon that can be used. Primarily the palmaris longus tendon is used, but this tendon can be difficult to palpate and is absent in 15% of the population. When the palmaris longus tendon is missing the plantaris longus tendon can be used instead. This tendon is not palpable and is also absent in 1% of people bilaterally and in 7–18% unilaterally.[30] Therefore, ultrasound can be helpful to prove the existence of these tendons.

Vessels

Venous Thromboses

Venous thromboses can be diagnosed with ultrasound. A normal vein, as mentioned earlier, is characterized by the ease with which it can be compressed. In a case of an acute thrombosis the vein

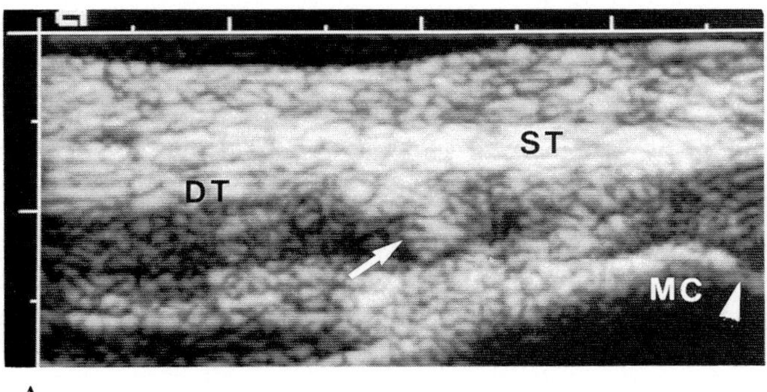

A

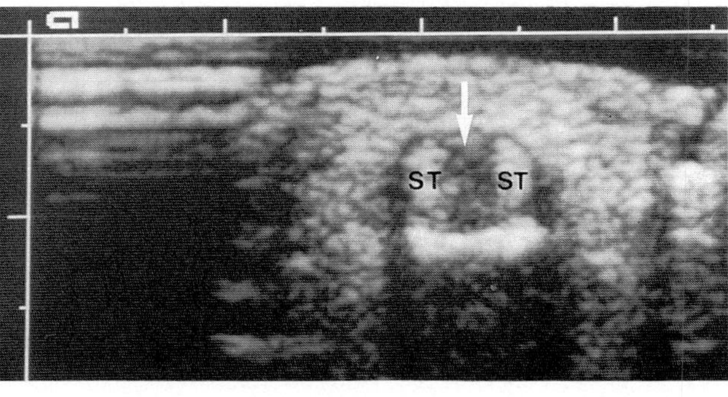

B

FIGURE 18–33. A: Palmar longitudinal view of a metacarpal bone (MC). The superficial flexor tendon (ST) is clearly evident passing over the joint (arrowhead), but the deep flexor tendon (DT) is totally ruptured, with its retracted end (arrow) located proximal to the joint. **B:** Palmar transverse view at the level of the proximal phalanx. Only the superficial flexor tendon (ST) is seen, and there is no tendon structure at the site (arrow) for the deep flexor tendon.

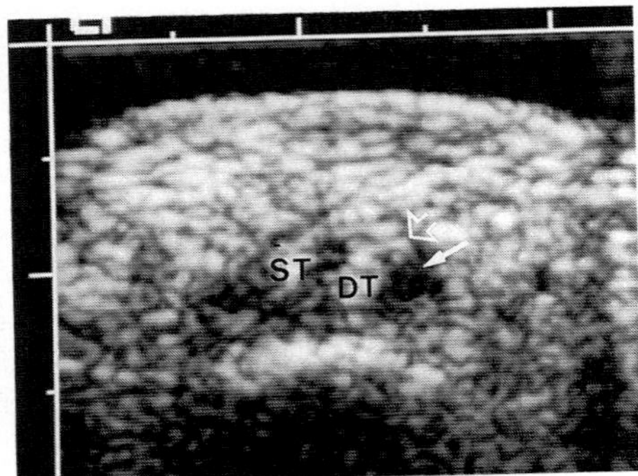

FIGURE 18–34. Palmar transverse view of a proximal phalanx. There is a thin anechoic layer of fluid due to tenosynovitis separating the tendons. The deep flexor tendon (DT) and the radial slip of the superficial flexor tendon (ST) are well seen. At the site of the ulnar slip there is a synovitis (arrow) and only a thin part of the tendon (open arrow) is seen, indicating a partial rupture.

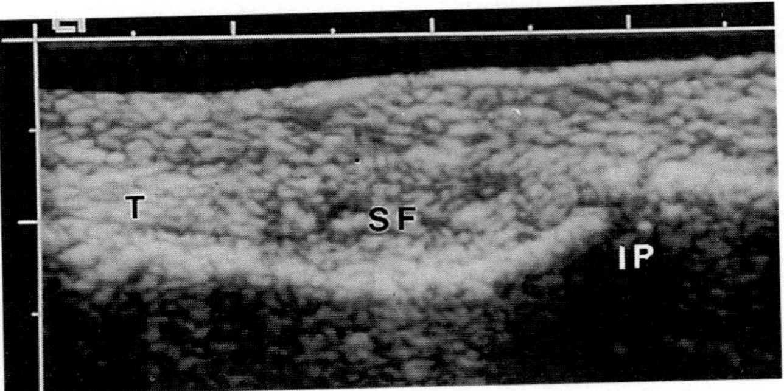

FIGURE 18–36. Palmar longitudinal view of the thumb. Six weeks earlier the flexor pollicis longus tendon had been sutured. Now tendon function is impaired; a rerupture was suspected. The interphalangeal joint (IP) is identified. The tendon (T) is clearly visualized lying close to the proximal phalanx and passing into an inhomogenous scar formation (SF) in which the tendon is caught. Thus there is no total rerupture that would lead to a retracted tendon.

cannot be compressed. In the acute stage of thrombosis, the vein has a larger diameter than expected and is filled with a hypoechoic mass representing the thrombus (Fig. 18–37). Even if the vein is not recanalized, it slowly regains its normal size and the thrombus becomes fibrotic and turns hyperechoic.

Arterial Occlusions

In the majority of cases arterial occlusions in the hand affect the ulnar artery in the hypothenar region. The etiology is probably repetitive localized trauma.[31] There is localized pain, but as a rule circulation to the fingers is not impaired because of the widespread collateral system. On ultrasound the artery can usually be followed from the wrist and distally through Guyon's canal until it branches into the palmar arcades. Because the diagnosis in a case of occlusion often is delayed, the artery is seen as a hyperechoic longitudinal band. Care must be taken that slow flow in an extremely narrow ulnar artery is not mistaken for an occlusion.

Mapping of Vessels

In cases of reconstructive surgery after major trauma and malformations, mapping of vessels is essential in planning surgical procedures.[32] In these cases an ultrasound examination can replace the invasive procedure of angiography and preoperatively give sufficient information about existing vessels to plan the reconstruction.

After microsurgical reconstruction with flaps, flow in the reconstructed vessels is commonly followed clinically or with conventional Doppler. With ultrasound equipped with Doppler, it is possible to direct the examination toward the arteries and veins of interest and evaluate the flow in each vessel.

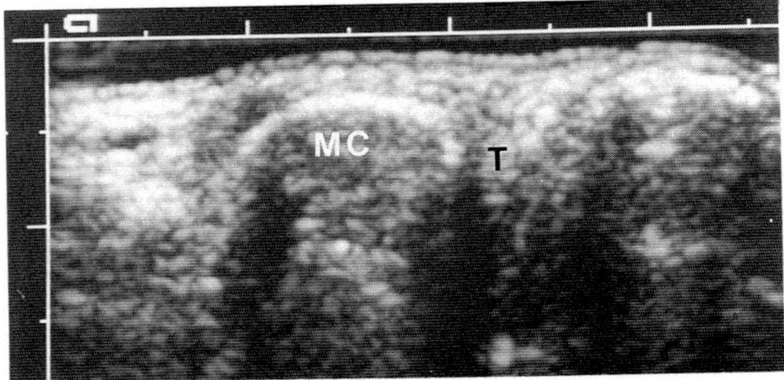

FIGURE 18–35. Dorsal transverse view at the level of a distal metacarpal bone (MC) in a patient with rheumatoid arthritis who is unable to extend the finger. The extensor tendon (T) is dislocated to the ulnar side of the metacarpal head.

Nerves

Compressions

Although nerve tumors are easily detectable with ultrasound, compressions of peripheral nerves are more difficult to visualize. It has not yet been possible to verify in a convincing way the often-described anatomic narrowing of the median nerve in connection with carpal tunnel syndrome.[25] In some cases of nerve entrapments with clinically more obscure symptoms, an ultrasound examination can be rewarding in demonstrating other causative factors, such as supplementary muscles, tenosynovitis, or tumors (Fig. 18–38).[33,34] A ganglion in Guyon's canal, which according to many reports is not rare, may have symptoms of ulnar nerve compression (Fig. 18–39).[35]

Injuries

Partial nerve injury to the median or ulnar nerve with uncharacteristic symptoms can be difficult to diagnose after wounds at the level of the wrist. These symptoms can also be caused by extrinsic compression from entities such as a foreign body or hematoma, or in a later stage, from scar formation. With ultrasound it is possible to rule out or demonstrate extrinsic causative factors and also to demonstrate a partial injury.

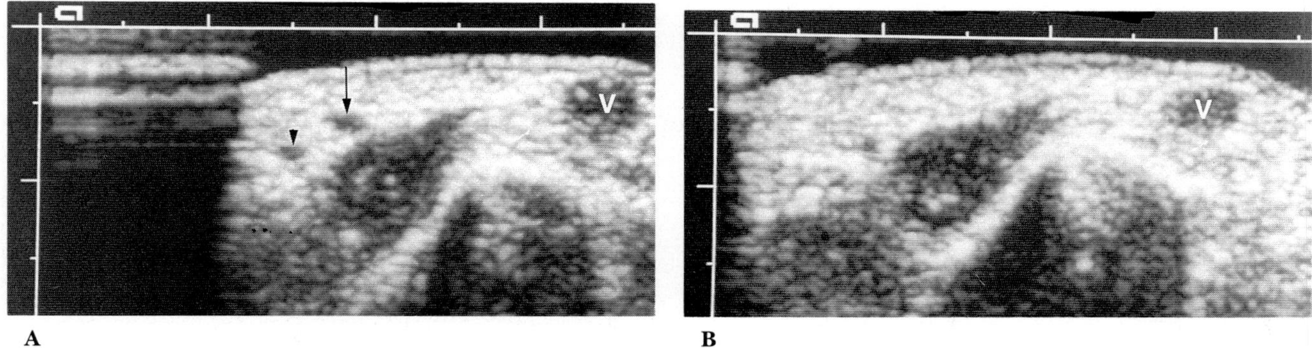

FIGURE 18–37. A: Transverse view of the wrist. An enlarged hypoechoic vein (V) 5 mm in diameter can be compared with a regularly sized vein (arrow) and an artery (arrowhead). **B:** The same view but with compression by the transducer. The enlarged vein (V) is not compressible, indicating an acute thrombosis, contrary to the normal vein, which is easily compressed.

Joints

Arthritis

Pyogenic arthritis demands prompt surgical intervention, and therefore an early diagnosis is important.[24] On ultrasound, in a case of joint effusion, there is periarticular edema. The capsule is swollen and an anechoic fluid space separates the capsule from the bone.[5] Because hemarthrosis has a similar appearance, this may be difficult to differentiate from other joint effusions (Fig. 18–40).

It is important for the clinician to diagnose *inflammatory arthritis* because it can subsequently destroy the cartilage. Mild arthritis is recognized as a hypoechoic area, thicker than normal, covering the joint and the adjoining bones (Fig. 18–41). This may correspond to an edematous synovial membrane. Extensive synovitis involving the joint, such as in *rheumatoid arthritis,* is characterized by large, almost anechoic masses bulging around the joints.

Ligaments

Ligament ruptures are common injuries and may be hazardous for future wrist function if they are not properly treated. For example, in connection with skiing, the *ulnar collateral ligament* of the first metacarpophalangeal joint is commonly injured, usually at its distal end. Radiographs are traditionally performed. These can demonstrate an avulsion fracture, however, they cannot depict ligament dislocation. An essential issue is the so-called Stener mechanism, the situation when the ulnar collateral ligament is dislocated outside the dorsal aponeurosis.[36] With a dislocated ligament an operation is considered necessary. After acute trauma effusion separates the ulnar collateral ligament from the capsule, and on ultrasound the ligament becomes visible. If the ligament is not dislocated, it is possible to identify the hyperechoic ligament in the anechoic fluid still in anatomic position under the capsule and dorsal aponeurosis. If the ligament is dislocated, it is not found under the capsule but is seen swollen and thickened, proximal or outside of the capsule and aponeurosis (Fig. 18–42).

FIGURE 18–38. Palmar transverse view of Guyon's canal. A medium-low–echoic villonodular synovitis (VS) lies next to the ulnar artery (arrow) that accompanies the ulnar nerve. The mass gives symptoms of nerve compression. In this color Doppler examination the artery is well demonstrated even on a black-and-white print.

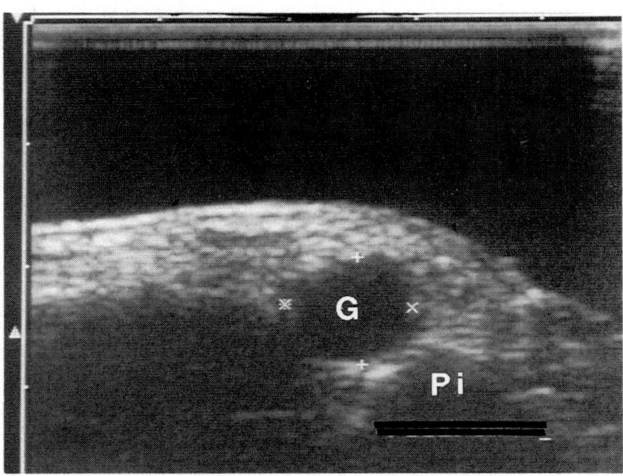

FIGURE 18–39. Palmar transverse view of Guyon's canal. Next to the pisiform bone (Pi) is an 8-mm anechoic ganglion (G) that causes symptoms of ulnar nerve compression.

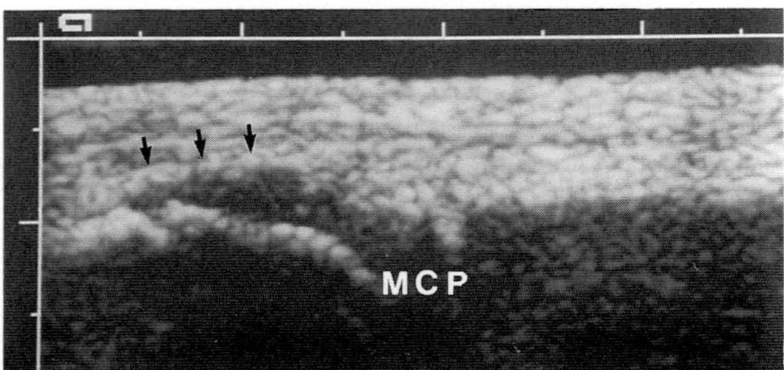

FIGURE 18–40. Longitudinal view of a metacarpophalangeal joint (MCP) with an anechoic fluid collection separating the capsule (arrows) from the bone. Because this is after acute trauma, this effusion most likely represents a hemarthrosis.

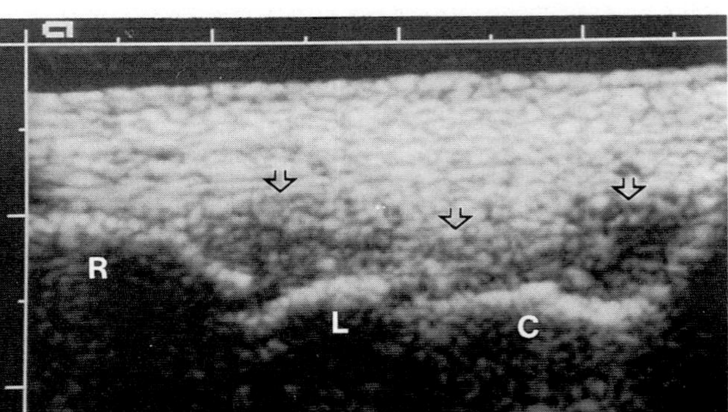

FIGURE 18–41. Dorsal longitudinal view of the carpal region with the radius (R), lunate (L), and capitate (C) bones at the bottom. Bulging up from the joints and partly covering the bones is an irregular low-echoic mass (arrows), representing a mild synovitis arising from the carpal joints.

The *scapholunate ligament* is sometimes seen with ultrasound. This is especially possible after trauma when there is fluid in the underlying joint, or when the ligament is delineated by an overlying ganglion. The degree of certainty with which ultrasound can diagnose an injury to this ligament has not yet been evaluated (Fig. 18–43).

Cartilage and Bones

Congenital Anomalies

Children with congenital anomalies of the hand are often referred to the hand surgeon at a very early age when all ossification centers are not yet calcified. Even when surgical intervention is not scheduled until later, it is of great importance that the parents be informed about the possibilities of future reconstructions.

The metacarpal bones should be well calcified at birth. The calcified part of a bone is seen as a hyperechoic structure with a distinct acoustic shadow underneath the structure. The epiphyses are rounded, and if not yet calcified, they are almost anechoic without any enhancement.

Calcification is often delayed in cases of congenital anomalies. With ultrasound it is possible to depict an uncalcified bone that has the same anechoic image as the uncalcified epiphysis. Even in small children it is possible to recognize the bones by their contours and localization. For example, if a baby has a rudimentary forearm and hand, it can be helpful in planning reconstructive surgery if ultrasound can demonstrate the presence of uncalcified forearm or metacarpal bones (Fig. 18–44).

Epiphyseolyses

Children who have uncalcified epiphyses with a history of trauma are at risk for epiphyseal displacement or dislocation that may be difficult or even impossible

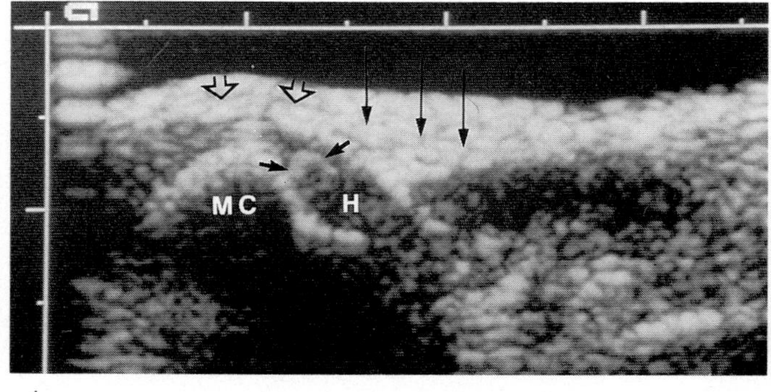

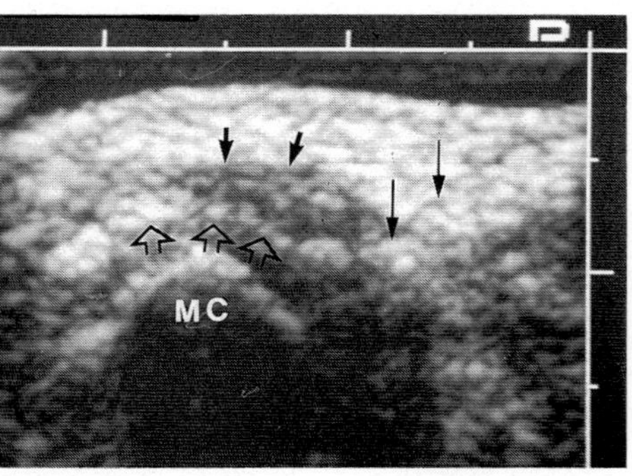

A B

FIGURE 18–42. A: Dorsal transverse view of the distal part of the first metacarpal bone (MC) after acute trauma. The joint capsule (open arrows) is separated from the bone by an anechoic effusion that is actually a hemarthrosis (H). The dorsal aponeurosis (long thin arrows) is seen as it merges into the capsule. In the hemarthrosis the ulnar collateral ligament (between short thick arrows) is in place and is not dislocated outside the capsule or aponeurosis. **B:** Dorsal transverse view of the distal part of the first metacarpal bone (MC) after acute trauma in another patient. The dorsal aponeurosis (long thin arrows) is seen as it merges into the capsule (open arrows). Here the ulnar collateral ligament (short thick arrows) is thickened and dislocated outside the capsule and aponeurosis.

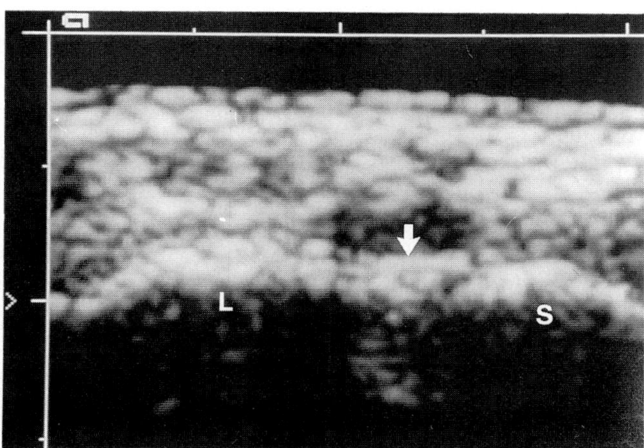

FIGURE 18–43. Magnified dorsal transverse view of the scapholunate joint with the lunate (L) and scaphoid (S) bones and the dorsal surface of the scapholunate ligament (open arrow) extending between these two bones.

to see on routine radiography. Because the cartilage is demonstrable on ultrasound, a possible displacement of epiphyses can be evaluated.

Dupuytren's Contracture

There is usually no problem in making the diagnosis of advanced Dupuytren's contracture. When located at an atypical site or in an early stage with only a small intracutaneous or subcutaneous nodule, the differential diagnosis of Dupuytren's contracture from other subcutaneous masses, such as epidermoid cysts or flexor tendon sheath ganglions, can be difficult. On ultrasound Dupuytren's contracture is seen as a hypoechoic mass without any capsule in close contact with the cutis. Commonly the mass is in close contact with the flexor tendons, but when the patient is asked to flex his or her fingers it is usually easy to see that the tendons move separately from the mass.

SUMMARY AND FUTURE OF HAND AND WRIST ULTRASOUND

As mentioned earlier, ultrasound is easily accessible, nonionizing, and is relatively inexpensive compared

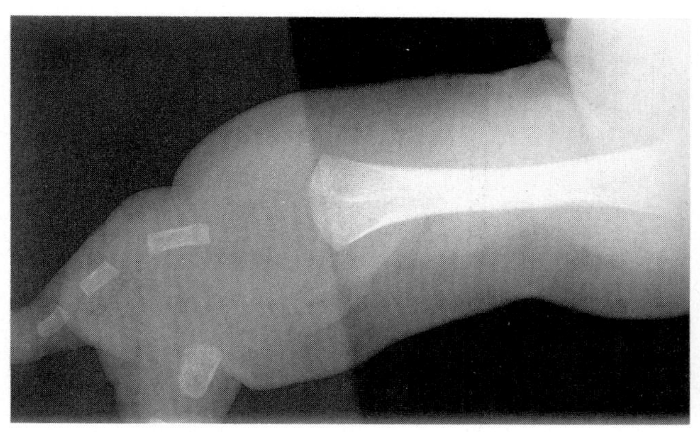

A

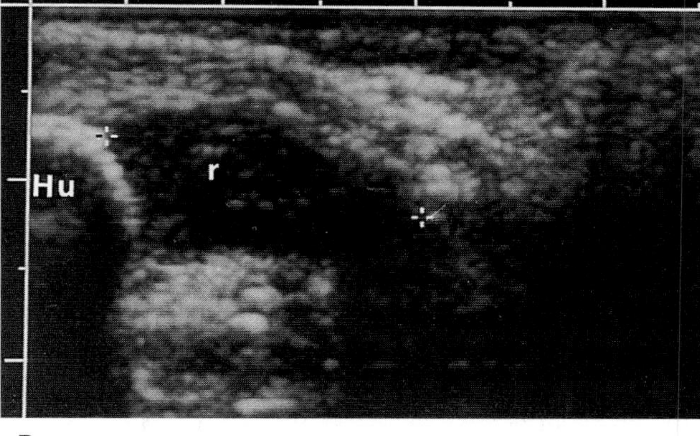

B

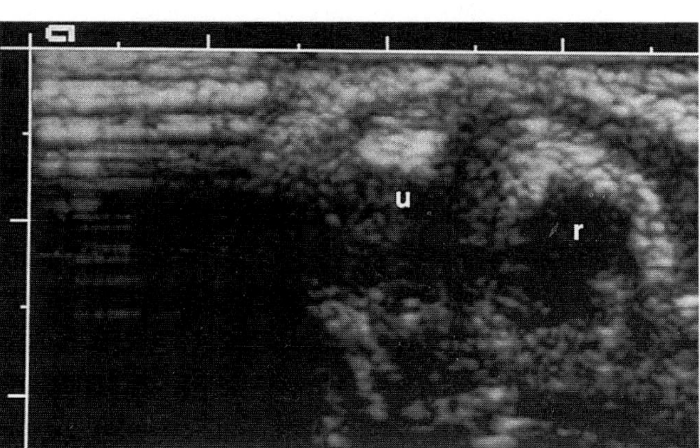

C

FIGURE 18–44. A: Anteroposterior radiograph of an upper extremity with a congenital malformation. The question was whether there were any forearm bones. **B:** Radial longitudinal view of the arm just below the distal humerus (Hu). A 2-cm–long anechoic mass (r) is present, which represents a noncalcified rudimentary radial bone. **C:** Palmar transverse view at the same level with two adjacent anechoic masses. This indicates that there is one ulnar (u) and one radial (r) rudimentary, noncalcified bone in the forearm.

with many other examinations. This should encourage many physicians to request an ultrasound examination for any questionable pathologic disorder of the soft tissues in the hand. Any palpable mass or infections, e.g., felons, can be evaluated as to the area involved and the depth and possible involvement of neighboring tissues. Masses cannot only be proved by ultrasound, they can also be excluded. Ligaments have not yet been thoroughly evaluated. With detailed evaluation and mapping of at least the extrinsic ligaments in the hand, ultrasound could be a possible way to diagnose pathology of ligaments.

Young children commonly need general anesthesia when CT or MRI is performed. This can be avoided many times if ultrasound is used as the method of choice when evaluating soft-tissue pathology in children. Since cartilage and noncalcified bones are readily depictable on ultrasound, this can be used to evaluate any articular surface with noncalcified cartilage structure. When a malformed epiphysis is suspected, such as in cases of delta phalanges, this epiphysis can be depicted on ultrasound. Tendons, vessels, and possibly even muscles can be thoroughly mapped in conditions such as malformations, before reconstructive surgery is performed.

As technology improves, higher-frequency transducers are being developed. Today these are mostly used in dermatology. With higher frequency the resolution is better but the penetration is shallower. When evaluating the soft tissues on the palmar aspect of the hand a penetration depth of up to 3 cm is commonly needed. However, on the dorsal aspect of the hand and on the phalanges the penetration depth needed for diagnostic purposes is usually not more than 1 cm. Therefore it should be possible to use higher-frequency ultrasound in thin parts to get better resolution. Such improved ultrasound would make it easier to better evaluate small and thin structures such as the extensor tendons, ligaments, and joint capsules. New areas and pathologic conditions will then be included in the diagnostic possibilities for ultrasound in the hand.

REFERENCES

1. Höglund M, Tordai P, Engkvist O. Ultrasonography for the diagnosis of soft tissue conditions in the hand. *Scand J Plast Reconstr Surg Hand Surg* 1991;25:225–231.
2. Fornage BD. Technique for sonography of muscles and tendons of the extremities. In: Fornage BD, ed. *Ultrasonography of muscles and tendons.* New York: Springer-Verlag, 1989:6–12.
3. Fornage BD, Rifkin MD. Ultrasound examination of tendons. *Radiol Clin North Am* 1988;26:87–107.
4. van Holsbeeck M, Introcaso JH. Sonography of the elbow, wrist and hand. In: van Holsbeeck M, Introcaso JH, eds. *Musculoskeletal ultrasound.* St. Louis: Mosby-Year Book, 1991: 285–296.
5. Fornage BD, Rifkin MD. Ultrasound examination of the hand and foot. *Radiol Clin North Am* 1988;26:109–129.
6. Russell RC, Williamson DA, Sullivan JW, et al. Detection of foreign bodies in the hand. *J Hand Surg* 1991;16A:2–11.
7. Greene RG. Soft tissue tumors of the hand and wrist. *J Med Soc NJ* 1964;61:495–498.
8. Nigst H. Einführung zum Thema "Tumoren der Hand." *Handchir Microchir Plast Chir* 1984;16(suppl 3–4):1–27.
9. Angelides AC. Ganglions of the hand and wrist. In: Green DP, ed. *Operative hand surgery,* 2nd ed. Vol III. New York: Churchill Livingstone, 1988:2281–2299.
10. Höglund M, Tordai P, Muren C. Diagnosis of ganglions in the hand and wrist by sonography. *Acta Radiol* 1994;35:35–39.
11. Leung PC. Tumours of the hand. *The Hand* 1981;13:169–176.
12. Angelides AC, Wallace PF. The dorsal ganglion of the wrist: Its pathogenesis, gross and microscopic anatomy, and surgical treatment. *J Hand Surg* 1976;1:228–235.
13. Greendyke SD, Wilson M, Shepler TR. Anterior wrist ganglia from the scaphotrapezial joint. *J Hand Surg* 1992;17A:487–490.
14. Johnson J, Kilgore E, Newmeyer W. Tumorous lesions of the hand. *J Hand Surg* 1985;10A:284–286.
15. Leffert RD. Lipomas of the upper extremity. *J Bone Joint Surg* 1972;54A:1262–1266.
16. Newmeyer WL. Vascular disorders. In: Green DP, ed. *Operative hand surgery,* 2nd ed. Vol III. New York: Churchill Livingstone, 1988:2391–2458.
17. Carroll RE, Berman AT. Glomus tumors of the hand. *J Bone Joint Surg* 1972;54A:691–703.
18. Madewell JE, Sweet DE. Tumors and tumor-like lesions in or about joints. In: Resnick D, Niwayama G, eds. *Diagnosis of bone and joint disorders,* 2nd ed. Vol. VI. Philadelphia: WB Saunders, 1988:3889–3943.
19. Rosai J. Soft tissues. In: Rosai J, ed. *Ackerman's surgical pathology,* 7th ed. Vol. II. St. Louis: CV Mosby, 1989:1547–1633.
20. Strickland JW, Stechen JB. Nerve tumors of the hand and forearm. *J Hand Surg* 1977;2:285–291.
21. Holdsworth BJ. Nerve tumours in the upper limb. A clinical review. *J Hand Surg* 1985;10B:236–238.
22. Ritt MJPF, Bos KE. A very large neurilemoma of the anterior interosseous nerve. *J Hand Surg* 1991;16B:98–100.
23. Rousseau A, Madinier JF, Favre A, et al. Tumeurs métastatiques des parties molles de la main. *Ann Chir Main Memb Super* 1992;11:57–61.
24. Von Reh-Plass S, Schaller E. Stellenwert der Frühintervention bei Handinfektionen. *Handchir Microchir Plast Chir* 1991;23: 214–217.
25. Kellerhouse LE, Reicher MA, Kursunoglu-Brahme S. Imaging of the wrist. In: Edelman RR, Hesselink JR, eds. *Clinical magnetic resonance imaging.* Philadelphia: WB Saunders, 1990: 1057–1075.
26. Bonnici AV, Spencer JD. A survey of "trigger finger" in adults. *J Hand Surg* 1988;13B:202–203.
27. Fahey JJ, Bollinger JA. Trigger-finger in adults and children. *J Bone Joint Surg* 1954;36A:1200–1218.
28. Ger E, Kapcha P, Ger D. The management of trigger thumb in children. *J Hand Surg* 1991;16A:944–947.
29. Trumble TE, Vedder NB, Benirschke SK. Misleading fractures after profundus tendon avulsions: A report of six cases. *J Hand Surg* 1992;17A:902–906.
30. Mackay IR, McCulloch AS. Imaging the plantaris tendon with ultrasound. *Br J Plast Surg* 1990;43:689–691.
31. DiBenedetto MR, Nappi JF, Ruff ME, et al. Doppler mapping in hypothenar syndrome: An alternative to angiography. *J Hand Surg* 1989;14A:244–246.
32. Mathes SJ, Alpert BS. Free skin and composite flaps. In: Green DP, ed. *Operative hand surgery,* 2nd ed. Vol II. New York: Churchill Livingstone, 1988:1151–1213.
33. Budny PG, Regan PJ, Roberts AHN. Localized nodular synovitis: A rare cause of ulnar nerve compression in Guyon's canal. *J Hand Surg* 1992;17A:663–664.
34. Regan PJ, Feldberg L, Bailey BN. Accessory palmaris longus muscle causing ulnar nerve compression at the wrist. *J Hand Surg* 1991;16A:736–738.
35. Seddon HJ. Carpal ganglion as a cause of paralysis of the deep branch of the ulnar nerve. *J Bone Joint Surg* 1952;34B:386.
36. Stener B. Displacement of the ruptured ulnar collateral ligament of the metacarpo-phalangeal joint of the thumb: A clinical and anatomical study. *J Bone Joint Surg* 1962;44B:869–879.

CHAPTER 19

ANGIOGRAPHIC AND INTERVENTIONAL PROCEDURES IN THE HAND

Wayne F. J. Yakes and Michael D. Dake

Angiographic studies of the hand and wrist are an integral part of the work-up of the vascular disorders that affect this complex organ. When considered in the context of the number and types of clinician requests for diagnostic and therapeutic vascular studies in a typical interventional/special procedures service, the request for angiographic evaluations of the hand and wrist is not that common. Perhaps for this reason, interventionalists are not completely familiar with appropriate superselective and pharmacoangiographic techniques that can result in superior examinations, reveal subtleties of vascular disorders, and aid in patient management strategies, rather than just a cursory vascular overview. Furthermore, these procedures can take much longer to perform appropriately. The purpose of this chapter is to discuss the various techniques used for the proper performance of angiographic studies, arteriographic and venographic anatomy of the hand and wrist, and the angiographic appearances of some of the disorders that affect the hand and wrist.

INDICATIONS AND TECHNIQUES

The most common indication for arteriography of the hand and wrist is related to a patient demonstrating ischemic symptoms. Ischemia can result from a wide range of etiologies: atherosclerosis, thromboembolic disease, autoimmune disorders, hypercoagulable states, trauma, and the like. In patients suffering from hand/digital ischemia of an unknown cause, a complete examination from the brachiocephalic arteries to the hand is mandatory. This allows a total evaluation to define the particular pathologic process and identify its extent. Using these studies, appropriate management strategies can be decided after consultation with medical and surgical specialists. The interventionalist may play a significant role in patient management with the use of endovascular procedures such as fibrinolytic therapy, transluminal angioplasty, and embolotherapy.

Noninvasive vascular assessment can be performed with color-Doppler imaging (CDI) and magnetic resonance angiography (MRA). Despite the abilities of these current imaging modalities, arteriography still remains the standard for full definition of the vascular pathologic process and ultimately therapy direction. CDI and MRA do, however, provide an extremely useful noninvasive adjunct to follow patient response to therapy, especially when follow-up studies can be compared with baseline studies before any intervention. Cut-film magnification arteriographic techniques and 512 × 512 or 1024 × 1024 matrices of digital subtraction arteriography (DSA) provide high-quality images with excellent detail. Cut-film techniques may have a slightly better spatial resolution overall, however.

One of the most difficult entities to arteriographically evaluate thoroughly is vascular malformation of the hand and wrist. Global injections can certainly make the diagnosis of a high-flow lesion such as an arteriovenous malformation (AVM) or arteriovenous fistula (AVF) or a low-flow lesion such as a venous malformation (VM). Selective and superselective catheterization arteriograms, however, are essential to fully define the arterial angioarchitecture before any contemplated surgical or endovascular therapy. In low-flow lesions, MRI is essential to fully delineate the extent of the VM as well as determine its anatomic relationships to muscles, tendons, and nerves.[1] VMs are only incompletely opacified by arteriography. Closed-system venography or direct puncture venography will give a better angiographic assessment of the VM compared with arteriography alone.[2]

Traumatic injuries, whether acute or chronic, that cause ischemia or distal embolism usually require arteriography to adequately assess the vascular injury. Arterial crush injuries, transections, dissections, thromboembolic occlusions, pseudoaneurysms, and various chronic injuries, such as the thenar and hypothenar hammer syndromes, are best evaluated arteriographically. Blunt trauma, fractures, penetrating injuries, crush injuries, as well as high-velocity bullet injuries, can cause any form of vascular injury.[3,4]

With the advent of current microvascular surgical techniques performed by hand surgeons and plastic and reconstructive surgeons, angiographic assessment before surgery is becoming essential and is being requested increasingly more often. Myocutaneous grafts, sacrificing the radial artery to use as a vascular pedicle for example, require arteriography to determine if the ulnar artery alone can totally perfuse the deep and superficial palmar arterial arches of the hand. Microvascular free flap grafts require not only that the arterial anastomotic site be evaluated, but also that an adequate venous phase be obtained to determine if the venous outflow anastomoses are adequate to support a delicate grafting procedure. Venography may be indicated if arteriography does not adequately opacify the veins.

The various vasculitides such as Buerger's disease, giant cell arteritis, and so on, may require hand arteriography to determine the extent of involvement. Follow-up arteriography may even be requested to evaluate the efficacy of medical management, correlating the arteriographic findings to the clinical findings. Furthermore, comparison arteroigrams to the contralateral upper extremity, lower extremities, and abdominal visceral arteries may also be required.[5–7]

Patients with renal failure from various causes who require placement of a Gortex arterial-to-vein fistula for dialysis often have undergone many upper extremity venipunctures and have "poor veins." To minimize cardiac consequences, the dialysis graft is initially placed in the distal forearm. In unusual circumstances, an arteriogram of the hand, in particular the radial artery and its distal runoff to the hand, may be requested. A closed-system venogram to identify the best forearm vein to perform the distal Gortex end-to-end anastomosis may also be requested in problematic cases.

Because the arteries of the hand react to various stimuli (pain, catheter/wire manipulations, ionic high osmolar contrast media, and so on) by becoming spastic and difficult to arteriographically visualize, the knowledge of selective catheter techniques, superselective microcatheter techniques, and the use of oral and intravascular vasodilators is required. With good technique, detailed arteriographic studies that are diagnostically useful to the referring clinician can be consistently obtained. The correct diagnosis can be determined from high-quality studies and appropriate management strategies can then be instituted.

Vasodilators have proved extremely useful for full visualization of digital arteries. With current hypoosmolar, isoosmolar, and nonionic contrast agents, problems related to vasospasm pain and digital artery nonvisualization have been much improved. Nonetheless, the use of vasodilators may still be required to produce a high-quality diagnostic arterial study. Before the study, 10 mg of nifedipine squirted sublingually is an excellent calcium channel antagonist to minimize vasospasm. One inch of nitropaste placed on the chest before the procedure could also be used to minimize vasospasm. An overzealous application, however, could lead to the patient suffering from a headache. Intraarterial spasmolytic agents may additionally be used as required. A premixed solution (in a glass bottle) of nitroglycerine at a concentration of 200 μg/mL (μg = microgram) is commercially available. Several boluses of 1 mL will usually overcome any vasospasm encountered. Blood pressure monitoring must be performed to prevent any unwanted hypotension from excessive nitroglycerine use. Tolazoline, a potent adrenergic blocking agent whose method of action is on the alpha receptors of postganglionic fibers, has a direct dilator effect predominantly at the arteriolar and capillary level. For maximal effectiveness in the hand, experience has proved that a slow injection of 25 mg of tolazoline over approximately 2 minutes in the distal brachial artery is much superior to rapid bolus injection. Although papaverine, lidocaine, prostaglandin E_1, tourniquet-induced hyperemia, and so on have also been reported, the previously mentioned drug protocols are the most common in current practice (Fig. 19–1).[3,8–10]

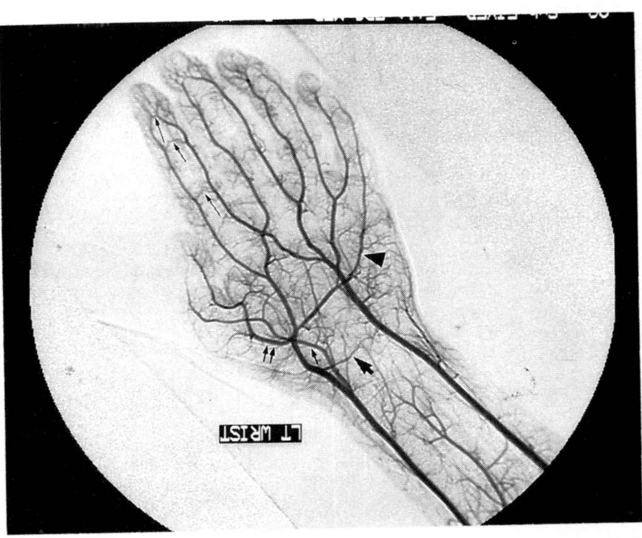

FIGURE 19–1. Anteroposterior (AP) brachial artery injection. Note prominent filling of the radial artery, ulnar artery, interosseous artery, and all palmar and digital branches after slow injection of 25 mg of tolazoline. The deep branch of the distal radial artery is not continuous with the deep palmar arch, but ends in a radial-side arterial branch to the thumb (small arrow). The ulnar-side branch to the thumb arises from the superficial palmar arch (compare to Fig. 19–5A) (double arrows). The deep palmar arch branch arises from the radial artery's superficial palmar branch (large arrow). The ulnar-side branch to the fifth digit arises from the superficial palmar arch (compare to Fig. 19–5A) (arrowhead). Note the digital transverse proximal arterial branches (proximal long arrow), digital transverse interphalangeal arterial branches (middle long arrow), and digital transverse distal arterial branches (distal long arrow).

In the total evaluation of the hand, the entire upper-extremity vascular tree from its origin at the aortic arch to the digits must be evaluated. Without meticulous adherence to this principle, incomplete examinations can lead to misdiagnoses and inadequate clinical management. Pathologic processes as well as arterial anatomic anomalies proximally can cause hand and digital ischemic symptoms. Access from the femoral route is the most common of percutaneous endovascular approaches. If various circumstances do not permit this, then contralateral upper extremity access, ipsilateral antegrade axillary, and brachial approaches can be performed. In unusual tortuous arterial anatomy, which may be encountered in vascular malformations, direct arterial access at the wrist or hand may be required during a diagnostic and/or therapeutic procedure.[11–16]

Current 5 to 5.5 Fr catheter systems have an 0.038 catheter lumen. In most adult patients these catheters, from the femoral route, will reach the distal brachial artery and at times the proximal radial, ulnar, and interosseous arteries. However, more distal catheterizations to the wrist can be very helpful to perform a superior examination of the palmar arches and digital branches. Distal selective catheterizations reduce the total contrast load required and therefore the pain of the arterial study. It is much easier for the patient to tolerate the procedure when distal catheterizations can be performed. This can be accomplished with coaxial placement of the Tracker-18 catheter and guidewire system through the 5 to 5.5 Fr seating catheter, which is advanced to the catheter hub in the groin. The Tracker-18 catheter is 175 cm in length and can usually reach the wrist in most patients, sometimes even more distally. If luerlock 1, 3, or 5 mL syringes are used to inject contrast material through the Tracker-18 catheter, good hand and digital arterial contrast opacification can be accomplished. Furthermore, if 1024 × 1024 DSA equipment is used, contrast diluted with saline can enhance the ease of contrast injection through the Tracker-18 catheter. Current 4 Fr catheter systems, with a 0.035 catheter lumen, can accommodate the Tracker-10 catheter/guidewire system and can be used in the same fashion as the 5 to 5.5 Fr catheter/Tracker-18 system described previously. However, the smaller inner lumen of the Tracker-10 catheter does not allow the flow rate by hand injection that the Tracker-18 catheter allows, but still may be adequate in many situations. It must be remembered that when coaxial systems are employed, a Tuohy–Borst valve must be attached to the hub of the seating catheter to allow saline infusion around the coaxially placed Tracker catheter to prevent unwanted thrombosis in the seating catheter residual lumen. The Tracker catheter is inserted through the back of the Tuohy–Borst with the valve tightened to allow advancement of the Tracker but prevent saline leakage around the Tracker. A pressure bag of heparinized saline is then attached via connecting tubing to the side port of the Tuohy–Borst valve to effect coaxial saline infusion through the seating catheter. A slow drip rate is usually preferred to prevent unwanted saline volume overload.

VASCULAR ANATOMY

Arterial System

The upper extremity can have multiple arterial variations that may be of more clinical consequence than arterial variations elsewhere in the body. The arterial anatomy and its variations have been well studied with regard to the upper extremity and hand. These variations are numerous, and a complete knowledge of every variant arterial anomaly need not be known in its entirety to perform an excellent study. Nonetheless, a list of references to direct the reader is provided.[17–22]

The arterial supply to the hand arises from the brachial artery branches, notably the ulnar and radial arteries. The major arterial supply to the hand is the ulnar artery, although the radial artery is more easily palpable. In the normal person the brachial artery usually branches in the elbow region. Published data reveal that variant brachial artery branches occur in approximately 15% of people. A superficial brachial artery that arises from the proximal brachial artery and distally rejoins the distal brachial artery can occur in 12% of individuals. Proximal brachial origin or "high" origin of the radial or ulnar artery can be seen in 14–17% of people. Of the two, the radial artery more commonly has this "high" variation (Figs. 19–2 to 19–4). The right extremity is slightly more affected than the left (1.2% greater). The radial artery lies ventral to the wrist and courses medially to be continuous with the deep palmar arch. The ulnar artery proximally gives rise to the interosseous artery. Distally, the ulnar artery branches into two vessels and is continuous with the deep branch of the deep palmar arch and the superficial branch of the superficial palmar (ventral) arch of the hand. The distal interosseous artery may give rise to a persistent median artery that contributes to the hand circulation in about 3% of patients. These arterial variants should be kept in mind, especially when distal selective arteriography or direct percutaneous catheter access are performed. Retrograde or antegrade brachial access in these smaller variant arteries could lead to arterial occlusion, loss of pulse, and hand ischemia. If distal selective catheter arteriography is performed without previous evaluation of the proximal vasculature, an erroneous diagnosis of radial or ulnar occlusion could be entertained.

In the ideal anatomic scenario the radial and ulnar arteries end in the formation of two palmar arches. This is obviously a developmental mechanism to minimize or prevent digital and hand ischemia in the event of arterial occlusion from whatever cause. The deep palmar branch of the radial artery (deep palmar arch) is formed by its termination. The distal

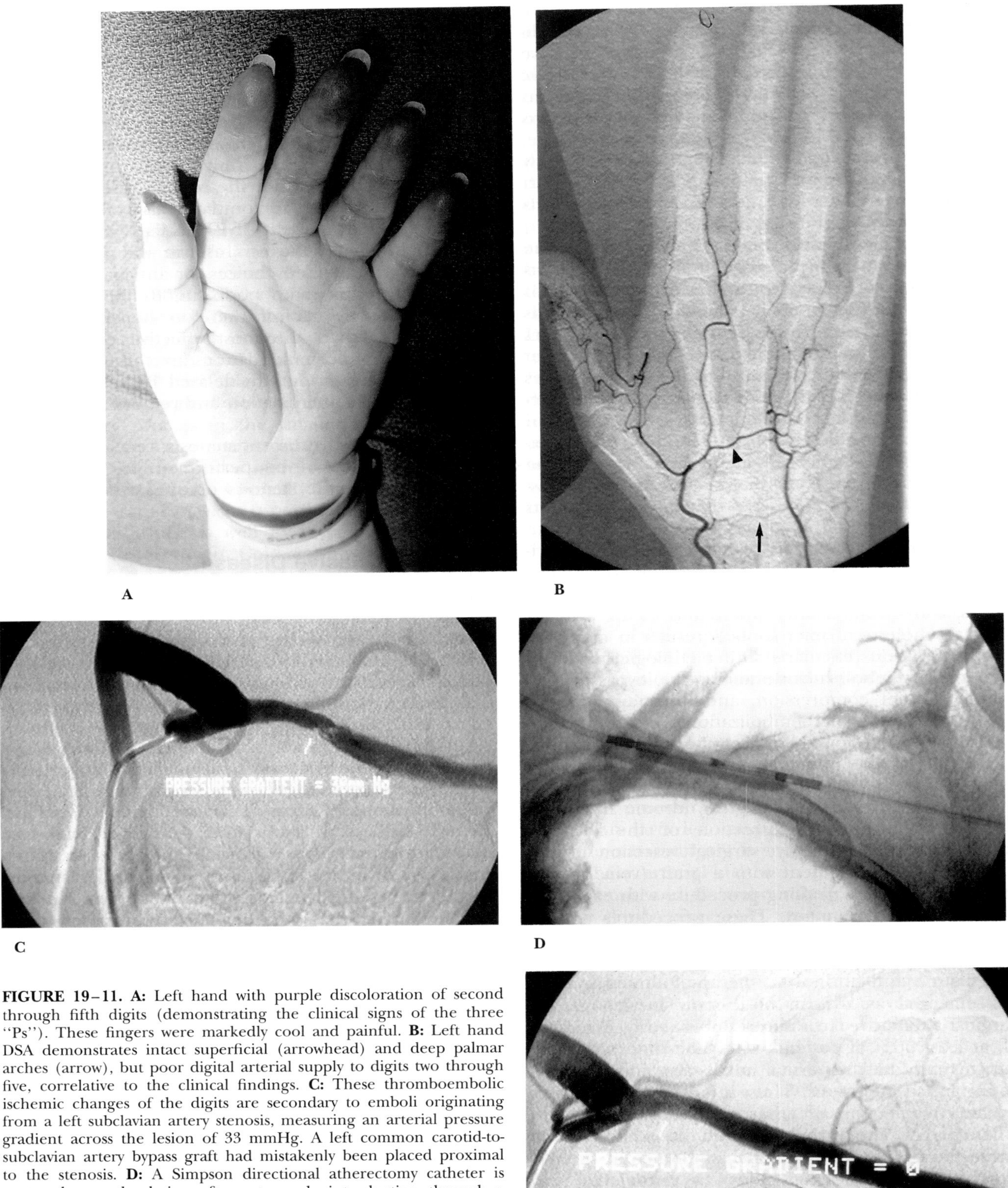

FIGURE 19–11. A: Left hand with purple discoloration of second through fifth digits (demonstrating the clinical signs of the three "Ps"). These fingers were markedly cool and painful. **B:** Left hand DSA demonstrates intact superficial (arrowhead) and deep palmar arches (arrow), but poor digital arterial supply to digits two through five, correlative to the clinical findings. **C:** These thromboembolic ischemic changes of the digits are secondary to emboli originating from a left subclavian artery stenosis, measuring an arterial pressure gradient across the lesion of 33 mmHg. A left common carotid-to-subclavian artery bypass graft had mistakenly been placed proximal to the stenosis. **D:** A Simpson directional atherectomy catheter is centered over the lesion after retrograde introduction through a brachial artery sheath. **E:** After the atherectomy procedure was performed, the postprocedure DSA showed an excellent morphologic result. No residual pressure gradient was identified. Because of the extensive digital embolization before therapy, multiple digital amputations were required.

syndrome. Conversely, 80% of patients with effort-related thrombosis have thoracic outlet compression.[47]

Venous occlusions related to systemic disease and hypercoagulable states are found in a group of patients who have a life-threatening illness, decreased tissue perfusion, hypercoagulability, venous endothelial injury, and may or may not be dehydrated. Overwhelming venous thrombosis can eventually result in arterial inflow restriction and occlusion, which eventually leads to tissue loss. The clinical syndrome of swelling, pain, cyanosis, and pallor associated with massive venous thrombosis and tissue loss is called phlegmasia cerulea dolens.[83]

Treatment of venous thrombosis includes elevation, anticoagulation, and treatment of the disorder inciting the thrombosis. If the venous thrombosis is devastating and tissue loss is a concern, thrombolytic therapy with urokinase may be added to heparin therapy. Conventional therapy may work too slowly to prevent significant morbidity and mortality, postphlebitic syndrome, tissue loss, and pulmonary embolism. Response rates are directly related to the early institution of catheter-directed fibrinolytic therapy and good success rates have been reported if thrombolytic therapy is initiated within 3 days of symptom onset.[86] In venous thrombosis refractory to urokinase fibrinolysis, particularly of the subclavian veins, innominate veins, and superior vena cava, endovascular stenting can "create" a vascular venous lumen whereby continued fibrinolysis can lead to complete vein recanalization and long-term patency.[87,88] The use of mechanical stents coupled with aggressive fibrinolytic therapy has ushered in a new era in patient management of large vein thrombosis that was refractory to treatment by any other procedure or combination of currently performed procedures.

Vascular Malformation Diagnosis and Management

Vascular malformations constitute some of the most difficult diagnostic and therapeutic dilemmas encountered in the practice of medicine. Vascular malformations were first treated by surgeons with the early approach of proximal ligations of the inflow arteries to the arteriovenous malformation (AVM). This experience proved totally futile as microfistulous connections enlarged and neovascular recruitment reconstituted arterial inflow to the AVM nidus. Surgical extirpation of the AVM is difficult, extremely hazardous, and impossible in many cases. Suboptimal partial resections may cause a good initial clinical response, but with time the malformation recurs with the patient's presenting symptoms frequently worse at follow-up.[89–91] According to D. Emerick Szilagyi,

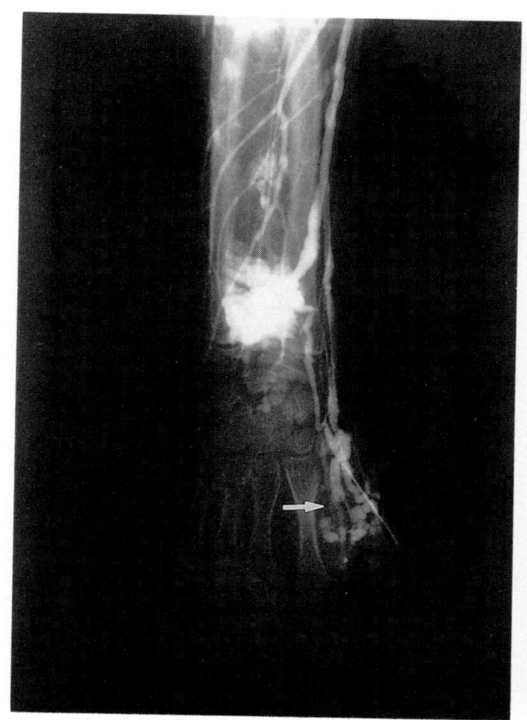

A

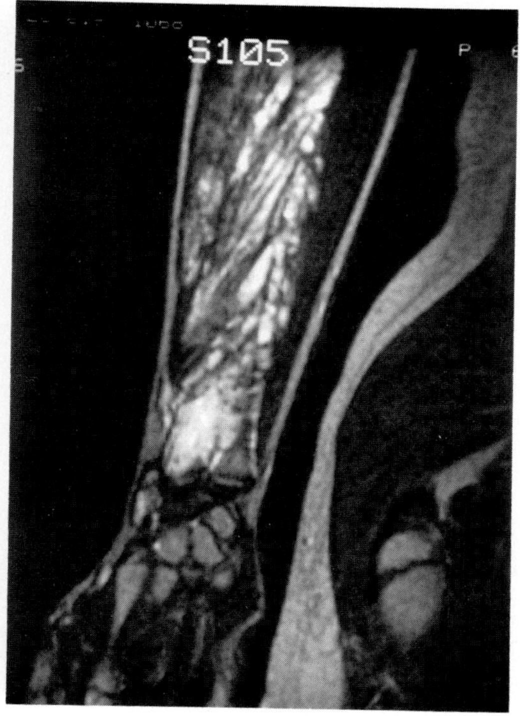

B

FIGURE 19–12. A: Closed-system venogram of the upper extremity reveals venous malformation of the thenar eminence (arrow) and forearm. **B:** MRI T-2 weighted sequence showing to advantage the diffuse nature of the forearm venous malformation not opacified by the closed-system venogram. (Reprinted with permission from Rak KM, Yakes WF, Ray RL, et al. MR imaging of symptomatic peripheral vascular malformations. *AJR* 1992;159:107–112.)

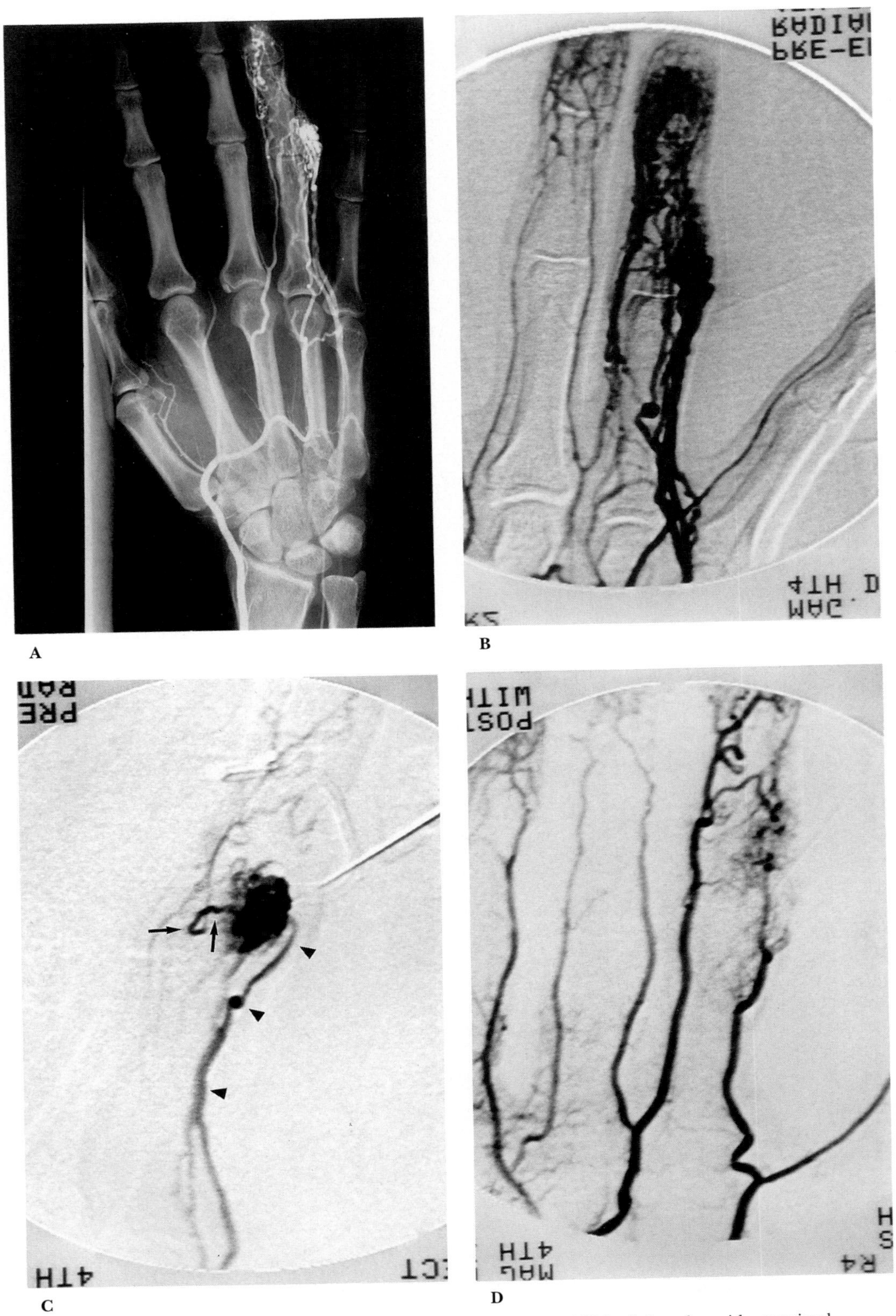

FIGURE 19–13. A: PA right hand arteriogram demonstrating an AVM of the ulnar-side proximal interphalangeal joint of the fourth digit. **B:** PA right hand DSA again demonstrating the hypertrophied inflow arteries, AVM, and outflow veins. **C:** Direct puncture DSA opacifying the AVM nidus demonstrating the outflow veins (arrowheads) and refluxing into the radial-side digital transverse interphalangeal arterial branch (arrows). **D:** Postethanol DSA demonstrating patency of digital arterial branches, absence of AVM filling, and no arteriovenous shunting into the outflow veins. The AVM is thrombosed. (Reprinted with permission from Yakes WF, Luethke JM, Parker SH, et al. Ethanol embolization of vascular malformations. *RadioGraphics* 1990;10:787–796.)

M.D., editor for the *Journal of Vascular Surgery* ". . . with few exceptions, their (vascular malformations) cure by surgical means is impossible. We intuitively thought that the only answer of a surgeon to the problem of disfiguring, often noisome, and occasionally disabling blemishes and masses, prone to cause bleeding, pain, or other unpleasantness, was to attack them with vigor and with the determination of eradicating them. The results of this attempt at radical treatment were disappointing." Of 82 patients seen in this series, only 18 patients were believed to be operative candidates. Of these 18 patients who underwent surgery, 10 patients improved, 2 were the same, and 6 were worse at follow-up.[90] It is a sobering fact that 64 patients were left untreated and without hope. This patient series points to the enormity of the problem posed by vascular malformations.

Classification of vascular malformations has always been difficult and misleading because the clinical and angiographic manifestations can be extremely varied. To compound the problem, a vast array of descriptive terms and eponyms have been applied to impressive clinical examples in the hopes of distinguishing them as distinct clinical syndromes. Based on the landmark work of Mulliken, Glowacki, and coworkers, a rational classification of hemangioma and vascular malformations has evolved that all physicians should incorporate into modern clinical practice.[92–97] This classification system, based on endothelial cell characteristics, has removed much of the confusion in terminology that exists in the literature today. Accurate terminology will eliminate ambiguity and lead to precise identification of clinical entities and enhanced patient care.

Pediatric cutaneous vascular lesions, and hemangiomas are usually not present at birth, become clinically manifested within the first month of life, exhibit a rapid growth (proliferative) phase in the first year, and involute and spontaneously regress to near complete resolution by age 7. Thus, the natural history of spontaneous involution suggests that aggressive procedures are not warranted and most patients should be managed conservatively.

Vascular malformations, on the other hand, are lesions that are present at birth and grow commensurately with the child into adulthood. Vascular malformations may be quiescent and cause no symptoms; however, once they become symptomatic they rarely revert to their asymptomatic state without therapy. Trauma, surgery, hormonal influences caused by birth control pills, and hormonal swings during puberty and pregnancy may cause the lesion to expand hemodynamically. They may be composed of any combination of primitive arterial, capillary, venous, or lymphatic elements with or without shunts. Vascular malformations are true developmental structural anomalies resulting from inborn errors of vascular morphogenesis. We categorize vascular malformations into high-flow or low-flow lesions. High-flow lesions include AVMs and congenital arteriovenous fistulae (AVF). Posttraumatic AVF are acquired lesions that are high flow. Chronic long-standing traumatic AVF may simulate an AVM and be misdiagnosed as an AVM until the proper history is obtained and super-

Text continued on page 519

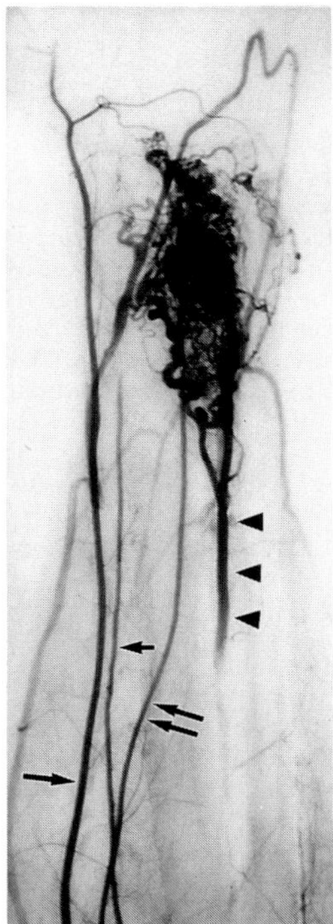

A

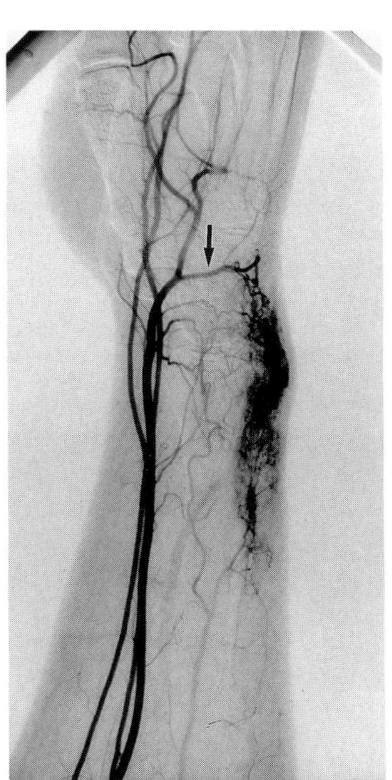

B

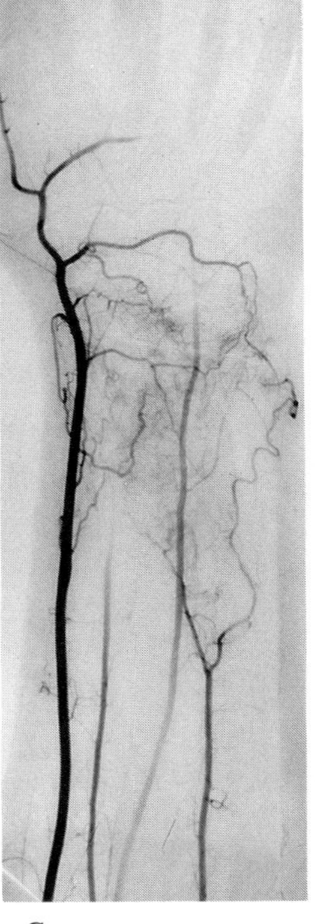

C

FIGURE 19–14. A: PA right forearm arteriogram. The normal radial artery (arrow), interosseous artery (small arrow), and ulnar artery (double arrows) are normal. The AVM dominant arterial supply is from a retained primitive branch arising from the brachial artery (arrowheads). The patient suffered from severe pain and swelling on the dorsum of the wrist. **B:** The lateral right forearm arteriogram demonstrates the dorsal wrist aspect of the AVM, and the palmar aspects of the radial interosseous and ulnar arteries. The collateral supply to the AVM (arrow) is from the radial artery. **C:** PA right forearm arteriogram 4 months posttherapy. The AVM remains occluded and the patient's pain syndrome cured. The patient remains stable without recurrence at 5-year follow-up. (Reprinted with permission from Yakes WF, Parker SH, Gibson MD, et al. Alcohol embolotherapy of vascular malformations. *Semin Intervent Radiol* 1989;6:146–161.)

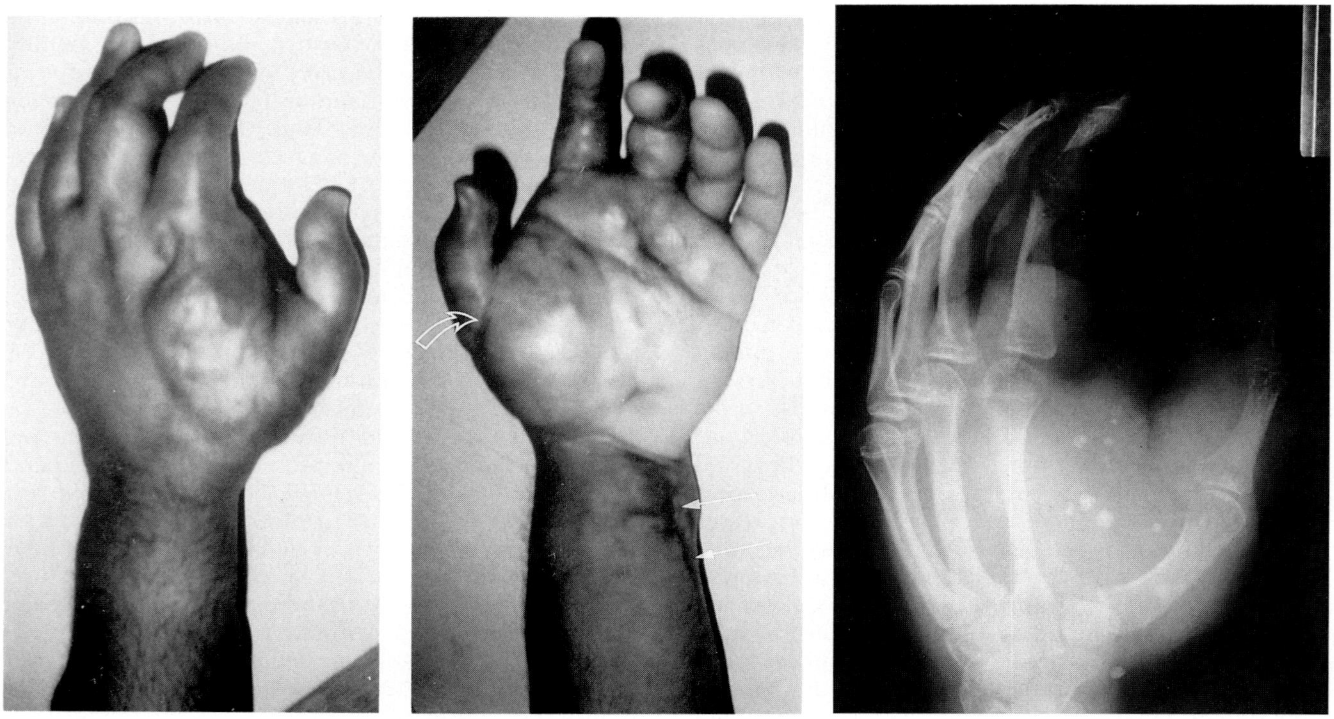

A

B

C

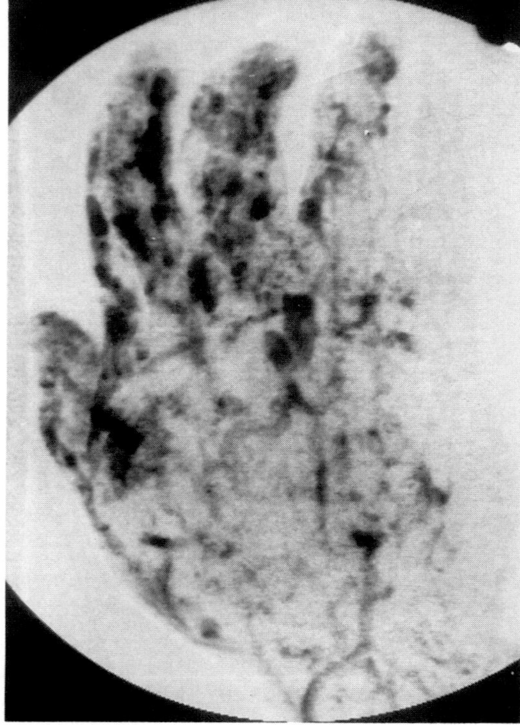

D

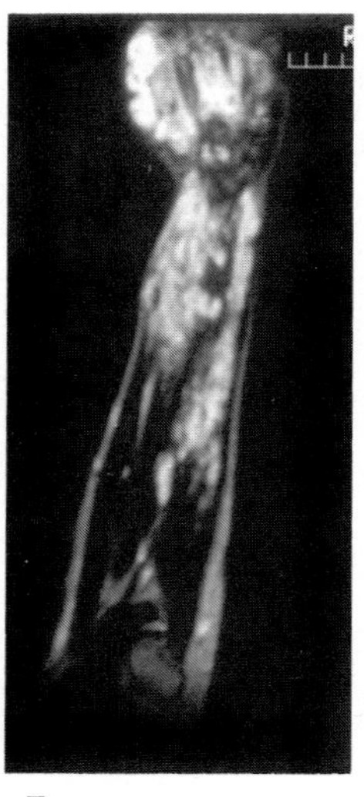

E

FIGURE 19–15. A: Dorsal view of the left hand demonstrates dilated bluish vascular lesions and swelling of the hand and digits. **B:** Palmar view of the left hand demonstrates bluish vascular lesions of the wrist, hand, and digits. Surgical scars are present on the forearm (arrows) and thumb (curved arrow). **C:** Plain film of the left hand demonstrates calcified phleboliths consistent with venous malformation. **D:** AP left hand DSA late phase demonstrating contrast pooling in multiple abnormal venous spaces in the digits and hand. **E:** Left forearm and hand MRI T-2 weighted. Increased signal present in hand and forearm is consistent with venous malformation diagnosis.

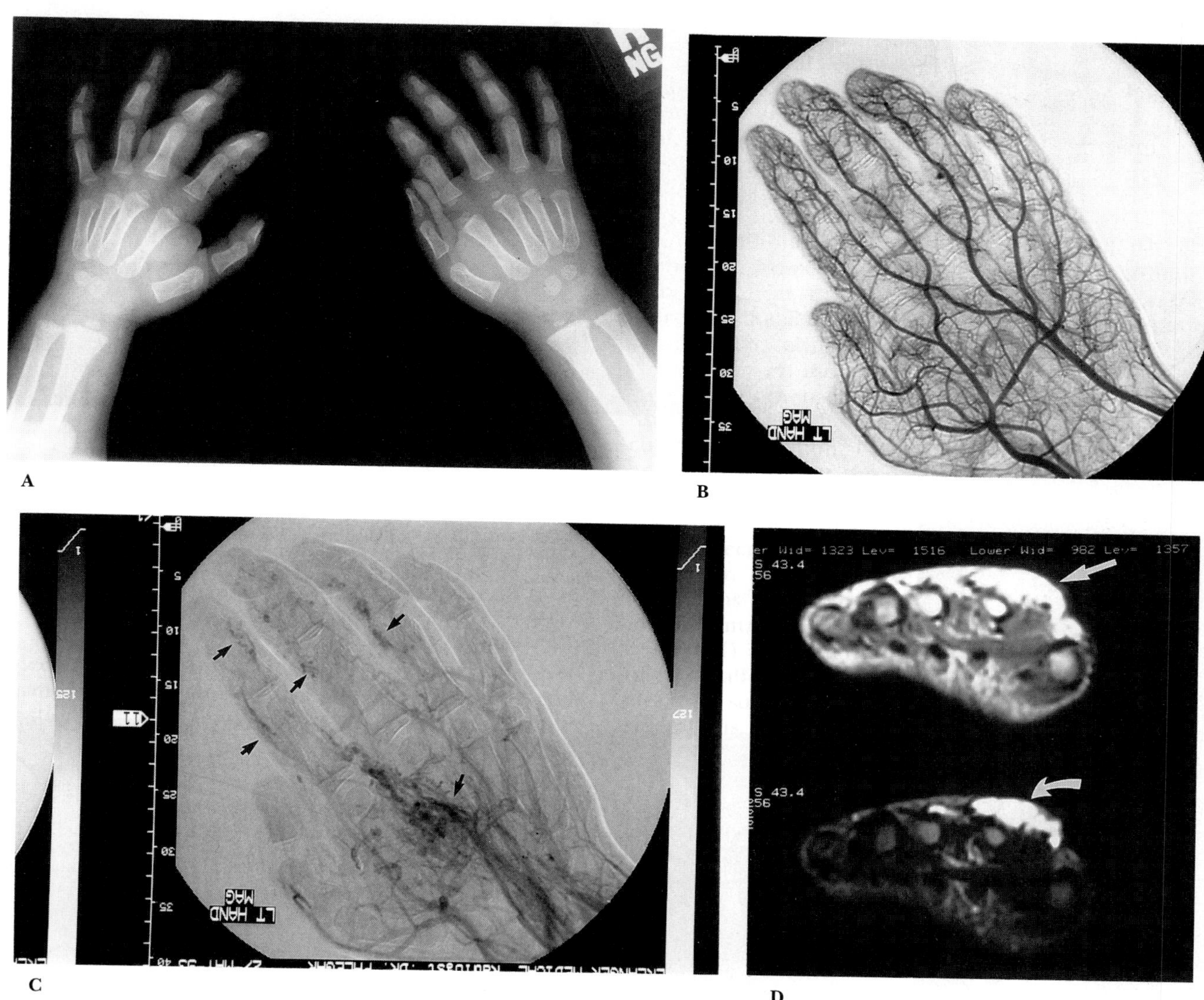

FIGURE 19–16. A: Bilateral plain films of both hands demonstrate swelling of hand and second and third digits of the left hand. Compare with right hand. **B:** AP left hand DSA arterial phase shows no AV shunts. **C:** AP left hand DSA late phase shows contrast pooling in venous malformation (arrows). **D:** Upper image is T-1 weighted axial MRI (arrow) through bases of the digits. Lower image is T-2 weighted axial MRI with fat suppression, whereby the area of increased signal (curved arrow) confirms that the digital soft-tissue prominence is caused by venous malformation. (Case contributed by Robert Phlegar, M.D., Chattanooga, TN.)

noses and poor patient outcomes. Vascular malformations are best treated in medical centers where afflicted patients are regularly treated in significant numbers and the team approach is used. The occassional embolizer will never gain enough experience to adequately treat these lesions. Moreover, when complications do occur, the morbidity is lessened in centers that have encountered these problems and deal with them regularly. It cannot be overemphasized that a cavalier approach will lead to significant complications and dismal patient outcomes. All too often the initial enthusiasm to treat one of these lesions gives way to the grim reality of complications and their inherent difficulties. When large numbers of patients are treated, significant experience will be gained, improved judgment in managing these lesions will develop, and definitive statements in the treatment of vascular malformations can evolve.

SUMMARY

The hand is a complex organ in which many disease states can be manifested. Diagnostic arteriography and venography can be important for accurate diagnosis of vascular manifestations of various disease states so that appropriate therapy can be instituted. Furthermore, interventional procedures can be a primary mode of therapy particularly when PTA, fibrinolysis, intraarterial antispasmodics, and embolotherapy may be appropriately used. It is hoped that after reviewing this chapter, referring clinicians will be aware of the diagnostic and therapeutic interventional radiologic procedures that are available to help them manage their patients.

REFERENCES

1. Rak KM, Yakes WF, Ray RL, et al. MR imaging of symptomatic peripheral vascular malformations. *AJR* 1992;159:107–112.
2. Geiser JH, Eversmam WW. Closed system venography in the evaluation of upper extremity hemangioma. *J Hand Surg* 1978;3:173–178.
3. Vogelzang RL. Arteriography of the hand and wrist. *Hand Clin* 1991;7:63–86.
4. Conn J, Bergan JJ, Bell JL. Hypothenar hammer syndrome: Posttraumatic digital ischemia. *Surgery* 1970;68:1122–1128.
5. Buerger L. Thrombo-angiitis obliterans: A study of the vascular lesions leading to presenile spontaneous gangrene. *Am J Med Sci* 1908;136:567–580.
6. Hagen B, Lohse S. Clinical and radiologic aspects of Buerger's disease. *Cardiovasc Intervent Radiol* 1984;7:283–293.
7. Zimmerman NB. Occlusive vascular disorders of the upper extremity. *Hand Clin* 1993;9:139–150.
8. Cohen MI, Vogelzang RL. A comparison of techniques for improved visualization of the arteries of the distal lower extremity. *AJR* 1986;147:1021–1024.
9. Levy JM, Joseph RB, Bodell LS, Nycamp PW, Hessel SJ. Prostaglandin E-1 in hand angiography. *AJR* 1983;141:1043–1046.
10. Jacobs JB, Hanafee WN. The use of priscoline in peripheral arteriography. *AJR* 1965;94:213–220.
11. Yakes WF, Pevsner PH, Reed MD, Donohue HJ, Ghaed N. Serial embolizations of an extremity AVM with alcohol via direct percutaneous puncture. *AJR* 1986;146:1038–1040.
12. Yakes WF, Haas DK, Parker SH, et al. Symptomatic vascular malformations: Ethanol embolotherapy. *Radiology* 1989;170:1059–1066.
13. Yakes WF, Parker SH, Gibson MD, et al. Alcohol embolotherapy of vascular malformations. *Semin Intervent Radiol* 1989;6:146–161.
14. Yakes WF, Luethke JM, Parker SH, et al. Ethanol embolization of vascular malformations. *RadioGraphics* 1990;10:787–796.
15. Yakes WF, Luethke JM, Merland JJ, et al. Ethanol embolization of arteriovenous fistulas: A primary mode of therapy. *Journal of Vascular and Interventional Radiology* 1990;1:89–96.
16. Yakes WF, Parker SH. Diagnosis and management of vascular anomalies. In: Castaneda-Zuniga WR, Tadavarthy SM, eds. *Interventional radiology*. 2nd ed. Baltimore: Williams & Wilkins, 1992;152–189.
17. Edwards EA. Organization of the small arteries of the hand and digits. *Am J Surg* 1960;99:837–846.
18. Coleman SS, Anson BJ. Arterial patterns in the hand based upon a study of 650 specimens. *Surg Gynecol Obstet* 1961;113:409–425.
19. Brockis JG. The blood supply of the flexor tendons of the fingers in man. *J Bone Joint Surg* 1953;35:131–140.
20. Janevski BK. Anatomy of the arterial system of the upper extremities. In: Janevski BK, ed. *Angiography of the upper extremity*. The Hague: Martinus Nijoff, 1982:41–122.
21. McCormack LJ, Cauldwell W, Anson BJ. Brachial and antebrachial arterial patterns: A study of 750 extremities. *Surg Gynecol Obstet* 1953:96:43–54.
22. Keller FS, Rosch J, Dotter C, et al. Proximal origin of radial artery: Potential pitfall in hand angiography. *AJR* 1980;134:169–170.
23. Adachi B. *Das arteriensystem der Japaner. Band 1.* Kyoto: Maruzen, 1928.
24. Tandler J. Zur anatomie der arterien der hand. *Anat Hefte* 1897;7:263–282.
25. Ettien JT, Allen JT, Vargas C. Hypothenar hammer syndrome. *South Med J* 1981;74:491–493.
26. Foster DR, Cameron DC. Hypothenar hammer syndrome. *Br J Radiology* 1981;54:995–996.
27. Vayssairat M, Debure C, Cormier JM. Hypothenar hammer syndrome: Seventeen cases with long term follow-up. *J Vasc Surg* 1987;5:838–843.
28. Janevski BK. Vascular injuries of the upper extremity. In: Janevski BK, ed. *Angiography of the upper extremity*. The Hague: Martinus Nijoff, 1982:123–140.
29. Kadir S. Athanousoulis CA. Peripheral vasospastic disorders: Management with intra-arterial infusion of vasodilatory drugs. In: Athanousoulis CA, Pfister RC, Greene RE, et al, eds. *Interventional radiology*, Philadelphia: WB Saunders, 1982:343–354.
30. Janevski BK. Arterial occlusive disease of the upper extremity. In: *Angiography of the upper extremity*. The Hague: Martinus Nijoff, 1982:179–220.
31. Yao JST, Bergan JJ, Neiman HL. Arteriography for upper extremity and digital ischemia. In: Neiman HL, Yao JST, eds. *Angiography of vascular disease*. New York: Churchill Livingstone, 1985:353–391.
32. Allen EV, Brown GE. Raynaud's disease: A critical review of minimal requisites for diagnosis. *Am J Med Sci* 1932;183:187–200.
33. Metzler M, Silver D. Vasospastic disorders. *Postgrad Med* 1979;65:79–88.
34. Rosch J, Porter JM. Hand angiography of Raynaud's syndrome. *Fortschr Rontgenstr* 1977;127:30–37.
35. Machleder H. Vasoocclusive disorders of the upper extremity. *Curr Probl Surg* 1988;25:7–67.
36. Dabich L, Bookstein JJ, Zweifler A, et al. Digital arteries in patients with scleroderma. *Arch Intern Med* 1972;130:708–714.
37. Rivers SP, Baur GM, Inahara T. Arm ischemia secondary to giant cell arteritis. *Am J Surg* 1982;143:554–558.
38. Winiwarter F. Uber eine eigentum liche Form von Endar-

teriitis mit Gangran des FuBes. *Arch Klin Chir* 1879;23:202–226.
39. Goodwin JN, Berne TV. Symmetrical peripheral gangrene. *Arch Surg* 1974;108:780–784.
40. Andrasch RH, Bardana EJ, Porter JM, et al. Digital ischemia and gangrene preceeding renal neoplasm. *Arch Intern Med* 1976;136:486–488.
41. Hawley PR, Johnston AW, Rankin JT. Association between digital ischaemia and malignant disease. *Br J Med* 1967;3:208–212.
42. Hoffman S, Valderrama E, Gribetz I, et al. Gangrene of the hand in a newborn child. *The Hand* 1974;6:70–73.
43. Billig DM, Hallman GL, Cooley DA. Arterial embolism: Surgical treatment and results. *Arch Surg* 1967;95:1–6.
44. Vohra R, Lieberman DP. Arterial emboli to the arm. *J R Cell Surg Edinb* 1991;36:83–85.
45. Conn J Jr. Thoracic outlet syndromes. *Surg Clin North Am* 1974;54:144–164.
46. Mathes SJ, Salam AA. Subclavian artery aneurysm: Sequelae of thoracic outlet syndrome. *Surgery* 1974;76:506–510.
47. Dunant JH. Effort thrombosis, a complication of thoracic outlet syndrome. *Vasa* 1981;10:322–324.
48. Banis JC, Rich N, Whelan TJ. Ischemia of the upper extremity due to noncardiac emboli. *Am J Surg* 1977;134:131–139.
49. Kleinert HE, Burget GC, Morgan JA, Kutz JE, Atasoy E. Aneurysms of the hand. *Arch Surg* 1973;106:554–557.
50. O'Connor RL. Digital nerve compression secondary to palmar aneurysm. *Clin Orthop* 1972;83:149–150.
51. McClinton MA. Tumors and aneurysms of the upper extremity. *Hand Clin* 1993;9:151–169.
52. Suzuki K, Takahashi S, Nakagawa T. False aneurysm in a digital artery. *J Hand Surg* 1980;5:402–403.
53. Swanson E, Freiberg A, Salter DR. Radial artery infections and aneurysms after catheterization. *J Hand Surg* 1990; 15A:166–171.
54. Thio RT. False aneurysm of the ulnar artery after surgery employing a tourniquet. *Am J Surg* 1972;123:604–605.
55. May JW, Grossman JAI, Costas B. Cyanotic painful index and long fingers associated with an asymptomatic ulnar artery aneurysm: Case report. *J Hand Surg* 1982;7A:622–625.
56. Melhoff TL, Wood MB. Ulnar artery thrombosis and the role of interpositional vein grafting: Patency with microsurgical technique. *J Hand Surg* 1991;16A:274–278.
57. Haimovici H. Peripheral arterial embolism: Study of 330 unselected cases of embolization of extremities. *Angiology* 1950;1:20–36.
58. Harris RW, Andros G, Dulawa LB, et al. Large vessel arterial occlusive disease in symptomatic upper extremity. *Arch Surg* 1984;119:1227–1282.
59. Fisher CM. A new vascular syndrome: The subclavian steal. *New Engl J Med* 1961;265:912–913.
60. Yakes WF, Kumpe DA, Parker SH, et al. Angioplasty of the infrarenal abdominal aorta. *Semin Intervent Radiol* 1989;6:129–137.
61. Yakes WF, Kumpe DA, Brown SB, et al. Percutaneous transluminal aortic angioplasty: Techniques and results. *Radiology* 1989;172:965–970.
62. Beebe HG, Stark R, Johnson ML, Jolly PC, Hill LD. Choices of operation for subclavian-vertebral arterial disease. *Am J Surg* 1980;139:616–623.
63. Becker GJ. Non-coronary angioplasty. *Radiology* 1989; 170:921–940.
64. Theron J. Angioplasty of supraaortic arteries. *Semin Intervent Radiol* 1987;4:331–342.
65. Vitek JJ. Subclavian artery angioplasty and the origin of the vertebral artery. *Radiology* 1989;170:407–409.
66. Motarjeme A, Keifer JW, Zuska AJ, Nabawi P. Percutaneous transluminal angioplasty for subclavian steal. *Radiology* 1985;155:611–613.
67. Burke DR, Gordon RL, Mishkin JD, McLean GK, Meranze SG. Percutaneous transluminal angioplasty of subclavian arteries. *Radiology* 1987;164:699–704.
68. Erbstein RA, Wholey MH, Smoot S. Subclavian artery steal syndrome: Treatment by percutaneous transluminal angioplasty. *AJR* 1988;151:291–294.
69. Tsai FY, Matovich V, Hieshima G, et al. Percutaneous transluminal angioplasty of the carotid artery. *AJNR* 1986;7:349–358.
70. Wingo JP, Nix ML, Greenfield LJ, Barnes RW. The blue toe syndrome: Hemodynamics and therapeutic correlates of outcome. *J Vasc Surg* 1986;3:475–480.
71. Karmody AM, Powers SR, Monaco VJ, Leather RP. "Blue toe" syndrome: An indication for limb salvage surgery. *Arch Surg* 1976;111:1263–1268.
72. Lee BY, Brancata RF, Thoden WR, Madden JL. Blue digit syndrome: Urgent indication for limb salvage surgery. *Am J Surg* 1984;147:418–422.
73. Kempezinski RF. Lower extremity arterial emboli from ulcerating atherosclerotic plaques. *J Amer Med Assoc* 1979;241:807–810.
74. Brenowitz JB, Edward WS. The management of atheromatous emboli to the lower extremities. *Surg Gynecol Obstet* 1976;143:941–945.
75. Roon AJ, Sauvage LR. Blue toe syndrome: A warning sign of unsuspected vascular injury. *Surgery* 1983;93:722–724.
76. Darsee JR. Cholesterol embolization: The great masquerader. *South Med J* 1979;72:174–180.
77. Harvey JC. Cholesterol crystal microembolization: A cause of the restless leg syndrome. *South Med J* 1976;69:269–272.
78. Mehigan JT, Stoney RJ. Arterial microemboli and fibromuscular dysplasia of the external iliac arteries. *Surgery* 1977;81:484–486.
79. Samuels PB, Katz DJ. Diagnosis and management of arterial mural thromboemboli. *Am J Surg* 1977;134:209–213.
80. Kumpe DA, Zwerdlinger S, Griffin DJ. Blue digit syndrome: Treatment with percutaneous transluminal angioplasty. *Radiology* 1988;166:37–44.
81. Brewer ML, Kinnison ML, Perler BA, White RI Jr. Blue toe syndrome: Treatment with anticoagulants and delayed percutaneous transluminal angioplasty. *Radiology* 1988;166:31–36.
82. Paletta FX. Venous gangrene of the hand. *Plast Reconstr Surg* 1981;67:67–69.
83. Smith BM, Shield GW, Riddell DH, et al. Venous gangrene of the upper extremity. *Am Surg* 1985;201:511–519.
84. Nemmers DW, Thorpe PE, Knibbe MA, et al. Upper extremity venous thrombosis: Case report and literature review. *Orthop Rev* 1990;19:164–172.
85. Horattas MC, Wright DJ, Fenton OH, et al. Changing concepts of deep venous thrombosis of the upper extremity: Report of a series and review of the literature. *Surgery* 1988;104:561–566.
86. Fraschini G, et al. Local urokinase infusion for the lysis of subclavian venous thrombi associated with central venous catheters. *Proc ASCO* 1992;11:788–793.
87. Semba CP, Dake MD. Aggressive therapy of iliofemoral deep venous thrombosis using catheter directed thrombolysis. *Radiology* 1994;191:487–494.
88. Putnam JS. Superior vena cava syndrome associated with massive thrombosis: Treatment with expandable wire stents. *Radiology* 1988;167:727–728.
89. Decker DG, Fish CR, Juergens JL. Arteriovenous fistulas of the female pelvis. *Obstet Gynecol* 1968;31:799–805.
90. Szilagyi DE, Smith RF, Elliott JP, Hageman JH. Congenital arteriovenous anomalies of the limbs. *Arch Surg* 1976; 111:423–429.
91. Flye MW, Jordan BP, Schwartz MZ. Management of congenital arteriovenous malformations. *Surgery* 1983;94:740–747.
92. Mulliken JB, Glowacki J. Hemangiomas and vascular malformations in infants and children: A classification based on endothelial characteristics. *Plast Reconst Surg* 1982;69:412–420.
93. Mulliken JB, Zetter BR, Folkman J. In vitro characteristics of endothelium from hemangiomas and vascular malformations. *Surgery* 1982;92:348–353.
94. Glowacki J, Mulliken JB. Mast cells in hemangiomas and vascular malformations. *Pediatrics* 1982;70:48–51.
95. Finn MC, Glowacki J, Mulliken JB. Congenital vascular le-

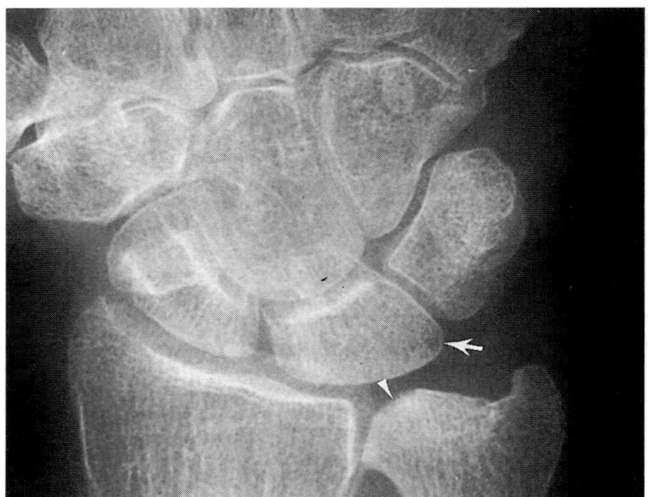

FIGURE 20–1. PA radiograph of the right wrist. Cortical loss and subchondral sclerosis involve the radial aspect of the distal articular surface of the ulna (arrowhead). An ovoid subcortical radiolucency is within the proximal ulnar corner of the lunate (arrow).

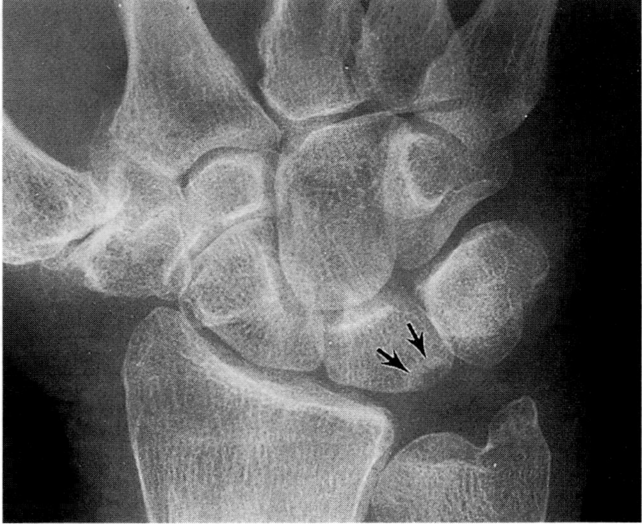

FIGURE 20–3. PA radiograph of the right wrist with the wrist held in slight radial deviation. In the proximal ulnar aspect of the lunate is a small subcortical lucency with sclerosis surrounding its distal margin (arrows). The small well-corticated avulsed bone fragment adjacent to the ulnar styloid process and deformity of the ulnar styloid process are due to previous trauma. Severe degenerative joint disease involves the first CMC joint space.

ulnar impaction syndrome may also occur in the presence of neutral ulnar variance.[1]

The causes of ulnar positive variance include congenital ulnar positive variance (most common), premature closure of the distal radial physis,[8] "normal variant long ulna with occupational overload" (in occupations or sports where rotational or ulnar deviation loading is required),[9] and trauma that involves the distal radius and ulna, such as Colles's fracture, Galeazzi's fracture, Essex–Lopresti fracture–dislocation, or radial head resection (from an abnormality of the interosseous membrane that allows shortening of the radius). Furthermore, patients with Colles's fractures may also develop altered biomechanical loading at the ulnocarpal articulation due to malunion of the fracture resulting in dorsal tilt of the distal radial articular surface.

Before determining a therapeutic regimen for ulnocarpal impaction, one must distinguish this entity from other disorders that cause ulnar-sided wrist pain, most commonly problems of the TFC, TFCC, LT ligament, or distal radioulnar joint (DRUJ) malfunction. Conservative treatment, consisting of abstinence from the activities that exacerbate the patient's discomfort and anti-inflammatory medication, is the initial therapeutic regimen employed.

If nonoperative treatment is unsuccessful, surgical options in those with a normal DRUJ include: (1) ulnar shortening in those with ulnar positive variance or ulnar neutral variance,[9] (2) distal radial osteotomy in those with a malunited distal radial fracture result-

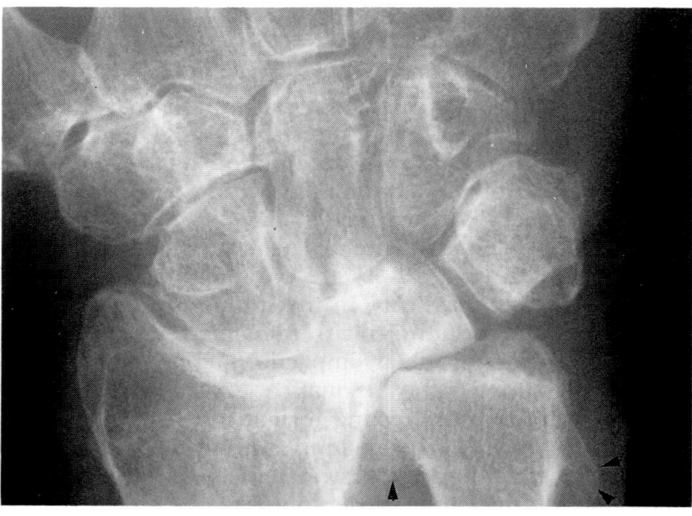

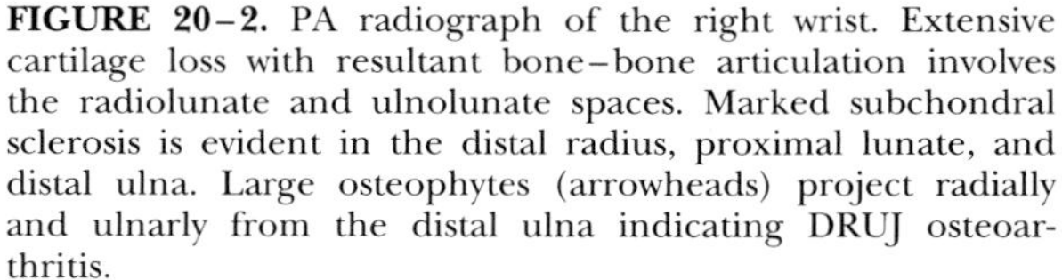

FIGURE 20–2. PA radiograph of the right wrist. Extensive cartilage loss with resultant bone–bone articulation involves the radiolunate and ulnolunate spaces. Marked subchondral sclerosis is evident in the distal radius, proximal lunate, and distal ulna. Large osteophytes (arrowheads) project radially and ulnarly from the distal ulna indicating DRUJ osteoarthritis.

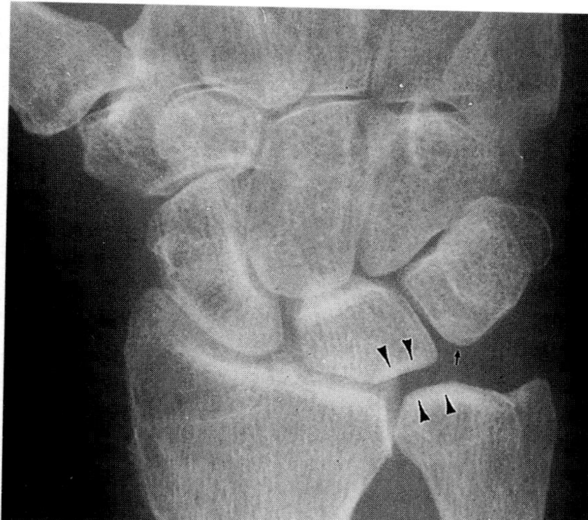

FIGURE 20–4. PA radiograph of the right wrist. Flattening and subcortical sclerosis are present at the proximal lunar and distal ulnar articular surfaces (arrowheads). Loss of normal cortical medullary junction associated with vague increased density in the radial edge of the triquetrum (small arrow) suggests that reactive bone formation from ulnar impaction also involves the triquetrum.

ing in dorsal tilt of the distal radial articular surface,[9] and (3) wafer procedure, consisting of resection of the distal part of the ulnar head that does not serve as the attachment for the TFC.[6,7] In those patients with painful DRUJ involvement, a matched ulnar resection of Bowers's type[9] or Suavé–Kapandji procedure, i.e., arthrodesis of the DRUJ with resection of a portion of the distal ulnar shaft, is the treatment of choice of some authors.[1]

In summary, ulnar impaction syndrome is a painful condition with abnormalities usually demonstrable with some type(s) of imaging study(ies). The presence of imaging changes characteristic of this syndrome does not mean the patient is symptomatic, since these changes can commonly develop as people age. Symptoms in the ulnocarpal area have to be analyzed closely in light of clinical findings for effective treatment.

ULNAR IMPINGEMENT

Although much of the literature uses the terms ulnar impingement and ulnar impaction interchangeably, they are two distinct entities that are mutually exclusive.[1] Whereas ulnar impaction is primarily due to

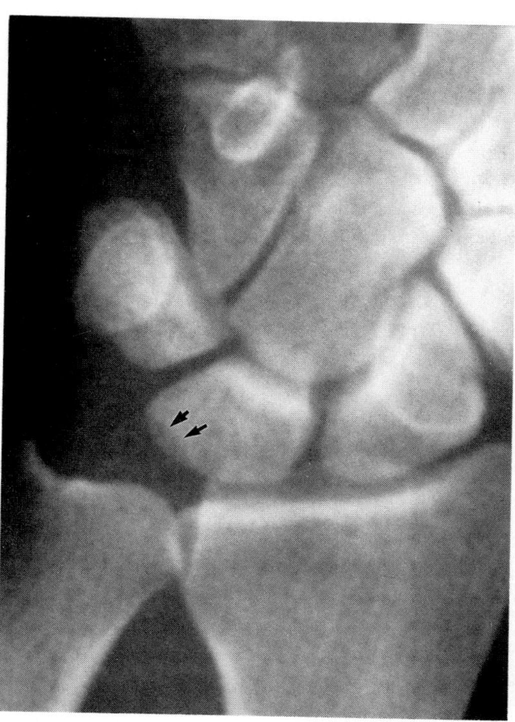

A

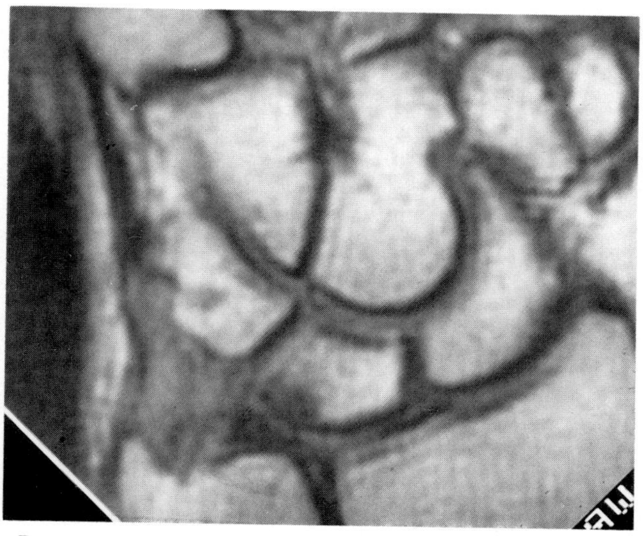

B

FIGURE 20–5. A: PA fluoroscopic spot of the left wrist with the wrist held in radial deviation. Subtle radiolucencies are present along the ulnar aspect of the proximal pole of the lunate (arrows). **B:** Coronal T1-weighted spin echo image of the left wrist, TR 500 msec, TE 30 msec, obtained 2 weeks after the plain radiographs in **A.** A focus of intermediate-signal intensity in the proximal pole of the lunate corresponds to the radiolucent area seen on plain radiography. This finding is characteristic of ulnar impaction changes and not avascular necrosis (see text).

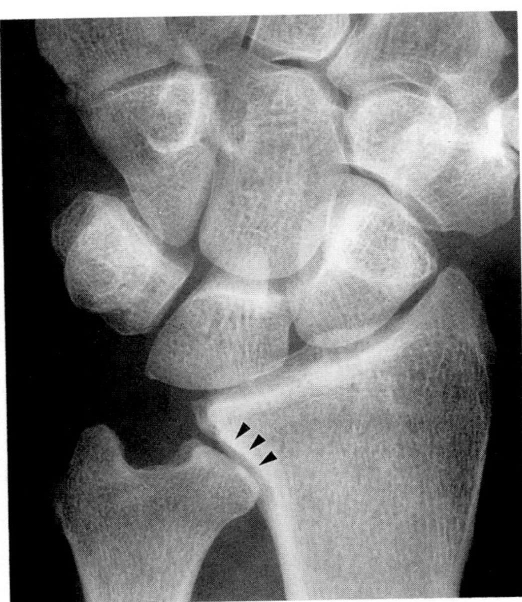

FIGURE 20–6. PA radiograph of the left wrist with the wrist held in minimal radial deviation. Prominent ulnar minus variance is present. Scalloping along the ulnar margin of the distal radius cephalad to the sigmoid notch represents the DRUJ. The fact that normal parallelism (arrowheads) exists between the radius and ulna with no obvious osteophytes, and the ulnar head has an unusual shape with a much larger fovea at the ulnar styloid base indicates these are congenital changes, or changes that developed very early in life.

ulnar positive variance with abnormalities between the adjacent articulating surfaces of the ulna and radius, lunate, and/or triquetrum, ulnar impingement is characterized by a shortened distal ulna that articulates with the distal radius proximal to the sigmoid notch (Fig. 20–6)[2,10] Perhaps the initial confusion has resulted from the similar clinical presentation of these two groups of patients. As in ulnar impaction, patients with painful ulnar impingement present with ulnar-sided wrist pain and there may be wrist clicking. However, in contrast to ulnar impaction patients, the latter group has been noted to have a narrow wrist on physical examination.[10]

Most often, a markedly shortened distal ulna results from prior surgical resection secondary to prior wrist trauma, rheumatoid arthritis, or correction of Madelung's deformity.[10] However, none of these entities results in the typical appearance shown in Fig. 20–6, since the DRUJ in Fig. 20–6 developed since childhood. Such development early in life is evidenced by alteration of the sigmoid notch without much, if any, osteoarthritis. Less commonly, ulnar impingement may be present in de novo cases of negative ulnar variance or premature fusion of the distal ulna secondary to prior trauma.

Most cases of ulnar impingement such as that shown in Fig. 20–6 are normal variants. When osteoarthritis involves the distal radioulnar articulation, and/or pain is localized at this joint, then a painful ulnar impingement may be present. Otherwise a major point to realize with this condition is that ulnar lengthening is contraindicated in this entity because it may create ulnar impingement syndrome. Slopes of the DRUJ vary considerably; therefore, whenever ulnar lengthening is contemplated, careful evaluation of the shape of the DRUJ on the plain PA radiograph should be performed to ensure that impingement will not be created surgically.

CARPAL BOSS, CARPE BOSSU, DORSAL BOSS

The carpal boss is a bony protuberance located on the dorsum of the wrist at the level of the second and third carpometacarpal (CMC) joints. Most often the deformity is caused by dorsal bony prominences on both sides of the CMC joints, but the prominence may also be caused by an os styloideum, an accesory ossicle, or by degenerative osteophytes.

Pain is the presenting symptom and is likely due to adjacent bursitis, osteoarthritis, extensor tendons slipping over the bony prominence, and/or a ganglion.[11] An additional cause of pain is a fracture of one of the bony prominences or osteophytes.

The carpal boss is most easily detected on a lateral roentgenograph with the wrist in 30 degrees of supination and ulnar deviation.[11] However, in some cases the carpal boss will be detectable on a conventional lateral roentgenograph of the wrist (Fig. 20–7). Oc-

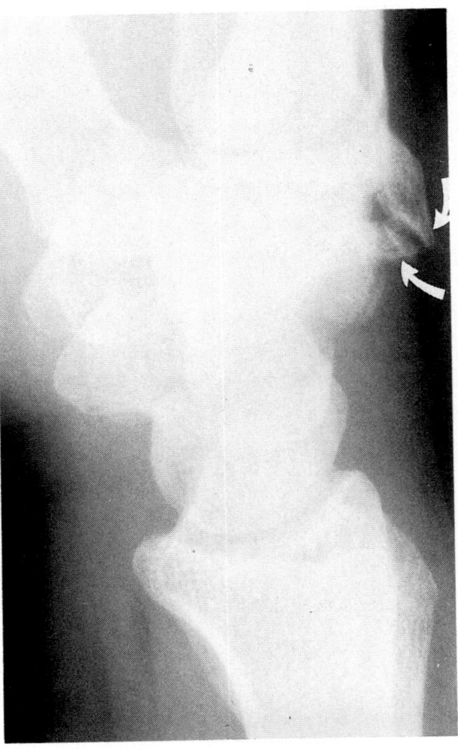

FIGURE 20–7. Lateral wrist radiograph. Two large osteophytes (arrows) project dorsally at the level of the CMC joint.

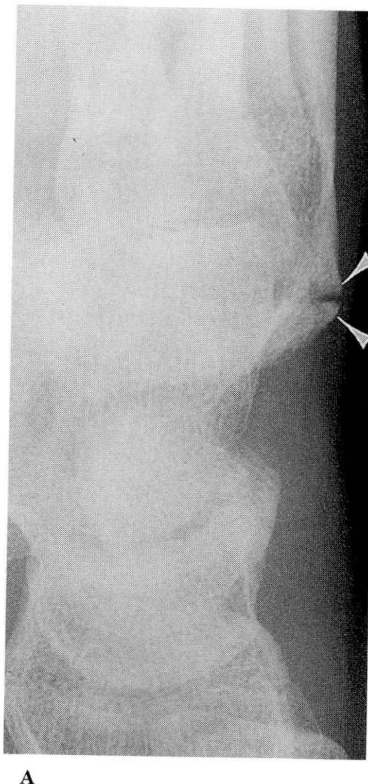

A

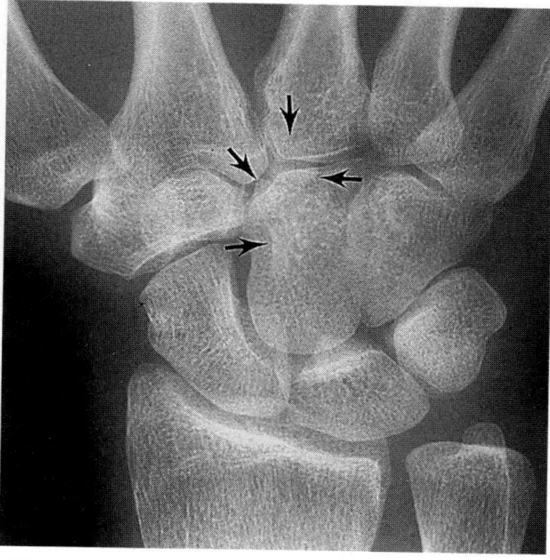

B

FIGURE 20–8. A: Lateral radiograph of the right wrist. Large bony prominences (arrowheads) project dorsally at the CMC joint level. **B:** PA radiograph of the right wrist in the same patient as in **A.** The large exostoses arise from the capitate and the third metacarpal base (arrows).

casionally, findings can be confirmed on the PA roentgenograph (Figs. 20–8A and 20–8B) but often no abnormality will be evident on the PA view.

If bone scintigraphy is performed with or without the presence of symptoms related to the boss, focal increased uptake may be detected in the dorsal carpal boss. Therefore, knowledge about this entity is helpful when interpreting bone scintigrams.

Conservative therapy consists of restricted use of the wrist coupled with the administration of nonsteroidal antiinflammatory medication. If this fails, surgical excision of the bony prominence or overlying bursa has been shown to yield excellent results.[12] If the pain results from a fracture and pain does not resolve with time, the fracture fragment may have to be removed.

KIENBÖCK'S DISEASE

Kienböck's disease, also known as lunatomalacia, refers to avascular necrosis (AVN) of the lunate. Its association with negative ulnar variance is controversial. Although several authors have reported an association with ulnar minus variance,[13] others have found a similar distribution of ulnar minus variance among those with lunatomalacia and in control subjects.[14] Other factors, including sports-related and work-related trauma[15] and the vascularity of the lunate,[16–18] have been implicated in lunatomalacia.

The clinical presentation consists of wrist pain, limited range of motion, decreased grip strength, and mild to marked synovial inflammation.[19]

Radiographically, four stages of lunatomalacia have been described by Decoulx and colleagues[20]: Stage I—osteosclerosis of the lunate with preservation of its shape (Fig. 20–9A); Stage II—cystic change within the lunate; Stage III—subchondral collapse and fragmentation of the lunate (Fig. 20–9B); and Stage IV—secondary perilunate osteoarthritis.

An alternative staging system, the modified Stahl classification, is based on the premise that Kienböck's disease results from devascularization of the lunate secondary to a stress fracture of the lunate. According to this scheme, the five roentgenographic stages of lunatomalacia are the following: Stage I—compression fracture of the lunate manifesting as either a radiolucent or a radiodense line; Stage II—rarefaction along the line of the compression fracture; Stage III—changes of Stages I and II, along with sclerosis of the proximal pole of the lunate; Stage IV—fragmentation or flattening of the lunate (Fig. 20–10); and Stage V—secondary perilunate arthritis.[20]

The third and probably most common classification used is that of Lichtman. Stage zero is radiographically occult on plain films but MRI or bone scan is abnormal; Stage I—linear or compression fracture, but otherwise normal; Stage II—abnormal density, without lunate collapse; Stage III—lunate collapse; and Stage IV—perilunate osteoarthritis.

Conventional roentgenographs may be sufficient to establish the diagnosis of lunatomalacia. However, in cases of roentgenographically occult disease, bone scintigraphy and MRI have been shown to be more sensitive.[21–24]

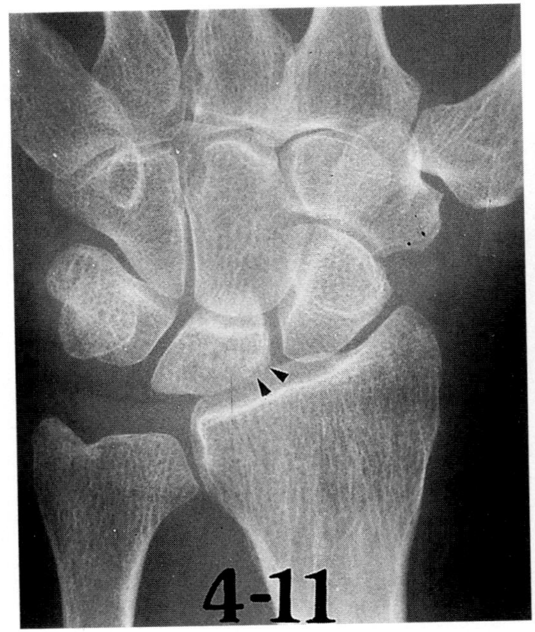

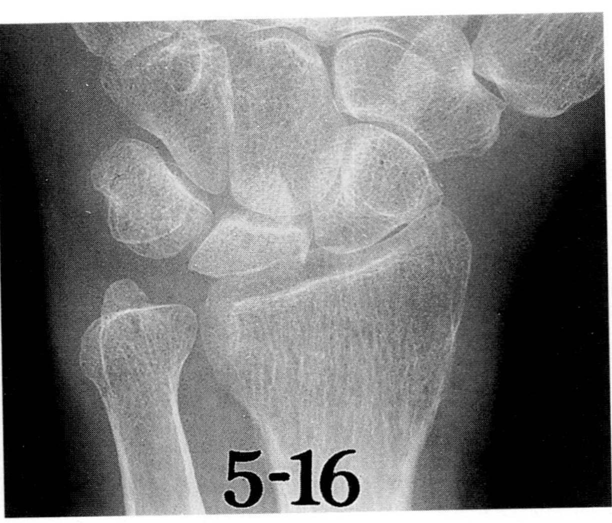

A B

FIGURE 20-9. A: PA radiograph of the left wrist. Mild diffuse sclerosis involves the lunate which makes this Stage I (Decoulx). However, the proximal curvature of the lunate has slight concavities (arrowheads) suggesting early collapse, which would make this Stage III (Decoulx or Lichtman). **B:** PA radiograph of the left wrist, same patient, approximately 1 month later. In the interim, osteosclerosis of the lunate has progressed, but some of this increased density may be due to interval development of marked collapse of the proximal articular surface of the lunate. This would be Decoulx Stage III, modified Stahl Stage IV, or Lichtman Stage III.

Traditionally, AVN has been described as an area of relatively low signal on both T1- and T2-weighted images. More recently, however, both low and high signal intensity have been seen with AVN of the lunate on T2-weighted images, depending on the stage of the disease. This parallels the Mitchell classification described for AVN of the femoral head.[24] However, the exact significance of lunate bone marrow edema with decreased signal on T1-weighted and increased signal on T2-weighted images is uncertain. It is not known if this pattern will act as a "bone bruise," as it does elsewhere in the body, or if Kienböck's disease will result (see Chapter 17). Furthermore, MRI may be helpful in assessing the lunate for revascularization during treatment.[25,26] In most instances, computed tomography (CT) has been replaced by MRI for establishing the diagnosis of lunatomalacia. An exception arises when additional bony detail of the lunate is required to separate focal patterns of lunate pathology from more diffuse disease. This will be discussed subsequently.

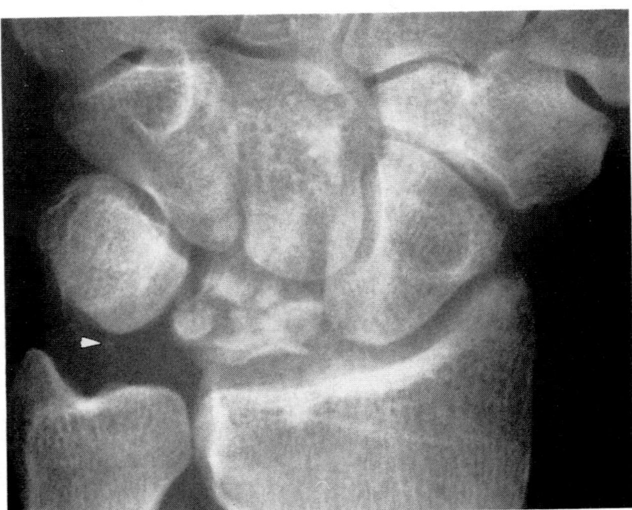

FIGURE 20-10. PA radiograph of the left wrist. The lunate is diffusely sclerotic and fragmented. A small unnamed ossicle (arrowhead) is adjacent to the triquetrum.

Radiographically, it is necessary to distinguish lunatomalacia from other pathology within the lunate. These conditions have different origins and treatments than Kienböck's disease. The distribution of these radiographic changes within the lunate is the key to distinguishing these conditions from Kienböck's disease (Fig. 20-11).

Several radiologic patterns of intraosseous lunate disease described by Gilula, Higgs, Hsieh, and Weeks[27] include: (1) a radial-sided lucency that communicates with the scapholunate joint space representing either a ganglion, fluid-filled cavity with or without a cyst wall, or collection of fibrous tissue (Figs. 20-12A to 20-12C); (2) a central proximal radiolucent defect that communicates with the radio-

Text continued on page 531

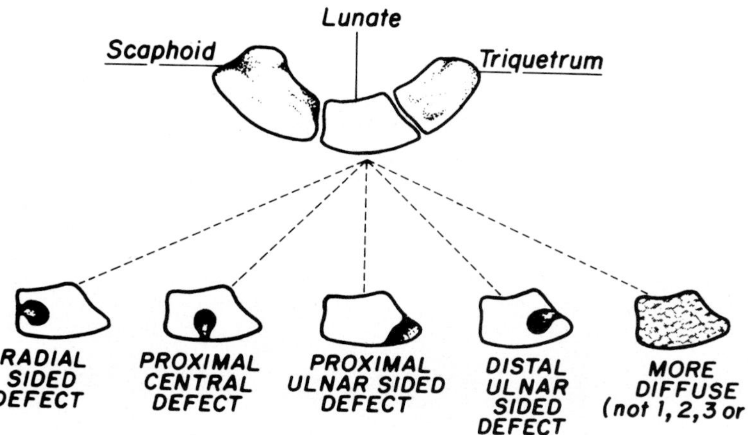

FIGURE 20–11. Five patterns of lunate abnormalities (see text).

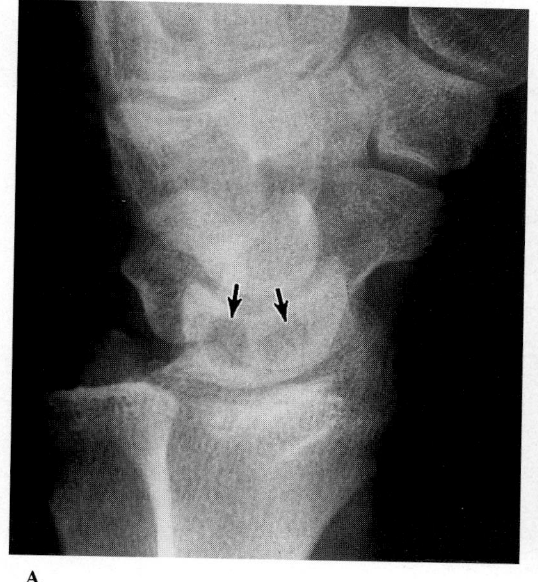

A

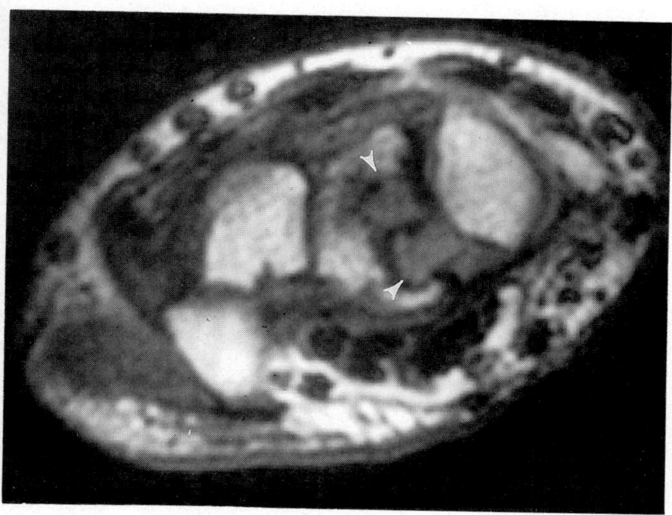

B

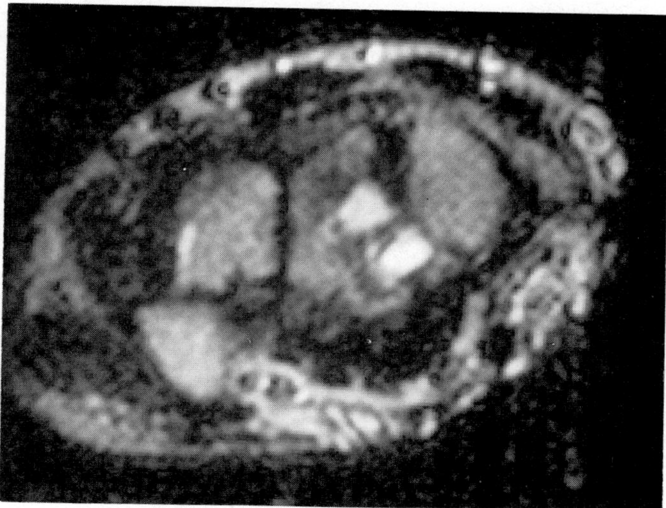

C

FIGURE 20–12. A: Off-lateral radiograph of the left wrist. Two well-circumscribed radiolucencies are present within the lunate (arrows). **B:** Axial T1-weighted MRI of the left wrist, TR 780 msec, TE 30 msec, same patient. A bilobed mass of intermediate signal intensity is present within the lunate (arrowheads). The lesion involves the radial aspect of the lunate and abuts the scapholunate joint space. **C:** Axial T2-weighted MRI of the left wrist, TR 3000 msec, TE 90 msec, same patient. High-signal intensity is present within the bilobed lunate lesion. The signal characteristics on T1- and T2-weighted images indicate that this is a fluid-filled lesion suggesting fluid or intraosseous ganglia. (Reprinted with permission from Gilula LA, Higgs PE, Hsieh P, Weeks PM. Imaging classification of lunate disease: An evolving spectrum. *Radiology* 1995, submitted.)

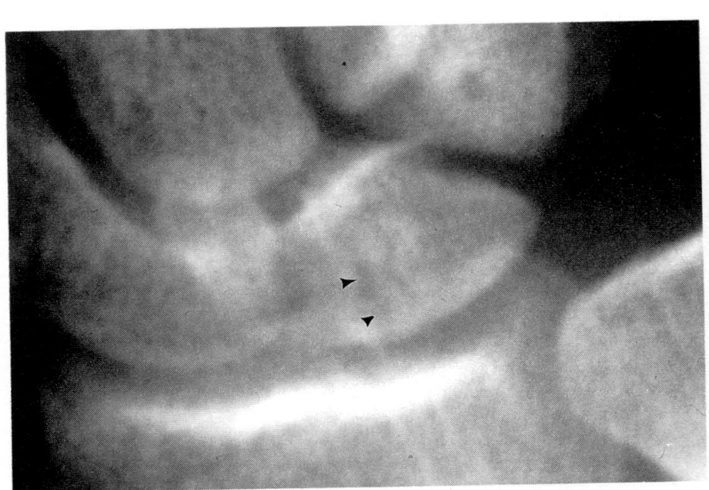

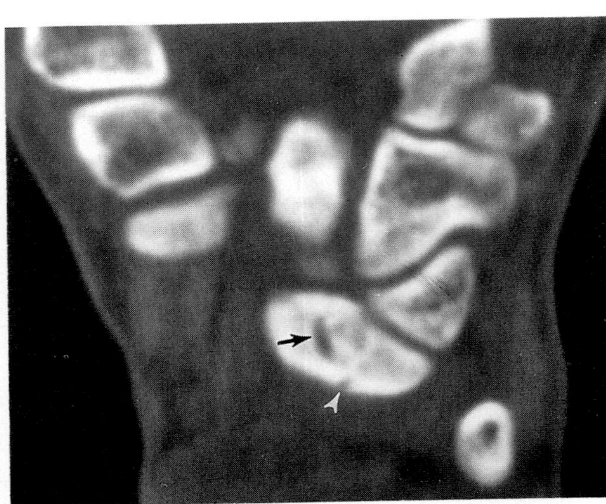

A B

FIGURE 20–13. A: Detailed obliqued PA fluoroscopic spot of the right lunate. A serpiginous radiolucency is present within the proximal pole of the lunate (arrowheads). **B:** Coronal CT of the right wrist. A central radiolucency within the proximal pole of the lunate possibly represents a vascular groove (arrow). A small subcortical triangular-shaped lucency probably indicates the connection of the more central radiolucency to the radiolunate joint (arrowhead). (Reprinted with permission from Gilula LA, Higgs PE, Hsieh P, Weeks PM. Imaging classification of lunate disease: An evolving spectrum. *Radiology* 1995, submitted.)

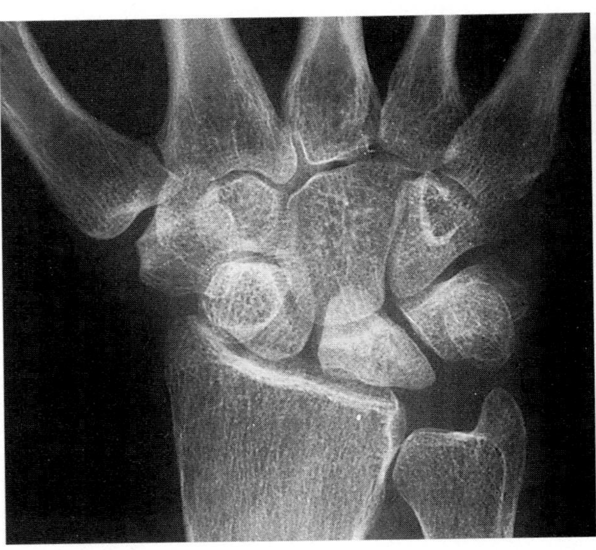

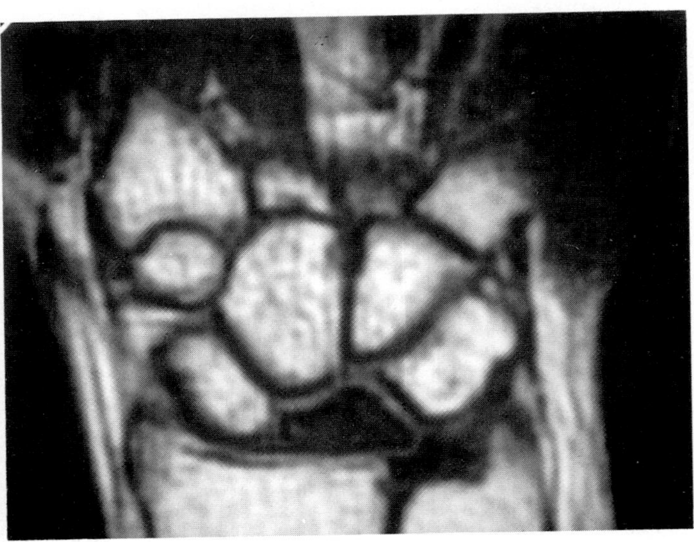

A B

FIGURE 20–14. A: PA radiograph of the right wrist. Uniform and diffuse sclerosis is present within a collapsed lunate compatible with Kienböck's disease. **B:** Coronal T1-weighted MRI of the right wrist, TR 500 msec, TE 23 msec, same patient, obtained 2 weeks after the plain radiograph performed for academic interest. Diffuse low to absent signal intensity is present within the lunate, consistent with Kienböck's disease. No T2 image was obtained since this was an old case and currently we do not routinely perform MRI on obvious cases like this. (Reprinted with permission from Gilula LA, Higgs PE, Hsieh P, Weeks PM. Imaging classification of lunate disease: An evolving spectrum. *Radiology* 1995, submitted.)

lunate joint space possibly representing a vascular groove (Figs. 20–13A and 20–13B); (3) a lucent or sclerotic focus within the proximal ulnar aspect of the lunate related to ulnar impaction syndrome (see Fig. 20–3) and/or aging; (4) a lucent defect within the distal ulnar aspect of the lunate that communicates with the LT joint space, possibly representing a fluid-filled cavity, fibrous defect, or ganglion similar to the radial-sided focal lunate defect; and (5) a more diffuse lucent or sclerotic defect within the lunate representing Kienböck's disease (Figs. 20–14A and 20–14B). Whereas a number of surgical options exist for Kienböck's disease, these first four entities require, at most, opening of the radiolucent defect or local curettage,[27] or a selection of treatment choices described earlier if ulnar impaction syndrome is deemed the cause of the lunate changes.

In addition to these five changes, other alterations have been recognized, and still others will undoubtedly be recognized, also. Figure 21–1C (see Chapter 21) shows a different pattern related to ulnar impaction syndrome. As mentioned above, it is uncertain if the MRI pattern of decreased signal in T1 and increased signal in T2 compatible with bone marrow edema will resolve or progress to obvious Kienböck's disease. We have personally seen this pattern of edema associated with the same pattern involving the capitate head. In one other symptomatic patient, we have seen thin tracks of decreased signal in T1 and increased signal in T2, suggesting edema in a vascular pattern. This pattern became normal on follow-up. We do not know the explanation for this final pattern.[27]

Management and prognosis of lunatomalacia depend on the stage at which it is detected.[22] The outcome for functional recovery is best for those patients presenting before collapse of the lunate.[26]

Some authors advocate immobilization for Stage I disease.[19] However, long-term studies have shown that these patients do progress to severe disease, often requiring arthrodesis later.[28,29] These results seem to suggest that surgical intervention is indicated even in the earliest stages of Kienböck's disease. However, with the advent of MRI and thus earlier detection of Kienböck's disease, anecdotal comments at wrist meetings query the appropriateness of casting or unloading with traction as a viable treatment plan.

The goal for treatment of Kienböck's disease before osteoarthritis is to unload the compressive forces on the lunate. This may be accomplished by any one of the following surgical options: (1) distal forearm osteotomy, particularly if significant negative ulnar variance is present.[19] Radial shortening or ulnar lengthening osteotomies have both been very successful, albeit not without complications[30–32]; (2) capitate–hamate fusion of Chuinard and Zeman[17]; (3) shortening of the capitate at its waist with capitohamate fusion[17]; and (4) triscaphe arthrodesis.[17]

Several salvage procedures exist for those patients who have later stages of Kienböck's disease; (1) excision of the lunate with or without placement of a tendon spacer[33,34]; (2) proximal row carpectomy[17,19,35]; (3) limited intercarpal fusion[19,35]; and (4) total wrist fusion.[17,19,35] Lunate silicone arthroplasty has become a less desirable treatment option because of subsequent particulate synovitis, prosthesis dislocation, and/or persistent pain after placement of the prosthetic device and the incidence of particulate synovitis.[36,37]

PARTICULATE SYNOVITIS

Many complications have been recognized with increasing frequency since the advent of silicone polymer implants. Synovitis, often more occult than subluxation, dislocation, or fracture of the prosthetic components, is now recognized as a common entity.[38] Detritic or foreign-body synovitis typically manifests with swelling and severe unexplained pain that may

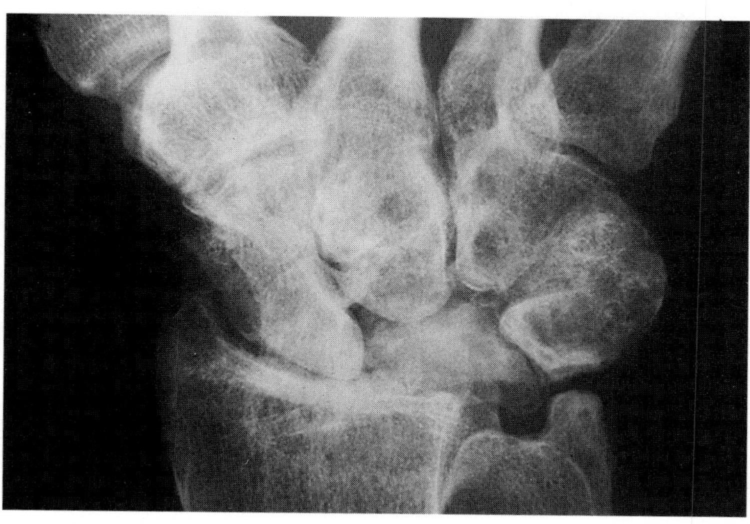

FIGURE 20–15. PA radiograph of the right wrist. A silastic prosthesis replaces the lunate. Large cyst-like defects are identified at least within the distal radius, ulnar styloid process, triquetrum, pisiform, capitate, and hamate, consistent with the diagnosis of detritic synovitis. Osseous densities overlying the amorphous lunate prosthesis are due to residual ventral bone fragments in extrinsic ligaments that attached to the lunate.

mimic infection and/or calcium pyrophosphate dihydrate deposition disease (CPPD).[39–42] Although synovitis is most often recognized as a late complication of arthroplasty, the literature does contain reports denoting its onset within a few months of arthroplasty.[41–43]

Radiographic features, first reported in 1985, include primarily lytic lesions that must be distinguished from degenerative lucent defects that may be a natural progression of the patient's underlying condition.[38,44] This diagnostic dilemma is exacerbated by the fact that the roentgenographic features of particulate synovitis also progress until the inciting object is removed. The lytic lesions may or may not appear in carpal bones directly adjacent to the implant.[38] Typically, the lytic lesions are well defined with thin, sclerotic margins (Fig. 20–15). Well-defined marginal articular erosions may also be present. Surrounding bone mineralization is normal.[45,46] When the treating surgeon desires preoperatively to determine extent of the particulate synovitis, CT can be used successfully to show more extensive involvement than plain radiographs. Deformity, dislocation, or decreased size of the implant may be present.[46] However, more typically the prosthesis will appear grossly intact.[43,47] Although many patients with radiographically evident lytic lesions will be symptomatic, some patients will have no painful clinical correlate for the radiographic changes.[38,48]

Synovitis is identified in areas of silicone debris. Abraded particles are believed to be directly related to repeated compressive loading and shearing.[49] Debris exists in both intracellular and extracellular locations.[50] Although many particles are in the immediate vicinity of the implant, debris is also detected at sites distant from the implant.[50] Histologically, multinucleated foreign-body giant cells surround shedded particulate debris.[49]

Removal of the implant and synovectomy of all involved tissues are indicated once the diagnosis of particulate synovitis is established.[41,46] Removal of the implant arrests the progressive destructive process.[46,47] Therefore, patients should be followed with radiographs for the earliest possible detection and treatment of synovitis.

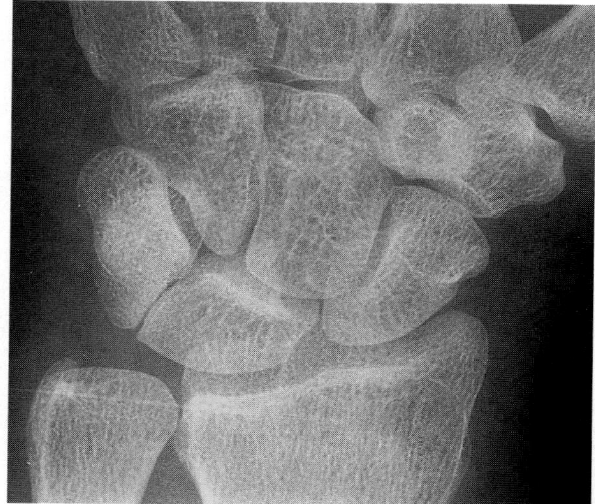

FIGURE 20–16. PA radiograph of the left wrist. Fibrous or cartilaginous LT coalition is present. This is coalition and not degenerative joint disease, as evidenced by the narrowed LT joint without associated osteophytes or subcortical sclerosis as would be found if this LT joint were narrowed because of osteoarthritis. This was considered to be an isolated form of carpal coalition, since the patient reported no other skeletal or extraskeletal abnormalities.

CARPAL COALITION (FAILURE OF SEGMENTATION)

Congenital coalition of the carpus may occur as part of a syndrome or as an isolated entity. Isolated carpal coalition tends to involve bones within the same carpal row and is usually limited to two bones (Fig. 20–16). When associated with a congenital syndrome, carpal coalition tends to involve more than two bones and tends to bridge bones within both carpal rows.[51,52]

Carpal coalition results from failure of segmentation or incomplete segmentation of the embryologic cartilaginous carpus.[51,52] The exception to this occurs with the extremely rare pisohamate coalition, which is probably due to metaplasia of the pisohamate ligament, the structure linking the sesamoid (pisiform) to the hamate.[53,54]

LT coalition is by far the most common carpal coalition. With an incidence of 0.1% to 9%,[56] it frequently is bilateral.[53] The Minaar classification describes four types of LT coalition: Type I—proximal pseudarthrosis; Type II—fusion proximally with a notch distally; Type III—complete fusion; Type IV—complete fusion with associated abnormalities (Figs. 20–17A to 20–17D).[51,52]

Although it is almost always an incidental finding, LT coalition Type I may be symptomatic at the level of the segmentation defect.[51] Bone scintigraphy, typically normal in the setting of carpal coalition, may demonstrate increased activity at the site of the coalition (Figs. 20–18A and 20–18B). Increased radiotracer activity on bone scintigraphy and pain are the distinguishing features that separate an uncomplicated carpal coalition from one complicated by the presence of a pseudarthrosis as can develop posttrauma. Symptomatic arthritis may develop in cases of incomplete coalition of the LT joint and may also contribute to the presence of increased radiotracer activity at the site of coalition on radionuclide imaging.[55]

A widened scapholunate joint space, with an intact scapholunate ligament, may occur as a normal variant in the presence of LT coalition.[56] Wrist arthrography may demonstrate any remnant of a LT joint space or a fracture of a developmental or congenital crevice at the site of the coalition (Fig. 20–18C).

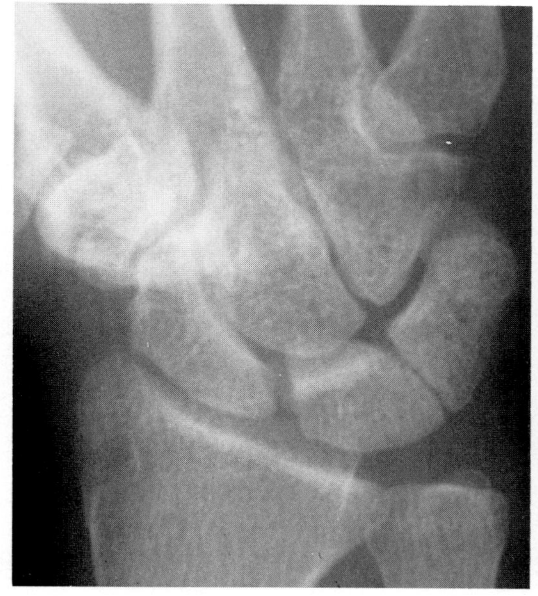

A

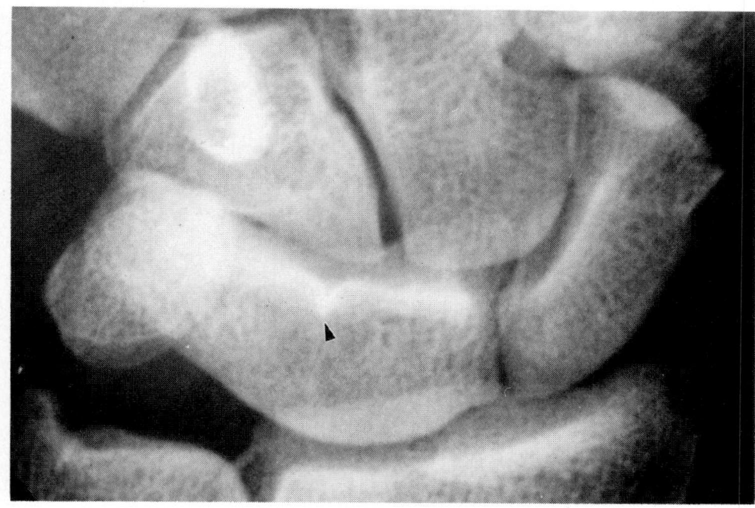

B

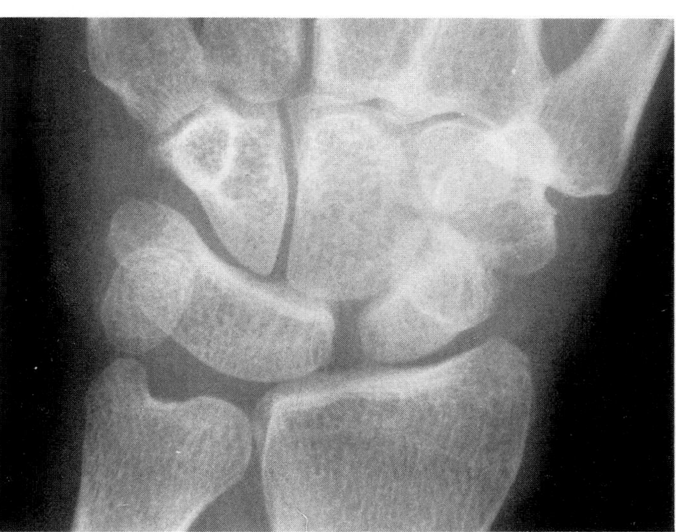

C

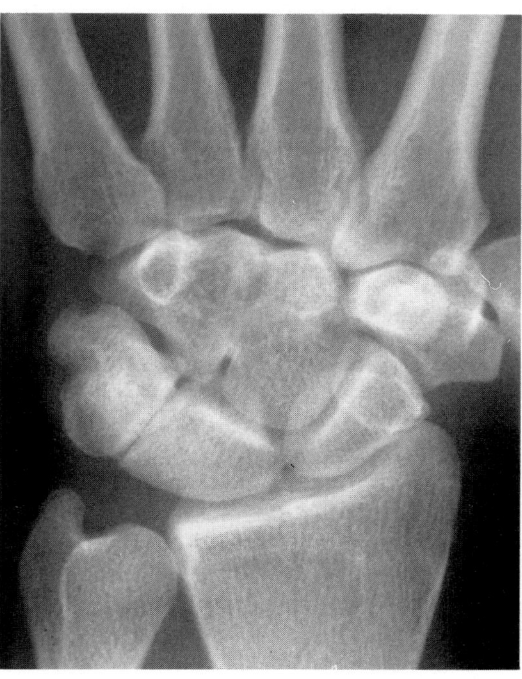

D

FIGURE 20–17. A: PA radiograph of the right wrist with the wrist held in radial deviation. A segmentation anomaly involves the LT joint. This represents a Type I carpal coalition with the proximal portion of the LT joint narrowed more than its distal portion, according to the Minaar classification. **B:** PA radiograph of the left wrist. Bony union is noted along the entire articular surface of the lunate and triquetrum, with the exception of the site of notching (arrowhead) at the distal cortical margin. This represents a Type II carpal coalition, Minaar classification. **C:** PA radiograph of the left wrist. Bony bridging is present along the entire length of the LT articular surface. The scapholunate joint is at least two times as wide as the capitolunate joint space. Such widening can be a normal variant when associated with LT coalition.[55] This represents a Type III carpal coalition, Minaar classification, since no other associated skeletal anomalies are present. **D:** PA radiograph of the left wrist. Segmentation anomalies are present at the LT and capitohamate joints. This represents a variant of the Type IV carpal coalition, Minaar classification, since complete osseous fusion of the LT joint is not present.

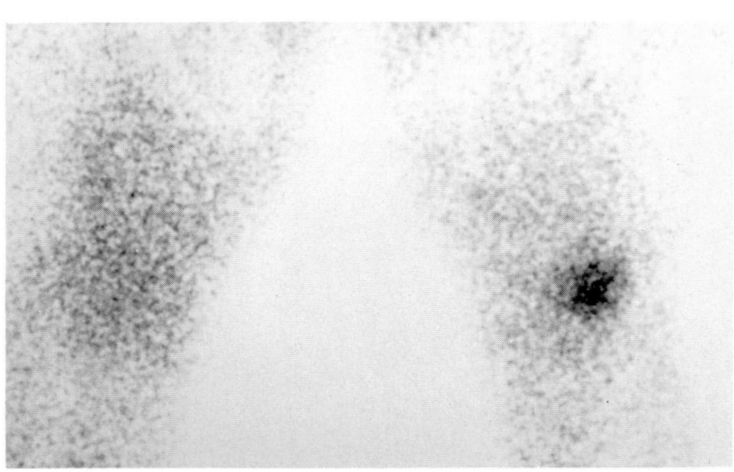

A

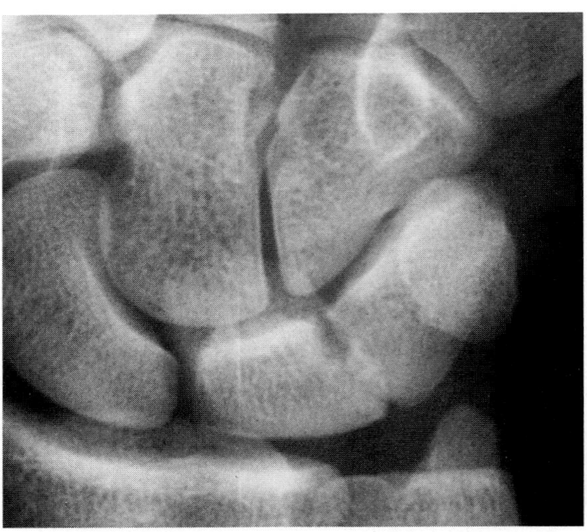

B

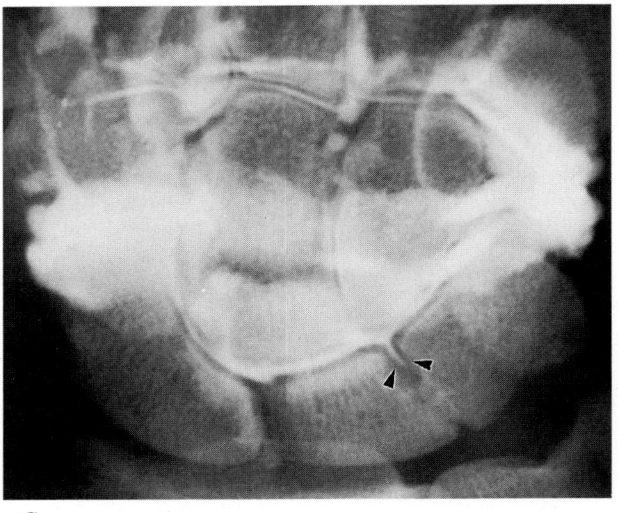

C

FIGURE 20–18. A: Bone scintigraphy, static PA images of both wrists. Focally increased radiotracer activity, Grades II to III of IV, is present in the vicinity of the proximal carpal row. **B:** PA radiograph of the right wrist. A Type I LT coalition corresponds to the site of increased radiotracer activity on bone scintigraphy. This corresponded to the site of the patient's pain and was presumed to be a fractured fibrous or cartilaginous coalition, or a pseudarthrosis. **C:** PA fluoroscopic spot view obtained after a midcarpal compartment injection at wrist arthrography. Contrast passes clearly only into the distal third of the LT joint. A thin column of contrast (arrowheads) such as what could be seen in a thin defect or crevice, which could be a normal variant or a fracture within the cartilaginous or fibrous LT coalition mass, is present.

CONGENITAL SCAPHOID ANOMALIES

Bipartite scaphoid is a rare anomaly resulting from the development of two ossification centers for the scaphoid.[57] Its key significance is that it must be distinguished from nonunion of the scaphoid and from stress fractures of the scaphoid, which require immobilization and/or surgical intervention.[58] The features that speak in favor of a bipartite scaphoid are: (1) bilaterality of the process, (2) equidistance between the scaphoid poles compared with the intercarpal distance between adjacent carpal bones, (3) absent history of trauma, and (4) the absence of periscaphoid osteoarthritis.[59] MRI has been reported to be helpful in distinguishing a bipartite scaphoid, in which each ossific density is surrounded by cartilage with a high signal on GRASS (gradient-recalled acquisition in the steady state) sequence, from a fibrous nonunion, in which low-signal intensity tissue, representing fibrous tissue, is seen between the two ossific fragments.[57]

Hypoplasia and aplasia of the scaphoid and rare anomalies of carpal development have been reported in association with other abnormalities of the thumb ray.[60] In most cases, other congenital anomalies are present, although no uniform pattern of anomalies has been described.

MADELUNG'S DEFORMITY

Although controversy exists as to the origin of this condition, Madelung's deformity describes the entity characterized by a deficiency of the ulnar aspect of the distal radial epiphysis, which results in a triangular shape of the distal radius and a triangular shape of the carpus with the lunate as its apex.[61] Additional radiologic features that are present in Madelung's deformity include a decreased length of the radius, both in absolute terms and relative to the ulna, and dorsal subluxation or dislocation of the ulna (Figs. 20–19A and 20–19B).[61]

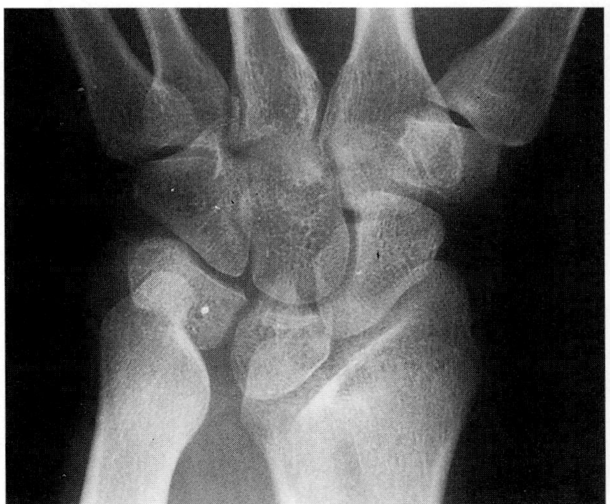

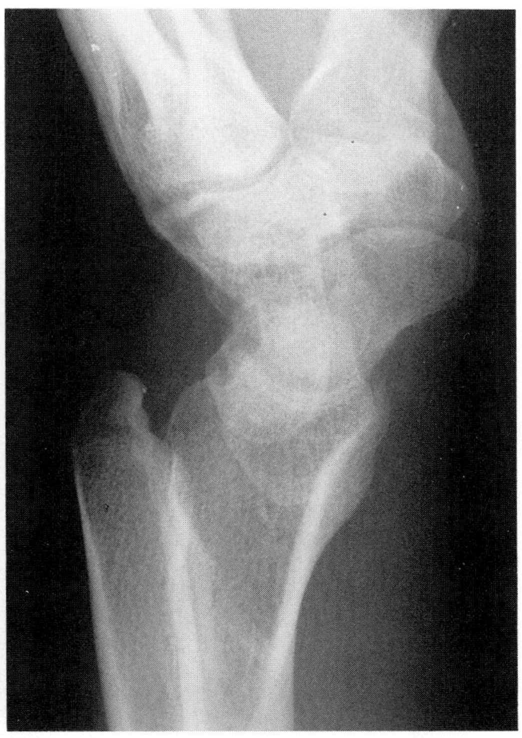

A B

FIGURE 20–19. A: Madelung's deformity. PA radiograph of the left wrist. The medial aspect of the distal radius is shortened relative to the lateral aspect of the radius. The carpal angle is reduced, measuring approximately 80 degrees. The length of the ulna is preserved. **B:** Lateral radiograph of the left wrist with the wrist held in slight extension. The ulna is dorsally subluxed.

Most often Madelung's deformity presents as a primary entity. Dyschondrosteosis, an autosomal dominantly inherited bone dysplasia with mild mesomelia, is the most common disorder associated with Madelung's deformity. Less frequently, Madelung's deformity may be associated with Turner's syndrome, nail-patella syndrome, or multiple hereditary exostoses.[61,62] Occasionally, a deformity with some of the features of Madelung's deformity may be the result of infection (Figs. 20–20A to 20–20C) or trauma occurring before the completion of skeletal maturation,[62] usually causing early closure of part or all of the distal epiphyseal plate of the ulna (Fig. 20–20) or the ulnar side of the radial epiphyseal plate.

Patients usually become aware of the deformity in adolescence.[62] If present, pain in younger patients is believed to originate from the capitolunate and ulnar collateral ligaments because of settling of the carpus proximally and palmarly. However, symptoms do not correlate with radiographic findings.[62] Discomfort in older patients is attributed to mechanical derangement at the DRUJ.

Although an exhaustive list of operative procedures, including epiphysiodesis of the ulna or radial portion of the radius, ulnar shortening, corrective radial osteotomy, or radiocarpal arthrodesis, can be performed to correct the deformity, most patients can be managed with a wrist support during the painful period.[62,63]

CALCIUM PYROPHOSPHATE DIHYDRATE DEPOSITION DISEASE

Deposits of calcium pyrophosphate dihydrate crystals into the joint are usually referred to as CPPD but could possibly more correctly be called "CPPDD." Commonly such deposits, especially into cartilages, are asymptomatic. When these crystals are deposited in the joints pain may occur, which is characterized by acute and chronic inflammatory joint disease.[64] Pseudogout refers to the acute or subacute painful form of this arthritis.[64]

CPPD frequently occurs in association with osteoarthritis[64] or as an aging process with no known underlying etiology. In a minority of patients, CPPD occurs in association with any one of several metabolic diseases, including hyperparathyroidism, hemochromatosis, gout, hypophosphatasia, hypomagnesemia, hypothyroidism, ochronosis, Wilson's disease, and amyloid.[64] A hereditary form of CPPD has also been described and may result in a severe, debilitating state.[64]

The initial site of crystal deposition is believed to

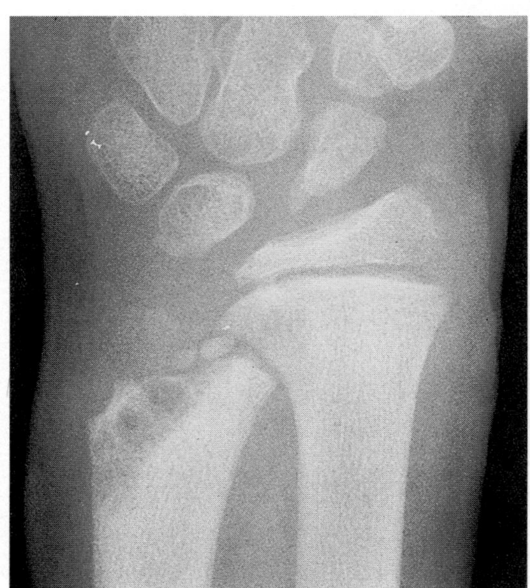

A

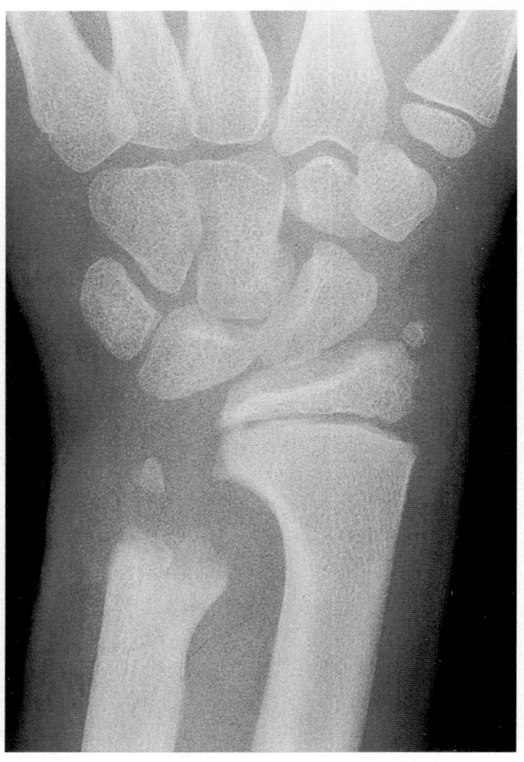

B

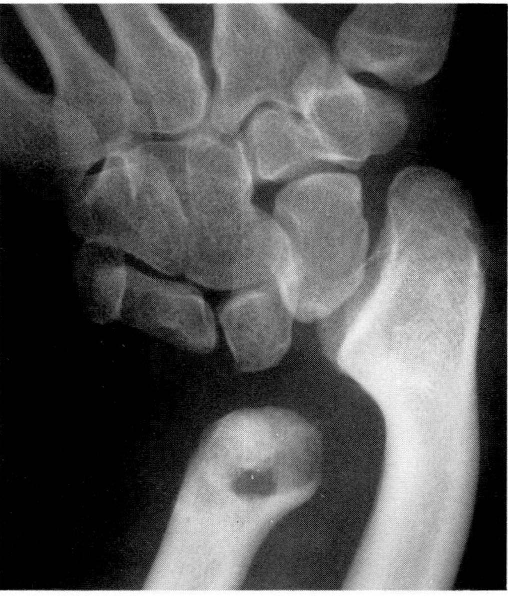

C

FIGURE 20–20. A: PA radiograph of the left wrist several months after a documented staphylococcus infection of the distal ulna. The ulna is shortened. Two well-corticated bony fragments probably represent the remains of the ulnar epiphysis. The radiolucency within the distal ulnar metaphysis represents the site of prior infection. New bone is attempting to fill in this radiolucency. **B:** PA radiograph of the left wrist several years after the radiograph in **A.** The ulna is shorter with respect to the radius than on the prior examination. Bony proliferation has occurred at the radiolucent defect previously seen within the distal ulnar metaphysis. The ulnar styloid epiphysis has ossified since the prior examination. An ossific fragment is seen adjacent to the distal radial epiphysis, which probably represents irregular ossification of the distal radius ossification center. Increased concavity of the ulnar aspect of the radius proximal to the distal radius epiphyseal plate indicates the site at which the distal end of the ulna is articulating with the radius. **C:** PA radiograph of the left wrist 7 years after the radiograph in **B.** The ulna remains markedly shortened. Furthermore, the ulnar aspect of the distal radius is relatively shortened with ulnar deviation of the distal end of the radius. The radial side of the scaphoid articulates with the radius in a grossly congruous fashion. Due to the marked deformity of the distal radius and ulna, much of the carpus projects ulnar to the ulna. Additionally, for this wrist to function or to simulate a more normal appearance, it must be held in a full or nearly full radial deviation position, which also moves the lunate ulnar to the radius.

be in cartilage.[64] With lowered amounts of calcium or pyrophosphate ions in synovial fluid, or as a result of cartilage degradation secondary to either mechanical stress or release of enzymes, the crystals are shed into the synovial fluid, where they incite an inflammatory response. Thus, crystals are most likely to be recovered from the synovial fluid only in the settings of an acute attack or pseudogout. Once recovered from the joint, synovial fluid demonstrates CPPD crystals, most often in an extracellular location. These crystals are weakly birefringent relative to sodium urate crystals when examined under polarized light, and stain with alizarin red S.[64]

The clinical presentation of pseudogout is frequently indistinguishable from that of gout and septic arthritis.[65] Intermittent attacks may be confined to a

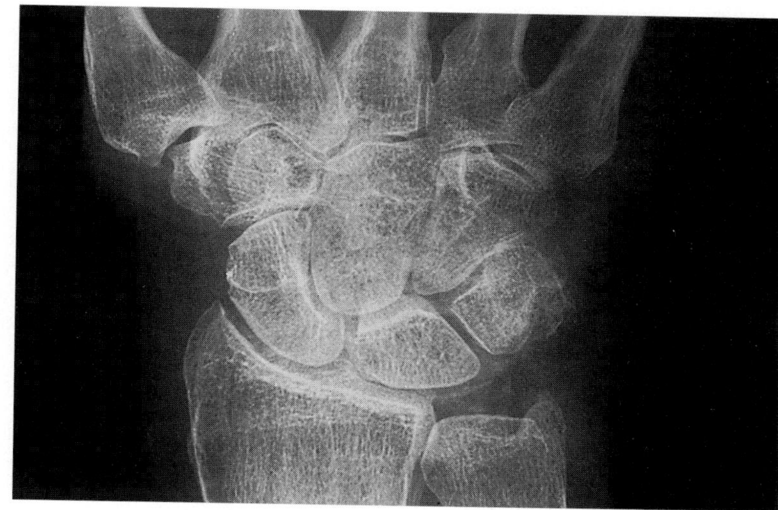

FIGURE 20–21. PA radiograph of the right wrist. Chondrocalcinosis is present within the LT ligament area, the articular cartilage of the proximal lunate, cartilage at the radioscaphoid joint, and the proximal surfaces of the TFC and triquetrum consistent with CPPD.

single joint, manifesting as a warm, swollen erythematous, painful joint.[64] However, CPPD is polyarticular in more than 60% of cases[64] and is most commonly asymptomatic.

Chondrocalcinosis refers to the radiologic appearance of calcification seen with CPPD. Chondrocalcinosis may occur within hyaline cartilage, fibrocartilage, ligaments, and/or joint capsule (Fig. 20–21). Although calcifications within articular cartilage have a linear configuration paralleling subchondral bone, they may appear more diffuse or punctate in the latter three locations.[64] Crystal deposition is found primarily in the cartilaginous portion of the TFC. Actually, the radial portion of the TFC is cartilaginous and the ulnar portion of the TFC is more fibrous, passing its attachments to the fovea at the base of the ulnar styloid. Furthermore, defects in the TFC and chondromalacia in the proximal ulnar aspect of the lunate correspond in general to the radial site of crystal deposition in the TFC.[66] Although the presence of chondrocalcinosis is presumptive of CPPD, chondrocalcinosis is not diagnostic of CPPDD. Chondrocalcinosis may occur in the setting of oxalosis, either primary or secondary.[64] Thus, the definitive diagnosis of CPPDD is made by demonstrating the characteristic crystals in synovial fluid or articular tissue.[64]

In addition to chondrocalcinosis, osteophytes, subchondral lucent defects, and cartilage loss occur at the MCP joints and wrist (Fig. 20–22).[67] Although the arthropathy associated with renal dialysis typically does not have an appearance similar to that of CPPDD and may or may not have CPPD, a report has described identical radiographic features occurring with an arthropathy associated with renal dialysis, hence the name pyrophosphate-like arthropathy.[68] Although rare, tophaceous deposits with CPPD crystals and deposition of CPPD crystals within tendon sheaths resulting in tendon sheath rupture have been reported.[69] In as many as 25% of cases of patients with known CPPDD, a scapholunate advanced collapse (SLAC) wrist pattern may develop (see next

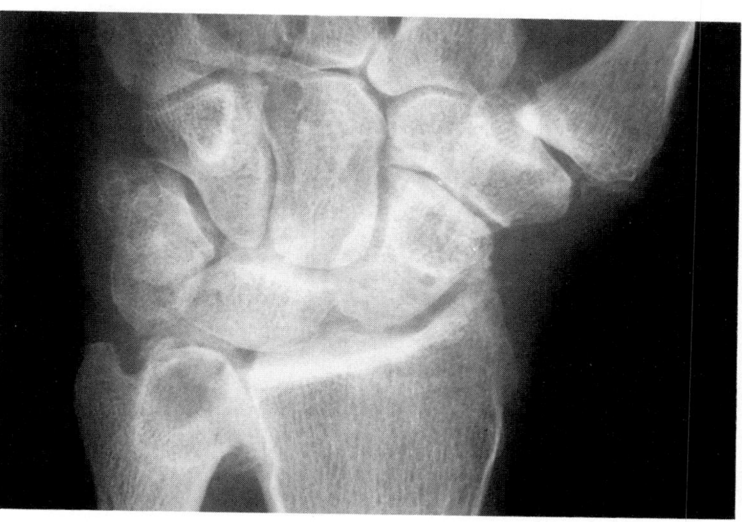

FIGURE 20–22. PA radiograph of the left wrist. A fluffy pattern of chondrocalcinosis is identified in the first CMC joint, within the TFC, radiocarpal joint, and just distal to the radial styloid, probably in the cartilage and synovium but perhaps within the joint capsule. A large radiolucency is within the ulnar head, and a smaller radiolucency is within the distal pole of the capitate, most likely representing subchondral cysts. However, the contents of the lucencies cannot be accurately identified because synovial tissue, fibrous tissue, and fluid without cyst walls all look the same on plain radiographs. A spur projects off the proximal articular surface of the ulna at the DRUJ. These changes are due to CPPDD. Mild narrowing and subchondral sclerosis at the scaphotrapeziotrapezoidal joint space is likely secondary to routine osteoarthritis, but CPPDD is also a consideration in light of the rest of the changes present.

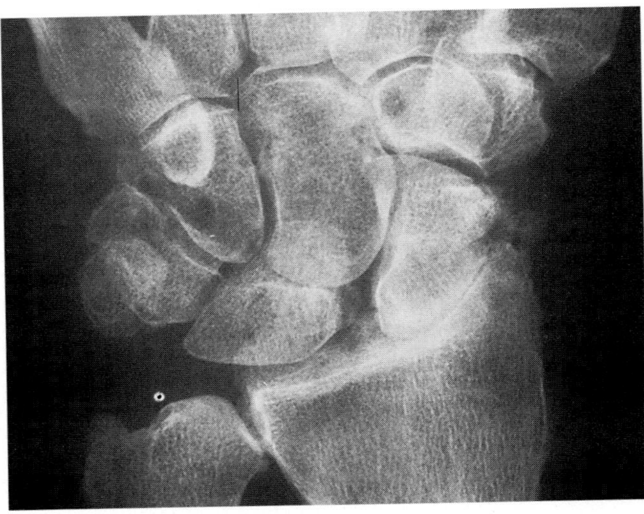

FIGURE 20–23. PA radiograph of the left wrist. Severe cartilage loss is present at the radioscaphoid and capitolunate joint spaces. Subchondral sclerosis is identified at the radioscaphoid joint space. The scapholunate joint space is twice as wide as the hamate–triquetral joint space, indicative of scapholunate diastasis. Multiple radiolucencies are present in the trapezoid, hamate, and lunate. The radiolunate joint space has been spared. These findings are indicative of SLAC wrist, possibly secondary to CPPDD, but the lack of chondrocalcinosis, and the lack of scaphoid fossa bone loss (increased concavity of the scaphoid fossa) suggests this is not related to CPPDD.

section).[70,71] However, typically when the SLAC wrist pattern develops in patients with known CPPDD, destructive changes resulting in a deep concave scaphoid fossa are typical (Fig. 20–25). Such destructive changes in the scaphoid fossa are not typical of SLAC wrist in patients without CPPDD (Fig. 20–23).

When the condition is painful, treatment consists of the administration of NSAIDs and the aspiration of synovial fluid, followed by the administration of intra-articular steroids.[64] Low-dose colchicine may be given as prophylactic treatment in those patients subject to recurrent attacks. Once the crystals are deposited, however, they cannot be removed by treatment. Hence, with repeated crystal deposition progressive arthritis may develop.

SLAC WRIST

Scapholunate advanced collapse (SLAC)[72] refers to the arthritic condition of the wrist primarily caused by laxness and malpositioning of the scaphoid and lunate. It may occur as an isolated entity or in association with triscaphe arthrosis.

SLAC is due to abnormal alignment between the articular surfaces of the radius and the scaphoid usually associated with scapholunate (SL) dissociation. This altered alignment may be ligamentous (through the SL joints) or bony (through a scaphoid fracture) in origin. Both trauma and CPPD have been implicated as causes of SLAC wrist.[70–72] The discrepancy in opinion about the relationship between SLAC and CPPD probably reflects the patient population seen. Rheumatologists or radiologists who see patients referred for systemic arthritis may have many more patients with CPPDD than with old trauma. As mentioned above, the pattern of SLAC with chondrocalcinosis seems to be associated with more bone destruction than that without chondrocalcinosis. Treating hand surgeons who see a lot of trauma rarely see SLAC associated with chondrocalcinosis.

With rotary subluxation of the scaphoid (Figs. 20–24A and 20–24B), edge-loading of the scaphoid against the radial aspect of the radius results in degenerative joint disease at this site. With continued motion at the radioscaphoid joint, degenerative joint disease develops along the remainder of the radioscaphoid joint. Simultaneously, due to scapholunate diastasis and gradual evolution from rotary subluxation of the scaphoid to dorsal intercalated segmental instability (DISI), the capitate migrates proximally, resulting in edge-loading of the capitate against the lunate.[72,73] Thus SLAC is characterized by the sequential progression of osteoarthritis initially at the radial aspect of the radioscaphoid joint, next at the ulnar aspect of the radioscaphoid joint, and then ultimately at the capitolunate joint. The absence of arthritic involvement of the radiolunate joint, even in the late stages of the condition (Fig. 20–25), is a hallmark of SLAC.[72,73]

Scaphoid nonunion is the primary bony condition that results in SLAC wrist. Some cases of scaphoid nonunion result in rotary subluxation of the distal pole of the scaphoid.[74] Through the mechanism described above, patients with scaphoid nonunion sequentially develop osteoarthritis in the same sequence described above.[75] However, the articulation between the proximal pole of the scaphoid and the distal radius, and the radiolunate joint do not develop osteoarthritis.[74] In other words, the proximal pole of the scaphoid acts as a small lunate. The distal scaphoid fragment needs the abnormal forces with the radius to develop degenerative joint disease between the scaphoid fossa and the distal scaphoid fracture fragment. Any condition predisposing to scaphoid nonunion and malalignment between fracture fragments, among them delayed diagnosis of a scaphoid fracture or unreduced angulation or displacement of the fracture fragments, will also predispose to development of SLAC wrist.

Retrospective studies have shown that SLAC wrist may be the end result of scaphoid nonunions treated nonoperatively.[74,75] Therefore some recommend early intervention, even in the asymptomatic patient. Either bone grafting with or without K-wire fixation or electrical stimulation serve as prophylactic treatment in cases of scaphoid nonunion.[75] Some people em-

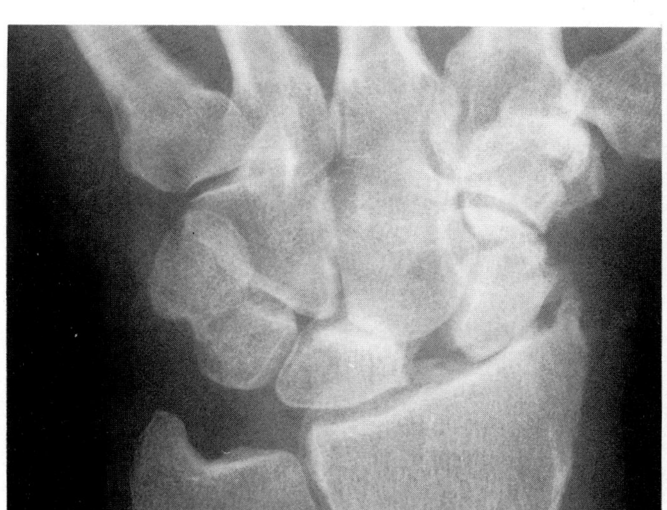

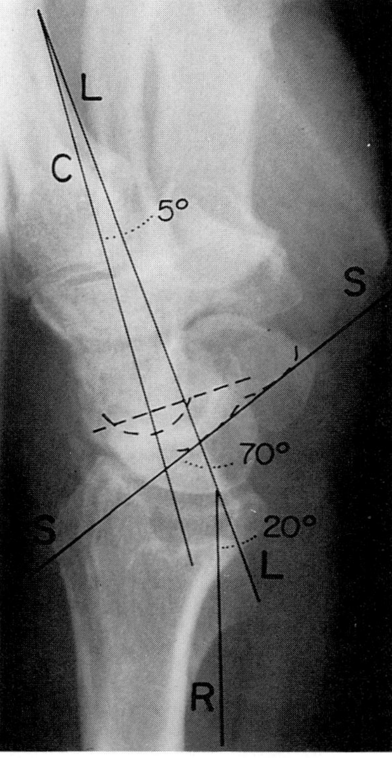

A B

FIGURE 20–24. A: PA radiograph of the left wrist with the wrist held in slight hyperextension, because the CMC joints are not in profile and the hamate hook is elongated. Degenerative spur formation is present at the radioscaphoid joint. Severe cartilage loss is present at the radioscaphoid and capitolunate joint spaces. The scapholunate joint space is nearly four times as wide as the scaphocapitate joint space indicating scapholunate diastasis. The radiolunate joint space appears normal, although a small spur involves the radial-proximal border of the lunate. These findings are consistent with a SLAC wrist. **B:** Lateral radiograph of the left wrist. The lunate is dorsiflexed. The scapholunate angle is 70 degrees, consistent with a DISI configuration. The capitolunate angle of 5 degrees is normal. C, capitate axis; L, lunate axis; S, scaphoid axis; R, radius axis.

phasize Herbert's screw fixation, but the important goal is to gain healing with fragments in the true anatomic position. Once arthritis has begun, treatment options include: (1) radial styloidectomy for those with radial-sided osteoarthritis only, (2) wrist denervation to maintain pain-free wrist function, (3) removal of the distal scaphoid fragment, entire scaphoid, or proximal row carpectomy, with or without soft-tissue interposition, in the setting of more advanced arthritis, or (4) limited intercarpal fusions including fusion of both scaphoid poles with the capitate, the proximal pole of the scaphoid with the lunate to the capitate while removing the distal scaphoid fragment, the original SLAC procedure (capitolunate fusion and removal of scaphoid), or four-bone fusion (capitohamatotriquetrolunate). Salvage procedures for the late stages of SLAC wrist include proximal row carpectomy and total wrist fusion.

Currently the more common SLAC procedure consists of four-bone fusion (capitate, lunate, hamate, triquetrum). Although the procedure initially included the replacement of the scaphoid with a silastic prosthesis, the present procedure includes excision of the scaphoid without insertion of a silastic prosthesis.[72,73] This avoids the possibility of a complicating particulate synovitis.

TRISCAPHE OSTEOARTHRITIS

The scaphotrapeziotrapezoidal (STT) or triscaphe joint[76] is probably the most common site of primary, noninflammatory arthritis in the wrist after first CMC degenerative joint disease. Often first CMC joint osteoarthritis accompanies STT osteoarthritis (Fig. 20–26).[77] Although no definite etiology is known, some believe that an unstable articulation at the STT joint may be a contributing factor in the development of osteoarthritis at this joint.[78]

Typical findings of osteoarthritis, including osteophyte formation, cartilage loss, and subchondral scler-

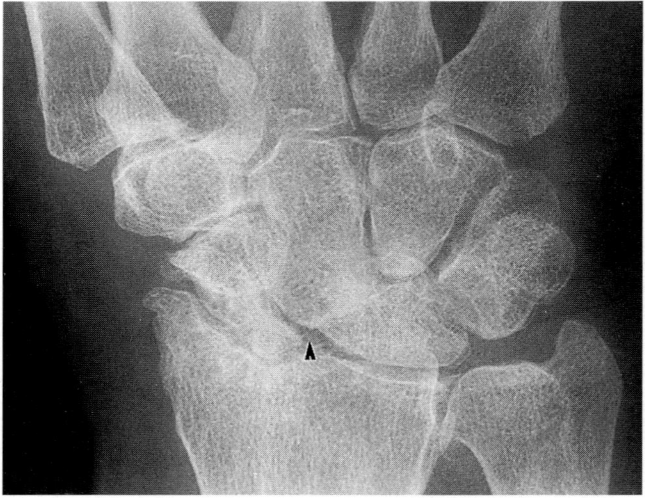

FIGURE 20–25. PA radiograph of the right wrist. The scaphoid fossa of the distal radial articular surface is markedly concave, and the scaphoid has lost volume in its proximal half and is irregular in its shape proximally. Degenerative spur formation is present at the radioscaphoid joint. The capitolunate joint space is completely obliterated with subchondral sclerosis. The radiolunate joint space is preserved. These findings are consistent with SLAC wrist in the typical pattern seen associated with CPPDD. Questionable chondrocalcinosis is at the ridge between the scaphoid and lunate fossae (arrowhead). An ossicle, presumably degenerative, is distal to the radial styloid.

osis and/or lucent cyst-like defects may be present in either a unilateral or bilateral distribution.[77] These changes are best demonstrated on a semisupinated oblique view of the wrist that profiles the STT joint.[79] Frequently the severity of a patient's symptoms bears no relation to the severity of radiologic findings[78]; patients may be asymptomatic in the presence of roentgenographically severe osteoarthritis and may be highly symptomatic in the presence of minimal or no roentgenographic changes.

Treatment is based on patient symptomatology rather than on radiographic appearance. Conservative treatment usually consists of rest, the oral administration of antiinflammatory agents, and/or the injection of corticosteroids locally.

The local administration of intraarticular anesthetic may have diagnostic implications. In those patients in whom operative management is being considered, response after the injection of intraarticular anesthetic may help confirm the exact source of pain. Corticosteroids may be injected with the anesthetic in attempt to get more long-lasting relief. Although those with pain at both the STT and first CMC joints may be candidates for a trapeziectomy, soft-tissue reconstruction, and/or placement of some type of tendon spacer, those with disease restricted to the STT joint may undergo a limited arthrodesis procedure such as triscaphe arthrodesis.[78]

FIRST CMC JOINT OSTEOARTHRITIS

Primary osteoarthritis of the first CMC joint typically manifests in the fifth and sixth decades, often accompanying osteoarthritis at the STT joint.[77,80] Factors that predispose to the development of arthritis at this site include the inherent laxity of this joint as well as the heavy stresses related to pinching and grasping that are placed on it. Predisposing factors to secondary arthritis at this site include Bennett's fractures, Rolando's fractures, and other intraarticular fractures of the first metacarpal base and/or trapezium.[81] Rarely, dislocation of the trapezium will be the inciting event resulting in arthritis at this site.

Physical examination often demonstrates swelling around the joint. The axial compression test, consisting of applying a rotational force while compressing the CMC joint, will be positive.[82] Because of the frequent association with other skeletal or soft-tissue pathology, careful examination of the surrounding soft-tissue structures is recommended. The term basal joint pain syndrome has been coined to reflect the

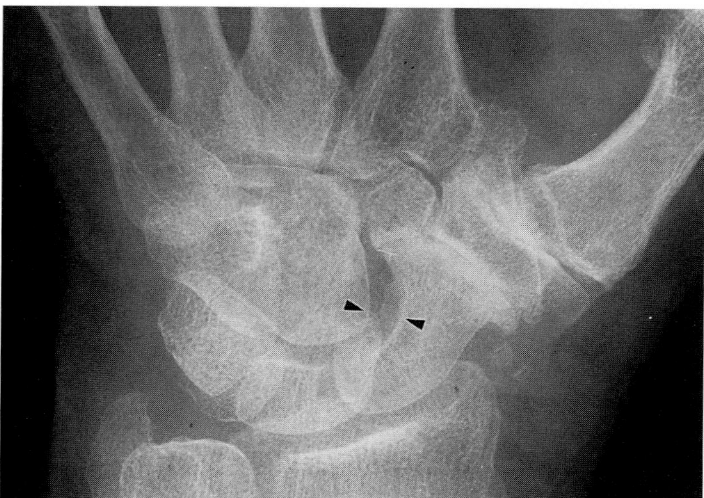

FIGURE 20–26. Supinated oblique PA radiograph of the left wrist. Severe cartilage loss, subchondral sclerosis, focal subcortical lucencies, and degenerative spur formation are present at the scaphotrapezial, scaphotrapezoidal, and first CMC joints consistent with degenerative joint disease. Most of or all of the trapeziotrapezoidal joint is normal on this view. The two ossific fragments just distal to the radial styloid may represent joint bodies, but more commonly are in the soft tissues at the margin of the joint. Scaphocapitate joint widening (between arrowheads) reflects abnormal alignment between these bones. An incidental finding of a benign focal lucency is suspected in the radial portion of the lunate.

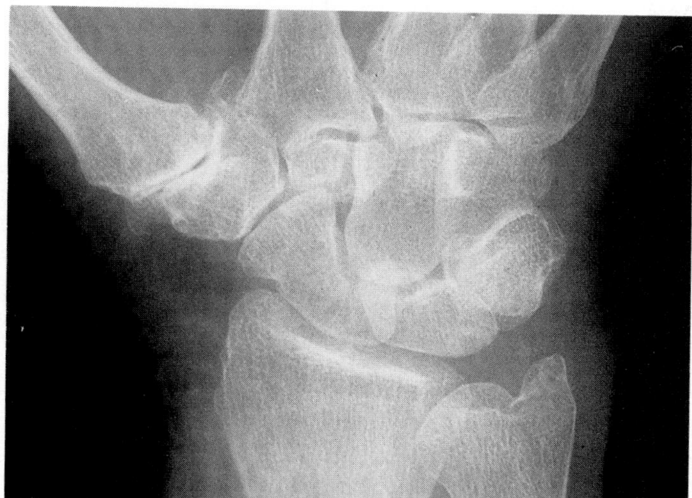

FIGURE 20–27. PA semipronated radiograph of the right wrist. Extensive cartilage loss, subchondral sclerosis, and osteophyte formation are indicative of osteoarthritis at the first CMC joint. Minimal cartilage loss may be present at the scaphotrapezial joint space, indicating early osteoarthritis.

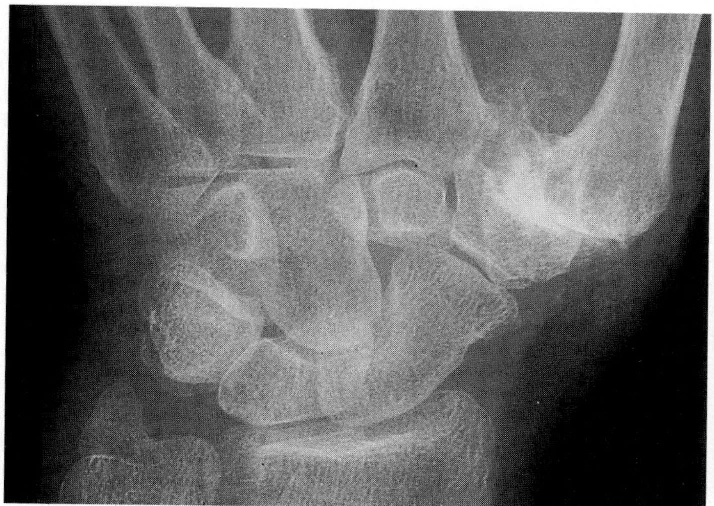

A

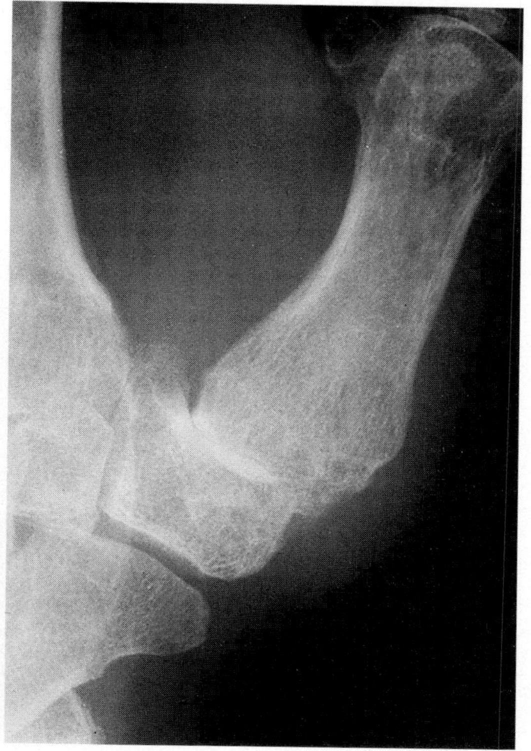

B

FIGURE 20–28. A: PA semipronated radiograph of the left wrist. Severe cartilage loss, subchondral sclerosis, osteophyte formation, and multiple para-articular ossific bodies, possibly intracapsular, indicate osteoarthritis of the first CMC joint. **B:** PA semipronated radiograph of the left thumb in another patient. Less-advanced osteoarthritis of the first CMC than in **A** is manifested by narrowing, subchondral sclerosis, subcortical lucencies, and smaller marginal osteophytes than those seen in **A.**

widespread inflammatory changes detected at the time of surgical intervention.[83]

Radiographic features include narrowing of articular cartilage, marginal osteophytes, subchondral cyst-like lucent defects, and subchondral sclerosis (Figs. 20–27, 20–28A and 20–28B).[84] PA views with the thumbs opposed may be helpful in detecting subluxation or dislocation at the first CMC joint.

Conservative treatment consists of rest, steroid injections, and/or anti-inflammatory medication. Indications for surgery include uncontrolled pain and/or an inability to perform the activities of daily living. Arthrodesis and arthroplasty are the mainstay of surgical intervention.[82] Arthrodesis has a high success rate and has the advantage of preserving grip strength; however, motion across the CMC joint is limited. Resection arthroplasty entails excision of the base of the first metacarpal, part of the trapezium, or the entire trapezium.[81] The surgical bed may be filled with a tendon spacer or left empty. The use of trapezial prostheses has been limited because of their attendant complications, e.g., subluxations, dislocations, and detritic synovitis.

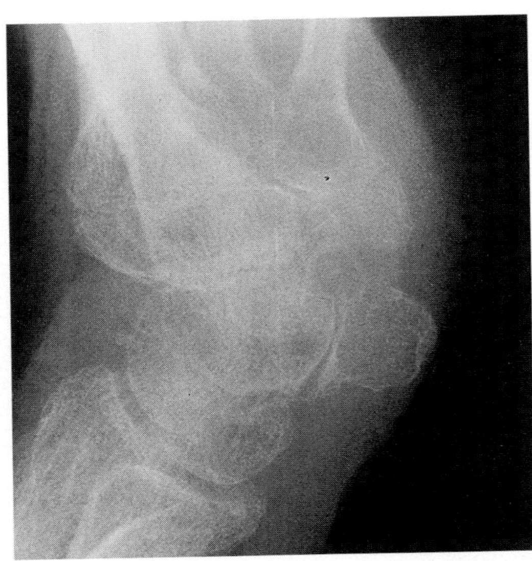

FIGURE 20–30. Off-lateral view of the left wrist for pisotriquetral joint. Mild subchondral sclerosis and marginal spurs are present along the articular margin of the pisiform, indicating pisotriquetral osteoarthritis. (Case courtesy of Don Resnick, M.D., San Diego, CA.)

PISOTRIQUETRAL ARTHRITIS

The pisiform, a sesamoid bone arising within the flexor carpi ulnaris tendon, articulates with the triquetrum through a synovial joint. Osteoarthritis of the pisotriquetral joint should be considered in any patient with ulnar-sided wrist pain. Although its onset may be insidious, it may occur in the setting of previous trauma such as a fracture, subluxation, or dislocation. Those who play racquet sports are particularly predisposed to this entity.[85] The diagnosis of dislocation or subluxation can be very difficult to make unless the pisiform is locked to the ulnar side of the triquetrum clinically. Radiographically the pisiform usually should move away from the triquetrum with flexion of the wrist, as the flexor carpi ulnaris tendon moves away from the triquetrum on wrist flexion. Also, with elevation of the ulnar side of the wrist off the x-ray film with the wrist in a PA position, the pisiform can normally project ulnar to the triquetrum.

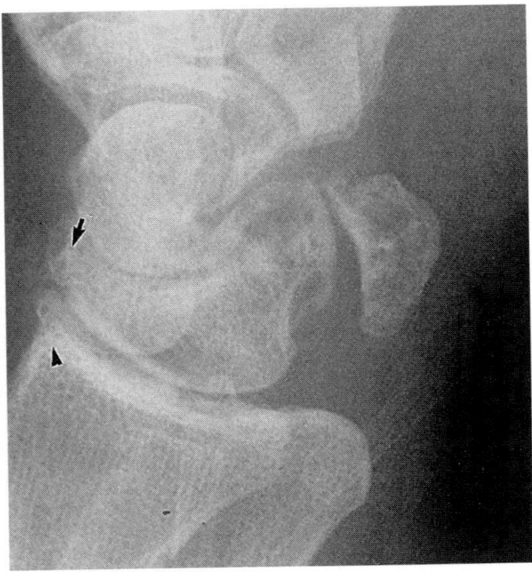

FIGURE 20–29. AP semisupinated radiograph of the left wrist. The pisotriquetral joint is narrowed most severely at its distal aspect. Subcortical lucent defects, subchondral sclerosis, and osteophyte formation indicate the presence of pisotriquetral osteoarthritis. Osteophytes also involve the dorsum of the radius (arrowhead) and scaphoid (arrow) indicative of radiocarpal osteoarthritis.

The major symptom of pisotriquetral arthritis is pain in the hypothenar eminence. Symptoms of ulnar neuropathy may be present in as many as one third of patients.[86] Clinical examination demonstrates focal tenderness to direct pressure over the pisiform. Side-to-side passive motion may reproduce pain and/or crepitus. When pain is focal to the pisotriquetral area, triquetral abnormalities such as fracture or other intraosseous pathology of the triquetrum must be considered. Hypothenar eminence symptoms are not unique to pisotriquetral osteoarthritis and may be produced by other ulnar-sided entities including ulnar collateral ligament injury, tendinitis of the flexor carpi ulnaris, ulnar styloid nonunion, or DRUJ subluxation.[86]

Pisotriquetral osteoarthritis or other arthritic conditions of this joint may be detected on an off-lateral radiograph obtained with the forearm and wrist in 10–30 degrees of supination (Figs. 20–29 and 20–30). Alternatively a carpal tunnel view may profile the pisotriquetral joint.[85,86] PA and lateral radiographs of the wrist do not usually aid in the diagnosis because they fail to profile the pisotriquetral joint.

Radiographic features are similar to those in other sites involved with osteoarthritis. An easy way to precisely profile this joint or evaluate this joint with motion is with fluoroscopic spot views. Axial plane CT provides an excellent way to image this joint, and MRI can show the intraosseous character of the pisiform and triquetrum and adjacent soft-tissue structures well.

Injection of intraarticular anesthetic to test the disappearance of pain may determine if pain is coming from this joint. Conservative treatment with immobilization, anti-inflammatory medications, and/or steroid injections may successfully relieve the symptoms. However, excision of the pisiform, the definitive treatment for this entity, may be indicated.[86–88]

CHONDROMALACIA OF THE HAMATE

Chondromalacia refers to the cartilage changes associated with arthrosis, including cartilage erosion. The proximal pole of the hamate has been described as the most common site of chondromalacia in the wrist.[89] In more than one quarter of dissected cadaveric wrists, chondromalacia was detected bilaterally and symmetrically.[89]

Earlier cadaveric work describing the changes of chondromalacia stated that these findings were radiographically occult.[90] However, a more recent study has described the radiologic features seen with degeneration of the proximal pole of the hamate. These changes include a Type II lunate (lunate with a radiologically evident hamate facet of the lunate), radiolucencies within the proximal pole of the hamate, and/or subchondral bone loss at the proximal pole of the hamate (Figs. 20–31A and 20–31B).[91] Accompanying changes may be seen on other imaging modalities as well, including bone scintigraphy, CT, and/or MRI (Figs. 20–32A to 20–32D).

One of the most prevalent features of chondromalacia of the hamate, a Type II lunate, has been detected in over 65% of individuals in cadaveric studies.[89,90] All Type II facets on gross-anatomic study were not evident on radiographs. A Type II lunate is one that has a separate facet, called the medial or hamate facet, which articulates with the hamate. Whereas over 25% of patients with a Type II lunate have been shown to have degenerative changes of the proximal pole of the hamate, no associated pathologic changes have been described in patients with a Type I lunate, a lunate without a medial facet.[89,90,92] Furthermore, similar degenerative changes have been described at the opposing articular surface of the lunate.[89,90,92]

Cadaveric dissection has also shown that chondromalacia of the proximal pole of the hamate may also be seen in association with tears of the lunotriquetral interosseous ligament.[89,92]

There seems to be a spectrum of clinical correlation with this finding. Patients may be asymptomatic and this may be just an incidental finding. In others there may be focal tenderness exactly over the proximal pole of the hamate. Depending on the severity of symptomatology, the patient can be treated with nothing, mild pain medications, or surgical evacua-

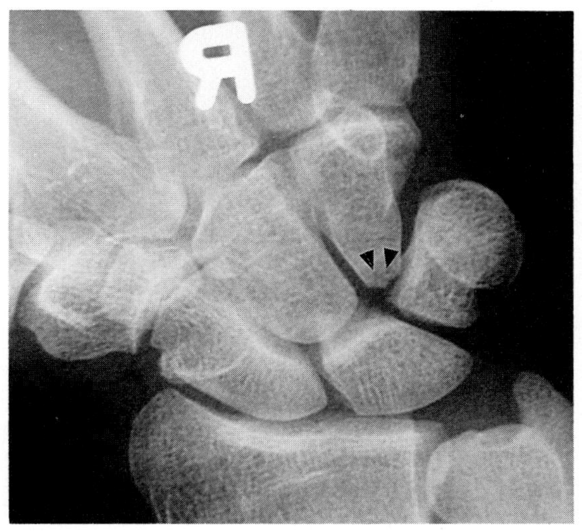

A

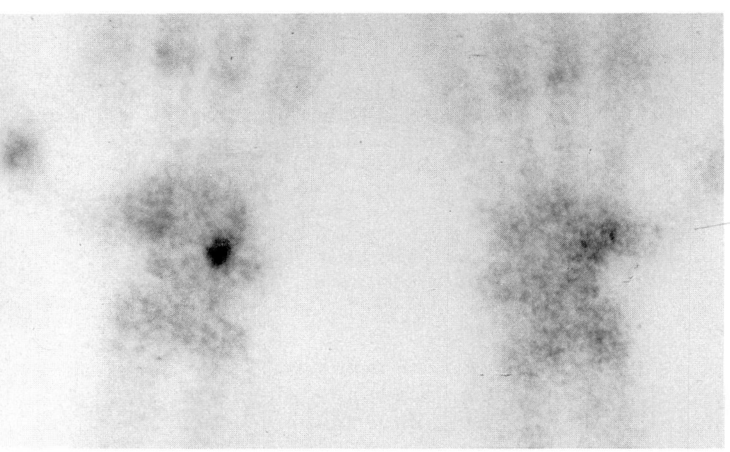

B

FIGURE 20–31. A: PA radiograph of the right wrist with the wrist held in radial deviation. Absence of the cortical margin and subcortical lucency (arrowheads) at the proximal pole of the hamate are consistent with chondromalacia. **B:** Bone scintigraphy: static delayed bone images of both wrists. Increased Tc^{99m} radiotracer activity, Grade III of IV, corresponds to the site of cortical loss at the hamate.

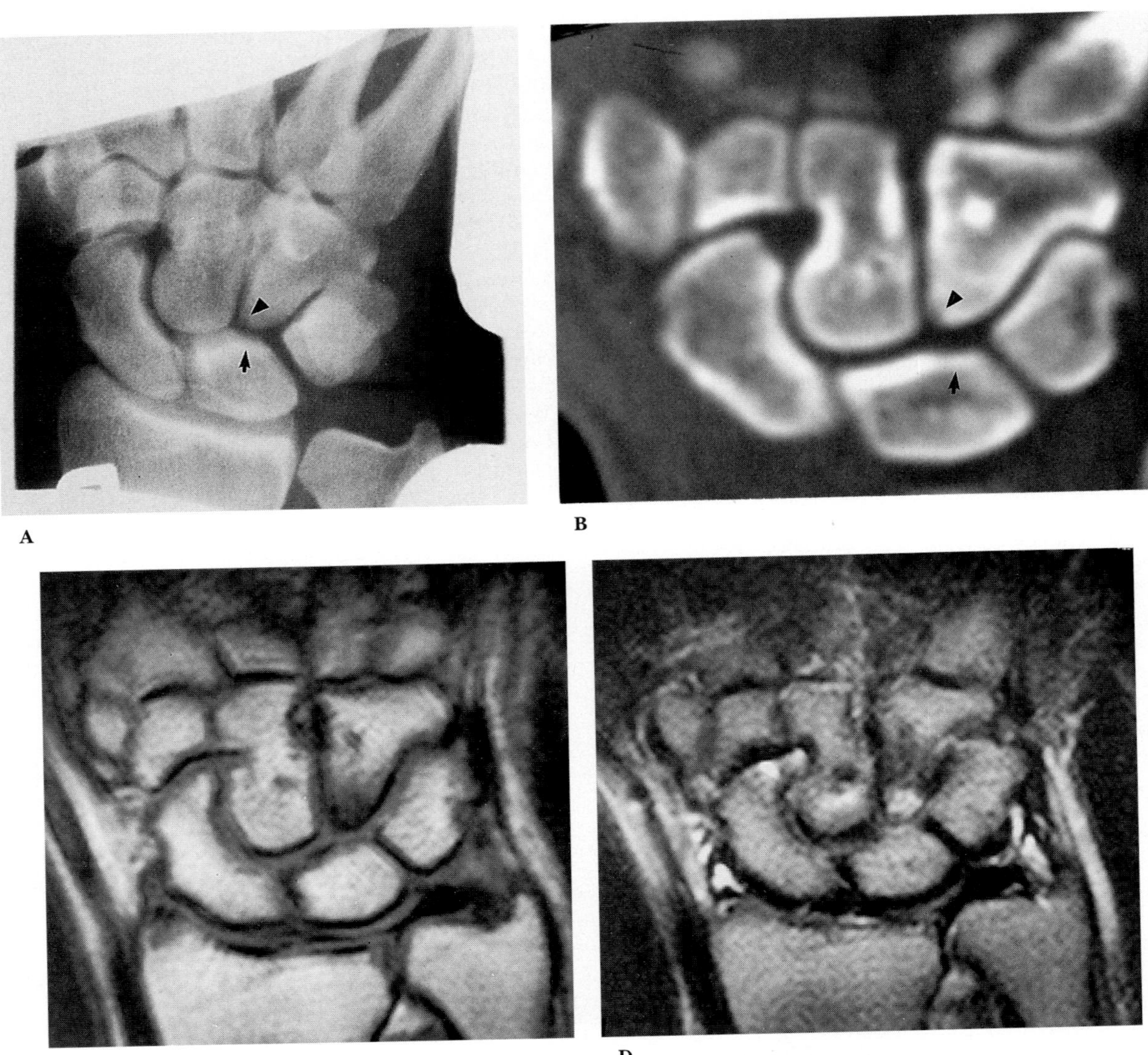

FIGURE 20–32. A: PA radiograph of the right wrist. A tiny subchondral lucency (arrowhead) is present within the proximal pole of the hamate. The radiolucency faces the hamate facet (arrow) of the lunate (Type II lunate). **B:** Coronal CT image of the right wrist, 2-mm slice thickness, 2-mm intervals. Cortical loss along the proximal pole of the hamate (arrowhead) and a Type II lunate (arrow) are consistent with the diagnosis of chondromalacia of the hamate. An enostosis is present within the hamate. **C:** Coronal MRI of the right wrist. TR 500 msec, TE 23 msec. A larger area of low-signal intensity in the proximal hamate corresponds to the site of abnormality seen on plain radiographs. **D:** Coronal MRI of the right wrist. TR 3000 msec, TE 90 msec. An area of high-signal intensity within the proximal pole of the hamate corresponds to a subcortical area of fluid or fluid-laden tissue, which most commonly represents degenerative alteration of the bone underlying an area of chondromalacia. (Parts **C** and **D** reprinted with permission from Peh WCG, Gilula LA, Viegas SF, et al. Degenerative lesions in the proximal pole of the hamate: Radiological features. *Radiology* 1995, submitted.)

tion of the defect.[91] In the one patient in the paper by Peh et al[91] treated surgically in this manner, symptoms were relieved. In another communication, similar results were obtained.[93]

REFERENCES

1. Friedman SL, Palmer AK. Problems of the distal radioulnar joint: The ulnar impaction syndrome. *Hand Clin* 1991;7:295–310.
2. Mann FA, Wilson AJ, Gilula LA. Radiographic evaluation of the wrist: What does the hand surgeon want to know? *Radiology* 1992;184:15–24.
3. Palmer AK, Werner FW. Biomechanics of the distal radioulnar joint. *Clin Orthop* 1984;187:26–35.
4. Epner RA, Bowers WH, Guilford WB. Ulnar variance: The effect of wrist positioning and roentgen filming technique. *J Hand Surg* 1982;7A:298–305.
5. Uchiyama S, Terayama K. Radiographic changes in the wrist with ulnar plus variance observed over a ten-year period. *J Hand Surg* 1991;16A:45–48.
6. Wnorowski DC, Palmer AK, Werner FW, et al. Anatomic and

biomechanical analysis of the arthroscopic wafer procedure. *Arthroscopy* 1992;8:204–212.
7. Feldon P, Terrono AL, Belsky MR. Wafer distal ulna resection for triangular fibrocartilage tears and/or ulna impaction syndrome. *J Hand Surg* 1992;17A:731–737.
8. Albanese SA, Palmer AK, Kerr DR, et al. Wrist pain and distal growth plate closure of the radius in gymnasts. *J Pediatr Orthop* 1989;9:23–28.
9. Bowers WH. The distal radioulnar joint. In: Green DP, ed. *Operative hand surgery,* 2nd ed. New York: Churchill Livingstone, 1988:939–989;1001–1004.
10. Bell MJ, Hill RJ, McMurtry RY. Ulnar impingement syndrome. *J Bone Joint Surg* 1985;67B:126–129.
11. Conway WF, Destouet JM, Gilula LA, et al. The carpal boss: An overview of radiographic evaluation. *Radiology* 1985; 156:29–31.
12. Kaulesar SDM, Steinberg PJ, Lichtveld PL. The carpal boss. *Neth J Surg* 1986;38:90–92.
13. Chen WS, Shih CH. Ulnar variance and Kienbock's disease: An investigation in Taiwan. *Clin Orthop* 1990;255:124–127.
14. Nakamura R, Tanaka Y, Imaeda T, et al. The influence of age and sex on ulnar variance. *J Hand Surg* 1991;16B:84–88.
15. Nakamura R, Imaeda T, Suzuki K, et al. Sports-related Kienbock's disease. *Am J Sports Med* 1991;19:88–91.
16. Amadio PC, Hanssen AD, Berquist TH. The genesis of Kienbock's disease. Evaluation of a case by magnetic resonance imaging. *J Hand Surg* 1987;12A:1044–1049.
17. Almquist EE. Kienbock's disease. *Hand Clin* 1987;3:141–148.
18. Gelberman RH, Bauman TD, Menon J, et al. The vascularity of the lunate bone and Kienbock's disease. *J Hand Surg* 1980;5A:272–278.
19. Alexander AH, Lichtman DM. Kienbock's disease. *Orthop Clin* 1986;17:461–472.
20. Taliesnik J. Kienbock's disease. In: Taliesnik J, ed. *The wrist.* New York: Churchill Livingstone, 1985:169–194.
21. Reinus WR, Conway WF, Totty WG, et al. Carpal avascular necrosis: MR imaging. *Radiology* 1986;160:689–693.
22. Jackson MD, Barry DT, Geiringer SR. Magnetic resonance imaging of avascular necrosis of the lunate. *Arch Phys Med Rehab* 1990;71:510–513.
23. Trumble TE, Irving J. Histologic and magnetic resonance imaging correlations in Kienbock's disease. *J Hand Surg* 1990;15A:879–884.
24. Cristiani G, Cerofolini E, Squarzina PB, et al. Evaluation of ischaemic necrosis of carpal bones by magnetic resonance imaging. *J Hand Surg* 1990;15B:249–255.
25. Viegas SF, Amparo E. Magnetic resonance imaging in the assessment of revascularization in Kienbock's disease: A preliminary report. *Orthop Rev* 1989;18:1285–1288.
26. Tamai S, Yajima H, Ono H. Revascularization procedures in the treatment of Kienbock's disease. *Hand Clin* 1993;9:455–466.
27. Gilula LA, Higgs PE, Hsieh P, Weeks PM. Imaging classification of lunate disease: An evolving spectrum. *Radiology* 1995, submitted.
28. Lichtman DM, Mack GR, MacDonald RI, et al. Kienbock's disease: The role of silicone replacement arthroplasty. *J Bone Joint Surg* 1977;59A:899–908.
29. Mikkelsen SS, Gelineck J. Poor function after nonoperative treatment of Kienbock's disease. *Acta Orthop Scand* 1987;58: 241–243.
30. Kinnard P, Tricoire JL, Basora J. Radial shortening for Kienbock's disease. *Can J Surg* 1983;26:261–262.
31. Trumble T, Glisson RR, Seaber AV, et al. A biomechanical comparison of the methods for treating Kienbock's disease. *J Hand Surg* 1986;11A:88–93.
32. Sundberg SB, Linscheid RL. Kienbock's disease: Results of treatment with ulnar lengthening. *Clin Orthop* 1984;187:43–51.
33. Kato H, Usui M, Minami A. Long-term results of Kienbock's disease treated by excisional arthroplasty with a silicone implant or coiled palmaris longus tendon. *J Hand Surg* 1986;11A:645–653.
34. Kawai H, Yamamoto K, Yamamoto T, et al. Excision of the lunate in Kienbock's disease: Results after long-term follow-up. *J Bone Joint Surg* 1988;70A:287–292.
35. Michon J. Kienbock's disease and complications of injuries to the lunate bone. In: Tubiana R, ed. *The hand.* Vol. II. Philadelphia: WB Saunders, 1985:1106–1116.
36. Alexander AH, Turner MA, Alexander CE, et al. Lunate silicone replacement arthroplasty in Kienbock's disease: A long-term follow-up. *J Hand Surg* 1990;15A:401–407.
37. Evans G, Burke FD, Barton NJ. A comparison of conservative treatment and silicone replacement arthroplasty in Kienbock's disease. *J Hand Surg* 1986;11B:98–102.
38. Carter PR, Benton LJ, Dysert PA. Silicone rubber carpal implants: A study of the incidence of late osseous complications. *J Hand Surg* 1986;11A:639–644.
39. Perlman MD, Schor AD, Gold ML. Implant failure with particulate silicone synovitis. *J Foot Surg* 1990;29:584–588.
40. Peimer CA, Medige J, Eckert BS, et al. Reactive synovitis after silicone arthroplasty. *J Hand Surg* 1986;11A:624–638.
41. Atkinson RE, Smith RJ. Silicone synovitis following silicone implant arthroplasty. *Hand Clin* 1986;2:291–299.
42. Shergy WJ, Urbaniak JR, Polisson RP. Silicone synovitis: Clinical, radiologic, and histologic features. *South Med J* 1989;82:1156–1158.
43. Yamashina M, Moatamed F. Peri-articular reactions to microscopic erosion of silicone-polymer implants: Light- and scanning electron-microscopic studies with energy-dispersive x-ray analysis. *Am J Surg Pathol* 1985;9:215–219.
44. Manes HR. Foreign body granuloma of bone secondary to silicone prosthesis: A case report. *Clin Orthop* 1985;199:239–241.
45. Rosenthal DI, Rosenberg AE, Schiller AL, et al. Destructive arthritis due to silicone: A foreign-body reaction. *Radiology* 1983;149:69–72.
46. Schneider HJ, Weiss MA, Stern PJ. Silicone-induced erosive arthritis: Radiologic features in seven cases. *AJR* 1987;148:923–925.
47. Christie AJ, Pierret G, Levitan J. Silicone synovitis. *Semin Arthritis Rheum* 1989;19:166–171.
48. Freeman GR, Honner R. Silastic replacement of the trapezium. *J Hand Surg* 1992;17B:458–462.
49. Smith RJ, Atkinson RE, Jupiter JB. Silicone synovitis of the wrist. *J Hand Surg* 1985;10A:47–60.
50. Eiken O, Ekerot L, Lindstrom C, et al. Silicone carpal implants. *Scand J Plast Reconstr Surg* 1985;19:295–304.
51. Simmons BP, McKenzie WD. Symptomatic carpal coalition. *J Hand Surg* 1985;110A:90–93.
52. Delaney TJ, Eswar S. Carpal coalitions. *J Hand Surg* 1992; 17A:28–31.
53. Berkowitz AR, Melone CP, Belsky MR. Pisiform-hamate coalition with ulnar neuropathy. *J Hand Surg* 1992;17A:657–662.
54. Ganos DL, Imbriglia JE. Symptomatic congenital coalition of the pisiform and hamate. *J Hand Surg* 1991;16A:646–650.
55. Gross SC, Watson HK, Strickland JW, et al. Triquetral-lunate arthritis secondary to synovitis. *J Hand Surg* 1989;14A:95–102.
56. Metz VM, Schimmerl SM, Gilula LA, et al. Wide scapholunate joint space in lunotriquetral coalition: A normal variant? *Radiology* 1993;188:557–559.
57. Doman AN, Marcus NW. Congenital bipartite scaphoid. *J Hand Surg* 1990;15A:869–873.
58. Engel A, Feldner-Busztin H. Bilateral stress fracture of the scaphoid. *Arch Orthop Trauma Surg* 1991;110:314–315.
59. Richards RR, Ledbetter WS, Transfeldt EE. Radiocarpal osteoarthritis associated with bilateral bipartite carpal scaphoid bones: A case report. *Can J Hand Surg* 1987;30:289–291.
60. van Goor H, Houpt P. Bilateral congenital hypoplasia of the carpal scaphoid bone. *J Hand Surg* 1989;14A:291–294.
61. Fagg PS. Wrist pain in the Madelung's deformity of dyschondrosteosis. *J Hand Surg* 1988;13B:11–15.
62. Thomas RD, Fairhurst JJ, Clarke NMP. Madelung's deformity masquerading as a bone tumour. *Skeletal Radiol* 1993;22:329–331.
63. Vickers D, Nielsen G. Madelung deformity: Surgical prophylaxis (physiolysis) during the late growth period by resection

of the dyschondrosteosis lesion. *J Hand Surg* 1992;17B:401–407.

64. Hoffman GS. Calcium pyrophosphate dihydrate (CPPD) deposition disease. In: Wilson JD, Braunwald E, Isselbacher KJ, et al., eds. *Harrison's principles of internal medicine.* 12th ed. New York: McGraw-Hill, 1991:1480–1481.
65. Jobanputra P, Gibson T. Diagnosis of pseudogout and septic arthritis. *Br J Rheumatol* 1987;26:379–380.
66. Berger RA, Buckwalter JA. Calcium pyrophosphate dihydrate crystal deposition patterns in the triangular fibrocartilage complex. *Orthopedics* 1990;13:75–80.
67. Resnik CS, Resnick D. Crystal deposition disease. *Semin Arthritis Rheum* 1983;12:390–403.
68. Braunstein EM, Menerey K, Martel W, Swartz R, Fox IH. Radiologic features of a pyrophosphate-like arthropathy associated with long-term dialysis. *Skeletal Radiol* 1987;16:437–441.
69. Jones A, Barton N, Pattrick M, et al. Tophaceous pyrophosphate deposition with extensor tendon rupture. *Br J Rheumatol* 1992;31:421–423.
70. Chen C, Chandnani VP, Kang HS, et al. Scapholunate advanced collapse: A common wrist abnormality in calcium pyrophosphate dihydrate crystal deposition disease. *Radiology* 1990;177:459–461.
71. Doherty W, Lovallo JL. Scapholunate advanced collapse pattern of arthritis in calcium pyrophosphate deposition disease of the wrist. *J Hand Surg* 1993;18A:1095–1098.
72. Watson HK, Ballet FL. The SLAC wrist: Scapholunate advanced collapse pattern of degenerative arthritis. *J Hand Surg* 1984;9A:358–365.
73. Watson HK, Ryu J. Evolution of arthritis of the wrist. *Clin Orthop* 1986;202:57–67.
74. Vender MI, Watson HK, Wiener BD, et al. Degenerative change in symptomatic scaphoid nonunion. *J Hand Surg* 1987;12A:514–519.
75. Osterman AL, Mikulics M. Scaphoid nonunion. *Hand Clin* 1988;14:437–455.
76. Watson KH, Dhillon HS. Intercarpal arthrodesis. In: Green DP, ed. *Operative hand surgery.* 3rd ed. Vol. 1. New York: Churchill Livingstone, 1993:113–130.
77. Resnick D, Niwayama G. Degenerative disease of extraspinal locations. In: Resnick D, Niwayama G, eds. *Diagnosis of bone and joint disorders.* 2nd ed. Philadelphia: WB Saunders, 1988:1402–1405.
78. Taliesnik J. Classification of carpal instability. In: Taliesnik J, ed. *The wrist.* New York: Churchill Livingstone, 1985:229–238.
79. Destouet JM, Gilula LA, Reinus WR. Roentgenographic diagnosis of wrist pain and instability. In: Lichtman DM, ed. *The wrist and its disorders.* Philadelphia: WB Saunders, 1988:82–95.
80. Flatt AE. Correction of arthritic deformities of the upper extremity. In: McCarty DJ, ed. *Arthritis and allied conditions.* 9th ed. Philadelphia: Lea & Febiger, 1979:551–552.
81. Gunther SF. The carpometacarpal joint of the thumb: Practical considerations. In: Lichtman DM, ed. *The wrist and its disorders.* Philadelphia, WB Saunders, 1988:187–198.
82. Milford L. Reconstruction after injury. In: Crenshaw AH, ed. *Campbell's operative orthopaedics.* 7th ed. St. Louis: CV Mosby, 1987:280–284.
83. Melone CP Jr, Beavers B, Isani A. The basal joint pain syndrome. *Clin Orthop* 1987;220:58–67.
84. Gold RH, Bassett LW, Seeger LL. The other arthritides: Roentgenologic features of osteoarthritis, erosive osteoarthritis, ankylosing spondylitis, psoriatic arthritis, Reiter's disease, multicentric reticulohistiocytosis, and progressive systemic sclerosis. *Radiol Clin North Am* 1988;26:195–212.
85. Belliappa PP, Burke FD. Excision of the pisiform in pisotriquetral osteoarthritis. *J Hand Surg* 1992;17B:133–136.
86. Carroll RE, Coyle MP. Dysfunction of the pisotriquetral joint: Treatment by excision of the pisiform. *J Hand Surg* 1985; 10A:703–707.
87. Palmieri TJ. Pisiform area pain treatment by pisiform excision. *J Hand Surg* 1982;7A:477–480.
88. Palmieri TJ, Grand FM, Hay EL, et al. Treatment of osteoarthritis in the hand and wrist: Nonoperative treatment. *Hand Clin* 1987;3:371–383.
89. Viegas SF, Patterson RM, Eng M, et al. Wrist anatomy: Incidence, distribution, and correlation of anatomic variations, tears, and arthrosis. *J Hand Surg* 1993;18A:463–475.
90. Viegas SF, Wagner K, Patterson R, et al. Medial (hamate) facet of the lunate. *J Hand Surg* 1990;15A:564–571.
91. Peh WCG, Gilula LA, Viegas SF, et al. Degenerative lesions in the proximal pole of the hamate: Radiological features. *Radiology* 1995, submitted.
92. Burgess RC. Anatomic variations of the midcarpal joint. *J Hand Surg* 1990;15A:129–131.
93. Palmer A. Personal communication with Dr. Louis Gilula, 1993.

CHAPTER 21

MISCELLANEOUS SURGICAL ENTITIES OF THE HAND AND WRIST

Douglas K. Smith and Alan Christensen

INTRODUCTION

Numerous surgical procedures are performed for treatment of hand and wrist disorders. Postoperative radiographs can provide important information about the patient's previous medical history and treatment. The radiographic appearance or "footprint" can frequently reveal which surgical procedure was performed and the most likely initial diagnosis. An abnormal appearance can explain a patient's recurrent symptoms or suggest that an additional procedure should be performed. The interpreter of postoperative radiographs must be familiar with both the normal and abnormal radiographic appearances of the surgical procedures performed by referring hand surgeons. The goal of this chapter is to show the radiographic appearances of several common and a few uncommon surgical procedures performed in the hand and wrist. The chapter will be divided into procedures performed on the distal radioulnar joint, arthroplasties, arthrodeses, skeletal fixation techniques, procedures for scaphoid fracture nonunions, and procedures performed for repair or reconstruction of complex hand injuries.

PROCEDURES INVOLVING THE DISTAL RADIOULNAR JOINT

The anatomic structures of the ulnocarpal joint are important contributors to the stability and normal function of the wrist. In the normal wrist the distal articular surface of the radius and the triangular fibrocartilage (TFC) (covering the head of the ulna) form a smooth, level articulating surface for the carpal bones.[1] The relative lengths of the articular surfaces of the distal radius and ulna determine relative distribution of forces transmitted through the radiocarpal and ulnocarpal joints.[2] If the head of the ulna bone projects distal to the articular surface of the radius (ulnar positive variance), the lunate may impact on the triangular fibrocartilage during ulnar deviation of the wrist, producing the clinical entity of ulnocarpal impaction syndrome (Fig. 21–1).[3,4] The radiographic features of ulnocarpal impaction syndrome include ulnar positive variance on a neutral rotation projection and bony sclerosis or subcortical radiographic lucencies that may be either cyst formation or fibrosis in the proximal ulnar aspect of the lunate. Magnetic resonance imaging (MRI) shows variable marrow signal in the same area of the lunate (either bright signal on T2-weighted images consistent with cyst formation or low signal on all sequences consistent with fibrosis or bone sclerosis) and thinning or perforation of the TFC (Fig. 21–1).[5,6] Ulnar impaction syndrome is treated surgically by shortening the ulna and repairing or debriding tears of the TFC. The length of the ulna can be shortened by resecting a segment of the diaphysis of the ulna by performing a transverse, step-cut, or oblique osteotomy (Fig. 21–2).[7–9] The osteotomy is usually stabilized with a plate and cortical screws. Feldon, Belsky, and Terrono described an ulnar shortening technique involving resection of a 2- to 4-mm thick wafer of cartilage and bone from the articular dome of the distal ulna (Fig. 21–3).[10] This surgical procedure is recognizable by the decreased ulnar length and flattening of the distal ulnar articular surface.

If the articular surface of the ulna is located proximal to the radius (ulnar minus variance), excessive force may be transmitted through the radiolunate articulation.[5] This excessive force may predispose the patient to developing Kienböck's disease or osteonecrosis of the lunate. The surgical goal for treatment of early Kienböck's disease (before collapse of the lunate and development of secondary carpal osteoarthritis) is to decrease the force transmitted through the radiolunate articulation by correcting the ulnar minus variance. The surgical options include length-

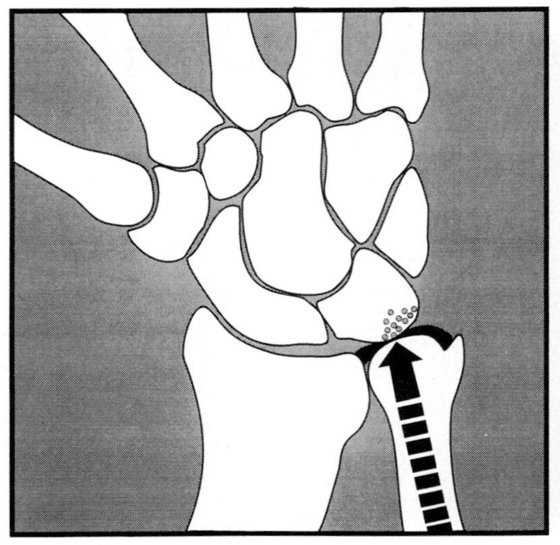

A

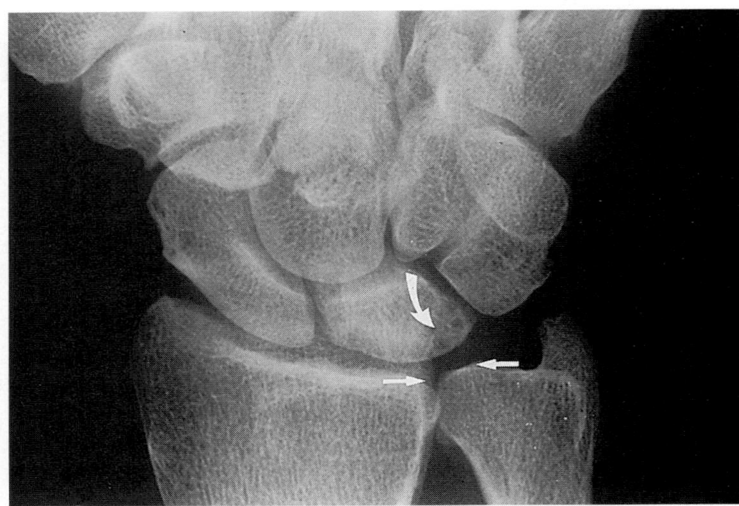

B

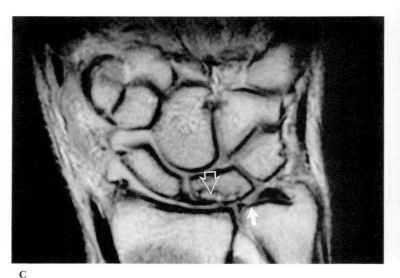

C

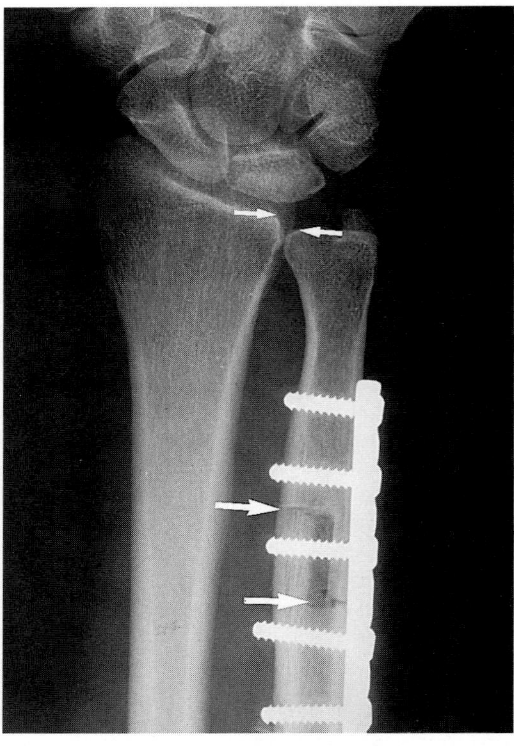

D

FIGURE 21–1. A: Mechanism of ulnocarpal impaction syndrome. Head of ulna projects distal to articular surface of radius (ulnar positive variance). Proximal carpal row impinges on soft tissues covering ulnar head during radial deviation of wrist (arrow). Intraosseous cysts, fibrosis, or sclerosis of the proximal ulnar aspect of the lunate bone may develop. **B:** Frontal radiograph of patient with ulnolunate impaction syndrome showing slight ulnar positive variance (between small arrows) with a few subchondral lucent defects at the site of impaction (curved arrow). **C:** Coronal T2-weighted (TR:TE = 2000/80 msec) shows increased marrow signal of subcortical bone of the proximal ulnar and radial aspects of the lunate (open arrow), thinning of triangular fibrocartilage (TFC) at site of impaction (white arrow), and ulnar positive variance. **D:** Postoperative radiograph shows ulnar minus variance (between small arrows) following transverse step-cut ulnar shortening osteotomy (between large arrows) with plate fixation.

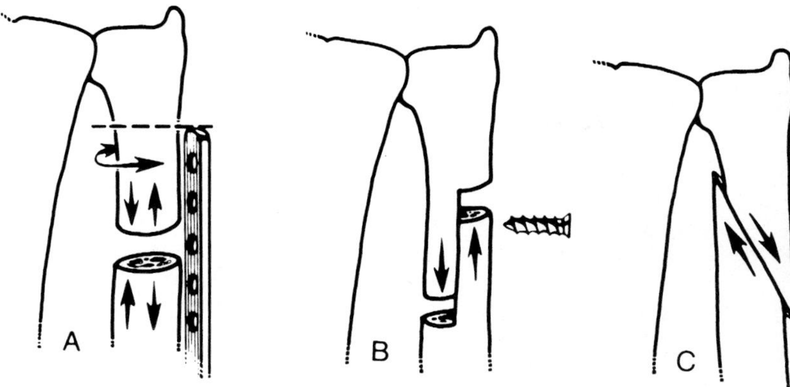

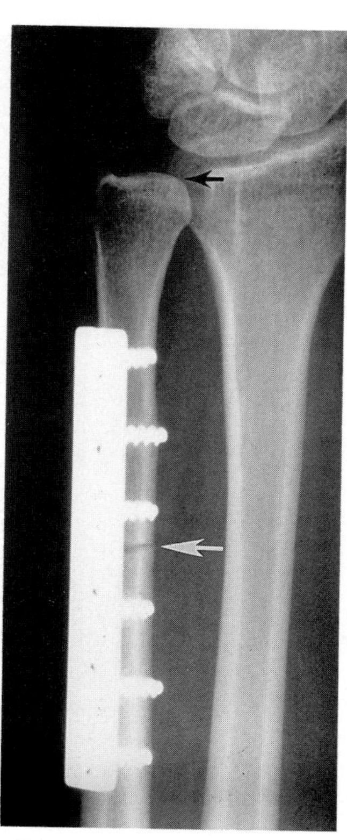

D

FIGURE 21–2. A–C: Techniques for ulnar osteotomy. Transverse osteotomy with side plate fixation **(A)** may be used for lengthening or shortening the ulna. Step-cut **(B)** and oblique osteotomy techniques **(C)** are also applicable for shortening the ulna and provide more bone surface for healing to decrease the incidence of nonunion. (Panels A–C reprinted with permission from Bowers WH. The distal radioulnar joint. In: Green DP, ed. *Operative hand surgery,* 3rd ed. Vol. 1. Churchill Livingstone, New York, 1993:973–1019.) **D:** Transverse ulnar shortening osteotomy (white arrow) with side plate fixation producing slight ulnar minus variance (black arrow). Distinguished from ulnar lengthening by absence of bone graft material and bone graft donor site. (Panel D reprinted with permission from Smith DK, Baker K, Gilula LA. Radiographic features of hand and wrist surgery excluding arthroplasties. *Eur J Radiol* 1990;10:85–91.)

ening of the ulna by insertion of a bone graft or shortening the radius by resecting a thin wafer of bone from the radial metaphysis or diaphysis.[7–9,11,12] The preoperative radiograph will show an ulnar minus variance and sclerosis of the lunate bone sug-

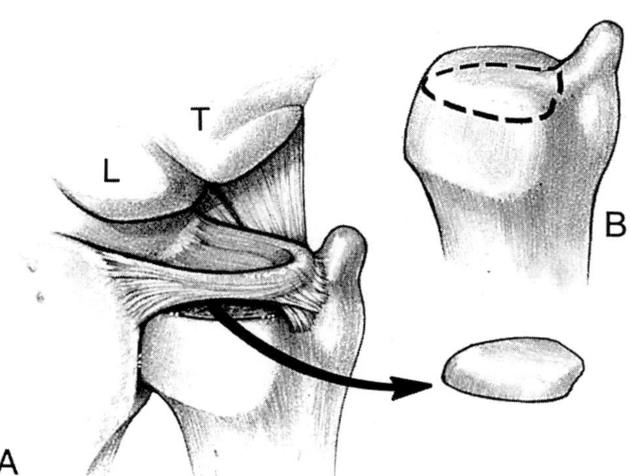

FIGURE 21–3. Feldon "wafer" osteotomy. Ulnar length is shortened by resecting a 2- to 4-mm thick wafer of bone and cartilage from articular surface of the ulnar head **(A).** The distal radioulnar joint is not disturbed. L, lunate bone, T, triquetral bone. Site of bone resection is shown in **B**. (Reprinted with permission from Bowers WH. The distal radioulnar joint. In: Green DP, ed. *Operative hand surgery,* 3rd ed. Vol. 1. Churchill Livingstone, New York, 1993:973–1019.)

gesting Kienböck's disease (Figs. 21–4 and 21–5). The ulna may be lengthened by performing a transverse osteotomy, distracting the two fragments, applying a fixation plate, and packing bone graft within the osteotomy site (Fig. 21–4).[7–9,12] The bone graft donor site may be visible as a rectangular lucency in the metaphysis of the distal radius (Fig. 21–4). A radial shortening osteotomy is performed by resecting a thin wafer of the radial metaphysis or diaphysis (Fig. 21–5).[11] Postoperative radiographs of a metaphyseal osteotomy usually show a slight size discrepancy between the distal and proximal metaphyseal fragments and no evidence of bone graft spacer or bone graft donor site.

The sigmoid notch of the distal radius rotates around the smooth articular surface of the distal ulna during pronation and supination of the forearm. Any incongruity of this articulation due to arthritis or traumatic deformity may produce painful or limited motion of the distal radioulnar joint. Surgical treatment options include resecting the distal radioulnar articular surfaces along with all or part of the ulnar head (Darrach's procedure), or arthrodesing the distal radioulnar joint and providing rotational forearm movement through a surgically created distal ulnar pseudarthrosis (Lauenstein or Suavé–Kapandji procedure) (Fig. 21–6).[13–16] In a Darrach procedure, the ulnar head and distal shaft are resected, leaving the TFC and its supporting ligaments intact (Fig. 21–7).[17] Several modifications of the Darrach technique have been proposed to prevent the ulnocarpal

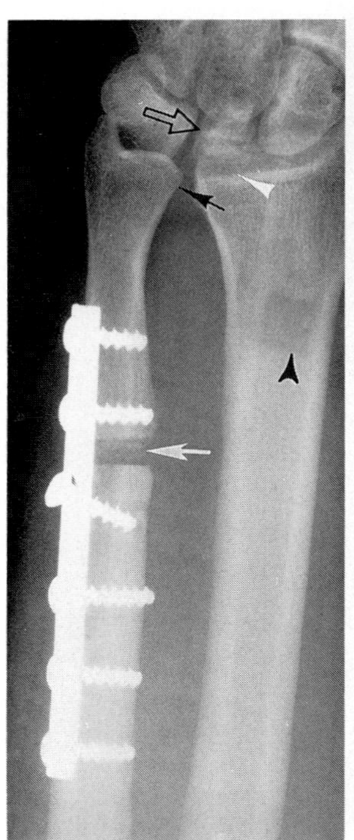

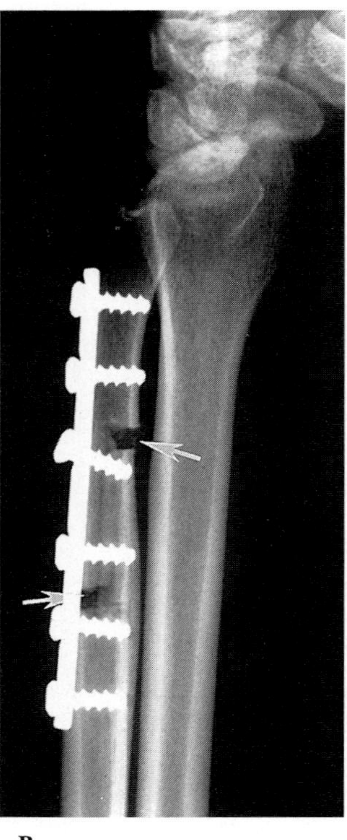

A B

FIGURE 21–4. A: Transverse ulnar lengthening osteotomy for treatment of Kienböck's disease (sclerotic fragmented lunate—open arrow and white arrowhead). Radiolunate joint stress transmission reduced by creation of ulnar positive variance (black arrow). Bone graft material in osteotomy site (white arrow) and bone graft donor site (black arrowhead) are visible. **B:** Sliding "step-cut" ulnar lengthening osteotomy (arrows) with bone graft visible within the bony defects. (Reprinted with permission from Smith DK, Baker K, Gilula LA. Radiographic features of hand and wrist surgery excluding arthroplasties. *Eur J Radiol* 1990;10:85–91.)

instability that can result from this procedure. Most of these modifications involve restraining the distal ulna with a tendon (tenodesis) or interposing soft tissue within the surgical defect. These soft-tissue procedures cannot be distinguished radiographically. Swanson advocated insertion of a silicone rubber spacer to fill the gap left by resection of the ulnar head. Most surgeons have abandoned the insertion of a silicone spacer because of the high rate of prosthetic fracture and dislocation and because of the risks of silicone (particulate) induced synovitis (Fig. 21–11C).[18,19]

Bowers popularized the "hemiresection interposition technique" or "HIT" distal radioulnar arthroplasty (Fig. 21–8).[20] Only the radial half of the ulnar head is resected, leaving the ulnar styloid and medial cortex intact. The surgical defect is filled with a roll of tendon to prevent painful impingement of the remaining ulna with the radius. Watson, Ryu, and Burgess described a technique of circumferential resection of the distal ulna (Fig. 21–9).[21] The distal ulna is sculpted into a tapered cone with a size and shape that matches the sigmoid fossa of the radius bone (Fig. 21–9).[21]

ARTHROPLASTIES OF THE HAND AND WRIST

The two most popular surgical treatment options for joints that are destroyed by arthritis or trauma are joint arthroplasty or arthrodesis. An arthroplasty is usually performed in patients with limited functional demands that require more motion than is obtainable with an arthrodesis.[22] An active individual with high functional demands would tend to wear out or fracture an arthroplasty. An arthrodesis is frequently a better long-term choice in such an individual.[23] If an arthroplasty is performed, the affected joint surfaces are resected. The resulting space may be filled with the patient's soft tissues, synthetic interpositional materials, or with a total joint replacement.[24]

Carpal arthroplasties may include replacement of joint surfaces with prosthetic material such as silicone rubber or titanium.[22,24] From the late 1960s until the mid-1980s, silicone rubber implants were inserted to resurface an articular surface or to replace a carpal bone destroyed by trauma or arthritis.[22,24] Silicone implants are used less frequently today because of concerns about long-term complications; however, since silicone implants were placed in thousands of patients, it is important to recognize both the normal and abnormal radiographic appearances of these procedures. Primary osteoarthritis frequently affects the carpometacarpal (CMC) joint of the thumb, and silicone implants were often used around the thumb CMC joint.[22] If the arthritis was isolated to the CMC joint, the base of the first metacarpal or distal surface of the trapezium was resected and replaced by a silicone implant (Fig. 21–10). If the arthritis involved both the scaphotrapezial and carpometacarpal joints, the trapezium was resected and replaced by a silicone trapezial prosthesis (Fig. 21–11).[25,26] Silicone implants in these locations were subjected to excessive mechanical stresses and tended to wear over time (releasing particulate silicone).[27,28] In some patients, an aggressive foreign-body mediated synovitis developed with a radiographic appearance similar to rheumatoid arthritis (Fig. 21–11).[27,28] Currently, most surgeons have abandoned silicone implants for treatment of osteoarthritis at the base of the thumb. Some surgeons perform an arthrodesis between the trapezium and the thumb metacarpal (Fig. 21–12). Other surgeons prefer to resect the trapezium and perform an "anchovy" interpositional arthroplasty by rolling up a ball of tendon and inserting it into the surgical defect (Fig. 21–13).[22,29,30] This procedure provides greater motion but less stability than the arthrodesis.

Prosthetic implants made of silicone rubber have also been used to replace a lunate bone deformed by Kienböck's disease or a scaphoid bone deformed by a scaphoid fracture malunion or avascular necrosis

Text continued on page 553

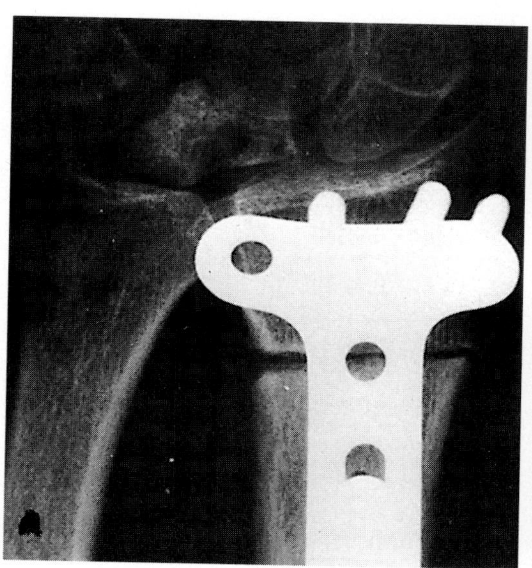
A

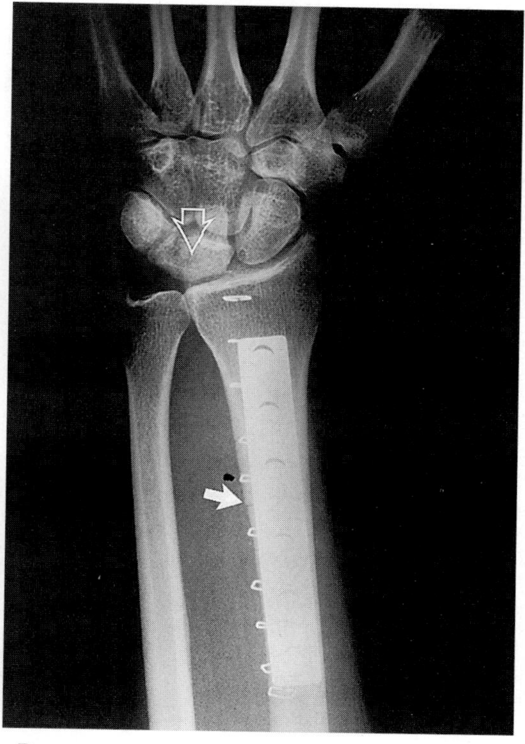
B

FIGURE 21–5. Radial shortening osteotomy for treatment of Kienböck's disease. **A:** Segmental resection of radial metaphysis with buttress plate fixation device. (Reprinted with permission from Taleisnik J. Kienböck's disease. In: Taleisnik J, ed. *The wrist.* Churchill Livingstone, New York, 1985.) **B:** Segmental resection of radial diaphysis as a radial shortening osteotomy (white arrow) for Kienböck's disease recognizable by lunate bone sclerosis (open arrow).

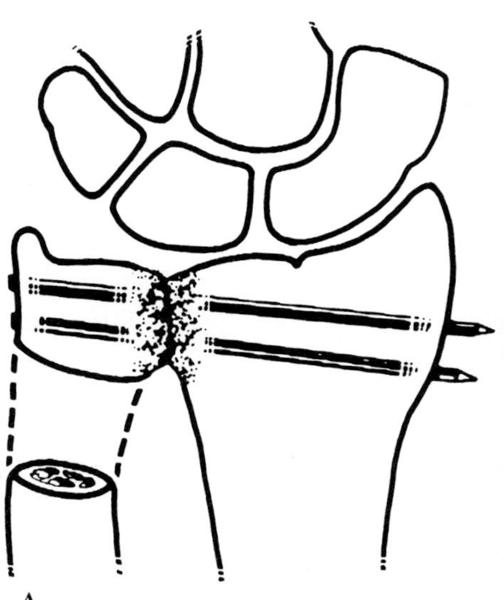
A

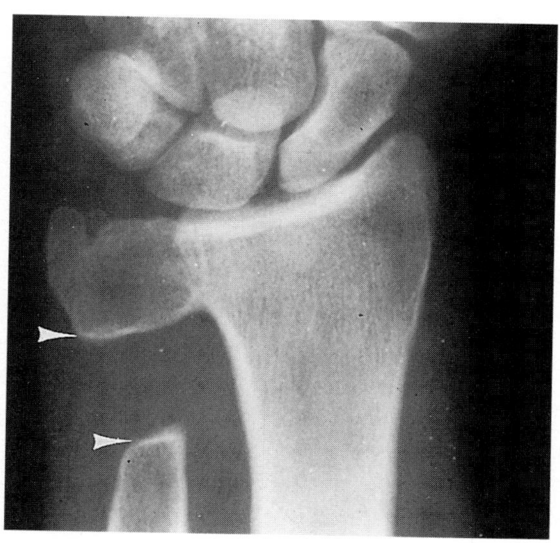
B

FIGURE 21–6. Suavé–Kapandji procedure (also known as Lauenstein's procedure). **A:** Drawing showing distal radioulnar joint arthrodesis with segmental resection of distal ulnar diaphysis and creation of ulnar pseudarthrosis. Forearm rotation takes place through ulnar pseudarthrosis. (Reprinted with permission from Bowers WH. The distal radioulnar joint. In: Green DP, ed. *Operative hand surgery.* Churchill Livingstone, New York, 1993.) **B:** Radiographic appearance of Suavé–Kapandji procedure. Segmental resection defined by arrowheads. (Reprinted with permission from Smith DK, Baker K, Gilula LA. Radiographic features of hand and wrist surgery excluding arthroplasties. *Eur J Radiol* 1990;10:85–91. Courtesy of Julio Taleisnik, M.D., Orange, CA.)

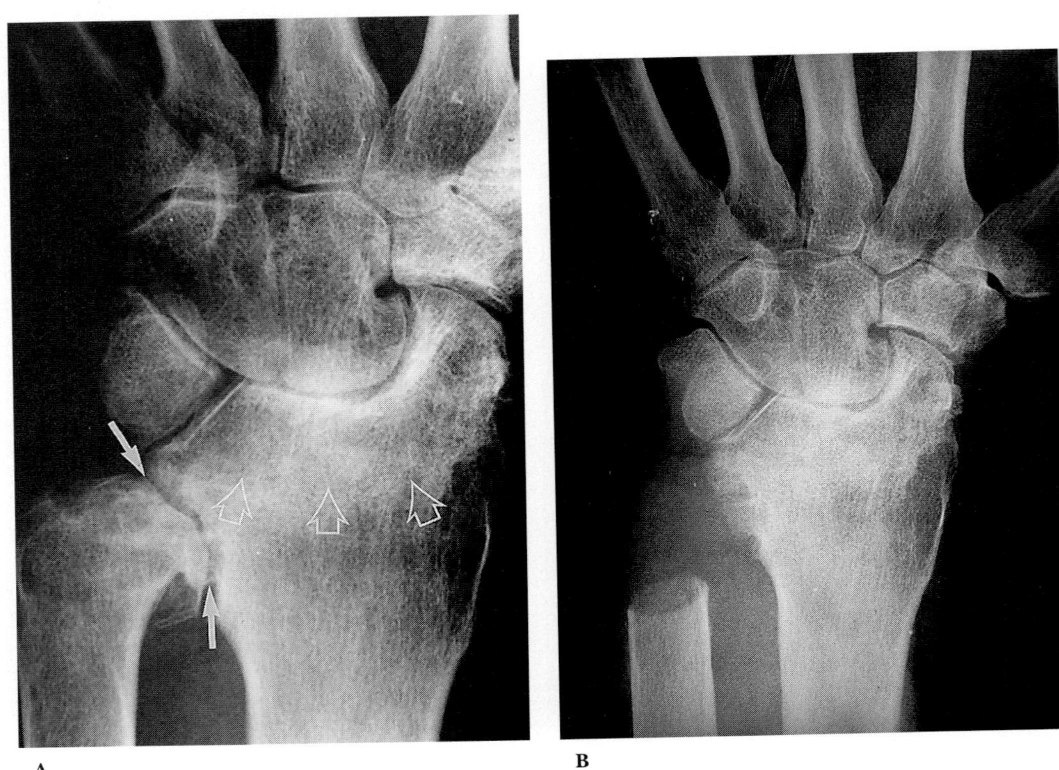

FIGURE 21–7. Darrach's procedure. **A:** Severe posttraumatic osteoarthritis of the distal radioulnar joint (closed arrows) following radioscapholunate arthrodesis (open arrows) for traumatic radiocarpal arthritis. **B:** Resection of ulnar head leaving TFC intact (Darrach's procedure) to decrease distal radioulnar joint pain. This procedure may be performed in association with radiocarpal arthrodesis, proximal row carpectomy, or silicone interposition arthroplasty to prevent impingement of the ulnar head with the carpus.

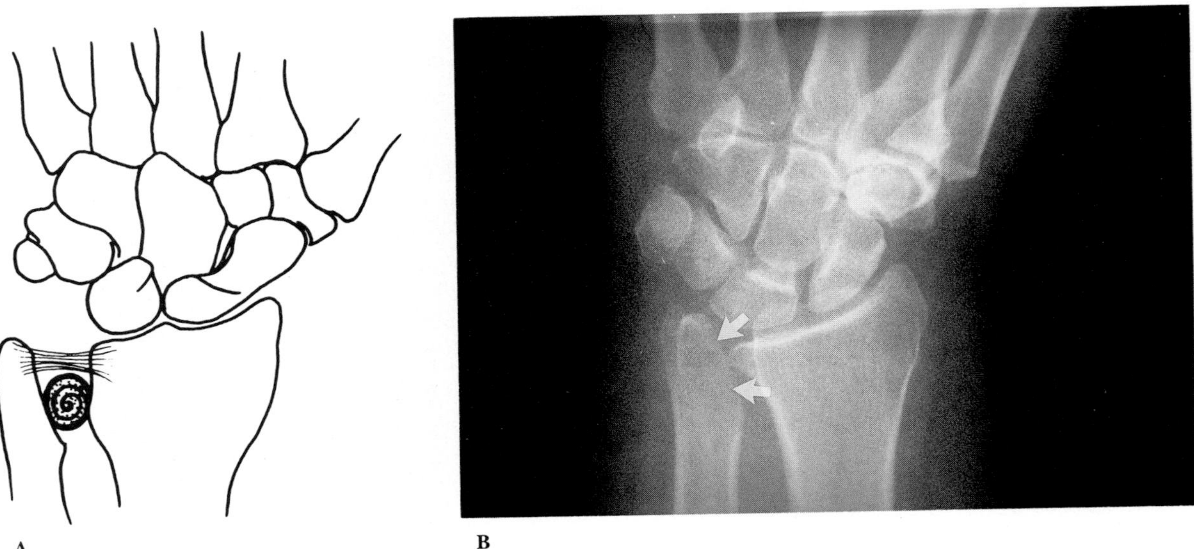

FIGURE 21–8. Hemiresection interposition technique (HIT) for distal radioulnar joint arthroplasty. **A:** Line drawing: resection of radial half of ulnar head with insertion of tendon "anchovy" within bony defect to prevent radioulnar impingement. **B:** Hemiresection of the distal ulna: resection of radial aspect of the distal ulna with concave defect (arrows). (Reprinted with permission from Smith DK, Baker K, Gilula LA. Radiographic features of hand and wrist surgery excluding arthroplasties. *Eur J Radiol* 1990;10:85–91.)

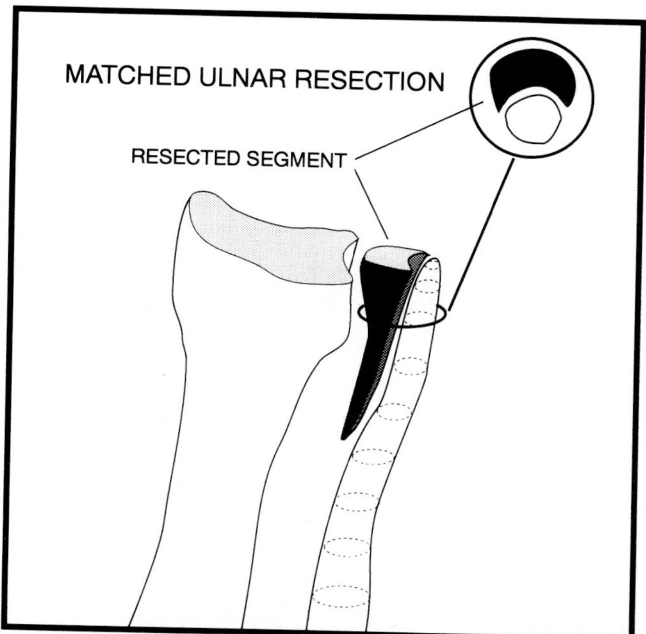

FIGURE 21–9. Watson "matched" ulnar resection. Resection of radial cortex of ulnar head producing cone-shaped ulna matching shape of sigmoid fossa of radius. Resected ulnar bone is in black.

with collapse (Figs. 21–14 and 21–15).[31] Most surgeons have abandoned the use of silicone carpal bones unless a limited carpal fusion is also performed to limit the stresses applied to the prosthesis (Figs. 21–14 and 21–15).[22] Some surgeons have used a titanium (metal alloy) scaphoid prosthesis while other surgeons have combined a silicone implant with some type of limited intercarpal arthrodesis (Fig. 21–16).[22,32,33]

A proximal row carpectomy can be performed for patients with deformity of the proximal carpal row (Kienböck's disease or collapsed scaphoid fracture) when the lunate fossa and the head of the capitate are relatively normal.[34] The scaphoid, lunate, and triquetral bones are resected, and the capitate articulates directly with the lunate fossa of the radius (Fig. 21–17). This procedure provides adequate function for many patients but may need to be converted to a wrist arthrodesis if radiocapitate osteoarthritis develops.[35] In older cases, the distal pole of the scaphoid bone may have been left in situ, but the entire scaphoid is now removed to prevent the painful impingement of the distal pole of the scaphoid with the radial styloid process (Fig. 21–17).[36]

Silicone implants are still frequently used in patients with rheumatoid arthritis.[24] In patients with severe erosion of the wrist, the distal radius and proximal carpal row are resected and replaced by a flexible silicone hinge (Fig. 21–18).[24] The silicone radiocarpal implant is held in place by fixation stems that are inserted into the medullary cavities of the third metacarpal and distal radius.[24] Smaller implants may be used to reconstruct the proximal interphalangeal joints (Fig. 21–19).[37] Late findings of silicone implants include migration or settling of the implant into the soft arthritic bone, fracture of the fixation stems at the site of bending, or dislocation of the stems from the medullary cavities (Figs. 21–18 and 21–19).[27,28] Newer models have incorporated metal flanges to protect the sites of bending (Figs. 21–18 and 21–19).[38] A Darrach resection or silicone prosthetic ulnar head may also be performed along with the silicone radiocarpal arthroplasty (Fig. 21–18).[22,31,38]

A total wrist arthroplasty is usually performed in patients with rheumatoid arthritis who are over the age of 50 and require more motion than that available with a wrist fusion and more stability than that available using a silicone radiocarpal implant.[22] Several models of prosthetic wrists have been developed with designs based on a hinge or ball and socket joint (with varying degrees of constraint).[22,39,40] All of the designs have fixation stems that are inserted into the distal radius and metacarpals, and most are fixed in place with methyl methacrylate (Fig. 21–20).[22] Potential complications include loosening or migration of the fixation stems, dislocation of the proximal and distal components, or fracture of the implant.[22]

ARTHRODESIS OF THE HAND AND WRIST

A wrist arthrodesis may be performed in various clinical settings: a patient with rheumatoid arthritis and the need for stability; a young, heavy-laboring man with advanced radiocarpal arthritis; or following failed total wrist arthroplasty.[23] Arthrodesis techniques vary as to the amount of carpal bone resected and the method of applied fixation.[23,41–43] In the cortical inlay technique, the dorsal cortex of the distal radius, carpal bones, and bases of the index and middle metacarpal bones are resected (Fig. 21–21).[23,41,42] A corticocancellous bone graft is harvested from the ilium and is sculpted to fit the dorsum of the wrist. The bone graft may be transfixed with cortical or cancellous screws. If the bone graft reabsorbs around the screws, the heads of the screws may project into the dorsal soft tissues without surrounding bone graft. In the Association for Osteosynthesis (AO) technique for wrist fusion only the scaphoid, lunate, capitate, and third metacarpal bones are decorticated and a dorsal fixation plate is applied (Fig. 21–22).[43] In a Nalebuff technique, a Steinman pin or large Kirschner wire is inserted in a retrograde fashion either from the third metacarpal or the second or third web space into the distal radius to maintain support until the fusion heals (Fig. 21–23).[44] The fixation pin can be easily removed using local anesthesia when the arthrodesis is healed. Because the fixation pin is not cemented, postoperative radiographs must be examined for signs of loosening or migration (Fig. 21–23).

When the carpal destructive process is more focal,

Text continued on page 556

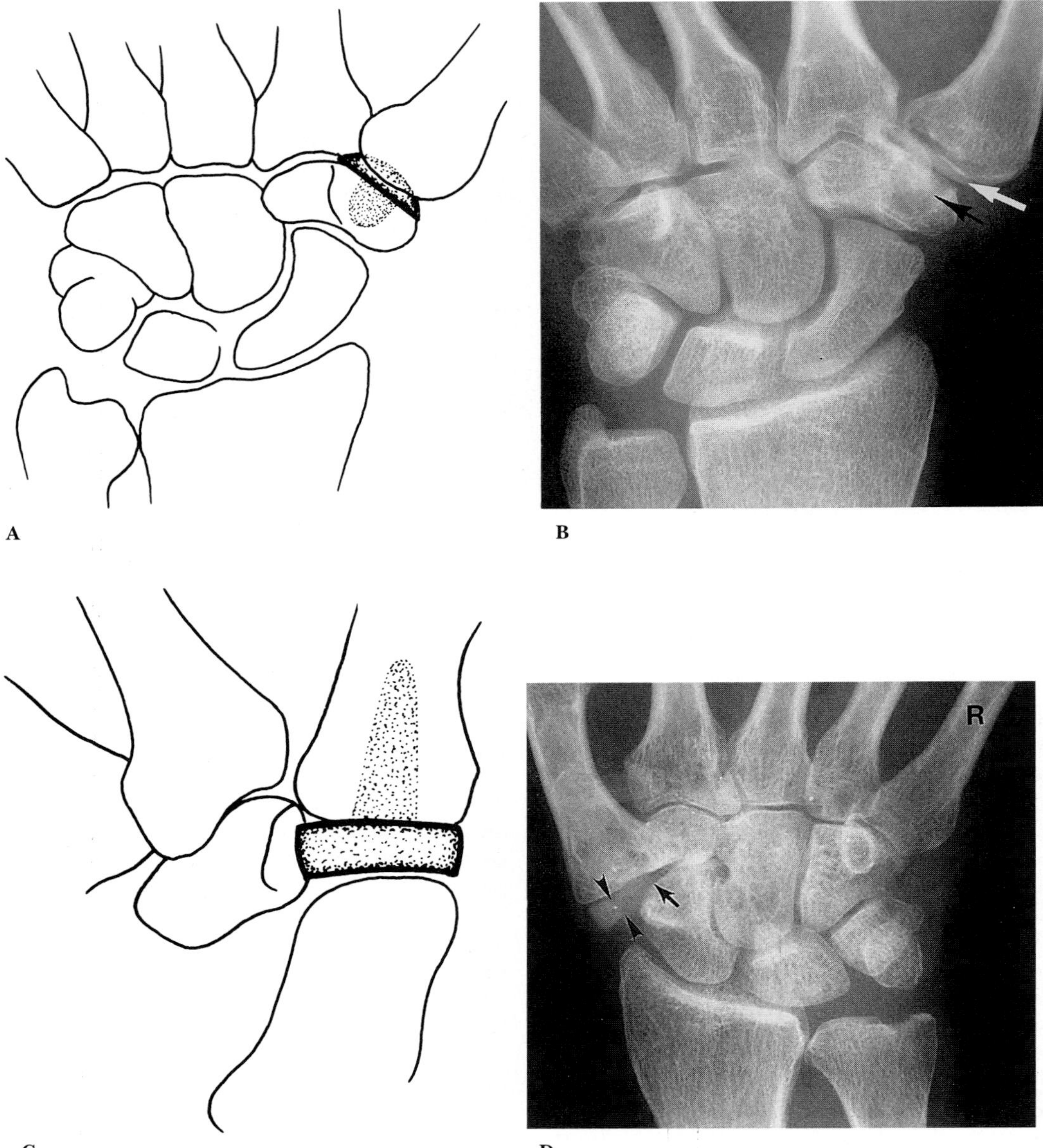

FIGURE 21–10. A: Line drawing: resection of distal articular surface of trapezium and resurfacing with implant made of silicone rubber. **B:** Progressive thinning of implant (white arrow) and lucency around the fixation stem (black arrow) may represent prosthetic loosening or early silicone-induced (particulate) synovitis. **C:** Line drawing of silicone "great toe" implant resurfacing base of first metacarpal. **D:** Prosthetic fracture (arrowheads) and uneven wear of the ulnar aspect of the prosthesis (arrow). (Figures A to D reprinted with permission from Smith DK, Baker K, Gilula LA. Radiographic features of hand and wrist arthroplasties. *Eur J Radiol* 1990;10:3–8.)

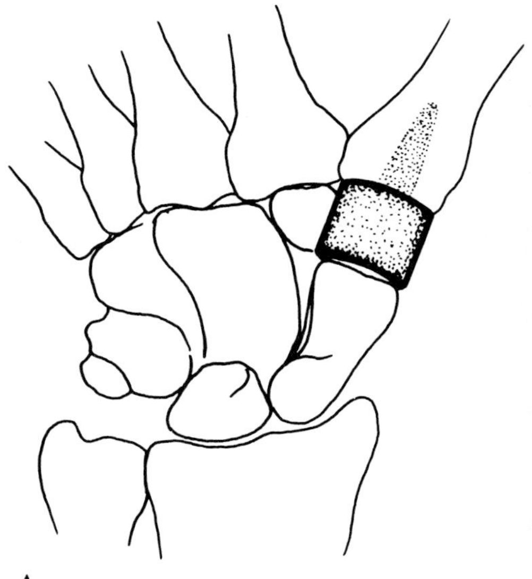

A

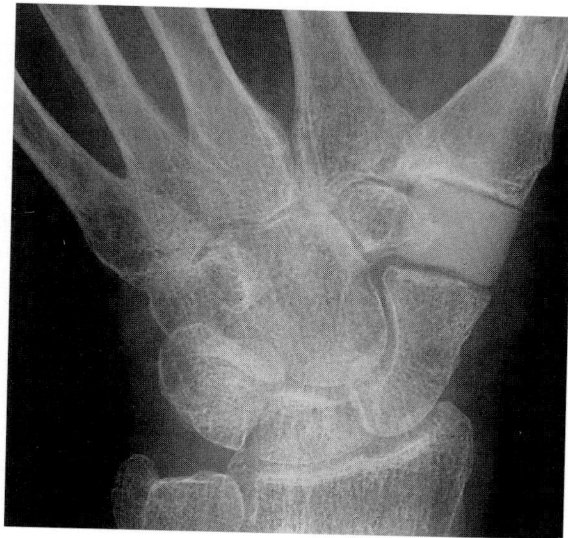

B

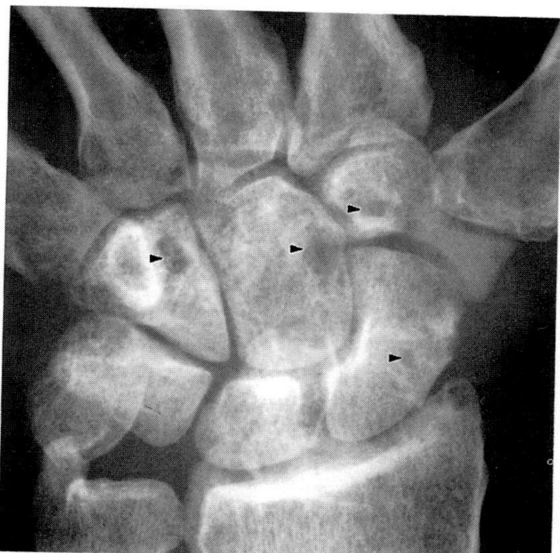

C

FIGURE 21–11. A: Line drawing of trapezial resection for osteoarthritis of both the scaphotrapezial and trapeziometacarpal joints with silicone trapezial prosthesis. **B:** Trapezial prosthesis with mild osteoarthritic changes of the distal scaphoid. **C:** Radiographic findings of pathologically proven silicone-induced (particulate) synovitis. Diffuse, progressive carpal lucencies (arrowheads) resembling rheumatoid arthritis developed in association with a worn silastic prosthesis. (Figures A to C reprinted with permission from Smith DK, Baker K, Gilula LA. Radiographic features of hand and wrist arthroplasties. *Eur J Radiol* 1990;10:3–8.)

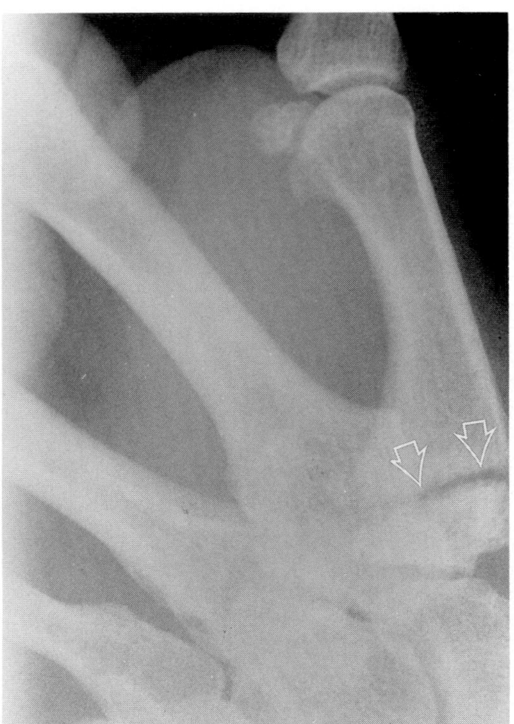

FIGURE 21–12. Arthrodesis of the CMC joint of the thumb for severe osteoarthritis. Trabecular bone crossed a portion of the fusion site and the joint was clinically fused despite a persistent radiographic lucency across much of the fusion site (open arrows).

a limited intercarpal arthrodesis may be performed.[33,45,46] Limited intercarpal fusions may be performed as treatment for deformities of carpal fractures, localized carpal arthritis, carpal instability, and as an adjunct to silicone carpal implants.[33,45,46] A scaphotrapeziotrapezoidal (STT) or triscaphe arthrodesis is usually performed for severe osteoarthritis of the STT joint or to correct the excessive ventral flexion of the scaphoid that occurs with rotary subluxation of the scaphoid (Fig. 21–24).[33,45–47] Scapholunate arthrodeses are rarely performed due to the high incidence of nonunions.[45] Radioscaphoid, radiolunate, and radioscapholunate arthrodeses are usually performed for posttraumatic deformities of the radiocarpal joints (Figs. 21–7 and 21–25).[33,45,46] A radiolunate arthrodesis may also be performed to prevent or correct ulnar translocation of the carpus in patients with rheumatoid arthritis.[45] A scaphocapitate fusion may be performed as an adjunct to silastic lunate implantation to decompress the prosthesis (Fig. 21–14).[33] A capitolunate fusion may be performed for arthritis of the capitolunate articulation or as an adjunct to prosthetic scaphoid implantation (Fig. 21–15).[45] A scapholunocapitate arthrodesis is a salvage procedure performed as treatment of advanced midcarpal arthritis with spared radiocarpal joints (Fig. 21–26).[33,45,46] Triquetrohamate and lunotriquetral arthrodeses are usually performed for ulnar-sided wrist instability.[45] The lunotriquetral arthrodesis is

Text continued on page 559

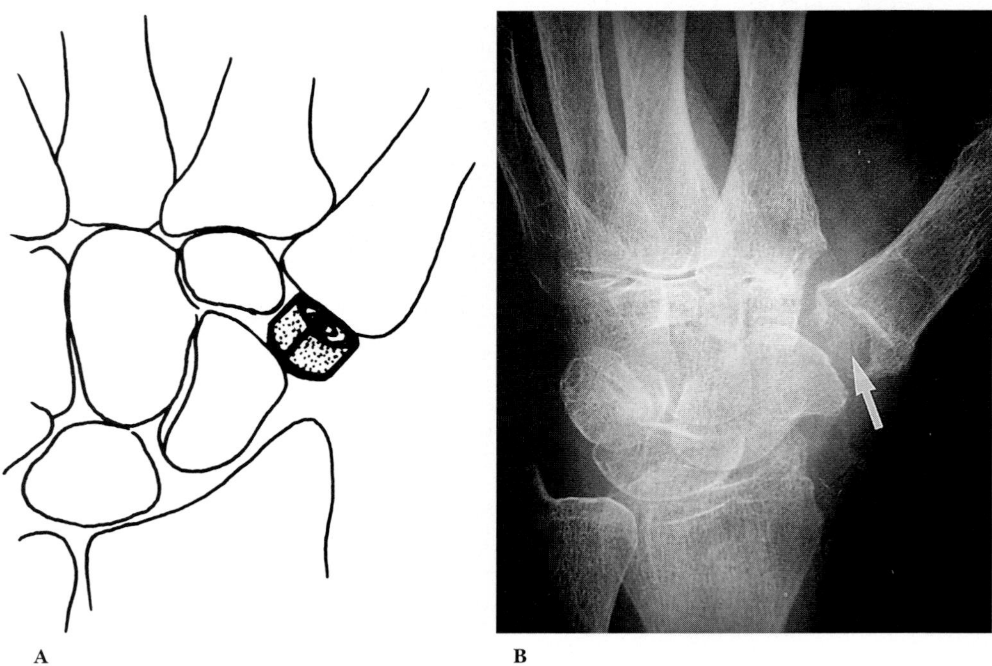

FIGURE 21–13. A: Line drawing: "anchovy" trapezial arthroplasty. Resection of trapezium with insertion of coiled flexor carpi radialis tendon (anchovy). **B:** Soft-tissue anchovy (arrow) faintly visible within bed of resected trapezium. (Reprinted with permission from Smith DK, Baker K, Gilula LA. Radiographic features of hand and wrist arthroplasties. *Eur J Radiol* 1990;10:3–8.)

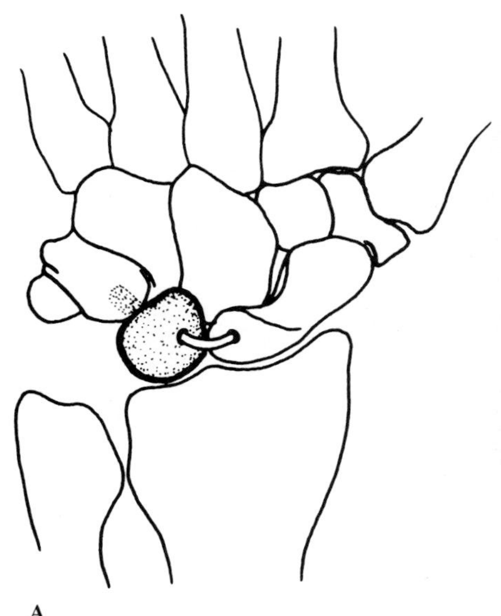
A

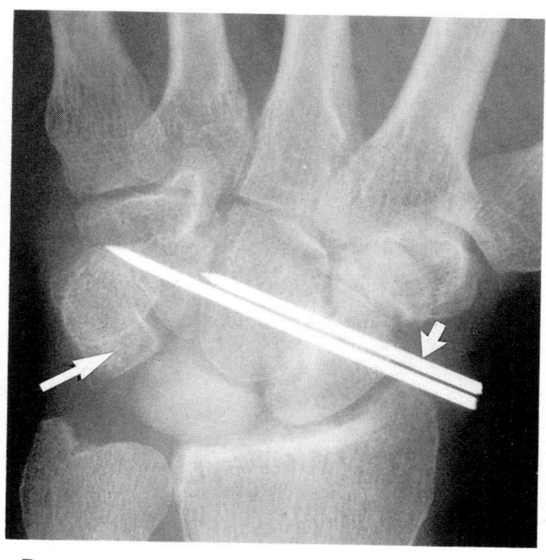
B

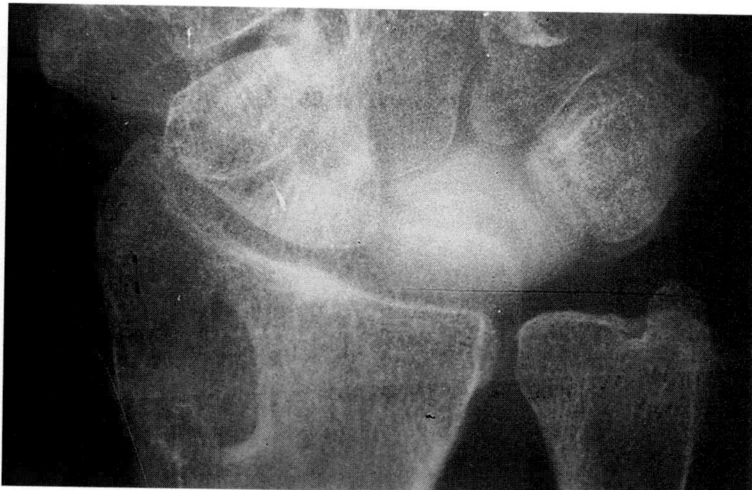
C

FIGURE 21–14. Silicone lunate prosthesis. **A:** Line drawing: silastic lunate prosthesis with fixation peg within triquetral bone and suture fixation to scaphoid. **B:** Silicone lunate prosthesis inserted after lunate resection for treatment of Kienböck's disease. Two parallel K-wires (short arrow) stabilizing recent scaphocapitate arthrodesis. Fixation peg of lunate prosthesis in the triquetrum (long arrow). (Figures A and B reprinted with permission from Smith DK, Baker K, Gilula LA. Radiographic features of hand and wrist arthroplasties. *Eur J Radiol* 1990;10:3–8.) **C:** Silicone lunate prosthesis implanted as treatment of Kienböck's disease. Scaphocapitate arthrodesis performed to decrease loading and wear of lunate prosthesis. (Reprinted with permission from Feldon P. Wrist fusions: Intercarpal and radiocarpal. In: Lichtman DM, ed. *The wrist and its disorders.* Philadelphia: WB Saunders, 1988:446–464.)

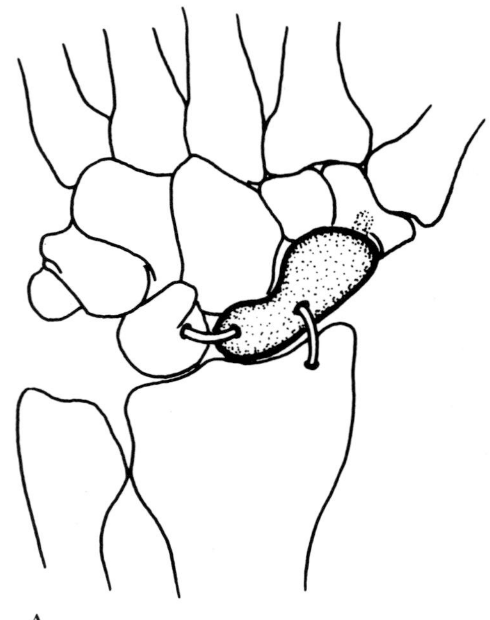

A

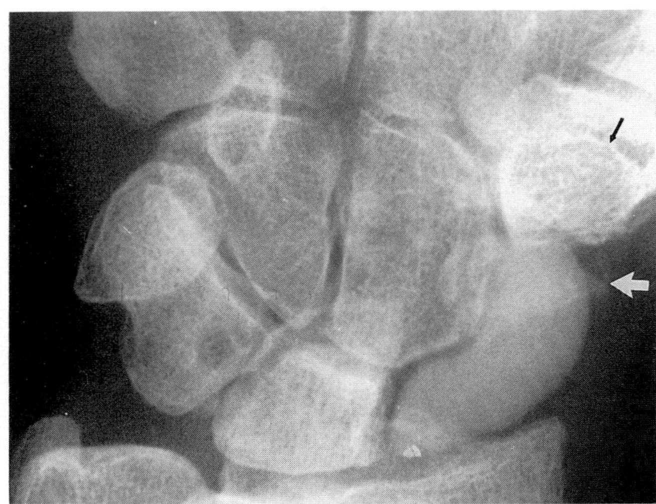

B

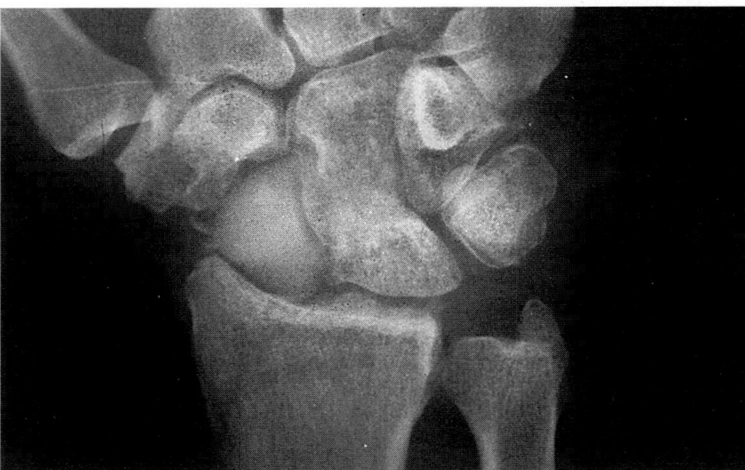

C

FIGURE 21–15. Silicone scaphoid prosthesis. **A:** Line drawing: silicone scaphoid prosthesis stabilized by fixation peg placed into trapezial bone and suture fixation in radius and lunate. **B:** Silicone scaphoid implant with fixation stem in trapezium (black arrow). Bone fragments (white arrow) are at insertion site of flexor carpi radialis tendon to native scaphoid and were left intentionally to avoid injuring the tendon. (Figures A and B reprinted with permission from Smith DK, Baker K, Gilula LA. Radiographic features of hand and wrist arthroplasties. *Eur J Radiol* 1990;10:3–8.) **C:** Silicone scaphoid prosthesis with adjunctive capitolunate arthrodesis to decrease mechanical stress applied to implant. (Figure C reprinted with permission from Feldon P. Wrist fusions: Radiocarpal and intercarpal. In: Lichtman DM, ed. *The wrist and its disorders.* Philadelphia: WB Saunders, 1988:446–464.)

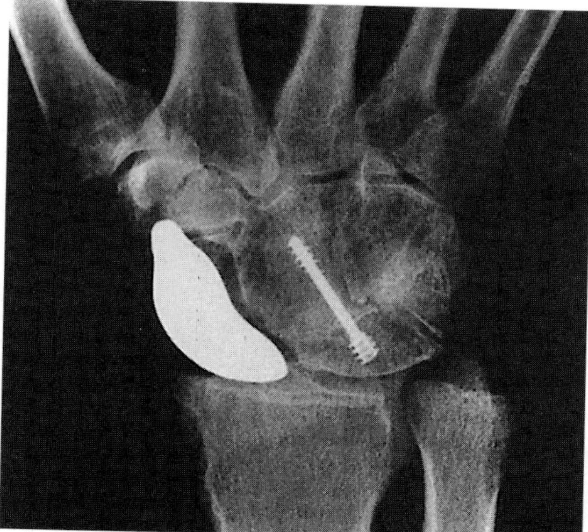

FIGURE 21–16. Titanium scaphoid prosthesis inserted in conjunction with capitolunotriquetrohamate arthrodesis. A Herbert screw is inserted to stabilize the arthrodesis until fusion healed. (Reprinted with permission from Beckenbaugh RD, Linscheid RL. Arthroplasty in the hand and wrist. In: Green DP, ed. *Operative hand surgery*. 3rd ed. Vol. 1. Churchill Livingstone, New York, 1993:143–187.)

predisposed to nonunions and a cancellous screw or Herbert screw is frequently used for additional fixation (Fig. 21–26).[33,45,46] A CMC arthrodesis is usually performed for posttraumatic arthritis of the index or long finger metacarpals, while arthroplasties are usually performed for the ring and small fingers (Fig. 21–27).[33]

SKELETAL FIXATION TECHNIQUES

Skeletal fixation techniques may be used for treatment of fractures or dislocations, or to maintain alignment until an arthrodesis, fracture, or soft-tissue reconstruction is healed.[36,48,49] It is important for radiologists to be aware of the generic names of these devices so that they can be properly described in reports and the normal and abnormal appearances of these devices can be recognized. External fixation devices are frequently used for immobilization of comminuted distal radial fractures (Fig. 21–28).[36,48,50] In some patients, especially the elderly, comminution of the dorsal cortex and metaphysis of the radius predisposes these fractures to collapse or apex ventral angulation using simple cast immobilization. The external fixator distracts the wrist and prevents fracture impaction, while percutaneously placed pins can be used to maintain the position of the fracture fragments until the fractures heal. Prolonged immobilization in an external fixator may predispose the patient to reflex sympathetic dystrophy that is recognizable as severe disuse osteopenia.[51] The external fixation is usually converted to cast immobilization after 4 to 10 weeks when the fracture is clinically united or "sticky," but perhaps before there is bridging callus or radiographic union.[51] On sequential radiographic examinations, it is important to check for change in fracture position or reduction loss, lucency around the fixation pins (loosening), or severe osteopenia (suggesting reflex sympathetic dystrophy).[52]

Fixation plates may be used to stabilize fractures and immobilize osteotomies (Figs. 21–1 to 21–4) or arthrodeses (Fig. 21–22).[36,43,48,49] A spe-

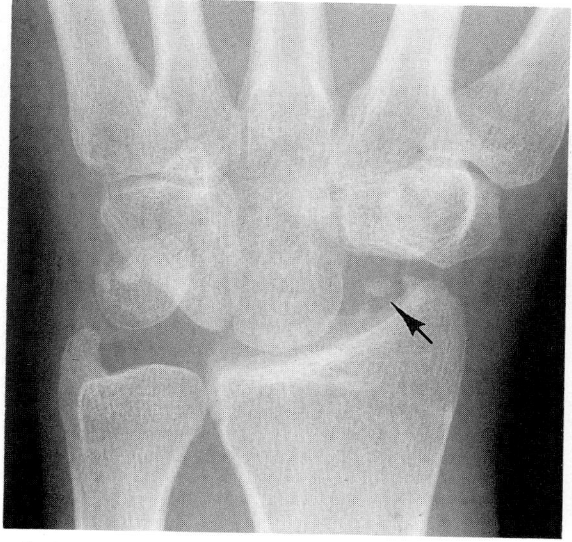

A

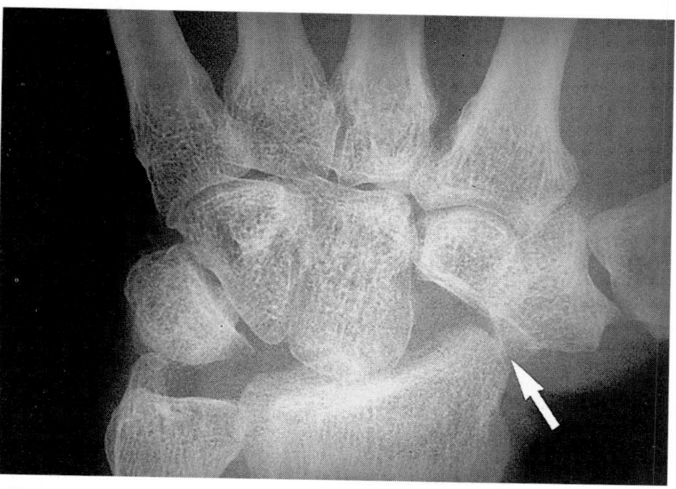

B

FIGURE 21–17. Proximal row carpectomy. **A:** Resection of scaphoid, lunate, and triquetral bones. Carpal bone fragments (arrow) are attached to ventral carpal ligaments and were left attached to avoid injuring the ligaments. (Reprinted with permission from Smith DK, Baker K, Gilula LA. Radiographic features of hand and wrist arthroplasties. *Eur J Radiol* 1990;10:3–8.) **B:** Resection of scaphoid and lunate with retention of triquetrum. In some cases the trapezium may impinge on the radial styloid during radial deviation of the wrist (arrow).

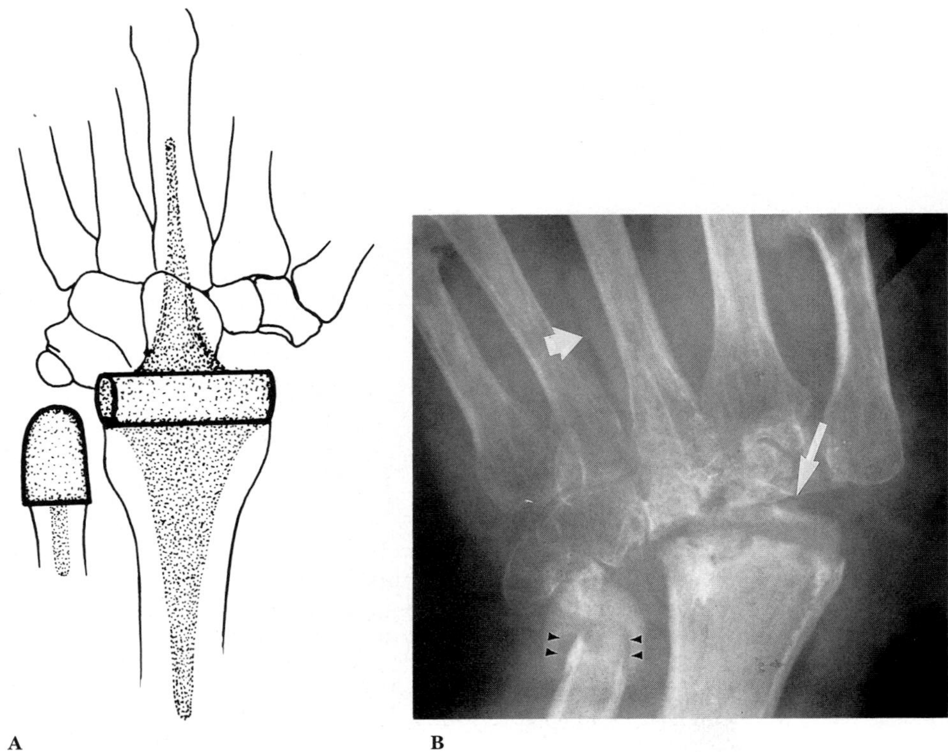

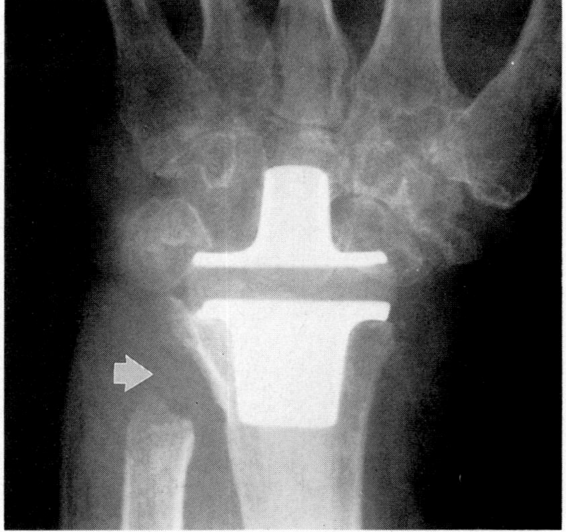

FIGURE 21–18. A: Drawing of Swanson silicone radiocarpal implant implanted following resection of distal radius, scaphoid, and lunate. Silastic ulnar styloid cap is inserted into diaphysis of distal ulna following a Darrach resection of distal ulna. **B:** Fracture of radiocarpal implant at stem/body junction (long arrow). Dislocation of the distal fixation stem (short arrow) out of the third metacarpal shaft. Distal ulnar fracture and bone resorption (double arrowheads) at the base of the ulnar cap. **C:** Newer model of silicone radiocarpal implant with metal flanges to protect the vulnerable stem/body junction. A Darrach resection without ulnar cap (arrow). (Panels A to C reprinted with permission from Smith DK, Baker K, Gilula LA. Radiographic features of hand and wrist surgery excluding arthroplasties. *Eur J Radiol* 1990;10:85–91.)

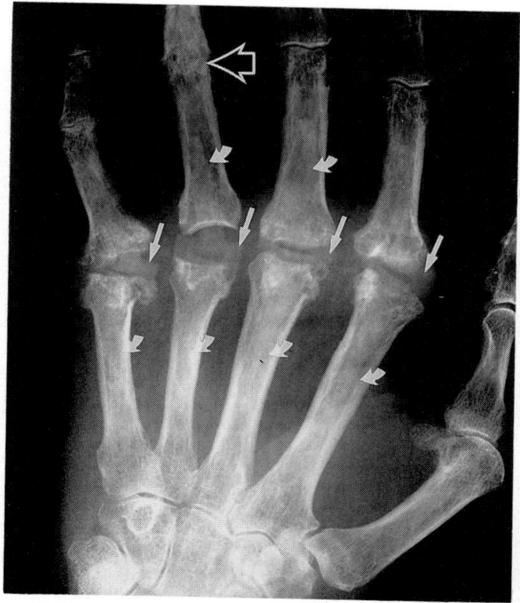

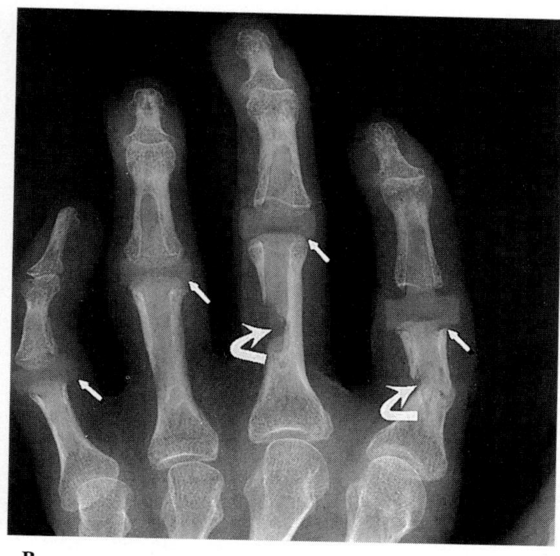

A B

FIGURE 21–19. A: Swanson silicone implants of metacarpophalangeal joint implants (straight arrows) in patient with rheumatoid arthritis. Fixation stems visible within medullary cavities of metacarpals and phalanges (curved arrows). Previous arthrodesis of proximal interphalangeal joint of ring finger (open arrow). **B:** Multiple silicone interphalangeal joint prostheses (straight arrows). Cortical defects along the fixation stems (curved arrows) were created during reaming of the medullary cavities (initially interpreted as metastatic disease by an unwary radiologist). (Panel B reprinted with permission from Smith DK, Baker K, Gilula LA. Radiographic features of hand and wrist arthroplasties. *Eur J Radiol* 1990;10:3–8.)

cial fixation plate with a broad flare at one end is called a buttress plate (Fig. 21–29).[43,48,49] This plate may be used for fixation of a distal radial osteotomy for radial shortening (Fig. 21–5), corrective osteotomy for fracture malunion (Fig. 21–29), or for primary fixation of a comminuted distal radial fracture.[43,48,49,51] In primary fracture fixation, this plate may be used to buttress against ventral displacement, and the distal screw holes may be left unfilled.

Fixation screws are available in varying styles and sizes to provide bone fixation in various applications.[43,48] Cortical screws are similar to wood screws and have narrow, closely spaced threads for attachment to dense cortical bone (Figs. 21–2D, 21–4A, 21–4B, 21–22B, and 21–30A).[43,48] Cancellous screws have large, widely spaced threads to maximize the surface area of fixation within weak trabecular bone (Figs. 21–22B and 21–30).[43,48] Cancellous screws may not be threaded proximally, so that a compressive force is applied as the screw is tightened (Figs. 21–22B, 21–26B, and 21–30). A Herbert screw is specially designed for fixation of scaphoid fractures or intraarticular fractures (Figs. 21–16, 21–26A, 21–30, 21–32D, and 21–35B).[53] This screw has cancellous threads at both ends but with varying pitch. The greater pitch of the distal end causes it to advance faster than the proximal end, producing a compressive force across the fracture. With each of these screws, it is not desirable for them to cross the fracture or fusion site, since this may produce undesirable distraction unless the size of the hole in the proximal fragment is over-drilled using a "lag screw" technique.[43,48]

Several fixation techniques use Kirschner wires (K-wires), metal wire, or suture material.[43] One of the most commonly used methods of bony fixation is percutaneous placement of K-wires.[35,43,48,49] Since these thin fixation wires can be inserted percutaneously using fluoroscopic guidance, they are particularly useful for maintaining bony alignment obtained with a closed reduction (Fig. 21–31). They may also be used to immobilize fragments that are too small for screw fixation. When there is enough room, K-wires are usually inserted in a crossing configuration ("crossed K-wires") (Figs. 21–28, 21–31, 21–35A, and 21–36A).[35,43,48,49] This configuration controls both axial rotation and translational movement. Parallel K-wires control axial rotation but do not control motion in the plane of the wires (Figs. 21–6A, 21–14B, and 21–31).[35,43,48,49] This configuration is used when the fragment is too small to use a crossed K-wire technique or when translational motion in the plane of the wires is not expected.[35,43,48,49] A stronger fixation configuration is the tension band wiring technique (Figs. 21–32 and 21–36A).[43,48,49] Two crossed K-wires are inserted, and a figure-eight configuration of wire is wrapped around the protruding ends of the K-wires. This configuration is

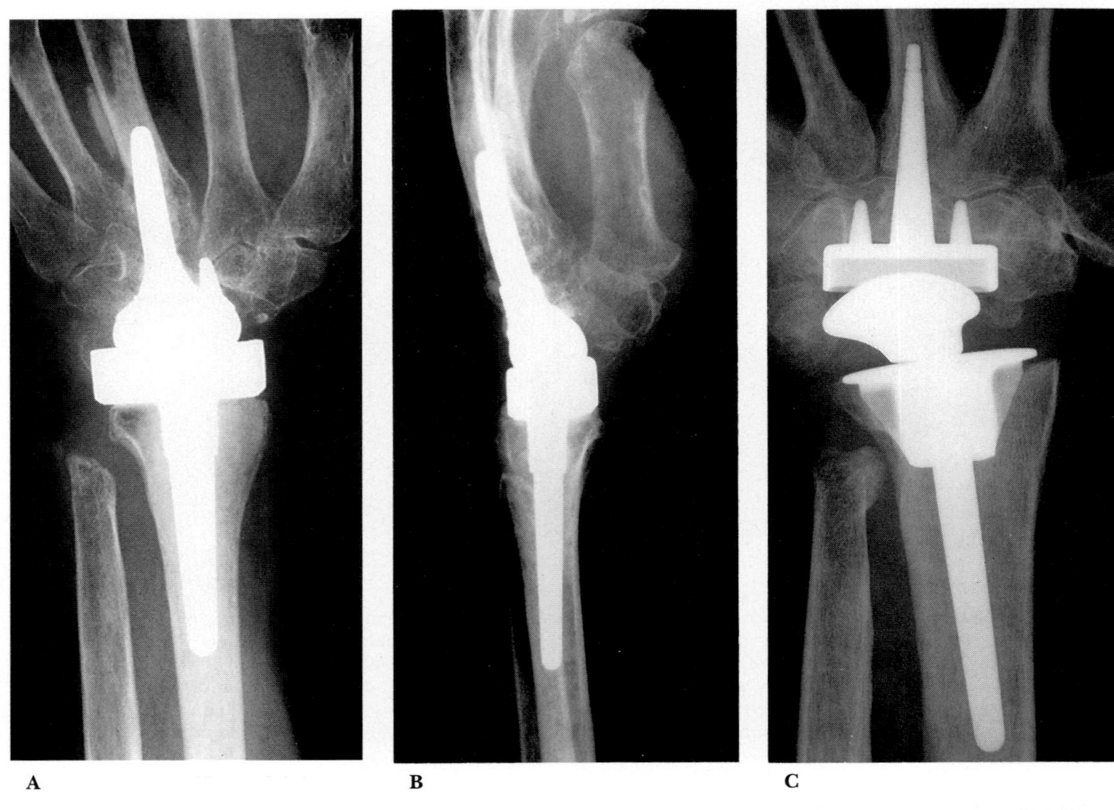

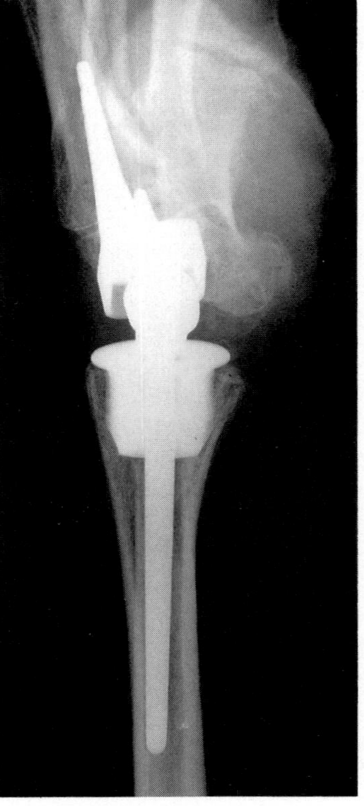

FIGURE 21–20. A and **B:** Cemented CFV total wrist prosthesis and Darrach's resection of distal ulna: PA and lateral radiographs. **C** and **D:** Porous coated Beckenbaugh's prosthesis: small fixation stems within the distal carpal row to prevent toggling of the distal component. (Panels A to D reprinted with permission from Smith DK, Baker K, Gilula LA. Radiographic features of hand and wrist arthroplasties. *Eur J Radiol* 1990;10:3–8.)

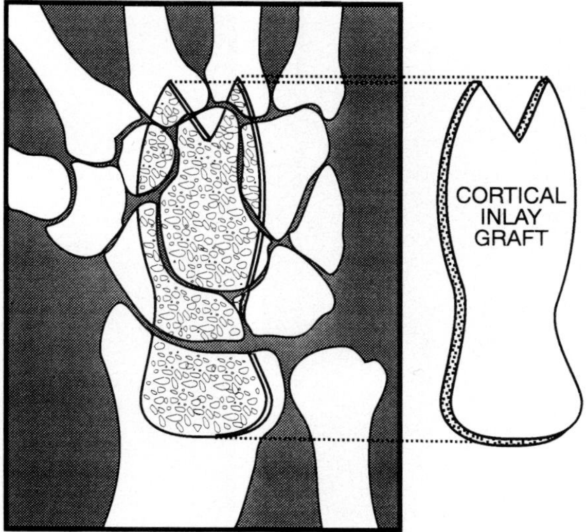

FIGURE 21–21. Drawing of cortical inlay wrist fusion technique. Dorsal aspect of radius, carpal bones, and metacarpals are decorticated. Corticocancellous bone graft from iliac crest is trimmed to fit decortication defect (graft may be held in place with screws). Cortical bone provides immediate stability and medullary bone improves graft healing.

biomechanically suited to take advantage of the natural tensile and compressive forces across the fracture.

Intraosseous wiring is an open procedure that may be used in stable (not comminuted) transverse fractures or for joint arthrodeses (Figs. 21–32A, 21–36, and 21–37).[35,43,48,49] A single loop of wire is passed through each bone and is twisted at one site. Intraosseous wiring provides axial compression and some degree of rotational control, but the wire may break with excessive stress. A specialized application of intraosseous wiring is a "pull-out" wire (Fig. 21–32D).[48,49] The two fragments are wired together but both ends of the wire are brought out through the skin and tied over a button. When the fracture is healed enough to remove the fixation, the wire is cut and pulled out through the skin without the need for another surgical procedure. In many cases a radiolucent suture may be used and only the button on the skin will be visible evidence of the "pull-out" fixation technique.

Kirschner wires can also be inserted across a joint to immobilize the joint (Figs. 21–31B and 21–32C). In some cases an intraarticular fragment may be too small to pin.[43,48,49] A K-wire may be in-

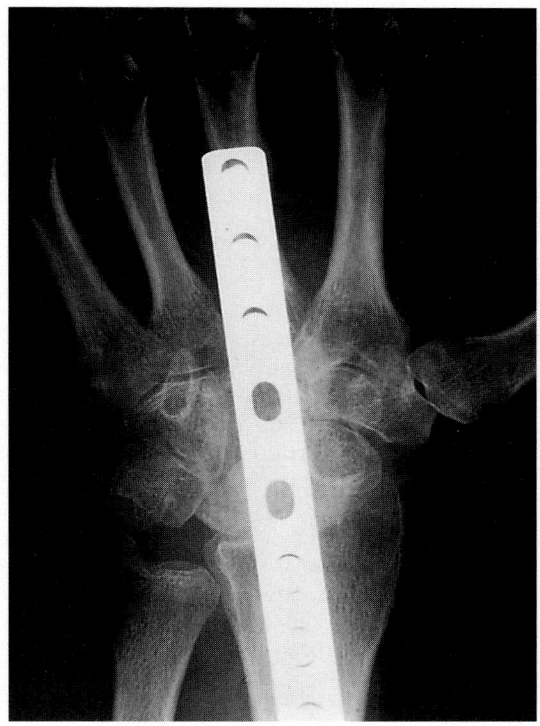

A

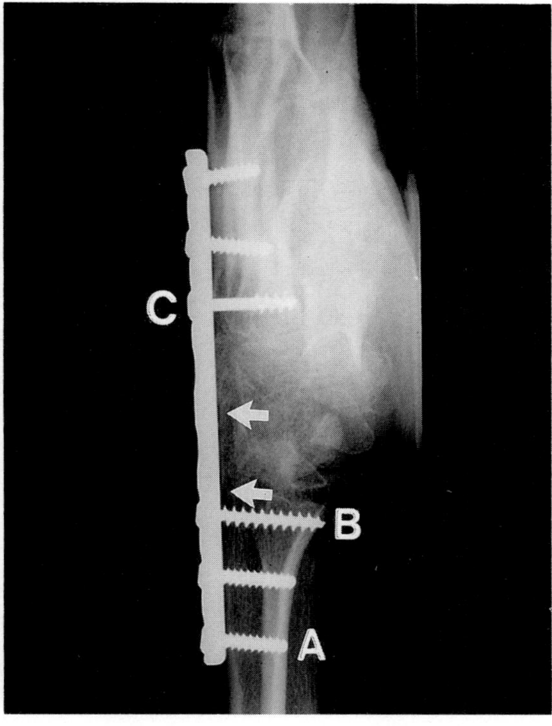

B

FIGURE 21–22. A and **B:** Association for Osteosynthesis (AO) technique for wrist fusion. The dorsal and articular surfaces of radius, lunate, capitate, and third metacarpal are decorticated. Cancellous bone graft is packed between the carpal bones and beneath the dorsal fixation plate (arrows). Combination of cortical screws (A) with closely spaced threads, fully threaded (B), and distally threaded (C) cancellous screws were used in this case.

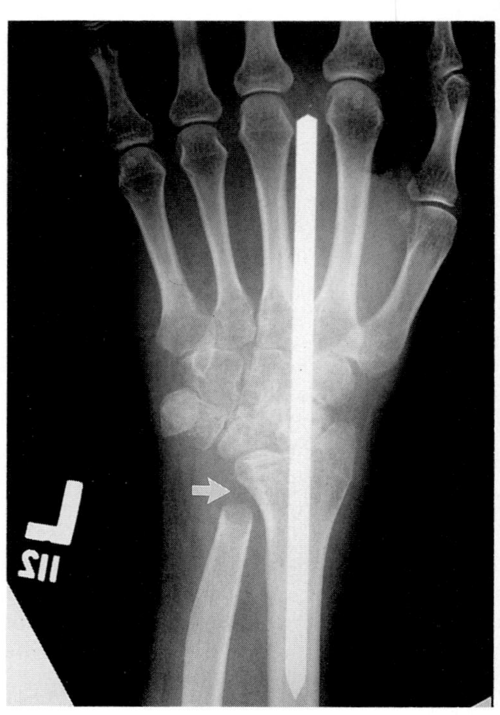

A

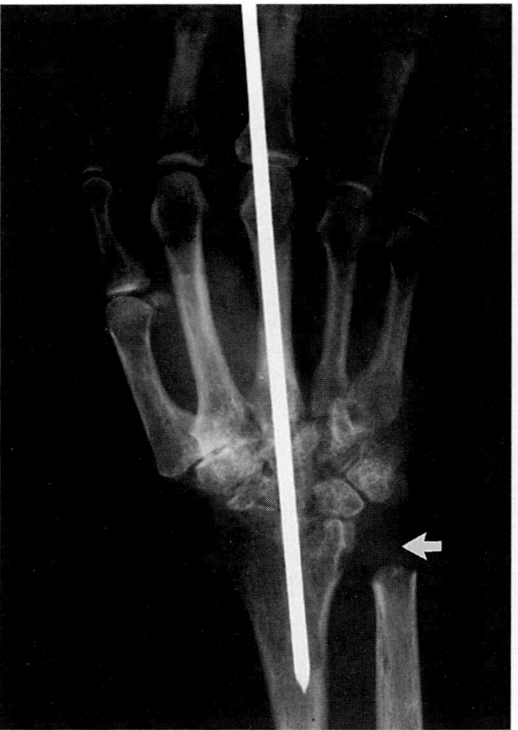
B

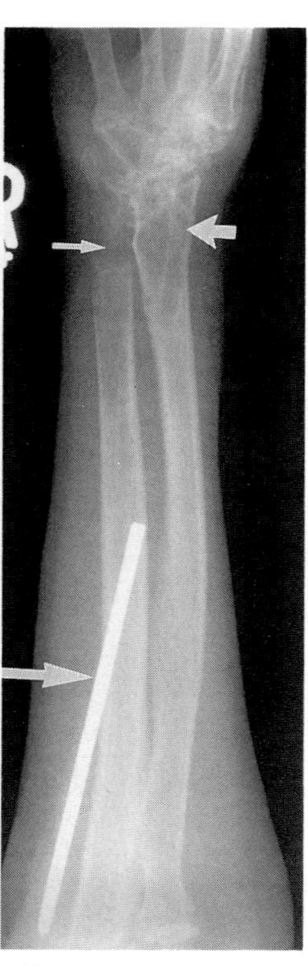
C

FIGURE 21–23. A and **B:** Nalebuff's technique for wrist fusion. The articular surfaces of the carpal bones are decorticated and bone grafted. A Steinman pin or large K-wire is inserted through either the second web space (A) or within the third metacarpal shaft (B) and traverses the wrist fusion. The fixation pin can be easily removed using local anesthesia when the fusion is healed. Darrach's resection of distal ulna (arrow). **C:** Abnormal migration of fixation pin into soft tissues of forearm (long arrow). Pin tract is still visible in distal radius (short arrow). Darrach's resection of distal ulna (small arrow).

serted to maintain reduction by immobilizing the larger articular fragment (this should not be misinterpreted that the surgeon missed the articular fracture fragment) (Fig. 21–32C).[49] Intramedullary K-wires can be inserted into the phalanges or across the wrist as part of a surgical arthrodesis (Figs. 21–23 and 21–38).[48,49] The ends of these wires may protrude through the skin or be positioned just beneath the skin surface and can be removed percutaneously.

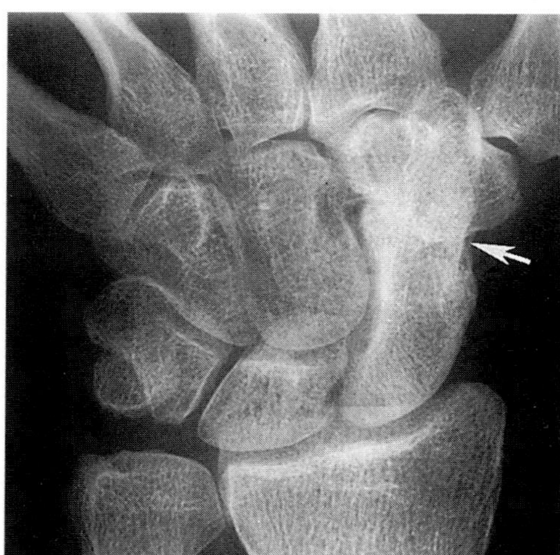

FIGURE 21–24. Triscaphe (scaphotrapeziotrapezoidal) arthrodesis (arrow) performed for rotary subluxation of the scaphoid. (Reprinted with permission from Smith DK, Baker K, Gilula LA. Radiographic features of hand and wrist arthroplasties. *Eur J Radiol* 1990;10:3–8.

Bone staples may be used to immobilize small bones with irregular shapes (Figs. 21–25C, 21–26C, and 21–27). A stapling gun is used to insert the staples. With time the staples are covered by callus and are difficult to remove.

Longitudinal skeletal traction may be used to treat comminuted intraarticular fractures of the phalanges. Miniature external fixation devices (Fig. 21–33) can immobilize a single joint while allowing continued motion of the adjacent joints. Skeletal traction can also be applied by inserting a small transverse fixation pin and attaching this pin to an "outrigger" by a rubber band (Fig. 21–33). This technique allows for both longitudinal traction and continuous joint motion.

TECHNIQUES FOR SCAPHOID FRACTURE NONUNIONS

Nonunited fractures of the carpal scaphoid bone are frequently encountered and can produce severe car-

Text continued on page 571

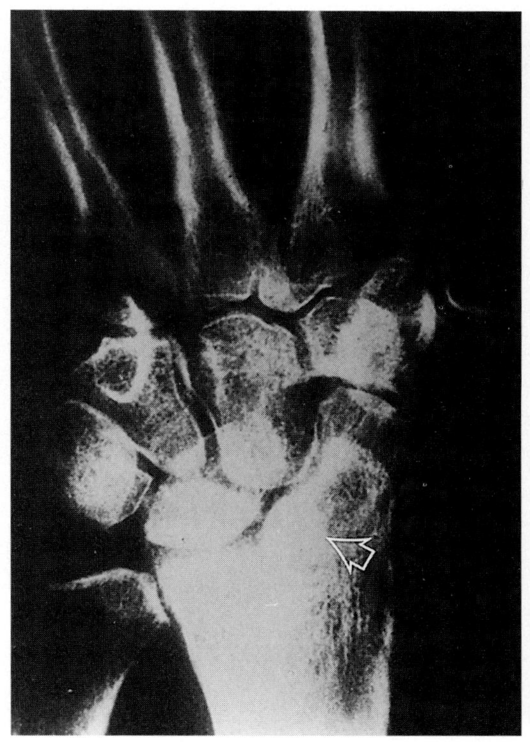

A

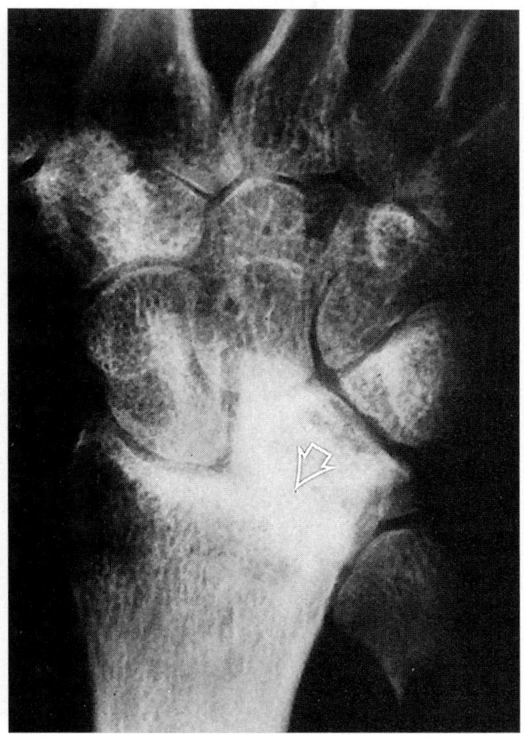

B

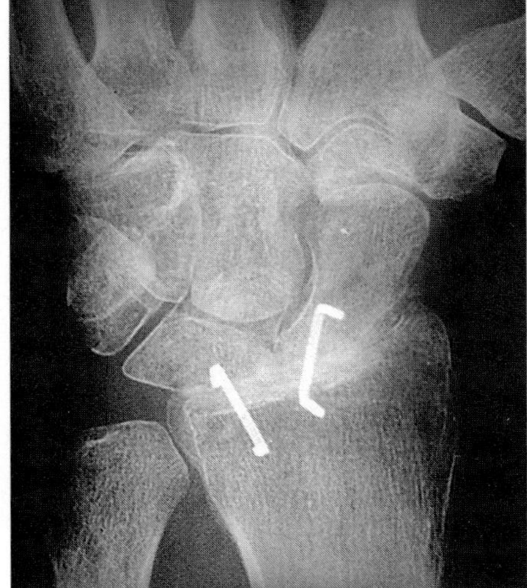

C

FIGURE 21–25. A: Radioscaphoid arthrodesis (open arrow) for treatment of depressed, central radial fracture with subsequent posttraumatic arthritis in manual laborer. **B:** Radiolunate arthrodesis (open arrow) for treatment of radiolunate joint destroyed in motorcycle accident. (Panels A and B reprinted with permission from Watson HK. Limited wrist arthrodesis. In: Tubiana R, ed. *The hand.* Vol. 2. Philadelphia: WB Saunders, 1985:737–747.) **C:** Radioscapholunate arthrodesis performed as treatment for scapholunate dissociation with radiocarpal arthritis. Bone staples used for stabilization prior to arthrodesis healing.

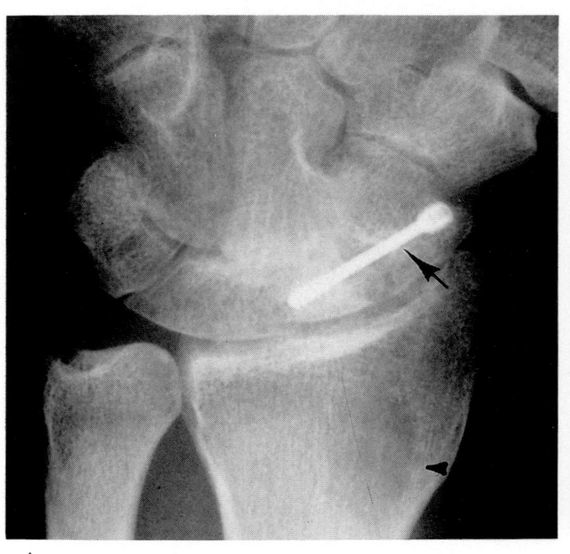

A

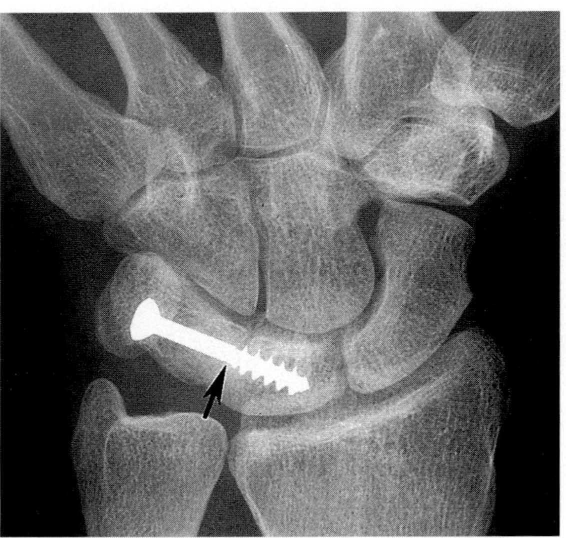

B

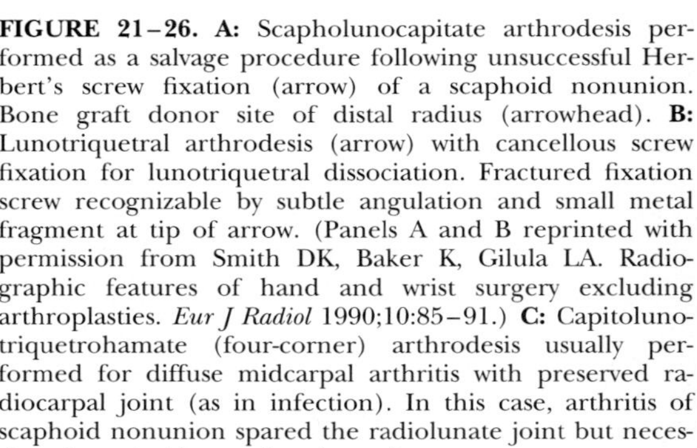

FIGURE 21–26. A: Scapholunocapitate arthrodesis performed as a salvage procedure following unsuccessful Herbert's screw fixation (arrow) of a scaphoid nonunion. Bone graft donor site of distal radius (arrowhead). **B:** Lunotriquetral arthrodesis (arrow) with cancellous screw fixation for lunotriquetral dissociation. Fractured fixation screw recognizable by subtle angulation and small metal fragment at tip of arrow. (Panels A and B reprinted with permission from Smith DK, Baker K, Gilula LA. Radiographic features of hand and wrist surgery excluding arthroplasties. *Eur J Radiol* 1990;10:85–91.) **C:** Capitolunotriquetrohamate (four-corner) arthrodesis usually performed for diffuse midcarpal arthritis with preserved radiocarpal joint (as in infection). In this case, arthritis of scaphoid nonunion spared the radiolunate joint but necessitated scaphoid resection (arrow).

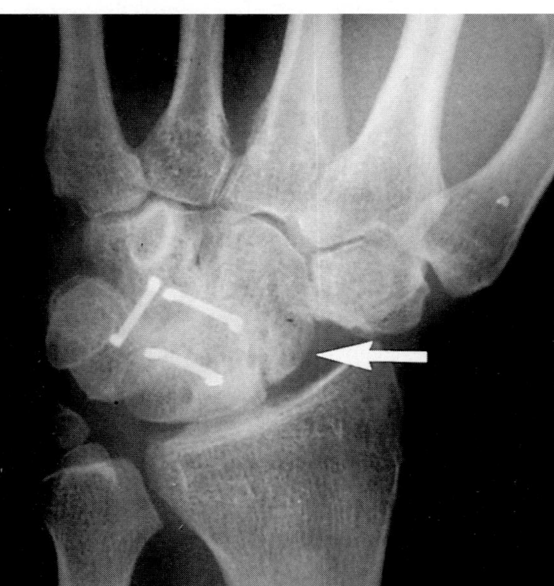

C

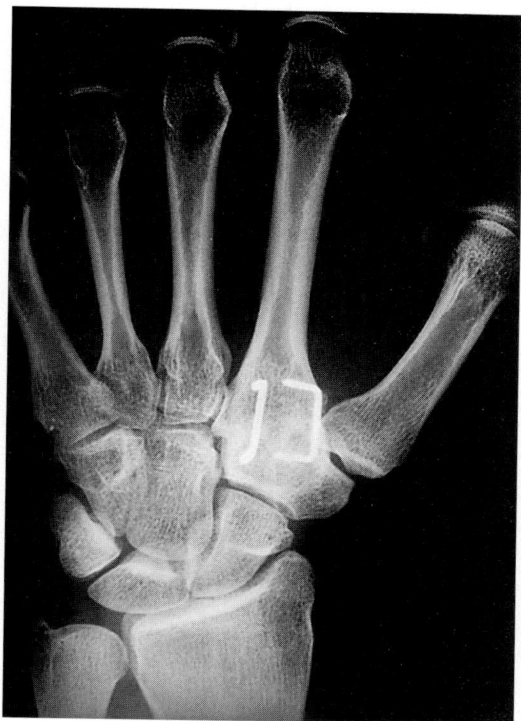

FIGURE 21–27. CMC arthrodesis of index finger performed for posttraumatic arthritis. Arthrodesis immobilized with bone staples.

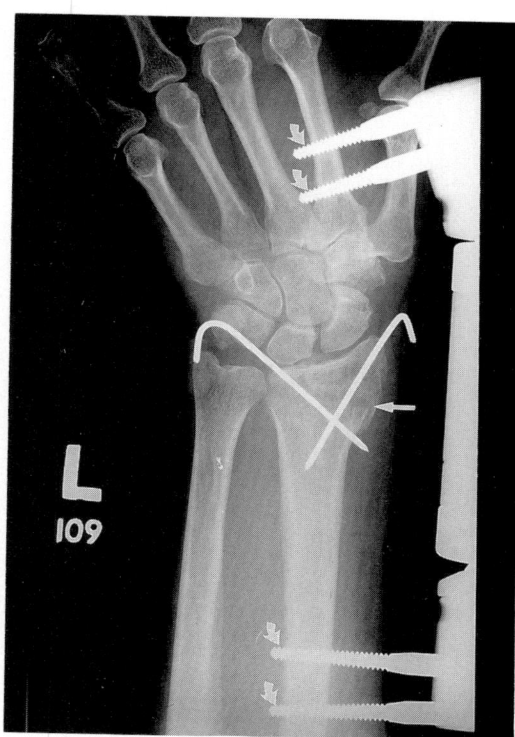

FIGURE 21–28. External fixation device with percutaneously placed pins within the index and middle metacarpals and distal radius (curved arrows) corrects impaction of radial fracture (straight arrow) by applying distraction force. Crossed K-wire fixation of fracture fragments following closed fracture reduction.

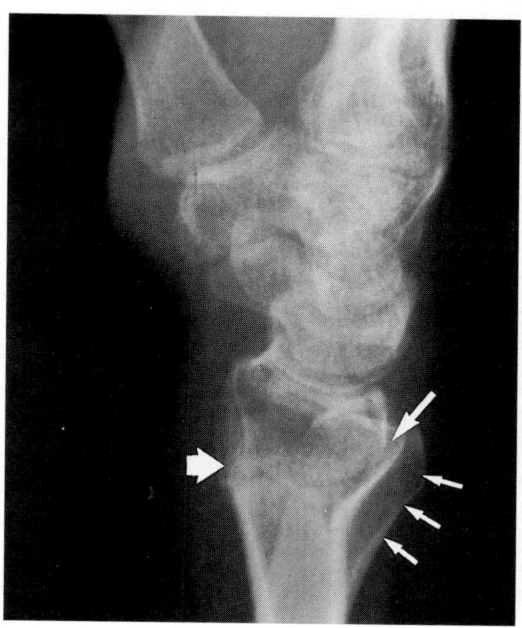

A

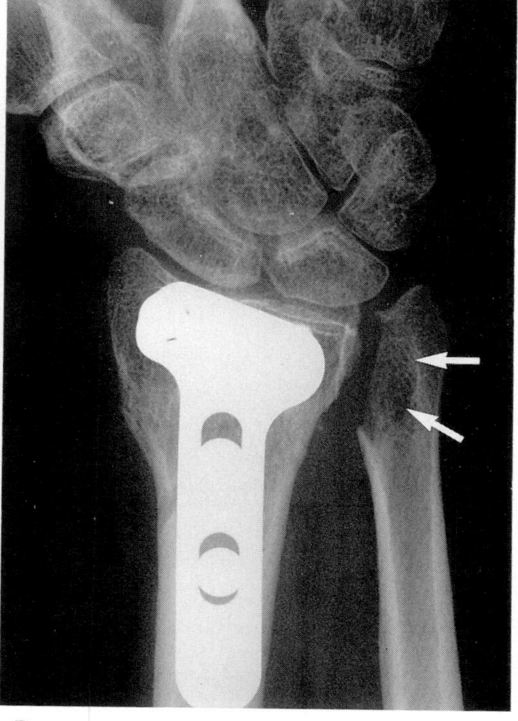

B

FIGURE 21–29. A: Lateral radiograph of distal radial fracture malunion with apex ventral angulation (thick arrow), impaction of dorsal radial cortex (long arrow), and dorsal subluxation of ulnar head (outlined by small arrows). **B:** Fracture malunion treated by corrective osteotomy and fixation with dorsal T-shaped buttress plate and cortical screws. Painful subluxation of ulnar head treated with hemiresection of distal ulna (outlined by arrows).

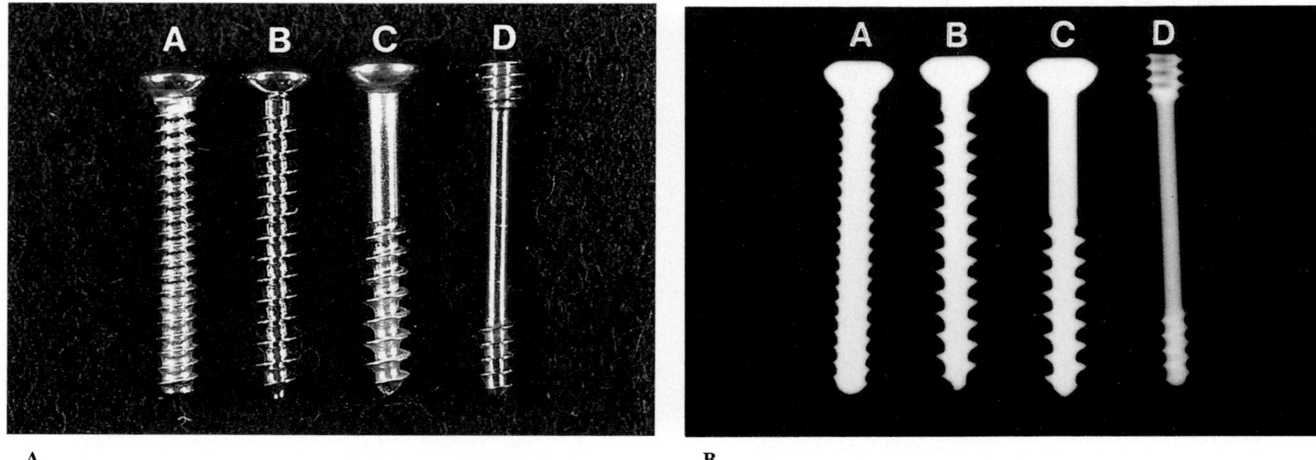

FIGURE 21–30. A: Photograph of cortical screw with thin, closely spaced threads (A); fully threaded cancellous screw with broad, widely spaced threads (B); cancellous screw with unthreaded proximal segment (C); and Herbert screw with wider distal pitch (below) than proximal (above) (D) to produce impaction across fracture or osteotomy. **B:** Radiograph of same four screws.

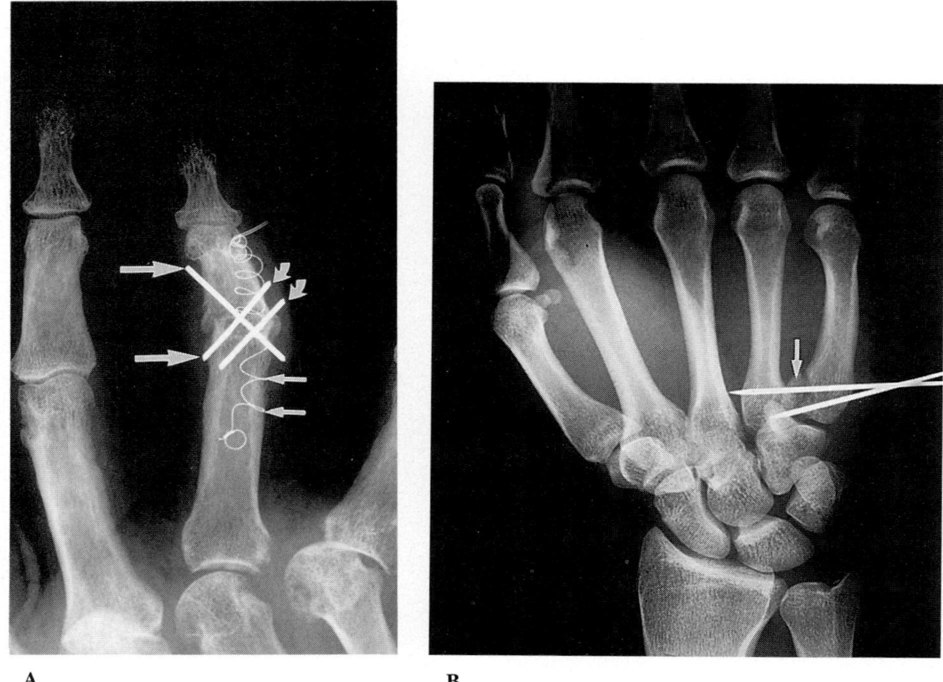

FIGURE 21–31. A: Combined parallel K-wire fixation technique (curved arrows) and crossed K-wire fixation technique (large straight arrows) for arthrodesis of a proximal interphalangeal joint in a patient with rheumatoid arthritis. Spiral wire suture (small straight arrows) was used to close skin and is removed when wound is healed. **B:** Nonparallel K-wire fixation of "baby Bennett's" fracture of fifth metacarpal base. K-wires are placed to maintain reduction of the metacarpal shaft with the hamate. K-wire may not necessarily transfix the smaller fracture fragment (arrow).

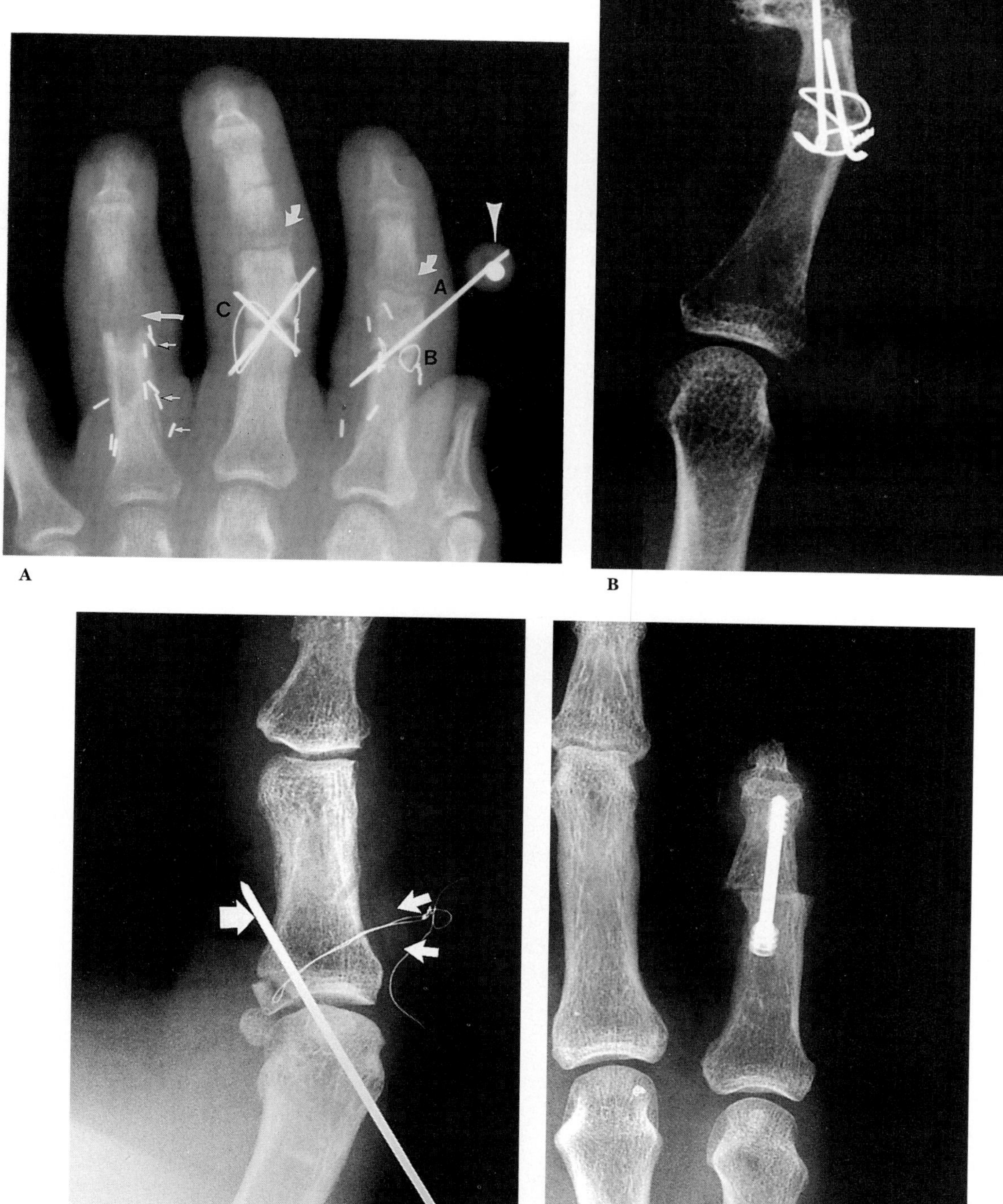

C D

FIGURE 21–32. A: Skeletal fixation techniques for amputations of the index, long, and ring fingers. Single oblique K-wire (A) used to supplement intraosseous wiring (B) of midshaft fracture of index finger proximal phalanx. Jergen's ball used to cover sharp end of K-wire (white arrowhead). Tension band wiring technique (C) with obliquely placed K-wires applies compressive force across the proximal phalangeal fracture of the long finger. Silicone implant (large arrow) inserted to replace destroyed proximal interphalangeal joint of the ring finger. Multiple vascular clips (small arrows) suggest previous vascular injury or replantation. Since bone requires blood supply to be resorbed, disuse osteopenia (curved arrows) of the phalangeal bases is a favorable prognostic sign. (Reprinted with permission from Smith DK, Baker K, Gilula LA. Radiographic features of hand and wrist surgery excluding arthroplasties. *Eur J Radiol* 1990;10:85–91.) **B:** Tension band wiring with longitudinal, intramedullary K-wire fixation technique of proximal interphalangeal joint arthrodesis for posttraumatic arthritis. **C:** "Pull-out" wiring technique for bony gamekeeper's injury of thumb. Single oblique K-wire (thick arrow) maintains reduction of metacarpophalangeal joint. Thin metallic wire suture crosses both fracture fragments and exits through skin. Wire suture is tied around a button (outlined by thin arrows) on surface of skin until fracture is healed. Wire can be easily removed in the office. Alternatively, a radiolucent suture may also be used and will not be seen on radiographs. In this case, it will appear that the surgeon "missed" the smaller fragment with the K-wire designed to maintain joint reduction. **D:** Intramedullary Herbert screw fixation of arthrodesis of proximal interphalangeal joint.

FIGURE 21–33. A: Miniature external fixation device used to immobilize comminuted intraarticular fracture of middle phalanx (arrow). **B:** Longitudinal traction applied to comminuted intraarticular fracture of middle phalanx (curved arrow) by means of a transverse skeletal fixation pin (thick solid arrows). Fixation pin attached by rubber bands (outlined by thin solid arrows) to a plaster outrigger (outlined by hollow arrows) or distal extension of the splint. Device applies longitudinal traction while allowing early motion.

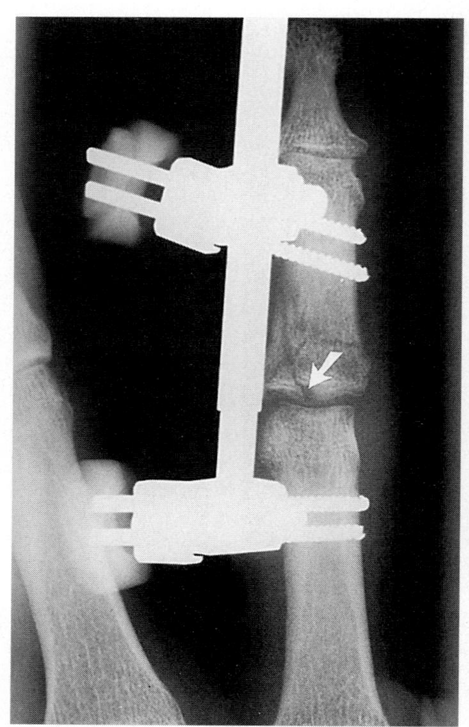

A

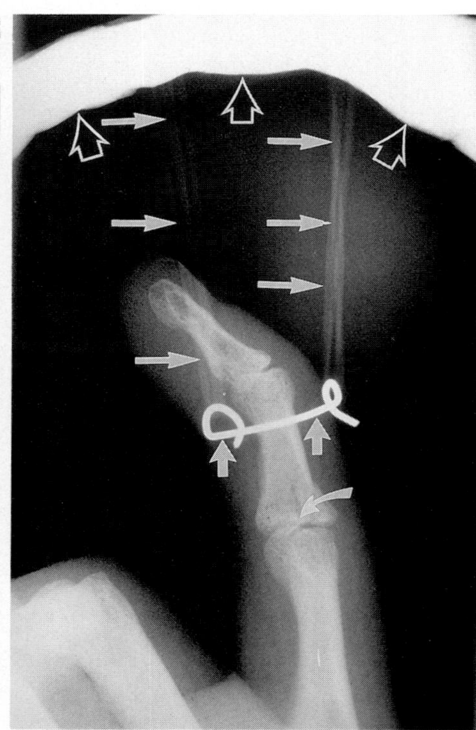

B

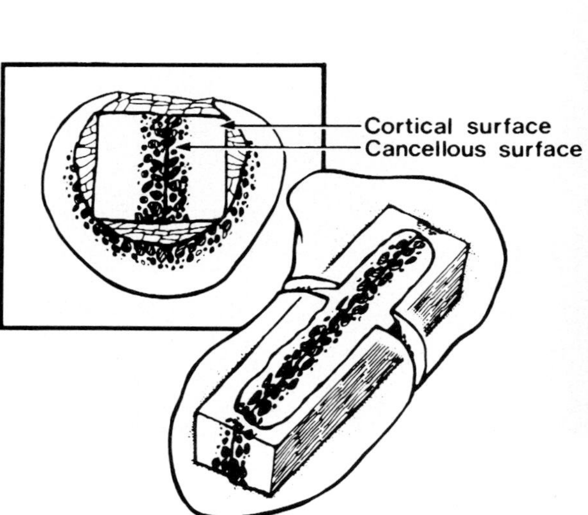

A

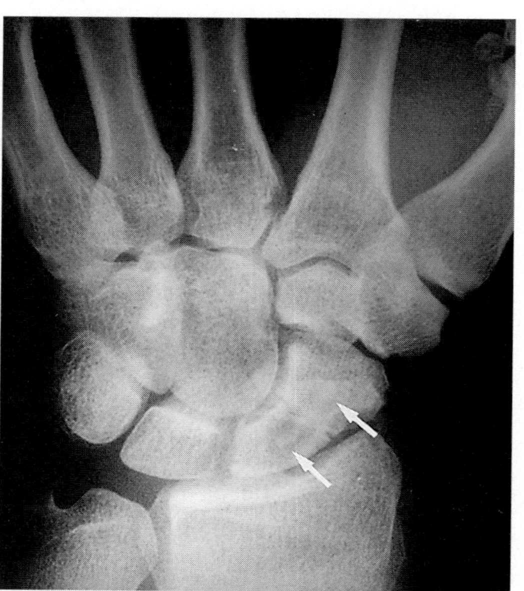

B

FIGURE 21–34. A: Russe volar bone grafting technique. Ventral trough is created in scaphoid and two corticocancellous strut grafts are inserted within trough with cancellous surfaces abutting. (Reprinted with permission from Green DP. The effects of avascular necrosis on Russe bone grafting for scaphoid nonunion. *J Hand Surg* 1985;10A:597–605.) **B:** PA radiograph of Russe bone grafting of scaphoid fracture nonunion. Cortical bone graft (arrows) visible within medullary cavity of scaphoid.

pal arthritis and disability if they are left untreated. The two most popular surgical techniques for treatment of scaphoid fracture nonunions include the Russe technique popularized by Green and the Fernandez technique (Figs. 21–34 and 21–35).[54–56] The Russe bone grafting technique is usually performed for minimally displaced fracture nonunions (see Fig. 21–34).[54,55] A trough is created in the ventral surface of both fragments. Two corticocancellous bone strips are harvested from the ventral surface of the radius and cut to length. The grafts are inserted into the trough with the cancellous surfaces abutting. A Russe graft is recognizable by the two parallel cortical segments traversing a scaphoid fracture nonunion. The graft may be supported by K-wire fixation, but frequently only a cast is used. Even when the graft is healed, normally a lucency may persist across the dorsal aspect of the fusion site, since no graft material traverses this area.

A Fernandez graft is used to correct the apex dorsal angulation (humpback deformity) that is frequently seen with scaphoid fracture nonunions (Fig. 21–35).[56,57] The magnitude and direction of the angular deformity can be measured using plain radiographs, complex motion tomograms, computed tomograms, or MRI techniques.[56–59] A wedge-shaped graft is inserted into the concave (ventral) side of the nonunion site to correct the foreshortening and angular deformity (Fig. 21–35).[56] The wedge-shaped graft is usually clearly visible on postoperative radiographs and the scaphoid bone is usually longer than on preoperative radiographs. The graft is usually supported by either percutaneously placed K-wires or a Herbert screw.[36] Postoperative radiographs must be analyzed for signs of graft extrusion or progressive angulation of the nonunion site. If this occurs with a Herbert screw in place, the screw may migrate through the proximal surface and can injure the radiocarpal joint (Fig. 21–35).

COMPLEX HAND INJURIES AND RECONSTRUCTIVE PROCEDURES

Amputated digits may be replanted or reconstructed using microvascular techniques. Most replantations involve several digits since the replantation of a single digit (except the thumb) is not commonly performed (Fig. 21–36A).[60,61] Surgical hemoclips within the soft tissues at the base of a digit suggest a previous replantation. The bones may be stabilized using any combination of the techniques described earlier.[35,43,48,49,51,61] After traumatic avulsion of the skin and neurovascular bundles of a digit ("degloving in-

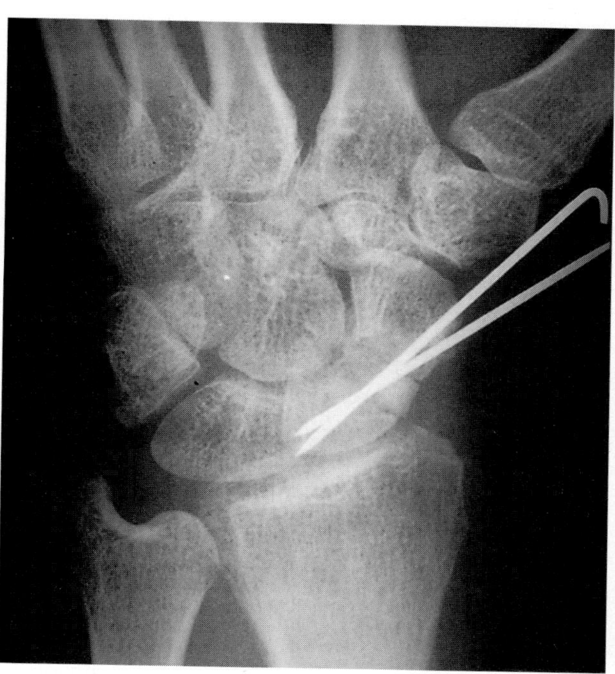

A

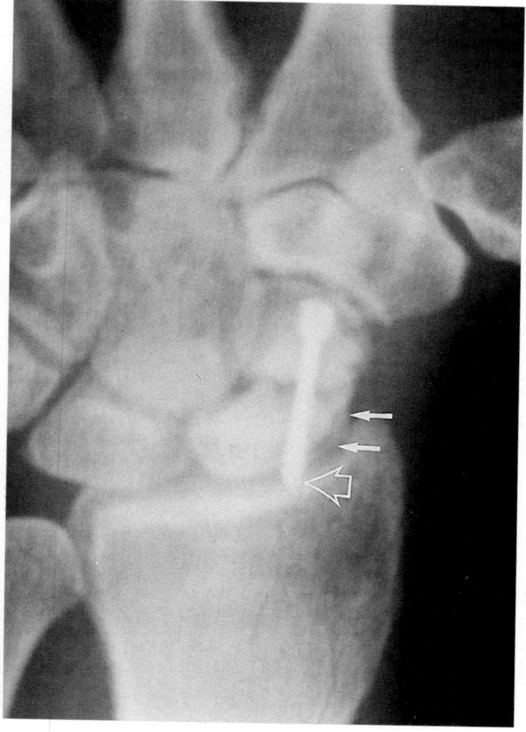

B

FIGURE 21–35. A: Fernandez-type bone grafting technique of scaphoid waist nonunion. Bicortical bone graft inserted within nonunion site to correct apex dorsal angulation and to restore normal scaphoid length. Graft may be stabilized by crossed K-wires (A) or a Herbert screw (B). **B:** Cortical bone graft has displaced (small arrows), allowing recurrent angulation and foreshortening of fracture. Herbert screw has migrated through proximal fragment and impinges on distal radius (open arrow).

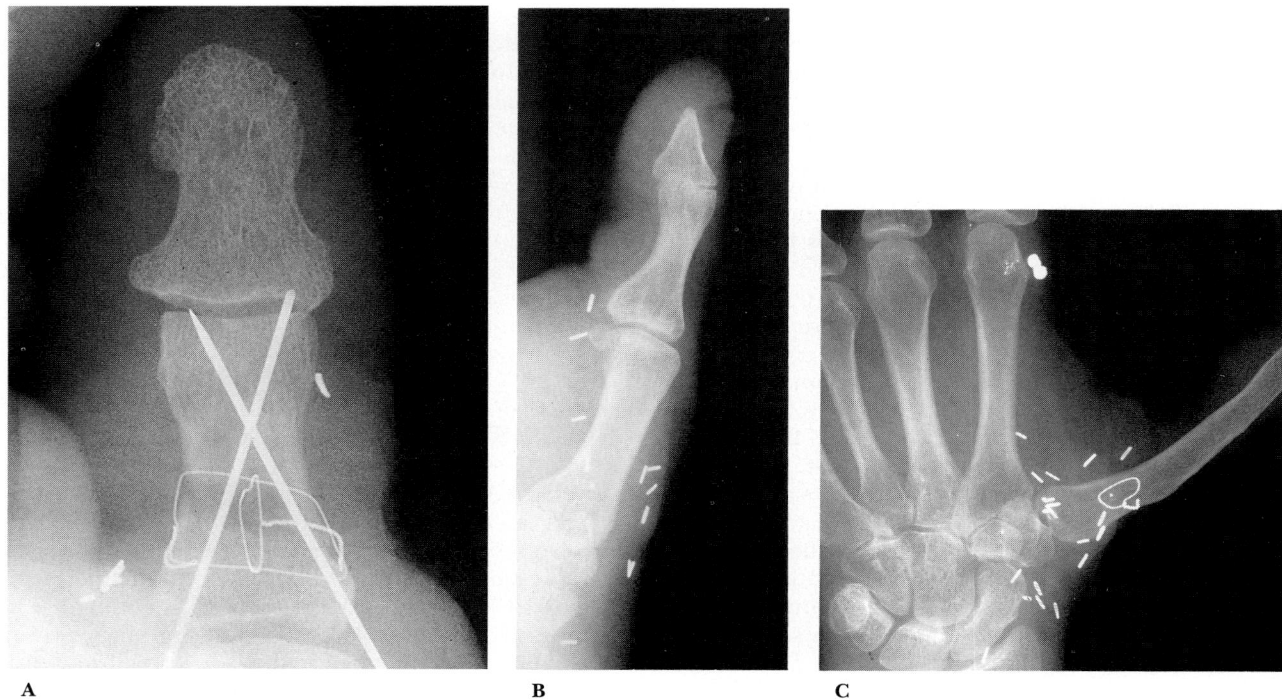

FIGURE 21–36. A: Thumb amputation with all tissues remaining. Thumb replanted using crossed K-wires and intraosseous wiring technique. **B:** Degloving injury. Soft tissues of second toe wrapped around bony stump of thumb to replace degloved soft tissues. Transplanted soft tissues are disproportionately smaller than the remainder of the thumb. **C:** Proximal complete amputation. Soft tissues of second toe wrapped around a piece of iliac crest bone graft to reconstruct a thumb. (Panels A to C reprinted with permission from Smith DK, Baker K, Gilula LA. Radiographic features of hand and wrist surgery excluding arthroplasties. *Eur J Radiol* 1990;10:85–91.)

jury"), the soft tissues of the great or second toe may be "wrapped around" the remaining bony stump of the digit (Fig. 21–36B).[60,62,63] If the thumb is amputated, a bony post can be created with an iliac crest bone graft, and the soft tissues can be "wrapped around" the bony post (Fig. 21–36C).[60,62] This wrap-around procedure combines a solid bony core with a relatively cosmetic soft-tissue appearance.

A toe-to-thumb transfer may be performed for thumb amputations at the perimetacarpophalangeal joint level (Fig. 21–37A).[60,62,63] The soft tissues and bone of the great or second toe are transferred to the thumb amputation site using microvascular techniques. If the site of thumb amputation is close to the base, a neighboring ray (frequently index or long finger) may be transferred with an intact neurovascular pedicle (Fig. 21–37B).[62] Since there is no microvascular anastomosis, vascular hemoclips may be absent. The "metacarpal head" of the reconstructed thumb is smaller than normal, since it actually represents a phalangeal head. In cases where a functionally important joint has been destroyed, a relatively normal joint in an expendable or unsalvageable ray may be used to replace the injured joint (Fig. 21–37C).

Skin grafts, pedicle flaps, or free flaps are used to provide skin coverage for hand wounds with deep soft tissue loss, exposed tendons, or exposed neurovascular structures.[64] Vascular pedicle or free flap grafts usually include skin and subcutaneous fat and are recognized radiographically by their bulky appearance, presence of subcutaneous fat, and associated vascular clips (Fig. 21–38).[64,65]

When extensive soft-tissue injury is associated with a flexor tendon laceration, a two-stage reconstruction of the flexor tendons may be performed.[65,66] In the first stage, the injured flexor tendon is resected and a silicone (Hunter's) rod is placed within the bed of the damaged flexor tendon (Fig. 21–39).[66] The silicone Hunter's rod is attached to the distal phalanx by a screw or suture and slides within the bed of the resected flexor tendon. This rod serves as a sliding stent until the tendon sheath is restored by granulation tissue. At that time, the rod is removed and a transplanted tendon (i.e., palmaris longus or plantaris tendon) is implanted.

SUMMARY

The radiographic appearances of all surgical procedures in the hand and wrist are too numerous to completely cover in a single chapter. It was our goal to show examples of some of the more commonly seen surgical procedures and their radiographic appearances. We hope that this information will be helpful for interpretation of postoperative radio-

Text continued on page 575

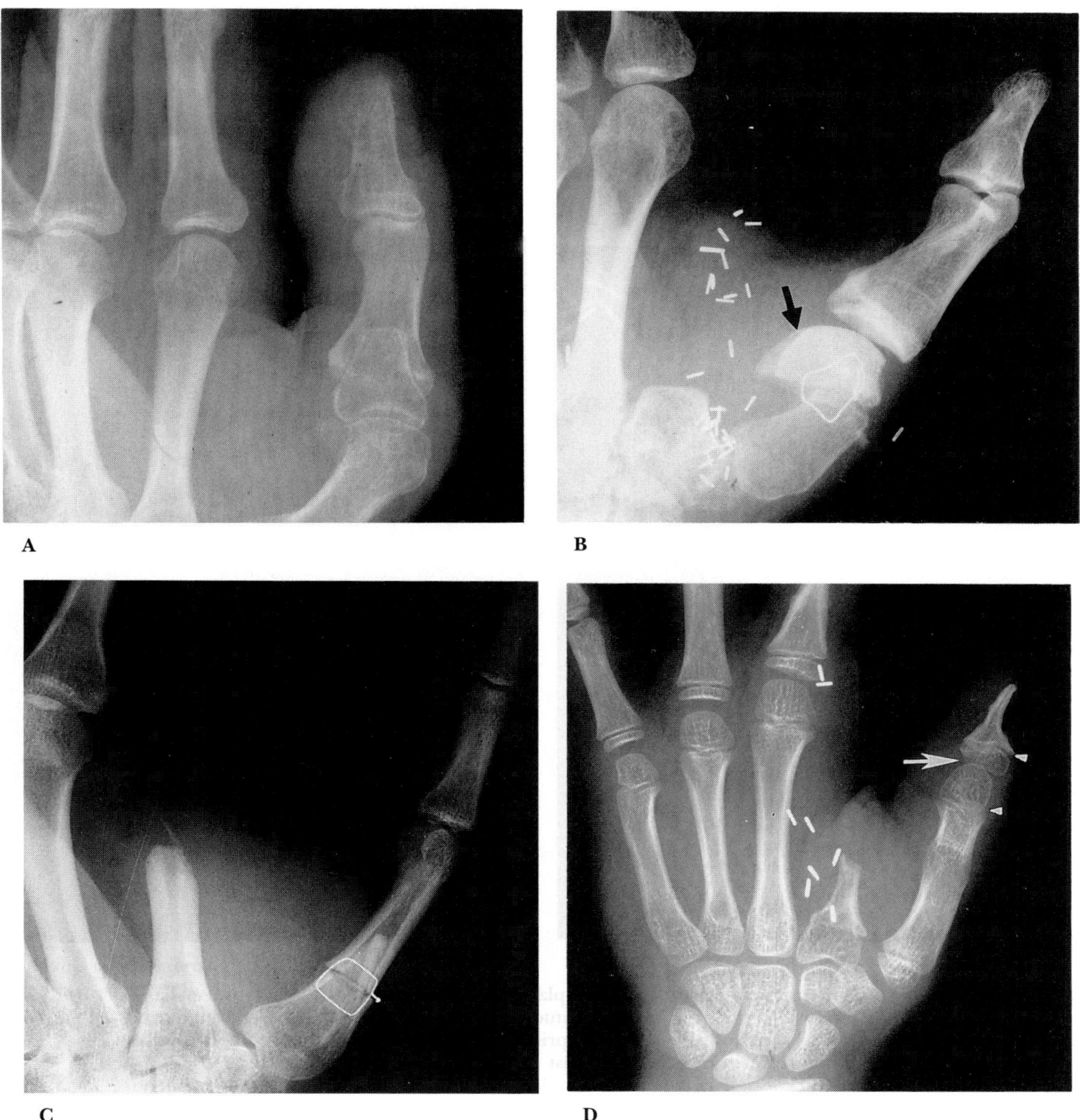

FIGURE 21–37. A: Great toe impaled on bony stump of an amputated thumb (arrow). Transplanted soft tissues of toe are bulkier than toe wrap-around graft or normal thumb. **B:** Great toe transplantation with relatively sclerotic (hypovascular) metatarsal head (arrow). Clues to toe transfer: vascular clips in thenar eminence, absence of sesamoid bones (retained in foot), and disproportionate size of bones in toe. **C:** Index finger to thumb transplantation on a vascular pedicle (no vascular clips). Disproportionately small "metacarpal head" from index finger. **D:** Metacarpophalangeal joint of index finger (arrow) used to replace missing segment of thumb in skeletally immature child. Transplanted growth plates (arrowheads) provide continued growth with remainder of hand. (Panels A to D reprinted with permission from Smith DK, Baker K, Gilula LA. Radiographic features of hand and wrist surgery excluding arthroplasties. *Eur J Radiol* 1990;10:85–91.)

ed. *Operative hand surgery.* 3rd ed. Vol. 1. New York: Churchill Livingstone, 1993:861–928.
36. Amadio PC, Taleisnik J. Fractures of the carpal bones. In: Green DP, ed. *Operative hand surgery.* 3rd ed. Vol. 1. New York: Churchill Livingstone, 1993:799–860.
37. Swanson AB. Silicone implants for replacement of arthritic or destroyed joints in the hand. *Surg Clin North Am* 1968;48: 1113–1127.
38. Swanson AB, de Groot Swanson G. Flexible implant resection in the upper extremity. In: Jupiter JP, ed. *Flynn's hand surgery.* 4th ed. Vol. 4. Baltimore: Williams and Wilkins, 1991:342–386.
39. Meuli HC. Reconstructive surgery of the wrist joint. *Hand* 1972;4:88–90.
40. Voltz RG. Total wrist arthroplasty: A new approach to wrist disability. *Clin Orthop* 1977;128:180–189.
41. Campbell CJ, Keokarn T. Total and subtotal arthrodesis of the wrist: Inlay technique. *J Bone Joint Surg* 1964;46A:1520–1533.
42. Carroll RE, Dick DM. Arthrodesis of the wrist for rheumatoid arthritis. *J Bone Joint Surg* 1971;53A:1365–1369.
43. Heim U, Pfeiffer KM. *Small fragment set manual: Technique recommended by the AO/ASIF group.* 3rd ed. New York: Springer-Verlag, 1982.
44. Millender LH, Nalebuff EA. Arthrodesis of the wrist in rheumatoid arthritis: An evaluation of sixty patients and a description of a different surgical technique. *J Bone Joint Surg* 1973;55A:1026–1034.
45. Watson HK. Limited wrist arthrodesis. In: Tubiana R, ed. *The hand.* Vol. 2. Philadelphia: WB Saunders, 1985:737–747.
46. Watson HK, Dillon HS. Intercarpal arthrodesis. In: Green DP, ed. *Operative hand surgery.* 3rd ed. Vol. 1. New York: Churchill Livingstone, 1993:113–142.
47. Watson HK, Ryu J, Akelman E. An approach to Kienbock's disease: Triscaphe arthrodesis. *J Hand Surg* 1985;10A:179–187.
48. Brennwald J. Principles and techniques of AO/ASIF fracture fixation. In: Green DP, ed. *Operative hand surgery.* 3rd ed. Vol. 1. New York: Churchill Livingstone, 1993:759–765.
49. Stern PJ. Fractures of the metacarpals and phalanges. In: Green DP, ed. *Operative hand surgery.* 3rd ed. Vol. 1. New York: Churchill Livingstone, 1993:695–765.
50. Anderson R, O'Neil G. Comminuted fractures of the distal end of the radius. *Surg Gynecol Obstet* 1944;78:434–440.
51. Palmer AK. Fractures of the distal radius. In: Green DP, ed. *Operative hand surgery.* 3rd ed. Vol. 1. New York: Churchill Livingstone, 1993:929–971.
52. Cooney III WP, Dobyns JH, Linscheid RL. Complications of Colles fractures. *J Bone Joint Surg* 1980;61A:613–619.
53. Herbert TJ, Fisher WE. Management of the fractured scaphoid using a new bone screw. *J Bone Joint Surg* 1984;66B:114–123.
54. Russe O. Fracture of the carpal navicular: Diagnosis, non-operative treatment and operative treatment. *J Bone Joint Surg* 1960;42A:759–768.
55. Green DP. The effects of avascular necrosis on Russe bone grafting for scaphoid nonunion. *J Hand Surg* 1985;10A:597–605.
56. Fernandez DL. A technique for anterior wedge-shaped grafts for scaphoid nonunions with carpal instability. *J Hand Surg* 1984;9A:733–737.
57. Smith DK, Gilula LA, Amadio PC. Dorsal lunate tilt (DISI configuration): A sign of scaphoid fracture angulation. *Radiology* 1990;176:497–499.
58. Smith DK. Anatomic features of the carpal scaphoid: Validation of biometric measurements and symmetry using three-dimensional magnetic resonance imaging. *Radiology* 1993; 187:187–191.
59. Smith DK, Linscheid RL, Amadio PC, et al. Evaluation of scaphoid anatomy by triaxial trispiral tomography. *Radiology* 1989;173:177–180.
60. Michon J. Complex hand injuries. In: Tubiana R, ed. *The hand.* Vol. 2. Philadelphia: WB Saunders, 1985:196–213.
61. Urbaniak JR. Replantation. In: Green DP, ed. *Operative hand surgery.* 3rd ed. Vol. 1. New York: Churchill Livingstone, 1993:1085–1102.
62. Strickland JW, Kleinman WB. Thumb reconstruction. In: Green DP, ed. *Operative hand surgery.* 3rd ed. Vol. 1. New York: Churchill Livingstone, 1993:2043–2156.
63. Gordon L. Toe-to-thumb transplantation. In: Green DP, ed. *Operative hand surgery.* 3rd ed. Vol. 1. New York: Churchill Livingstone, 1993:1253–1282.
64. Lister GD. Free skin and composite grafts. In: Green DP, ed. *Operative hand surgery.* 3rd ed. Vol. 1. New York: Churchill Livingstone, 1993:1103–1158.
65. Smith DK, Baker K, Gilula LA. Radiographic features in hand surgery excluding arthroplasties. *Eur J Radiol* 1990;10:85–91.
66. Schneider LH, Hunter JM. Flexor tendons—Late reconstruction. In: Green DP, ed. *Operative hand surgery.* 3rd ed. Vol. 1. New York: Churchill Livingstone, 1993:1925–1954.
67. Taleisnik J. Kienböck's disease. In: Taleisnik J, ed. *The wrist.* New York: Churchill Livingstone, 1985:183.
68. Bowers WH. Surgical procedures for the distal radioulnar joint. In: Lichtman DM, ed. *The wrist and its disorders.* Philadelphia: WB Saunders, 1988:242.
69. Smith DK, Baker K, Gilula LA. Radiographic features of hand and wrist arthroplasties. *Eur J Radiol* 1990;10:3, 4.

CHAPTER 22

ARTHROSCOPIC FINDINGS OF LIGAMENTS AROUND THE WRIST

Terry L. Whipple and Daniel J. Pereles

Of all the human diarthrodial joints, the wrist has by far the most complicated anatomy. Through a linkage of 8 bones, 45 articular surfaces, and a myriad of ligaments, the wrist allows motion in 6 directions around 3 independent axes.[1] Few motions involve a single articulation, and, for most movement, a coordinated symphony of gliding and rolling must occur. Consequently, it is often difficult to distill clinical symptoms and attribute pain to a single area of pathology. To help in this respect, magnetic resonance imaging (MRI) and arthrography are added to the history and physical examination. These techniques are helpful in diagnosis, however, they often lead to more questions than answers. In addition, sophisticated imaging techniques can be expensive and inconvenient. Physicians should ensure that a patient's symptoms justify the cost of pursuing an elusive diagnosis.

MRI combined with arthrography offer considerable information about the wrist without the morbidity of surgery. However, with MRI, the information obtained is very machine- and interpreter-dependent. Arthrography has limits in that it is really an indirect assessment of ligamentous structure, even when performed in a fluoroscopic mode. In short, there is presently no substitution for the actual physical investigation of the wrist in assessing the integrity of intraarticular anatomy. A minimally invasive and extremely informative method of direct examination of the wrist is arthroscopy. Wrist arthroscopy today represents over 60 years of refined arthroscopic surgical technique. Most of the effective developments for this procedure have occurred in the past decade, however.

The increasing number of indications for wrist arthroscopy reflects the rapid rise in technology combined with a better understanding of wrist mechanics and anatomy. As with other joints, arthroscopic surgical procedures for the wrist offer reduced treatment morbidity, faster recuperation, and earlier return to function than conventional open surgical procedures. It has proven valuable in three general circumstances: intraarticular soft-tissue disorders, intraarticular fractures, and symptomatic wrists with unconfirmed diagnoses. In this chapter, we will concentrate on arthroscopic evaluation of intraarticular soft-tissue disorders —specifically pathology involving the triangular fibrocartilage complex (TFCC), intrinsic and extrinsic ligaments, and the wrist capsule.

ARTHROSCOPY PORTALS

There are 10 useful portals for wrist arthroscopy: 5 for the radiocarpal space, 3 for the midcarpal space, and 2 for the distal radioulnar joint (DRUJ).[1,2] These portals allow access to specific intraarticular regions and pass between nerves, vessels, and tendons. For the radiocarpal space, the portals are described by the extensor compartments between which they lie, or to which they relate most closely (Table 22–1). In the midcarpal space, the portals are less precisely named and correspond to the region where they enter the joint (Table 22–2).

The DRUJ is often difficult to access arthroscopically unless its supporting structures have been damaged. Ordinarily, the interosseous membrane holds the ulna in close apposition to the radius. However, when the forearm is supinated, the dorsal capsule of the DRUJ becomes lax. The joint can then be distended using a hypodermic needle introduced dorsally between the fourth and fifth extensor compartments just proximal to the sigmoid notch of the radius. With distention, the arthroscope can be inserted more easily in the same place and direction as the needle. A second DRUJ portal can be established if negative ulnar variance is present. In this more distal portal, the arthroscope is placed just proximal to the TFCC and distal to the ulna between tendons of the extensor digitorum communis (EDC) (Table 22–3).

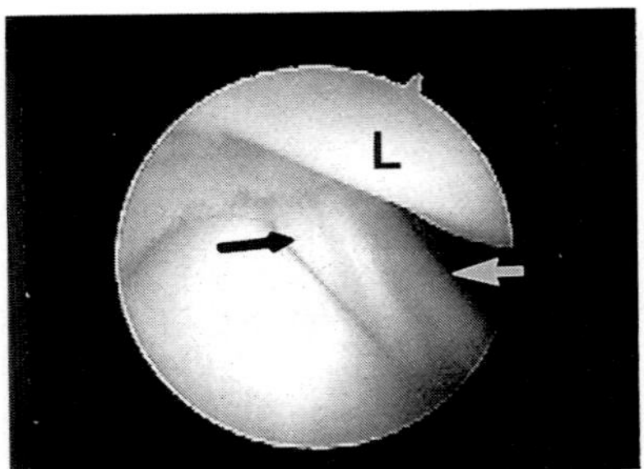

FIGURE 22–3. View of ventral radiocarpal ligaments, left wrist. On the right is the radioscaphocapitate (RSC) ligament (white arrow); on the left, the radiolunotriquetral (RLT) ligament (black arrow). The lunate (L) is seen above the ligaments.

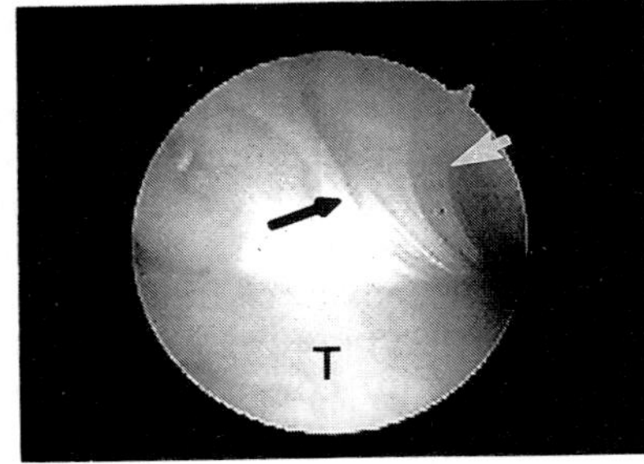

FIGURE 22–5. Ulnocarpal ligaments seen from the 6–R portal, right wrist. On the right is the ulnotriquetral (UT) ligament (white arrow); on the left, the ulnolunate (UL) ligament (black arrow). Below is the TFCC central disk (T).

from the ventral margin of the TFCC as a single ligament and bifurcate distally to insert on the lunate and triquetrum. By switching to the 6–U portal, one can track the ulnocarpal ligaments to their respective distal insertions. The most ulnar margin of the ulnotriquetral (UT) ligament defines the palmar extent of the prestyloid recess. The dorsal radiocarpal ligaments cannot be differentiated arthroscopically and blend into what is seen as the dorsal capsule. This confluence is best seen from either the 1–2 or the 6–U portal, but is adequately visualized from the 3–4 portal.

Looking distally, the proximal carpal row and associated ligaments can be examined. Farthest ulnar is the articular surface of the triquetrum, which appears convex. If the proximal row has a large radius of curvature, the triquetrum will lie more transversely and a large surface of articular cartilage will be exposed in the radiocarpal joint. The proximal pole will be more easily visualized as well. In a petite wrist, this curvature is smaller and the proximal pole will have less articular cartilage and be lesss accessible to arthroscopic examination. Placing the wrist in ulnar deviation can improve triquetral visualization somewhat.

As the arthroscope pans across the triquetrum in an ulnar-to-radial direction, the surface will become briefly concave. This concavity is the location of the lunotriquetral (LT) ligament. Like most ulnar pathology, the LT ligament is best seen from the 4–5 or 6–R portal (Fig. 22–6), but may be visualized from the 3–4 portal in a routine scan of the joint. The LT ligament will be nearly the same color as the adjacent cartilage of the lunate and triquetrum. In addition, its fibers blend imperceptibly into a smooth confluence with the lunate and triquetrum. Therefore, the only way to locate this ligament in normal individuals is to note the change in articular contour from convex to concave. Both palmar and dorsal aspects of the ligament may be examined by flexing and extending the wrist.[1]

Moving the scope radially, the lunate comes into view. Its surface is firm and slippery. With the wrist in a neutral position, one half of the lunate articulates with the TFCC and the other half articulates with the lunate facet of the distal radius. At the radial edge of the lunate, the surface again changes from convex to concave. This concavity represents the scapholunate (SL) ligament. The scapholunate and lunotriquetral ligaments are the only intrinsic ligaments visible to arthroscopic examination.[3]

Like the LT ligament, the SL ligament is nearly the same color and texture as the surrounding cartilage. It may be followed palmarly by flexing the wrist,

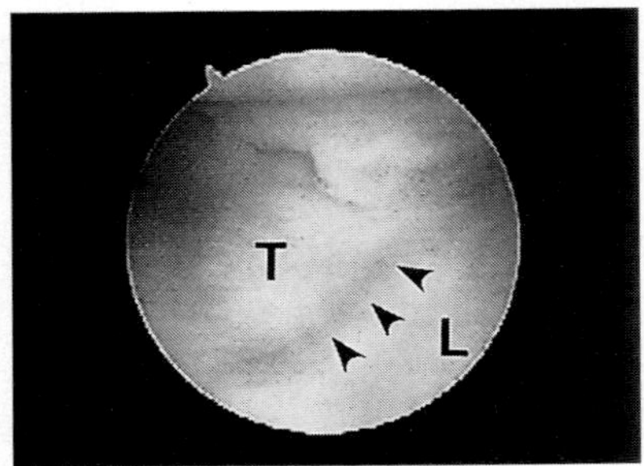

FIGURE 22–4. View of TFC attachment to sigmoid notch of the radius (arrowheads), left wrist. The TFC central disk (T) merges with the articular cartilage of the lunate facet (L).

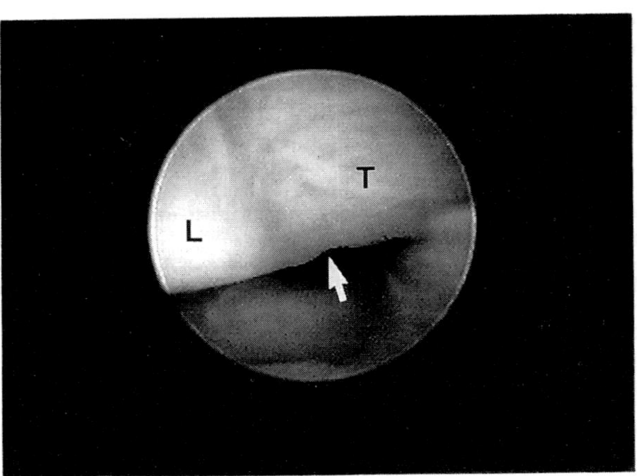

FIGURE 22–6. LT intrinsic ligament, right wrist, seen from the 6–R portal. The lunate (L) is on the left and triquetrum (T) on the right of a slight concavity on the horizon of the proximal carpal row, which represents the LT ligament (arrow).

and ends in a synovial tuft. Extending the wrist allows the dorsal aspect of the SL ligament to be seen as it blends with the dorsal wrist capsule. The SL and LT ligaments may have slight folds or redundancy, especially in older individuals or those with ligamentous laxity. Folds can also be artificially produced by wrist flexion and extension where the scaphoid usually extends more than the lunate and the triquetrum flexes more than the lunate, contributing to the normal supination of the radiocarpal interval in extension and pronation of the radiocarpal interval in flexion. These folds must be differentiated from those of true pathology. Discerning normal variants from pathologic stretch of these ligaments becomes a function of experience, judgment, and clinical correlation.

Farther radially, the joint capsule attaches to the scaphoid along a thin dorsal ridge, and the synovium can be seen at the edge of the attachment site. The normal synovial lining is smooth and thin. If inflamed, a lacy pattern of capillaries can be seen within thickened synovial villi. These villi can be spectacular in size and color, appearing like sea anemone in shades of pink and red.

EXAMINATION OF THE MIDCARPAL SPACE

Pathology is encountered much less frequently in the midcarpal space than in the radiocarpal space.[4] However, much information can be gathered from an examination of the region. There are three useful portals for midcarpal arthroscopy. The radial midcarpal (RMC) portal, found between the scaphoid and the capitate on a line extended from the radial border of the third metacarpal, is usually used for arthroscopic viewing. The ulnar midcarpal portal is most convenient for accessory instruments and is at the same level as the RMC portal, between the capitate, hamate, lunate, and triquetrum, and in line with the fourth metacarpal. The scaphotrapeziotrapezoidal (STT) portal, located ulnar to the extensor pollicis longus (EPL), in line with the radial margin of the second metacarpal, is the tightest and is only used for work on the STT joint. It allows access to the distal scaphoid, trapezium, and trapezoid. Normally there is no communication between the radiocarpal and midcarpal spaces; therefore fluid is introduced through the arthroscope sheath. One ominous sign of pathology is the leakage of saline from the midcarpal space after finishing radiocarpal space arthroscopy. A systematic evaluation of the midcarpal space may then shed light on more proximal radiocarpal pathology.[2]

Looking through the RMC portal, the interval between the scaphoid and capitate is clearly seen. Unless the scaphoid is fractured, the articular surface is smooth and concave. Distally, at the STT junction, the articular surface of the scaphoid is transverse. The trapezium can be seen in the background, and the trapezoid is in the foreground.

The STT portal is located at the level of the distal pole of the scaphoid just ulnar to the EPL tendon. As the arthroscope is moved proximally down the scaphoid surface, a clear definition between the scaphoid and lunate will be seen. There are no intrinsic intercarpal ligaments in the midcarpal space, so this scapholunate interval is easily recognized. Marginal fraying of articular cartilage along the SL interval may be indicative of rotary subluxation of the scaphoid, and further examination is warranted (Fig. 22–7).

The LT interval is also clearly seen as the arthroscope moves ulnarly in the midcarpal space. This interval should be symmetrical in its spacing from anterior to posterior. The triquetrum and lunate can be manipulated with external pressure, and this action will cause them to rock in the sagittal plane. However, there should not be any motion in the coronal plane between the two bones.

Likewise, the articulation between the hamate and triquetrum should be tight, held in place by the palmar triquetrohamate capitate (THC) ligament.[2] If the THC ligament tears and midcarpal instability occurs, the hamate and triquetrum can be distracted by axial traction or radial deviation. In such cases, the palmar triquetrohamate and triquetrocapitate ligaments can be seen. These ligaments are usually not visible and, if they can be seen, midcarpal instability is most likely present (Fig. 22–8).[2] Another sign of midcarpal instability is an articular defect on the extreme proximal pole of the hamate.[1] This lesion occurs as the hamate is forcefully driven into the ulnar edge of the lunate in ulnar wrist deviation. The lunate moves from a volar (ventral) intercalated segmental instability (VISI) position to a dorsal intercalated segmental instability (DISI) position as the wrist is ulnarly deviated, and the shearing of the lunate against the hamate causes the articular lesion.[4,5]

WRIST PATHOLOGY

Intrinsic Ligament Injury and Carpal Instability

The intrinsic ligaments of the wrist link together the bones of the proximal and distal carpal rows. By

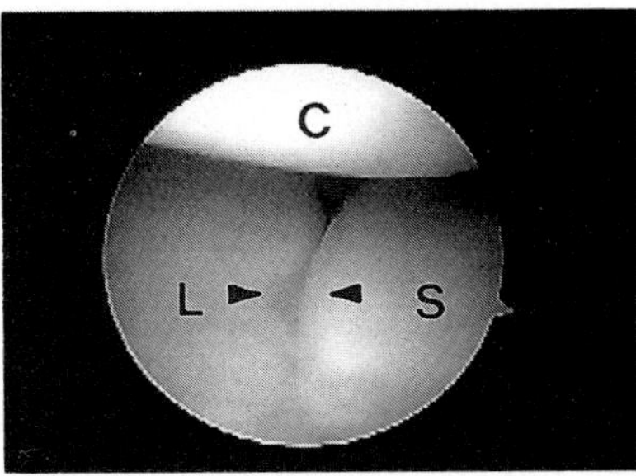

FIGURE 22–7. The SL articulation is seen from the radial midcarpal (RMC) portal of a left wrist. Articular cartilage fraying in the foreground (between arrowheads) is evidence of SL instability, even though the joint space is not widened. S, scaphoid; L, lunate; C, capitate.

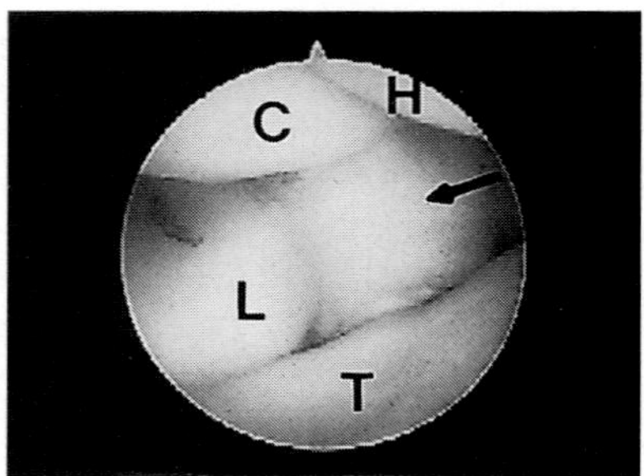

FIGURE 22–8. From the ulnar midcarpal (UMC) portal of a right wrist, the intersection of the capitate (C), hamate (H), triquetrum (T), and lunate (L) is seen. The space between the hamate and triquetrum is wider than normal, and in the center of the field fibers of the triquetrocapitate ligament (arrow) can be seen behind a synovial veil.

keeping the bones in a perfectly articulated relationship, they allow loads to be transferred smoothly from the hand to the forearm and elbow. Only two intrinsic ligaments can be viewed through the arthroscope: the SL and the LT ligaments. They maintain the radiocarpal joint and the midcarpus as two separate fluid compartments.[6,7] The fibers of these ligaments blend into the proximal articular surfaces of the scaphoid, lunate, and triquetrum. Dorsally and palmarly, they blend into the wrist capsule. The palmar and ulnar aspects of each ligament are much thicker than their dorsal and radial counterparts. Therefore, when disruption occurs from trauma, the tear or perforation usually occurs at the dorsal and radial side.

Normally, during axial loading, the capitate and hamate squeeze into the distal articular surface of the proximal row. The intrinsic ligaments keep the scaphoid from flexing and the triquetrum from extending while transferring the force to the lunate and the distal radius. With loss of intrinsic integrity, the midcarpus collapses on the proximal row and the ability to transfer axial load is reduced.[8] Pancarpal arthritis and a painful nonfunctioning wrist eventually result. When arthroscoping the wrist, hemorrhage, synovitis, and specific patterns of articular degeneration are secondary signs of ligament pathology, and the intrinsic ligaments need to be carefully examined when these signs are found.

Scapholunate Instability

Injury to the SL ligament can result from chronic stretch, attritional tearing, or acute rupture. The mechanism may be either hyperextension, hyperflexion, or axial overloading, but especially in conjunction with radial deviation. Hyperflexion tears may be associated with scaphoid fracture. Hyperextension tears may accompany rupture of the RSC extrinsic ligament or Colles's fractures of the distal radius, and often go unnoticed for some time as the attention is drawn to the more obvious fracture.

Stretch injuries may occur where the RSC ligament is elongated without frank rupture, allowing increased motion to occur between the scaphoid and lunate. The excessive motion causes cartilage degeneration and pain. This injury pattern manifests as dynamic instability—one in which plain films and an arthrogram are normal, but stress views or fluoroscopic examination reveals excessive scaphoid flexion. The wrist bothers the patient only when he or she grips an object tightly or radially deviates the wrist. Arthroscopically, stretch injuries appear as SL ligament redundancy, but there may be early fibrillation changes seen at the articular margins of the scaphoid and lunate in the midcarpal space.

In an acute rupture, the SL fibers are usually pulled off the scaphoid or shredded in the midsubstance of the ligament. Plain x-rays may show a widened SL interval likened to gapped teeth. This finding is known as the Terry Thomas (or it could be called the David Letterman) sign, named after the famous late British comedian and current American talk-show host, respectively, who are known for their gapped front teeth. With SL widening, an arthrogram will usually show communication between the radiocarpal and midcarpal spaces through the SL space.

Additional clues to a SL disruption or perforation are DISI orientation of the lunate on a lateral x-ray and an excessive SL angle of more than 70 degrees.[5] The lunate's orientation in the lateral plane is determined by its attachments to the scaphoid radially and to the triquetrum ulnarly. The scaphoid exerts a palmar flexion force and the triquetrum exerts an extension force. If the SL ligament is disrupted, then the triquetral force goes unchecked, and the lunate rocks into extension—the so-called DISI pattern.

With the arthroscope in the 3–4 portal of the radiocarpal space, a torn SL ligament looks like a shredded weed patch with dorsal and palmar synovial hypertrophy. A stretched ligament is less obvious, but SL motion can be observed when stressing the wrist. Articular degeneration on the proximal pole of the scaphoid and the scaphoid facet of the radius might also be seen. In a wide-open tear, a small arthroscope can pass between the scaphoid and the lunate into the midcarpal space, where the base of the capitate is seen. Looking proximally from the midcarpal space, abnormal separation will be seen between the scaphoid and lunate. There are no intrinsic ligaments in the midcarpal space, and the edges of the scaphoid and lunate are clearly visible. The intercarpal gap should be roughly equal to that between the lunate and triquetrum. Wrist flexion or ulnar deviation may accentuate an abnormally wide SL interval. In chronic SL tears, shearing from incongruent and excessive motion causes fibrillated cartilage changes along the articular margins of the scaphoid and lunate.[1]

Lunotriquetral Ligament Instability

Like the SL ligament, the LT ligament is a short flexible link between the lunate and triquetrum, which blends into articular cartilage proximally and merges with the fibers of the dorsal and palmar capsules. Injury to this ligament can occur with forceful pronation or with severe force to the pisiform directed dorsally. The latter mechanism commonly occurs as a fall on an outstretched hand where the trauma is applied to the palmar ulnar side of the wrist directly under the pisiform forcing it into the triquetrum and shearing the triquetrum dorsally away from the lunate.

The LT ligament usually ruptures in its midsubstance, but can stretch or avulse off the weaker lunate attachment. Disruption of this ligament can represent a continuum of injury to the palmar ulnocarpal ligaments.[1,9] For instance, as the palmar UT ligament supporting the ulnar side of the wrist is torn from violent hyperpronation or extension, the triquetrum gains excess mobility in the anteroposterior (AP) plane with respect to the lunate. Continuing force will propagate through the more mobile triquetrum, and shear it from the lunate. Another associated injury pattern with LT ligament rupture is midcarpal instability.[1,4] In this case, the palmar THC ligament, which is an extension of the palmar UT ligament, is injured through a similar loading pattern. The midcarpus becomes unstable as the capitate and triquetrum become uncoupled in addition to the triquetrum and lunate.

Arthroscopically, a torn LT ligament is best viewed through the 4–5 or 6–R portal. Unlike an SL tear, the arthroscope cannot pass from the radiocarpal space distally into the midcarpus through an LT tear. Triangular fibrocartilage (TFC) tears can sometimes be seen with an associated LT tear, as this also is an injury of hyperpronation. Viewing in the radiocarpal space, a shredded LT ligament will be seen with a widened LT interval.

Volar (Palmar) Extrinsic Ligament Injuries

The extrinsic ligaments of the wrist maintain the longitudinal relationship of the carpus to the forearm proximally and the metacarpals distally.[10] They determine the limits of motion in all planes and are therefore commonly sprained. The radial originating palmar extrinsic ligaments are the RSC, RLT, and the short radioscapholunate (RSL) ligaments. Arthroscopically, the RSC and RLT ligaments are seen as distinct bands passing through the radiocarpal space. The short RSL ligament is hidden behind a tuft of synovial tissue at the palmar edge of the SL intrinsic ligament. Its orientation is transverse, nearly perpendicular to the RSC and RLT ligaments. Most injuries to these ligaments heal spontaneously with proper splinting, but if the ligaments are ruptured, the carpus becomes unstable and repair should follow arthroscopic evaluation.[1]

Extension is generally the mechanism of injury to the palmar extrinsic wrist ligaments. In ulnar deviation, hyperextension or axial load may tear the short RSL ligament, and in extremes may tear or stretch the RSC ligament. Hyperextension or axial load in radial deviation is more likely to fracture the distal radius and tear or stretch the RLT ligament. The reason for ligament vulnerability in radial versus ulnar deviation is that the axis of rotation for radial and ulnar deviation passes sagittally through the head of the capitate. Therefore, radial deviation displaces the lunate and triquetrum farther from the point of origin of the RLT ligament on the radial styloid tightening the short RSL ligament while shortening the RSC ligament. Conversely, if the wrist is ulnarly deviated when subjected to axial load, the RSC ligament comes under stretch and may ultimately fail. These two ligaments work in complementary fashion, stabilizing the carpus in radial and ulnar deviation.[10]

Arthroscopically, these ligaments are best seen through the 3–4 or 1–2 portal. When injured, the overlying synovium will be swollen, boggy, and hemorrhagic. Torn or stretched ligaments feel soft or lax when probed, even in positions of wrist extension. Acutely, the fibers may be separated or hemorrhagic. If avulsed, they usually tear from the carpus rather than the radius, and the loose end may fold into the radiocarpal space.

Volar (Palmar) Ulnocarpal Ligament Injuries

Major sprains of the palmar ulnocarpal ligaments occur rarely. The mechanism of injury is hyperextension and radial deviation or hypersupination pulling the carpus dorsally away from the head of the ulna. Usually, the distal radius and other ligaments fail before the ulnolunate (UL) and UT ligaments rupture. However, when they do fail, it is almost always at their origin from the fossa of the ulnar head.[1]

Assessment of the palmar ulnocarpal ligaments is best done with the arthroscope in the 6–U portal.[2] Accessory instruments can be introduced through the 4–5 portal for palpation and debridement of torn or impinging structures. The wrist should be placed in extension and slight radial deviation to place these ligaments under stress. If they do not tighten with wrist extension, significant stretch or avulsion injury must be suspected.

Avulsion of the palmar ulnocarpal ligaments from the ulna allows the TFC articular disc to fold distally. Deviating the wrist radially may allow the arthroscope to be introduced into the DRUJ proximal to the torn TFCC. If the ligaments are acutely avulsed, an area of prolific hypertrophic synovium will be present and appear as a hemorrhagic mass. Blood can be aspirated from the DRUJ in this circumstance.

Volar (Palmar) Midcarpal Ligament Injuries

In midcarpal instability, when looking in the midcarpal space, radial deviation will open the saddle joint of the triquetrohamate articulation, exposing the palmar triquetrohamate ligament. The ligament appears redundant and hemorrhagic in the acute setting. There may be an associated palmar chip fracture of either the triquetrum or lunate. Disruption of the triquetrohamate and triquetrocapitate ligaments is thought to be the essential lesion for midcarpal instability.

Dorsal Capsular Injuries and Ganglia

Dorsal capsule injuries are a result of hyperflexion or hypersupination. The capsule does not usually rupture. Instead it avulses from the distal radius or carpus. When looking through the arthroscope, a bare area of exposed bone will be seen where the avulsion occurred. Hemorrhagic synovitis highlights these injuries as well, and occurs more frequently on the dorsum of the wrist. The dorsal radiocarpal ligaments are best seen through the 1–2 portal with the wrist in extension. The capsule originates from the dorsal radius and inserts distally at the proximal and distal carpal rows.

The floor of the ECU is the main dorsal capsular ligament on the ulnar side of the wrist.[10] Injury to this structure can be difficult to differentiate from tendinitis or subluxation. When the dorsal ulnocarpal ligaments are injured, hemorrhagic synovitis can be seen along the dorsal ulnar capsule from the dorsum of the TFCC to the prestyloid recess. A probe is often needed to lift redundant capsule away from the suspected injury sites. With the capsule pushed aside, a recess between the TFC articular disc and the dorsal capsule can be seen. This recess may communicate with the DRUJ, but does not always extend so proximally.

If the dorsal capsule is avulsed completely from the proximal carpal row, the arthroscope can be passed between the radiocarpal and midcarpal spaces. Best viewed through the 3–4 portal, the capsule is commonly avulsed from the dorsal rim of the lunate or waist of the scaphoid. Extending the wrist allows more room dorsally to maneuver the arthroscope. If any part of the hamate, capitate, or STT joint can be seen through this portal, the dorsal capsule has been avulsed.

Capsular injuries at the level of the distal carpal row usually occur on the ulnar side of the wrist. Looking from the RMC portal, large bare areas of the capitate or hamate may be observed. Normally, the capsule attaches to these bones along the margin of articular cartilage. However, there is a variable degree of exposed bone within the realm of normal capsular insertion, and the arthroscopic examination needs to be closely correlated with the clinical examination to determine what represents true pathology. Rarely, the entire dorsal capsule is stripped from the distal carpal row, and the ulnar three carpometacarpal joints can be seen. If the clinical examination suggests this injury as well, then repair is indicated.[1]

Dorsal Ganglia

Dorsal ganglia usually arise from the radiocarpal aspect of the SL interval, but occasionally are found in the midcarpal interval as well. Their presence is associated with degenerative wear of bones or ligaments. Rarely, intraarticular ganglia occur as grape-like cysts within the joint itself. Ganglion cysts are located arthroscopically by noting the accompanying synovial hypertrophy present. This synovium is redundant but uninflamed and without villi. Resection of the hypertrophic synovium will expose the palmar wall of the ganglion at the 3–4 interval. Dorsal ganglia can be decompressed into the radiocarpal space by careful resection of a portion of the dorsal wrist capsule.

TFCC Tears

The central disc (TFC) of the TFCC can be torn in a number of ways, through either acute trauma or attritional wear. Attritional tears rarely cause symptoms, but any TFCC tear might cause pain with ulnar axial loading in wrist extension. Extremes of pronation and supination can tear the disc as well. Arthrography is the best imaging technique for identifying TFCC perforations.[6] Contrast material injected into the radiocarpal space will be seen passing into the DRUJ, and the reverse will occur if the DRUJ is injected. Occasional false-negative arthrograms occur when a valve effect is created by a flap tear.[6] To avoid this possibility, both the radiocarpal space and DRUJ should be examined sequentially when doing a contrast (“dye”) study. MRI has not proven to be accurate in identifying all TFCC perforations because these tears are often very small and may exist between the MRI cuts.

The arthroscopic appearance of a TFCC tear depends on which part of the disc is torn. The central portion of the TFCC is thinnest and is most likely to tear. Older discs are more yellow and stiffer than younger ones. In addition, discs vary greatly in their thickness. Tears in thinner discs are more evident than tears in thicker discs, where probing may be required to reveal the lesion.

The TFCC is best examined through the 3–4 portal with accessory instruments introduced through the 4–5 portal. Some perforations may not be readily visible, therefore it is wise to thoroughly probe the TFCC for loss of its normal taut resiliency. Squeezing the DRUJ may also open a hidden tear as irrigating fluid is forced distally from the DRUJ into the radiocarpal space. Tears need to be distinguished from the normal prestyloid recess on the palmar ulnar side of the wrist and the occasionally present capsular opening into the pisotriquetral space adjacent to the palmar UT ligament.

Dorsal peripheral detachment of the TFCC should be considered a ligamentous injury. It may appear with synovial hypertrophy as a crevice between the dorsal capsule and the dorsal margin of the articular disc. It usually extends dorsally and radially from the prestyloid recess. This type of tear can and should be repaired if clinical correlation warrants.[1] Experience is required to differentiate this type of tear from an unusually large, but normal, opening into the prestyloid recess. Typically, the prestyloid recess does not extend dorsally past the ulnar edge of the ECU. The symptomatic tear can be reduced with slight pronation and wrist flexion and can be repaired with an outside-to-inside suture technique, aided by arthroscopic visualization.

REFERENCES

1. Whipple TL. *Arthroscopic surgery: The wrist.* Philadelphia: JB Lippincott, 1992.
2. Whipple TL, Marotta JJ, Powell JH III. Techniques of wrist arthroscopy. *Arthroscopy* 1986;2:244.
3. Palmer AK, Levinsohn EM, Kuzma GR. Arthroscopy of the wrist. *J Hand Surg* 1983;8A:15.
4. Cooney WP, Dobyns JH, Linscheid RL. Arthroscopy of the wrist: Anatomy and classification of carpal instability. *Arthroscopy* 1990;6:133.
5. Watson HK, Black DM. Instabilities of the wrist. *Hand Clin* 1987;3:103–111.
6. Roth JH, Haddad RG. Radiocarpal arthroscopy and arthrography in the diagnosis of ulnar wrist pain. *Arthroscopy* 1986;2:234.
7. Taleisnik J. *The wrist.* New York: Churchill Livingstone, 1985:247.
8. Fisk GR. An overview of injuries of the wrist. *Clin Orthop* 1980;149:137.
9. Bottke CA, Louis DS, Braunstein EM. Diagnosis and treatment of obscure ulnar-sided wrist pain. *Orthopaedics* 1989;8:1075.
10. Kauer JM. Functional anatomy of the wrist. *Clin Orthop* 1988;149:9.

CHAPTER 23

ALGORITHMIC APPROACH TO WRIST PAIN

Yuming Yin, Frederick A. Mann, and Louis A. Gilula

Wrist pain has many causes, and patients may have wide varieties of clinical history and symptoms. These disparate clinical presentations can be divided into the following three categories according to clinical history at presentation: (1) acute trauma, (2) chronic wrist pain with a history of remote trauma, or (3) atraumatic continuous or intermittent wrist pain. There are many imaging techniques available to evaluate the underlying causes of wrist pain, including plain radiography, conventional tomography, computed tomography (CT), magnetic resonance imaging (MRI), ultrasound, nuclear scintigraphy, arthrography, cineradiography, and videofluoroscopy. The specific imaging approach for each clinical category is different. However, the imaging evaluation of each category begins with a general survey, routine radiography. In most cases, conventional radiography can provide enough information for management.[1]

There are many variations concerning the number and types of exposures for a routine examination. The number and specific projections of radiographic exposures should be tailored to the clinical problems. Our routine examination is composed of four radiographic exposures (posteroanterior [PA], 45-degree pronated oblique, PA obtained in ulnar deviation, and a neutral lateral) and is designed to survey the wrist for gross abnormalities (Fig. 23–1). We consider these four views to be the most important for both diagnosis and selection of further imaging studies.[1–3] In patients with a history of possible synovial arthritis, such as rheumatoid arthritis, only two views, PA and lateral, may provide most of the information. The PA wrist view is particularly important (Fig. 23–2). Often fluoroscopic "spot" films allow the best profile of symptomatic sites for evaluation of a possible abnormality (Fig. 23–3).

Scintigraphy (bone scan) is valuable to exclude metabolically active osseous abnormalities that are not evident on plain radiographs.[2,3] In general, if the bone scan is "hot" diffusely, synovitis, reflex dystrophy, or disuse osteoporosis should be considered (Fig. 23–4). If there is a very hot focal abnormality corresponding to the location of the patient's symptom complex, additional imaging techniques should be performed to define osseous and soft-tissue pathology. Depending on the preference of the imager and the available technique, CT, conventional polytomography, or MRI may be used next. CT has the advantage of being less expensive than MRI and routinely shows cortical and trabecular detail better than MRI (Fig. 23–5). Although conventional polytomography also clarifies planar anatomy without the confusion caused by overlapping structures, polytomography blurs the bone detail (Fig. 23–6). Because CT does not have the blur present with polytomography, it is much easier to make definitive statements with CT than with polytomography.

Compared with MRI, sometimes CT may be better at showing a fracture line in the cortex or the osseous trabecular anatomy of a finding, especially when one is looking for fine cortical detail between two adjacent cortical surfaces such as adjacent bone, healing fracture site, or arthrodesis site. MRI can demonstrate marrow edema, cysts, avascular necrosis, and other marrow processes including fractures within the marrow space better than any other technique.[4–6] MRI has developed rapidly as a diagnostic tool in evaluation of the wrist. Wrist evaluation is facilitated by an understanding of the anatomy of the carpal ligaments, triangular fibrocartilage (TFC) complex (TFCC), carpal tunnel, and anatomic features of the distal radioulnar joint (DRUJ). With proper attention to technique and an understanding of wrist pathophysiology, MRI is a valuable diagnostic tool.

CT can be complementary to MRI. When the cause of an MRI abnormality is ambiguous, CT can often provide the precise osseous anatomy to explain it. An example of this is a focal defect in the lunate. When it is uncertain on MRI if the defect is actually avascular necrosis (AVN), the shape of the defect can be clarified with CT. Currently, the best imaging

Text continued on page 590

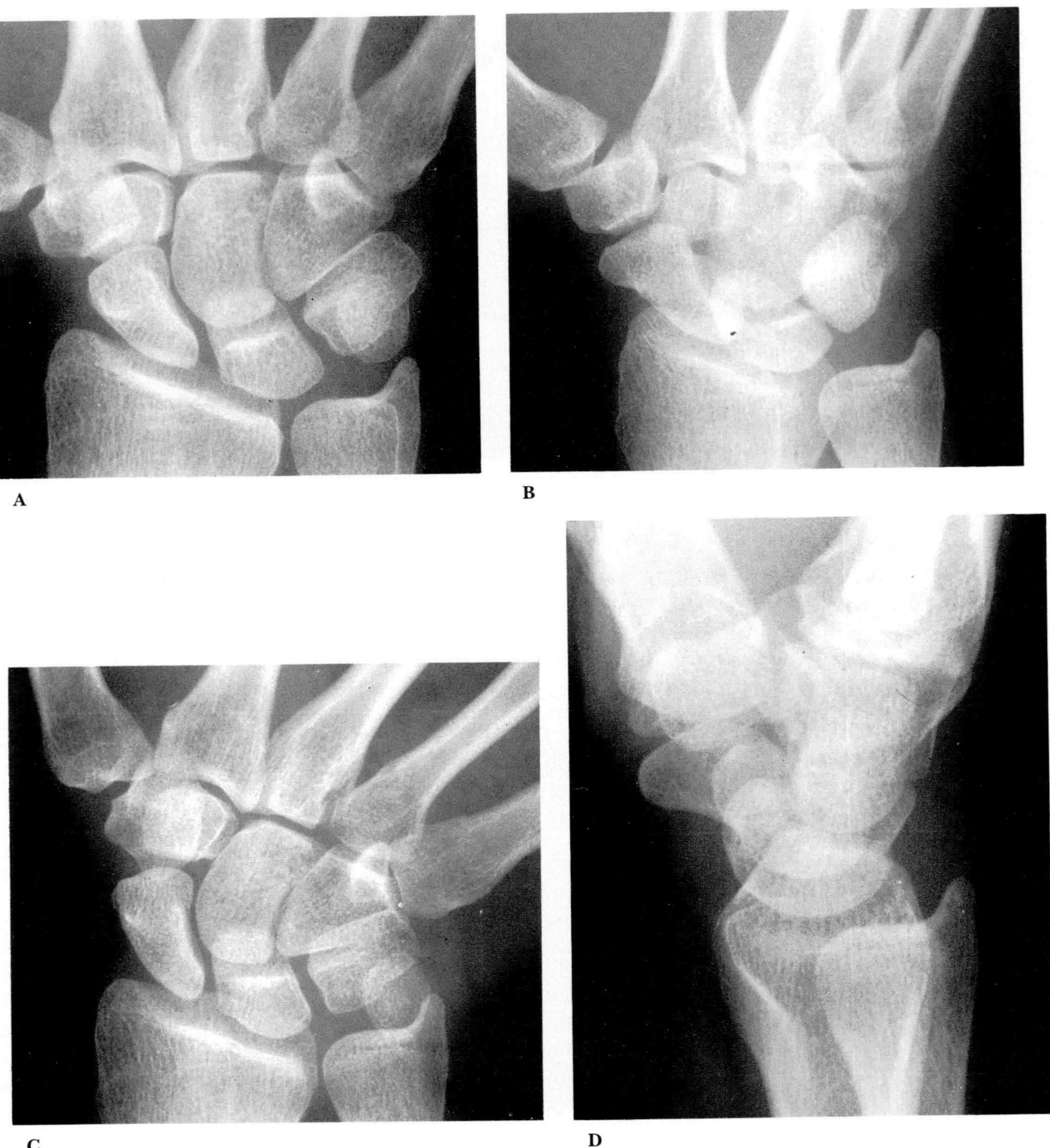

FIGURE 23–1. Four views of an apparently normal wrist (see Fig. 23–10). **A:** PA in neutral position. **B:** 45-degree pronated oblique. **C:** PA in ulnar deviation. **D:** Lateral view of the right wrist in neutral position. The fact that the ulnar styloid is in similar profile as the PA projection indicates that the lateral wrist view was taken with the elbow in the same position as the PA view, at the shoulder height. The pisiform is lined up correctly between the capitate and distal pole of the scaphoid (see Chapter 5).

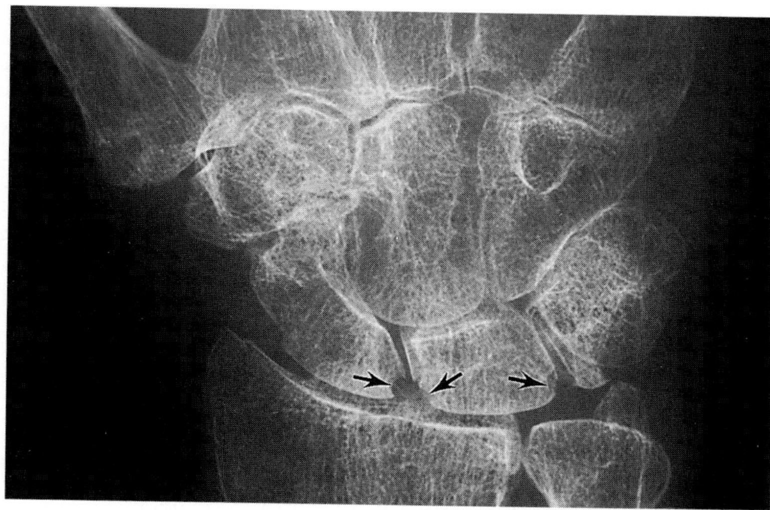

FIGURE 23–2. Rheumatoid arthritis. PA view of the right wrist demonstrates generalized osteopenia of the entire wrist. Multiple bone erosions involve the edges of the scapholunate and lunotriquetral joints (arrows). Diffuse joint space loss is present at the scaphotrapeziotrapezoidal joint. Soft-tissue swelling is present around the wrist but is not obvious on this figure.

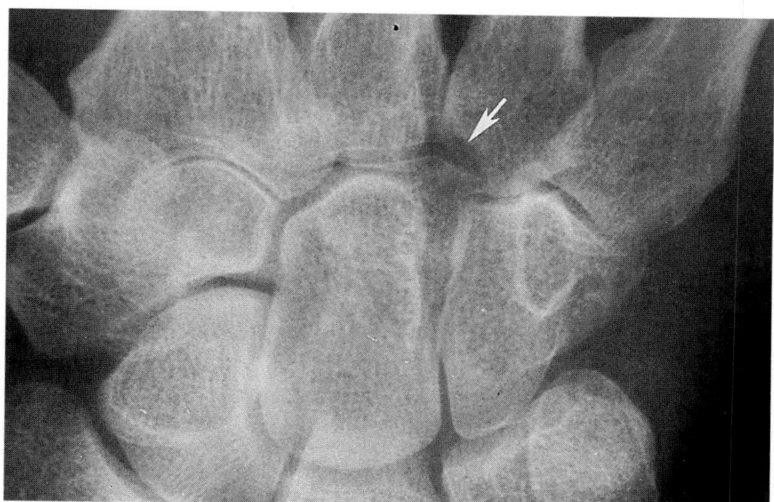

A

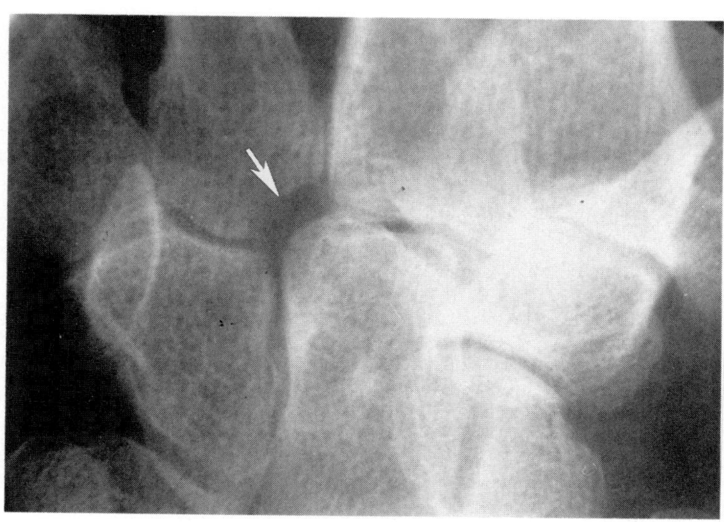

B

FIGURE 23–3. Focal erosion at fourth metacarpal base. **A:** PA view of the wrist demonstrates a questionable radiolucency at the radial side of the fourth metacarpal base (arrow). **B:** On a fluoroscopic spot obtained in supination with minimal obliquity, an erosion at the radial side of the fourth metacarpal base is clearly shown (arrow).

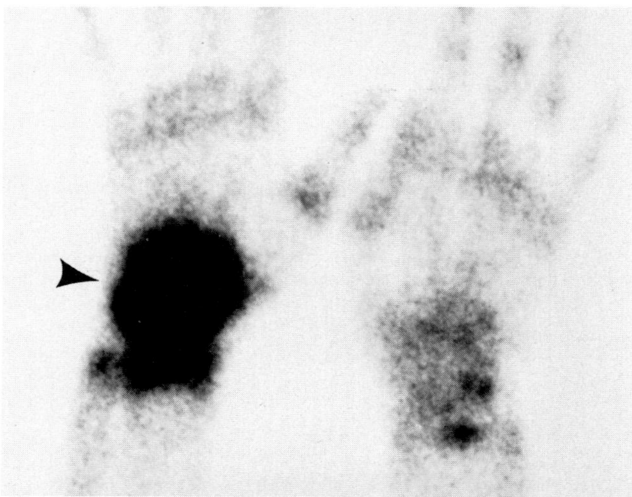

FIGURE 23-4. Synovitis. Bilateral wrist bone scan demonstrates diffuse increased uptake in the left wrist (arrowhead) including the distal radius and ulna and carpometacarpal joints.

technique to demonstrate a ligament or capsule disruption in the wrist is arthrography.[4,7] Arthrographically demonstrable ligament or capsule defects, however, do not always correlate with patient symptoms and signs. Bilateral symmetric defects correlate infrequently with the clinical picture and are probably degenerative or congenital in nature. Thus, if an abnormal finding is found on an arthrogram of the symptomatic wrist, the asymptomatic wrist should also be studied arthrographically to exclude fortuitous association of symptoms with either developmental, old posttraumatic, or degenerative changes. Although it is unproven, potentially the asymmetric arthrographic defects that correlate with the patient's history and physical findings may be more likely to be the cause of wrist pain (Fig. 23-7).

The following algorithms are not meant to be clinically exhaustive but are designed to give perspective to imaging of the painful wrist. Careful clinical history, physical examination, and plain radiography are the most important and fruitful explorations and are certainly necessary before any other imaging studies.[4,8] The major concerns of physical examination are to localize the site(s) of maximum tenderness, produce stresses that cause the symptoms, and identify any association with underlying anatomic structures. Once a painful and tender spot is found, the next step is to identify its anatomic and physiologic character.

IMAGING ALGORITHM FOR DIFFERING PATIENT PRESENTATIONS

Before any kind of imaging study is begun, a clinical history and physical examination are necessary to determine what kind of imaging approach should be used (Fig. 23-8). When a patient has a history of acute trauma, a traumatic injury to bone or soft tissue should be the major consideration. If the patient has a history of a subacute or remote trauma with wrist pain, a subtle fracture, TFC injury, or carpal instability due to ligament injury should be the major concerns. The algorithm for subacute or remote trauma is designed to approach the above abnormalities. If the patient has chronic pain without a history of trauma, infection, synovitis, AVN, tumor, chondromalacia, osteoarthritis, and other nontraumatic causes should be considered.

ALGORITHM FOR ACUTE TRAUMA TO THE WRIST

Acute Trauma (Fig. 23-9)

When a history of acute trauma is present, careful physical examination is usually important to deter-

Text continued on page 593

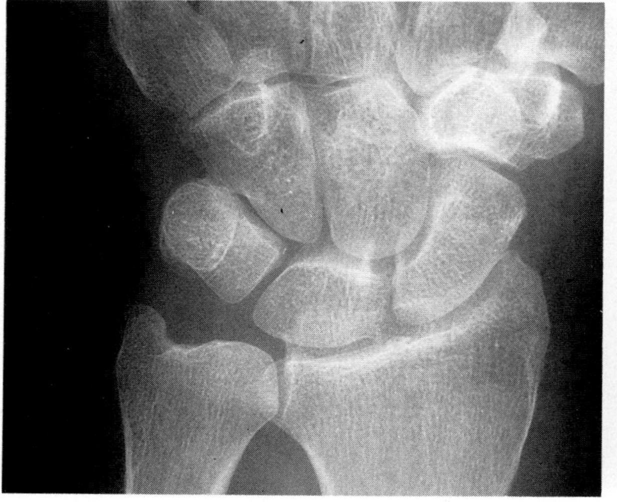

A

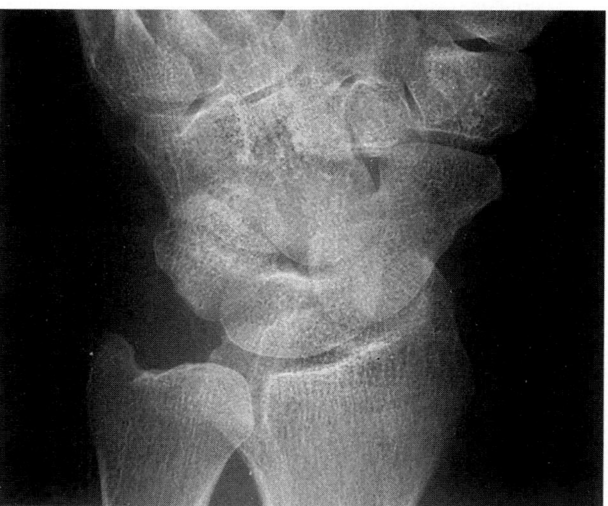

B

FIGURE 23-5. (panels **A** and **B**) *See legend on opposite page*

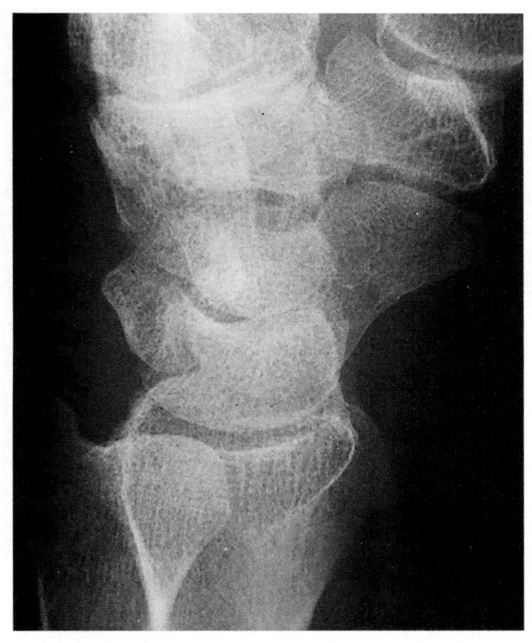

C

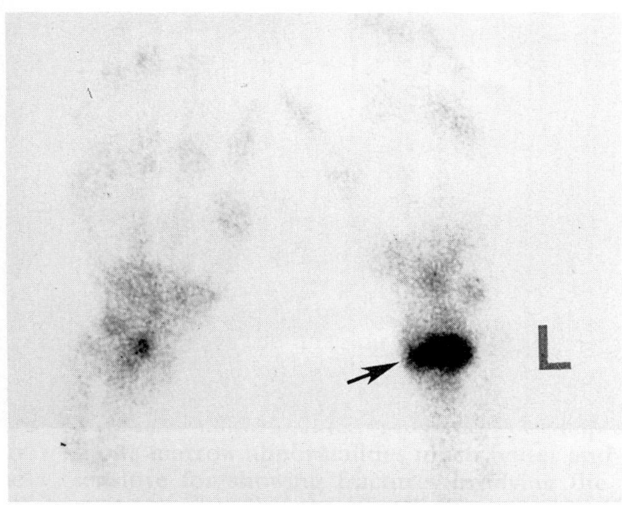

D

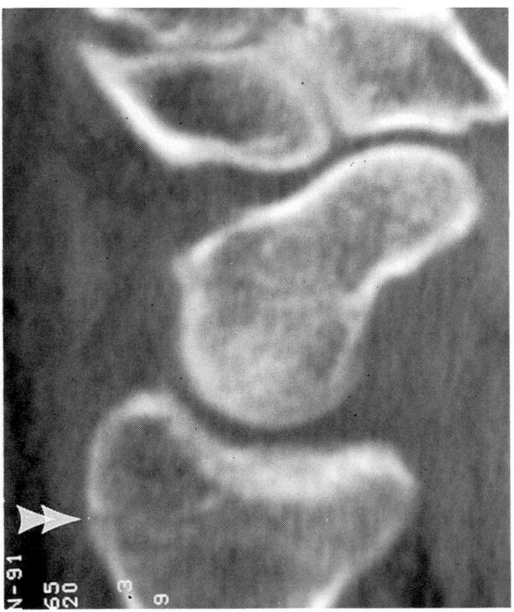

E

FIGURE 23–5. Nondisplaced fracture of the radius in a patient with clinical question of scaphoid fracture. Neutral PA **(A)**, 45-degree pronated oblique **(B)**, and slightly pronated lateral views **(C)** of the left wrist are normal. **D:** Bone scan demonstrates a linear band of increased uptake in the distal left radius (arrow). **E:** Sagittal CT image demonstrates a subtle fracture line at the dorsal aspect of the distal radius (double-tailed arrowhead). Clinical correlation confirmed the maximal tender site to be the distal radius.

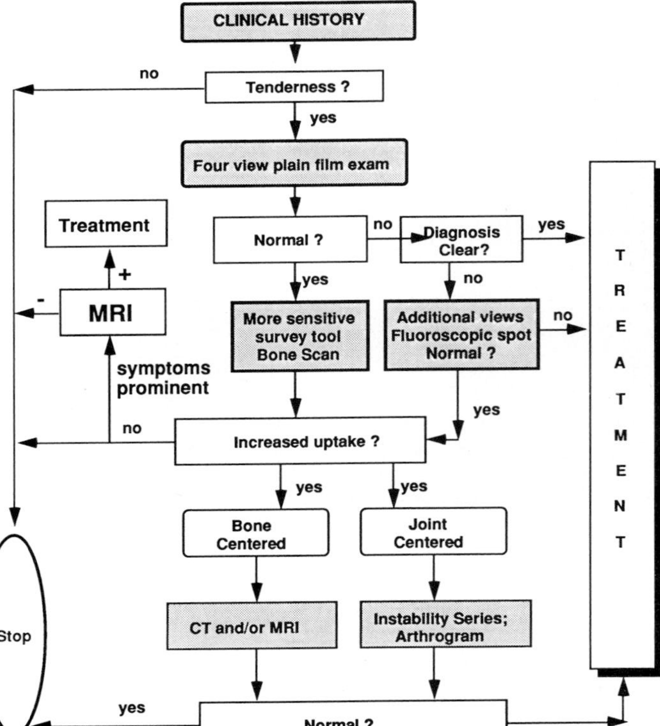

FIGURE 23–9. Imaging algorithm for acute trauma to the wrist. (+), definitive diagnosis; (−), normal; (±), indeterminate/equivocal. (Modified with permission from Linn MR, Mann FA, Gilula LA. Imaging the symptomatic wrist. *Orthop Clin North Am* 1990;21:515–543.)

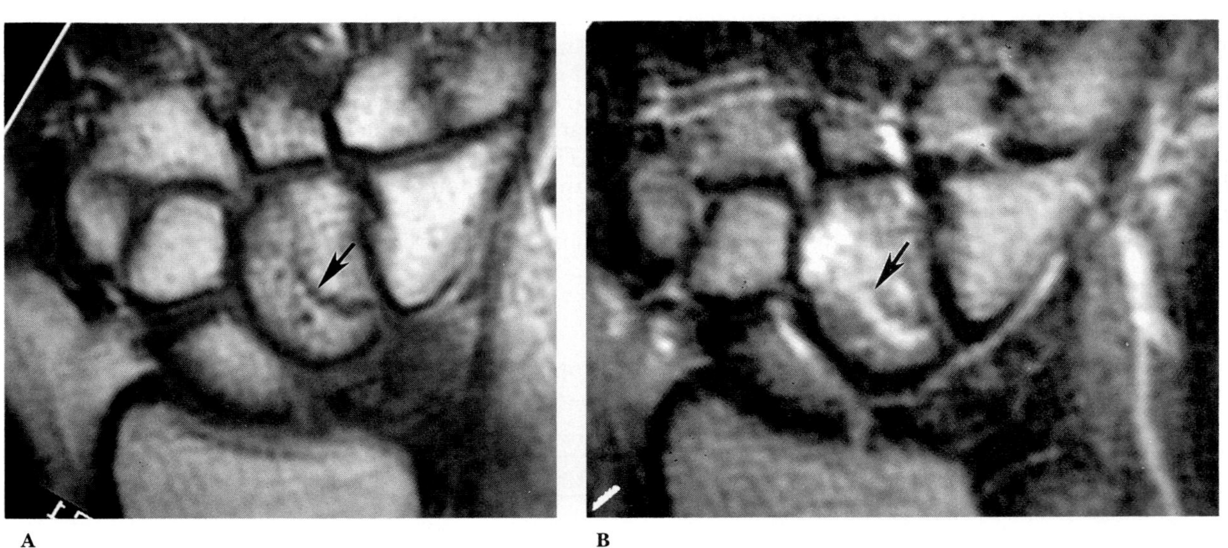

FIGURE 23–10. Nondisplaced fracture of the capitate. Same case as Fig. 23–1. Coronal T1 (500/23) weighted image **(A)** demonstrates a curvilinear pattern of decreased signal in the body of the capitate (arrow), **(B)** which demonstrates increased signal of fluid on the T2 (3000/90) weighted image (arrow) indicative of a fracture. This fracture would not be identified on CT, even in retrospect. (Reprinted with permission from Peh WCG, Gilula LA, Wilson AJ. Detection of occult wrist fractures by magnetic resonance imaging. *J Hand Surg*, submitted.)

(see Chapter 17). With higher resolution, these images may be helpful in examining the integrity of intercarpal ligaments and evaluate dynamic instability. However, a good prospective study with a large number of patients that compares MRI with arthrography to see if it is as accurate as arthrography has not yet been performed.

TFC perforations, which represent an important cause of ulnar-sided wrist pain, can be evaluated well on thin-section high-resolution MRI (see Chapter 17). On the short repetition time/echo time (TR/TE), proton density weighted spin echo, or gradient echo images, these defects or perforations appear as a linear band of increased signal extending to the surface of the TFC. Increased signal within the substance of the TFC may be normal in both adolescents and older patients; however, it may represent presenescent degenerative change in patients 20 to 40 years old.

ALGORITHM FOR SUBACUTE AND REMOTE WRIST TRAUMA

Subacute or Remote Trauma (Fig. 23–11)

With patients who have persistent pain of a subacute (4 to 36 weeks) or chronic (longer than 36 weeks) duration, a slight variation of the acute patient approach may be used. After the history is taken and physical examination is performed, regardless of whether there is focal tenderness, a routine four-view plain-film examination remains the most valuable initial imaging study. If there is an abnormality, such as a previously unrecognized fracture, imaging studies could stop at this point. If there is a questionable fracture that is not clearly profiled, additional films, especially fluoroscopic spot films, may demonstrate a subtle fracture or subluxation. If there is abnormal intercarpal alignment, symptoms at the scapholunate joint, or symptoms of capitolunate instability pattern (CLIP), a tailored instability series is the next appropriate test to see if there is associated abnormal intercarpal motion (see Chapter 7).[9] Abnormal carpal alignment in association with abnormal intercarpal motion is supportive of a "carpal instability." An instability series with plain films may be the first choice to demonstrate whether there is an abnormal gap or motion within the carpal joints. Integrity of the intrinsic ligaments (e.g., scapholunate and lunotriquetral) and the TFC are most accurately assessed by wrist arthrography (Fig. 23–12). An abnormal arthrogram may allow subclassification of instability patterns into carpal instability dissociated (CID) (see Chapter 8), support the clinical diagnosis, and lead to treatment.

If the additional studies are normal, a bone scan may be used as survey tool to find the abnormal site. Again, if the abnormal increased uptake is centered in a bone, CT or MRI may help demonstrate the abnormal bone pathology.

If an intracarpal abnormality, such as an intraosseous lucency associated with focal tenderness, is identified on the instability series or arthrogram, an MRI may be valuable for determining the nature and extent of the lesion (Fig. 23–13). In other words, is the lesion fluid containing, is it consistent with a ganglion, is its location palmar or dorsal to dictate

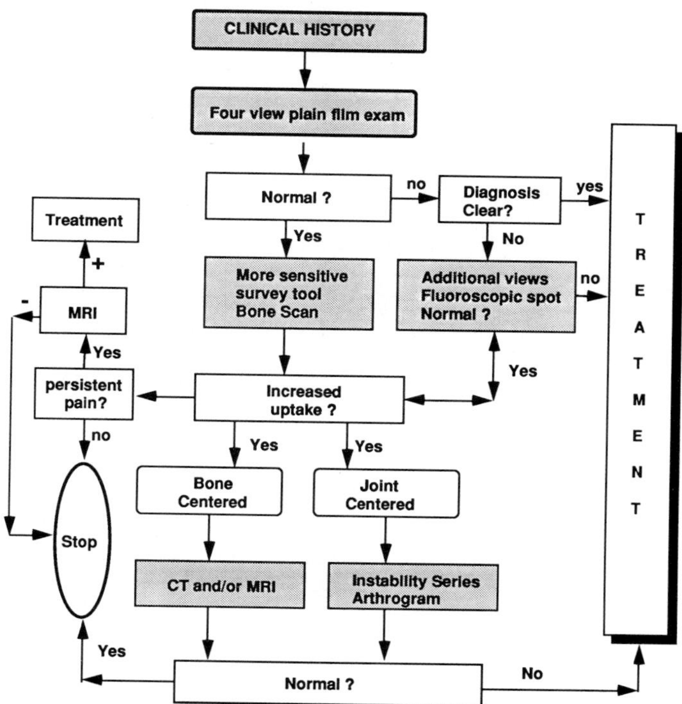

FIGURE 23–11. Algorithm for subacute and remote trauma to the wrist. (+), definitive diagnosis; (−), normal; (±), indeterminate/equivocal. (Modified with permission from Linn MR, Mann FA, Gilula LA. Imaging the symptomatic wrist. *Orthop Clin North Am* 1990;21:515–543.)

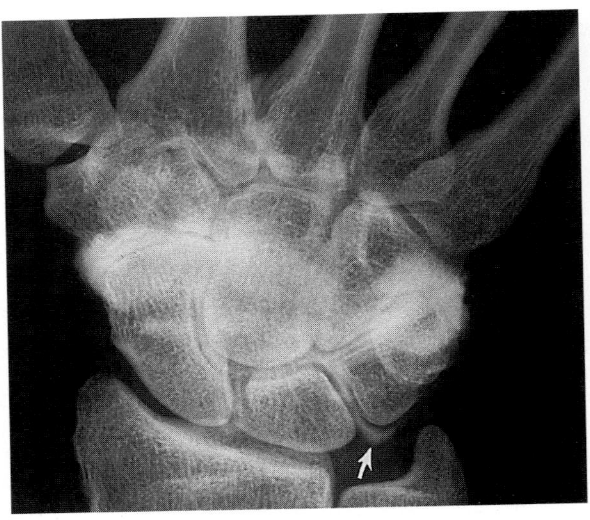

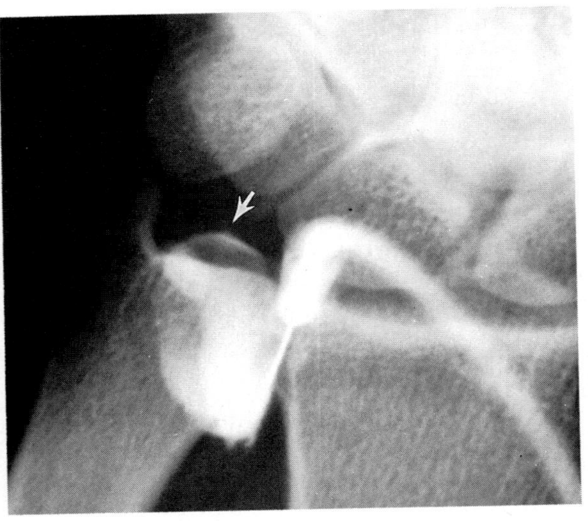

A B

FIGURE 23–12. A: Midcarpal joint arthrogram shows a noncommunicating lunotriquetral perforation or defect (arrow). Contrast passing around the proximal surface of the triquetrum with no contrast passing into the radiocarpal joint is supportive of lunotriquetral ligament avulsion from its attachment to the triquetrum. **B:** DRUJ arthrogram demonstrates a noncommunicating defect (arrow) in the proximal midsurface of the TFC.

the operative approach,[10,11] and what is the extent of the lesion? CT may be valuable when additional information is desired about anatomic cortical and trabecular detail. When an intracarpal lesion is identified, bone scintigraphy is valuable for determining if the lesion is physiologically active. Bone scintigraphy can be used at any stage in this algorithm to survey the wrist for evidence of an active osteochondral abnormality not shown on routine radiographs. It is also valuable to assess the physiologic activity of a previously documented osseous abnormality. Finally, bone scintigraphy can be used to see if there is a diffuse abnormality, such as from synovitis or reflex sympathetic dystrophy. If focal increased uptake is centered around a joint, a ligamentous abnormality may be suspected, and this could be confirmed or rejected by an arthrogram. However, it may be difficult to separate activity from a solitary bone or from that which is centered about a joint. It has been our experience that a focally moderately hot or very hot spot on scintigraphy suggests clinically relevant pathology that may be demonstrated on additional imaging studies (e.g., MRI or CT).

ALGORITHM FOR OSTEONECROSIS

Osteonecrosis (Fig. 23–14)

Other entities can cause a painful wrist. These may be suspected clinically or can be detected on plain radiographs. One of these is osteonecrosis or AVN. AVN is known to occasionally involve the proximal pole of the scaphoid after a fracture and to affect the entire lunate without history of trauma. Idiopathic AVN of the entire lunate is called Kienböck's disease, lunomalacia, or lunatomalacia. Again, the standard four-view plain-film series is the first imaging examination performed. If that is positive (shows AVN), treatment can be instituted (Fig. 23–15). If the plain-film examination is normal, scintigraphy, CT, or MRI can be performed next. Controversy exists about which of these three procedures should be used next. Bone scintigraphy has the advantage of surveying the entire carpus for physiologically abnormal activity and may demonstrate early avascular changes (see Chapter 12).[12] If this examination is normal, usually CT should not be of any value. However, MRI can potentially still be of value. In rare cases in which the amount of healing and dead bone are in balance, the scintigram can be normal and the MRI can show an abnormality. If the scintigram is abnormal, treatment can be instituted at this time. However, generally, the abnormal scintigram is not specific enough to differentiate among such diverse conditions as fracture, AVN, bone marrow edema, painful focal intracarpal defects, and so on. MRI is valuable to show intramedullary abnormality and help detect pathology that can objectively support the patient's claim that the wrist is painful. Sometimes when such an abnormality is found on MRI, the anatomic structure of the abnormality must be clarified further to separate a painful carpal hole or ulnar impaction syndrome from AVN of the lunate. Then CT examination can help more precisely define the anatomic details of the lesion and support the diagnosis of AVN or a painful carpal hole. If both the MRI and bone scintigram are normal, then for practical purposes AVN has been excluded.[13]

INDEX

Note: Page numbers in *italics* indicate figures; page numbers followed by t indicate tables.